Ma and Mateer's
Emergency Ultrasound

Ma and Mateer's
Emergency Ultrasound

Third Edition

O. John Ma, MD
Professor and Chair
Department of Emergency Medicine
Oregon Health & Science University
Portland, Oregon

James R. Mateer, MD, RDMS
Clinical Professor of Emergency Medicine
Department of Emergency Medicine
Medical College of Wisconsin
Milwaukee, Wisconsin
Attending Emergency Physician
Waukesha Memorial Hospital
Waukesha, Wisconsin

Robert F. Reardon, MD
Department of Emergency Medicine
Hennepin County Medical Center
Associate Professor of Emergency Medicine
University of Minnesota Medical School
Minneapolis, Minnesota

Scott A. Joing, MD
Department of Emergency Medicine
Hennepin County Medical Center
Assistant Professor of Emergency Medicine
University of Minnesota Medical School
Minneapolis, Minnesota

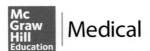

New York Chicago San Francisco Athens London Madrid
Mexico City Milan New Delhi Singapore
Sydney Toronto

Ma and Mateer's Emergency Ultrasound, Third Edition

Copyright © 2014 by McGraw-Hill Education. All rights reserved. Printed in China. Except as permitted under the United States Copyright Act of 1976, no part of this publication may be reproduced or distributed in any form or by any means, or stored in a data base or retrieval system, without the prior written permission of the publisher.

Previous editions copyright © 2008, 2003 by The McGraw-Hill Companies, Inc.

1 2 3 4 5 6 7 8 9 0 CTP/CTP 18 17 16 15 14 13

Set ISBN   978-0-07-179215-8
Set MHID   0-07-179215-5
Book ISBN   978-0-07-179214-1
Book MHID   0-07-179214-7
DVD ISBN   978-0-07-179213-4
DVD MHID   0-07-179213-9

This book was set in Times Roman by Aptara, Inc.
The editors were Anne M. Sydor and Robert Pancotti.
The production supervisor was Catherine H. Saggese.
The illustration manager was Armen Ovsepyan.
Project management was provided by Amit Kashyap, Aptara, Inc.
China Translation & Printing Services, Ltd. was the printer and binder.

Library of Congress Cataloging-in-Publication Data

Ma and Mateer's emergency ultrasound / editors, O. John Ma ... [et al.]. – 3rd ed.
      p. ; cm.
   Emergency ultrasound
   Rev. ed. of: Emergency ultrasound. 2nd ed. c2008.
   Includes bibliographical references and index.
   ISBN 978-0-07-179215-8 (set) – ISBN 0-07-179215-5 (set) – ISBN 978-0-07-179214-1 (book) –
ISBN 0-07-179214-7 (book) – ISBN 978-0-07-179315-5 (ebook) – ISBN 0-07-179315-1 (ebook) –
ISBN 978-0-07-179213-4 (DVD) – ISBN 0-07-179213-9 (DVD)
   I. Ma, O. John. II. Emergency ultrasound. III. Title: Emergency ultrasound.
   [DNLM: 1. Ultrasonography–methods. 2. Emergencies. 3. Emergency Medical
Services–methods. WN 208]
      616.07'543–dc23   2012051400

McGraw-Hill Education books are available at special quantity discounts to use as premiums and sales promotions or for use in corporate training programs. To contact a representative, please visit the Contact Us pages at www.mhprofessional.com.

To Julius and Sabrina: many thanks for your love and companionship during the writing of this textbook.
— O. John Ma —

I am dedicating this third edition to all practitioners who are investing the effort required to learn and utilize point of care ultrasonography. Acquiring this skill will help you provide a safer, faster, and more cost-effective method for diagnosis and management of many patients. These elements coincide with the evolving current and future needs of our health care system.
—James R. Mateer —

To my beautiful wife Julianne, my children Kylie, Kate and Shea, and my parents Mary and Fran. I thank them for their love, support, and tolerance while I took time away from them to work on this project.
— Robert F. Reardon —

To my wonderful wife, Elizabeth, and our two energetic boys, Micah and Owen.
— Scott A. Joing —

CONTENTS

CONTRIBUTORS

Alyssa M. Abo, MD
Assistant Professor
Department of Emergency Medicine
Hofstra North Shore-LIJ School of Medicine
Hempstead, New York
Pediatric Applications

Srikar Adhikari, MD, MS, RDMS
Associate Professor
Department of Emergency Medicine
University of Arizona Medical Center
Tucson, Arizona
Testicular

Frédéric Adnet, MD
Universite Paris XIII
Hopital Avicenne
Bobigny, France
Ultrasound in Prehospital and Austere Environments

Gernot Aichinger, MD
Department of Anesthesiology and Intensive Care
Medicine
Medical University of Graz
Graz, Austria
*Ultrasound in Prehospital and Austere
Environments*

Aaron E. Bair, MD, MSc
Professor
Department of Emergency Medicine
University of California, Davis School of Medicine
Sacramento, California
Vascular Access

Raoul Breitkreutz, MD
Associate Professor
FINeST, Simulation Centre
University Hospital of Frankfurt am Main
Frankfurt, Hessen, Germany
*Ultrasound in Prehospital and Austere
Environments*

Franziska Brenner, MD
Department of Trauma, Hand and Reconstructive
Plastic Surgery
Johann Wolfgang Goethe - University Hospital
Frankfurt/Main, Germany
*Ultrasound in Prehospital and Austere
Environments*

Gavin R. Budhram, MD
Assistant Professor
Department of Emergency Medicine
Tufts University School of Medicine
Boston, Massachusetts
Critical Care

Donald V. Byars, MD, RDMS, FACEP
Director, Emergency Ultrasound Fellowship
Associate Professor
Eastern Virginia Medical School
Norfolk, Virginia
Second and Third Trimester Pregnancy

Marco Campo dell'Orto, MD
Department of Cardiology
Kerckhoff Heart Centre
Bad Nauheim, Germany
*Ultrasound in Prehospital and Austere
Environments*

Liberty V. Caroon, RDMS
Sonographer
Department of Emergency Medicine
Hennepin County Medical Center
Minneapolis, Minnesota
First Trimester Pregnancy

Michelle E. Clinton, MD
Ultrasound Fellow
Department of Emergency Medicine
Hennepin County Medical Center
Minneapolis, Minnesota
Abdominal Aortic Aneurysm

Thomas P. Cook, MD
Program Director
Department of Emergency Medicine
Palmetto Health Richland Medical Center
Columbia, South Carolina
Abdominal Aortic Aneurysm

Thomas G. Costantino, MD
Associate Professor
Department of Emergency Medicine
Temple University School of Medicine
Philadelphia, Pennsylvania
Deep Venous Thrombosis

Innes Crawford, MBChB, BSc
University of Aberdeen
Aberdeen, Scotland
Ultrasound in Prehospital and Austere Environments

Andreas Dewitz, MD, RDMS
Associate Professor of Emergency Medicine
Department of Emergency Medicine
Boston University School of Medicine
Boston, Massachusetts
*Musculoskeletal, Soft Tissue, and Miscellaneous
   Applications*
Additional Ultrasound-Guided Procedures

Jason W. Fischer, MD, MSc
Assistant Professor of Pediatrics
Department of Paediatrics
University of Toronto
Toronto, Ontario
Pediatric Applications

J. Christian Fox, MD, RDMS
Professor
Department of Emergency Medicine
University of California, Irvine
Irvine, California
Equipment
Gynecologic Concepts

Harry J. Goett, MD
Assistant Professor
Department of Emergency Medicine
Temple University School of Medicine
Philadelphia, Pennsylvania
Deep Venous Thrombosis

Corky Hecht, BA, RDMS, RDCS, RVT
Program Director
Cardiovascular Sonography
Sanford-Brown Institute
Jacksonville, Florida
Physics and Image Artifacts

William G. Heegaard, MD, MPH
Department of Emergency Medicine
Hennepin County Medical Center
Associate Professor of Emergency Medicine
University of Minnesota Medical School
Minneapolis, Minnesota
*Ultrasound in Prehospital and Austere
   Environments*

Jamie Hess-Keenan, MD
Assistant Professor
Department of Emergency Medicine
University of Wisconsin School of Medicine
Madison, Wisconsin
First Trimester Pregnancy

Jeffrey D. Ho, MD
Department of Emergency Medicine
Hennepin County Medical Center
Associate Professor of Emergency Medicine
University of Minnesota Medical School
Minneapolis, Minnesota
*Ultrasound in Prehospital and Austere
   Environments*

Timothy Jang, MD
Associate Professor of Clinical Medicine
Department of Emergency Medicine
David Geffen School of Medicine at UCLA
Los Angeles, California
Training and Program Development

Scott A. Joing, MD
Department of Emergency Medicine
Hennepin County Medical Center
Assistant Professor of Emergency Medicine
University of Minnesota Medical School
Minneapolis, Minnesota
Cardiac
First Trimester Pregnancy

Robert A. Jones, DO
Associate Professor
Department of Emergency Medicine
Case Western Reserve University
Cleveland, Ohio
Additional Ultrasound-Guided Procedures

Andrew W. Kirkpatrick, MD, MHSC
Professor of Critical Care Medicine and Surgery
Foothills Medical Centre
Calgary, Alberta
Ultrasound in Prehospital and Austere Environments
Trauma

Thomas Kirschning, MD, DESA
Attending Physician
Department of Anaesthesiology and Intensive Care
University Medical Centre Mannheim
Mannheim, Germany
Ultrasound in Prehospital and Austere Environments

Barry J. Knapp, MD, RDMS
Associate Professor
Department of Emergency Medicine
Eastern Virginia Medical School
Norfolk, Virginia
Second and Third Trimester Pregnancy

Dietrich von Kuenssberg Jehle, MD, RDMS
Professor and Director of Emergency Ultrasonography
Department of Emergency Medicine
SUNY at Buffalo
Buffalo, New York
Ocular

Michael J. Lambert, MD
Department of Emergency Medicine
Advocate Christ Medical Center
Oak Lawn, Illinois
Training and Program Development
Gynecologic Concepts

Frédéric Lapostolle, MD
Universite Paris XIII
Hopital Avicenne
Bobigny, France
Ultrasound in Prehospital and Austere
  Environments

Andrew Laudenbach, MD
Department of Emergency Medicine
Hennepin County Medical Center
Assistant Professor of Emergency Medicine
University of Minnesota Medical School
Minneapolis, Minnesota
Cardiac

Resa E. Lewiss, MD, RDMS
Assistant Clinical Professor of Medicine
Columbia University College of Physicians and
  Surgeons
New York, New York
Hepatobiliary

Matthew Lyon, MD
Associate Professor
Department of Emergency Medicine
Georgia Health Sciences University
Augusta, Georgia
Ocular

O. John Ma, MD
Professor and Chair
Department of Emergency Medicine
Oregon Health & Science University
Portland, Oregon
Trauma

Frank Madore, MD
Ultrasound Fellow
Department of Emergency Medicine
Hennepin County Medical Center
Minneapolis, Minnesota
Abdominal Aortic Aneurysm

William Manson, MD, RDMS
Assistant Professor
Department of Emergency Medicine
Emory University School of Medicine
Atlanta, Georgia
Physics and Image Artifacts

Ingo Marzi, MD
Department of Trauma Surgery
University of Saarland
Hamburg, Germany
Ultrasound in Prehospital and Austere Environments

James R. Mateer, MD, RDMS
Clinical Professor of Emergency Medicine
Department of Emergency Medicine
Medical College of Wisconsin
Milwaukee, Wisconsin
Attending Emergency Physician
Waukesha Memorial Hospital
Waukesha, Wisconsin
Trauma

Paul B. McBeth, MD, MASc
Department of Surgery
Foothills Medical Centre
Calgary, Alberta, Canada
Ultrasound in Prehospital and Austere Environments

Lisa D. Mills, MD
Associate Professor
Department of Emergency Medicine
University of California, Davis
Sacramento, California
Pulmonary

Masaaki Ogata, MD
Director
Department of Emergency Medicine and Surgery
Kobe City Medical Center West Hospital
Kobe, Japan
General Surgery Applications

Aman K. Parikh, MD
Associate Professor
Department of Emergency Medicine
University of California, Davis
Sacramento, California
Vascular Access

Michael A. Peterson, MD
Professor
Department of Medicine
David Geffen School of Medicine at UCLA
Los Angeles, California
Deep Venous Thrombosis

Tomislav Petrovic, MD
Attending Physician
Prehospital Emergency Department
SAMU 93 - Hôpital AVICENNE
Bobigny, France
*Ultrasound in Prehospital and Austere
    Environments*

David W. Plummer, MD
Department of Emergency Medicine
Hennepin County Medical Center
Associate Professor of Emergency Medicine
University of Minnesota Medical School
Minneapolis, Minnesota
Critical Care

Gerhard Prause, MD
Associate Professor
Department of Anaesthesiology and Intensive Care
Medical University of Graz
Graz, Austria
Ultrasound in Prehospital and Austere Environments

Daniel D. Price, MD
Director of International Ultrasound
Department of Emergency Medicine
Alameda County Medical Center - Highland Hospital &
    Trauma Center
Oakland, California
Ultrasound in Prehospital and Austere Environments

Robert F. Reardon, MD
Department of Emergency Medicine
Hennepin County Medical Center
Associate Professor of Emergency Medicine
University of Minnesota Medical School
Minneapolis, Minnesota
Cardiac
Critical Care
Abdominal Aortic Aneurysm
First Trimester Pregnancy

Jessica G. Resnick, MD
Assistant Professor
Emergency Medicine
Case Western Reserve University School of Medicine
Cleveland, Ohio
Additional Ultrasound-Guided Procedures

Chad E. Roline, MD
Staff Physician
Department of Emergency Medicine
North Memorial Medical Center
Robbinsdale, Minnesota
First Trimester Pregnancy

John S. Rose, MD
Professor
Department of Emergency Medicine
University of California, Davis
Sacramento, California
Vascular Access

William Scruggs, MD, RDMS
Director of Emergency Ultrasound
Department of Emergency Medicine
Hawaii Emergency Physicians Associated
Kailua, Hawaii
Equipment

Dina Seif, MD, MBA, RDMS
Assistant Professor
Department of Emergency Medicine
Los Angeles County-USC Medical Center
Los Angeles, California
Renal

Fernando R. Silva, MD, MSc
Attending Physician
Department of Emergency Medicine
Kaiser Permanente Northern California
Vallejo/Vacaville, California
Pulmonary

Adam B. Sivitz, MD
Clinical Assistant Professor
Department of Emergency Medicine
Newark Beth Israel Medical Center
Newark, New Jersey
Pediatric Applications

Michael B. Stone, MD
Chief, Division of Emergency Ultrasound
Emergency Ultrasound Fellowship Director
Department of Emergency Medicine
Brigham and Women's Hospital
Boston, Massachusetts
Additional Ultrasound-Guided Procedures

Stuart P. Swadron, MD
Associate Professor
Department of Emergency Medicine
Keck School of Medicine of the University of
  Southern California
Los Angeles, California
Renal

Daniel L. Theodoro, MD, MSCI
Assistant Professor
Division of Emergency Medicine
Washington University School of Medicine
St. Louis, Missouri
Hepatobiliary

Corina Tiruta, MSc
Regional Trauma Services
Foothills Medical Centre
Calgary, Alberta, Canada
Ultrasound in Prehospital and Austere Environments

Felix Walcher, MD, PhD
Department of Trauma Surgery
University Hospital Frankfurt
Hamburg, Germany
Ultrasound in Prehospital and Austere Environments

Gernot Wildner, MD
Attending Physician
Department of Anesthesiology and Intensive Care
  Medicine
Medical University of Graz
Graz, Austria
Ultrasound in Prehospital and Austere Environments

Peter M. Zechner, MD
Resident
Department of Internal Medicine
LKH Graz West
Graz, Austria
Ultrasound in Prehospital and Austere Environments

FOREWORD

In this third edition of *Ma and Mateer's Emergency Ultrasound*, Drs. Ma, Mateer, Reardon, and Joing have again delivered the definitive text for emergency medicine ultrasound. They have included the most relevant topics for practitioners and have enlisted nationally and internationally recognized clinicians and educators as contributing authors. All authors have demonstrated that they were up to the challenge of delivering the latest information on their topics in a clear, comprehensive manner, including the significant advances since the last edition. New chapters and topics in cardiac, critical care, and musculoskeletal ultrasound have been included and reflect the expansion of clinical applications of point-of-care ultrasound as well as the expanding role of ultrasound outside of the emergency medicine setting.

Since the last edition of this text, the practice of point-of-care ultrasound has become accepted as an important adjunct to the clinician's armamentarium. Originally advanced by emergency medicine physicians and other specialists, the recognition that this noninvasive technology can improve the rapidity and accuracy of patient diagnoses and treatment has led to the potential for its use by a broad spectrum of providers. Thus, this text, like point-of-care ultrasound itself, will find enthusiasts across multiple frontline practitioners including primary care physicians, emergency medical technicians, nurse practitioners, and physician assistants. In addition, specialists and subspecialists from many disciplines will find particular chapters of immense value to their practices, such as the chapters *Musculoskeletal, Soft Tissue, and Miscellaneous Applications* and *Additional Ultrasound-Guided Procedures* for medical and surgical subspecialists.

The chapter format that includes anatomical considerations, physiological explanations, scanning techniques, normal and pathological findings, case studies, and pitfalls lends itself well to the education of students, trainees, and practitioners at all levels from the ultrasound novice to the experienced user who wants to expand their knowledge and skill of point-of-care ultrasound. The high-quality embedded figures and the accompanying DVD provide learners with the best in ultrasound education. Each chapter is thoroughly referenced and grounded in the emergency medicine literature as well as specialty-based evidence.

The editors and all contributing authors are to be congratulated on this major contribution to the advancement of point-of-care ultrasound and ultimately for the role this text will play in improving patient care and safety; and in increasing access to health care through the use of point-of-care ultrasound across the globe.

Jeanette Mladenovic, MD, MBA, MACP
Provost and Executive Vice President
Professor of Medicine
Oregon Health and Science University
Portland, Oregon

Richard Hoppmann, MD, FACP
Dean
Professor of Medicine
Director of the Ultrasound Institute
University of South Carolina School of Medicine
Columbia, South Carolina

PREFACE

Ultrasonography has been demonstrated to improve the quality of patient care and enhance patient safety. Its applications transcend any one medical specialty or hospital location. Medical centers, both large and small, along with medical and nursing schools have incorporated ultrasound into their clinical pathways and educational curriculums in a multidisciplinary and transprofessional manner. Ultrasound is used by medical providers working in austere environments and on the frontlines of war zones. Clinician investigators from nearly all medical specialties and from across the globe have published research on the applications of point-of-care ultrasound.

This textbook was written by and for clinicians who are actively engaged in patient care at the bedside. We have selected topics that represent those problems most commonly encountered in the emergency or acute care setting. Our aim was to address the needs of clinicians with varied backgrounds and training. Emergency physicians certainly will find this book applicable to their daily practice. Physicians who practice in family medicine, internal medicine, hospital medicine, critical care, pediatrics, and general surgery will use many of these ultrasound examinations to optimize their patient care. We trust that mid-level providers who practice in related fields will also find this textbook useful.

We would like to thank the readers of previous editions of this textbook who offered us excellent feedback. New topics or chapters on cardiac, pulmonary, critical care, and musculoskeletal ultrasound applications are included. More color figures are embedded throughout the book. Finally, we feel that if a picture is worth a thousand words, then a video may be worth several hundred thousand. A DVD that demonstrates common emergency ultrasound examinations is enclosed with this textbook; these videos include expert commentary, multiple camera angles, and video images of numerous normal and abnormal findings.

Experts from several countries and numerous medical specialties have contributed to this textbook. We would like to express our warmest appreciation to the chapter contributors for their commitment and hard work in helping to produce this textbook. We also would like to thank them for helping us collect the more than 900 figures that are included in this textbook. We would like to thank Lori Green and Gulfcoast Ultrasound for their support of this project and for providing us with ultrasound images from their library. We are indebted to a number of individuals who assisted us with this project; in particular, we would like to thank Anne M. Sydor, Sarah M. Granlund, and Robert Pancotti for their invaluable contributions.

O. John Ma, MD

James R. Mateer, MD

Robert F. Reardon, MD

Scott A. Joing, MD

CHAPTER 1

Training and Program Development

Michael J. Lambert and Timothy Jang

Establishing a training program in point-of-care ultrasound is an exciting and rewarding experience. The impact of ultrasound on the clinical practice of medicine becomes so clear that many clinicians, after acquiring basic ultrasound skills, wonder how they got along without this technology. This chapter outlines the process for developing a point-of-care ultrasound training program and addresses the common questions encountered when starting a new program.

Point-of-care ultrasound examinations are performed in real time at the bedside by clinicians to answer specific questions in order to expedite care and improve patient care. These studies are not intended to provide comprehensive surveys of anatomical areas nor are they mere extensions of the physical examination.[1] Point-of-care ultrasound provides imaging to rule in or rule out specific disease entities for which timely treatment is crucial (e.g., ruptured abdominal aortic aneurysm, ruptured ectopic pregnancy, and cardiac tamponade) or for whom invasive intervention could be especially unsafe (e.g., paracentesis, abscess drainages, and foreign body removal). As such, these studies require the highest levels of competence, accuracy, and clinical acumen.

► STEPS TO ESTABLISHING A POINT-OF-CARE ULTRASOUND PROGRAM

In order to establish a high-quality point-of-care ultrasound program, ultrasound directors must:

1. Determine type of examinations to be performed.
2. Develop a program implementation plan.
3. Obtain leadership approval of the implementation plan.
4. Acquire an ultrasound machine.
5. Train the group.
6. Incentivize group members to complete training and credentialing.
7. Perform problem solving, quality assurance, and ongoing training.

A critical factor in the timely implementation and success of an ultrasound program is to have the full support and active assistance of the department leadership. Also, appointing a dedicated ultrasound director with protected time is the best approach because each step in program implementation is very time intensive.

▶ DETERMINE TYPE OF EXAMINATIONS TO BE PERFORMED

Ultrasound use continues to expand along with technological advances and improvement in individual operator expertise. It makes sense to start with applications that will get the most use in a particular practice setting. For example, in a small community hospital, evaluation of cardiac arrest may be more pertinent than trauma evaluations. Likewise, in centers without 24-hour ultrasound services, it may be important to learn ultrasound for the evaluation of ectopic pregnancy and cholecystitis. We recommend starting with applications unique to the ED for which timely diagnosis and intervention are critical. This includes the focused assessment with sonography for trauma (FAST) examination, evaluation of cardiac arrest states, and evaluation of hypotension. In addition, procedural applications, such as intravenous line placement, paracentesis, thoracentesis, and abscess localization and drainage, are becoming standard of care.[2] Training in emergency medicine residency programs, however, should cover all of the primary applications and include exposure to emerging applications (Tables 1-1 and 1-2).

A new point-of-care ultrasound program should strive to identify all of the ultrasound examinations that are of interest, both now and in the future. Making this decision early allows the program to seek leadership approval for all of these examinations from the beginning instead of having to apply for additional approval later. It also allows the program to define equipment needs prior to initial equipment purchase. Otherwise, additional purchases may have to be made as new applications are brought online.

Some medical centers may choose to focus on just one or two ultrasound applications at a time. This allows everyone time to concentrate their efforts on becoming

▶ TABLE 1-1. CORE EMERGENCY ULTRASOUND APPLICATIONS

Trauma
Intrauterine pregnancy
Abdominal aortic aneurysm
Cardiac
Biliary
Urinary tract
Deep venous thrombosis
Soft tissue/musculoskeletal
Ocular
Thoracic
Procedural guidance

Adapted from American College of Emergency Physicians: Emergency ultrasound guidelines. *Ann Emerg Med* 53:550–570, 2009.

▶ TABLE 1-2. EMERGENCY ULTRASOUND— ADDITIONAL APPLICATIONS

	Additional Applications
Abdominal	Appendicitis
	Bladder volume
	Hernias
	Intussusception
Obstetrics/ gynecology	Adnexal masses
	Trauma in pregnancy
	Intrauterine device localization
	Fetal viability
Cardiothoracic	Gross wall motion
	Severe valvular disease
	Pleural effusion
	Pneumothorax
Soft tissue/orthopedic	Foreign body diagnosis
	Cutaneous abscess diagnosis
	Peritonsillar abscess diagnosis
Vascular	Deep venous thrombosis
	Inferior vena cava—assess volume status
Ophthalmologic	Retinal detachment
	Vitreous hemorrhage
Procedural	Bladder aspiration
	Fracture reduction
	Transvenous pacemaker placement
	Abscess drainage
	Foreign body removal
	Lumbar puncture
	Arthrocentesis
	Thoracentesis
	Paracentesis
	Peripheral nerve blocks
	Vascular access

proficient with each application and to learn the technical pitfalls inherent in those particular applications. By keeping the entire training group on the same application(s), the ultrasound director can focus quality improvement (QI) efforts on those specific applications, using reviews of specific cases to educate and train everyone involved. After quality performance levels are achieved, new applications can be introduced in a similar fashion one at a time until all of the applications are taught. In our experience, this is the most effective means for starting a program and allows for a safe and effective implementation of ultrasound into clinical care.

Since point-of-care ultrasound focuses on critical questions or interventions, rather than requiring "minimal training," the clinicians actually require the best training and highest standards of competence. In our experience, this is best accomplished by focused and appropriately directed program implementation and training.

► DEVELOP A PROGRAM IMPLEMENTATION PLAN

The program implementation plan defines all aspects of the ultrasound training program. The plan guides the ultrasound director through all the administrative and teaching aspects of the program and serves as a reference for requirements in training. The most straightforward way to develop a plan is to model it after another group or institution's plan, adapting it for the local clinical and political environment. Many residency programs are willing to share their program plans. The program plan should, at a minimum, include the following elements:

- Definition of specific privileges.
- Training and credentialing.
- Method of recording results.
- Performance improvement plan.
- CME requirements.

DEFINITION OF SPECIFIC PRIVILEGES

This section defines exactly how focused ultrasound examinations will be used. For example, a specific privilege may be: "Documentation of free abdominal fluid in trauma patients." This could also be shortened to "Documentation of free abdominal fluid" if there is an additional desire to diagnose ascites. Some institutions allow graduated privileges, meaning that clinicians can do more with their ultrasound examinations as they gain experience (Table 1-3). This approach is beneficial in that it allows earlier implementation of point-of-care ultrasound into patient care while establishing ongoing quality control parameters. Earlier implementation helps maintain momentum in the training program as clinicians see the benefits of their training sooner; however, graduated privileges create a more complex training program.

Privileges and training should be constructed toward the identification of *specific findings* (e.g., presence or absence of gallstones) and not toward the general evaluation of disease processes or anatomic structures (e.g., evaluation for "cardiac disease" or "right upper quadrant abdominal pain") consistent with existing guidelines. A useful resource for defining a particular examination is the Emergency Ultrasound Imaging Criteria Compendium.[3]

TRAINING AND CREDENTIALING

Training

Multiple guidelines for training in ultrasound have been published.[3–8] The American College of Radiology (ACR) and the American Institute of Ultrasound in Medicine (AIUM) have established guidelines[4,5] for learning comprehensive examinations, but have not published guidelines for point-of-care ultrasound. In 1994, a model curriculum for training in emergency ultrasound was published by the Society for Academic Emergency Medicine (SAEM) and subsequently modified as new evidence and experience emerged.[6] In 2001, the American College of Emergency Physicians (ACEP) published initial emergency ultrasound guidelines outlining utilization for six "primary applications" plus use for procedural guidance. The Council of Emergency Medicine Residency Directors (CORD) outlined ultrasound training standards for emergency medicine residency programs in 2008. They listed four primary applications (FAST, emergent cardiac, abdominal aortic aneurysm, intrauterine pregnancy) plus procedural guidance as the minimum skill set, but highly recommended training in at least six additional applications. ACEP published revised guidelines on ultrasound training that have expanded the list of "Core Applications" to a total of 11 applications[1] (Table 1-1). Although this expanded list provides support for additional uses, it is recognized that not all facilities may have the need to utilize all of these applications in their specific clinical practice setting. Specific didactic and experiential training criteria are outlined with a minimum of 25 training cases documented for each core application of interest. The ACEP

► TABLE 1-3. **EXAMPLES OF LEVELS OF PROFICIENCY**

Level I	This level is for the practitioner who has completed the introductory training.
Level II	This level is for the practitioner who is in the process of completing credentialing examinations.
	Credentialing examinations must be recorded and contain follow-up documentation. Each examination is to be reviewed by the ED ultrasound coordinator. Straightforward examinations may be used in some clinical situations if reviewed by a Level III sonographer. In general, these examinations will not be used to make patient-care decisions unless reviewed by a Level III sonographer.
Level III	This level is for the practitioner who is approved to use emergency ultrasound in the ED for patient-care decisions. This physician may supervise Level I and II practitioners.

Adapted from American College of Emergency Physicians. ACEP emergency ultrasound guidelines-2001. *Ann Emerg Med* 38(4):470–81, 2001.

guidelines are recognized as the current standard for training in point-of-care ultrasound.[7,8] Ultrasound directors still have some degree of latitude in designing their individual programs, but should consider CORD as well as ACEP guidelines when designing minimum training criteria. A program should also include minimum requirements for each of the following areas:

- Minimum overall didactic hours.
- Minimum overall didactic content.
- Minimum number of overall ultrasound examinations performed.
- Minimum didactic content pertaining to the specific examination.
- Minimum number of examinations performed to look for the specific finding (either positive or negative).
- Minimum number of abnormal examinations.

Credentialing

Credentialing applies mainly to hospital-based or clinic-based clinicians who wish to perform focused ultrasound examinations on patients in the hospital. Standard methods of credentialing are crucial to safely and effectively implement a successful ultrasound program. The cornerstone of the credentialing processes revolves around a required number of technically proficient scans and interpretations, as outlined in the training requirements. However, as a minimum number of exams may not ensure competency, some centers may choose to use other means of establishing competency such as proctoring and submission of a case portfolio. Noncredentialed clinicians should not discuss any of their results with either patients or consultants during the training period to avoid any misunderstandings about the accuracy of results. Well-intentioned clinicians could place their patients at risk by doing so and would be legally liable for any misinterpretations or outcomes that resulted from such communications. Once clinicians are credentialed by the hospital they may begin using examinations for patient care. If a graduated credentialing program is used, the clinician may be able to use some findings for patient care, but is considered "in training" for other findings.

Incentives for Completion of Training and Credentialing

Most busy physicians will not complete credentialing requirements in a timely manner (or ever) unless it is considered mandatory. The ultrasound director typically has little authority to compel other group members to complete "mandatory" training. This is why an ultrasound program must have full support and active assistance of the department leadership. Only department leaders can compel members to complete any manda-

tory activity. There should be consequences for those who choose not to put forth the effort to complete the credentialing process. This may sound draconian, but it is the only practical way to get all members credentialed in a timely manner, especially in a large group. For practicing physicians, incentives could include tying financial bonuses to completion of the credentialing process.

METHOD OF RECORDING RESULTS

Numerous methods are available to document the results of the ultrasound examinations. Two questions that need to be answered are as follows: (1) How will interpretations be documented and (2) How will images be saved? The answer to the latter question is especially important, as it will influence the type of ultrasound equipment purchased. Documentation of interpretations can be as straightforward as writing results on the chart or as comprehensive as entering them in the hospital information system so they are available to all interested health-care providers. For billing purposes, a "separately identifiable written report" must be generated for each ultrasound examination performed, although this report can be part of the ED record.[9] One solution is to develop a form for the sole purpose of reporting emergency ultrasound results. These forms can then be included in the medical record. The advantage of the form is that it can be devised so as to restrict interpretations to those findings that clinicians are privileged and help clinicians avoid making interpretations beyond their level of skill. An example of such a report form is shown in Figure 1-1.

Several options exist for the saving of images, including thermal printing and myriad of digital recording options. If results are to be included in the medical record, thermal images provide the easiest option, although with the growing use of electronic medical records, it may be possible to incorporate digital images into the medical record. For some applications, images need to be posted on the medical record in order to bill.[9] If images are to be archived separately from the medical record, digital storage or videotaping can be used; however, archiving images outside the medical record creates compliance problems with medical record confidentiality and lack of access by other clinicians. Some programs use digital video recording for quality assurance and teaching purposes only.

QUALITY IMPROVEMENT PLAN

Any department implementing a new ultrasound program should place a strong emphasis on QI. No other area of emergency ultrasound training will provide as

---

LIMITED EMERGENCY ULTRASOUND EXAM
Emergency Department, _____ Medical Center

Date: _____

Provider: _____
          (PRINT NAME)

          _____
          (SIGN)

LEVEL I

Trauma
- ☐ Intra-abdominal fluid
- ☐ Indeterminate
- ☐ No fluid noted

Gallbladder
- ☐ Gallstones
- ☐ Indeterminate
- ☐ No gallstones noted

Cardiac
- ☐ Pericardial fluid
- ☐ Indeterminate
- ☐ No pericardial fluid noted

Pelvic
- ☐ Definite IUP
      (IU fetal pole or IU cardiac activity)
- ☐ Indeterminate

Aorta
- ☐ Aneurysm_____cm
- ☐ Indeterminate
- ☐ No AA noted

(ATTACH IMAGES TO REVERSE SIDE OF MEDICAL RECORD COPY ONLY)

LEVEL II

Trauma
- ☐ **Visualization adequate**
- ☐ **Visualization inadequate**
- ☐ Intra-abdominal fluid
- ☐ No free fluid

Gallbladder
- ☐ **Visualization adequate**
- ☐ **Visualization inadequate**
- ☐ Gallstones
- ☐ Pericholecystic fluid
- ☐ None of above
      CBD _____ mm
      Wall thickness _____ mm

Cardiac
- ☐ **Visualization adequate**
- ☐ **Visualization inadequate**
- ☐ Pericardial fluid
- ☐ No pericardial fluid

Pelvic
- ☐ **Transabdominal**
- ☐ **Transvaginal**
- ☐ **Visualization adequate**
- ☐ **Visualization inadequate**
- ☐ Definite IUP
      (IU fetal pole or IU cardiac activity)
- ☐ Definite ectopic
      (Ectopic fetal pole or cardiac activity)
- ☐ Adnexal mass
- ☐ Pelvic/abdominal fluid
- ☐ None of above findings

Aorta
- ☐ **Visualization adequate**
- ☐ **Visualization inadequate**
- ☐ Aneurysm_____cm
- ☐ No aneurysm detected

Hydronephrosis
- ☐ **Visualization adequate**
- ☐ **Visualization inadequate**
- ☐ Hydronephrosis present R/L
- ☐ No hydronephrosis

Additional Comments:
(Findings in this section are preliminary and require confirmation when clinically indicated)

_____

_____

_____

All Emergency Ultrasounds are considered "Limited Exams."
Exams do not exclude findings other than those recorded above.
Practitioners should procure *comprehensive ultrasound*
examinations when findings not listed here or findings listed under
"additional comments" are of concern.

Figure 1-1. Example of bedside ultrasound report form.

many teaching opportunities as a well-run QI program. If the resources or experience are lacking initially to overread all of the program's ultrasound images, then finding a trained colleague in another location to assist with this endeavor is an option. There are pitfalls common to every application of ultrasound that can serve as a springboard for providing feedback and teaching within the program. This is clearly one of the most advantageous methods of enhancing both the technical and interpretative skills of clinicians.

The cornerstone of the QI program is review of examinations by the program's director. For a very active group of clinicians performing focused ultrasound examinations, it will be logistically difficult to review every ultrasound examination so a method for selecting examinations for review must be decided upon. Examinations can be reviewed on either an *indicated* basis or a *random* basis. Indicated reviews occur when a certain indicator is met, such as a reported discrepancy between the focused ultrasound examination and another definitive study or procedure, or when a case is referred by a colleague because of questions regarding the accuracy of the examination. Random reviews are conducted by randomly selecting a predetermined number, or percentage, of examinations to assess the overall performance of the group.

Problems that are encountered during the QI process should be categorized as to their importance. The following represents one method of categorization.

Level I: Minor

Level I deviations usually consist of some problem with the technical component of the examination (e.g., gain too high) or disagreement on diagnostic criteria (e.g., labeling a common bile duct as mildly dilated at 6.5 mm when for the patient's age, this was a normal measurement). Level I problems have no direct bearing upon the medical management of the patient. Typically, when this level of disagreement is found, a documented written or electronic copy of the disagreement is sent to the recipient.

Level II: Moderate

Level II deviations consist of discrepancies in interpretation between the clinician's recorded image(s) and the QI review. In these cases, the undiagnosed or misdiagnosed pathology is nonemergent. For example, the clinician may record a gallbladder examination in which gallstones were diagnosed. Upon review, the QI review discovers a classic novice pitfall of a hyperechoic duodenal area that is mistaken for gallstones. Typically, when this level of disagreement is found, a chart review is undertaken to determine if subsequent care of the patient was appropriate. Depending on the follow-up that was provided and the patient's clinical condition at the time of disposition, the action taken can range considerably.

Level III: Major

These problems consist of significant discrepancies between the clinician's recorded image(s) and the QI review. For example, clinician records a pelvic ultrasound examination on a pregnant patient as an intrauterine pregnancy. The QI review finds no evidence of an intrauterine pregnancy, but does note free fluid in the pelvis and a 3 × 4 cm adnexal mass. In this case, the chart is immediately pulled and reviewed. Depending on the follow-up provided or whether a confirmatory study was obtained, the patient may be immediately contacted. The patient is then given follow-up instructions appropriate to the changed diagnosis.

Feedback on reviews, both positive and negative, should be provided to the clinician, along with constructive suggestions for improvement. On occasion, mandated remedial education or training may be appropriate at the discretion of the program's director. Records should be kept on providers so that concerning trends can be recognized and addressed. Actions taken to address such problems as well as the outcome of such actions should be recorded. These records are confidential peer review in nature and should be labeled as such. Results of QI activities should be regularly reported to the appropriate QI organization in the department, hospital, or clinic.

CONTINUING MEDICAL EDUCATION

As with training requirements, there are no well-established guidelines to dictate the amount of CME one needs to maintain competency in focused ultrasound. A reasonable number of education hours, along with continued bedside ultrasound use, should easily maintain skill levels and, preferably, even advance them. "Reasonable" should be determined in light of all the other requirements for continuing education within a specialty. If physicians normally receive 50 hours a year of continuing education in all areas of their specialty, then it would seem excessive to insist that 20 or even 10 of those hours be specific to ultrasound. Likewise, in a residency program, it does not make sense to require 15–20 hours a year of ultrasound didactic education if the entire didactic curriculum is only 200 hours per year. In a survey of 42 academic ED ultrasound programs, the question was asked, "How much CME is needed to keep ultrasound skills up"? Responses varied from 0 to 30 hours, with a median of 8 hours.[10] Ultrasound directors should consider all the above factors when making a decision about CME requirements.

▶ SELECTING THE ULTRASOUND DIRECTOR(S)

The ultrasound program's director is an individual with expertise in focused ultrasound that oversees the training program at an institution or a clinic. This should ideally be a physician who has completed a fellowship in emergency point-of-care ultrasound in order to ensure the highest level of expertise. When this is not possible, a physician with comparable experience (>1000 ultrasound examinations performed, training in image review and program administration) should be carefully recruited, as this person would represent the program as a liaison to the department of radiology and all other clinical departments. Because of the administrative duties required to maintain a successful point-of-care ultrasound program, many departments spread the ultrasound director's duties among several clinicians.

In some instances, the ultrasound director is someone from outside the group who is hired on an hourly basis. Whenever possible, it is advantageous to establish this role within the group because the process of training other group members is continuous and easier to accomplish when the ultrasound director is readily available. The group should acknowledge that the ultrasound director will invest a considerable amount of time on initial training, and this time should be fairly compensated.

▶ OBTAIN HOSPITAL APPROVAL OF THE PROGRAM

When performing focused ultrasound examinations in a hospital setting, the program must be hospital approved and credentialing must be in place. Going through such an approval process increases the scrutiny of the program by individuals outside the department and may generate valuable additional input into the program structure. Closer scrutiny by others will also lead to a more careful internal review of the program before presentation to the hospital, invariably leading to a better program. Approval also ensures that in the event of a significant problem, it will be more difficult for others outside the department to unilaterally persuade hospital governance to restrict the ultrasound program's activities. As with the overall program design, a hospital proposal can be modeled after a successful one from another institution.

Obtaining hospital approval of an ultrasound program should be seen as a political process, especially since there has been some resistance to point-of-care ultrasound programs from other imaging specialists.[11–14] Knowing which physician groups side with the proposal and which oppose it before open discussion occurs may guide the process. Clinicians who tend to be most supportive are those who also want to establish ultrasound programs. This group includes emergency physicians, intensivists, hospitalists, internists, surgeons, nephrologists, and family physicians, among others. However, ultrasound allies and enemies vary from hospital to hospital, and making assumptions without investigation is not prudent. Clinicians who already use ultrasound in their practice, such as cardiologists, obstetricians, and gynecologists, may also be allies in this process.

The following are helpful to refer to in a proposal:

1. Specialty society policy statements regarding the use of focused ultrasound. In emergency medicine, for example, SAEM, the American Academy of Emergency Medicine, and ACEP have supported focused ultrasound use in the ED.[15–17]

2. The American Medical Association's Policy H-230.960 states that individual specialties have the right to determine how to appropriately use ultrasound in their practice.[18]

3. The percentage of residency programs in the individual specialty, as well as clinicians in the region and nationally, who are training in and using ultrasound. Has ultrasound become or is it becoming the norm locally or regionally? Is it a resident training requirement? Performing and interpreting point-of-care ultrasound is considered part of the core curriculum in emergency medicine.[19]

4. Numerous articles attesting to the safety and efficacy of focused ultrasound, especially in comparison to ultrasound examinations performed by traditional imaging specialists.[20–23]

▶ ACQUIRE AN ULTRASOUND MACHINE

This subject is covered in detail in Chapter 2, "Ultrasound Equipment." When making the decision on a purchase of an ultrasound machine, the best advice is to compare different ultrasound machines as you would compare cars. There are a variety of bells and whistles on different systems. Likewise, the cost can vary significantly with each manufacturer. You need to kick the tires and "drive" each system to find what is right for your department. This can usually be accomplished at annual emergency medicine conferences or specialty society meetings.[24–27] Another approach is to simply have two or three companies loan an ultrasound machine to you for several days. Asking a trusted and experienced colleague is another option. Determine what they liked and disliked about their machines. What equipment did they get that they do not use and what do they wish they had gotten? What kind of service do they get from the manufacturer? The relationship with the manufacturer is almost as important as the machine itself. Company representatives may assist with scheduled maintenance, urgent repairs, equipment upgrades, and in many instances, actual training within the program. Renting or leasing equipment may be a wise option while deciding on a particular manufacturer.

► TRAINING THE ULTRASOUND DIRECTOR

Several training options are available for the ultrasound director. Many directors completed one of many emergency ultrasound fellowships in the United States.[29] Others may fill the needs of their department with solid training obtained during their residency and additional educational courses given by various specialty societies.[24,25,27] There are numerous web-based ultrasound educational and CME sites to gain new knowledge, or polish up on specific didactic and case studies for various ultrasound applications.[27,28]

In the past, some emergency physicians learned ultrasound with the help of an experienced sonographer in their own hospital. It may be possible for the director-in-training to sit with a sonographer and perform examinations during normal working hours. This approach has the advantage of minimal cost, but is less time efficient since the trainee will be required to sit through many examinations that may not be applicable to the interests of that trainee. In addition, there are many examinations, like the FAST examination, that are not routinely performed by sonographers in the ultrasound suite. A better alternative is to hire an ultrasound-trained clinician on an hourly basis to individually teach in the ultrasound director's own clinical setting. The ultrasound director may require several months of training before they attain the expertise needed to train others within their group. It is imperative that the ultrasound director be well established before the rest of the group begins training. This is important to help facilitate the group through the "training doldrums," when the frustrations of training tend to peak. It should be emphasized that the learning curve is quite steep at the beginning of training but is actually relatively short in length so that examination competency can be achieved with a manageable number of ultrasound examinations.

► TRAINING THE GROUP

Initial training can be either brief or extensive, depending on the training approach that is taken. One training model is the "parallel" model, where individuals are trained in several ultrasound examinations simultaneously. The other method is the "serial" model, where training occurs with one ultrasound examination at a time, without proceeding to another examination until a certain level of proficiency is achieved. The parallel model works best when individual trainees are able to dedicate a larger portion of their time away from patient care to learn a new set of skills, as is typical in residency training programs. The serial model has the advantage of requiring less time input to get a trainee to a minimum level of competency for one particular examination. Serial training is ideal for community-based practitioners who have less time for training and want to incorporate one set of ultrasound skills into their practice as rapidly as possible.

All training programs generally have the following components:

- An initial block of didactic instruction.
- An initial "hands-on" exercise.
- A required number of proctored examinations performed on actual patients.

In addition, the ultrasound director should consider some type of competency assessment after the completion of training with a written test, observed examinations, or both.

INITIAL DIDACTIC INSTRUCTION

The initial didactic instruction is where members of the physician group get their "jump start" in training. Initial training may consist of anywhere from several hours of instruction, if training in only one examination type, to several days of instruction, if training in multiple examinations. At a minimum, an introduction to the basic physics of ultrasound is required to understand the capabilities and limitations of the technology. Understanding ultrasound physics, even at a basic level, is essential for acquiring and interpreting ultrasound images. In addition, there should be some specific didactic instruction on the examination(s) being taught. It is feasible for the ultrasound director to develop and perform the initial training block, especially if only a few applications are to be covered. If several applications are being taught, then it may be more practical to have group members attend one of the commercially available introductory ultrasound courses. Planning and giving a large hands-on ultrasound instruction block is time consuming. It is important, however, that the ultrasound director ensure that any outside course meets the training requirements established for their program. At an ultrasound course, 1–2 hours is generally spent on ultrasound physics and equipment instrumentation, and an additional hour or two on each specific examination type. Lectures should include discussions of the specific indications for the examination and review of the anatomy, including normal, normal variant, and abnormal ultrasound findings. Teaching should focus on surface transducer positioning to obtain the best "windows" for each application and minimize artifacts. Sonographic landmarks (key anatomical landmarks in a specific plane visible by ultrasound) for each application should be repeatedly stressed. The major finding for each application type (e.g., gallstones) as well as other pathology (e.g., common bile duct dilation, pericholecystic fluid, or thickened gallbladder wall) should be demonstrated, and the appropriate ways to use these findings for clinical decision-making should be discussed. Indications for outpatient referral for more comprehensive imaging or a confirmatory study should be covered. A comprehensive listing of suggested content for didactic sessions is available in the Model Curriculum for Emergency Ultrasound and the Emergency Ultrasound Imaging Criteria Compendium.[2,5] Guidelines for an introductory course are outlined in the ACEP training guidelines.[1] The problem- and symptom-based approach utilized by emergency medicine has quickly been adapted in other clinical specialties such as critical care, hospital medicine, and internal medicine.

INITIAL HANDS-ON EXERCISE

The initial hands-on exercise is usually combined with the initial didactic instruction. During this exercise, image acquisition is practiced on normal models in a non-stressful, non–patient-care environment. Ideally, there should be no more than four learners and one instructor per ultrasound machine to maximize learner scanning time. Topics covered should include operation of the ultrasound machine controls, techniques for maximizing image quality, normal ultrasound anatomy, and systematic approaches to each application. Specific "pelvic" models are employed when endovaginal ultrasound is taught, and chronic ambulatory peritoneal dialysis (CAPD) patients may be employed to demonstrate free intraperitoneal fluid on ultrasound examination. CAPD patients can simulate a positive examination by infusing fluid into their peritoneal cavity at will, and can even vary the amount of fluid to give different appearances. In instances where budgetary or planning constraints exist, these sessions can be run with trainees examining each other. Although pathology will not (usually) be demonstrated using this approach, learners can effectively acquire techniques for good image acquisition and systematic examination. Repetitive hands-on scanning with normal patients will help learners discern normal and anatomical variants for each application. Knowing what normal looks like sonographically will help tremendously when it is time to interpret pathological findings. A newer teaching method is the ultrasound simulator that uses a mannequin and a computer to sim-

ulate scanning. The advantage of a simulator is that it can be programmed to simulate pathology, thus giving the trainee a more varied, yet standardized training experience. Finding enough patients with actual pathology to examine is one of the biggest challenges during training. Simulator technology holds great promise for the future of ultrasound training. Future privileging will likely be based on objective data obtained by scanning these mannequins. There are also various training "phantoms" and models, which are commercially available and can be used to practice skills such as vessel cannulation, peripheral nerve blocks, and foreign body localization. Models can also be homemade. Good phantoms can be created with various materials, such as rubber tubing, gelatin, or even raw chicken or beef. There are even homemade models for pericardial effusions.[23]

PROCTORED EXAMINATIONS

Proctoring is the longest phase of training, often taking several months to complete. This is the part of the training process that often leads to significant delays or outright failure. The biggest challenge for an ultrasound director is to help learners maintain enthusiasm and focus during the proctoring process. This is the time when it is critical to have the full support of the department leadership and clear incentivized goals and expectations.

Proctoring is when most of the practical learning occurs, and the most important part of the educational process. The goals of proctoring are to help establish basic ultrasound skills, solidify the approach to examination, verify the quality of images produced, and verify the accuracy of the examinations. As the clinician begins scanning a variety of patients in his or her own clinical environment, the relative complexity of the skill will become evident. The learner needs to be mentally prepared for this predictably difficult period so that frustration will not inhibit training. "Real-time" proctoring is extremely helpful in assisting the clinician through this period. Real-time proctoring involves having the proctor sit with and guide the trainee through examinations and is the best way to learn ultrasound. Ultrasound directors should perform proctoring in their department on real patients. This is the ideal situation, and applications can be added in stepwise fashion. Unfortunately, if the number of clinicians who need to be trained is quite large, this can also be quite time consuming. Another time-tested approach is to use real-time proctoring with sonographers within your hospital.

Some programs choose to do "delayed" proctoring, meaning trainees perform examinations independently, and then an experienced individual judges the quality and accuracy of the examinations at a later time.

A common delayed proctoring technique is to videotape or record digital clips of examinations. This method results in slower training, but is usually less expensive than hiring a clinician for real-time proctoring and saves the ultrasound director from doing all of the real-time proctoring themselves. Another delayed proctoring option is to keep track of how trainee ultrasound results compare with other clinical information, including ultrasound examinations performed by traditional imaging specialists, other imaging studies (such as CT), or procedures. This method accomplishes verification of accuracy but does not fulfill the other goals of proctoring. Reviewing static sonographic images generated by trainees as the sole method to delayed proctoring is problematic, especially for negative examinations. Pathology may be visible in one imaging plane but not in another, and the inexperienced operator may simply fail to find and document the pathology. Static images that are clearly positive can be used for proctoring in a limited manner since it is more difficult to "create" a false positive image (though not at all impossible). If delayed proctoring is chosen as the predominant means of training, it would be wise to have the ultrasound director provide some real-time proctoring on an intermittent basis. This would include a hands-on skills session to teach trainees to document specific landmarks in each application as well as demonstrate technical skills and avoid common errors in these examinations. Proctoring is the longest phase of training, often taking several months to complete. The biggest challenge an ultrasound director faces is helping trainees to maintain enthusiasm for the training program as they begin to climb the steep learning curve.

QUALITY ASSURANCE

One of the best education tools available to the ultrasound director is quality assurance. As ultrasound examinations are reviewed for quality, it is also an ideal time to discuss the appropriate landmarks for each application, how the acquired image might be improved, and the diagnostic interpretation of each study. Carrying out this process with colleagues, trainees, residents, or students can be extremely valuable. Almost any pathologic study can be difficult to interpret if adequate landmarks or appropriate images are not documented. Likewise, capturing only still images can make it difficult to differentiate normal from pathologic findings. For example, documenting a live pregnancy with just still images can be difficult. Documentation has to tell a story. Images of a live pregnancy have to verify where the pregnancy is located. There must be views of the endometrial echo of the uterus demonstrating the gestational sac of the live pregnancy within its borders. Otherwise, one cannot rule out an extrauterine gestation. The repetitive nature of reviewing multiple images and video helps the trainee understand the correct documentation of an examination.

▶ PERFORM PROBLEM SOLVING

Ultrasound directors often experience two major problems with their programs. The first is difficulty in convincing all members of the group to participate in training. The second is maintaining trainee enthusiasm during the long proctoring phase. Emergency physicians, faced with the difficulty of integrating ultrasound-training examinations with patient care during busy ED shifts, will find it tempting to put off using ultrasound. The following are some strategies to help avoid these problems:

1. *Maintain easy access.* The easier the use of the ultrasound machine, the more it will be used. An ultrasound machine in a "safe" but inconvenient place will not be used. The ultrasound machine should be kept in close proximity to patient rooms and in full view. Not only will this remind clinicians to use the machine, it will assist with security of the ultrasound machine since its absence will be noticeable. This is especially important in critical care settings, such as with hypotensive and cardiac arrest patients, where a machine that is not close at hand is infinitely far away.

2. *Examination efficiency.* Point-of-care ultrasound examinations can add 5–10 minutes to a patient encounter (although they typically reduce overall length of stay in the ED), which can add up over the course of a shift. If clinicians perceive the ultrasound examination as a major time drain, they will not perform them. Bringing the machine to the patient's room at the time of first contact, if an ultrasound examination is anticipated, can reduce examination times. The examinations should be focused. If it is clear early in the examination that the examination will be technically difficult, the examination should be terminated and referred to a traditional imaging specialist. The goal of focused ultrasound is not to do all examinations, but to do those where immediate answers are necessary and/or those that can be performed efficiently.

3. *Make it easy to keep track of training examinations.* If trainees are required to bring or keep track of individual logbooks or digital storage, then the program will likely flounder. Books or thumb drives may be forgotten or lost, creating frustration on the part of trainees.

It is imperative in the digital age to have all of the group's ultrasound studies available for review immediately on the ultrasound system (so colleagues/consultants can review scans) and/or the DICOM workstation. A designated computer and office space to review, store, and backup studies is paramount.

4. *Introduce competition.* Competition is an effective motivating factor if applied appropriately. Clinicians tend to be competitive. Periodically publishing the progress of trainees so that they can see how they compare with their peers can encourage those who might otherwise be ambivalent. At a minimum, it serves to remind everyone to continue practicing their ultrasound skills. Introducing a stepped system of achievement is also beneficial, especially if the first level can be achieved in a reasonably short period of time. Being allowed to proctor less experienced trainees can also reward trainees who have achieved designated levels of training.

5. *Provide individual feedback for documented studies.* A few motivational words can boost ultrasound numbers. Capturing images in which the trainee has documented good landmarks or pathology correctly and letting them know is uplifting. A screen capture of the image and "a good job documenting...." emailed to the trainee frequently inspires further positive results.

► REGISTERED DIAGNOSTIC MEDICAL SONOGRAPHER

Registered Diagnostic Medical Sonographer (RDMS) is a certification that can be achieved after a prescribed period of training or experience and satisfactory performance on a standardized examination. The RDMS certification is recognized nationally as the standard of training for sonographers. This certification is available to physicians as well and some propose it as a logical step in the acquisition of ultrasound skills. Tests are given in several specialty areas including the abdomen, adult echocardiography, and obstetrics and gynecology. This certification, however, is directed toward comprehensive examinations rather than focused examinations. In order to be certified, an individual must pass both physics and instrumentation examinations and at least one specialty area examination. The advantage of RDMS certification is that it is a credential with which hospitals are familiar, and it may lend weight to the physician seeking credentialing in focused ultrasound. Information regarding RDMS certification can be found online (http://www.ardms.org/credentials_examinations).[29]

► ELECTIVE TRAINING

An elective in ultrasound during medical school or residency is a superb way to accelerate ultrasound learning. Electives are typically 2–4 weeks long and offer a trainee dedicated time to learn ultrasound without the distraction of other patient-care responsibilities. Setting objectives is the key to elective design. The elective director should be able to answer the question, "What should the trainee be able to do with ultrasound by the end of the elective?" Often, the objective is to perform a certain number of ultrasound examinations or it may be to meet the requirements for a particular privilege level. The goals should be made clear to the trainee at the outset of the elective.

Example activities include the following:

1. Performance of a certain number of examinations under direct supervision or by post hoc review of video or static images.
2. Assigned reading, either from texts or from journals.
3. Involvement with administrative aspects of the ultrasound-training program, including ultrasound machine maintenance, supplies, record keeping, and proctoring of other trainees. This is the contribution the trainee makes in return for the teaching time they receive. It is also an essential exercise for anyone considering directing an ultrasound program in the future.
4. Involvement with other special projects, including research, teaching, or creating teaching materials, such as an ultrasound teaching file.
5. Testing, both written and practical.

Here are example requirements for a 2-week elective:

1. A pre-elective meeting outlining the objectives of the elective.
2. Four to six hours of directly supervised scanning distributed over the elective period.
3. An additional 56 hours of time spent independently scanning.
4. Assigned readings from an ultrasound textbook.
5. A written examination at the end of the elective.
6. Tape review sessions as needed for item (3) above.
7. Special projects amounting to an additional 4–8 hours (e.g., submit two cases to the ultrasound teaching file).

Ultrasound is a skill of great interest to residents in emergency medicine as well as medical students applying for emergency medicine residencies. Anecdotally, the enjoyment and satisfaction residents have received while doing emergency ultrasound electives has made it one of the most popular rotations in many departments.

► FELLOWSHIP TRAINING

To master the skills necessary to integrate this powerful imaging modality into clinical practice, and especially for those considering a position as an ultrasound program director, a fellowship in ultrasound should be considered. Fellowships provide a means for intensive ultrasound training beyond that which is possible within the curriculum of an existing residency program. In order for a fellow to obtain a quality educational experience, programs will need a solid commitment from their departments to provide the necessary resources. Several vital elements are needed to foster this learning experience. First, there must be a physician who is qualified to mentor an ultrasound fellow. This person should invariably have an extensive experience in clinical ultrasound, along with a passion to teach. They should have research experience and academic involvement in one or more of their specialty's ultrasound committees. Second, the fellowship director's department must fully support their efforts to advance ultrasound education and provide protected academic time to mentor each fellow and train physicians within their own department. Departments should provide financial support for a quality ultrasound system and equipment, and administrative support for research. Third, the patient volume and demographics should be sufficient to provide the fellow with experience in all applications of focused ultrasound.[30]

While the curriculum may vary somewhat, the foundation of each ultrasound fellowship program is fairly similar. They provide each ultrasound fellow with a core content of subject matter that is covered within the 1-year program along with several other educational experiences covered in the preceding sections. Incoming fellows may have extreme variations in ultrasound education based on where they trained during their residency and how much experience they have accrued. The ultrasound director may focus on "core" content with a particular fellow, while only covering advanced applications with another.

CORE CONTENT OF THE FELLOWSHIP

The core content refers to the primary ultrasound applications, but can expand into additional applications, as the fellow's time and interest allow (see Tables 1-1 and 1-2). There are always new applications or different technical components of an existing application to learn. Like almost everything else in medicine, it is a dynamic process. The fellow can become the

teacher in applications that are recently discovered or updated.

QUALITY IMPROVEMENT

Fellows should be involved in the department's ultrasound QI program. This activity offers a high educational return for time invested since the mistakes of the group become lessons for the fellow. It also allows the fellow to see the structure and function of a QI program. The repetitive nature of reviewing multiple images helps the fellow understand the appropriate landmarks, image quality, and text annotation to properly document and interpret an ultrasound examination.

JOURNAL CLUB

Reviewing the literature is an important component of an ultrasound fellowship. Although the structure in which this is accomplished may vary, a working knowledge of the pertinent literature is an integral part of the educational process. Structured journal clubs throughout the year serve to educate the fellow, resident, and students as well as provide an avenue to formulate other research ideas. A plan to include literature of core applications and advanced applications keep the fellow focused on the basic fundamentals as well as cutting-edge information.

TEACHING RESPONSIBILITIES

The ultrasound fellow should also be responsible for educating students, residents, and attending physicians. Protected clinical time for teaching is of great importance. Depending on the experience of the ultrasound fellow, this duty may vary considerably throughout the year. Some fellows may benefit from staying with the ultrasound directors group and observing teaching skills early on in their fellowship. There are several levels of ultrasound teaching steps. Step one includes having a solid knowledge of the didactic skills of each application being taught. Step two is to master the equipment being utilized to educate the students. Step three, which is the most difficult, is to educate course participants on the technical portion of the examination without removing the transducer from their hands. The best teachers are able to verbally walk the participants through the hands-on sessions without taking the transducer away to demonstrate what they are attempting to convey.

FUTURE DIRECTORS

Most ultrasound fellows will start or direct an ultrasound program after graduating from the fellowship. This may involve implementing or enhancing an ultrasound program at an existing residency program or private hospital. The fellowship experience should include a road map for this important step. The administrative portion of the fellowship is customarily covered during the second half of the fellowship. This includes the likes of departmental policies on credentialing, ultrasound system maintenance, billing, QI discrepancies, and intradepartmental policies. They will need assistance in developing lectures, training courses, and various training aides for their program. The fellowship should also include networking with other leaders in their field who will provide them with an opportunity to share ideas, research projects, and shape the future of ultrasound.

► COST OF A POINT-OF-CARE ULTRASOUND PROGRAM

One of the most common questions posed by physician groups about ultrasound is, "How much will it cost us?" Little has been published about the costs of an ultrasound program. Some of the costs are easy to define (e.g., equipment and supply costs and price of training courses) and some are not as easy to define (e.g., time spent developing a program plan or performing practice ultrasound examinations). The bottom line is that the use of point-of-care ultrasound to aid in the diagnosis and the care of patients is starting to become the standard of care in the ED. Physicians who are trained in ultrasound understand the advantage of this technology.

► CODING AND REIMBURSEMENT

The second most common question asked by those who must make the balance sheet work for an office or department is, "Can we bill for this service?" The short answer is "yes." A detailed discussion of the financial side of ultrasound is beyond the scope of this chapter, but there are certain issues worth mentioning. Performing and billing for a focused examination does not exclude a traditional imaging specialist from performing and charging for a comprehensive examination of the same area, even on the same visit. Serial focused ultrasound examinations, if medically indicated, can be billed individually (e.g., serial FAST examinations in a deteriorating patient) at this time. Emergency physicians do not have to meet the same reporting standard as radiologists in order to charge for ultrasound examinations, but they may, in some instances, be required to record images to receive full reimbursement. Hospital-based clinicians generally cannot own an ultrasound machine and charge a "technical" fee in addition to their usual "professional" fee for an ultrasound examination.

Extensive and up-to-date information about ultrasound coding and reimbursement can be found on the ACEP website (www.acep.org).

REFERENCES

1. American College of Emergency Physicians: Emergency ultrasound guidelines. *Ann Emerg Med* 53:550–570, 2009.
2. Monico EP: The state of emergency ultrasound and the standard of care. ED Legal Letter October 2007:114–116.
3. Kendall JL, Bahner DP, Blaivas M, et al.: Emergency ultrasound imaging criteria compendium. American College of Emergency Physicians. *Ann Emerg Med* 48(4):487–510, 2006.
4. American College of Radiology: *Resolution 22, Standard for Performing and Interpreting Diagnostic Ultrasound Examinations. American College of Radiology.* Reston, VA: 1996.
5. American Institute of Ultrasound in Medicine: *Training Guidelines for Physicians Who Evaluate and Interpret Diagnostic Ultrasound Examinations.* Official Statement. September 2003. Available from: www.aium.org/publications/statements/statementSelected.asp?statement= 14. Accessed June 2, 2006.
6. Mateer J, Plummer D, Heller M, et al.: Model curriculum for physician training in emergency ultrasonography. *Ann Emerg Med* 23:95–102, 1994.
7. Witting MD, Euerle BD, Butler KH: A comparison of emergency medicine ultrasound training with guidelines of the Society for Academic Emergency Medicine. *Ann Emerg Med* 34:604–609, 1999.
8. Lanoix R, Leak LV, Gaeta T, et al.: A preliminary evaluation of emergency ultrasound in the setting of an emergency medicine training program. *Am J Emerg Med* 18:41–45, 2000.
9. Hoffenberg: Emergency ultrasound coding and reimbursement. Available from: www.acep.org/NR/rdonlyres/9ECB1EA2–0EFB-496F-ABE4–0D7C41144065/0/emerg UltrasoundCodingReimb.pdf. Accessed May 16, 2006.
10. Peterson M, Fischer T, Blaivas M: Survey: Cost of an ultrasound program. Preliminary results presented at the Ultrasound Section Meeting, Society for Academic Emergency Medicine Annual Meeting, May 2000.
11. Merritt CR: ER ultrasound services—some points to consider. Society of Radiologists in Ultrasound Newsletter, July 1999.
12. Hamper UM: Commentary on "Hertzberg BS, Kliewer MA, Bowie JD, Carroll BA, DeLong DH, Gray L, Nelson RC. Physician training requirements in sonography: How many cases are needed for competence. *AJR* 174(5):1221–1227, 2000." Society of Radiologists in Ultrasound Newsletter, June 2000.
13. Unknown author: Who can perform ultrasound imaging? Society of Radiologists in Ultrasound Newsletter, March 2000.
14. Hertzberg BS, Kliewer MA, Bowie JD, et al.: Physician training requirements in sonography: How many cases are needed for competence? *AJR Am J Roentgenol* 174:1221–1227, 2000.

15. Society for Academic Emergency Medicine: *Ultrasound position statement.* October 2004. Available from: www.saem.org/publicat/ultrasou.htm. Accessed June 2, 2006.

16. American Academy of Emergency Medicine: *Performance of emergency screening ultrasound examinations. Position Statement.* February 1999. Available from: www.aaem.org/positionstatements/ultra.shtml. Accessed June 2, 2006.

17. American College of Emergency Physicians: *Use of ultrasound imaging by emergency physicians. Policy Statement.* June 2001. Available from: www.acep.org/webportal/PracticeResources/PolicyStatements/pracmgt/Useof UltrasoundImagingbyEmergencyPhysicians.htm. Accessed June 2, 2006.

18. American Medical Association: *Privileging for ultrasound imaging.* House of Delegates Policy H-230.960, 2000. Available from: www.ama-assn.org/apps/pf_new/pf_online?f_n=browse&doc=policyfiles/HnE/H-230.960.HTM. Accessed June 2, 2006.

19. Allison EJ Jr, Aghababian RV, Barsan WG, et al.: Core content for emergency medicine. Task Force on the Core Content for Emergency Medicine Revision. *Ann Emerg Med* 29:792–811, 1997.

20. Milling TJ, Rose J, Briggs WM, et al.: Randomized, controlled clinical trial of point-of-care limited ultrasonography assistance of central venous cannulation: The Third Sonography Outcomes Assessment Program (SOAP-3) Trial. *Crit Care Med* 33:1764–1769, 2005.

21. Melniker LA, Leibner E, McKenney MG, et al.: Randomized controlled clinical trial of point-of-care limited ultrasonography for trauma in the emergency department: The First Sonography Outcomes Assessment Program Trial. *Ann Emerg Med* 48:227–235, 2006.

22. Moore CL, Copel JA: Point-of-care ultrasonography. *N Engl J Med* 364:749–757, 2011.

23. Girzadas D, Zerth H, Harwood R: An Inexpensive, Easily Constructed, Reusable Task Trainer for Simulating Ultrasound-Guided Pericardiocentesis. *Acad Emerg Med* 16, supp1:S279.

24. AAEM: www.aaem.org

25. ACEP: www.acep.org

26. RSNA: www.rsna.org

27. AIUM: www.aium.org

28. Sonoguide: www.sonoguide.com

29. RDMS: www.ardms.org

30. Emergency ultrasound fellowships: www.eusfellowships.com/index.php

CHAPTER 2

Equipment

William Scruggs and J. Christian Fox

Point-of-care ultrasound has grown rapidly over the last two decades. Practitioners in virtually all fields of medicine have moved ultrasound image acquisition and interpretation out of imaging suites and to the patient's bedside in a multitude of clinical settings. Not unexpectedly, the ultrasound equipment market has developed at an astonishing rate, leading to a wide range of choices of ultrasound equipment available to clinicians.

► GENERAL CONSIDERATIONS

PORTABILITY

Manufacturers have pushed the boundaries of ultrasound equipment creating a range of sizes. Top-end machines found in radiology suites are still generally larger machines best suited as stationary pieces of equipment (though even these may be moved fairly easily by a single individual). Smaller and lighter machines are now commonly found throughout hospital and outpatient settings. Durable handheld units are used in the prehospital and military combat settings.[1,2] Recently, ultrasound devices small enough to fit into the pocket of a clinician's white coat have been brought to market.

The size of a system should play an important role in purchasing decisions. Cart-based, handheld, and hybrid systems all deserve consideration depending on the clinical environment. Hybrid systems offer a cart from which a handheld component may be removed for easy transport. In general, cart-based systems are higher-end machines offering better imaging and more software options. However, the performance gap between cart-based machines and handheld machines is narrowing.[3]

The ED and critical care unit generally require some form of cart-based system. Several transducers are necessary for the growing number of applications that emergency and critical care physicians utilize; finding places to set a handheld machine while scanning can be difficult. Cart-based machines have varying amounts of storage space for commonly used adjunct equipment, such as ultrasound gel, transducer sheaths, printers, recording devices, and cleaners.

A removable component is beneficial when other areas of the hospital are covered for "code" situations or when a cart will not fit into the nooks and crannies of a treatment room overflowing with equipment and patients. Handheld-only options may be more appropriate for office-based practices, prehospital providers, and military providers who perform a more limited range of studies in a setting where the importance of small size trumps improved functionality.

POWER

Power is generally not the first consideration for clinicians when purchasing ultrasound equipment. However, the ultrasound machine battery power options and boot-up time may make the difference between a tool that is used regularly in practice and one that sits in the corner collecting dust.

Many companies offer products that are powered both via wall outlets and rechargeable battery packs. Most products with batteries allow for seamless use of the device as it is unplugged, which can be a huge advantage in situations where clinicians move quickly between patients.

The boot-up time of a machine is an important consideration. Ultrasound machines that take more than 30 seconds from power-switch to general use are impractical in the ED and critical care units. Beyond the obvious drawbacks in critical situations, machines with long boot-up times lead to physician aggravation and less use of the machine. No clinician wants to wait for their machine to start while other responsibilities await.

Another important consideration is the power cord itself. Machines in the ED are moved rapidly between patients by many different people with varying levels of concern for the machine. The power cord and its connection to the machine take a lot of abuse when it is run over or pulled from the wall. Devices should have a specific place to store the cord or the ability to retract it completely.

POWER FOR ANCILLARY DEVICES

Most devices provide outlets that are used to power ancillary devices (thermal printers, video recorders, or gel warmers) and some require specialized adapters. Specialized adapters may not be a problem if you plan to store images/video on the hard drive of the machine or other devices such as a USB drive, but realize that if the outlets are too few or too specialized, your options may be limited.

TRANSDUCER CHANGERS

Different ultrasound applications require different transducers so the ability of a clinician to instantly switch between transducers is important. Many cart-based systems have several "active" ports that allow the user to switch between transducers at the push of a button. Machines that only allow one transducer to fit into the machine at any given time have one "active" port, and several "storage" ports where other transducers are held while not in use.

Multiple active ports are essential for full use of an ultrasound machine in an ED or critical care setting. Emergency physicians perform many types of scans and often in rapid succession. Untangling cords and physically changing transducers between patients and scans is frustrating and time consuming. This is particularly evident when clinicians care for a trauma patient and need to seamlessly move between the linear transducer (to assess for a pneumothorax and obtain central venous access) and the small footprint phased array transducer (to assess for hemoperitoneum, hemopericardium and hemothorax).

▶ BASIC KNOBOLOGY

There are many different ultrasound machines, but they all have the same basic controls. Any practitioner with ultrasound experience should be able to operate any machine, no matter where it is found in the hospital or how many knobs are found on the control panel. The next section identifies the basic controls that are present on every ultrasound machine, from a single-transducer device found in a clinician's pocket to the fully loaded models found in a radiology suite.

CONTROL PANEL

Control panels on ultrasound machines vary widely. Machines with more bells and whistles tend to have more buttons and knobs compared with very portable machines with only the essentials. More complex control panels may intimidate clinicians who are novice to ultrasound. As the graphical user interface of tablet devices and other handheld electronic devices moves in a direction lacking buttons, so too will the portable ultrasound units. Touch screens employing no physical "buttons" will likely become the norm.

The durability testing manufacturers undertake should be considered. Machines with more buttons and knobs may also have more cracks and crevices through which fluids may enter and disrupt function. Another minor question relates to the difference between trackballs and track pads. Trackballs may work more quickly and precisely than a track pad (especially with gel-laden gloves). However, they also may become clogged with gel or other substances necessitating removal and cleaning.

ACOUSTIC POWER

The acoustic power (also called output power) relates to the amplitude of sound waves produced by the transducer and helps determine the brightness and quality of the image. Increasing the acoustic power results in higher transmitted amplitudes and stronger returning echoes. Greater acoustic power may improve image quality by increasing the contrast between light and dark areas on the display. However, if the power is too high, lateral and longitudinal resolution will decrease.

Acoustic power is directly related to intensity. The intensity of the ultrasound beam, meaning the amount of energy in a given area, determines the bioeffects of ultrasound. As the intensity increases, the amount of heat produced in the tissue increases, which potentially could cause tissue injury. While no studies have provided concrete evidence that diagnostic ultrasound has deleterious effects on tissues, including fetal tissue, practitioners using ultrasound work by the ALARA (**A**s **L**ow **A**s **R**easonably **A**chievable) principle, meaning we use the lowest possible power setting necessary for creation of the appropriate image.[4] Potential bioeffects are especially important when scanning pregnant women and

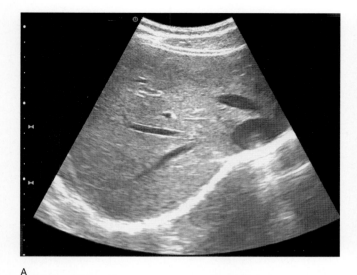

A

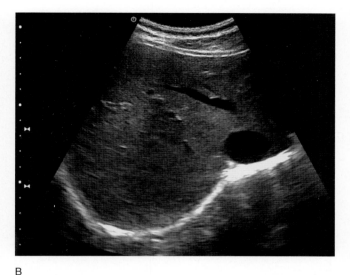

B

C

Figure 2-1. Gain—over, under, correct. (A) (Over) The image has too much gain applied to the image. Compared with image C, echoes are found where there should be none. (B) (Under) The image is under-gained. The periphery of the image is very dark, potentially making an accurate diagnosis very difficult. (C) (Correct) Appropriately gained. (Courtesy of Ultrasonix)

the eye. The obstetrics and ocular presets on a given machine appropriately adjust the power output to FDA-approved levels for these tissue types.

Most machines do allow the clinician to adjust the power. However, the controls for acoustic power are generally not found on the primary control panel on portable machines. With some more basic machines, the power is only adjusted by toggling the presets.

GAIN

The primary control clinicians use to adjust brightness is gain. When an echo returns from the body to the transducer, it does so within an amplitude range. The ultrasound device translates that amplitude range to a brightness, which is displayed on the monitor. The overall gain allows the clinician to adjust the brightness of all returning echoes, thereby adjusting brightness over the entire screen. Care should be taken not to over-gain images. Despite the perception of many novice ultrasound operators that brighter is better, increased gain can lead to loss of subtle findings.

Both acoustic power and gain change the brightness of the image. Power changes the brightness by changing the strength of sound entering the body, thereby increasing the strength of returning echoes. Gain changes the brightness by adjusting the amplification of the electronic signals after the echoes have returned to the transducer (Figure 2-1). Therefore, when an image is not bright enough, the user should first adjust the gain to improve the image.

TIME GAIN COMPENSATION

Time gain compensation (TGC) allows the clinician to adjust the brightness of the image at different depths. To

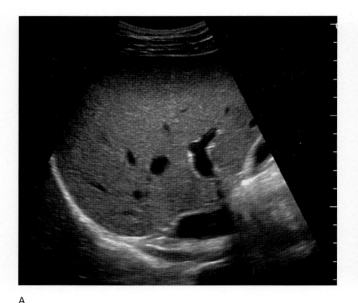

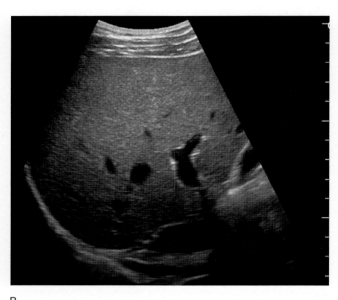

A   B

Figure 2-2. TGC—near field, far field. (A) The near field is under-gained. (B) The far field is under-gained. Compare with Figure 1c— an appropriately gained image that is uniformally "bright" from top to bottom. (Courtesy of Zonare)

understand TGC, one must understand attenuation. Attenuation is the progressive weakening of the ultrasound beam as it passes through tissue. Attenuation occurs due to absorption, reflection, and scattering of sound energy away from the transducer. If the ultrasound device were to display the actual amplitude of returning echoes, the image would become progressively darker from superficial to deep. Accordingly, ultrasound devices are built to compensate for attenuation by increasing the brightness that is displayed for structures that are deeper in the body in order to create an image with the same echogenicity from top to bottom.

Ultrasound devices often make this adjustment with slight inaccuracies because structures attenuate sound at different rates. As an example, the very bright image that is typically displayed posterior to a bladder in a transabdominal pelvic window occurs because sound does not weaken much as it passes through fluid such as urine. Echoes therefore return with a much higher amplitude than sound waves that pass through soft tissue. The ultrasound machine interprets that to mean that there are stronger reflectors posterior to the bladder and display them much more brightly.

Clinicians can adjust the TGC to correct for inaccurate assumptions made by the device (Figure 2-2). The simplest method of adjustment is two knobs: one dedicated to the near field and the other dedicated to the far field. More complex machines have a series of sliding levers that correspond the various depths on the display. Users are thus able to adjust the gain more smoothly through the image. Newer technology now allows some machines to evaluate and

better self-correct image brightness at the push of a button.

DEPTH

The most frequently used button or knob on any ultrasound machine is depth. The depth function adjusts how far into the body the machine images. There are two important reasons to optimize the depth. First, the size of the display is finite and imaging to a greater depth means structures are made smaller to present more on the display. If the deeper structures are not important to the user, that area of the display is simply "wasted real-estate." When the depth is reduced, less area is displayed making the presented structures relatively larger on-screen (Figure 2-3).

Second, adjusting the depth changes the amount of time the machine listens for returning echoes. If the depth is increased, the machine listens longer to collect data before displaying information reducing the displayed frame rate. Decreasing the frame rate may diminish the temporal resolution making the stream of images displayed less smooth to the eye, which may have a negative effect on diagnostic accuracy and procedure guidance.

The depth refresh time refers to how long it takes a machine to create a new image after the clinician adjusts the depth knob. Most machines will refresh the image almost seamlessly, but some machines may have a noticeable delay. While it may not be clinically relevant, a slow refresh rate can be frustrating to the user.

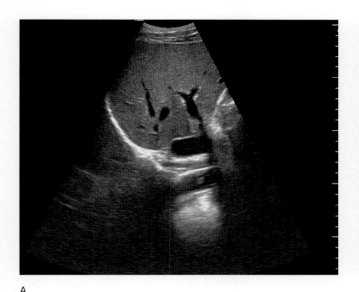 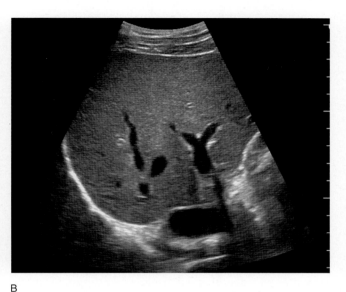

A   B

Figure 2-3. Depth—deep, correct. (A) Note the depth is set too deep, wasting valuable space on the display. (B) The depth is set correctly providing a balance between all important structures, while utilizing the entire display. (Courtesy of Zonare)

ZOOM

Most ultrasound machines offer a zoom function. The zoom function magnifies one section of the display. Importantly, the resolution remains the same, meaning the number of pixels does not change. Rather, they are magnified to create the larger image. The zoom function is most useful when the clinician wants to focus on deeper structures (Figure 2-4).

Zoom and depth work through entirely different mechanisms and, whenever possible, the depth should be altered first to optimize the image. The zoom function magnifies the original data that are collected (postprocessing). The depth function actually changes the way the image is acquired (preprocessing). Decreasing the depth allows the machine to dedicate more pixels to a smaller area, thereby improving the resolution. Only use zoom when deeper structures need to be magnified.

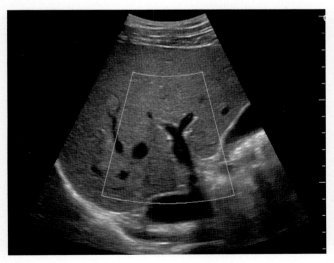 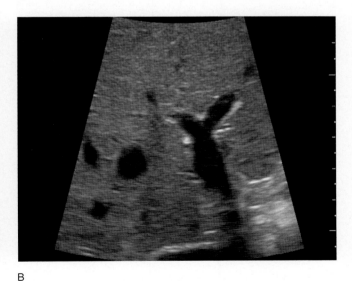

A   B

Figure 2-4. Zoom. (A) A sector of the image is selected prior to the zoom function activation. (B) The zoom function is activated, effectively magnifying the hepatic vein and surrounding structures. (Courtesy of Zonare)

FREEZE

The freeze button holds an image on the display. Most devices keep the last several seconds of images in memory (referred to as a "cine loop"), so when clinicians freeze the display, they are allowed to move through those saved images. The exact number of images saved in current memory varies with the device.

MEASUREMENTS AND CALCULATIONS

The ability to measure structures is very important for any machine in any clinical setting. Almost all ultrasound devices produce electronic calipers that allow the clinician to make accurate measurements. Many machines also offer packages that will use the measurements made to make clinically important calculations such as area, volume, crown-rump length, biparietal diameter, cardiac output, and others.

▶ ADVANCED KNOBOLOGY

M-MODE

M-mode (motion-mode) ultrasound is used to graph the movement of structures within the body. The clinician focuses the machine on a narrow area of returning echoes. The machine maps the returning echoes on the y-axis with time graphed on the x-axis (Figures 2-5 and 2-6). Cardiologists use M-mode ultrasound to precisely

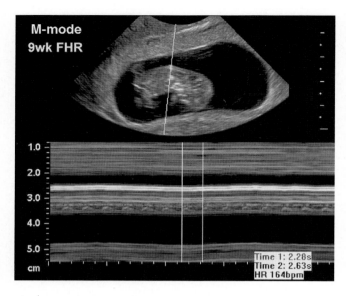

Figure 2-6. M-mode fetal heart. The M-mode line is placed through the fetal heart in this image. The movement of the heart is charted against time and can be seen at approximately 3.4 cm on the resulting graph. The movement calculates to 164 bpm. (Courtesy of Zonare)

evaluate the movement of heart valves. Common uses in emergency settings include evaluation for pneumothorax and quantifying fetal heart tones.

DOPPLER

Doppler ultrasound uses the frequency shift created by the reflection of sound off a moving body to observe and describe that movement. Doppler shift is the change from the original frequency that occurs when the sound reflects off a moving structure. The amount of shift relates to the velocity of that structure. The simplest form of Doppler ultrasound audibilizes the Doppler shift. Palm-sized machines that "whoosh" in time with the pulsating flow of blood through peripheral vessels or the fetal heart are used in many areas of the hospital. Diagnostic ultrasound devices offer more advanced Doppler that visually displays Doppler shift.

COLOR FLOW AND POWER DOPPLER

Bidirectional Doppler is probably the most recognizable form of Doppler ultrasound. Doppler shift is detected and movement toward and away from the transducer is displayed in different colors—generally in red and blue (but not limited to those colors). The color image is placed on the backdrop of the gray scale image so flow can be assessed related to the surrounding anatomy (Figure 2-7).

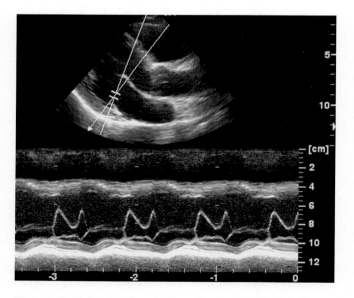

Figure 2-5. M-mode cardiac. The cursor has been placed over the mitral valve. The graph below demonstrates the motion of the mitral valve at the cursor over time. (Courtesy of GE Medical)

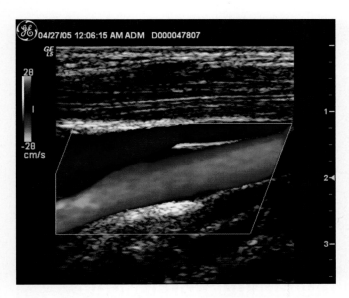

Figure 2-7. Color Doppler. Color Doppler measures the frequency shift and displays it as color over the gray scale image. Note the color scale to the left of the ultrasound image. The blue color at the top of the scale indicates that flow toward the transducer is labeled blue. (Courtesy of GE Medical)

For inexperienced users of color Doppler ultrasound, it is important to note that red and blue have nothing to do with arteries and veins. The ultrasound device will display a graph in one corner of the display when color Doppler is activated that demonstrates one color corresponding to flow toward the transducer

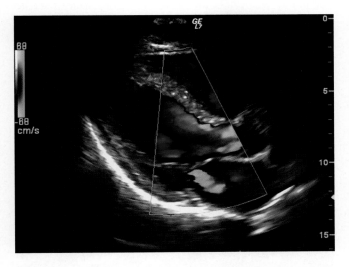

Figure 2-8. Variance mode. In the upper left corner of the display, there is a legend referencing the colors to the echocardiogram. The left side of the legend shows that red color indicates flow toward the transducer and blue color flow away from the transducer. The right side of the legend demonstrates that green color indicates turbulent flow. (Courtesy of GE Medical)

and one color corresponding to flow away from the transducer. The color displayed at the top of the graph refers to flow toward the transducer, while the color at the bottom of the graph corresponds to flow away from the transducer. Velocity and variance modes may be available within Doppler ultrasound. Velocity mode demonstrates the speed of movement toward or away from the transducer. The lighter shades of each color on the Doppler graph (generally red and blue) represent higher flow rates. Variance mode demonstrates the presence or absence of turbulence (Figure 2-8). Devices display turbulence on the same chart as the velocity on the horizontal axis. The color to the right indicates more turbulent flow, while the color to the left is laminar. Variance mode is commonly used by cardiologists to evaluate blood flow through the valves of the heart or by radiologists and vascular surgeons to evaluate flow through blood vessels.

Power Doppler displays flow without regard to direction. Rather than two colors distinguishing the direction of flow, the same color (frequently orange) with a range of hues is applied to a gray scale image wherever a Doppler shift is identified (Figure 2-9). Power Doppler is more sensitive, thereby showing slower flow, but comes at the expense of more motion artifact. Additionally, power Doppler is less affected by the angle of the ultrasound beam to the direction of flow than is bidirectional Doppler.

Doppler ultrasound is optimized by various means, some of which are very complicated. Common methods include adjusting the color gain, pulse repetition frequency (PRF), steering, and wall filtering. Color gain adjusts the amount of color displayed in color Doppler mode in the same way the gain adjusts the brightness of the image in B-mode ultrasound. The method used to adjust color gain varies by machine, but often involves turning the "Gain" knob on the machine while in color Doppler mode. If the color gain is set too high, excessive noise is displayed and detracts from the image. If the color gain is set too low, flow may not be displayed at all.

PRF is the frequency at which the transducer emits pulses of sound. Relative to Doppler ultrasound, the PRF affects the sensitivity of Doppler to flow. A low PRF will better display low-flow states such as blood flow through veins. However, using a low PRF for arterial flow may cause significant aliasing (an artifact that limits the ability to accurately measure flow velocity). A high PRF setting will appropriately demonstrate faster movement without aliasing, but may not display lower velocity flow. Fortunately, most manufacturers allow for a choice of optimization for low, medium, or high-flow states.

Steering of the ultrasound beam is necessary because Doppler ultrasound will not display flow if the ultrasound beam is perpendicular to the direction of flow. Therefore, devices allow for the clinician to change the

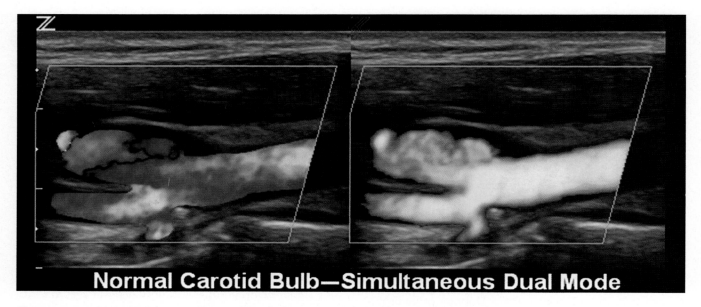

Figure 2-9. Power Doppler versus color Doppler. The image on the left demonstrates normal flow in the carotid sinus with bidirectional Doppler. The image on the right uses Power flow. Note the single color for all flow in the power Doppler image versus the color Doppler image that uses two colors to indicate flow toward and away from the transducer. (Courtesy of Zonare)

angle the ultrasound beam is emitted from the transducer.

Wall filtering is used to optimize the clarity of Doppler imaging at vessel walls. When Doppler demonstrates blood flow, the movement of the blood vessel walls creates artifact. Wall filters reduce artifact by rejecting the low level Doppler shifts caused by that movement.

PULSE WAVE OR SPECTRAL DOPPLER

Pulse wave is a type of spectral (or quantitative) Doppler that displays the velocity of moving structures (such as blood cells) on the vertical axis of a graph with time on the horizontal axis (Figure 2-10). The resulting graph accurately quantifies the flow. It is commonly used to

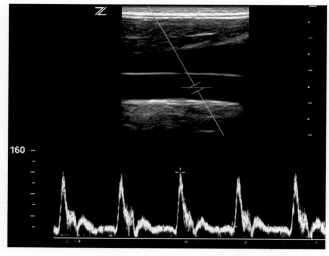

A

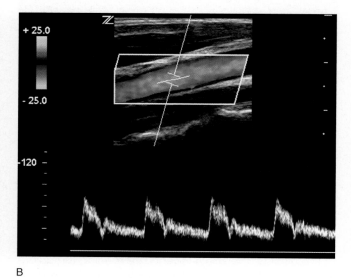

B

Figure 2-10. Duplex and triplex ultrasound. (A) Duplex ultrasound consists of either the gray scale image with color, or the gray scale image with the spectral Doppler graph. (B) Triplex ultrasound displays consist of a gray scale image, color Doppler, and spectral Doppler graph on the same display. (Courtesy of Zonare)

provide detailed evaluation of blood flow through the vasculature and heart.

The terms duplex and triplex ultrasound refer to how many "layers" of ultrasound imaging are displayed with Doppler ultrasound. Duplex ultrasound combines the anatomic image of two-dimensional (2D) ultrasound with either color Doppler or the graph representing the spectral Doppler analysis on the same display. Triplex scanning demonstrates the spectral Doppler waveform, the color Doppler image, and the gray scale ultrasound image on the same display. The screen is split into two sections with the gray scale and color Doppler image overlaid and the spectral Doppler graph found elsewhere on the screen. Duplex and Triplex ultrasound are useful tools in determining the location and flow patterns of vasculature.

FOCUS

Ultrasound transducers effectively transmit an hourglass-shaped cone of sound. The greatest resolution is found at the narrowest portion of that hourglass shape—the focal zone. Many devices offer the ability to electronically adjust one or more focal zones. The focus is represented by a small arrow or line to the left or right of the image. It is moved up or down the screen by the track pad or ball. The greatest lateral resolution will be found at the level identified by the arrow. High-end machines offer the ability to create multiple focal zones within the image. Multiple arrows will be displayed and the overall lateral resolution of the image will improve. However, while increasing the number of focal zones may improve lateral resolution, it will also decrease temporal resolution as the device spends more time listening for returning echoes and processing each image.

HARMONICS

All ultrasound devices send pulses of sound into the body at a primary frequency and then listen for echoes at that same frequency. Ideally, each crystal in the transducer will only "hear" returning echoes that they emitted. However, they also receive signals scattered from surrounding tissue decreasing the overall quality of the image.

When echoes are reflected, they return at the primary frequency and at harmonic frequencies, which are at multiples (2×, 4×, 8×, etc.) of the original frequency. Harmonic frequencies produce less scatter and side-lobe artifacts creating cleaner images. They are attenuated less by tissue than the primary frequency. Thus, higher frequency waves can reach further through the

tissue and potentially yield a higher resolution image. Tissue harmonic imaging (THI) filters echoes returning at the primary frequency and uses the harmonic frequencies to create the image. THI can be very useful in difficult-to-scan patients. However, in some patients the image quality may actually decrease. Clinicians should be just as willing to turn it off as they are to turn it on.

OPTIMIZATION BUTTON

Many machines offer an "Optimization" button. This function may be noted by several other terms, but they all refer to the same basic idea. This feature allows the processor within the device to use all of the above functions as well as a few more advanced techniques to create the "ideal image." This can be a very simple and effective way to improve image quality. It should not, however, be the sole means to improve image quality. Any clinician should be able to adjust the image using the above functions separately.

PRESETTINGS

Presets use adjustments of acoustic power, gain, focal zones, lines per sector, sector size, and other settings to create an image generally most useful for that particular type of imaging. Obstetrical settings are notable in that they decrease the power output to FDA accepted levels for ultrasound of the fetus. Cardiac settings work to increase the frame rate at the expense of image quality to maximize the ability to evaluate cardiac motion. Aside from imaging differences, some machines allow for different calculations while using certain presets such as biparietal diameter and crown-rump length in obstetrics mode. Many machines also allow the user to create their own presets.

VOLUMETRIC ULTRASOUND/ THREE-DIMENSIONAL ULTRASOUND

Technological advances in volumetric and three-dimensional (3D) ultrasound are being made as the speed of computer processors improves. In a volume scanning protocol (volumetric ultrasound), the transducer is held in place while an ultrasound beam is steered through a wide scanning plane and data collected through the entire volume through which the beam passes (Figure 2-11). The data are then processed and can be manipulated and viewed from any angle. The technology has the potential to revolutionize ultrasound in the same way CT image reconstruction has revolutionized computed tomography.

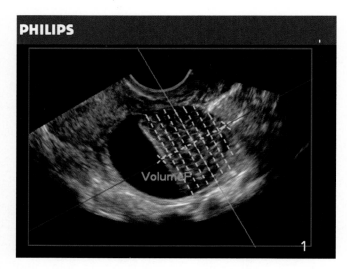

Figure 2-11. Volumetric scanning. Volume scan collects data over an entire volume rather than a single slice. The resulting data set can be manipulated to display an image through any plane in the volume. (Courtesy of Philips)

Three-dimensional ultrasound imaging for diagnostic purposes and procedure guidance is a budding technology in many fields, but clinical use is still very limited (Figure 2-12). There is limited research available for point-of-care ultrasound using 3D technology. The American Institute of Ultrasound in Medicine (AIUM) considers 3D ultrasound to be an adjunct to 2D ultrasound.[5]

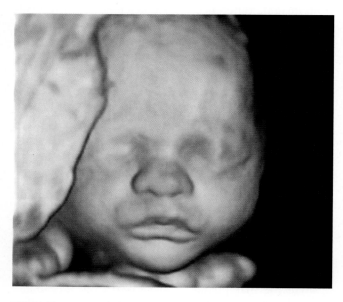

Figure 2-12. 3D ultrasound. Three-dimensional technology provides incredible ultrasound images, such as this image of the face of a fetus, but has little diagnostic value at this time. (Courtesy of Philips)

► TRANSDUCERS

BASICS

There are several layers to an ultrasound transducer. Piezoelectric crystals form the active element of the transducer, converting electrical to mechanical energy in the form of sound waves when transmitting and the reverse when sound energy returns. A matching layer directly covers the piezoelectric crystals and provides an impedance (resistance to movement of sound through a substance) layer between the crystals and the body. The matching layer is important because large differences in impedance cause reflection. Piezoelectric crystals have an impedance 20 times that of tissue. Such a difference would cause 80% of sound to be reflected away from the body.[6] The matching layer drastically reduces this effect.

The backing material suppresses crystal vibration. By damping the vibration caused by the application of electricity to the crystal, the backing material improves the ability of the crystal to listen. Finally, the covering to the transducer protects the internal mechanisms within the transducer from trauma and insulates the patient and user from electrical shock.

Transducer maintenance is very important. Never use a transducer when its covering is cracked. A compromised cover may expose the clinician and patient to electrical current. Return any damaged transducer to the manufacturer for repair.

Durability is a very important factor in transducer selection, especially in rougher environments such as an ED. Ask the company how they test their transducers and machines for durability. Transducers are expensive and it is important to consider whether or not they fit well into a specific practice setting.

TRANSDUCER CLEANING

Never autoclave ultrasound transducers. Piezoelectric substances are polarized and stabilized at high heats and pressures, meaning they will no longer change shape, rendering them useless.

Ultrasound transducers that only contact intact skin are considered noncritical items and should be cleaned with soap and water, a low or intermediate-level disinfectant such as quaternary ammonium sprays, or wipes as directed by the manufacturer.

Ultrasound transducers that contact bodily fluids, nonintact skin, and/or mucus membranes (endocavitary transducers) are considered semicritical items and require more stringent measures. Clean these transducers with nonabrasive soap and water, followed by a high-level disinfectant such as glutaraldehyde products,

Cidex OPA, or 7.5% hydrogen peroxide.[7-9] More information regarding FDA-approved high-level disinfectants can be found at the FDA website.[10] Cover transducers in contact with mucus membranes with an impermeable barrier prior to use. Manufacturers supply a list of allowable cleaning solutions that will not damage their transducers.

FREQUENCY

Most diagnostic ultrasound transducers are broadband devices made to work over a range of frequencies. General-purpose transducers allow users to toggle between two and three preset frequencies. An example of this would be a 2–4 MHz abdominal transducer that can be switched to 2 MHz, 3 MHz, or 4 MHz. Higher frequencies yield greater resolution and a cleaner image, but reduced penetration. A lower frequency transducer will image deeper into the body, but sacrifice resolution. Use the highest possible frequency that will allow imaging at the required depth.

FOOTPRINT

The footprint is the area through which sound leaves and subsequently returns to the transducer. Larger footprints allow for better deep imaging, but have difficulty working around sound-resistant barriers at the skin surface, such as the ribs in abdomino-thoracic scanning (Figure 2-13). Smaller footprint transducers pass the

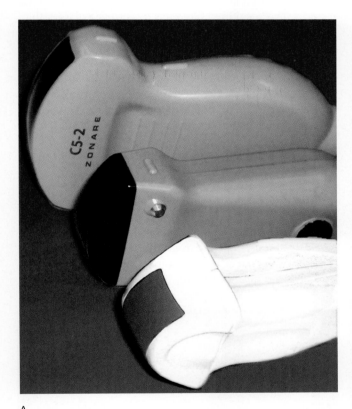

A

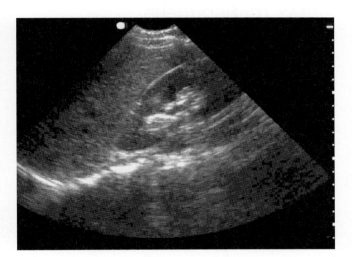

B

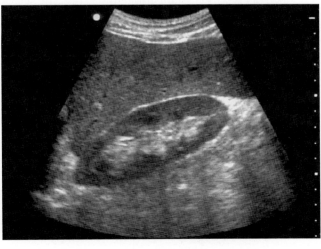

C

Figure 2-13. Convex array transducers: 60 mm, 30 mm, 15 mm. These three curved array transducers have different footprint sizes (A). Note the smaller footprint transducers have a tighter curvature. The sector created by each is pie shaped. The smaller footprint transducer (B) has a much smaller near-field image making it easier to scan between the ribs than the larger footprint transducer (C).

ultrasound beam through a smaller aperture making it easier to direct the beam between structures such as the ribs, but sacrifice resolution in the far fields as the beam diverges from the focus.

MECHANICAL TRANSDUCERS

Mechanical sector transducers are used on many older machines. A single piezoelectric element is moved across the scanning plane while pulses of electrical energy are applied, producing and receiving echoes. The transducer palpably vibrates due to the movement of the crystal. Mechanical transducers are not extensively used in newer machines.

ARRAY TRANSDUCERS

Modern ultrasound transducers use electronic array technology. Array transducers sequentially arrange crystals or groups of crystals along the footprint of the transducer.[11] By varying the timing of activation of groups of crystals, the ultrasound device can electronically steer and focus the ultrasound beam. Precise timing is required and malfunction of a single group of crystals can alter the direction and focus of the entire beam. Array transducers are produced in multiple forms, each with their own advantages or disadvantages.

LINEAR ARRAY TRANSDUCERS

Linear array transducers have a flat face along which a sequence of crystals is arranged (Figure 2-14). The sector

size of the linear transducer is identical to the footprint of the transducer itself. Linear transducers are generally used to view superficial structures and are therefore constructed to produce higher frequencies. However, larger linear transducers producing lower frequencies are sometimes used for deeper abdominal examinations. Transducers solely used for procedure guidance are generally smaller (~25 mm in width), and produce frequencies greater than 8 MHz. General use linear transducers used for the full spectrum of point-of-care ultrasound applications are closer to 40 mm, with frequencies ranging from 5 to 10 MHz.

CONVEX ARRAY TRANSDUCERS

The crystals in a convex array are arranged in a curved fashion. The resulting image has a sector size larger than the footprint of the transducer (Figure 2-13). There are many variations in convex array transducers. Lower frequency curved transducers are used for deep imaging in the thorax, abdomen, and bladder. Higher frequency curved transducers are used for endocavitary scanning, such as transvaginal and transrectal applications. Larger footprint transducers typically provide better lateral resolution. However, smaller footprint transducers with a tighter curvature allow for easier access through the intercostal spaces.

Endocavitary transducers are basically curved array transducers on a stick (Figure 2-15). They can be inserted into an orifice to get closer to the organ(s) of interest. They have a very wide field of view, up to 180 degrees, and are higher frequency transducers (8–13 MHz) because they require little tissue penetration to access the desired organs. The resolution is generally

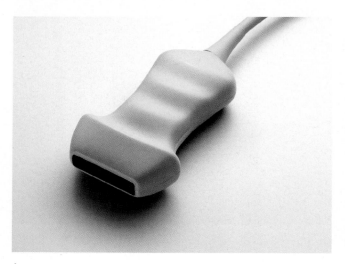

A

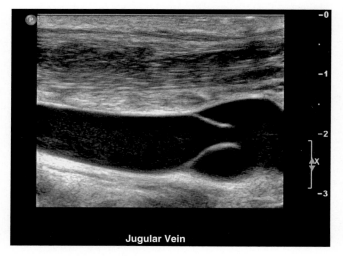

B

Figure 2-14. (A, B): Linear array transducer, linear image. The linear transducer with high frequency provides excellent superficial resolution. Note the sector size is equal to the footprint of the transducer. (Courtesy of Philips)

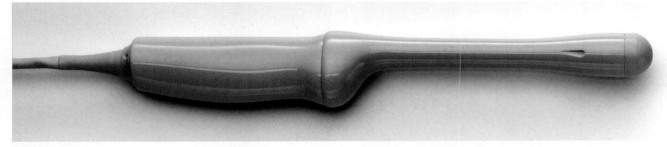

A

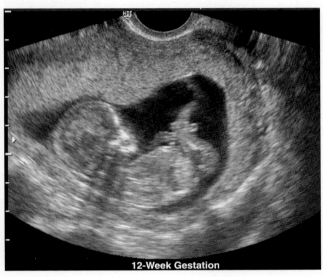

12-Week Gestation

B

Figure 2-15. (A, B): Endocavitary transducer, endovaginal image. The endocavitary transducer has a very wide field of view. Note the near 180 degrees of imaging in this ultrasound of a 12-week fetus. (Courtesy of Philips)

outstanding. While endovaginal scanning is the most common use of endocavitary transducers, urologists use similar transducers to evaluate the prostate. In the emergency setting, intraoral ultrasound for the diagnosis of peritonsillar abscess and procedure-guided drainage are other uses for the endocavitary transducer.[17]

PHASED ARRAY TRANSDUCERS

Phased array transducers have a flat footprint much like linear array transducers (Figure 2-16). The crystals are grouped into a very small cluster and every element activates with each ultrasound pulse. The device varies the timing and sequence of electrical pulses to the crystals to create a sector-shaped image. Phased array transducers are often used in echocardiography as the small footprint allows for easy intercostal imaging and the small, flat transducer makes excellent skin contact with minimal pressure. Furthermore, phased array transducers provide excellent deep imaging and Doppler capabilities making them useful to clinicians in a wide range of fields.[11] Limiting factors of phased array transducers include a small superficial field of view, prominent near-field arti-

fact that limits superficial imaging, and somewhat limited deep focusing capabilities.

VECTOR ARRAY TRANSDUCERS

Vector array transducers are linear transducers that steer and focus the ultrasound beam to create a sector that is trapezoidal in shape and wider than the footprint of the transducer (Figure 2-17). Vector array transducers are useful for superficial structures that are larger than the footprint of the linear transducer, such as imaging the thyroid gland, testicles, large abscesses, or other superficial structures.

► ACCESSORIES

GEL

Gel is used between ultrasound devices and the skin or mucus membranes to decrease the amount of air between the transducer and the patient. Air has a very different impedance than both the transducer and

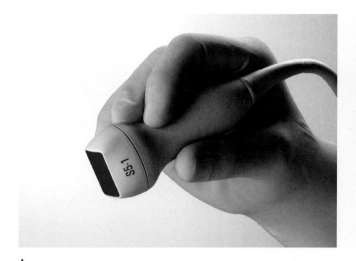

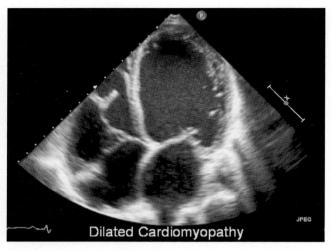

A   B

Figure 2-16. (A, B): Phased array transducer, phased array image. Phased array transducers have a small, flat footprint and create a pie-shaped sector. The resulting image has a very narrow superficial field-of-view with a large far field. (Courtesy of Philips)

the skin, causing tremendous reflections and a "white out" on the screen. By providing a medium with an impedance between the matching layer and the skin, gel allows more sound waves to pass from the transducer into the body, similar to the way the matching layer improves transmission of sound from the crystal.

There are two situations when standard ultrasound gel should not be used. First, commercially available gels may be irritating to mucous membranes.[12] They are for external use only. Sterile, nonirritating gels should be used for endocavitary exams. Gels that are made for contact with mucous membranes, such as sterile packets used for rectal and pelvic exams, are more appropriate. Second, gels for standard ultrasound use are not sterile.[13] Several companies offer sterile gels for ultrasound-guided procedures.

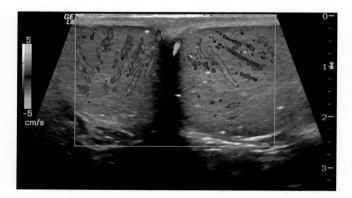

Figure 2-17. Vector array. Vector array technology creates a trapezoidal image from a linear transducer. This image views both testicles with Doppler. (Courtesy of GE Medical)

SHEATHS

Transducer sheaths are an essential part of ultrasound when performing sterile procedures and endocavitary scanning. Low rates of perforation and contamination have been found with standard latex condoms, making them an inexpensive and useful adjunct.[14] Commercial sheaths are available, but have been associated with higher rates of perforation and contamination.[15] Whatever cover is to be used, care should be taken to identify the latex allergic patients as severe reactions can occur if latex comes in contact with the mucous membranes of allergic patients.[16]

STERILITY

Standard sterile precautions such as gowns, masks, and gloves should be used for ultrasound-guided procedures. Packets containing sterile covers and gels are commercially available. Ultrasound-guided procedures are most easily performed with covers and gels specific to that purpose and are particularly helpful as they most often extend to cover the cord connecting the transducer to the machine (Figure 2-18).

NEEDLE GUIDANCE

Many companies offer disposable accessories that attach to ultrasound transducers and provide directional and depth assistance with needles during procedures (Figure 2-19). The attachments direct the needle to the middle of the transducer in the long axis, enabling the operator

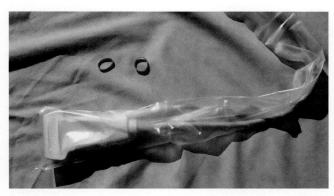

A

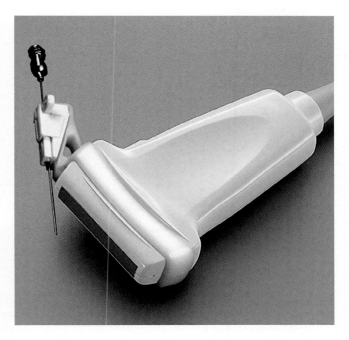

Figure 2-19. Needle guide attachment. Many companies offer attachments that provide needle guidance to their small parts transducers. (Courtesy of SonoSite)

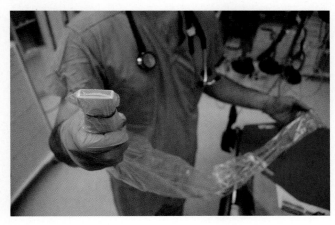

B

Figure 2-18. (A, B): Sterile sheaths. Sterile sheaths specifically made for ultrasound transducers will extend over the ultrasound transducer and cord. (B: Courtesy of Nicholas Jubert, MD)

to more easily see the entire length of the needle. In the short axis, different attachments are used for structures at different depths so the tip of the needle will not pass beyond the plane of the ultrasound beam.

Manufacturers are working to make needle visualization easier for medical professionals performing ultrasound-guided procedures. Needle manufacturers are attempting to make their needles more echogenic (brighter) on-screen. The holy grail of procedure guidance is the ability to demonstrate the entire needle on a single display. 3D/4D ultrasound holds promise, but is limited by several factors.[17] Another technology uses a special introducer needle and catheter, sensors embedded within the transducer, and an external sensor to demonstrate the location of the needle relative to the transducer on a single display (Figure 2-20).

HEAD-MOUNTED DISPLAYS

Procedure-guidance can be very cumbersome and technically challenging. In the single-operator method, the

clinician has the transducer in one hand, the needle in the other, and must frequently turn their head between the skin and the ultrasound machine. Head-mounted displays are available that minimize head turning and the potential for complications due to excessive movement.

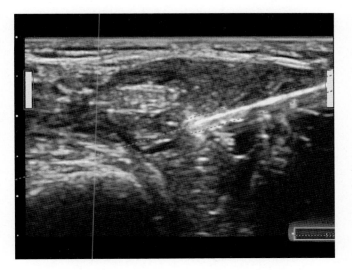

Figure 2-20. Needle guidance system. Numerous companies are trying to improve needle guidance. This image visualizes the needle in the long axis while providing a directional representation. The needle is also represented in relation to the transducer with the image of the transducer on the right lower quadrant of the screen. (Courtesy of Ultrasonix)

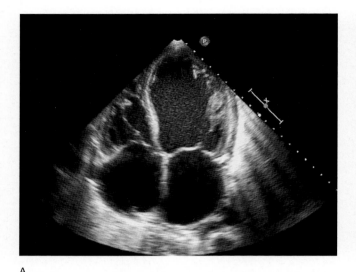

A

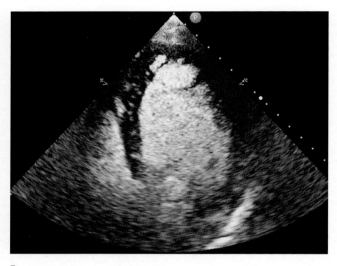

B

Figure 2-21. Ultrasound contrast agents. Ultrasound contrast agents are composed of small bubbles that are extremely echogenic. Image (A) represents an apical echocardiogram without contrast. Image (B) demonstrates an apical view of the left ventricle with IV contrast. (Courtesy of Philips)

The image is displayed onto a small monitor positioned just above the eyes. The eyes can move between the skin and display without moving the head and shoulders to visualize the screen.

ULTRASOUND CONTRAST AGENTS

Ultrasound contrast agents are air-filled microbubbles administered intravenously. Microbubbles are very reflective of ultrasonic energy and increase the overall contrast of the image improving both gray scale images and Doppler signals. Contrast-enhanced ultrasound is commonly used in echocardiography laboratories to better evaluate cardiac structures and in radiology suites to evaluate solid organ lesions (Figure 2-21). There is also great potential for contrast use in trauma to evaluate for solid organ injury. Studies suggest clinicians can accurately identify solid organ injury, even without the presence of hemoperitoneum, when contrast agents are used.[18,19]

▶ IMAGE VIEWING AND DATA STORAGE

The ability to view and store images is essential to any ultrasound program. Monitor attributes are important to consider as they affect the quality of imaging and the number of people who may view the image at a given time. Storing images or video is important for quality assurance, archiving for patient records, and teaching.

Digital storage is becoming more prevalent and convenient for archiving and quality assurance.

MONITORS

High-quality monitors are available on most machines. Considerations include flat panel versus cathode-ray tube (CRT) monitors, viewing angle, and overall monitor size. Flat-panel displays can offer high-quality images and weigh much less than CRT monitors. However, they tend to cost more than CRT monitors of similar quality.

Particularly with flat-panel monitors, the angle at which you can view the display is important. Lower quality machines may make it difficult for those at the periphery of the screen to view the image. Higher quality machines can offer almost 180 degrees of viewing.

The size of the display varies greatly among machines. Handheld machines have small, liquid crystal displays 5–8 inches in size. Larger machines offer 12–15 inch displays that are much easier to view. Some handheld machines are able to connect to larger monitors when on the cart.

Regardless of the monitor used, it is important to remember to adjust the room lighting to a low setting when performing a point-of-care ultrasound examination. A bright room may make subtle findings difficult to identify. Turning the lights down may not be an option when treating a critically ill or injured patient; B-color ultrasound may help visualization in these scenarios. B-color ultrasound assigns various shades of color to the gray scale image that can provide better recognition of more subtle pathology.

PRINTERS

Portable ultrasound machines are usually limited to thermal printers. Thermal printers offer low-cost and high-quality copies of ultrasound images that can be maintained for review, teaching, or archiving in medical records. Color printers are also available. Anecdotally, typical films used in thermal printing will save a high-quality image for 10 or more years if stored correctly. Films used in radiology departments are much more costly, but have a much longer shelf life. With the digital age and the electronic medical record, printing an ultrasound image is quickly becoming obsolete.

VIDEO STORAGE

Most machines allow users to record cine loops ranging from several seconds to minutes. Videos are typically stored in the memory of the machine that can be uploaded to an external server through a hardwired or, more conveniently, a wireless connection, thereby keeping the storage on the ultrasound device available for new studies. Alternatively, an older format for capturing videos is through connection to an external device such as a DVD recorder. It bears mentioning that video allows those reading the scans later to experience the ultrasound examination in the same way the clinician saw the images, which can be valuable in education, credentialing, and quality assurance.

ELECTRONIC STORAGE AND TRANSMISSION

Virtually all ultrasound machines manufactured today support a variety of means to transfer data. Whereas older machines were limited to analog data transfer through S-video or VGA ports, newer models support digital data transfer via USB, IEEE, HD ports, and even wireless systems. Such a variety of communication ports allows users a seemingly limitless number of electronic storage options including CD, DVD, digital video, CF/SD cards, and picture archiving and communication systems (PACS).

PACS is a collection of digital technologies used to store and transmit medical imaging.[20] Radiology departments are the primary users of PACS but other clinicians are integrating their ultrasound images into hospital-wide systems at many institutions. The technology allows clinicians to share images and interpretations of their ultrasound examinations with other health-care professionals. Digital Imaging and Communication in Medicine (DICOM) is a standard format to which images and data can be coded for transmission and electronic storage.[21] It is a standard format used within PACS. Many of the new generation of portable ultrasound machines are manufactured with the ability to encode in the DICOM format along with many others.

REFERENCES

1. Walcher F, Weinlich M, Conrad G, et al.: Prehospital ultrasound imaging improves management of abdominal trauma. *Br J Surg* 93(2):238–242, 2006.
2. Rozanski TA, Edmondson JM, Jones SB: Ultrasonography in a forward-deployed military hospital. *Mil Med* 170(2):99–102, 2005.
3. Blaivas M, Brannam L, Theodoro D: Ultrasound image quality comparison between an inexpensive handheld emergency department (ED) ultrasound machine and a large mobile ED ultrasound system. *Acad Emerg Med* 11(7):778–781, 2004.
4. Barnett SB, Haar Ter GR, Ziskin MC, Rott HD, Duck FA, Maeda K. International recommendations and guidelines for the safe use of diagnostic ultrasound in medicine. *Ultrasound Med Biol* 26(3):355–366, 2000.
5. AIUM. AIUM Statement: 3D Technology [Internet]. 2005. Available from: http://www.aium.org/publications/statements.aspx
6. Kremaku FW: *Diagnostic Ultrasound: Principles and Instruments.* 7th ed. St Louis, MO: Elsevier Saunders, 2005.
7. DHQP/C: *Guideline for Disinfection and Sterilization in Healthcare Facilities* 1–158, 2008.
8. AIUM. AIUM Statement: Recommendations for Cleaning Transabdominal Transducers [Internet]. 2005. Available from: http://www.aium.org/publications/statements.aspx
9. AIUM. AIUM Statement: Guidelines for Cleaning and Preparing Endocavitary Ultrasound Transducers Between Patients [Internet]. 2003. Available from: http://www.aium.org/publications/statements.aspx
10. US Food and Drug Administration: FDA-Cleared Sterilants and High Level Disinfectants with General Claims for Processing Reusable Medical and Dental Devices—March 2009. 2010.
11. Middleton WD, Kurtz AB: *Ultrasound: The Requisites.* 2nd ed. Requisites in Radiology Series. St Louis, MO: Mosby, 2003.
12. Villa A, Venegoni M, Tiso B: Cases of contact dermatitis caused by ultrasonographic gel. *J Ultrasound Med* 17(8): 530, 1998.
13. Wooltorton E: Medical gels and the risk of serious infection. *CMAJ* 171(11):1348, 2004.
14. Amis S, Ruddy M, Kibbler CC, Economides DL, MacLean AB: Assessment of condoms as probe covers for transvaginal sonography. *J Clin Ultrasound* 28(6):295–298, 2000.
15. Milki AA, Fisch JD: Vaginal ultrasound probe cover leakage: implications for patient care. *Fertil Steril* 69(3):409–411, 1998.
16. Fry A, Meagher S, Vollenhoven B: A case of anaphylactic reaction caused by exposure to a latex probe cover

in transvaginal ultrasound scanning. *Ultrasound Obstet Gynecol* 13(5):373, 1999.

17. French JLH, Raine-Fenning NJ, Hardman JG, Bedforth NM: Pitfalls of ultrasound guided vascular access: The use of three/four-dimensional ultrasound. *Anaesthesia* 63(8):806–813, 2008.

18. Catalano O, Aiani L, Barozzi L, et al.: CEUS in abdominal trauma: Multi-center study. *Abdom Imaging* 34(2):225–234, 2009.

19. Blaivas M, Lyon M, Brannam L, Schwartz R, Duggal S: Feasibility of FAST examination performance with ultrasound contrast. *J Emerg Med* 29(3):307–311, 2005.

20. Doi K: Diagnostic imaging over the last 50 years: Research and development in medical imaging science and technology. *Phys Med Biol* 51(13):R5–R27, 2006.

21. Graham RNJ, Perriss RW, Scarsbrook AF: DICOM demystified: A review of digital file formats and their use in radiological practice. *Clin Radiol* 60(11):1133–1140, 2005.

APPENDIX

Ultrasound Manufacturers with Offices in the United States

Hitachi Aloka Medical—www.aloka.com
BK Medical—www.bkmed.com
Esaote North America—www.esaoteusa.com
GE Healthcare—www.gehealthcare.com
Samsung Medison—www.samsungmedison.com
Philips Healthcare—www.healthcare.philips.com
Siemens Healthcare—www.healthcare.siemens.com
SonoSite—www.sonosite.com
Terason Ultrasound—www.terason.com
Toshiba Medical—www.medical.toshiba.com
Ultrasonix—www.ultrasonix.com
Zonare—www.zonare.com

CHAPTER 3
Physics and Image Artifacts

Corky Hecht and William Manson

Diagnostic ultrasound has experienced tremendous technological advances. Over the past 50 years, ultrasound has evolved from a single specialty tool with large bulky machines to a technology that is highly compact and portable. The development of smaller, less expensive ultrasound systems has increased the number of medical specialties utilizing ultrasound. Many are discovering the benefits of "point-of-care" diagnostic ultrasound. Medical students, nurses, mid-level providers, and physicians have embraced ultrasound as a tool to facilitate patient evaluation and improve outcomes of invasive procedures. The operator must have a basic understanding of the physical principles of ultrasound. It is these principles upon which ultrasound bases its ability to be an effective tool in medical imaging.

▶ UNDERSTANDING SOUND AND ULTRASOUND

The simplest way to describe ultrasound is in the pulse-echo principle. Sonar can be used as an example of the forerunner of diagnostic ultrasound. A submarine that possesses sonar capability can precisely control when an acoustic pulse is generated. It assumes a relative propagation speed as it travels through a specific medium (water). The amount of elapsed time required for the "echo" to return subsequent to striking an object allows the relative distance to be calculated to the target of interest.

Diagnostic ultrasound uses the same concept of the pulse-echo principle. Electric current is passed through crystals in the transducer and generates a sound wave. This piezoelectric effect generates a constant pulse of high-frequency, longitudinal, mechanical sound waves

that can be measured and used in calculations. This pulse travels at a relatively constant speed until it encounters a reflective surface, which causes a fraction of the sound to reflect back toward the transducer crystal. When the returning sound wave strikes the crystal, it generates an electrical impulse that is processed into a diagnostic image. Based on the assumption that sound travels at the same speed through all tissues (1540 m/s), a computer measures the round-trip time and intensity of each returning "echo." The amount of time required for the returning echo determines its relative distance from the transducer while the returning intensity is proportional to the grayscale assignment of the pixel. Each returning echo is presented as a pixel (dot) of information on the display device.

Sound waves are actually a series of repeating mechanical pressure waves that propagate through a medium (Figure 3-1). These pressure waves are measured in hertz (cycles/second). Typically, audible sound ranges between 16,000 and 20,000 Hz. Ultrasound is technically defined as a "sound" having a frequency in excess of 20,000 Hz. In medicine, ultrasound used for diagnostic purposes incorporates frequencies that generally range between 2 and 15 million cycles/second, or 2 and 15 MHz, well above the range of human hearing.

▶ PRINCIPLES OF ULTRASOUND PHYSICS

AMPLITUDE

Amplitude is the peak pressure of the wave (height). This may be simply interpreted as the loudness of the

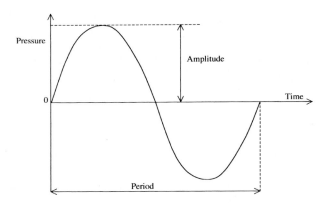

Figure 3-1. Time versus pressure graph of a sound wave. Amplitude: peak pressure of a wave. Period: time required to complete a single cycle. (Courtesy of SonoSite)

wave. Amplitude correlates with the intensity of the returning echo. A loud sound has large amplitude while a soft sound has small amplitude (Figure 3-1).

PERIOD

Period is the time required to complete a single cycle.

FREQUENCY

Frequency is the number of times per second the wave is repeated. The range of frequencies typically discussed here is between 2 and 15 MHz.

SPATIAL PULSE LENGTH

A diagnostic ultrasound transducer generates an image by sending and receiving ultrasound waves. It receives the returning, or reflected, ultrasound waves; the generation of ultrasound waves usually occurs less than 1% of the time. The period where it generates ultrasound waves is termed a pulse. Spatial pulse length is the distance or length of each pulse. Spatial pulse length is determined by the frequency and pulse duration.

Transducer technology is based on the piezoelectric effect. *Piezoelectric* is defined as "pressure-electricity" and refers to materials that have a dual function of converting electric energy into mechanical energy (pressure) and conversely mechanical energy (returning echo) into electrical energy. While quartz is a naturally occurring crystal, the crystal elements in modern transducers are synthetic. The arrangement and the number of crystals within a transducer vary depending on the

manufacturer, transducer design, and its intended application.

Transducer frequency has a direct effect on image quality and resolution. In general, high frequencies result in higher resolution and enhanced image quality. While resolution may increase, tissue penetration will decrease. Lower frequencies result in lower resolution, but have better tissue penetration.

Resolution is the result of the spatial pulse length as well. Higher frequency provides more reference points or pixels over a similar spatial distance and thus produces higher resolution by displaying smaller tissue segments. However, the trade-off is that the higher frequency will not travel as far or penetrate deep tissue.

BANDWIDTH

Historically, ultrasound transducers emitted only one frequency. As ultrasound equipment became more sophisticated, each transducer could generate multiple different frequencies, but could only send one frequency at a time. Modern ultrasound transducers emit a "center" frequency during the transmit portion of the cycle. A range of frequencies exists on either side of the center frequency and is known as the bandwidth (Figure 3-2). The resulting frequency is actually an average of the frequencies in the bandwidth.

Many ultrasound systems make use of these bandwidth frequencies during the received portion of the cycle and thus incorporate broadband transducers. Technology may allow the operator to select one of multiple "center" frequencies available from a single transducer. This selection allows the operator to easily maximize the transmit frequency of the transducer that offers the best resolution or best penetration for the area of interest. Regardless of which type of transducer technology is utilized, the highest frequency should be used that will penetrate the area of interest and that offers the best resolution.

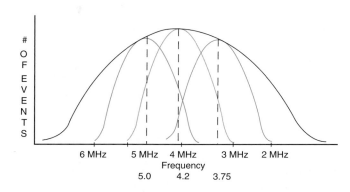

Figure 3-2. Broad bandwidth or multifrequency selectable transducers.

Image resolution is based on many transducer factors including the spatial pulse length of the wave. The spatial pulse length is dependent on specific transducer characteristics set by the manufacturer. This may explain why simply increasing the transmit frequency of a transducer may not consistently result in improved resolution or improved image quality.

VELOCITY

Velocity of sound is defined as the speed of the wave. The velocity of sound is dependent on the material through which the wave is traveling. Velocity is independent of frequency. Since the speed of ultrasound through a given medium is constant, the closer the molecules are in position to one another, the better the propagation. Therefore, sound travels faster in bone than in human soft tissue. When molecules become less dense (gases), the velocity of the sound slows even further or may not propagate at all as is the case with a vacuum.

WAVELENGTH

Wavelength (propagation speed/frequency) is the distance the wave travels in a single cycle.

ATTENUATION

The attenuation of sound begins the instant the pulse is generated within the transducer and it continues throughout its round-trip path until the sound pulse returns to the transducer to be recorded as an "echo." There are several factors that contribute to attenuation. These factors include the wavelength of the emitted sound, the medium through which the sound is traveling, and the number of interfaces it encounters.

The type and density of tissue combined with its degree of homogeneity or heterogeneity contribute to the rate of attenuation. Tissue of the same type and density facilitates the transmission of sound. Ultrasound travels best, with the least attenuation, through homogeneous fluid-filled structures. This is why transabdominal ultrasound of the uterus and ovaries is facilitated by a distended urinary bladder. The fluid inside the bladder provides an acoustic window for the sound wave and allows an efficient use of the transmitted sound to visualize the posterior anatomy.

Reflection is a form of attenuation. It is the redirection of part of the sound wave back to its source. Reflection is the foundation upon which ultrasound scanning is based. The ultrasound beam should evaluate the anatomy of interest at 90 degrees to maximize the re-

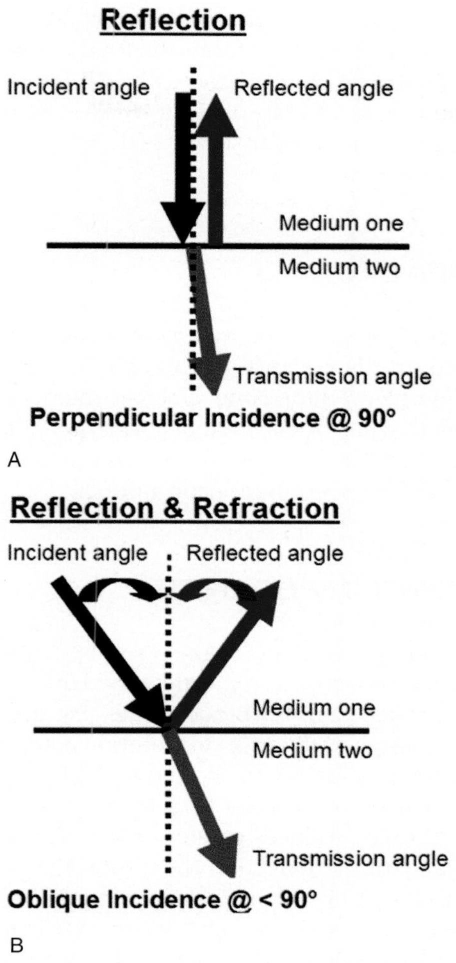

Figure 3-3. Reflection and refraction.

flection and visualize the anatomical structures. Manipulating the transducer so the area of interest is positioned directly under the transducer in the center of the display offers improved visualization and the ability to better appreciate the surrounding anatomical structures.

Refraction is the redirection of part of the sound wave as it crosses a boundary of mediums possessing different propagation speeds. This condition worsens with non-perpendicular incidence (Figure 3-3).

Scattering occurs when the ultrasound beam encounters an interface that is smaller than the sound beam or irregular in shape. The term *Rayleigh scattering* is specific to red blood cells (RBC) (<5 microns) that are not normally seen unless they are clustered together making a larger surface area. This may occur when blood movement slows during stasis, early clot formation, or asystole. *Spontaneous contrast* is another term used to describe this phenomenon, which is best noted during real-time B-mode imaging

Absorption occurs when the energy of the sound wave is contained within the tissue. When the acoustic energy is converted into thermal energy, it dissipates as heat within the tissue. This forms the foundation for therapeutic ultrasound. For instance, physiatrists use therapeutic ultrasound to help patients recover from injuries by using an output power significantly greater than that of diagnostic ultrasound.

INTERFACES

When sound crosses a boundary of tissues having different acoustic impedance, an interface is said to occur. In emergency ultrasound, a classic interface is Morison's pouch, where the liver abuts the hyperechoic renal fascia. This interface becomes more pronounced when anechoic fluid is seen in Morison's pouch.

ACOUSTIC IMPEDANCE

Acoustic impedance refers to the resistance of the tissue to molecular movement. Acoustic impedance is directly related to tissue density. Blood, urine, fat, and muscle all have enough difference in acoustic impedance to generate a reflection when the ultrasound wave passes from one tissue to the next. Greater density difference between tissues produces greater or stronger reflection. The intensity of the reflection (how loud the echo is) is determined by how much of a difference in impedance exists between the tissues in contact. A small density difference (acoustic impedance) results in a small echo being generated. A large difference in density results in

a large echo generated with much of the energy lost to reflection. Therefore, little energy remains available to continue for visualization of deeper structures. This explains why diagnostic ultrasound cannot "see" through bowel gas or bone, as there is too large a difference in acoustic impedance between these types of interfaces and soft tissue. This phenomenon is referred to as "acoustic mismatch" and will be covered further in the section on artifacts.

IMAGE RESOLUTION

Resolution refers to the quality of the image produced by the machine. It is the ability to differentiate the details of anatomical structures. While there are several factors that contribute to the overall image quality, we will limit our discussion to axial, lateral, temporal, and contrast resolution.

AXIAL RESOLUTION

Axial resolution is the ability to differentiate two closely spaced structures that lie in a plane parallel to the direction of sound wave propagation; that is, objects above one another on the viewing screen.

There are several factors that contribute to the quality of the axial resolution; however, the rate-limiting step under control by the operator is the ultrasound beam and transducer frequency. In general, higher transducer frequency produces better axial resolution and resultant image quality (Figure 3-4).

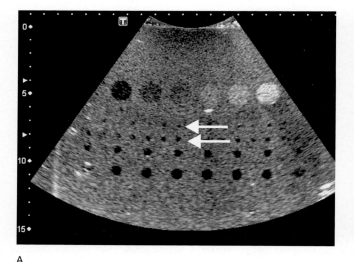
A

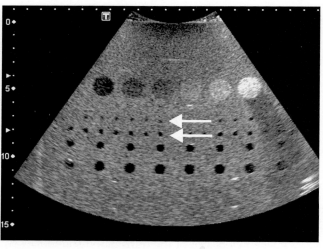
B

Figure 3-4. Axial resolution is improved by increasing the transducer frequency as the illustration demonstrates. Note how grainy and pixilated the lower frequency (1.9 MHz) image (A) is compared with the smoother characteristics of the higher resolution (5.0 MHz) image (B). Also, note the better visualization of the entire row of small cysts (top arrow) and the next row of slightly larger cysts (bottom arrow), along the "axis" of the transmitted beam. Both images were obtained using a multipurpose phantom. (Courtesy Model 539 Multipurpose, ATS Laboratories, Inc.)

LATERAL RESOLUTION

Lateral resolution is the ability to differentiate two closely spaced structures that are positioned perpendicular to the direction of propagation of the ultrasound beam; that is, objects that are side by side on the viewing screen. Generally, lateral resolution will be inferior to axial resolution. The primary equipment control that improves lateral resolution is adjusting the "focal zone" to the area of interest. However, some popular point-of-care ultrasound machines do not have the ability to separately adjust the focal zone. On these machines, adjusting the depth or resolution mode will indirectly adjust the focal zone. Additionally, ultrasound beam width contributes to this side-to-side resolution. The beam may be as wide as 5–10 mm at the surface of the transducer, but tapers to as little as approximately 1–1.5 mm at the focal zone depth. If this "focal zone" is positioned on the screen adjacent to the area of interest, then the ultrasound beam will in theory be the narrowest at this point, allowing for improved lateral resolution. Multiple focal zones may be selected on a single ultrasound image in an attempt to maximize the resolution at specific depths. Since this action requires additional processing time, a slower frame rate will occur and the image will begin to appear "choppy." Single focal zone capabilities are generally sufficient for most abdominal and cardiac examinations. Multiple focal zones are often of greater value when examining superficial structures when transducer movement is at a minimum and additional signal processing time is of less concern.

Adjusting the focal zone also narrows the "in and out of plane dimension" of the beam or the "slice thickness." The ultrasound beam is not quite two dimensional (2D), but has a thickness similar to a credit card. Adjusting the focal zone can prevent "slice thickness artifacts" that result from the beam being thicker than the structure being imaged and averaging larger volumes of tissue than intended. For instance, when trying to visualize a blood vessel (like the inferior vena cava), if the beam thickness is wider than the blood vessel, it may get reflected signal from the tissue on either side of the blood vessel and the averaged signal display may make the lumen appear to have some tissue component producing a slice thickness artifact (Figure 3-5). The operator can also affect frame rate by adjusting the width of the sector from wide to narrow or vice versa. As the sector width narrows, the frame rate increases (Figure 3-6). This adjustment can be especially important when scanning to detect motion such as in early pregnancy using a wide-angled endovaginal transducer.

TEMPORAL RESOLUTION

Temporal resolution refers to the acquisition rate of a composite frame expressed as frame rate (frames per second) or sometimes expressed as hertz (cycles per second). A frame rate of 15 Hz is required to see structures move in "real time" such as a fetal heartbeat or other adult cardiac structures. Adjusting sector width or decreasing line density will have the greatest impact on increasing temporal resolution or frame rate because in both situations the system is scanning fewer lines that require less time, making the image appear less choppy.

CONTRAST RESOLUTION

Contrast resolution refers to the ultrasound system's ability to assign a grayscale value to returning echoes of varying amplitudes. Most modern diagnostic ultrasound systems use 256 shades of gray, which allows recognition of subtle changes in tissue density. A higher contrast (less shades of gray) may be more pleasing to the human eye but may, in fact, contain less diagnostic information. This dynamic range of information (measured in decibels or db) is often a programmable feature and may be examination specific. The optimum setting allows a clear differentiation between the area of interest and the surrounding anatomy and typically the more shades of gray the better the contrast resolution. Abdominal imaging often uses a wide dynamic range with many shades of gray. Cardiac imaging uses a narrow dynamic range to create clarity between the moving endocardium and the anechoic blood (Figure 3-7).

▶ MODES

A-mode, or "amplitude-mode," provided one of the original evaluations of the human body using sound. A-mode ultrasound included an oscilloscope display for returning amplitude information and the traditional image did not exist. The peak amplitude information on the horizontal axis provided information regarding the strength or "loudness" of the wave, while the vertical axis provided reflector distance information from the transducer (Figure 3-8A). A-mode imaging is used in ophthalmology when measuring precise distances to the retina for calculating intraocular lens implantation. A-mode is generally not used in emergency ultrasound.

B-mode, or "brightness-mode," converts the amplitude of the returning echo into a grayscale image allowing better correlation with anatomical structures. This "2D" tomographic slice is what most emergency ultrasound exams use and is referred to as B-mode imaging (Figure 3-8A).

M-mode, or "motion-mode," permits a simultaneous display of the 2D B-mode image and a characteristic waveform (Figure 3-8B). This waveform depicts the motion or deflection of the tissue relative to the transducer on the vertical axis and represents time or changes in the cardiac cycle on the horizontal axis. M-mode

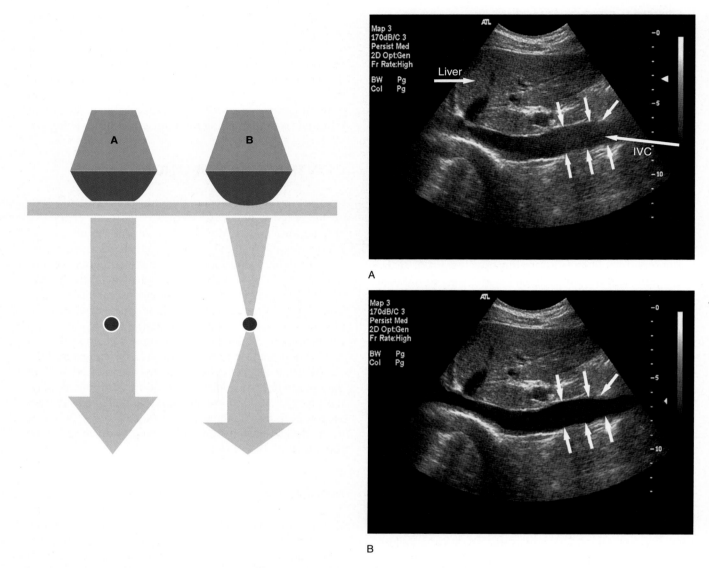

Figure 3-5. (Left) Slice thickness illustration. Beam profiles seen from side view. Beam is unfocused in image (A), creating a thicker beam than the focused beam in image (B). (Right) In image (A), the tomographic slice is imaging the IVC (small arrows) and some adjacent liver tissue creating the artifact (long arrow) because of the volume averaging that occurs. In image (B), the tomographic slice is thin and focused and therefore isolates only the IVC without the apparent artifact from volume averaging.

technology can be of value in the emergency and acute care setting during pregnancy examinations and permits measurement and documentation of fetal cardiac activity. It can also be useful to demonstrate timing of events during changes in the cardiac cycle such as identifying right ventricular diastolic collapse secondary to cardiac tamponade. Similarly, documentation of lung sliding can also be achieved using M-mode.

DOPPLER

Doppler is presented in a few different forms. Doppler technology relies on the interpretation of the "frequency shift" that exists between the transmitted and received Doppler signal, while the anatomy (blood within the vessel) is moving as it is imaged. For example, as a train whistle is engaged, the pedestrian at the crossing will experience an increase in the pitch (Doppler shift) of the whistle as the train approaches and a decrease in the pitch as the train continues to move away.

Doppler ultrasound technology makes use of this "frequency shift." Sources (e.g., RBC) moving toward the receiver (transducer) produce a higher reflected frequency, while sources moving away produce a lower reflected frequency, allowing the system to display flow direction and velocity. The angle of interrogation of

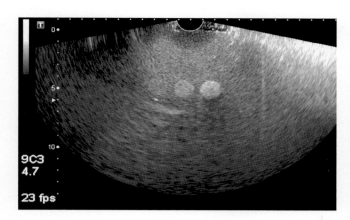

A

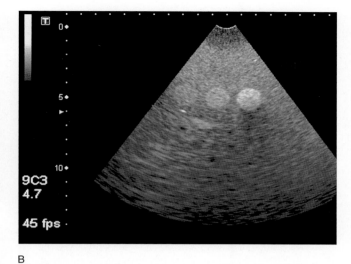

B

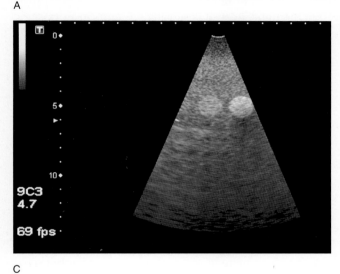

C

Figure 3-6. Sector width versus frame rate. The more narrow the sector, the faster the frame rate as noted for wide sector (A) frame rate = 23 fps, medium sector (B) frame rate = 45 fps, narrow sector (C) frame rate = 69 fps.

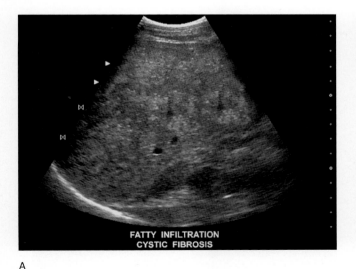

A

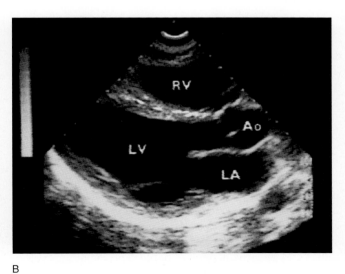

B

Figure 3-7. Contrast resolution. In image (A) the pathology in the liver parenchyma is best visualized using a wide dynamic range. In image (B) a narrow dynamic range is optimal for visualization of the rapidly moving cardiac anatomy.

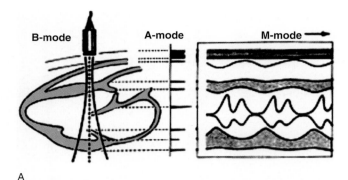

A

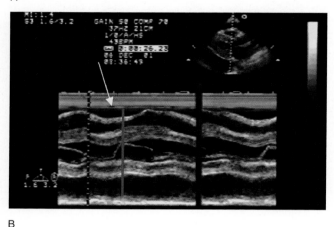

B

Figure 3-8. Comparison of modes. The diagram (A) depicts the image display for each of three modes: B-mode, A-mode, and M-mode. The mitral valve is open during ventricular diastole and closed during systole. M-mode ultrasound of pericardial effusion (B). The arrow shows that the RV collapses during early diastole (MV open on right as indicated by red time line).

blood flow is a prominent factor in the quality and accuracy of the Doppler signal.

Spectral Doppler provides a characteristic waveform and allows a quantitative assessment for blood flow analysis consisting of continuous wave or pulsed wave technologies. Pulsed wave Doppler produces short bursts of sound. It uses the same crystal to generate and receive the signal. By the transducer listening at specific intervals, it can control precisely where the reflected sound is coming from and thus has "range gate resolution." The limitation of pulsed wave techniques is that it can only display certain maximum or peak velocities (known as the Nyquist limit) before the signal will alias and become nonquantifiable. The maximum velocity it can display is limited by the transducer's Doppler frequency and the depth of the moving target. Aliasing or wraparound occurs if the velocity is too high to display. The peaks are cut off and displayed below baseline. Continuous wave Doppler uses different crys-

tals to send and receive signals. One crystal constantly sends signals while another receives the reflected signal. Therefore, a live B-mode image is not seen on the viewing screen. Continuous wave Doppler has no depth or range gate resolution but it does not alias and can quantify much higher velocities.

Color Doppler utilizes the pulse-echo principle to generate color images. The color image is superimposed on the 2D image. The red and blue displays provide information regarding direction and *mean* velocity of flow. It cannot display instantaneous peak velocities and is not truly quantifiable. The color at the top of the display represents flow toward the transducer, and color at the bottom of the display represents flow away from the transducer. It is sensitive to transducer position (Figure 3-9).

Whether using pulsed wave Doppler or color Doppler imaging, if the sound pulse strikes the blood vessel or blood flow at an angle over 60 degrees, it can result in inaccurate velocity readings and may even suggest that there is no flow when in fact it is due to poor Doppler angle.

Power Doppler images are based on amplitude or strength of the motion. Color maps in power Doppler are represented by one continuous color. It provides better sensitivity for slow flow or low blood volume states like ovarian or testicular torsion. It accomplishes this because it compares or averages several frames storing the accumulated flow over a number of cardiac cycles. This does take additional processing time and slows the acquisition frame rate. It is less angle dependent, but more sensitive to motion artifacts.

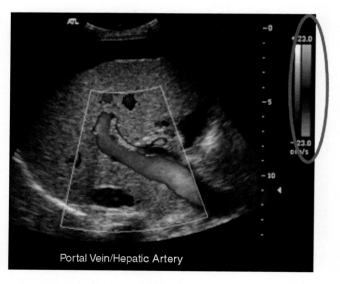

Figure 3-9. Color Doppler of portal vein. Red circle emphasizes color key for direction and/or mean velocity of flow.

Each form of Doppler consists of benefits and limitations; however, its operation appears deceptively simple. A comprehensive discussion of Doppler physics and velocity measurements is beyond the scope of this chapter.

► TWO-DIMENSIONAL IMAGING

Two-dimensional images (also referred to as B-mode or grayscale images) are created when the computer places pixels on a two-dimensional monitor based on the direction from which the signal was received and the time interval between emission and return of the signal. Echogenicity refers to the amplitude (brightness) of the signals reflected from a given structure compared to the amplitude of the signals from surrounding structures. If a structure presents as hyperechoic, it is said to be more echogenic (of increased amplitude) than the surrounding anatomy. Conversely, hypoechoic structures appear less echogenic (of decreased amplitude). Isoechoic information has the same echogenicity as the surrounding structures. Finally, anechoic refers to the absence of echoes. Typically, fluid-filled structures appear anechoic (devoid of echos or black) (Figures 3-10 and 3-11).

► IMAGE ARTIFACTS

Unrecognized artifacts are frequently the source of misleading information and misdiagnosis. However, some artifacts are the key to identifying certain pathologies. Accurate interpretation of ultrasound images requires recognition of anatomical reflections that we expect to

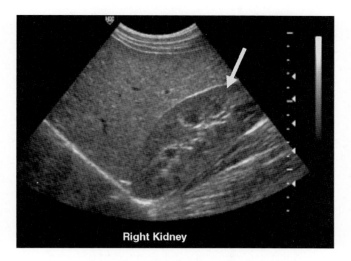

Figure 3-11. Renal parenchyma texture (arrow) is slightly hypoechoic as compared with the adjacent liver texture.

visualize as well as non-anatomic signals that appear as the result of artifacts. Artifacts will be defined as any echo information that does not correspond to accurate anatomical information. The origin of these artifactual echoes may occur from within the patient, as a result of attenuation or refraction, from an external source, or as the result of operator error.

SHADOWING

Acoustic shadowing is one of the most common and frequently encountered imaging artifacts in diagnostic ultrasound. Acoustic shadowing frequently occurs

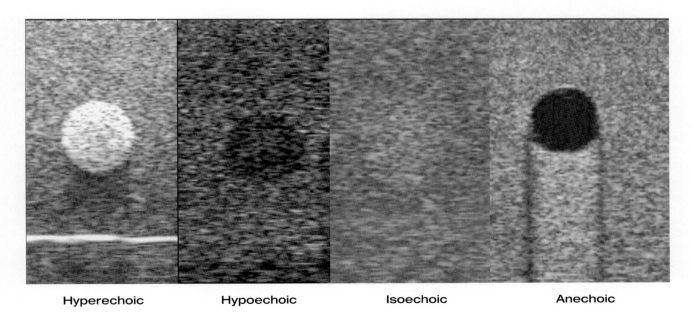

Hyperechoic   Hypoechoic   Isoechoic   Anechoic

Figure 3-10. Echogenicity. Note the edge artifact seen in the anechoic example. (Courtesy of SonoSite)

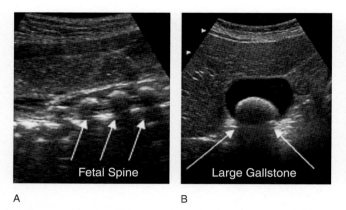

A   B

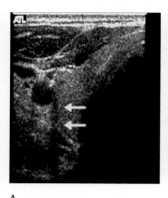 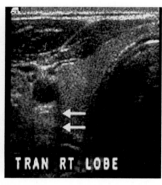

A   B

Figure 3-12. Clean shadowing from attenuation. Bone density objects, such as this fetal spine and a large gallstone, generally result in a darker more homogenous ("clean") shadow (arrows).

Figure 3-14. Transverse view of the thyroid. The arrows indicate the "edge artifact" that is seen in both images despite moving away from the density seen on the first image of the carotid artery. The sound is refracted off the side of the vessel, thus creating the acoustic shadow.

when the sound encounters a highly reflective (high-attenuation) surface. The reflected energy is returned to the transducer with little acoustic energy available to continue traveling to deeper structures. "Clean shadows" are caused by ribs, gallstones, and other calcified structures. "Dirty shadows" result from acoustic mismatch at tissue–air interfaces and are most commonly caused by bowel gas (Figures 3-12 and 3-13).

REFRACTION—"EDGE ARTIFACT"

Shadows may also occur because of changes in the ultrasound beam. A change in the sound beam direction

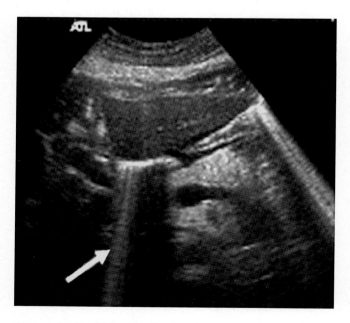

Figure 3-13. Dirty shadowing from air (arrow). Gas density objects such as bowel gas produce a shadow containing lighter, irregular gray level ("dirty") echoes.

results when there is an oblique incidence of the sound beam as it crosses a boundary of tissue with different propagation speeds or strikes a curved structure. As the sound crosses this boundary, a change in the beam direction occurs and an acoustic shadow results (Figure 3-10 and Figure 3-14).

ACOUSTIC ENHANCEMENT

Sound waves traveling through areas of lower attenuation cause posterior acoustic enhancement. The effects of acoustic enhancement are quite simply the opposite of high-attenuating objects. As sound passes through ultrasound-friendly structures (e.g., simple cysts, distended normal gallbladder filled with bile, urinary bladder, and some types of solid tissue), less attenuation of the signal occurs, which results in a greater amount of acoustic energy available to continue its journey along the same path. This increase in acoustic energy results in a similar increase in echogenicity (hyperechoic) immediately posterior to the area where less attenuation of the signal occurred. This type of imaging artifact is commonly used to confirm the presence of areas suspected to be fluid-filled, such as hemorrhage, joint effusions, and tissue necrosis or abscess and can be used to see the spread of anesthetic as it is injected. It is most commonly referred to as increased through-transmission or posterior acoustic enhancement (Figure 3-15).

GAS

The presence of gas is often the enemy of ultrasound. The large difference in density that exists between gas and soft tissue disperses the sound waves. Diagnostic

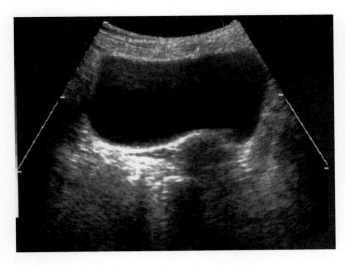

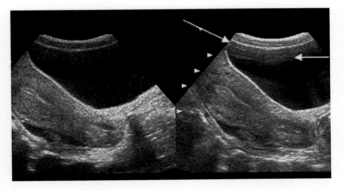

Figure 3-17. Longitudinal suprapubic view of the bladder and uterus. The arrows on the right image indicate a reverberation artifact. The TGC was adjusted on the left image to reduce this artifact.

Figure 3-15. Posterior acoustic enhancement. This echogenic (bright) artifact is seen below the left side of the image of the bladder (transverse view), and is also referred to as "increased through transmission." As this artifact is particularly common with a full bladder, it is imperative to reduce the far field gain in this setting, to avoid missing free fluid distal to the bladder.

ultrasound is not equipped to handle large differences in density and much of the acoustic energy is scattered with little or no appreciable diagnostic information visualized. Often, bowel gas can prevent visualization of some portion of the abdominal aorta. Transducer pressure or a change in patient and/or transducer positioning may minimize this obstacle (Figure 3-16).

REVERBERATION

When sound "bounces" between two highly reflective objects, reverberation artifacts appear as recurrent bright

arcs displayed at equidistant intervals from the transducer. This artifact will frequently appear when performing procedural guidance, with distal replication of the needle. This reverberation artifact may be severe enough to obliterate the B-mode image distally. Adjusting the depth, time gain compensation (TGC), transducer positioning, patient positioning, or transducer transmit frequency may reduce the appearance of reverberation artifacts. However, their presence is not likely to be confused with a pathologic condition (Figure 3-17).

Reverberation is also seen when imaging the pleural line of the lung. In the setting of normal lung, this reverberation produces horizontal hyperechoic lines distal to the pleural line, termed A-lines. In the setting of the interstitial syndrome, the dominant reverberation artifact becomes B-lines, or comet-tail artifacts, that originate from the pleural line and extend to the far field of the image (see Trauma, Figure 5-15).

MIRRORING

Mirror artifacts are displayed as objects that appear on both sides of a strong reflector. These artifacts can be confusing in appearance and occur because of changes in the reflected beam. Ultrasound assumes that sound is traveling in a straight line and the distance (or depth) of the reflector is proportional to the travel time necessary to make the return trip. When the ultrasound beam undergoes multiple reflections as it returns, an incorrect interpretation of the signal timing ensues and results in a duplication of structures. The more posterior echo information is the "false" echo. Mirror artifacts are common around the diaphragm and may depict hepatic structures appearing on both sides of the diaphragm. During the FAST exam, mirror artifact of the liver or spleen above the diaphragm argues against a pleural effusion or hemothorax. Changes in transducer

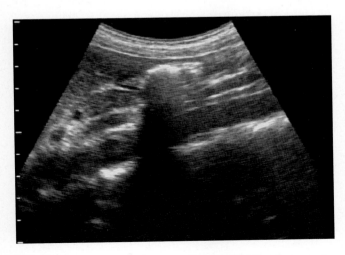

Figure 3-16. Longitudinal aorta is partially obscured by bowel gas. (Courtesy of SonoSite)

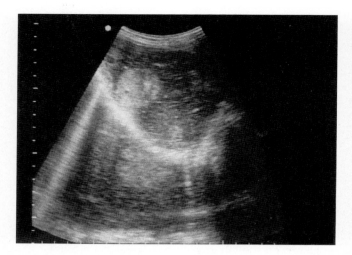

Figure 3-18. Mirror image artifact. Liver tissue and hyperechoic liver lesion are duplicated above the diaphragm. (Courtesy of SonoSite)

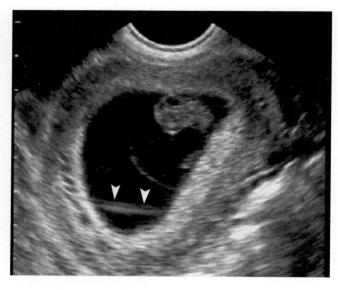

Figure 3-19. Side lobes. Endovaginal image reveals intrauterine gestation with embryonic pole and thin amniotic membrane. Side lobe artifact is demonstrated within the gestational sac (arrowheads). (Courtesy of SonoSite)

or patient positioning should alleviate the potential for misdiagnosis (Figure 3-18).

SIDE LOBES

It is easy to envision one ultrasound beam being emitted from the transducer as the thickness of a credit card. In reality, ultrasound beams of lower intensity, called "side lobes," may originate at angles to the primary beam and are generally of little consequence. Highly reflective interfaces return echoes via this pathway of side lobes and present as false information. This false information may be introduced as an oblique line of acoustic reflection. Changes in the scanning angle often confirm these returning echoes as side lobes (Figure 3-19).

▶ MAINTENANCE AND QUALITY ASSURANCE

Ultrasound system and transducer performance may change over time. Diagnostic ultrasound phantoms exist in part to allow a reproducible standard to be documented, to ensure that the ultrasound system and its components are operating at the performance level defined by the product manufacturer. Ultrasound phantoms allow evaluation of transducer parameters, measurement calibration, focal zone, axial and lateral resolution, sensitivity, functional resolution, grayscale displays, transducer beam profile, and Doppler measurements.

▶ BIOLOGICAL EFFECTS

Risks associated with diagnostic ultrasound are merely theoretical and clinically significant adverse effects have not been reported. Nonetheless, the American Institute of Ultrasound in Medicine (AIUM) has adopted an acronym termed ALARA: As Low As Reasonably Achievable. The term reminds operators that the amount of time for an examination, along with equipment settings, contributes to prudent use of diagnostic ultrasound. The receiver controls (i.e., TGC and Gain) need to be optimized before increasing acoustic power capabilities in an attempt to secure or improve the desired image. Some point-of-care ultrasound machines with simplified controls do not allow the user to independently adjust the acoustic power. The power may be automatically reduced when certain presets are selected such as "Early Obstetrical" setting.

Further reading materials include the AIUM publications listed below on ultrasound safety and are available by contacting AIUM:

American Institute of Ultrasound in Medicine
www.aium.org
800-638-5352
14750 Sweitzer Lane Suite 100
Laurel, MD 20707

ULTRASOUND SAFETY PUBLICATIONS

Bioeffects and Safety of Diagnostic Ultrasound

Evaluation of Research Reports: Bioeffects Literature Reviews (1962–1982)

Evaluation of Research Reports: Bioeffects Literature Reviews (1985–1991)

Evaluation of Research Reports: Bioeffects Literature Reviews (1992–1998)

How to Interpret the Ultrasound Output Display Standard for Higher Acoustic Output Diagnostic Ultrasound Devices (technical bulletin)

Mechanical Bioeffects from Diagnostic Ultrasound: Consensus Statements

Medical Ultrasound Safety

What You Should Know about the Safety of Your Ultrasound Examination (patient pamphlet).

SUGGESTED READING

Gill K: *Abdominal Ultrasound: A Practitioner's Guide.* Philadelphia, PA: WB Saunders, 2000.

Goodsit MM, Carson JY, Witt TG, et al.: Real-time B-mode ultrasound quality control test procedures. Report of AAPM Ultrasound Task Group No. 1. *Am Assoc Phys Med* 27:23–25, 1998.

Kremkau FW: *Diagnostic Ultrasound: Principles and Instruments.* 6th ed. Philadelphia, PA: WB Saunders, 2002.

Kurtz AB, Middleton AB: *Ultrasound: The Requisites.* Philadelphia, PA: WB Saunders, 1996.

Lin GS, Milburn DT, Briggs S: Power Doppler: How it works, its clinical benefits and recent technological advances. *JDMS* 14:45–48, 1998.

Nielsen TJ, Lambert MJ: Physics and instrumentation. In: Ma OJ, Mateer JR, eds. *Emergency Ultrasound.* New York, NY: McGraw Hill, 2003.

Nilsson A, Ingemar Loren I, Nirhov N, et al.: Power Doppler sonography: Alternative to computed tomograph in abdominal trauma patients. *JUM* 18:129–132, 1999.

Rumack CM, Charboneau JW, Wilson SR: *Diagnostic Ultrasound.* 2nd ed. Philadelphia, PA: WB Saunders, 1998.

Stephen E, Felkel S: Ultrasound safety mechanical and thermal indices: A primer. *JDMS* 15:98–100, 1999.

Tempkin BB: *Ultrasound Scanning: Principles and Protocols.* 2nd ed. Philadelphia, PA: WB Saunders, 1998.

CHAPTER 4

Ultrasound in Prehospital and Austere Environments

William G. Heegaard, Felix Walcher, Franziska Brenner, Marco Campo dell'Orto,
Thomas Kirschning, Ingo Marzi, Raoul Breitkreutz, Peter M. Zechner, Gernot Aichinger,
Gernot Wildner, Gerhard Prause, Tomislav Petrovic, Frédéric Lapostolle, Frédéric Adnet,
Jeffrey D. Ho, Andrew W. Kirkpatrick, Paul B. McBeth, Innes Crawford,
Corina Tiruta, and Daniel D. Price

The term "out-of-hospital ultrasound" refers to sonographic examinations performed in a wide variety of settings outside of traditional hospital departments, laboratories, and freestanding imaging centers. "Prehospital ultrasound" is synonymous, even though this term is mostly used in reference to EMS and tactical medicine applications. Prehospital ultrasound examinations are generally not performed by radiologists or clinicians; caregivers incorporate the use of ultrasound into the initial patient assessment at the point of care in the prehospital setting. The images obtained provide real-time morphologic and functional clinical information. In the emergency and critical care literature, "point-of-care ultrasound" most commonly refers to "bedside emergency ultrasound" since the scientific debate has been originally focused on patients being cared for in the ED; the resuscitation, operative, or recovery room; the intensive care unit; the diagnostic imaging department; or other medical and surgical wards. Diagnostic and therapeutic advances have allowed "critical care" to be taken outside of the hospital setting to the scene of illness and injury in a wide variety of settings (Table 4-1).

In all of these settings, ultrasonography provides a visual extension of the clinical examination, permitting more accurate assessment of anatomic and physiologic integrity in complex states of illness and injury (Figures 4-1 and 4-2). Prehospital applications are generally incorporated into defined problem-based clinical pathways rather than organ-based categorizations (i.e., "shock assessment" rather than "liver assessment").

Clinical accuracy and timeliness are essential for successful decision making and problem-solving in the prehospital environment. The prehospital use of ultrasonography can improve initial data gathering, which enhances the delivery of acute care in a timely and effective fashion. Efforts are being made to identify its most appropriate applications in the prehospital setting, the technical feasibility and reliability of its use, prehospital provider training and competency requirements, and the impact of prehospital ultrasound on patient outcomes and community health.[1–10]

To highlight the growing evidence in support of prehospital ultrasound, this chapter will review the experience of the German, Austrian, French, and American helicopter and ground-based EMS. This chapter will also review ultrasound in tactical medicine, remote telementored ultrasound, and the use of ultrasound in under-resourced settings.

► **TABLE 4-1. OUT-OF-HOSPITAL ULTRASOUND SETTINGS AND PROVIDERS**

ULTRASOUND SETTINGS	ULTRASOUND PROVIDERS
Prehospital care	Emergency physicians
Accident scenes	Critical care physicians/intensivists
Aboard helicopters, planes, ambulances	Anesthesiologists
Mass casualties and disaster medicine	Emergency/trauma surgeons
Natural catastrophes	Orthopedists
Building collapses	Sports Medicine physicians
Car, train, air crashes	Other "system-based" specialists
Explosions, terrorist attacks	General practitioners
Remote, austere, wilderness medicine	Nurses
Mountain, rural, forest, desert areas	Midwives
Cruise ships, air flights, space flights	Paramedics
Scarce-resource health services	Emergency medical technicians
Humanitarian operations	Lay personnel
Tactical medicine	
Combat fields	
Field hospitals	
Peacekeeping operations	
Sports medicine	
Sports stadiums, Olympic Games	
Primary care	
General practice	
Primary health care	

Germany

Felix Walcher, Franziska Brenner, Marco Campo dell'Orto, Thomas Kirschning, Ingo Marzi, and Raoul Breitkreutz

The German emergency system takes advantage of a close alliance between emergency physicians and the rescuing service staff prior to transportation to the hospital. The overriding principle of on-scene care is "stay and play" in nontraumatized patients and "treat and run" in traumatized patients; however, this is in contrast to the "scoop and run" principle of most international prehospital systems. The implementation of ultrasonography into such a system is supported by the development of two major concepts and training programs: Prehospital Focused Assessment with Sonography for Trauma (P-FAST) and Focused Echocardiographic Evaluation in Life Support (FEEL) for emergency and critical care physicians, and partially paramedics. Those protocols are embedded as "understand, treat and run" into the prehospital workflow.

► PREHOSPITAL FOCUSED ASSESSMENT WITH SONOGRAPHY FOR TRAUMA

P-FAST is related to prehospital trauma care. Clinical estimates of intraperitoneal bleeding at the trauma scene are difficult to accurately assess. A blunt trauma patient with normal vital signs and an unremarkable physical examination may have massive intraperitoneal bleeding that requires urgent operative management for hemorrhage control. Data from several studies support the role of prehospital ultrasound in enhancing detection of intraperitoneal hemorrhage.[10,11]

The 2001 Frankfurt/Main pilot study and a subsequent prospective multicenter study of P-FAST investigated its feasibility in trauma care.[10,11] Five air rescue centers in southwestern Germany and one ground ambulance rescue team in Frankfurt/Main took part in these studies. The entire P-FAST examination took about 2 minutes when results were negative, whereas positive intraperitoneal sonographic findings could be detected within seconds. Prehospital diagnosis of intraperitoneal injury by ultrasound was made approximately half an hour prior to arrival at the ED. In more than 90% of the cases, there was enough time to complete the P-FAST examination on the scene or during transportation.

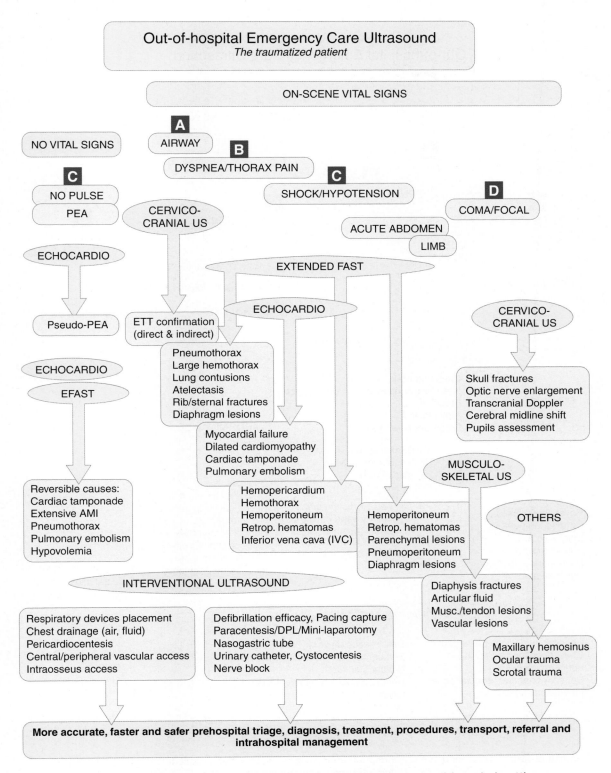

Figure 4-1. ABCD-conformed ultrasound applications in out-of-hospital setting.

In a few cases, ultrasound could not be completed because of suboptimal conditions (e.g., subcutaneous emphysema, patient obesity, or lack of time). The P-FAST examination had a sensitivity of 93% for the detection of intraperitoneal hemorrhage. The investigators concluded that P-FAST had potential as a useful, reliable diagnostic tool in surgical triage at the trauma scene.[11]

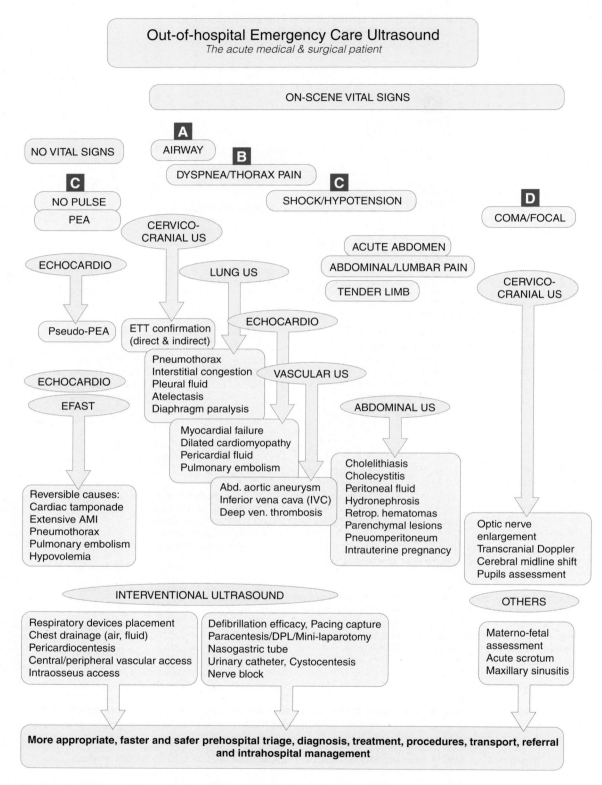

Figure 4-2. Current level 1 ultrasound applications in out-of-hospital setting: ABCD-conformed pathways for the acute medical and surgical patient.

All rescue teams involved in the multicenter study stated that P-FAST had an important impact on decision making. In approximately one-third of the cases, the findings of P-FAST had an influence on trauma management at the scene. Whenever intraperitoneal bleeding was detected, the prehospital phase of care was minimized to enable immediate transportation, either by ground or by helicopter. In contrast, if the findings of P-FAST were negative, the routine algorithm for trauma care at the scene was followed by completion of the primary and secondary surveys in accordance with the principles of advanced trauma life support (ATLS). The ultrasound findings led to a change in the choice of admitting hospital in approximately 20% of the cases. In addition, the results of P-FAST gave surgeons additional information that allowed appropriate planning of the hospital phase of care.

▶ FOCUSED ECHOCARDIOGRAPHIC EVALUATION IN LIFE SUPPORT

FEEL is an ACLS-compliant echocardiographic assessment and also addresses the development of skills for acute and critical care physicians in time-dependent scenarios.[1] The aim of FEEL is to elucidate treatable conditions and not to terminate CPR. Entities such as pulmonary embolism, pericardial tamponade, global left ventricular failure, and hypovolemia should be identified during the initial resuscitation. A major challenge is recognizing return of spontaneous circulation when no central pulse is palpable and differentiating pulseless electrical activity (PEA) states with or without wall motion. New evidence suggests that echocardiography can identify a "subclinical" return of spontaneous circulation (i.e., mechanical cardiac output).

The FEEL algorithm is a structured workflow within the ACLS clinical management approach that can be applied in real time. The 2010 American Heart Association resuscitation guidelines recommend high-quality CPR with minimal interruptions to reduce no-flow intervals. The 2010 European Resuscitation Council guidelines have now incorporated suggestions for ultrasound concepts for identification and treatment of reversible causes or complicating factors and training of ALS-conformed ultrasound.

Studies have evaluated the FEEL concept for its ease of implementation into the CPR process and its ability to identify characteristic pathologies.[12–14] The FEEL examination is a 10-step procedure (Table 4-2) designed to be performed during CPR cycles in order to reduce unwanted interruptions. Prehospital indications for performing FEEL are listed in Table 4-3.

A prospective, observational trial in the prehospital setting tested (a) the capability of FEEL to differentiate PEA states and (b) the feasibility of FEEL using a mobile, battery-powered ultrasound system. Trained emergency physicians applied the FEEL examination as described. A total of 230 patients were included, with 204 undergoing a FEEL examination during ongoing cardiac arrest (100) and in a shock state (104). Images of diagnostic quality were obtained in 96%. In 35% of those with an ECG diagnosis of asystole, and 58% of those with PEA, cardiac motion was detected, and associated with increased survival. Echocardiographic findings altered management in 78% of cases.[12]

▶ **TABLE 4-2. THE 10-STEP FOCUSED ECHOCARDIOGRAPHIC EVALUATION IN LIFE SUPPORT (FEEL) ALGORITHM**

PHASE	FEEL STEP
High-quality CPR, preparation, team information	1. Perform immediate and accurate BLS and ACLS according to AHA guidelines, at least five cycles of chest compression/ventilation 2. Tell the CPR team: "I am preparing an echocardiogram" 3. Prepare portable ultrasound 4. Accommodate situation (e.g., best position of patient and doctor, and removal of clothes), be ready to start
Execution, obtaining the echocardiogram	5. Tell CPR team to count 10 seconds and to perform a pulse check simultaneously 6. Command: "Interrupt at the end of this cycle for echocardiography" 7. Put the transducer gently onto the patient's subcostal region during chest compressions 8. Perform a subcostal (long axis) echocardiogram as quickly as possible. If you cannot identify the heart after 3 seconds, stop the interruption and repeat again after five cycles with or without the parasternal approach 9. "Continue CPR"
Resuming CPR interpretation and consequences	10. Communicate (after continuation of chest compressions only): the findings to the CPR team (e.g., "wall motion, heart is squeezing," "cardiac stand still," "(massive) pericardial effusion," "no conclusive finding," "suspected pulmonary artery embolism," "hypovolemia" and explain consequences as well as follow-up procedures)

▶ **TABLE 4-3. PREHOSPITAL INDICATIONS TO PERFORM FOCUSED ECHOCARDIOGRAPHIC EVALUATION IN LIFE SUPPORT (FEEL)**

"Pre-resuscitation" care, shock assessment
    Penetrating trauma, blunt trauma
    Postcardiotomy due to cardiac surgery
    Hypotension, shock of unknown origin
    Unconsciousness, unresponsiveness
    Acute severe dyspnea
    Syncope in young adults
    Vein thrombosis
    AMI, mechanical complications of AMI
"Atypical" chest pain: suspected aortic-dissection, suspected aortic abdominal or thoracic aneurysm, nontraumatic cardiac rupture
Iatrogenic complications following invasive procedures (e.g., insertion of an artificial pacemaker, pulmonary artery catheter, and electrophysiologic investigative procedures)
Great-vessel disease
CPR
    PEA
    Bradycardia-asystole, pacemaker-ECG
    Suspected cardiac tamponade
    Early detection of return of spontaneous circulation
    Effectiveness of chest compressions
Postresuscitation care
    Hypotension, adaptation of vasopressors

▶ EDUCATION AND TRAINING

Before 2001, a uniform course to teach P-FAST was unavailable in Germany or other parts of Europe. Prior to the P-FAST studies, it was necessary to set up a structured educational program for emergency physicians and paramedics. A P-FAST course concept was developed on the basis of several studies that had been performed in the 1990s with respect to the use of ultrasound in the clinical setting. Some groups had investigated which type of education programs were required to gain competency in performing the FAST examination and had assessed the learning curve. The recommended duration of didactic training, including hands-on experience, ranged from 2 to 30 hours.

The main goal of the P-FAST training is to prepare participants for uncommon situations in trauma scenarios under field conditions. The 1-day course in P-FAST includes both didactic and hands-on training. The didactic session includes a general introduction to ultrasound, physics of ultrasound, and the causes and relevance of artifacts and shadows that may be encountered during an ultrasound examination. Participants are introduced to the rationale for performing ultrasound as part of trauma management and are taught how to integrate P-FAST into the prehospital algorithm for trauma care. Numerous images and videos provide an overview

of the physiologic and pathologic situations. Hands-on training is the main focus of the course. Participants perform the P-FAST examination under the supervision of clinicians experienced with ultrasound. The ratio of instructors to students is 1:2 or 1:3. During the course, a trainee performs 30–40 ultrasound examinations under the supervision of the instructors.

In the first part of hands-on training, participants perform the standardized procedure of P-FAST on healthy and patient volunteers. Patient volunteers have positive findings for free intraperitoneal fluid secondary to peritoneal dialysis or ascites. In the second part of the hands-on training, students learn how to perform the ultrasound examination under difficult circumstances, such as on patients found in challenging prehospital conditions. In the third part, real-time scenarios are presented with healthy or patient volunteers found in critical situations following a traumatic event. These scenarios include surgical triage of three or more victims or volunteers trapped in the wreckage of a vehicle. Evaluation of the course program is consistent with data from other training evaluations in the literature, which have shown that these programs produce competent examiners and are associated with a steep learning curve. No significant differences were found between emergency physicians and paramedics in terms of sensitivity, specificity, and accuracy of P-FAST examinations.

A 1-day course was established on focused echocardiography for emergency physicians and critical care physicians who had no previous experience in performing echocardiography.[13] The course emphasizes basic echocardiography, rapid evaluation, and communication skills. In addition, a real-time 3D-ultrasound simulation combined within a full-scale ACLS training system as well as web-based learning and tests are included. We also evaluated an emergency physician's ability to obtain a correct subxiphoid 4-chamber view and to interpret a 5-second echocardiogram of normal and pathologic findings. We found that emergency physicians could learn to identify some simple pathologic findings on very short video clips, and for the combined ultrasound and ACLS trainer there were high positive ratings. In 2011, P-FAST and FEEL became incorporated into the nationwide certified training programs of the German Society of Ultrasound in Medicine (DEGUM) and German Society of Anesthesiology, Intensive and Emergency Care (DGAI) as extended-FAST (E-FAST) (including lung ultrasound) and cardiosonography modules.

▶ MOBILE ULTRASOUND DEVICES

Prior to the German P-FAST multicenter study, the fire department of the city of Frankfurt and the Department of Trauma Surgery at the University of Frankfurt used a device based on Esaote Tringa. The compact ultrasound machine SonoSite 180 Plus is used by the German Army and in the MedEvac system operating worldwide. The SonoSite NanoMaxx is standard of care in an increasing number of prehospital care services. Up to 35 German air rescue helicopter services, Lufthansa German Airline, and fire department-based emergency services of several metropolitan areas are equipped with General Electric Vscan.

These mobile devices can be held with one hand; the adjustments necessary during an examination can be made with the thumb. It is now very well received that our concepts also apply to many acute care settings for point-of-care exams within the hospital.

▶ PROPAGATION OF PREHOSPITAL ULTRASOUND IN AIR AND GROUND RESCUE SERVICE

Since 2003, the German Air Rescue Organization (Deutsche Rettungsflugwacht) has incorporated P-FAST into the algorithm for trauma management. By 2012, 35 helicopters and 3 fixed-wing aircrafts were equipped with portable ultrasound devices and most of the emergency physicians and paramedic crews were trained. The other main provider of air rescue services, the German Automobile Club, also partially adopted P-FAST.

Some air rescue centers of the German federal police have implemented P-FAST; in addition, the German Air Force also have equipped their international mobile medical crews and supplied their aircraft for multi-national flights with mobile ultrasound devices. Their crews have been trained in our courses.

P-FAST and FEEL have been integrated into ground-based services as well. The region of Darmstadt adopted the prehospital FEEL examination in 2002. In Frankfurt/Main, the five ground-based ambulances staffed by emergency physicians have been equipped with portable ultrasound devices with financial support from the city's public health department.

Austria

Peter M. Zechner, Gernot Aichinger, Raoul Breitkreutz, Gernot Wildner, and Gerhard Prause

In Austria, physicians, who staff ambulances, treat prehospital patients. As a result, prehospital portable ultrasound as well as other specialized point-of-care diagnostic tools, such as blood gas analysis systems, invasive blood pressure monitoring, and fiberoptic bron-

choscopy, have become available. The first emergency vehicle in Graz was equipped with portable ultrasound (SonoSite 180 Plus) in 2000. Today, up to three emergency vehicles in Graz are equipped and some other emergency systems have also implemented its use. While prehospital ultrasound was almost exclusively applied to detect free intraabdominal fluid in trauma patients in the initial years, its applications have been extended. An increasing number of emergency physicians have begun using prehospital ultrasound for differentiation between cardiac and pulmonary causes of dyspnea with the evaluation of B-lines, the prediction of outcome in cardiac arrest patients, the detection of pneumothorax, and ultrasound-guided venous and arterial line insertion. A report published by the Graz group studied the prognostic value of prehospital emergency echocardiography in cardiac arrest and the ability of optic nerve ultrasound to detect elevated intracranial pressure.[14] Although prehospital emergency ultrasound is still in its infancy in Austria, the results and improvement in patient care have been promising and groundbreaking.

France

Tomislav Petrovic, Frédéric Lapostolle, and Frédéric Adnet

The feasibility and usefulness of prehospital ultrasound have expanded since the early 1980s in France. Bulky ultrasound machines requiring very skilled operators were used back then; as a result, they had limited applicability to most prehospital systems. In the early 1990s, technological advances produced lighter ultrasound machines that were much more practical to use in the prehospital setting.

French prehospital clinicians have been interested in broad applications of prehospital ultrasound. Investigators have studied the detection of free intraperitoneal fluid, assessment of cardiac function in shock and arrest states, evaluation of thoracic injuries, detection of deep venous thrombosis, assessment of long diaphysis fractures, and detection of optic nerve enlargement.

The methods of training and the level of performance of emergency physicians using ultrasound in prehospital settings in France were evaluated. The ultrasound training was scheduled for one half-day session that included didactic and practical instruction. Like our German colleagues, didactic sessions reviewed the guiding principles of ultrasonography and normal and pathological images. The practical training consisted of performing examinations on healthy subjects or on patients with pertinent findings on ultrasound examinations (e.g., patients with ascites). The training focused on examinations pertinent to the French prehospital setting, which included the assessment for pneumothoraces, pleural effusions, abdominal or pericardial effusions, or deep venous thrombosis of the lower limbs.

Eight physicians of the SAMU 93 (EMS department) were trained on the emergency use of a portable ultrasound device (SonoSite 180). The number of training sessions varied from 1 to 6, according to the experience level of the operators. Each operator determined a clinical diagnostic probability (before ultrasonography) noted on an analog visual scale from 0 (*absence of lesion*) to 10 (*presence of lesion*). According to the same principle, the operator determined a second probability after ultrasound. The hospital follow-up of the patients made it possible to obtain the final diagnosis (0 for absent and 10 for present lesion) that was compared with the pre- and posttest probabilities.[3]

The initial analysis of 83 ultrasound examinations carried out on 40 patients revealed a median time of examination of 5 minutes, 100% sensitivity, 98% specificity, a positive predictive value of 92%, and a negative predictive value of 100%. In our analysis of the learning curve for ultrasound proficiency by prehospital providers, we found that the number of ultrasound examinations required to achieve desired proficiency was approximately 25 examinations.

The absolute difference between the probabilities before and after ultrasound was calculated and compared with the final diagnosis (0 or 10). When ultrasound had brought the operator closer to it, a positive value was allotted to the obtained number; conversely, a negative value was allotted when ultrasound had moved the operator away from the final diagnosis. For example, if a diagnostic probability was 3 before and 8 after ultrasonography, the absolute difference was 5 (8 − 3). If the final diagnosis was positive (presence of a lesion), ultrasound would have brought the operator closer to the final diagnosis. The value allotted to ultrasound would then be + 5. Conversely, if the final diagnosis was negative (absence of lesion), ultrasound would not have been helpful in making the final diagnosis. The value allotted to ultrasound would then be − 5.

The results of 302 ultrasound examinations were analyzed. The median impact of ultrasound on the final diagnosis was + 2. The diagnostic performance was improved by ultrasound in 67% of the cases; it was not modified in 25% of the cases and it was degraded in 8% of the cases. Our results were consistent with the use of ultrasound as a "complement" to the clinical assessment.[3]

In France, prehospital ultrasound has established itself as a legitimate clinical adjunct. Just as the stethoscope serves as an extension of the physician's ears, the ultrasound transducer serves as an extension of her

hands and eyes. If the indications are focused, the procedure is codified, and the operators are properly trained, then the level of performance approaches that of a medical imaging expert. The rapidity of the examinations provides additional diagnostic information without delaying transport or definitive care. As experience with this modality increases and technological advances produce improved portability and resolution, we believe that the use of ultrasound will gain broad acceptance in prehospital venues around the world.

United States of America
William G. Heegaard

The advancement of prehospital ultrasound in the United States has been significant. While no large randomized prehospital study has yet to be completed in the United States, the body of literature is increasing. Four broad areas are utilizing prehospital ultrasound: helicopter EMS, ground EMS, tactical, and tele-transmission of ultrasound. While the American EMS system has not swayed from expeditiously transporting ill or injured patients to the receiving medical center for definitive care, ultrasound may expand the traditional tools that prehospital providers use in their care of patients.

▶ AIR AND GROUND MEDICAL TRANSPORT

Point-of-care ultrasound use in helicopter EMS is growing. This growth is not surprising given the critical and time-sensitive nature of helicopter EMS patients. Helicopter EMS transport in the United States has consistently grown each year for the past two decades. Approximately 867 rotor-wing air ambulances currently operate out of 714 bases across the country.[15] For millions of rural Americans prompt emergency care is only accessible through the use of helicopter EMS.

Numerous United States helicopter EMS programs are now utilizing or have utilized ultrasound. Some programs include Oregon Health & Science University, Portland, Oregon; MetroHealth Medical Center, Cleveland, Ohio; Medical College of Georgia, Augusta, Georgia; University of San Diego, San Diego, California; several USA-based military helicopter EMS programs; and Life Link III, Minneapolis, Minnesota.

It has been demonstrated that the FAST examination can be performed rapidly and with relative ease in the helicopter.[8] Using a SonoSite 180 ultrasound machine with a 3.5 MHz transducer, 10 flight clinicians

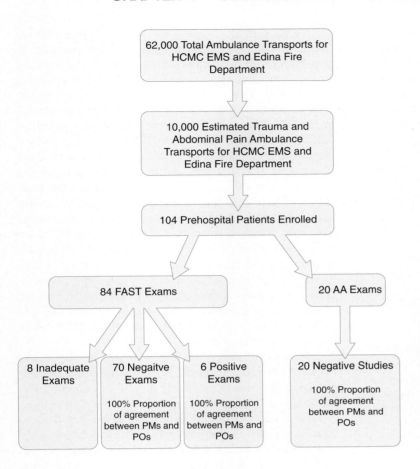

Figure 4-3. Flow diagram of patients included in Ultrasound study. AA, abdominal aortic; FAST, Focused Assessment with Sonography for Trauma; HCMC, Hennepin County Medical Center; PM, paramedic; PO, physician overreader. Reprinted with permission from Heegaard W, Hildebrandt D, Spear D, Chason K, Nelson B, Ho J. Prehospital ultrasound by paramedics: results of field trial. *Acad Emerg Med* 17(6):624–630, 2010.

performed 21 FAST examinations on 14 patients. Nine patients were simulated. They reported no effect on avionics and were able to complete the standard FAST examination in a mean time of 3 minutes. In 2004, Heegaard and coinvestigators applied a focused template for didactic ultrasound training with additional hands-on training in an ED.[2] They found that flight clinicians could perform a wide variety of ultrasound examinations with good long-term retention (>90%) over 1 year. Ultrasound examinations were performed proficiently in the helicopter, although time and space constraints limited the clinicians' ability to perform the complete FAST examination. One study analyzed the use of ultrasound to perform a screening examination on obstetric patients transported by helicopter.[7] The Fetal Evaluation for Transport with Ultrasound (FETUS) is a screening examination that evaluates fetal heart rate, position, and movement and general condition of the placenta. The examination can be performed serially in flight with no acoustic distortion from rotor noise. In 2011, a study examined the feasibility of using M-mode to detect pneumothoraces during helicopter transport.[16] Earlier studies on helicopter EMS ultrasound in the United States utilized the SonoSite 180, a 2.4-kg compact ultrasound machine with 3.5 MHz transducer. One helicopter EMS

program (Life Link III, Minneapolis, Minnesota) utilized the SonoSite iLook ultrasound machine (1.4 kg) with a 3.5 MHz transducer, which was mounted in the helicopter for ease of use. Other studies have been utilizing newer generation ultrasound machines that have both M-mode and video recording capability.

Ultrasound use in ground ambulances has gained traction. In 2010, Heegaard reported on 104 FAST and abdominal aortic ultrasound examinations performed by 9-1-1 paramedics in the prehospital environment (Figure 4-3).[17,18] Of the FAST exams performed, 7.1% were positive for intraperitoneal/pericardial fluid. Paramedics were unable to obtain adequate images in 7.7% (8/104) patients. All exams recorded 6-second video clips of each portion of the exam. FAST and aortic ultrasound exams performed by the paramedics had a 100% agreement with an independent emergency medicine physician ultrasound expert.

It remains to be seen whether the European experience will impact the implementation of ultrasound in ground ambulances in the United States. The first American ground EMS system to utilize prehospital ultrasound was in Odessa, Texas. Currently, there are multiple United States prehospital agencies utilizing ultrasound in various capacities on their ground ambulances.

Obstacles to implementing prehospital ultrasound programs include lack of reimbursement for ultrasound imaging, difficulty in maintaining ultrasound competency among numerous EMS personnel, and the cost of ultrasound machines.

Potential applications of helicopter EMS and ground ambulance ultrasound in the United States include, but are not limited to:

- E-FAST examination on trauma patients to expedite definitive care and early operating/radiological intervention suite activation, especially in rural areas;
- Focused cardiac ultrasound examination in hypotensive patients to place them in one of four shock states (severe hypovolemia, cardiogenic, pericardial tamponade, or right ventricular obstruction), which helps guide therapy;
- Fetal monitoring and evaluation in obstetrical patients;
- Early detection of mainstem intubations;
- Early detection of pneumothorax with the E-FAST examination;
- Early evaluation of cardiac arrest and PEA;
- Confirmation of out-of-hospital death (cardiac standstill).

Tactical Medicine

Jeffrey D. Ho

Tactical Medicine, often referred to as Tactical Emergency Medical Support (TEMS), is an evolving niche of out-of-hospital medical practice with origins based on military medical knowledge. TEMS is specifically designed for use in austere, often hostile situations, usually in support of high-risk civilian law enforcement operations (LEOs).[19] TEMS has become important because of decades of experience demonstrating a breakdown in standard operations by EMS personnel during high-risk, unsecured situations. One only has to search the Internet for "active shooter incidents" to find numerous examples of situations with multiple casualties where standard civilian EMS personnel were not able to enter the scene to treat, evacuate, or transport the injured. In situations such as these, the only personnel generally operating within a secured perimeter are suspects, innocents, LEOs, and specially-trained TEMS personnel. Depending on the type of incident, the perimeter can be as small as a few hundred yards to as large as several miles around. Without TEMS availability, especially during prolonged operations, it is likely that casualties within these perimeters will go untreated.

TEMS providers can come from different training backgrounds, ranging from basic first aid provider to physician levels of training. Many TEMS physicians may already have adequate ultrasound training. Paramedic-level providers can also be trained to perform prehospital ultrasound.[18] Regardless of medical training background, TEMS personnel are generally taught specialized topics not normally found in standard care and resuscitation classes.[20] These areas of competency may seem obscure to most but are vital in tactical situations and include topics such as Remote Patient Assessment, Evaluation of Injury due to Lethal and Less-Lethal Weapons, and Care Under Fire. These topics generally assume that treatment decisions may need to be made rapidly based on consideration of risk versus survival, ability to perform immediate lifesaving interventions, as well as ability to evacuate in a timely manner to an appropriate facility. The introduction of ultrasound into the prehospital care setting is beginning to gain support and is likely to have significant ramifications for use in the TEMS arena as this support increases.

Ultrasound use in a TEMS scenario by a qualified operator for rapid diagnosis of pneumothorax or pericardial tamponade is extremely helpful in shortening decision time to perform a potentially lifesaving procedure. A FAST exam performed within the perimeter demonstrating rapidly worsening intraperitoneal hemorrhage would likely cause a specific hasty evacuation plan to be followed, leading to an appropriate trauma-receiving destination. These skills and preplans are generally put in place by TEMS providers before an operation unfolds, but may not be acted upon unless absolutely necessary because of the danger to the providers if they are enacted unnecessarily (e.g., if actively under fire, it may be safer to leave a person with minor injuries in place behind cover rather than attempt a rescue extraction and evacuation that places numerous LEOs at unnecessary risk)

The working environment of a TEMS operator is foreign to most clinicians. They carry large amounts of portable medical equipment, cumbersome protective gear, and often tools of law enforcement that may include a firearm. They may have their attention divided between patient care and personal safety/security during an operation. The development of small, portable ultrasound machines has recently made the use of ultrasound in the tactical medical practice arena even more of a reality. Because of the amount of equipment carried by TEMS operators and the environment for use, any ultrasound machine needs to be lightweight, durably rugged, battery-operated, and rapid and simple to use. A single microconvex transducer could suffice for almost every necessary field application. An ultrasound machine that cannot tolerate being knocked around in a field pouch or one that requires numerous keystrokes or time delays to function is not acceptable.

The niche specialty of TEMS is growing as the benefit of having TEMS providers present is recognized to improve casualty outcomes.[21,22] Use of ultrasound by TEMS providers is an emerging area of diagnostic interest. It has the potential for enabling more rapid, accurate decisions to be made about diagnostic uncertainties. This, in turn, allows for more informed decisions to be made with regard to injury care, taking into account risk versus benefit in high-risk tactical situations.

Remote Telementored Ultrasound

Andrew W. Kirkpatrick, Paul B. McBeth, Innes Crawford, and Corina Tiruta

Ultrasound offers an almost unlimited scope for enhancing the bedside care of the critically ill or injured patient. With the ever-increasing availability of ultrasound machines, however, there is often a gap between the education and experience of care providers and the needs of the critical patient. This paradigm is no more pertinent than in space medicine, where a state-of-the-art ultrasound machine is the only potential imaging capability onboard the International Space Station (ISS), yet a nonphysician such as a geologist may be required to make time-sensitive critical diagnoses and provide invasive therapies to a fellow crewmate.[23-25] This quandary has led investigators working on behalf of the National Aeronautics and Space Administration (NASA) to pioneer remote guidance techniques wherein a novice care provider onboard the ISS is mentored to obtain meaningful ultrasound images that can be interpreted by terrestrial experts to guide diagnosis and therapy. Using such an approach a wide variety of specific ultrasound examinations have been conducted, including the FAST examination, demonstrating that with advanced informatics, even inexperienced but motivated novice operators can generate meaningful images.[26-28]

Terrestrially, although telemedicine, and specifically tele-ultrasound, becomes more extensively utilized every year in clinical care,[29,30] its use in real-time trauma resuscitation remains limited. One study examined guiding paramedics remotely via two-way radio communication through solely viewing the ultrasound images without viewing the on-site examiner's hand or transducer movements.[31] The study noted that 51 paramedics were able to generate 100% of the required FAST views, after 20-minute didactic sessions without hands-on scanning.[31] Another study utilized the Net-Meeting software application from the Microsoft Corpo-

ration to transmit 50 patient images from Serbia to the United States, concluding that there was potential to further investigate these techniques.[32] To our knowledge the first use of real-time remote telementored ultrasound for trauma resuscitation was reported in 2008.[33] This involved trauma surgeons at a tertiary care trauma center viewing the resuscitative bay of a rural referral center in the Rocky Mountains with both a macro-field camera and real-time display of the rural ultrasound machine on a console in the ED. Using this somewhat complex system, remote telementored ultrasound was found to be not only feasible and accurate, but it also impacted patient triage, educated novice operators, and increased collegiality.[33,34] The system, however, was unsustainable for 24/7 immediate responses, as it required the responding trauma surgeons who mentored the remote examiners to physically respond to the tele-ultrasound console.

Newer efforts have centered on attempting to make tele-ultrasound simpler and to reduce the infrastructure required to facilitate communication. One group has championed the use of a stand-alone video compression device to stream through a secure satellite modem to allow one-way ultrasound and video transmissions and two-way audio from challenging environments such as Mount Everest and the Canadian Arctic.[35-37] In this manner, remote lung examinations for high altitude pulmonary edema and joint examinations were performed by novice operators, guided by Henry Ford Medical Center in Detroit, Michigan.[35-37] Efforts in Calgary, Alberta, have attempted to simplify remote telementored ultrasound even further. This group has used freely available but password protected voice over Internet Protocol (VOIP) software to transmit from a portable head mounted video camera and portable handheld ultrasound devices, thus providing the remote mentor with an ultrasound image produced by the novice and simultaneous real-time views of the novice's handling of the ultrasound transducer.[38-40]

Once the macro scene and ultrasound images have been assembled and transmitted using VOIP, the device used by the remote mentor can be any that receives a password-protected secure Internet signal such as desktop or laptop computer, a tablet device, or a smartphone. Pilot investigations have demonstrated the ease of using such systems from essentially anywhere that the Internet can be received through fixed lines, wireless networks, or tethered to cellular phone networks. Thus, remote telementored ultrasound can be conducted from rural mountainsides, within small airplanes, and from buildings while remote mentors can respond from anywhere they can use a smartphone.[40] While technically feasible, the next level of evaluation is to demonstrate that such technologies benefit decision making and patient outcomes. As a great percentage of the developing world lacks adequate medical services, including medical imaging, the ability to remotely diagnose, teach, and guide seems to offer a remote outreach with limitless potential.

Ultrasound in Under-Resourced Settings

Daniel D. Price

According to the United Nations, over 60% of the world's population has no access to medical imaging.[41] Most people will never have access to plain film radiography, let alone CT, MRI, or PET. In challenging under-resourced settings, ultrasound offers a solution.

- Ultrasound systems can be hand-carried, which allows them to go to the patient. Ultrasound systems have been carried on horseback, motorcycles, boats, and on long hikes to extremely remote areas. Virtually all other imaging systems are built for stationary and controlled environments.
- Ultrasound systems can be battery operated, so patient care doesn't have to stop when the power is out. Patient care can also take place in health-care centers that have no electricity.
- Ultrasound is relatively straightforward to learn, but adequate training and experience are essential. Ultrasound has been used successfully by nurses, midwives, clinical officers (similar to physician assistants), and even health promoters with limited formal education, most of whom operate independently of physicians. Other imaging modalities require significantly more training.
- Ultrasound images are more accessible. Printing radiographs and CT images require film, silver, and other expensive and caustic ingredients, which add cost and complexity. Electronic viewing systems, such as PACS, are expensive and rely on unreliable infrastructure and vulnerable technology. Ultrasound images and clips can be viewed on the device and can be easily transferred wirelessly or via removable media.
- Ultrasound imaging is dynamic and can evaluate physiology over time, which is important in echocardiography, obstetrics, and other applications. Other imaging modalities provide only static images.
- In resource-limited settings, cost is paramount. An ultrasound system has only the fixed cost of purchase, which is much less than other imaging modalities. Furthermore, the costs of other imaging options are ongoing with respect to supplies and maintenance.
- Maintenance of a rugged ultrasound system is minimal, compared with the complexity and vulnerability of other imaging options. In many areas of the world, dust is ubiquitous and can easily damage equipment. This is also true for ultrasound systems not designed for austere environments, making maintenance an important consideration in purchasing decisions.
- Technical support can be challenging in under-resourced settings, which are generally remote. Lightweight, hand-carried ultrasound systems can be easily shipped to servicing centers, in contrast to other systems that require site visitation by a technician. Many health-care facilities in developing countries have broken devices sitting in closets. If a system becomes nonfunctional, the ultrasound program at that facility will be at risk for ceasing to function as well, as practitioners' skills degrade from lack of use and the flame of their enthusiasm dims.

▶ APPLICATIONS

The differential diagnosis in resource-limited settings often varies from the differential in more developed settings. Tropical diseases and illnesses related to tuberculosis, malaria, and HIV/AIDS are much more prominent on a differential, because prevalence is so high. Bedside ultrasound can help establish a firm diagnosis and guide appropriate management.[42-44]

One of the advantages of ultrasound is that it can help in the evaluation of many conditions. Appropriate ultrasound applications have been well elucidated in the Partners In Health *Manual of Ultrasound for Resource-Limited Settings*, which is available online free of charge.[45] There is an excellent review of the literature regarding the use of ultrasound in the developing world[46] and the breadth of applications. Novel applications of ultrasound not used in highly developed countries are emerging from under-resourced settings.[42-44] An important factor in considering the use of specific applications is that the information gained be actionable and lead the provider along a management algorithm.

▶ IMPACT

A central question in the decision of whether to implement ultrasound in under-resourced settings is, "What difference does it make?" Studies have found that ultrasound led to changes in management in 17-68% of patients.[47-52] Changes included the decision to perform a surgical procedure, medication changes, clinic referral, and canceling of a planned surgical procedure.[47]

Treatment in resource-limited settings may be more expensive, difficult, and dangerous to the patients than if they were treated in resource-rich settings. For example, a patient with tuberculosis misdiagnosed as having a pulmonary embolism could die from the use of heparin or warfarin.

Even if the use of blood thinners was correct, the warfarin may be expensive and difficult to find, and monitoring costly when available. For these reasons, it is necessary to have a high degree of diagnostic certainty before undertaking such treatment. A study in the Amazon found that the physician's differential diagnosis narrowed after the ultrasound results in 72% of cases, with diagnostic certainty achieved in 68%.[50] In a study in Cameroon, about half of the confirmed diagnoses made by ultrasound had not been previously considered.[52]

A "magnet effect" has also been observed. The compelling nature of ultrasound draws patients from outside the health-care system to facilities where they can receive public health interventions known to be of benefit, such as immunization, HIV screening, and education. A study in Mali observed that women came to a health center from farther and farther away as word of the use of ultrasound spread.[53]

Ultrasound empowers health-care providers at the point of care. New skills with ultrasound have been shown to improve job satisfaction[53] and can lead to better retention of skilled personnel, a common problem in under-resourced settings.

REFERENCES

1. Breitkreutz R, Walcher F, Seeger FH: Focused echocardiographic evaluation in resuscitation management: concept of an advanced life support-conformed algorithm. *Crit Care Med* 35(5 suppl):S150–S61, 2007.
2. Heegaard W, Plummer D, Dries D, et al.: Ultrasound for the air medical clinician. *Air Med J* 23(2):20–23, 2004.
3. Lapostolle F, Petrovic T, Catineau J, et al.: Out-of-hospital ultrasonographic diagnosis of a left ventricular wound after penetrating thoracic trauma. *Ann Emerg Med* 43:422–423, 2004.
4. Lenoir G, Petrovic T, Galinski M, et al.: Influence de l'échographie préhospitalière sur le diagnostic porté par le médecin urgentiste. *Congres Urgences* 2003 (Paris), *JEUR* 16:1S49, 111, 2003.
5. Melanson SW, McCarthy J, Stromski CJ, et al.: Aeromedical trauma sonography by flight crews with a miniature ultrasound unit. *Prehospital Emerg Care* 5:399–402, 2001.
6. Plummer D, Brunette D, Asinger R, et al.: Emergency department echocardiography improves outcome in penetrating cardiac injury. *Ann Emerg Med* 21:709–712, 1992.
7. Polk JD, Merlino JI, Kovach BL, Mancuso C, Fallon WF, Jr: Fetal evaluation for transport by ultrasound performed by air medical teams: A case series. *Air Med J* 23(4):32–34, 2004.
8. Price DD, Wilson SR, Murphy TG: Trauma ultrasound feasibility during helicopter transport. *Air Med J* 19:144–146, 2000.
9. Rodgerson J, Heegaard W, Plummer D, et al.: Emergency department right upper quadrant ultrasound is associated with a reduced time to diagnosis and treatment of ruptured ectopic pregnancies. *Acad Emerg Med* 8:331–336, 2001.
10. Walcher F, Kortüm S, Kirschning T, et al.: Optimierung des Traumamanagements durch präklinische Sonographic [Optimized management of polytraumatized patients by prehospital ultrasound]. *Der Unfallchirurg* 105(11):986–994, 2002.
11. Walcher F, Weinlich M, Conrad G, et al.: Prehospital ultrasound imaging improves management of abdominal trauma. *Br J Surg* 93:238–242, 2006.
12. Price S, Ilper H, Uddin Sh, et al.: Peri-resuscitation echocardiography: training the novice practitioner. *Resuscitation* 81: 1534–1539, 2010.
13. Breitkreutz R, Price S, Steiger HV et al.: Focused echocardiographic evaluation in life support and peri-resuscitation of emergency patients: a prospective trial. *Resuscitation* 81:1527–1533, 2010.
14. Aichinger G, Zechner PM, Prause G, et al.: Cardiac movement identified on prehospital echocardiography predicts outcome in cardiac arrest patients. *Prehosp Emerg Care* PMID:22235765, 2012.(in press)
15. *Atlas and Database of Air Medical Services* 7th ed. In: Flanigan M BA, Mancuso D eds, ed.: Association of Air Medical Services (AAMS) and the Calspan University of Buffalo Research Center (CUBRC), 2009.
16. Lyon M, Shiver SA, Walton P: M-mode ultrasound for the detection of pneumothorax during helicopter transport. *Am J Emerg Med* 2011.
17. Heegaard W, Hildebrandt D, Reardon R, Plummer D, Clinton J, Ho J: Prehospital ultrasound diagnosis of traumatic pericardial effusion. *Acad Emerg Med* 16(4):364, 2009.
18. Heegaard W, Hildebrandt D, Spear D, Chason K, Nelson B, Ho J: Prehospital ultrasound by paramedics: Results of field trial. *Acad Emerg Med* 17(6):624–330, 2010.
19. Carmona RH: The history and devolution of tactical emergency medical support and its impact on public safety. *Top Emerg Med* 25:277–281, 2003.
20. Swatz RB, McManus JG, Croushorn J, et al.: Tactical medicine-competency-based guidelines. *Prehosp Emerg Care* 15:67–82, 2011.
21. Gildea JR, Janssen AR: Tactical emergency medical support: Physician involvement and injury patterns in tactical teams. *J Emerg Med* 35:411–414, 2008.
22. Metzger JC, Eastman AL, Benitez FL, Pepe PE: The lifesaving potential of specialized on-scene medical support for urban tactical operations. *Prehosp Emerg Care* 13:528–531, 2009.
23. Kirkpatrick AW, Jones JA, Sargsyan A, et al.: Trauma sonography for use in microgravity. *Aviat Space Environ Med* 78(4 suppl):A38–A42, 2007.
24. Kwon D, Bouffard JA, van Holsbeeck M, et al.: Battling fire and ice: remote guidance ultrasound to diagnose injury on the International Space Station and the ice rink. *Am J Surg* 193(3):417–420, 2007.

25. Kirkpatrick AW, Hamilton DR, Nicolaou S, et al.: Focused assessment with sonography for trauma in weightlessness: a feasibility study. *J Am Coll Surg* 196(6):833–844, 2003.

26. Sargsyan AE, Hamilton DR, Jones JA, et al.: FAST at MACH 20: Clinical ultrasound aboard the International Space Station. *J Trauma* 58(1):35–39, 2005.

27. Fincke EM, Padalka G, Lee D, et al.: Evaluation of shoulder integrity in space: first report of musculoskeletal US on the International Space Station. *Radiology* 234(2):319–322, 2005.

28. Chiao L, Sharipov S, Sargsyan AE, et al.: Ocular examination for trauma; clinical ultrasound aboard the International Space Station. *J Trauma* 58(5):885–889, 2005.

29. Sutherland JE, Sutphin HD, Rawlins F: A comparison of telesonography with standard ultrasound care in a rural Dominican clinic. *J Telemed Telecare* [Comparative Study Randomized Controlled Trial Research Support, Non-U.S. Gov't]. 15(4):191–195, 2009.

30. Chan FY, Soong B, Lessing K, et al.: Clinical value of real-time tertiary fetal ultrasound consultation by telemedicine: preliminary evaluation. *Telemed J* 2000 6:237–242, 2000.

31. Boniface KS, Shokoohi H, Smith ER, Scantlebury K: Tele-ultrasound ad paramedics: Real-time remote physician guidance of the Focused Assessment with Sonography for Trauma. *Am J Emerg Med* (in press).

32. Popov V, Popov D, Kacar I, Harris RD: The feasibility of real-time transmission of sonographic images from a remote location over low-bandwidth Internet links: a pilot study. *AJR Am J Roentgenol* 188(3):W219–W222, 2007.

33. Dyer D, Cusden J, Turner C, et al.: The clinical and technical evaluation of a remote telementored telesonography system during the acute resuscitation and transfer of the injured patient. *J Trauma* 65(6):1209–1216, 2008.

34. Al-Kadi A, Dyer D, Ball CG, et al.: User's perceptions of remote trauma telesonography. *J Telemed Telecare* 15(5): 251–254, 2009.

35. Otto C, Hamilton DR, Levine BD, Hare C, Sargsyan AE, Altshuler P, et al.: Into thin air: Extreme ultrasound on Mt Everest. *Wilderness Environ Med* 20(3):283–289, 2009.

36. Otto C, Comtois JM, Sargsyan A. The Martian chronicles: Remotely guided diagnosis and treatment in the Arctic Circle. *Surgical endoscopy* 24(9):2170–2177, 2010.

37. O'Connell K, Bouffard AJ, Vollman A, et al.: Extreme musculo-skeletal ultrasound: training of non-physicians in the Arctic Circle. *Crit Ultrasound J* 3:19–24, 2011.

38. Crawford I, Tiruta C, Kirkpatrick AW: Big brother could actually help quite easily: Telementored "just-in-time"

39. Crawford I, McBeth PB, Kirkpatrick AW: Telementorable "just-in-time" lung ultrasound on an iPhone. *J Emerg Trauma Shock* 4(4):526–527, 2011.

40. McBeth PB, Crawford I, Hamilton T, et al.: Simple, almost anywhere, with almost anyone: Remote low-cost telementored resuscitative lung ultrasound. *J Trauma* (in press).

41. Mindel S: Role of imager in developing world. *Lancet* 349:426–429, 1997.

42. Levine AC, Shah SP, Umulisa I, et al.: Ultrasound assessment of severe dehydration in children with diarrhea and vomiting. *Acad Emerg Med* 17(10):1035–1041, 2010.

43. Murphy S, Cserti-Gazdewich C, Dhabangi A, et al.: Ultrasound findings in Plasmodium falciparum malaria: A pilot study. *Pediatr Crit Care Med* 12(2):e58–e63, 2011.

44. Agarwal D, Narayan S, Chakravarty J, Sundar S: Ultrasonography for diagnosis of abdominal tuberculosis in HIV infected people. *Indian J Med Res* 2010132:77-80.

45. Shah S, Price D, eds.: *Partners in Health Manual of Ultrasound for Resource-Limited Settings*. 1 ed. Boston, MA: Partners In Health, 2011. http://parthealth.3cdn.net/3ad982b2456f524cf8_kxvm6qpr9.pdf

46. Sippel S, Muruganandan K, Levine AC, Shah S: Review Article: Use of ultrasound in the developing world. *Int J Emerg Med* 4:72, 2011.

47. Shah SP, Epino H, Bukhman G, et al.: Impact of the introduction of ultrasound services in a limited resource setting: Rural Rwanda 2008. *BMC Int Health Hum Rights* 9:4, 2009.

48. Kimberly H, Murray A, Mennicke M, et al.: Focused maternal ultrasound by midwives in rural Zambia. *Ultrasound Med Biol* 36(8):1267–1272, 2010.

49. Kotlyar S, Moore CL: Assessing the utility of ultrasound in Liberia. *J Emerg Trauma Shock* 1(1):10–14, 2008.

50. Blaivas M, Kuhn W, Reynolds B, Brannam L: Change in differential diagnosis and patient management with the use of portable ultrasound in a remote setting. *Wilderness Environ Med* 16(1):38–41, 2005.

51. Spencer JK, Adler RS: Utility of portable ultrasound in a community in Ghana. *J Ultrasound Med* 27(12):1735–1743, 2008.

52. Steinmetz JP, Berger JP: Ultrasonography as an aid to diagnosis and treatment in a rural African hospital: A prospective study of 1119 cases. *Am J Trop Med Hyg* 60(1):119–123, 1999.

53. Eckardt M., Ahn R, Reyes R, et al.: "The impact of maternal ultrasound in Mali." American Public Health Association Annual Meeting. *Poster Presentation* November 1. Washington, DC, 2011.

CHAPTER 5

Trauma

O. John Ma, James R. Mateer, and Andrew W. Kirkpatrick

Over the past 30 years, trauma surgeons in Europe and Japan have demonstrated the proficient use of ultrasonography in evaluating blunt trauma patients.[1-9] During the 1990s, emergency physicians and trauma surgeons in North America have prospectively evaluated the applications of ultrasonography in trauma and have presented results comparable with those of other investigators worldwide.[10-18]

The focused assessment with sonography for trauma (FAST) examination is a bedside screening tool to aid clinicians in identifying free intrathoracic or intraperitoneal fluid. The underlying premise behind the use of the FAST examination is that clinically significant injuries will be associated with the presence of free fluid accumulation in dependent areas. The FAST examination was originally developed as a limited ultrasound examination, focusing primarily on the detection of free fluid, and was not designed to universally identify all sonographically detectable pathology. Over the last decade many groups have proposed additions or modifications to the standard FAST examination. However, the essence of the FAST examination is identifying findings that can be interpreted by clinicians within a clinical context. As this approach has grown to the extent that some propose integrating ultrasound completely within the advanced trauma life support (ATLS) sequence,[19] the challenge for the future is to capitalize on the information point-of-care ultrasound provides, while not delaying critical interventions.[20]

▶ CLINICAL CONSIDERATIONS

The rapid and accurate diagnosis of injuries sustained by trauma patients can be difficult, especially when they are associated with other distracting injuries or altered mental status from head injury or drug or alcohol use. In the United States, the three generally accepted diagnostic techniques for evaluating abdominal trauma patients are diagnostic peritoneal lavage (DPL), CT of the abdomen, and ultrasonography. Each of these diagnostic modalities has its own advantages and disadvantages.

DPL remains an excellent screening test for evaluating abdominal trauma. Table 5-1 reviews the advantages and disadvantages of DPL.

▶ TABLE 5-1. **ADVANTAGES AND DISADVANTAGES OF DIAGNOSTIC PERITONEAL LAVAGE**

Advantages
Sensitivity for detecting hemoperitoneum
Availability of equipment
Relative speed with which it can be performed
Low complication rate with an experienced operator
Ability to detect early evidence of bowel perforation

Disadvantages
Potential for iatrogenic injury
Misapplication for evaluation of retroperitoneal injuries
Lack of specificity

CT of the abdomen has a greater specificity than DPL, thus making it the initial diagnostic test of choice at all trauma centers. IV contrast material should be given to provide optimal resolution. Table 5-2 reviews the advantages and disadvantages of CT.

Ultrasonography offers several advantages over DPL and abdominal CT. Numerous studies have demonstrated that the FAST examination, like DPL, is an accurate screening tool for abdominal trauma.[1-18] Advantages of the FAST examination are that it is accurate, rapid, noninvasive, repeatable, and portable, and involves no nephrotoxic contrast material or radiation exposure to the patient. There is limited risk for patients who are pregnant, coagulopathic, or have had previous abdominal surgery. The average time to perform a complete FAST examination of the thoracic and abdominal cavities is 4.0 minutes or less.[12] However, investigators have demonstrated that a massive hemoperitoneum may be quickly detected with a single view of Morison's pouch in 82–90% of hypotensive patients,[18,21] and this required an average of only 19 seconds in one study.[18] One major advantage of the FAST examination compared with DPL or abdominal CT is the ability to

▶ TABLE 5-2. **ADVANTAGES AND DISADVANTAGES OF CT**

Advantages
Ability to precisely locate intra-abdominal lesions preoperatively
Ability to evaluate the retroperitoneum
Ability to identify injuries that may be managed nonoperatively
Noninvasive

Disadvantages
Expense of the study
Time required to perform the study
Need to transport the trauma patient to the radiology suite
Need for contrast materials
Ionizing radiation exposure to patient

also evaluate for free pericardial or pleural fluid and for pneumothorax. The main disadvantage of the FAST examination compared with CT has been the inability to determine the exact etiology of the free intraperitoneal fluid. This limitation has the potential for significant change as a growing number of studies have reported the utility of contrast-enhanced ultrasonography for the identification and treatment of solid organ injuries.[22-24] Other potential disadvantages of the FAST examination are the operator-dependent nature of the examination, the difficulty in interpreting the images in patients who are obese or have subcutaneous air or excessive bowel gas, and the inability to distinguish intraperitoneal hemorrhage from ascites. The FAST examination also cannot evaluate the retroperitoneum as well as CT, making these complementary rather than competing technologies when time permits and the potential benefits of CT outweigh the risks.

In light of the evolving nonoperative approach to certain types of solid-organ injuries, a positive DPL by itself is becoming less of an indication for immediate exploratory laparotomy than the amount of hemorrhage and the clinical condition of the patient. Since the FAST examination can reliably detect small amounts of free intraperitoneal fluid and can be used to estimate the rate of hemorrhage through serial examinations, ultrasonography has essentially replaced DPL for blunt abdominal trauma in the majority of North American trauma centers.

▶ CLINICAL INDICATIONS

Generally accepted clinical indications for performing the FAST examination include

- acute blunt or penetrating torso trauma,
- trauma in pregnancy,
- pediatric trauma,
- subacute torso trauma, and
- undifferentiated hypotension.

▶ ACUTE BLUNT OR PENETRATING TORSO TRAUMA

At Level 1 trauma centers, the primary utilization of the FAST examination has been for the rapid detection of free intraperitoneal fluid in patients who have sustained significant blunt torso trauma. More recently, trauma programs have begun to incorporate the FAST examination into the primary patient assessment for detecting the presence, amount, and location of intracavitary hemorrhage in general. It is likely that these indications will greatly expand as an ever-increasing numbers of clinicians adopt resuscitative ultrasound into their daily practice. This will increase the responsibility for these clinicians to ensure the use of ultrasound as an adjunct will expedite, and not delay, therapy.

With blunt trauma, the FAST examination is particularly useful for patients who (1) are too hemodynamically unstable to leave the ED for CT scanning; (2) have a physical examination that is unreliable secondary to drug intoxication, distracting injury, or central nervous system injury; and (3) have unexplained hypotension and an equivocal physical examination.

With penetrating trauma patients, the FAST examination should be performed when it is not certain that immediate surgery is indicated. In patients with multiple wounds, the FAST examination can be used to quantify and locate the source of internal hemorrhage. When the trajectory of a penetrating wound is uncertain, the FAST examination may quickly identify the course by the presence of free fluid within the compartments involved. This is particularly helpful when the entry location is the precordium, lower chest, or epigastrium. Inappropriate surgical sequencing has been reported to occur in 44% of patients with wounds in multiple body cavities.[25] In a review of patients with injuries to both the thoracic and abdominal cavities, the investigators regretted their limited use of early FAST examinations in directing surgical sequencing and strongly recommended its increased use in the initial patient evaluation.[25] The FAST examination can therefore be used to prioritize such lifesaving interventions as pericardiocentesis, pericardiotomy, thoracostomy, thoracotomy, laparotomy, or sternotomy. The FAST examination is useful in evaluating patients who have sustained stab wounds to the abdomen where local wound exploration indicates that the superficial muscle fascia has been violated. Also, the FAST examination may be useful in confirming a negative physical examination when tangential or lower chest wounds are involved.

In non-Level 1 trauma centers, emergency physicians and surgeons may lack the immediate availability of CT scans and formal two-dimensional (2D) echocardiograms. The use of bedside ultrasonography by physicians trained to perform the FAST examination in these settings will significantly improve patient evaluation, initial treatment, consultation, and the timely transportation of patients to trauma centers when indicated. When the FAST examination demonstrates intracavitary fluid in these settings, surgeons and operating room personnel can be consulted immediately and/or transportation to a Level 1 trauma center can be initiated. When the diagnostic imaging personnel and surgeons are out of the hospital, and the severity of the patient's injuries is not clinically evident, a positive FAST examination could save up to an hour or more of time to definitive surgical treatment.[26-28]

Although the FAST examination is used most commonly to detect free intraperitoneal fluid, it may also aid in the rapid identification of pneumothorax and free pericardial or pleural fluid, and the evaluation of the fetus in the pregnant trauma patient. In addition, the FAST examination has been evaluated in the management of pediatric trauma patients and can be utilized in patients who present with subacute trauma but with a significant mechanism of injury or concerning physical examination.

DETECTION OF FREE INTRAPERITONEAL FLUID

By the latter half of the 1990s, for patients who had sustained blunt or penetrating abdominal trauma, the FAST examination's utility for detecting free intraperitoneal fluid had been universally recognized. While CT remained the gold standard for detecting specific intra-abdominal pathology, the FAST examination had gained acceptance as a rapid screening tool for identifying free intraperitoneal fluid.

During the 1980s, surgeons in Germany developed bedside utilization of ultrasonography for evaluation of trauma patients. Although excellent results were reported in early studies, with the sensitivity ranging from 84% to 100% and the specificity from 88% to 100%, these findings went largely unnoticed in the United States as the articles were not initially translated into English.[2-7]

In the 1990s, a number of prospective studies (with study sizes greater than 100 patients) had been reported on this issue in the English literature.[1,8-18] The majority of these studies focused on the FAST examination for the evaluation of free intraperitoneal fluid in blunt abdominal trauma patients only. These studies reported the sensitivity and the specificity to range from 69% to 90% and 95% to 100%, respectively.

Tiling and colleagues were the first investigators to suggest that the FAST examination could provide comprehensive evaluation for significant areas of hemorrhage, including pericardial, pleural, intraperitoneal, and retroperitoneal. Their prospective study of 808 blunt trauma patients found a sensitivity of 89% and a specificity of 99% for free intraperitoneal fluid. Their clinical algorithm incorporates the FAST examination during the initial patient evaluation.[1]

One of the first North American trauma ultrasound studies demonstrated the FAST examination to have an overall sensitivity of 79% and specificity of 95.6%. They concluded that appropriately trained surgeons could rapidly and accurately perform and interpret FAST examinations and that ultrasound was a rapid, sensitive, and specific diagnostic modality for detecting intraperitoneal fluid and pericardial effusion.[10] Ultrasound has been used as the primary adjuvant modality to detect hemoperitoneum and pericardial effusion in injured patients (Figure 5-1). After finding that the FAST

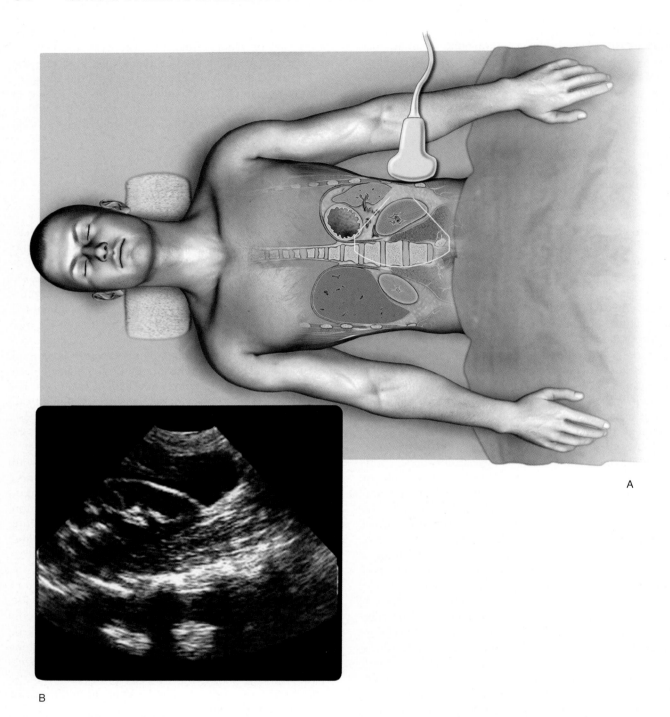

A

B

Figure 5-1. Examination of the abdomen to assess for free intraperitoneal fluid. Transducer position for the coronal view of the left upper quadrant (A) and corresponding ultrasound image (B) with free fluid in the paracolic gutter adjacent to the lower pole of the kidney.

examination had an 81.5% sensitivity and 99.7% specificity, the investigators stated that ultrasound should be the primary adjuvant instrument for the evaluation of injured patients because it was rapid, accurate, and potentially cost-effective.[11]

In 1995, Ma and Mateer prospectively demonstrated that the FAST examination could serve as a sensitive, specific, and accurate diagnostic tool in the detection of free intraperitoneal and thoracic fluid in patients who had sustained major blunt or penetrating trauma. Overall, the FAST examination had a sensitivity of 90%, specificity of 99%, and accuracy of 99%. In evaluating the subgroup of blunt trauma patients, which consisted of 165 of the 245 patients, the FAST examination was 90% sensitive, 99% specific, and 99% accurate. In evaluating the subgroup of penetrating trauma victims, which consisted of 80 of the 245 patients, the FAST examination was 91% sensitive, 100% specific, and 99% accurate.[12] Since emergency physicians performed all the FAST examinations, it became the first prospective study to support that appropriately trained emergency physicians could accurately perform and interpret FAST examinations. The results reiterated that a FAST examination of the entire torso could successfully provide early and valuable information for the presence of free fluid in both the peritoneal and thoracic cavities. In addition, the FAST examination was found to be equally sensitive, specific, and accurate for both blunt and penetrating torso trauma. Penetrating trauma patients could benefit from the rapid and accurate information yielded by ultrasonography.[18] The identification and localization of significant hemorrhage in penetrating trauma patients would allow physicians "to prioritize resources for resuscitation and evaluation."[10] Most studies have utilized a multiple-view FAST examination for evaluation of trauma patients. Some investigators have employed a single-view technique, examining only Morison's pouch for free intraperitoneal fluid.[29-31] In one study, all patients were placed in the Trendelenburg position and the perihepatic (Morison's pouch) was the single area examined. The results of this technique were reported to be 81.8% sensitive, 93.9% specific, and 90.9% accurate.[29]

The single-view (perihepatic) imaging technique was compared with the multiple-view technique of the FAST examination for the identification of free intraperitoneal fluid in patients who had sustained major blunt or penetrating torso trauma. For detecting free intraperitoneal fluid, when comparing the multiple-view FAST examination of the abdomen to the gold standard, the multiple-view FAST examination technique had a sensitivity of 87%, a specificity of 99%, and an accuracy of 98%. When comparing the perihepatic single view of the abdomen to the gold standard, the single-view FAST examination technique had a sensitivity of 51%, a specificity of 100%, and an accuracy of 93%.[13] Based on

this and other studies, the more sensitive and accurate FAST examination method for detecting free intraperitoneal fluid was determined to be the multiple-view technique.[13]

DETECTION OF SOLID ORGAN INJURY

The use of contrast-enhanced ultrasonography may help clinicians identify specific organ injuries on the FAST examination.[32-35] Contrast-enhanced ultrasonography is the application of ultrasound contrast agents to complement or augment traditional sonography. Newer second-generation ultrasound contrast agents contain perflutren microbubbles that when administered IV can pass through the pulmonary circuit into the systemic vasculature. The microbubbles vibrate strongly at the high frequencies used in diagnostic ultrasonography, which makes them several thousand times more reflective than normal body tissues. This characteristic allows microbubbles to enhance both gray scale images and flow-mediated Doppler signals. Although an initial FDA black box warning has slowed widespread utilization in the United States, microbubble contrast agents have subsequently been found to be as safe as conventional agents used in radiography and magnetic resonance imaging.[22-24]

Contrast-enhanced ultrasonography has been shown to be a promising tool for detecting solid organ (liver and spleen) injuries after blunt abdominal trauma. When an ultrasound contrast agent was administered immediately before performing the traditional FAST examination, the examination has correlated appreciably better than unenhanced sonography for detecting hepatic and splenic injuries and estimating the extent of their injuries.[32-34] One study reported their 5-year experience with 133 blunt abdominal trauma patients. When compared with CT, contrast-enhanced ultrasonography had a sensitivity and specificity of 96.4% and 98%, respectively. The authors concluded that "contrast enhanced ultrasonography is an accurate technique for evaluating traumatic lesions of solid abdominal organs . . . . is able to detect active bleeding and vascular lesions, and avoids exposure to ionizing radiation."[23]

Another study analyzed 392 patients with liver and/or spleen injuries and demonstrated no significant difference in detection rate for active bleeding between contrast-enhanced ultrasonography and contrast CT.[24] As clinicians continue to explore the uses for contrast-enhanced ultrasonography in trauma, there is great potential for reducing the costs and radiation exposure associated with CT while identifying patients requiring immediate operative intervention compared with those who may benefit from nonoperative management of solid organ injuries.

CLINICAL ALGORITHMS

Clinical pathways and protocols have been derived from the use of the FAST examination and incorporated with other diagnostic methods commonly used for trauma evaluation in North America (Figure 5-2). Inclusion of the FAST examination into a protocol for the management of patients sustaining torso trauma has been found to decrease time to operative intervention and improve resource utilization by reducing CT usage, hospital days, and total patient charges.[36] Another ultrasound-based key clinical pathway has been shown to reduce the number of DPL procedures and CT scans required to evaluate blunt abdominal trauma without increased risk to the patient (Figure 5-3). Cost savings were estimated to be $450,000 per year using this key clinical pathway.[37] The issue of cost savings of the FAST examination has also been addressed in another study. For blunt trauma patients, the FAST examination was found to be more efficient and cost-effective than CT scanning or DPL. There was a significantly shorter time to disposition at approximately one-third the cost in the ultrasonography group.[38]

An ultrasound-based scoring system has been developed to quantify the amount of intraperitoneal blood in blunt abdominal trauma patients and to assess the need for therapeutic exploratory laparotomy. Scores ranged from 0 to 8. The system assigned two points for significant fluid collections ≥2 cm and one point for fluid collections ≤2 cm. A score of 3 correlated with 1000 mL of fluid. In the study, of those patients who had

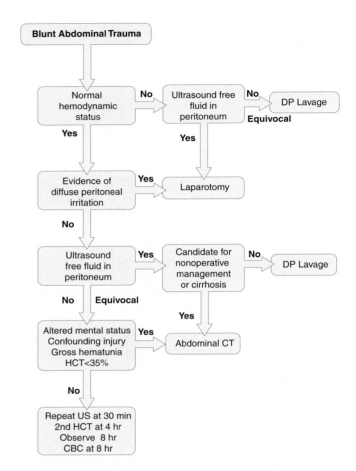

Figure 5-3. Key clinical pathway for the evaluation of blunt abdominal trauma. (From Branney SW, Moore EE, Cantrill S, et al.: Ultrasound-based key clinical pathway reduces the use of hospital resources for the evaluation of blunt abdominal trauma. *J Trauma* 42:1086–1090, 1997, with permission.)

a score of 3 or more, 24 of 25 patients (96%) required therapeutic laparotomy. Of those who had a score of less than 3, therapeutic laparotomy was required in only 9 of 24 patients (38%). The FAST examination was found to be a useful adjunct in helping to make clinical decisions during the resuscitation period.[39] In another study evaluating the role of the FAST examination in determining the need for therapeutic laparotomy, none of the patients with negative FAST examination results died or sustained identifiable mortality as a consequence of their negative scans.[40]

DETECTION OF PERICARDIAL FLUID

In the hypotensive patient who has sustained penetrating trauma to the torso, the echocardiographic portion of the FAST examination may prove to be the most beneficial aspect. Echocardiography remains the gold standard

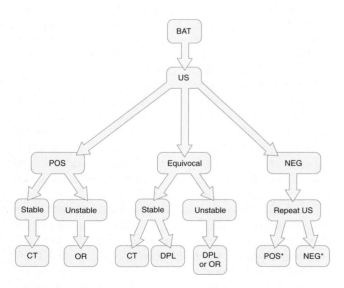

Figure 5-2. Suggested algorithm for the use of ultrasonography in the evaluation of the patient with blunt abdominal trauma. (From Rozycki GS, Shackford SR: Ultrasound: what every trauma surgeon should know. *J Trauma* 40:2, 1996, with permission.)

diagnostic procedure for detecting pericardial effusions. The classic physical examination findings of acute cardiac tamponade—distended neck veins, hypotension, and muffled heart tones—are present in less than 40% of patients with surgically proven cardiac tamponade.[41] Timely ED procedures and expeditious transportation of the patient to the operating room may be accomplished by ultrasound diagnosis of hemopericardium.

In 1992, Plummer and coinvestigators evaluated the effect of bedside echocardiography performed by emergency physicians on the outcome of 49 patients with penetrating cardiac injuries over a 10-year period. Compared with a retrospective control group, the use of bedside echocardiography significantly reduced the time of diagnosis and disposition to the operating room from 42.4 ± 21.7 minutes to 15.5 ± 11.4 minutes while the actual survival improved from 57.1% to 100%.[42]

The accuracy of point-of-care ultrasound has been evaluated after it was introduced into five Level I trauma centers for the diagnosis of acute hemopericardium. Surgeons or cardiologists (four centers) and technicians (one center) performed pericardial ultrasound examinations on patients with penetrating truncal wounds. By protocol, patients with positive examinations underwent immediate operation. In 261 patients, pericardial ultrasound examinations were found to have a sensitivity of 100%, specificity of 96.9%, and accuracy of 97.3%. The mean time from ultrasound to operation was 12.1 ± 5 minutes. This further demonstrated that ultrasound should be the initial modality for the evaluation of patients with penetrating precordial wounds because it is accurate and rapid.[43]

Over the years, numerous studies have examined the role of echocardiography in blunt cardiac trauma. The utility and role of ultrasound, particularly with the diagnosis of cardiac contusion, remain unclear (see Chapter 6, "Cardiac," for a comprehensive review of this topic).

DETECTION OF PLEURAL FLUID

Since patients who have sustained major trauma routinely present to the ED immobilized on a long spine board, clinicians may have difficulty identifying bilateral hemothoraces or a small unilateral hemothorax on the initial supine chest radiograph. The FAST examination can detect hemothorax before the completion of a chest radiograph or can be used as additional information when the chest radiograph is equivocal. Thus, tube thoracostomy for trauma patients may be expedited with the use of ultrasonography.

Ma and Mateer demonstrated that the FAST examination could serve as a sensitive, specific, and accurate diagnostic tool in detecting hemothorax in major trauma patients. When comparing the FAST examination

and the chest radiograph with the criterion of standard definitions, both diagnostic tests had an equal sensitivity (96.2%), specificity (100%), and accuracy (99.6%) for detecting pleural fluid. They concluded that ultrasonography was comparable to the chest radiograph for identifying hemothorax.[44]

Ultrasonography can detect smaller quantities of pleural fluid than the chest radiograph. It is estimated that an upright chest radiograph can accurately detect a minimum of 50–100 mL of pleural fluid[45] and that a supine chest radiograph can detect a minimum of 175 mL of pleural fluid.[46] By contrast, it is estimated that ultrasonography can detect a minimum of 20 mL of pleural fluid.[9] Also, ultrasonography can help differentiate between pleural fluid and pleural thickening or pulmonary contusion when the supine chest radiograph is equivocal.

Although the FAST examination cannot completely replace the chest radiograph, it can complement chest radiograph findings by rapidly identifying hemothorax in the supine patient. Of the six anatomic areas scanned by the FAST examination, only two are required to identify the presence of free pleural fluid in the two pleural cavities. By utilizing the FAST examination to initially identify hemothorax, the standard chest radiograph of the trauma patient can be performed after tube thoracostomy, thereby sparing the patient an additional chest radiograph.

DETECTION OF PNEUMOTHORAX

Not only can the FAST examination detect a hemothorax, it can also identify a pneumothorax before the completion of a chest radiograph. This is especially relevant since the reported proportion of pneumothoraces that are occult compared with those actually seen on the chest radiograph ranges from 29% to 72%.[47–52] The concept of using ultrasound to exclude the presence of a pneumothorax relies on the simple premise that if the two pleural surfaces are normally in apposition, then an intrapleural collection of air (pneumothorax) cannot be separating them. The focused goal is to identify the contiguity of the visceral and parietal pleura using simple sonographic signs to exclude the presence of a pneumothorax. This diagnostic test is considered to be an extended FAST (E-FAST) examination.[51] With experience and always appreciating the clinical setting, a pneumothorax can be expeditiously excluded in the vast majority of cases.[53]

Detecting a pneumothorax with ultrasound may initially appear to be paradoxical since air has the highest acoustic impedance of normal body substances, with almost complete reflectance of sound waves at commonly used frequencies.[54] Thus, only artifacts are normally seen deep to the pleural interface in the normal

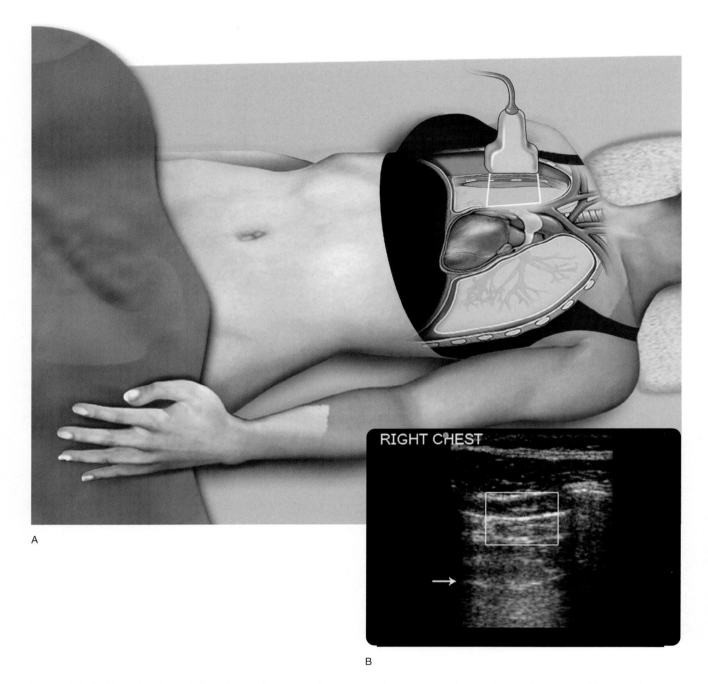

A

RIGHT CHEST

B

Figure 5-4. Examination of the pleural interface to assess for pneumothorax. Transducer position on the anterior chest with the patient in the supine position (A). Ultrasound image of the pleural interface (bright horizontal line in center of box) and normal A-line artifact (arrow) deep to the pleural interface (B).

lung.[55] Both hemothoraces and pneumothoraces, however, are superficial pleural-based diseases and, therefore, lend themselves to sonographic examination (Figure 5-4).

Unless there are pleural adhesions from previous disease or injury (a condition that reduces the risk of pneumothorax), normal respiration is associated with a physiologic sliding of the two pleural surfaces upon one another. The most common normal sign on sonography is lung sliding, which in essence excludes the presence of a pneumothorax in the area that has been imaged.[48,51,53] For this physiologic "lung sliding" along the visceral–parietal pleural interface to be seen, both surfaces must be accessible for imaging and must be either contiguous or separated by a layer of fluid.[50,51,56] Conceptually, this sign represents the visual depiction of breathing. It does not comment upon ventilator adequacy or exclude serious pulmonary pathology other than ruling out a pneumothorax; it simply indicates that the patient has ventilatory efforts when it is seen. This movement is better visualized at the lung bases and less so at the apices.[53] It is important to consider that free air within the thorax will usually seek the point of maximum elevation, so that a normal sliding sign seen in the lung bases cannot exclude a partial pneumothorax in a supine patient (the anterior and apical areas must be imaged as well). A notable exception for viewing a normal sliding sign is when subcutaneous emphysema superimposes itself between the skin and the parietal pleura, but this clinical situation is also associated with a specificity of 98% for underlying occult pneumothorax and is usually evident on physical examination.[57]

Examining the pleural interfaces with the color power Doppler mode can enhance the depiction of this sliding movement due to power Doppler's ability to detect motion, a finding that has been designated the "Power Slide."[49] Power Doppler is superior to conventional color Doppler in determining the presence or absence of flow at the expense of direction and speed information and thus has the ability to identify low-velocity and low-volume flow (or motion).[49,58,59] It also documents a real-time physiologic process in a single still image, allowing for simpler archiving and tele-transmission. In a similar way, the use of M-mode imaging documents either the presence of lung sliding ("seashore sign") or its absence when a pneumothorax is present ("stratosphere sign") since the pleural movement will normally generate a homogenous granular pattern in this mode.[53,60] An intermediate sign that is best documented in M-mode is the "lung point" sign, which is visualized when the lung intermittently contacts the parietal pleura with inspiration, thus alternating between the seashore and stratospheric signs.

Other commonly seen artifacts are B-lines, which are also referred to as the comet-tail artifact. This is a reverberation artifact thought to arise from distended water-filled interlobular septae under the visceral pleura. Comet-tail artifacts are presumed to be the ultrasound equivalents of Kerley B-lines seen on a chest radiograph.[53,61] Thus, this sign represents the visual equivalent of hearing lung crepitations. Being related to the visceral pleura, B-lines can be seen only when the visceral pleura is in apposition to the parietal pleura. When a pneumothorax is present, the intrapleural air will separate the two pleural surfaces, and B-lines will be absent. Instead, the only artifacts that will appear to be deep to this level are horizontal reverberation artifacts, which are often seen as a "mirror image" of the chest wall.

Lichtenstein and coworkers have described a standardized, but hierarchal thoracic examination whose scope depends on the clinical status and mobility of the patient. They designate the A-line as a brightly echogenic line between the rib shadows recurring at an interval that exactly replicates the interval between the skin and pleural line, and represents the horizontal reverberation artifact generated by the parietal pleura.[53]

If both lung sliding and B-lines are present, then the clinician can confidently exclude the presence of a pneumothorax. If lung sliding and B-lines are not visible, then the examiner should suspect the presence of a pneumothorax, a suspicion further heightened by the presence of the horizontal reverberation artifact (A-line).[62,63] The absence of lung sliding alone had 100% sensitivity, but only 78% specificity for diagnosing an occult pneumothorax. When an A-line was seen with absent lung sliding, there was 95% sensitivity and 94% specificity for diagnosing an occult pneumothorax.[60] The presence of a lung point had 100% specificity for an occult pneumothorax. This is a critical distinction. No sliding does *not* mean a pneumothorax is present, only that a pneumothorax *might* be present. The pleura will not "slide" normally when there is pleural symphysis from adhesions or there is apnea, either voluntary or induced, such as with paralysis. Thus, if lung sliding is not seen, then B-lines are sought next. If these are not seen, then a lung point should be sought by progressively scanning laterally on the supine chest or inferiorly on an upright chest. Clinical context is always important. The lung point implies intermittent contact of the underlying lung against the parietal pleura, meaning a so-called "partial pneumothorax." If there is a very large pneumothorax, the lung will never contact the parietal pleura and no lung point will be detected. Thus, diagnosis requires interpretation within the clinical context, which is what empowers point-of-care sonography in the clinician's hands.[64]

Kirkpatrick and coinvestigators prospectively evaluated a handheld ultrasound device in the real-time resuscitation of critically ill patients.[51] This study focused on the most difficult-to-diagnose subset of pneumothoraces, as any patient with a clinically evident pneumothorax was treated without any imaging and those patients with clear-cut pneumothoraces on chest radiograph were excluded as well. In the remaining clinically stable patients, when comparing E-FAST directly with chest radiography, the E-FAST examination was more sensitive for the detection of occult pneumothoraces after trauma (49% versus 21%). Using CT corroboration, there were 22 false negative studies with E-FAST compared with 34 with chest radiography.[51] Another study analyzed 176 patients by systematically examining four thoracic locations, ranging from the 2nd intercostal space in the midclavicular line to the 6th intercostal space at the posterior axillary line. The authors searched for lung sliding, supplemented by color power Doppler when lung sliding was not easily detected, and assessed the relative size of the pneumothorax by correlating the relative topography of lung sliding. Overall, the sensitivity and specificity of ultrasound were noted to be 98% and 99%, respectively, compared with 76% and 100%, respectively, for chest radiography in this setting.[65]

Reflecting on basic principles, the E-FAST technique has an inherent advantage over chest radiography due to the physiologic behavior of pneumothoraces in the supine patient. Because of the effect of gravity, the supine lung tends to hinge dorsally, with free air collecting anteromedially.[66–69] Supine pneumothoraces are reported to be most commonly located at the anterior (84%), apical (57%), basal (41%), medial (27%), lateral (24%), and never posterior (0%) lung locations.[70] The standard imaging anatomic sites for the E-FAST were chosen to correspond to the recommended auscultatory locations from the ATLS course.[71]

Despite the fact that pneumothoraces are often a dynamic process, clinical management is often based on the perceived size of a pneumothorax. Allowing for other factors such as the need for transport and positive pressure ventilation, many small pneumothoraces are managed expectantly, whereas larger ones are more aggressively treated. Thus, it is pertinent to ask whether ultrasound may be of help in determining the size of pneumothoraces. While it was once believed that sonography was of no use in determining the volume of a pneumothorax,[55] it is now suggested that sonography may actually have utility in determining not only the presence but also the actual extent of a pneumothorax.[68]

The presence of a "lung point" sign is not only 100% specific for pneumothorax but also the location of this sign roughly correlates with the radiographic size of the pneumothorax.[63] A "partial sliding" sign has been described to represent the same phenomenon whereby smaller or occult pneumothoraces might be detected.[72] Also, a good correlation between the estimates of pneumothorax size and CT findings using the relative thoracic topography of lung sliding has been noted.[64]

▶ TRAUMA IN PREGNANCY

Trauma continues to be one of the leading causes of nonobstetrical mortality in pregnant patients.[73] Moreover, it contributes to fetal death more frequently than maternal death.[74–78] Ultrasonography may be a valuable adjunct for rapid diagnosis of traumatic injuries for both the mother and the fetus.[79–81]

The pregnant trauma patient presents unique diagnostic and management issues for the emergency physician and trauma surgeon. Maternal shock carries a high fetal mortality rate.[77] Although there are two lives at stake, proper assessment and stabilization of the mother will provide the best opportunity for fetal stability. Therefore, rapid assessment of the pregnant trauma patient is essential for early identification of life-threatening injuries. The FAST examination clearly may play a role in the timely assessment of pregnant trauma patients.

In this setting, ultrasonography offers several advantages over abdominal CT scan and DPL. The FAST examination may aid in the timely identification of pregnant trauma patients who need exploratory laparotomy immediately, and may help avoid delays in management while other diagnostic tests are obtained. The FAST examination can be performed at the bedside and involves no contrast material or radiation exposure to the mother or the fetus. Sonography can rapidly assess the pregnant trauma patient for hemoperitoneum and intrathoracic hemorrhage, and can assess the fetus for fetal heart tones, activity, and approximate gestational age. While ultrasonography is useful for identifying fetal heart tones and fetal movement, it is not as accurate in diagnosing uterine rupture or placental abruption, and it may be more technically difficult for advanced third-trimester pregnancy.[82]

The identification of free intraperitoneal fluid may be related to hemorrhage from solid organ injuries or amniotic fluid from uterine rupture or both. Ultrasonography should not be considered a reliable method for the specific identification of uterine rupture. The presence of an intrauterine organized hematoma and/or oligohydramnios, however, may suggest this diagnosis. Finally, although ultrasonography can be utilized to confirm immediate fetal viability, it cannot be used to rule out fetal–placental injury. While ultrasonography is used as an adjunct for the diagnosis of placental abruption, it is not sufficiently sensitive to exclude this diagnosis.[82] Continuous cardiotocographic monitoring, which has been demonstrated to accurately detect significant placental abruption, should be utilized as early as possible for all pregnant patients with significant blunt trauma.[83] (Please see Chapter 15, "Second- and Third-Trimester Pregnancy," for further reading.)

PEDIATRIC TRAUMA

The role of the E-FAST examination in evaluating pediatric trauma patients is discussed in Chapter 20, "Pediatric Applications."

▶ SUBACUTE TORSO TRAUMA

Patients occasionally present one or more days after the traumatic event with complaints of chest or abdominal pain. The issues of evolving hemothorax, hemoperitoneum, or subcapsular organ hemorrhage should be considered. When solid organ injuries are strongly considered, CT scanning is the preferred diagnostic method. When the index of suspicion is lower, bedside ultrasonography can be utilized to confirm the absence of unexpected abnormalities. A common scenario is a patient with suspected left-sided rib injuries who has left upper quadrant abdominal tenderness on examination. With subacute trauma, a splenic injury is likely to have evolved to the point where it could be detected by ultrasonography. The confirmation of a normal perisplenic ultrasound examination (without hemoperitoneum or subcapsular hemorrhage) would validate the clinician's suspicion of an isolated rib cage injury. In this case, an unexpected abnormal ultrasound examination would significantly alter the patient's treatment and disposition. It is likely that contrast-enhanced ultrasonography will be utilized in the future as an adjunct for identifying patients with occult injuries from subacute trauma.

UNDIFFERENTIATED HYPOTENSION

The role of the E-FAST examination in evaluating undifferentiated hypotension is discussed in Chapter 8, "Critical Care."

▶ ANATOMIC CONSIDERATIONS

The shape of the peritoneal cavity provides three dependent areas when a patient is in the supine position. These areas are divided by the spine longitudinally and the pelvic brim transversely. The site of accumulation of intraperitoneal fluid is dependent on the position of the patient and the source of bleeding.[13] Free intraperitoneal fluid has the propensity to collect in dependent intraperitoneal compartments formed by peritoneal reflections and mesenteric attachments (Figure 5-5).

The main compartment of the peritoneal cavity is the greater sac, which is divided into the supramesocolic and inframesocolic compartments. These two compartments are connected by the paracolic gutters. The right paracolic gutter connects Morison's pouch with the pelvis. Morison's pouch is the potential space between the liver and the right kidney. The left paracolic gutter is more anterior than the right, and its course to the splenorenal recess is blocked by the phrenicocolic ligament. Thus, free fluid will tend to flow via the right paracolic gutter since there is less resistance. In the supine patient, the most dependent area of the supramesocolic compartment is Morison's pouch. Overall, however, the rectovesical pouch is the most dependent area of the supine male, and the pouch of Douglas is the most dependent area of the supine female.[84]

In the supine patient, free intraperitoneal fluid in the right upper quadrant will tend to accumulate in Morison's pouch first before overflowing down the right paracolic gutter to the pelvis. In contrast, free intraperitoneal fluid in the left upper quadrant will tend to accumulate in the left subphrenic space first, and not the splenorenal recess, which is the potential space between the spleen and the left kidney. Free fluid overflowing from the left subphrenic space will travel into the splenorenal recess and then down the left paracolic gutter into the pelvis. Free fluid from the lesser peritoneal sac will travel across the epiploic foramen to Morison's pouch. Free intraperitoneal fluid in the pelvis will tend to accumulate in the rectovesical pouch in the supine male and the pouch of Douglas in the supine female (Figure 5-6).[84]

Positioning of the patient during the FAST examination may allow redistribution of free fluid in some cases but it may require patient angles of 30° to 45° (decubitus or Trendelenburg) for fluid to flow completely over the spine or pelvic brim. In addition, intraperitoneal hemorrhage often results in a combination of liquid and clotted blood. The organized hemorrhage may not redistribute to another compartment with patient repositioning.

If an initial abbreviated FAST examination is required, the data from one study suggest that for supine patients, an isolated pelvic view may provide a slightly greater yield (68% sensitivity) than does an isolated view of Morison's pouch (59% sensitivity) in the identification of free intraperitoneal fluid.[13]

The quantity of free intraperitoneal fluid that can accurately be detected on ultrasound has been reported to be as little as 100 mL.[8] Tiling considered a small anechoic stripe in Morison's pouch to represent about 250 mL of fluid and a 0.5-cm anechoic stripe to correspond to more than 500 mL of fluid within the peritoneum.[1]

▶ GETTING STARTED

The FAST examination consists of multiple ultrasound views of the abdomen and lower thorax. The standard examination is performed with the patient in the supine position. In general, the clinician should stand on the right side of the patient's bed next to the ultrasound machine. Left-handed dominance, room configuration, or other ongoing procedures may alter this arrangement. The patient's torso should be exposed from the clavicles to the symphysis pubis.

A standard 3.5 MHz microconvex or phased array transducer is commonly used because the footprint of the transducer can scan between the ribs during the evaluation of the thorax and upper quadrant views. Although they may have some limitations for this examination, a mechanical sector or standard curved array transducer may also be used. A sweeping motion of the transducer should be used for each view to maximize the information obtained. The scan planes are longitudinal (sagittal), transverse, and coronal. Figure 5-7 demonstrates the six areas of the basic FAST examination protocol. The clinician should perform each FAST examination in a systematic manner. We recommend

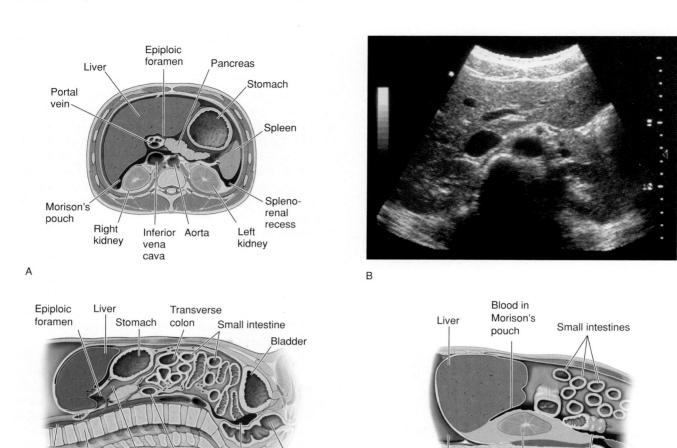

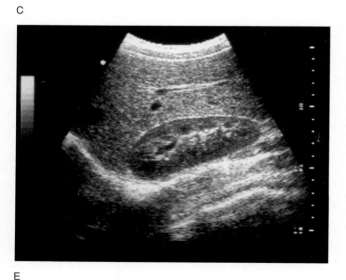

Figure 5-5. Transverse illustration of the upper abdomen that demonstrates the dependent compartments where free intraperitoneal fluid may collect (A). A transverse ultrasound view of the normal upper abdomen is depicted for comparison (B). Longitudinal illustration of the midline (C) and right paramedian abdomen (D) demonstrate the dependent compartments where free intraperitoneal fluid may collect. A longitudinal ultrasound view of the normal right upper abdomen is depicted for comparison (E). (B, E: Courtesy of *Gulfcoast Ultrasound*; A, C, D: Adapted from Mark Hoffmann, MD)

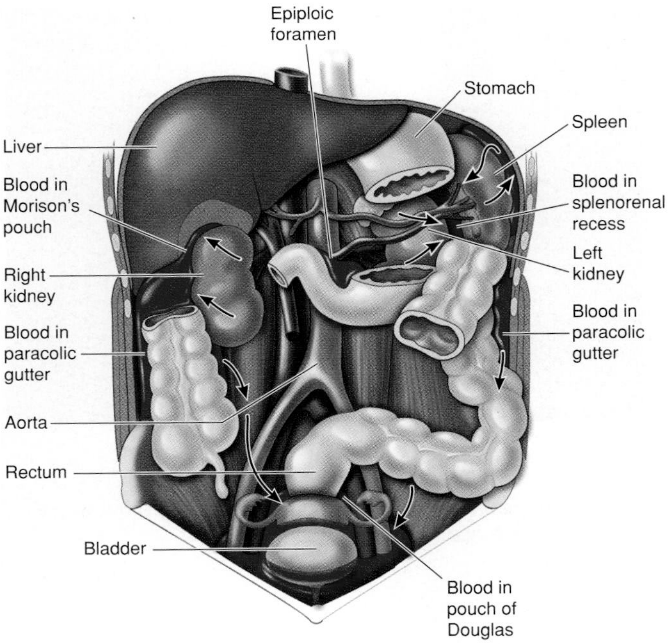

Liver

Blood in Morison's pouch

Right kidney

Blood in paracolic gutter

Aorta

Rectum

Bladder

Epiploic foramen

Stomach

Spleen

Blood in splenorenal recess

Left kidney

Blood in paracolic gutter

Blood in pouch of Douglas

Figure 5-6. Movement patterns of free intraperitoneal fluid within the abdominal cavity. (Adapted from Mark Hoffmann, MD)

that the FAST examination be performed using a standard sequence whenever possible: begin by examining the subxiphoid four-chamber view of the heart, move next to the right intercostal oblique and right coronal views, then examine the left intercostal oblique and left coronal views, and conclude by examining the pelvic (longitudinal and transverse) views. For the E-FAST examination, the transthoracic views should be assessed after these standard views.

The sensitivity of the FAST examination may be influenced by a number of factors, which include the experience of the clinician, type of equipment, timing of the FAST examination during the resuscitation, performance of serial examinations, the number of anatomical areas examined, and the position of the patient.

▶ TECHNIQUE AND NORMAL ULTRASOUND FINDINGS

The subxiphoid four-chamber view of the heart (Figure 5-7, area 1) should be used to examine for free pericardial fluid (Video 5-1 Trauma Cardiac). For this pericardial view, the ultrasound transducer is placed in the subxiphoid area and angled toward the patient's left shoulder. A coronal section of the heart should provide an adequate four-chamber view of the heart. From this view, global cardiac function and chamber size can be inspected briefly. The normal pericardium is seen as a hyperechoic (white) line surrounding the heart and,

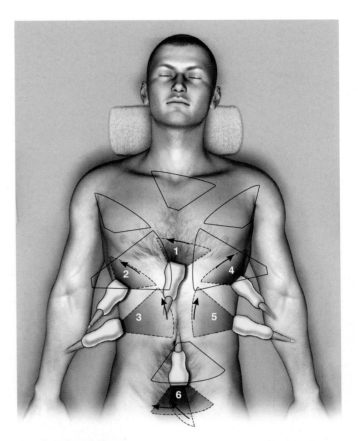

Figure 5-7. Ultrasound transducer positions for the focused assessment with sonography for trauma (FAST) examination. (Reproduced with permission from Ma OJ, Mateer JR, Ogata M, et al.: Prospective analysis of a rapid trauma ultrasound examination performed by emergency physicians. *J Trauma* 38:879–885, 1995.)

by using an anterior to posterior sweeping motion, the pericardium can be fully evaluated (Figure 5-8).

Next, the right intercostal oblique and right coronal views (Figure 5-7, areas 2 and 3, respectively) should be used to examine right pleural effusion, free fluid in Morison's pouch, and free fluid in the right paracolic gutter (Video 5-2 Trauma Right Upper Quadrant). From these views, the right diaphragm, the right lobe of the liver, and the right kidney also should be inspected briefly. For these perihepatic views, the ultrasound transducer is placed in the mid-axillary line between the 8th and 11th ribs with an oblique scanning plane. The transducer indicator should be pointed toward the right posterior axilla at the proper angle to keep the image plane between the ribs. The liver, right kidney, and Morison's pouch should be readily identified (Figure 5-9). The angle of the transducer can be directed more cephalad to examine for pleural fluid superior to the right diaphragm. The right diaphragm appears as a hyperechoic structure; pleural fluid can be identified as an anechoic

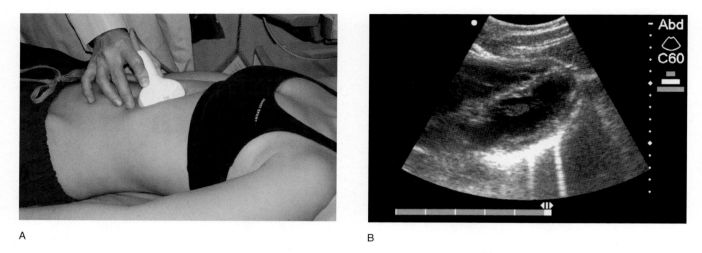

Figure 5-8. Subxiphoid four-chamber view of the heart. Transducer position (A) and corresponding ultrasound image (B). The normal pericardium is seen as a hyperechoic (white) line surrounding the heart.

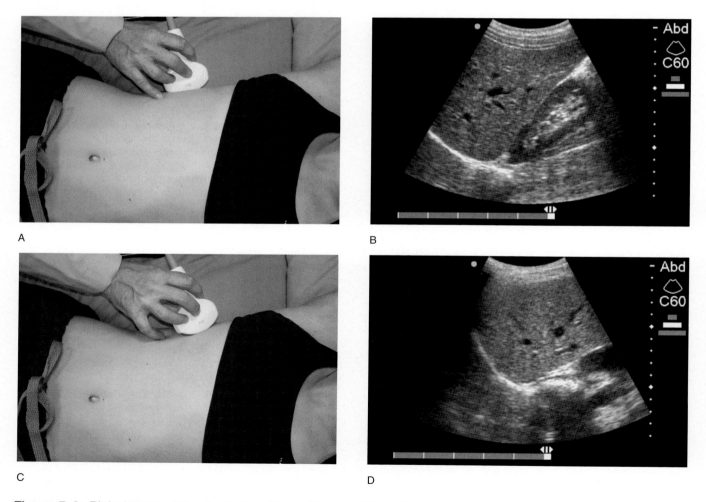

Figure 5-9. Right intercostal oblique view. Transducer position (A) and corresponding ultrasound image (B). The liver, right kidney, and Morison's pouch are readily identified. Right intercostal oblique view. Transducer position (C) and corresponding ultrasound image (D). The right diaphragm appears as a hyperechoic structure.

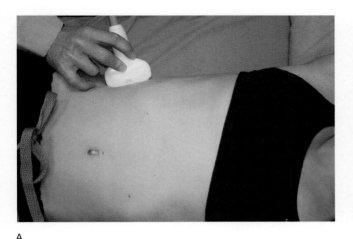
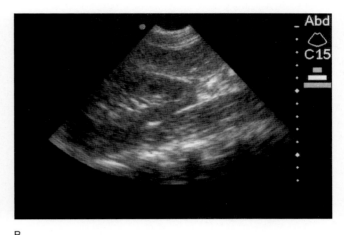

A   B

Figure 5-10. Right coronal view. Transducer position (A) and corresponding ultrasound image (B). The right pararenal retroperitoneum and paracolic gutter areas are identified above the psoas muscle in this view.

stripe superior to the diaphragm. The right pararenal retroperitoneum and paracolic gutter are viewed by rotating the transducer to the coronal imaging plane (transducer indicator toward the axilla) and positioning the transducer caudally below the 11th rib in the mid- to posterior axillary line (Figure 5-10).

The left intercostal oblique and left coronal views (Figure 5-7, areas 4 and 5, respectively) should be used to examine left pleural effusion, free fluid in the subphrenic space and splenorenal recess, and free fluid in the left paracolic gutter (Video 5-3 Trauma Left Upper Quadrant). From these views, the left diaphragm, the spleen, and the left kidney also should be inspected briefly. For these perisplenic views, the ultrasound transducer is placed at the left posterior axillary line between the 8th and 11th ribs with an oblique scanning plane. The transducer indicator should be pointed toward the

left posterior axilla. If the left kidney is identified first, then the transducer should be directed slightly more cephalad to locate the spleen (Figure 5-11). The angle of the transducer can then be directed more cephalad to examine for pleural fluid superior to the left diaphragm. The left diaphragm appears as a hyperechoic structure; pleural fluid can be identified as an anechoic stripe superior to the diaphragm. The left pararenal retroperitoneum and paracolic gutter are viewed by rotating the transducer to the coronal imaging plane (transducer indicator toward the axilla) and positioning the transducer caudally below the 11th rib in the mid- to posterior axillary line. The left kidney is often more difficult to visualize than the right kidney because it is positioned higher in the abdomen and can be obscured by overlying gas in the stomach and colon (Figure 5-12). Another reason why the left kidney may be more difficult to visualize

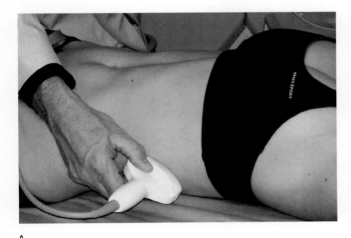
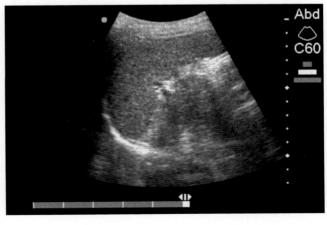

A   B

Figure 5-11. Left intercostal oblique view. Transducer position (A) and corresponding ultrasound image (B). A longitudinal view of the spleen, a portion of the diaphragm, and surrounding areas are visualized.

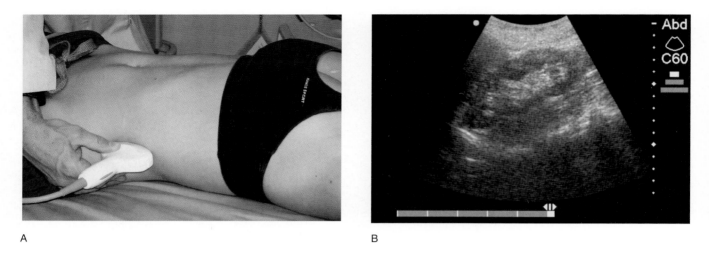

A

B

Figure 5-12. Left coronal view. Transducer position (A) and corresponding ultrasound image (B). The left pararenal, paracolic gutter areas, and kidney are examined in this view.

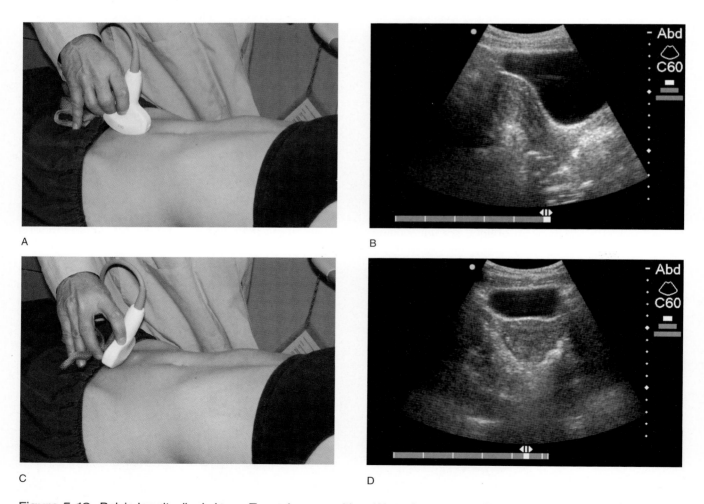

A

B

C

D

Figure 5-13. Pelvic longitudinal views. Transducer position (A) and corresponding ultrasound image (B). Ideally, these pelvic views should be obtained before the placement of a Foley catheter. Pelvic transverse views. Transducer position (C) and corresponding ultrasound image (D). In addition to potential fluid spaces, the bladder, the prostate or uterus, and the lateral walls of the pelvis can also be inspected briefly.

is that the spleen is a smaller organ than the liver, thus providing a much smaller acoustic window. Renal imaging may be facilitated in some patients by initiating a deep inspiration during this portion of the examination.

The pelvic (longitudinal and transverse) views (Figure 5-7, area 6) should be used to examine for free fluid in the anterior pelvis or cul-de-sac (pouch of Douglas) (Video 5-4 Trauma Pelvis). Ideally, these views should be obtained before the placement of a Foley catheter. From these views, the bladder, the prostate or uterus, and the lateral walls of the pelvis also should be inspected briefly (Figure 5-13). For these pelvic views, the ultrasound transducer should be placed 2 cm superior to the symphysis pubis along the midline of the abdomen with the scanning plane oriented longitudinally and the transducer aimed caudally into the pelvis. The transducer indicator should be pointed toward the patient's head. The transducer is then rotated 90° counterclockwise to obtain transverse images of the pelvis. Fluid in a filled bladder appears as a well-circumscribed and contained fluid collection that appears anechoic. In women, the uterus will be seen posterior to the bladder. A partially filled bladder can be differentiated from free peritoneal fluid by emptying the bladder (Foley catheter) or by retrograde bladder filling and repeating the examination.

Finally, to evaluate for a pneumothorax in the E-FAST examination (Figure 5-14), the use of a high-frequency

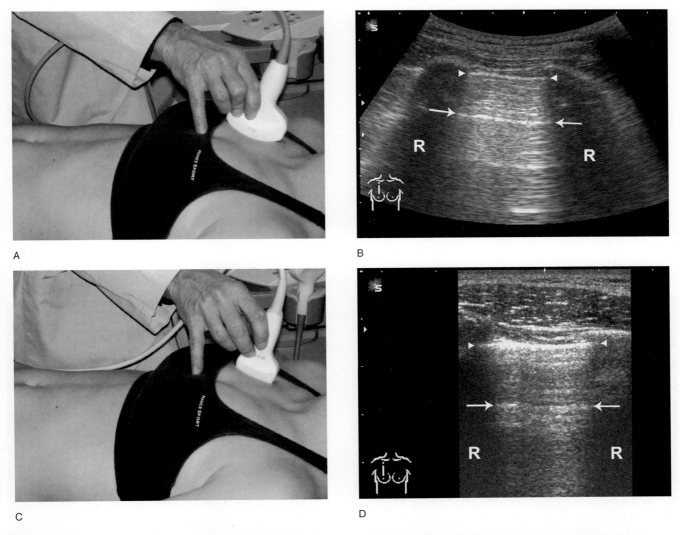

A

B

C

D

Figure 5-14. Longitudinal views of the normal lung surface demonstrating the "bat sign" described by Lichtenstein. Transducer position using a 3.5 MHz curved array transducer (A) and corresponding ultrasound image (B). This transducer allows visualization of more than one rib interspace and demonstrates normal artifacts more consistently. Transducer position using a 7.5-10 MHz linear array transducer (C) and corresponding ultrasound image (D). This transducer makes the pleural interface easier to recognize. In B and D the pleural line is visualized directly between the ribs (arrowheads) and A-lines (arrows) are the repeating horizontal artifacts deep to the pleural line. R = rib shadow

linear array transducer whose footprint fits well between the rib spaces is advisable since it provides the best resolution of the pleural interface (Video 5-5 Trauma Thoracic). However, the performance of the E-FAST examination for pneumothorax is most practically initiated using the same transducer as was used for the FAST examination. In fact, some diagnostic artifacts are more obvious with a lower frequency transducer (3.5 MHz) as opposed to the high-frequency linear array (7.5 + MHz) (Video 5-6 Trauma Complete Exam).

Regardless of which transducer is selected, the transducer should first be oriented longitudinally on the anterior chest wall at the midclavicular line. This produces an image perpendicular to the ribs to identify the echogenic pleural interface in reference to the overlying (and acoustically impervious) ribs (Figure 5-14). The image of the two ribs separated by the pleural line is known as the "bat-sign" and is a basic landmark of lung sonography. Once this view is obtained, the clinician should look for respiratory motion at the pleural interface (lung sliding) and for the presence of normal comet-tail artifacts and A-lines (Figure 5-15). Power Doppler (Figure 5-16) and M-mode analysis (Figure 5-17) may further document normal lung sliding. Estimating the size of a pneumothorax can be facilitated by rotating the transducer orientation parallel to the ribs and sliding the transducer laterally within successive rib interspaces (Figure 5-18). Detection of an image where partial sliding or a lung point is present marks the lateral aspect of a pneumothorax. For some patients, use of a high-frequency linear array transducer (when available) may enhance visualization of the pleura and detection of normal lung sliding.

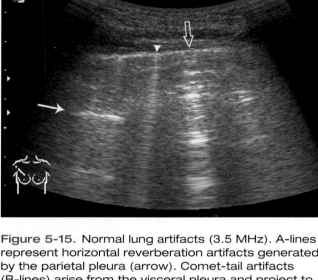

Figure 5-15. Normal lung artifacts (3.5 MHz). A-lines represent horizontal reverberation artifacts generated by the parietal pleura (arrow). Comet-tail artifacts (B-lines) arise from the visceral pleura and project to the depth of the image. They move back and forth along with the pleura with respirations and may vary between a narrow (arrowhead) or wider (open arrow) appearance.

► COMMON AND EMERGENT ABNORMALITIES

On ultrasound images, free fluid appears anechoic (black) or hypoechoic (if the blood is clotted) and, since it is not contained within a viscus, will have sharp edges as opposed to rounded edges.

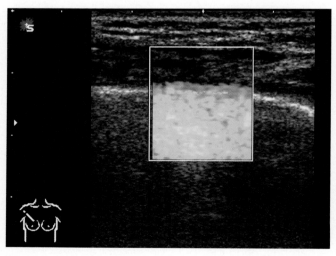

A

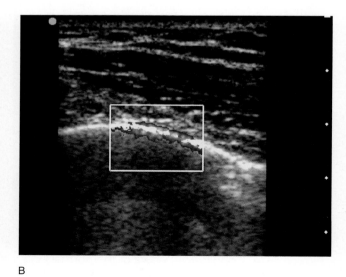

B

Figure 5-16. Power Doppler of normal lung (7.5–10 MHz). Power Doppler is very sensitive to movement. In (A) the color gain is set higher and both pleural and lung movement artifact are detected (entire color box is filled in below pleural line). In (B), the color gain is low so that only movement along the pleural interface is demonstrated. Avoid setting the gain too high, as general patient respiratory motion will be detected.

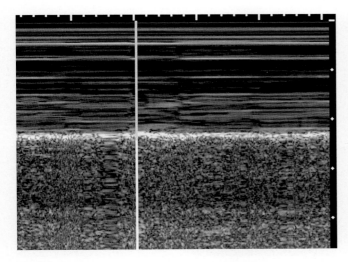

Figure 5-17. M-mode ultrasound of normal lung at 7.5–10 MHz ("seashore sign"). Granular artifacts below the bright pleural line represent normal pleural sliding and lung motion on M-mode.

HEMOPERICARDIUM

Free pericardial fluid is identified as an anechoic stripe surrounding the heart within the parietal and visceral layers of the bright hyperechoic pericardial sac (Figure 5-19).

FREE PLEURAL FLUID

The right or left diaphragm appears as a bright hyperechoic structure; free pleural fluid can be identified as an anechoic stripe superior to the diaphragm (Figure 5-20).

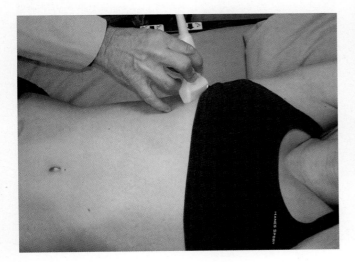

Figure 5-18. Extended lung examination. In a supine patient, the extent of a pneumothorax can be outlined by orienting the transducer parallel to the ribs and sliding it laterally along successive rib interspaces.

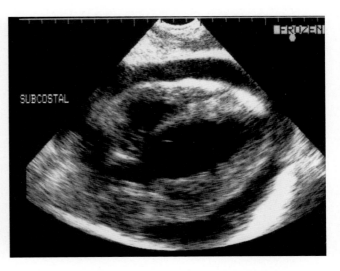

Figure 5-19. Hemopericardium. Pericardial fluid is identified as an anechoic stripe surrounding the heart between the parietal and visceral layers of the bright hyperechoic pericardial sac.

HEMOPERITONEUM

Morison's pouch is a common site for blood to accumulate when any solid intra-abdominal organ has been injured. Free fluid appears as an anechoic stripe in Morison's pouch (Figure 5-21) or within the right paracolic

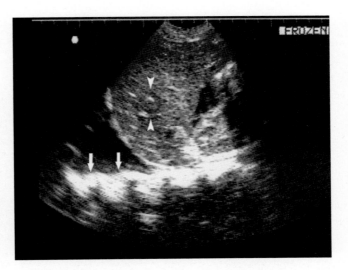

Figure 5-20. Free pleural fluid. The right diaphragm appears as a bright hyperechoic structure along the border of the liver. Free pleural fluid can be identified as an anechoic stripe superior to the diaphragm. The pleural fluid allows visualization of the posterior chest wall (arrows) that cannot be visualized when the air-filled lung is normally present. The patient also has a circular defect in the liver (arrowheads) from a bullet wound, and fluid in Morison's pouch.

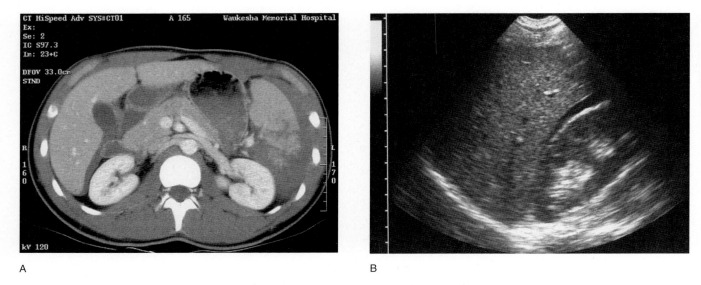

A   B

Figure 5-21. Hemoperitoneum. The abdominal contrast CT (A) demonstrates a fractured spleen with surrounding hematoma but a small stripe of fluid is also present above the right kidney in Morison's pouch. A right intercostal oblique ultrasound view from the same patient reveals a thin stripe of free fluid in Morison's pouch (B).

gutter (adjacent to the lower pole of the right kidney) (Figure 5-22A). For comparison, fluid contained within the retroperitoneal pararenal space appears as a hypoechoic stripe adjacent to the psoas muscle (Figure 5-22B).

In the perisplenic region, free fluid appearance and location are similar to the description for the perihepatic area (Figure 5-23). Free intraperitoneal fluid appears as an anechoic stripe in the subdiaphragmatic space, splenorenal recess, or the left paracolic gutter. Since

the splenorenal recess is not the most common site for free intraperitoneal fluid to accumulate in the left upper quadrant, it is essential to visualize the left diaphragm and left subphrenic space.

Free intraperitoneal fluid often accumulates in the pelvis because it is the most dependent area of the peritoneal cavity (Figure 5-24). Liquid blood or ascites floats above the bowels and will be located adjacent to the bladder and anterior peritoneum. Blood clots in the

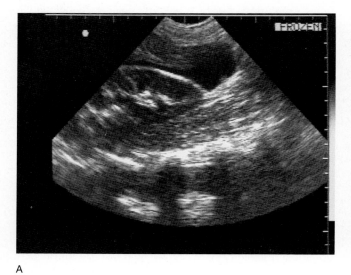

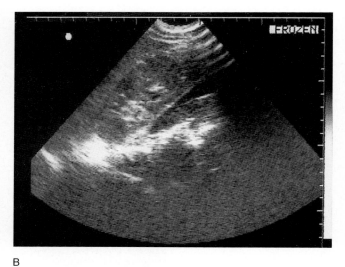

A   B

Figure 5-22. Free intraperitoneal fluid versus retroperitoneal fluid. Right coronal views. Image (A) demonstrates free peritoneal fluid in the paracolic gutter (adjacent to the lower pole of the right kidney). For comparison, image (B) shows contained retroperitoneal fluid (pararenal space) overlying the psoas muscle stripe and medial to the kidney.

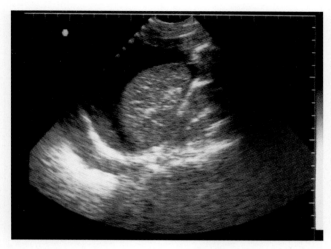
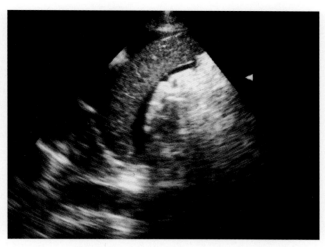

A   B

Figure 5-23. Left intercostal oblique views reveal the spleen surrounded by hypoechoic fluid in the subdiaphragmatic space (A). A small amount of clotted blood is also noted adjacent to the bright curvilinear diaphragm. Image (B) shows free intraperitoneal fluid as an anechoic stripe in the splenorenal recess. The tubular fluid-filled object at the bottom of the image is the aorta. (B: Courtesy of Lori Sens, Gulfcoast Ultrasound.)

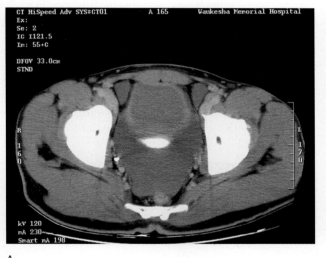

A

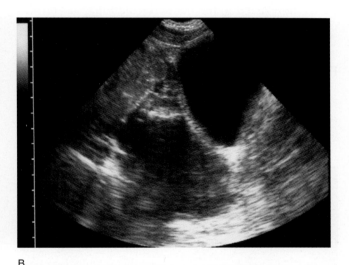

B

Figure 5-24. Pelvic hematoma. A pelvic CT shows dependent pelvic blood below the contrast-enhanced bladder (A). Longitudinal midline ultrasound view of the same patient demonstrates the partially clotted blood below the bladder (B) and a paramedian view reveals liquid density blood floating above the bowels and located adjacent to the bladder and anterior peritoneum (arrows) (C).

C

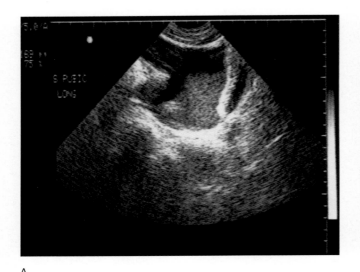

A

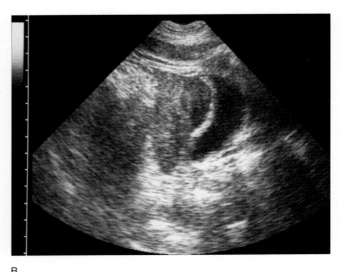

B

Figure 5-25. Longitudinal pelvic views demonstrate a collapsed bladder and dependent clotted blood in the rectovesical pouch with liquid blood above (A). Blood clots in the pelvis may distort the contour of the bladder. The uterus-like object in the center of the image in this male patient is actually a hematoma (B).

pelvis are located in the cul-de-sac and may distort the contour of the bladder (Figure 5-25).

PNEUMOTHORAX

Ultrasound diagnosis of a pneumothorax is based on the *absence* of the normal findings—sliding sign and comet-tail artifacts—along the pleural interface (see Figures 5-14 to 5-16). When these are absent, the specificity for the diagnosis may be further enhanced by document-ing the presence of an A-line (a reverberation artifact from the pleural interface that is found at twice the dis-tance from the skin to pleura) (Figure 5-26). In one study, lung sliding alone had 100% sensitivity, but only 78% specificity for diagnosing an occult pneumothorax. When an A-line was seen with absent lung sliding, there was 95% sensitivity and 94% specificity for diagnosing an

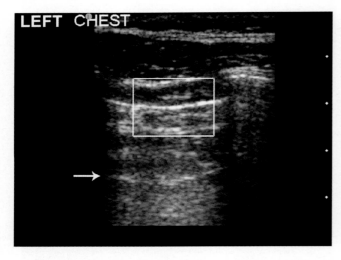

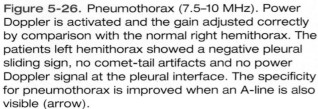

Figure 5-26. Pneumothorax (7.5–10 MHz). Power Doppler is activated and the gain adjusted correctly by comparison with the normal right hemithorax. The patients left hemithorax showed a negative pleural sliding sign, no comet-tail artifacts and no power Doppler signal at the pleural interface. The specificity for pneumothorax is improved when an A-line is also visible (arrow).

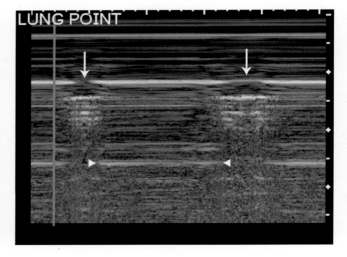

Figure 5-27. Lung point. The transducer is located on the chest at the edge of a pneumothorax. During the M-mode sweep the patient has taken two breaths allowing normal pleural movement to be documented briefly (arrows) as the "seashore sign." The remainder of the M-mode sweep shows the "stratosphere sign" of pneumothorax. Note: A-line (arrowheads).

occult pneumothorax.[60] The size of the pneumothorax may be estimated if the ultrasound examination reveals the lung point. This represents the lateral aspect of the pneumothorax in a supine patient and may be seen in real time as intermittent normal findings with respiration and documented with M-mode (Figure 5-27). The presence of a lung point had 100% specificity for an occult pneumothorax.[60]

▶ COMMON VARIANTS AND SELECTED ABNORMALITIES

When performing the FAST examination, it is essential to recognize common normal variants that may mimic positive findings. When examining the perihepatic views, fluid in the gallbladder, duodenum, hepatic flexure of the colon and other regions of the bowel, or inferior vena cava (IVC) may be erroneously identified as free intraperitoneal fluid. When examining the perisplenic views, fluid in the stomach or splenic flexure of the colon or blood within the vena cava or portal veins may be erroneously identified as free intraperitoneal fluid (Figure 5-28). When examining the pelvic views, fluid within a collapsed bladder or an ovarian cyst may be incorrectly identified as free intraperitoneal fluid. In the male patient, the seminal vesicles may be incorrectly identified as free intraperitoneal fluid. Also, premenopausal women occasionally may have a small baseline amount of free fluid in the pouch of Douglas.[85]

Occasionally, when performing the FAST examination, the clinician may directly detect injury in a solid organ, which is usually the spleen or liver. While this is not the specific goal of the FAST examination, it is helpful to understand some of the sonographic features of solid organ injury. When the patient is stable and serial follow-up examinations (control examinations) are being performed, the clinician has more time to evaluate for possible obvious solid organ injuries. Acute solid organ lacerations may appear as fragmented areas of increased or decreased echogenicity. Contained intraparenchymal or subcapsular hemorrhages may appear initially as isoechoic or slightly hyperechoic; this can make them difficult to reliably detect (Figure 5-29). The examiner must pay close attention to contour and organ tissue irregularities to observe these injuries (Figure 5-30). CT is more sensitive for acute organ injuries and should be ordered when these are suspected (Figure 5-21B). Contrast-enhanced ultrasonography may evolve as a useful alternative to CT diagnosis for solid organ injuries with the added advantages of reduced exposure to radiation and a lower cost (Figures 5-31 and 5-32). Over time, contained hemorrhage will become hypoechoic, with the area lacking sharp margins. A subcapsular hemorrhage may appear as a crescent-shaped hypoechoic stripe surrounding the organ (Figure 5-33).

Intraperitoneal fat is usually hyperechoic but in some cases is relatively hypoechoic. When the fat is present in the perinephric areas, it can be mistaken for intraperitoneal fluid or hematoma. Intraperitoneal fat (as opposed to hematoma) will be a consistent density throughout and will not move independently with respirations compared with the adjacent organ. Intraperitoneal hematoma contains gray level echoes but often will be accompanied by hypoechoic fluid areas as well. Clotted blood tends to move with respirations independent of surrounding structures.

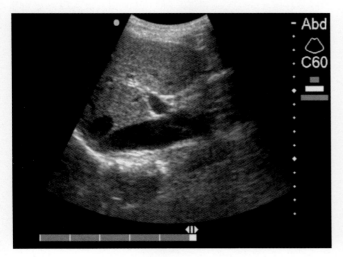

A

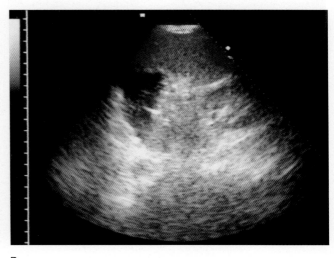

B

Figure 5-28. Fluid pitfalls. Oblique view of the liver shows fluid that is contained within the IVC (A). When examining the perisplenic views, fluid in the stomach (or bowel) may be erroneously identified as free intraperitoneal fluid (B).

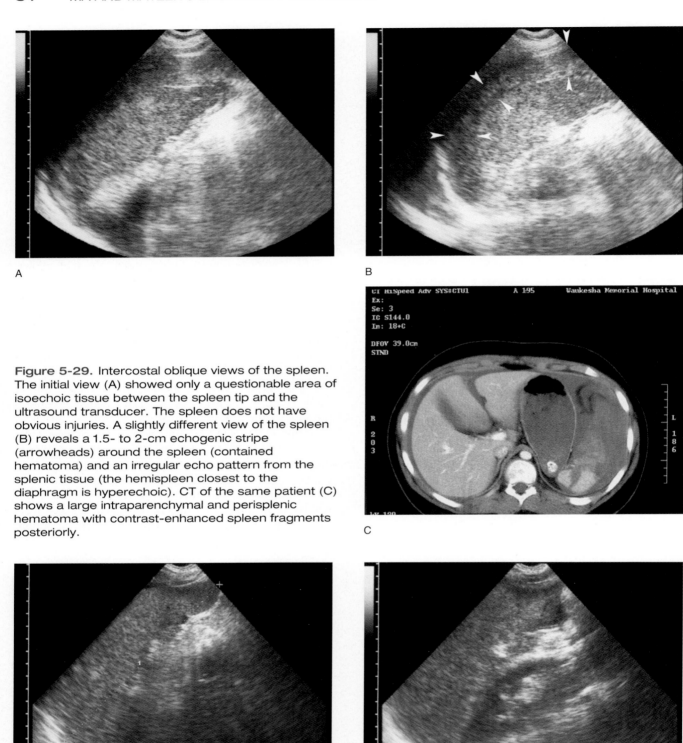

Figure 5-29. Intercostal oblique views of the spleen. The initial view (A) showed only a questionable area of isoechoic tissue between the spleen tip and the ultrasound transducer. The spleen does not have obvious injuries. A slightly different view of the spleen (B) reveals a 1.5- to 2-cm echogenic stripe (arrowheads) around the spleen (contained hematoma) and an irregular echo pattern from the splenic tissue (the hemispleen closest to the diaphragm is hyperechoic). CT of the same patient (C) shows a large intraparenchymal and perisplenic hematoma with contrast-enhanced spleen fragments posteriorly.

Figure 5-30. Initial oblique view of the spleen (A) showed enlargement (long axis is 17 cm) and a contour irregularity (narrow inferior tip). A slightly different view of the same patient revealed clots and liquid blood near the spleen tip (B). Compare these ultrasound findings with the CT findings from the same patient in Figure 5-21a. The splenic fractures were not apparent on the ultrasound views.

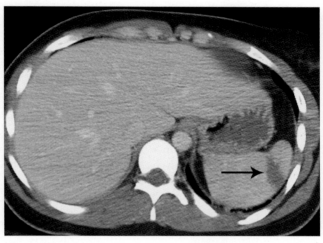

A

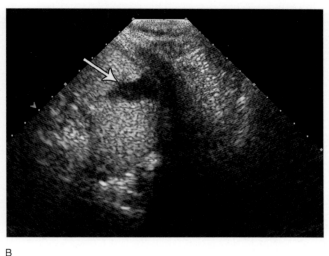

B

Figure 5-31. Contrast-enhanced ultrasound of splenic laceration in a 20-year-old woman. CT scan of the abdomen (A) shows a well-demarcated splenic laceration (arrow). Noncontrast-enhanced sonogram was interpreted as showing normal findings, whereas this axial contrast-enhanced sonogram (B) shows a well-demarcated hypoechoic splenic laceration (arrow), which correlated with the contrast-enhanced CT. (From McGahan JP et al. Appearance of Solid Organ Injury with Contrast-Enhanced Sonography in Blunt Abdominal Trauma: Preliminary Experience. *AJR* 187:658–666, 2006.)

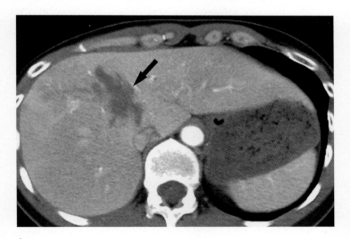

A

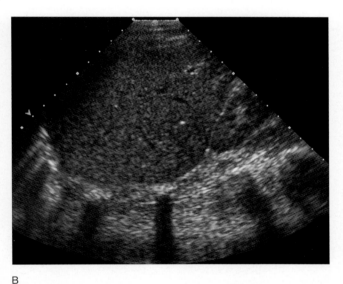

B

C

Figure 5-32. Liver laceration in 46-year-old woman. CT scan of liver (A) shows fairly well-demarcated region of decreased density within liver (arrow) corresponding to area of injury. Longitudinal noncontrast-enhanced sonogram (B) was interpreted as normal. Axial contrast-enhanced sonogram (C) shows central hypoechoic region (straight arrow). Hypoechoic region was surrounded by perfused hyperechoic region (curved arrow). (From McGahan JP et al. Appearance of Solid Organ Injury with Contrast-Enhanced Sonography in Blunt Abdominal Trauma: Preliminary Experience. *AJR* 187:658–666, 2006.)

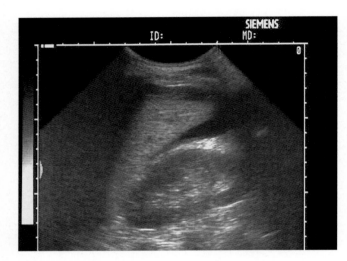

Figure 5-33. Subcapsular hemorrhage. This intercostal oblique view of the liver appears to have free fluid in Morison's pouch and a hypoechoic stripe between the transducer and the liver tissue. There was no other evidence for free fluid on ultrasound. The patient's CT revealed a contained subcapsular hematoma of the liver and no free fluid.

A pericardial fat pad can be hypoechoic or contain gray level echoes. The pericardial fat pad is almost always located anterior to the right ventricle and is not present posterior to the left ventricle (Figure 5-34). Pericardial fluid or hemorrhage will be located in both the anterior and posterior pericardial spaces. A small amount of fluid (<5 mm) may be present within the dependent pericardium, but is usually considered

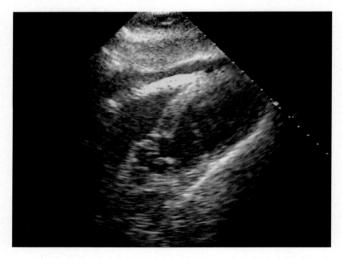

Figure 5-34. Subcostal long axis view of the heart and pericardium. A pericardial fat pad can be hypoechoic or contain gray level echoes. The pericardial fat pad is almost always located anterior to the right ventricle and is not present posterior to the left ventricle.

to be physiologic when it is visualized during systole only.

▶ PITFALLS

1. **Contraindication.** The only absolute contraindication to performing the FAST examination is when immediate surgical management is clearly indicated, in which case the FAST examination could delay patient transportation to the operating room.

2. **Overreliance on the FAST examination.** A clinical pitfall is the overreliance of an initial negative FAST examination in caring for the trauma patient. There is still no substitute for sound clinical judgment. Each FAST examination is a single data point in the overall clinical picture of the trauma patient. When mandated by the mechanism of injury or an evolving physical examination, serial FAST examinations or an abdominal CT scan should be performed on the patient. Serial FAST examinations are a common practice in Germany and are gaining acceptance in the United States.[86] They are used to determine if new intraperitoneal fluid has developed or if existing intraperitoneal fluid is expanding.

3. **Limitations of the FAST examination.** Limitations include difficulty in imaging patients who are morbidly obese or have massive subcutaneous emphysema. Also, in a patient at risk for ascites, it may be difficult to determine whether the free intraperitoneal fluid is ascites or blood. To help distinguish between the two, general ultrasound findings that point to ascites secondary to chronic liver disease include nodular cirrhosis of the liver, a contracted and hyperechoic liver, generalized thickening of the gallbladder wall, enlargement of the caudate lobe, enlargement of the spleen, or engorgement of the portal venous system (Figure 5-35). The clinician could also clarify the issue by performing an ultrasound-directed needle paracentesis of the fluid to distinguish ascites from hemoperitoneum. Another limitation is that ultrasound is not as reliable as CT in distinguishing and grading precise solid organ injury. Contrast-enhanced ultrasonography has been reported to improve identification of specific organ injuries on the FAST examination.

4. **Limitations associated with pregnancy.** There are limitations of the FAST examination in pregnant trauma patients that should be noted. Evaluating the pouch of Douglas for hemoperitoneum in the presence of a gravid uterus requires careful consideration. The distortion of

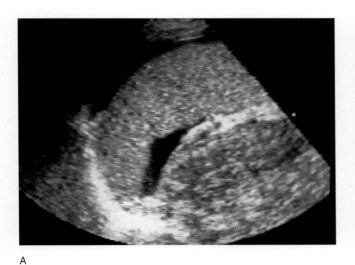

A

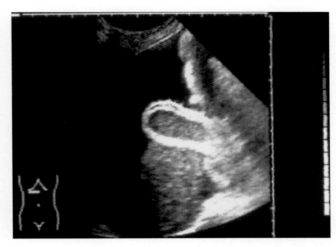

B

Figure 5-35. Cirrhosis of the liver. This oblique view of the right lobe demonstrates the findings of contracted size, increased echogenicity, and irregular texture of the liver (A). There is surrounding echo-free ascites. An oblique right upper quadrant view of the abdomen (B) shows a contracted liver, massive ascites, and generalized thickening of the gallbladder wall. This gallbladder finding is common with chronic liver disease and ascites. Long axis view of the spleen (C) measures more than 17 cm. (C: Courtesy of Lori Sens.)

C

usual landmarks and the difficulty with differentiating between intrauterine versus extrauterine fluid can make this a challenging examination for the inexperienced clinician. Also, the dependent portions of the peritoneal cavity may become further distorted with advanced third-trimester pregnancy, making the diagnosis of free intraperitoneal fluid versus intrauterine fluid more difficult.[81] As previously discussed, the FAST examination alone cannot exclude uterine rupture or placental abruption.

5. **Technical difficulties with the FAST examination.** (A) Most clinicians have little difficulty locating Morison's pouch but have greater difficulty locating the splenorenal recess and left pleural space. One common technical error is not placing the ultrasound transducer posterior or superior enough. The transducer often must be placed in the posterior axillary line at the 8–9th intercostal space to visualize these structures. (B) With some patients, visualizing the pericardium can be difficult. Placing the transducer as close to the xiphoid as possible and depressing the transducer toward the spine can facilitate the subcostal cardiac view. Even so, the patient may have to take a deep breath or the depth of the image adjusted to visualize the entire pericardium. If subcostal views are ineffective, then parasternal or apical views should be attempted (see Chapter 6, "Cardiac"). (C) Breathing or ventilation can interfere with the examination (from lung or rib artifact) or enhance the examination when it brings organs closer to the ultrasound transducer (diaphragm, heart, liver, spleen, or kidneys). (D) Fluid in a partially emptied bladder can be mistaken for free intraperitoneal fluid. This scenario can be clarified with complete catheter emptying of the bladder or by retrograde bladder filling and repeat examination.

6. **Injuries undetected by ultrasound.** Certain injuries may not be detected initially by the FAST examination. These include perforation of a viscus, bowel wall contusion, pancreatic trauma, or renal pedicle injury. Newer ultrasound imaging techniques such as power color Doppler or contrast-enhanced ultrasonography may be used to evaluate renal tissue perfusion in patients with suspected renal pedicle injury. The entire diaphragm also cannot be visualized using ultrasonography.

► CASE STUDIES

CASE 1

Patient Presentation

A 48-year-old man presented to the ED after he slid into a telephone pole when his motorcycle skidded on a patch of ice. He was wearing a helmet but lost consciousness at the scene of the crash. The patient complained of abdominal pain but denied any chest pain, shortness of breath, headache, or nausea and vomiting. He admitted to drinking "at least a dozen" beers earlier in the evening.

On physical examination, his blood pressure was 88/48 mm Hg, pulse rate 122 beats per minute, respirations 18 per minute, and temperature 37.0°C. He was arousable but drowsy and slurring his words. He had a strong odor of alcohol on his breath. His head, neck, pulmonary, and CV examinations were unremarkable. The abdominal examination was soft, diffusely tender, and without peritoneal signs. His extremities revealed diffuse deep abrasions but without bony injury. His neurologic examination was unremarkable except for his depressed mental status.

Management Course

After being infused 2 L of IV crystalloid fluid, the patient's blood pressure was 92/60 mm Hg and his pulse was 116 beats per minute. A supine chest radiograph was normal. Urinalysis revealed gross hematuria. His serum ethanol level was 342 mg/dL. A FAST examination of the abdomen performed by the emergency physician revealed a large quantity of free intraperitoneal fluid in Morison's pouch (Figure 5-36), in the right paracolic gutter, and in the pelvic cul-de-sac. The decision to perform an abdominal CT scan or DPL was deferred by the attending trauma surgeon. Instead, a head CT scan was performed in 10 minutes, which was negative for intracranial pathology. The patient was then taken directly to the operating room for an exploratory laparotomy, which revealed large liver and right kidney lacerations and 1.5 L of hemoperitoneum.

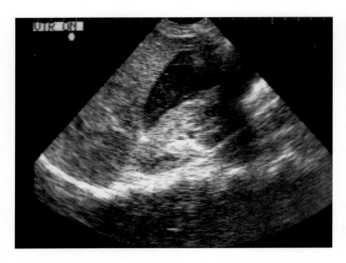

Figure 5-36. Case 1. A large quantity of free intraperitoneal fluid is present in Morison's pouch. The fluid is mildly echogenic because of the clotting of the blood.

Commentary

Case 1 was an example of a patient presenting to the ED hypotensive after sustaining blunt abdominal trauma. His profound alcohol intoxication and possible closed head injury complicated his examination and evaluation. Since the patient was too hemodynamically unstable to leave the trauma room, the FAST examination was an ideal diagnostic study to evaluate the patient. The FAST examination revealed gross free intraperitoneal fluid. The information provided by the FAST examination in this case negated the need for an abdominal CT scan or DPL. Instead, time was saved by the expeditious use of a head CT scan to evaluate for intracranial pathology followed by the direct transport of the patient to the operating suite.

CASE 2

Patient Presentation

An air medical crew responded to a scene call of a 43-year-old man who struck a pole while riding his motorcycle. The scene of the crash was 25 miles away from the nearest trauma center. His blood pressure was 92/60 mm Hg, heart rate 120 beats per minute, and respiratory rate 28 breaths per minute. The flight nurse found the patient's airway to be unstable and she intubated him at the scene. On initial survey, no obvious chest deformity or subcutaneous emphysema was noted, but the patient had diminished breath sounds in the left chest after intubation. The flight nurse withdrew the endotracheal tube 1 cm; breath sounds, however, remained diminished in the left chest.

Management Course

With a handheld ultrasound machine, an E-FAST examination by the flight nurse revealed an absence of lung sliding, no moving comet-tail artifacts, or power Doppler pleural movement in the left chest (Figure 5-26). The air medical crew made the decision to perform a left tube thoracostomy at the scene prior to air transport to the medical center. The patient was found to have multiple left-sided rib fractures and subcutaneous air of the chest wall upon arrival at the trauma center.

Commentary

Case 2 demonstrated the utility of the E-FAST examination in environments where more traditional medical imaging is not readily available. The sonographic findings of absent sliding and comet-tail artifacts after traumatic injury should be promptly addressed. When found on the left chest, the positioning of the endotracheal tube should be quickly verified. If the patient is unstable, particularly prior to air medical transport, chest tube insertion should be performed. The complications of chest tube insertion are not negligible, but are far outweighed by the consequences of an untreated tension pneumothorax during air medical transport.

CASE 3

Patient Presentation

An 18-year-old woman presented to the ED after sustaining a gunshot wound to her right flank. She complained only of abdominal pain. She denied any other complaints and reported no other injuries. The patient believed that she was about 4 months pregnant and had not received any prenatal care. She denied any significant past medical history.

On physical examination, her blood pressure was 128/78 mm Hg; pulse 94 beats per minute; respirations 18 per minute; and temperature 37.0 C. She was comfortable and appeared in no acute distress. Her pulmonary and cardiac examinations were normal. The abdominal examination was soft, nontender, and without peritoneal signs. A gravid uterus, 3 cm below the umbilicus, was noted. The rectal examination revealed normal sphincter tone and guaiac negative brown stool. A small entrance wound was noted in the right flank region, approximately 40 cm below the right scapula, and the exit wound was found on the right, lateral abdominal wall, at the level of the umbilicus.

Management Course

The patient remained hemodynamically stable in the ED. An upright chest radiograph was normal. Her urinalysis showed no RBCs. As arrangements were being made by the trauma surgeon to take the patient to the operat-

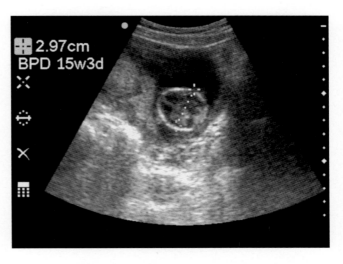

Figure 5-37. Case 3. Suprapubic longitudinal view of the uterus and a transverse view of the fetal head demonstrate a gestational age of 15.5 weeks by biparietal diameter.

ing room for an exploratory laparotomy, a FAST examination of the abdomen performed by the emergency physician revealed no evidence of hemoperitoneum, fetal heart tones present at 140 beats per minute, the fetus moving actively within the uterus, and a fetal gestational age of 15.5 weeks by biparietal diameter (Figure 5-37). The obstetrics consultant agreed with the emergency physician's clinical and ultrasonographic findings. Because of the patient's unremarkable abdominal examination and the normal FAST examination, the trauma surgeon opted to defer exploratory laparotomy in favor of admission and observation of the patient. After admission, a CT scan of the patient's abdomen confirmed the absence of intra-abdominal pathology. The patient was observed for 2 days and serial abdominal examinations remained unremarkable. She was discharged with the diagnosis of an extraperitoneal gunshot wound to the abdomen. The patient went on to deliver a healthy, 2655-gram baby girl.

Commentary

Case 3 was an example of penetrating trauma to the abdomen in a pregnant patient. Based on the mechanism of injury, the trauma surgeon initially believed that the patient needed exploratory laparotomy to investigate for possible intraperitoneal or retroperitoneal injury. The FAST examination demonstrated no evidence of intra-abdominal fluid and an active, viable fetus. Based on this information, the surgeon opted to obtain further imaging studies and observe the patient instead of performing exploratory laparotomy. The information provided by the FAST examination in this case negated the need for a nontherapeutic laparotomy and any associated morbidity to the mother or fetus.

REFERENCES

1. Tiling T, Bouillon B, Schmid A, et al.: Ultrasound in blunt abdomino-thoracic trauma. In: Border JR, Allgoewer M, Hansen ST, et al. eds. *Blunt Multiple Trauma: Comprehensive Pathophysiology and Care.* New York, NY: Marcel Dekker, 1990:415–433.
2. Halbfass HJ, Wimmer B, Hauenstein K, et al.: Ultrasonic diagnosis of blunt abdominal injuries. *Fortschr Med* 99:1681, 1981.
3. Aufschnaiter M, Kofler H: Sonographic acute diagnosis in polytrauma. *Aktuel Traumatol* 13:55, 1983.
4. Hoffman R, Pohlemann T, Wippermann B, et al.: Management of blunt abdominal trauma using sonography. *Unfallchirurg* 92:471, 1989.
5. Seifert M, Petereit U, Ortmann G: Sonographs of the diagnostic multi-system trauma patients. *Zentrlbl Chir* 114:1012, 1989.
6. Kohlberger VEJ, Strittmatter B, Waninger J: Ultrasound diagnostic technique after abdominal trauma. *Fortschr Med* 107:244, 1989.
7. Wening JV: Evaluation of ultrasound, lavage and computed tomography in blunt abdominal trauma. *Surg Endosc* 3:152, 1989.
8. Kimura A, Otsuka T: Emergency center ultrasonography in the evaluation of hemoperitoneum. A prospective study. *J Trauma* 31:20–23, 1991.
9. Rothlin MA, Naf R, Amgwerd M, et al.: Ultrasound in blunt abdominal and thoracic trauma. *J Trauma* 34:488–495, 1993.
10. Rozycki GS, Ochsner MG, Jaffin JH, et al.: Prospective evaluation of surgeons' use of ultrasound in the evaluation of the trauma patient. *J Trauma* 34:516–527, 1993.
11. Rozycki GS, Ochsner MG, Schmidt JA, et al.: A prospective study of surgeon-performed ultrasound as the primary adjunct modality for injured patient assessment. *J Trauma* 39:492–500, 1995.
12. Ma OJ, Mateer JR, Ogata M, Kefer MP, et al.: Prospective analysis of a rapid trauma ultrasound examination performed by emergency physicians. *J Trauma* 38:879–885, 1995.
13. Ma OJ, Kefer MP, Mateer JR, et al.: Evaluation of hemoperitoneum using a single- vs multiple-view ultra-sonographic examination. *Acad Emerg Med* 2:581–586, 1995.
14. Hoffman R, Nerlich M, Muggia-Sullam M, et al.: Blunt abdominal trauma in cases of multiple trauma evaluated by ultrasonography. A prospective analysis of 291 patients. *J Trauma* 32:452–458, 1992.
15. Tso P, Rodriquez A, Cooper C, et al.: Sonography in blunt abdominal trauma: A preliminary progress report. *J Trauma* 33:39–44, 1992.
16. Lentz KA, McKenney MG, Nunez DB, et al.: Evaluating blunt abdominal trauma: Role for ultrasonography. *J Ultrasound Med* 15:447–451, 1996.
17. McElveen TS, Collin GR: The role of ultrasonography in blunt abdominal trauma: A prospective study. *Am Surg* 63:184–188, 1997.
18. Rozycki GS, Ochsner MG, Feliciano DV, et al.: Early detection of hemoperitoneum by ultrasound examination of the right upper quadrant: A multicenter study. *J Trauma* 45:878–883, 1998.
19. Neri L, Storti E, Lichtenstein D: Toward an ultrasound curriculum for critical care medicine. *Crit Care Med* 35:S290–S304, 2007.
20. Matsushima K, Frankel HL: Beyond focused assessment with sonography for trauma: Ultrasound creep in the trauma resuscitation area and beyond. *Curr Opin Crit Care* 17:606–612, 2011.
21. Wherrett LJ, Boulanger BR, McLellan BA, et al. Hypotension after blunt abdominal trauma: The role of emergent abdominal sonography in surgical triage. *J Trauma* 41:815–820, 1996.
22. Khawaja OA, Shaikh KA, Al-Mallah MH: Meta-analysis of adverse cardiovascular events associated with echocardiographic contrast agents. *Am J Cardiol* 106:742–747, 2010.
23. Valentino M, Ansaloni L, Catena F, et al.: Contrast-enhanced ultrasonography in blunt abdominal trauma: Considerations after5 years of experience. *Radiol Med* 114:1080–1093, 2009.
24. Lv F, Tang J, Luo Y, et al.: Contrast-enhanced ultrasound imaging of active bleeding associated with hepatic and splenic trauma. *Radiol Med* 116:1076–1082, 2011.
25. Asensio JA, Arroyo H, Veloz W, et al.: Penetrating thoracoabdominal injuries: Ongoing dilemma—Which cavity and when? *World J Surg* 26:539–543, 2002.
26. Kirkpatrick AW, Simons RK, Brown DR, et al.: Digital handheld sonography utilised for the focussed assessment with sonography for trauma: A pilot study. *Ann Acad Med Singapore* 30:577–581, 2001.
27. Kirkpatrick AW, Sirois M, Laupland KB, et al.: The handheld FAST exam for blunt trauma. *Can J Surg* 48:453–460, 2005.
28. Brooks A, Davies B, Connolly J: Prospective evaluation of handheld ultrasound in the diagnosis of blunt abdominal trauma. *J R Army Med Corps* 148:19–21, 2002.
29. Jehle D, Guarina J, Karamanoukian H: Emergency department ultrasound in the evaluation of blunt abdominal trauma. *Am J Emerg Med* 11:342–346, 1993.
30. Hilty WE, Wolfe RE, Moore EE, et al.: Sensitivity and specificity of ultrasound in the detection of intraperitoneal fluid. *Ann Emerg Med* 22:921, 1993.
31. Branney SW, Wolfe RE, Moore EE, et al.: Quantitative sensitivity of ultrasound in detecting free intraperitoneal fluid. *J Trauma* 39:375–380, 1995.
32. Valentino M, Serra C, Zironi G, et al.: Blunt abdominal trauma: Emergency contrast-enhanced sonography for detection of solid organ injuries. *AJR* 186:1361–1367, 2006.
33. Catalano O, Lobianco R, Raso MM, et al.: Blunt hepatic trauma: Evaluation with contrast-enhanced sonography: Sonographic findings and clinical application. *J Ultrasound Med* 24:299–310, 2005.
34. Catalano O, Lobianco R, Sandomenico F, et al.: Splenic trauma: Evaluation with contrast-specific sonography and a second-generation contrast medium. *J Ultrasound Med* 22:467–477, 2003.
35. Blaivas M, Lyon M, Brannam L, et al.: Feasibility of FAST examination performance with ultrasound contrast. *J Emerg Med* 29:307–311, 2005.
36. Melniker LA, Leibner E, McKenney MG, et al.: Randomized control trial of point-of-care, limited ultrasonography for trauma in the emergency department. *Ann Emerg Med* 48:227–235, 2006.

37. Branney SW, Moore EE, Cantrill S, et al.: Ultrasound-based key clinical pathway reduces the use of hospital resources for the evaluation of blunt abdominal trauma. *J Trauma* 42:1086–1090, 1997.

38. Arrillaga A, Graham R, York JW, et al.: Increased efficiency and cost-effectiveness in the evaluation of the blunt abdominal trauma patient with the use of ultrasound. *Am Surg* 65:31–35, 1999.

39. Huang MS, Liu M, Wu JK, et al.: Ultrasonography for the evaluation of hemoperitoneum during resuscitation: A simple scoring system. *J Trauma* 36:173–177, 1994.

40. Porter RS, Nester BA, Dalsey WC, et al.: Use of ultrasound to determine the need for laparotomy in trauma patients. *Ann Emerg Med* 29:323–330, 1997.

41. Carrel R, Shaffer M, Franaszek J: Emergency diagnosis, resuscitation and treatment of acute penetrating cardiac trauma. *Ann Emerg Med* 11:504–517, 1982.

42. Plummer D, Brunette D, Asinger R, et al.: Emergency department echocardiography improves outcome in penetrating cardiac injury. *Ann Emerg Med* 21:709–712, 1992.

43. Rozycki GS, Feliciano DV, Ochsner MG, et al.: The role of ultrasound in patients with possible penetrating cardiac wounds: A prospective multicenter study. *J Trauma* 46(4):543–551, 1999.

44. Ma OJ, Mateer JR: Trauma ultrasound examination versus chest radiography in the detection of hemothorax. *Ann Emerg Med* 29:312–316, 1997.

45. Rubens MB: The pleura: Collapse and consolidation. In: Sutton D ed. *A Textbook of Radiology Imaging*, 4th ed. Edinburgh: Churchill Livingstone, 1987:393.

46. Juhl JH: Diseases of the pleura, mediastinum, and diaphragm. In: Juhl JH, Crummy AB, eds. *Essentials of Radiologic Imaging*. 6th ed. Philadelphia, PA: JB Lippincott Company, 1993:1026.

47. Dulchavsky SA, Schwarz KL, Kirkpatrick AW, et al.: Prospective evaluation of thoracic ultrasound in the detection of pneumothorax. *J Trauma* 50:201–205, 2001.

48. Kirkpatrick AW, Nicolaou S: The sonographic detection of pneumothoraces. In: Kharmy-Jones R, Nathens A, Stern E, eds. *Thoracic Trauma and Critical Care*. Boston, MA: Kluwer Academic Publishers, 2002:227–234.

49. Cunningham J, Kirkpatrick AW, Nicolaou S, et al.: Enhanced recognition of "lung sliding" with power color Doppler imaging in the diagnosis of pneumothorax. *J Trauma* 52:769–771, 2002.

50. Kirkpatrick AW, Nicolaou S, Rowan K, et al.: Thoracic sonography for pneumothorax: The clinical evaluation of an operational space medicine spin-off. *Acta Astronautica* 56:831–838, 2005.

51. Kirkpatrick AW, Sirois M, Laupland KB, et al.: Handheld thoracic sonography for detecting post-traumatic pneumothoraces. The extended focused assessment with sonography for trauma (EFAST). *J Trauma* 57:288–295, 2004.

52. Rowan KR, Kirkpatrick AW, Liu D, et al.: Traumatic pneumothorax detection with thoracic US: Correlation with chest radiography and CT—Initial experience. *Radiology* 225:210–214, 2002.

53. Lichtenstein DA: Pneumothorax and introduction to ultrasound signs in the lung. In: *General Ultrasound in the Critically Ill*. 1st ed. Berlin: Springer, 2002:105–115.

54. Merritt CRB: Physics of ultrasound. In Rumak CM, Wilson SR, Charboneau JW, eds. *Diagnostic Ultrasound*. 2nd ed. St. Louis, MO: Mosby, 1998:3–33.

55. Sistrom CL, Reiheld CT, Gay SB, et al.: Detection and estimation of the volume of pneumothorax using real-time sonography: Efficacy determined by receiver operating characteristic analysis. *AJR* 166:317–321, 1996.

56. Kirkpatrick AW, Ng AK, Dulchavsky SA, et al.: Sonographic diagnosis of a pneumothorax inapparent on plain chest radiography: Confirmation by computed tomography. *J Trauma* 50:750–752, 2001.

57. Ball CG, Kirkpatrick AW, Laupland KB, et al.: Incidence, risk factors, and outcomes for occult pneumothoraces in victims of major trauma. *J Trauma* 59:917–925, 2005.

58. Lencioni R, Pinto F, Armillotta N, et al.: Assessment of tumour vascularity in hepatocellular carcinoma: Comparison of power Doppler US and color Doppler US. *Radiology* 201:3583–358, 1996.

59. Rubin JM, Bude RO, Carson PL, et al.: Power Doppler US: A potentially useful alternative to mean-frequency based color Doppler US. *Radiology* 190:853–856, 1994.

60. Lichtenstein DA, Meziere G, Lascols N, et al.: Ultrasound diagnosis of occult pneumothorax. *Crit Care Med* 33:1231–1238, 2005.

61. Lichtenstein D, Meziere G, Biderman P, et al.: The comet-tail artifact: An ultrasound sign of alveolar-interstitial syndrome. *Am J Respir Crit Care Med* 156:1640–1646, 1997.

62. Lichtenstein D, Meziere G, Biderman P, et al.: The comet-tail artifact: An ultrasound sign ruling out pneumothorax. *Intensive Care Med* 25:383–388, 1999.

63. Lichtenstein D, Meziere G, Biderman P, et al.: The "lung point": An ultrasound sign specific to pneumothorax. *Intensive Care Med* 26:1434–1440, 2000.

64. Volpicelli G, Elbarbary M, Kirkpatrick AW, et al. International evidence-based recommendations for point-of-care lung ultrasound. *Intensive Care Med* 38:1-15, 2012.

65. Blaivas M, Lyon M, Duggal S: A prospective comparison of supine chest radiography and bedside ultrasound for the diagnosis of traumatic pneumothorax. *Acad Emerg Med* 12:844–849, 2005.

66. Rhea JT, vanSonnenberg E, McLoud TC: Basilar pneumothorax in the supine adult. *Radiology* 133:593–595, 1979.

67. Lams PM, Jolles H: The effect of lobar collapse on the distribution of free intrapleural air. *Radiology* 142:309–312, 1982.

68. Cooke DA, Cooke JC: The supine pneumothorax. *Ann R Coll Surg Engl* 6(9):130–134, 1987.

69. Tocino IM, Miller MH, Fairfax WR: Distribution of pneumothorax in the supine and semirecumbent critically ill adult. *AJR* 144:901–905, 1985.

70. Ball CG, Kirkpatrick AW, Laupland KB, et al.: Factors related to the failure of radiographic recognition of occult posttraumatic pneumothoraces. *Am J Surg* 189:541–546, 2005.

71. American College of Surgeons. *Advanced Trauma Life Support Course for Doctors*. Committee on Trauma. Instructors Course Manual. Chicago, IL, 1997.

72. Sargsyan AE, Hamilton DR, Nicolaou S, Kirkpatrick AW, et al.: Ultrasound evaluation of the magnitude of pneumothorax: A new concept. *Am Surg* 67:232–236, 2001.

73. Varner MW: Maternal Mortality in Iowa from 1952 to 1986. *Surg Gynecol Obstet* 168:555–562, 1989.

74. Lane PL: Traumatic fetal deaths. *J Emerg Med* 7:433–435, 1989.

75. Agran PF, Dunkle DE, Winn DG, et al.: Fetal death in motor vehicle accidents. *Ann Emerg Med* 16:1355–1358, 1987.

76. Pepperell RJ, Rubinstein E, MacIsaac LA: Motor-car accidents during pregnancy. *Med J Aust* 1:203–205, 1977.

77. Stafford PA, Biddinger PW, Zumwalt RE: Lethal intrauterine fetal trauma. *Am J Obstet Genecol* 159:459–459, 1988.

78. Crosby WM, Costiloe JP: Safety of lap-belt restraint for pregnant victims of automobile collisions. *N Engl J Med* 284:632–636, 1971.

79. Pearlman MD, Tintinalli JE, Lorenz RP: Blunt trauma during pregnancy. *N Engl J Med* 323:1609–1613, 1990.

80. Sherer DM, Schenker JG: Accidental injury during pregnancy. *Obstet Gynecol Surg* 44:330–338, 1989.

81. Drost TF, Rosemury AS, Sherman HF, et al.: Major trauma in pregnant women: Maternal/fetal outcome. *J Trauma* 30:574–578, 1990.

82. Ma OJ, Mateer JR, DeBehnke DJ: Use of ultrasonography for the evaluation of pregnant trauma patients. *J Trauma* 40:665–668, 1996.

83. Pearlman MD, Tintinalli JE, Lorenz RP: A prospective controlled study of outcome after trauma during pregnancy. *Am J Obstet Gynecol* 162:1502–1510, 1990.

84. Meyers MA: The spread and localization of acute intraperitoneal effusion. *Radiology* 94:547–554, 1970.

85. McKenney KL, Nunez DB, McKenney MG, et al.: Ultrasound for blunt abdominal trauma: Is it free fluid? *Emerg Radiol* 5:203–209, 1998.

86. Henderson SO, Sung J, Mandavia D: Serial abdominal ultrasound in the setting of trauma. *J Emerg Med* 18:79–81, 2000.

CHAPTER 6

Cardiac

Robert F. Reardon, Andrew Laudenbach, and Scott A. Joing

Echocardiography is the gold standard for the diagnosis of many cardiac abnormalities. Point-of-care echocardiography (or focused cardiac ultrasound), performed and interpreted by clinicians, was described 25 years ago.[1–3] Since then, there has been a significant amount of accumulated data to demonstrate that this practice changes management and improves patient care.[4–73] Clinician-performed echocardiography is now a well-accepted part of the practice of emergency medicine.[43,74,75] In addition, clinicians who manage critically ill or injured patients in other clinical settings are adopting the practice of focused cardiac ultrasound.[76–115]

Focused cardiac ultrasound is not meant to replace comprehensive echocardiography; it is a completely different paradigm in which a goal-directed examination is meant to answer specific clinical questions, not to detect all possible cardiac pathology. Some clinicians may use cardiac ultrasound to answer just one clinical question and others may use it for a wide variety of applications. Regardless, most focused cardiac ultrasound applications are relatively straightforward to learn because they rely on simple two-dimensional (2D) imaging and pattern recognition.[116]

► CLINICAL CONSIDERATIONS

Focused transthoracic echocardiography is an ideal diagnostic tool for detecting life-threatening cardiac conditions in the ED. Some of the information obtained from focused cardiac ultrasound could be obtained by invasive monitoring techniques, but it is not practical to use invasive techniques on all patients with potentially life-threatening conditions. In addition, placement of invasive monitoring devices is time consuming and is associated with complications.

Without bedside echocardiography, clinicians are left to manage critically ill patients with only indirect information about cardiac structure and function. "Classic" physical examination findings are often absent and unreliable for making critical diagnoses. Electrocardiograms (ECGs) are very helpful in patients with certain cardiac problems, but the majority of critically ill patients have nonspecific ECG findings. Chest radiographs provide very limited information about cardiac structure and function.

In cardiac arrest with pulseless electrical activity (PEA), it is critical to determine whether the patient has true electromechanical dissociation (EMD) with cardiac standstill or pseudo-EMD with mechanical cardiac contractions too weak to generate a palpable blood pressure.[117] Many patients with PEA have severe hypovolemia, while others have cardiac tamponade, massive pulmonary embolism (PE), or severe left ventricular dysfunction. All of these conditions can be detected with bedside transthoracic echocardiography. Echocardiography can be performed serially during a critical resuscitation as long as the examination itself does not interfere with resuscitative efforts.

Point-of-care cardiac ultrasound is also useful in stable patients with a wide variety of presentations. Pericardial effusions often cause nonspecific or minimal symptoms until tamponade develops. Focused echocardiography is the most efficient method to evaluate for a "silent" pericardial effusion since it is not reasonable to order a comprehensive echocardiographic examination on every patient with vague complaints who may have a pericardial effusion. Also, about 6% of all patients over 45 years of age have "silent" heart failure.[118,119] Many patients also have "silent" valvular disease and may benefit from focused echocardiography, even if the valves are not fully evaluated and the only information gained is the presence or absence of gross chamber enlargement. Transesophageal echocardiography (TEE) is used widely in the perioperative and intensive care settings and has the potential to be very useful in the hands of emergency physicians.[7]

▶ CLINICAL INDICATIONS

Any patient at risk of significant CV compromise is a candidate for a focused bedside echocardiographic examination. Patients with significant disease have widely varying presentations, from cardiac arrest to vague symptoms of dizziness, shortness of breath, or chest discomfort.[6,40] The challenge is to determine which echocardiographic findings can be readily recognized by noncardiologists with minimal training and which patients need comprehensive echocardiography.

Primary indications for focused cardiac ultrasound include:

- Cardiac arrest
- Pericardial effusion and tamponade
- Massive pulmonary embolism
- Left ventricular structure and function
- Volume status and fluid responsiveness
- Unexplained hypotension
- Guidance of emergency cardiac pacing

Other indications for focused cardiac ultrasound include:

- Valvular abnormalities
- Proximal aortic dissection
- Myocardial ischemia and infarction

CARDIAC ARREST

Bedside echocardiography is invaluable for directing management in cardiac arrest or near cardiac arrest states. Prior to the 1980s, all patients who had an organized electrical rhythm but no pulse were thought to have EMD. In the mid-1980s, using arterial catheters and echocardiography, physicians discovered that many patients with apparent EMD have mechanical contractions that are too weak to produce a blood pressure detectable by palpation.[1,2,10,117,120]

A 1988 study described two very different categories of EMD, those with "true" EMD and those with mechanical cardiac contractions. It observed that those with "true" EMD, or cardiac standstill, have a dismal prognosis, similar to the prognosis for asystole.[2] Several studies reported that more than half of patients with PEA have mechanical cardiac contractions.[10,13,63,121] In addition, multiple studies reported that patients initially thought to be in asystole may have cardiac contractions.[13,63,122]

Studies have confirmed that palpation of pulses is an unreliable means of assessing cardiac function and blood pressure. One study questioned whether carotid, femoral, or radial pulses correlated with certain blood pressure measurements.[123] They attempted to palpate pulses in 20 hypotensive patients who had arterial lines and invasive blood pressure measurement already established. They found that as systolic blood pressure declined the radial pulse always disappeared before the femoral pulse, which always disappeared before the carotid pulse. Surprisingly, the absence of pulses from a specific location did not correlate with an absolute blood pressure but was widely variable; for instance, several patients had palpable carotid pulses with a measured systolic blood pressure between 30 and 60 mm Hg. More worrisome was the finding that about 10% of these patients had no palpable carotid pulse with measured systolic blood pressures between 50 and 80 mm Hg.[123]

Since carotid pulses have been shown to be an unreliable means for determining true cardiac arrest, basic life support guidelines put forth by the American Heart Association have de-emphasized carotid pulse checks for both lay rescuers and health-care providers.[124] One study found that health-care providers are often inaccurate and unsure of themselves when doing carotid pulse checks during CPR.[121] Bedside echocardiography allows clinicians to directly visualize the heart and determine the presence and quality of mechanical cardiac function during a cardiac arrest. If a carotid pulse is absent but echocardiography shows reasonable mechanical cardiac function, then clinicians should proceed with aggressive resuscitation.

Several studies have examined whether bedside echocardiography in PEA can predict the outcome of cardiac arrest resuscitation. A 2001 study reported that 56% of patients presenting to two community hospitals with PEA had cardiac contractions on bedside echocardiography; 26% of those with contractions and 4% (one patient) with cardiac standstill survived to hospital admission.[63] A 2012 study reported that 24% of cardiac arrest patients had cardiac movement; 40% of those with contractions and 3% (one patient) with cardiac standstill survived to hospital admission.[125] In a multicenter trial from four academic medical centers, 32% of patients with PEA had mechanical contractions; 73% of those with mechanical contractions had return of spontaneous circulation and no patient with cardiac standstill had return of spontaneous circulation.[62] A 2010 study showed that 35% of those initially thought to have asystole and 58% of those with PEA had coordinated cardiac motion. They also reported that early echocardiography altered management in 78% of patients with cardiac arrest or shock.[13]

In current practice, many emergency physicians use echocardiography to confirm cardiac standstill before terminating resuscitation in all cardiac arrests. It may be reasonable to consider terminating resuscitative efforts in patients with PEA and cardiac standstill (true EMD). However, it is important to understand that some studies have shown that PEA with cardiac standstill is uniformly fatal, but others show a 3–8% survival to hospital admission after initial cardiac standstill.[8,13,62,63,125] This discrepancy is probably due to varying definitions of the term "cardiac standstill."

Beyond predicting the outcome of resuscitation, echocardiography is essential to rapidly identifying the cause of the cardiac arrest. Pulseless patients with non-shockable rhythms often have reversible conditions and can be treated successfully if those conditions are identified early.[117] The most common causes of PEA are listed in Table 6-1.[117] Hypovolemia, cardiac tamponade, massive PE, and massive myocardial infarction can be detected by bedside echocardiography so that early aggressive management of these abnormalities can be instituted.[13,38,125–128]

Cardiac ultrasound should be used in an advanced life support (ALS) conformed manner, so that ultrasound does not interrupt or delay standard ALS care.[13,14,129,130] This is accomplished by performing cardiac ultrasound only during scheduled pulse checks according to the ALS protocol.[14]

The first question to answer using bedside echocardiography is whether the etiology of the arrest is likely to be cardiac or noncardiac. Severe left ventricular dysfunction will be apparent. Some investigators have reported using a similar approach to determine whether hypotension had a cardiac or noncardiac etiology. The authors compared 2D echocardiography with hemodynamic measurements from pulmonary artery catheters and found that in 86% of cases echocardiography correctly determined whether the etiology of shock was cardiac or noncardiac.[131] In addition, studies have shown that emergency physicians can accurately estimate left ventricular function, especially when left ventricular dysfunction is severe.[44,52,58]

One prospective study used cardiac ultrasound in an ALS-conforming manner to identify patients with "pseudo-PEA" (cardiac contractions but no palpable pulses).[130] When cardiac contractions were noted, they extended the 10-second pulse check to 25 seconds and immediately administered 20 units of vasopressin, and then rechecked for pulses. Fifteen of 16 (94%) of these patients had return of spontaneous circulation and 8 patients (50%) had good neurologic outcome.

Patients in cardiac arrest with PEA as a result of severe hypovolemia will have a small, empty-appearing heart on bedside echocardiography.[126] Both the right and left ventricles will be poorly filled and the right ventricle will be almost completely collapsed. The left ventricle will usually be vigorous. The inferior vena cava (IVC) will have a small diameter and its lumen will disappear completely during inspiration (or expiration when positive pressure ventilation is being used). These findings on bedside echocardiography should prompt the clinician to aggressively replace volume and consider the etiology of hypovolemia.

One of the most straightforward applications of bedside echocardiography during cardiac arrest is evaluating for a pericardial effusion.[2,56,57] A pericardial effusion presents as an anechoic stripe surrounding the heart and should be obvious if it is large enough to cause cardiac tamponade. This finding should prompt the clinician to perform an immediate pericardiocentesis using ultrasound guidance (See Chapter 8, "Critical Care" and Chapter 22 "Additional Ultrasound-Guided Procedures,"). Pericardiocentesis can be life-saving and the removal of just a small amount of fluid may result in significant improvement in cardiac output.[1,2,41,127]

Massive PE is responsible for about 10% of cardiac arrests in cases where a primary cardiac etiology is clinically suspected.[132,133] The routine use of bedside echocardiography in cardiac arrest may allow immediate detection of massive PE, even in cases where the diagnosis is not clinically suspected.[26,32,38,39,134,135] It is important to immediately recognize that PE is the cause of a cardiac arrest because early thrombolytic therapy has been shown to significantly improve the chance of return of spontaneous circulation. A review of 60 cases of cardiac arrest caused by massive PE found that 81% of patients who received early thrombolytic therapy had

▶ **TABLE 6-1. MOST COMMON CAUSES OF PULSELESS ELECTRICAL ACTIVITY**

Hypovolemia
Hypoxia
Acidosis
Hypo/hyperkalemia
Hypoglycemia
Hypothermia
Drug overdose
Cardiac tamponade
Tension pneumothorax
Massive myocardial infarction
Massive pulmonary embolism

return of spontaneous circulation compared with 43% for those who did not receive the therapy.[132]

There is some evidence that TEE may be an attractive alternative to the transthoracic approach for patients in cardiac arrest. Image quality is better with transducer placement in the esophagus due to its proximity to the heart and lack of artifacts caused by interpositioned lung or bone tissue. It is not affected by body habitus or subcutaneous air. Perhaps the biggest advantage is the ability to minimize the interruption of chest compressions for transthoracic imaging. The TEE transducer may be left in place during the entire resuscitation and usually does not require changes in position, allowing the entire team to continuously view the heart. In addition, it is electrically isolated, so it can even be left in place during defibrillation.

A 2008 publication reviewed six cases where TEE offered distinct advantages over transthoracic echo, including detection of occult pathology in two patients who had aortic dissection and PE.[7] A 2009 study showed that TEE can be used to evaluate the effect of chest compressions and reported inadvertent compression of the aortic root or left ventricular outflow tract (LVOT) resulting in a 19–83% incidence of outflow obstruction during chest compressions.[136] TEE is generally considered a very safe imaging modality and the incidence of esophageal injury is extremely low (0.03%).[137] The additional equipment costs, learning curve, and maintenance issues associated with this technique may limit generalized use of TEE in point-of-care sonography.

PERICARDIAL EFFUSION AND TAMPONADE

In 1992, Plummer reported 100% sensitivity for recognizing pericardial effusion in the first 6 years after his group of emergency physicians began screening penetrating trauma patients with bedside echocardiography. More importantly, the use of bedside echocardiography significantly reduced the time to diagnosis and disposition to the operating room from 42 minutes to 15 minutes, while patient survival improved from 57% to 100%.[55] Bedside focused echocardiography is now the standard of care for patients with potential penetrating cardiac injuries (Figure 6-1).[108,138,139]

Patients with nontraumatic pericardial effusions are more difficult to identify because clinical signs and symptoms are inconsistent. Most patients with clinically significant pericardial effusions have nonspecific symptoms such as tachycardia, dyspnea, chest pain, cough, or fatigue.[140–144] Since cardiac tamponade can develop rapidly, even in those with chronic pericardial effusion, it is prudent to make the diagnosis as early as possible. Table 6-2 lists the disease processes that place patients at risk of pericardial effusion.[142,145] Effusions

associated with neoplastic disease or bacterial, fungal, or HIV infections have a higher risk of progressing to tamponade.[145] In addition, patients who have had recent catheter-based cardiac procedures, like coronary angiography or pacemaker/defibrillator placement, or cardiothoracic surgery, are at increased risk of a pericardial effusion that progresses to tamponade.[143,146]

Any patient with a pericardial effusion is at risk of developing cardiac tamponade, which is a life-threatening condition that occurs when a pericardial effusion causes significant compression of the heart leading to a decrease in cardiac output. When a pericardial effusion develops acutely, tamponade can occur with as little as 150 mL of fluid. Because the parietal pericardium can stretch over time, a chronic effusion can have a volume of >1000 mL without causing tamponade. The rate of pericardial fluid accumulation relative to pericardial stretch is the critical factor (Figure 6-2). The steep rise in the pericardial pressure–volume curve makes tamponade a "last-drop" phenomenon; the last few milliliters of fluid accumulation produce critical cardiac compression and the first milliliters of drainage produce the largest relative decompression.[142,145] Cardiac tamponade can present with nonspecific signs and symptoms and rapidly progress to hypotension, PEA, and death if not rapidly diagnosed and treated.[140–144,147] Echocardiography is the best imaging modality to evaluate for pericardial effusion or tamponade.[74,144,146,148] In addition, ultrasound-guided pericardiocentesis is the gold standard for percutaneous drainage of significant pericardial effusions (see Chapter 8, "Critical Care" and Chapter 22, "Additional Ultrasound-Guided Procedures").[144,146,148]

Pericardial effusions are often asymptomatic or associated with nonspecific symptoms. One study evaluated bedside echocardiography on 103 patients with unexplained dyspnea and found that 14 had pericardial effusions. Four had large effusions requiring pericardiocentesis and three had moderate-sized effusions that were treated conservatively. The authors recommended that ED patients with unexplained dyspnea should be evaluated for pericardial effusion.[6] Another study evaluated the accuracy of bedside echocardiography performed by emergency physicians to detect pericardial effusions. High-risk symptoms included unexplained hypotension or dyspnea, congestive heart failure, cancer, uremia, lupus, or pericarditis. They found 103 pericardial effusions in this high-risk population and determined that bedside echocardiography by emergency physicians was 97.5% accurate for making this diagnosis.[40]

Historically, the diagnosis of tamponade is a clinical diagnosis based on symptoms and physical exam findings.[142] However, symptoms and physical exam findings of cardiac tamponade are variable.[149] Pulsus paradoxus may be the most useful sign, but is not perfectly accurate for making the diagnosis. Pulsus paradoxus may be absent in patients with tamponade who

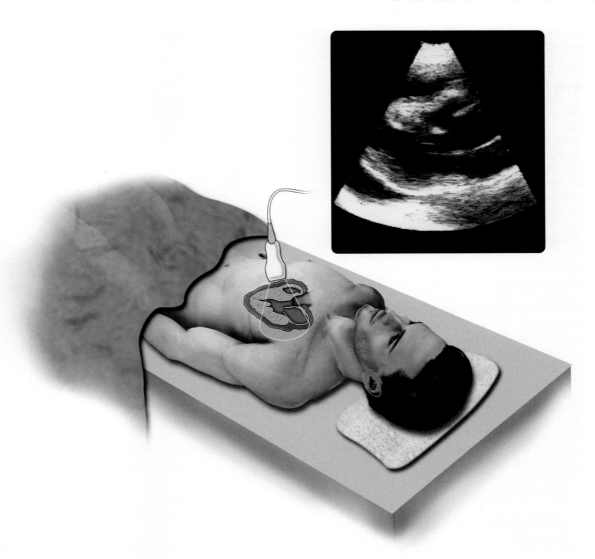

Figure 6-1. Pericardial effusion/tamponade. Ultrasound techniques and findings are outlined in the corresponding sections of this chapter.

also have left ventricular dysfunction and intubated patients who are receiving positive pressure ventilation.[150] Patients with loculated pericardial effusions may develop regional tamponade of the left ventricle. This tends to occur following cardiac surgery, does not result in pulsus paradoxus, and may be missed by point-of-care ultrasound if multiple cardiac views are not assessed.[23] In addition, pulsus paradoxus may be present in patients with emphysema in the absence of tamponade.[150] Therefore, physical exam findings of tamponade are often misleading and may be inadequate for making decisions regarding intervention. Both physical exam and echocardiographic signs need to be considered when making the diagnosis of tamponade (Table 6-3).

Most nonhemorrhagic pericardial effusions that cause tamponade are moderate to large (300–600 mL) in size.[142] Therefore, an indication for emergent pericardiocentesis is the finding of a moderate or large effusion in a patient with clinical signs of tamponade. Large pericardial effusions surround the entire heart while small effusions may collect first around the more dependent, mobile ventricles.[57] Effusions can be categorized by the maximal width of the anechoic pericardial stripe. A stripe <10 mm is small, 10–15 mm is moderate, and >15 mm is large.[6] These are gross measurements and do not correlate perfectly to the volume of the effusion. Also, hemorrhagic effusions can occur outside the setting of trauma and tend to accumulate rapidly and cause tamponade even when they are small.

► **TABLE 6-2. COMMON CAUSES OF CARDIAC TAMPONADE AND RISK FACTORS**

Common Causes of Cardiac Tamponade

Neoplasm: Involved in >50% of all tamponade cases
  Lung: Involved in >70% of neoplastic cases
  Breast
  Renal
  Lymphoma
  Leukemia
Viral infection
Human immunodeficiency virus (HIV):
  In young adults, particularly when the HIV is symptomatic
Coxsackievirus group B
Influenza
Echoviruses
Herpes
Bacterial infection
  Staphylococcus aureus
  Mycobacterium tuberculosis
  Staphylococcus pneumoniae: Rarely a cause
Fungal infection
  Histoplasma capsulatum
  Histoplasmosis
  Blastomycosis
Drug-induced
  Hydralazine
  Procainamide hydrochloride
  Isoniazine
  Minoxidil
Trauma: In 2% of all penetrating injuries of the thorax
Myocardial infarction. <7 Days after infarction—wall rupture, Dressler's syndrome
Connective-tissue disease
  Lupus
  Rheumatoid arthritis
  Dermatomyositis
Iatrogenic causes
  CV surgery: Postoperatively
  Central venous catheters
  Coronary intervention: Coronary dissection, perforation
  Pacemaker leads
  Pericardiocentesis
  Radiation therapy
Uremia
Idiopathic cause
Pneumopericardium
  Mechanical ventilation
  Gastric or esophageal fistula
Hypothyroidism

Common Risk Factors

  History of pericarditis
  Blunt or penetrating chest trauma
  Open-heart surgery or cardiac catheterization
  Known or suspected intrathoracic neoplasm
  Suspected dissecting aortic aneurysm
  Renal failure or dialysis

Reprinted with permission from Ariyarajah V, Spodick DH. Cardiac tamponade revisited: A postmortem look at a cautionary case. *Tex Heart Inst J* 34:347–351, 2007.

Rapid Pericardial Effusion

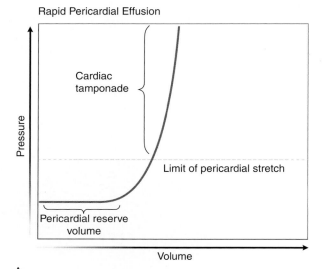

A

Slow Pericardial Effusion

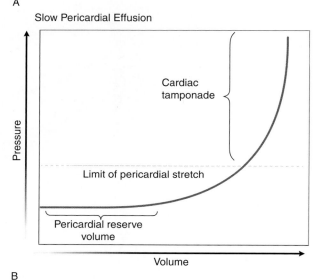

B

Figure 6-2. Physiology of cardiac tamponade. Pressure–volume curves in rapid and slow effusions in cardiac tamponade. (A) In cases of rapid accumulation of pericardial fluid, the cardiac reserve (the initial flat segment on the curve) is quickly exceeded and pressure thereafter rises with small increases in pericardial fluid. (B) When a pericardial effusion occurs gradually, the pericardium is able to adapt and stretch; with time, however, the limit of pericardial stretch is met and additional fluid accumulation results in increasing intrapericardial pressure. (Reprinted with permission from Ariyarajah V, Spodick DH. Cardiac tamponade revisited: A postmortem look at a cautionary case. *Tex Heart Inst J* 34:347–351, 2007.)

► **TABLE 6-3. ECHOCARDIOGRAPHIC SIGNS OF CARDIAC TAMPONADE[46,150]**

- Abnormal respiratory changes in ventricular dimensions
- Right atrial compression
- Right ventricular diastolic collapse
- Abnormal respiratory variation in tricuspid and mitral flow velocities
- Dilated IVC with lack of inspiratory collapse
- Left atrial compression
- Left ventricular diastolic compression
- Swinging heart

MASSIVE PULMONARY EMBOLISM

It is estimated that there are 300,000–600,000 cases of deep vein thrombosis (DVT) or PE each year in the United States.[151] In 25% of patients with DVT or PE there are no symptoms prior to cardiac arrest, and PE accounts for 60,000–100,000 deaths per year.[152] Patients who are hemodynamically stable at the time of PE diagnosis have a good prognosis, but those with a massive PE with hemodynamic compromise have a mortality rate of 25–50%.[153] Patients who present in extremis require rapid intervention since 70% of patients who die from PE do so within the first hour. Early thrombolytic therapy or embolectomy is required and rapid treatment often precludes obtaining time-consuming imaging studies.[154–161]

Bedside echocardiography can be used to rapidly confirm or refute the diagnosis of massive PE and shorten the time between patient presentation and treatment.[26,32,39,135] The echocardiographic findings in massive PE are not subtle and include massive right ventricular dilatation and right-sided heart failure with a small, vigorously contracting left ventricle (Figure 6-3).[38] In some cases, thrombus can actually be seen in the right atrium or ventricle. Point-of-care ultrasound can also help point to an alternative diagnoses in patients with symptoms that mimic PE, such as cardiac tamponade, pneumothorax, or left ventricular dysfunction.[74] It is important to understand that patients may have other underlying diseases that cause chronic right-sided heart strain, thus making the diagnosis of acute cor pulmonale in these patients difficult and unreliable.[162]

In patients with a high pretest probability of PE, ultrasound findings of overt right ventricular failure clinch the diagnosis and put the patient into a high-risk group that may benefit from thrombolytic therapy or surgical embolectomy.[163,164] Patients with massive PE often present with syncope, hypotension, cardiogenic shock, and cardiac arrest. The 2008 American College of Chest Physicians (ACCP) evidence-based clinical practice guidelines recommend fibrinolysis (Grade 1B evidence) for patients with acute PE and hemody-

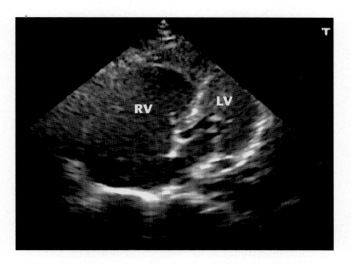

Figure 6-3. Massive pulmonary embolism. Apical view (centered over RV apex) shows severely decompensated right ventricle that is round in shape and much larger than the left ventricle. RV = right ventricle, LV = left ventricle. (Courtesy of Hennepin County Medical Center)

namic compromise.[165] They also warn that delaying fibrinolytic therapy may result in irreversible cardiogenic shock.[165] Investigators who performed a randomized trial of thrombolytic therapy for massive PE stopped their study early due to ethical concerns after enrolling only eight patients. Four patients who received streptokinase and heparin lived and did not have significant pulmonary hypertension on 2-year follow-up. All four patients treated with heparin alone died within 3 hours after arrival to the ED.[166]

The management of hemodynamically stable PE with echocardiographic findings of severe right ventricular failure (submassive PE) is controversial.[167] Although the ACCP guidelines recommend against thrombolytic therapy in patients with submassive PE, they note that thrombolytics are an option (Grade 2B evidence) for normotensive patients with an acute PE and right ventricular dysfunction who have a low risk of bleeding. The key point is that patients with echocardiographic findings of overt right heart failure have a massive clot burden and are at very high risk of death, regardless of whether they are hypotensive. A prospective study of 200 patients with submassive PE found that those treated with thrombolytic therapy had a much lower incidence of severe pulmonary hypertension 6 months after treatment.

There is good evidence that surgical embolectomy in patients with massive and submassive PE reduces mortality.[163,168–171] The drawback of surgical embolectomy is that it requires mobilization of significant resources and is not an option at most institutions. If surgical embolectomy is an option, point-of-care cardiac ultrasound is important for making a rapid diagnosis, so that resources can be quickly mobilized before the patient develops irreversible heart failure.

The use of bedside echocardiography to diagnose massive PE should not be confused with using echocardiography to evaluate stable patients suspected of having PE. There is a wealth of data demonstrating that echocardiography has poor accuracy when used to rule out PE in stable patients without severe symptoms or hemodynamic compromise.[172,173]

ASSESSMENT OF LEFT VENTRICULAR STRUCTURE AND FUNCTION

Echocardiography is the preferred first-line test for patients with symptoms or signs consistent with left ventricular dysfunction.[174] Patients who present with non-specific complaints may have unexpected left ventricular failure. More than half of patients with moderate-to-severe diastolic or systolic dysfunction have never been diagnosed with heart failure.[119] Patients with moderate-to-severe left ventricular dysfunction are at higher risk of complications regardless of their presentation.[119,175] In addition, when patients present with cardiogenic shock both short- and long-term mortality correlate with the degree of initial left ventricular systolic dysfunction and the degree of mitral regurgitation.[176]

Simple visual estimation of left ventricular ejection fraction is a reliable method of determining left ventricular systolic function.[177-179] Several studies have demonstrated that emergency physicians can use visual estimation to accurately assess left ventricular ejection fraction, even with as little as 3 hours of training.[44,52,73,90,101,180-182] It has been suggested that bedside echocardiography could be used to differentiate patients with primary pump failure from those with other potential causes of hypotension.[92]

One study showed that emergency physicians can reliably use qualitative visual estimates to assess left ventricular systolic function in hypotensive ED patients.[73] They compared their visual estimates of left ventricular ejection fraction to measurement of fractional shortening, which is known to be a reliable method for assessment of left ventricular systolic function, and found good agreement. They also showed that their fractional shortening measurements and their visual estimates of systolic function were reproducible on serial exams.

In addition to visual estimation, there are several techniques that can be used to obtain quantitative measurements of left ventricle function. E-point septal separation (EPSS) and fractional shortening are simple measurements that can be obtained quickly. Measurement of left ventricular volumes by the biplane method of discs or calculation of stroke volume and cardiac output by measuring Doppler flow through the LVOT are more complex techniques and require advanced training.

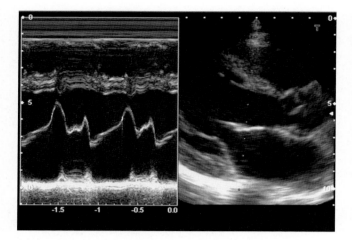

Figure 6-4. E-point septal separation (EPSS). EPSS is the distance between the anterior leaflet of the mitral valve and the septum during passive filling of the left ventricle. Decreased left ventricular function causes decreased valve opening and increased EPSS. EPSS is ≤6 mm if left ventricular function is normal. (See sections "Two-Dimensional Measurements," "M-Mode," Figure 6-33 for more details).

EPSS is a simple and rapid measurement that reliably estimates left ventricular function (Figure 6-4).[67,183-185] A 2011 study showed that emergency physicians with limited echocardiography experience could obtain measurements of EPSS in acutely dyspneic patients.[67] These measurements correlated closely with visual estimates of left ventricular ejection fraction by clinicians with extensive echocardiography experience. In general, EPSS >7 mm indicates left ventricular dysfunction, and EPSS >13 mm indicates severe dysfunction.[67,183,186,187] EPSS can reliably estimate left ventricular function in patients with aortic stenosis, but is usually misleading in patients with significant mitral stenosis or aortic regurgitation.[184]

Fractional shortening is a simple technique for assessing cardiac contractility based on one-dimensional (1D) measurements of the left ventricle during diastole and systole. Measurements of the left ventricular end-diastolic diameter (LVEDD) and end-systolic diameter (LVESD) with M-mode at the level of the papillary muscles are guided by 2D parasternal long- or short-axis images to calculate fractional shortening (FS) = (LVEDD-LVESD)LVEDD.[52,73,188] Measurement of FS by emergency physicians has been shown to be reproducible and accurate compared with cardiology overreads.[52,73]

Fractional shortening should not be confused with ejection fraction. A normal value for fractional shortening is >25%, whereas a normal left ventricular ejection fraction is >55%.[189] Also, fractional shortening <15% is consistent with severe left ventricular dysfunction and this correlates with a left ventricular ejection fraction of <30%.[189] Most modern ultrasound machines can calculate left ventricular ejection fraction when fractional shortening is measured. These calculations assume that the left ventricle has a "normal" shape and symmetrical function, so this method of determining left ventricular ejection fraction may be inaccurate in patients with regional wall motion abnormalities or oddly shaped ventricles. This method can also be inaccurate if the M-mode cursor is not exactly perpendicular to the septum and posterior wall.

The optimal method to measure left ventricular ejection fraction is using the method of discs (modified Simpson's rule).[189] This involves tracing the endocardial border during diastole and systole, so that the computer can calculate the change in left ventricular volume. It is most accurate if measurements are performed in two orthogonal planes (apical four-chamber and apical two-chamber views), which is known as the biplane method of discs.[189] Some modern ultrasound machines can calculate the left ventricular ejection fraction from one plane (usually the apical four-chamber view), which may be more practical in the point-of-care setting.

Calculation of left ventricular ejection fraction by the method of discs will be inaccurate if true apical views are not obtained and foreshortened (oblique) views of the left ventricle are measured. Also, it is often difficult to visualize the endocardial border, even if good images are obtained. Many echocardiography labs routinely use contrast agents to improve endocardial border detection. Contrast echocardiography significantly improves the accuracy and reproducibility of measuring left ventricular ejection fraction.[190,191] Contrast is especially useful in obese patients and those with lung disease.[192] This has not been well studied in the setting of clinician-performed focused cardiac ultrasound, but it has been found in ICU patients that the left ventricular ejection fraction was uninterpretable on 23% of exams using standard echocardiography, 13% using harmonic echocardiography, and 0% with contrast echocardiography (Figure 6-5).[191]

It is important to realize that fractional shortening and left ventricular ejection fraction are measurements of left ventricular dimension variation and not measurements of stroke volume and cardiac output. Patients with significant mitral regurgitation may have a hypercontractile left ventricle but a very low cardiac output, and patients with dilated cardiomyopathy may have a good stroke volume despite a low ejection fraction. When these clinical conditions are known or suspected it may be reasonable to correlate left ventricular ejection fraction with measurements of stroke volume. Stroke volume can be measured by obtaining two variables: (1) the area of the LVOT and (2) the velocity time integral (VTI) of the flow through the aortic valve during systole. Measuring stroke volume and cardiac output is not a routine part of point-of-care ultrasound, but it is not

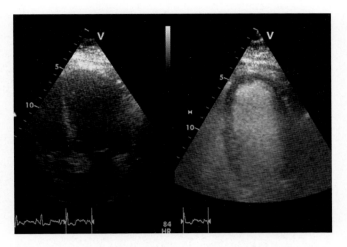

Figure 6-5. Contrast echocardiography. These images show apical views of the left ventricle before (left image) and after infusion (right image) of an IV contrast agent (Definity). The improved visualization of the endocardial border, left ventricle cavity, and myocardium is striking. Contrast echocardiography is especially important in critically ill patients, so that the greatest amount of information can be obtained when conditions (positioning, equipment, personnel) are suboptimal.

difficult for practitioners who have learned to obtain the standard echocardiographic views.

Although significant left ventricle systolic dysfunction (left ventricular ejection fraction <30%) is usually obvious in cases of cardiogenic shock and severe heart failure, it is important to understand that cardiac function includes more than just left ventricular contractility. Left ventricular ejection fraction may not be a good indicator of cardiac output in patients with aortic stenosis, mitral regurgitation, and concentric left ventricular hypertrophy (LVH).[193] Also, isolated left ventricular diastolic dysfunction is a significant cause of heart failure. Approximately 50% of patients with overt congestive heart failure have isolated left ventricular diastolic dysfunction, with normal left ventricular systolic function.[119,194,195]

Assessing for diastolic dysfunction usually requires Doppler measurements and was previously considered an advanced cardiac ultrasound skill. However, a 2010 study showed that emergency physicians with limited training could rapidly and accurately use pulsed Doppler to evaluate diastolic function in patients presenting with acute dyspnea.[48] The investigators performed simple Doppler measurements of transmitral velocity and noted whether a restrictive filling pattern was present or absent. They found that a restrictive filling pattern was more sensitive and specific than visual estimation of reduced left ventricular ejection fraction, the Boston criteria, or N-terminal prohormone brain natriuretic peptide for identification of left ventricular heart failure.

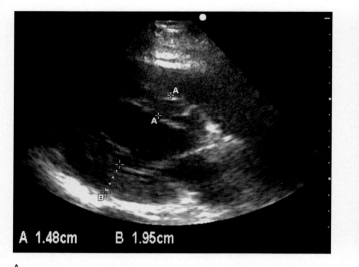

A 1.48cm   B 1.95cm

A

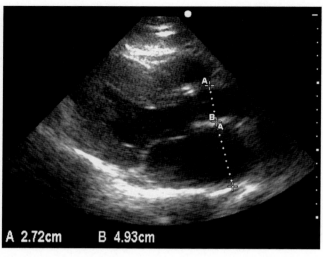

A 2.72cm   B 4.93cm

B

Figure 6-6. (A) Left ventricular hypertrophy, parasternal long-axis views. The septum (1.48 cm) and the posterior wall (1.95 cm) are >12 mm when measured during diastole. (B) Left atrial enlargement. Measurement of the aorta and left atrial dimension (Ao/LA=2.7/4.9) in a patient with left atrial enlargement (LA >4 cm).

A complete assessment of left ventricular diastolic function and filling pressures requires a combination of pulsed Doppler transmitral and tissue Doppler mitral annular measurements.[194,196–199] This is not difficult to learn and may be reasonable for emergency physicians with significant ultrasound experience.[45,200] Using pulsed Doppler to assess for simple indices, such as transmitral peak E velocity alone, may allow less experienced clinicians to assess for elevated filling pressures associated with diastolic heart failure.[201] Also, simple M-mode measurement of left atrial emptying fraction may be a practical technique for determining diastolic dysfunction.[202]

Left atrial enlargement (LAE) is an important marker of left-sided heart disease and a strong predictor of congestive heart failure, hospitalization, stroke, and mortality.[189,203–206] LAE is usually the result of elevated filling pressures caused by left ventricular diastolic dysfunction, but can also be caused by volume overload from valvular regurgitation and high output states like chronic anemia.[189,207–210] LAE may be obvious on multiple cardiac views and can be quickly confirmed by measuring the end-systolic atrial diameter in the parasternal long-axis view. If this measurement is >4 cm or significantly larger than the proximal aortic diameter, then LAE is likely (Figure 6-6).[183,189,211–219] A single-plane area can also be measured, but the optimal way to evaluate for LAE is measurement of left atrial volume using the biplane area-length method or the Simpson's method of discs.[189,220]

LVH is an important finding and there is a strong correlation between ultrasound measurements of left ventricular mass and subsequent coronary artery disease, sudden death, and other adverse clinical events.[221–224] The sensitivity of ECG for LVH is poor and does not detect the majority of cases.[221,225,226] Concentric LVH, an increase in wall thickness with normal chamber size, is usually the result of pressure overload from systemic hypertension. Eccentric hypertrophy, chamber enlargement with relatively normal wall thickness, is more common in patients with volume overload from regurgitant valvular lesions.[227] Left ventricular mass can be determined by more complicated methods or by simple measurements in the parasternal long-axis view plotted on a nomogram.[228,229] Normal left ventricular mass is variable depending on patient size and sex, but in general left ventricular internal chamber diameter >5.5–6.0 cm or wall thickness ≥ 12 mm, measured at the end of diastole, is suggestive of LVH (Figure 6-6).[189,212,214,218,219,229]

VOLUME STATUS AND FLUID RESPONSIVENESS

Fluid therapy is a critical part of shock management, especially in sepsis. Aggressive early fluid resuscitation is encouraged and appropriate in most cases.[230] However, not all patients benefit from aggressive fluid resuscitation and there is growing evidence that fluid overload may increase morbidity and mortality.[82,110,231–236] Therefore, it is best to give fluid in a goal-directed manner using some objective parameters to help guide therapy.[237,238] Point-of-care ultrasound is one of many tools that can be used to guide fluid therapy in shock because it allows a rapid noninvasive estimate of intravascular volume status and a prediction of fluid responsiveness.[76,79,93,113,238–241] In addition to guiding fluid management decisions in septic shock, ultrasound assessment of intravascular volume can be used in a variety of other clinical settings, such as hemodialysis, pediatric dehydration, trauma, and heart failure.[9,17,37,42,238,242–250]

Estimating central venous pressure (CVP) with point-of-care ultrasound is important because historically cardiac filling pressures [CVP and pulmonary capillary wedge pressure (PCWP)] were the clinical gold standard for determining volume status and guiding fluid resuscitation. The current guidelines for the Surviving Sepsis Campaign suggest fluid resuscitation based on CVP as well as central venous oxygen saturation.[251] The use of ultrasound to estimate CVP in the acute care setting, where invasive monitoring is not convenient or possible, has been one of the most important applications of point-of-care ultrasound.[3,57,58,73,74]

Despite the widespread use of CVP monitoring, there is significant data showing that cardiac filling pressures (CVP and PCWP) are relatively poor predictors of fluid responsiveness.[107,233,252–260] Fluid responsiveness is a relatively new concept that describes a positive hemodynamic response (increase in cardiac output) to fluid therapy.[76,79,93,233,237–239] The standard definition of fluid responsiveness is a >15% increase in cardiac output with a fluid bolus (500–1000 mL).[240] This concept is important because not all patients who are in shock benefit from aggressive fluid therapy and several studies demonstrate that fluid overload can lead to increased morbidity and mortality.[110,231,232,234–236,241] Fluid responsiveness can be predicted by measuring variations in IVC size or by assessing changes in cardiac output with the respiratory cycle or passive leg raising. Finally, an assessment of the left ventricular function and size can be used to estimate intravascular volume and the need for fluid therapy. Hyperdynamic cardiac function, small left ventricular end-diastolic area or left ventricular systolic collapse are reliable predictors of hypovolemia.[79,261]

Inferior Vena Cava Size and Degree of Collapse to Estimate CVP and Volume Status

The size and the magnitude of respiratory variations in the IVC correlate with CVP (Table 6-4).[58,64,266,262,267–269,263,270–277] In spontaneously breathing (nonintubated) patients with a normal CVP (<10 mm Hg), the IVC collapses significantly (≥50%) with passive inspiration. IVC diameter (during expiration) is generally large (>2 cm) in patients with elevated CVP (>15 mm Hg) and small (<1 cm) in patients who are hypovolemic.[47,85,248,262,263,276,278,279]

The utility of using IVC indices to estimate CVP in mechanically ventilated patients is controversial.[277] With mechanical ventilation, the IVC is typically less dynamic and does not exhibit significant variation with the respiratory cycle. However, a small IVC diameter (<10 mm) reliably predicts a low CVP.[64,85,246,248,249,279]

IVC diameter and degree of collapse correlate with volume status in the setting of hemorrhagic shock, heart failure, acute dehydration, and pre- and post-hemodialysis.[37,85,86,242,246,248,249] One study found that the IVC diameter was a better predictor of recurrent shock than blood pressure, heart rate, or arterial base excess.[246] Another study concluded that IVC diameter was a more accurate predictor of shock than the shock index and other commonly used noninvasive predictors of blood loss.

In the setting of hemodialysis, ultrasound assessment of the IVC has been used to help evaluate intravascular fluid volume and optimize dry weight.[245,247,250,280] One study found that IVCe ≤8 mm and collapsibility ≥90% was consistent with optimal dry weight and that IVCe ≥22 mm and collapsibility ≤10% were warnings of fluid overload. Another study found that lowering the dry weight so that interdialytic IVCe was <16 mm improved volume overload and cardiac function.

In the setting of acute dyspnea, IVC measurements can be used to help support the diagnosis of heart failure. In one study of ED patients presenting with acute dyspnea, IVC collapsibility of <33% had a sensitivity of 80% (but poor specificity) for the diagnosis of acute heart failure. IVC collapsibility of <15% and an IVC diameter to aorta diameter (IVC/aorta) ratio >1.2 were both highly specific for the diagnosis of acute heart failure (both 96% specific).[42]

IVC/aorta ratio is also used in pediatrics because it is thought to be a more valid measurement of IVC size that is independent of patient size in smaller patients.[17,36,243] The IVCe/aorta ratio may be useful for evaluating significant dehydration in children. One study

▶ TABLE 6-4. INFERIOR VENA CAVA (IVC) ESTIMATES OF RIGHT ATRIAL (RA) PRESSURE[189,262-265]

RA Pressure	IVC Size*	Change with Inspiration/Sniff	Hepatic Vein
0–5 mm Hg	<2.0 cm	≥50% collapse	Normal
6–10 mm Hg	>2.0 cm	≥50% collapse	Normal
10–15 mm Hg	>2.0 cm	<50% collapse	Normal
>15 mm Hg	>2.0 cm	No collapse	Dilated

IVC assessment may be misleading in patients with COPD or other causes of chronically elevated RA pressure.
*In children, normal IVC size is ≥aortic diameter, and an IVC/aorta ratio ≤0.8 correlates with low CVP.[17,243]

found that children requiring IV hydration had a mean IVC/aorta ratio of 0.75 compared with a mean of 1.01 for controls. The IVC/aorta ratio increased to a mean of 1.09 after hydration. An IVC/aorta ratio of ≤0.8 has been found to be a relatively good indicator of significant dehydration, with a sensitivity of 86%, but a specificity of only 56%.

All IVC studies are consistent on one point: measurements of size and collapsibility are more accurate at the extremes. A small collapsing IVC is a very reliable indicator of a low CVP, and a very large IVC with no inspiratory collapse is a reliable predictor of elevated CVP. Clinicians should realize that IVC indices are only one piece of evidence and should not be used in isolation, but in combination with calculations of pretest probability and other clinical factors. Also, there are little data on following serial IVC indices, but this is a very useful technique.[73] When a patient presents with hypotension, the initial treatment often involves a fluid challenge, and serial monitoring of the IVC can help clinicians evaluate changes in CVP related to fluid therapy. Serial monitoring may also help guide decisions about when to limit fluid therapy. In general, if the IVC remains flat and collapsible, more fluid can be given. When the IVC becomes large and noncollapsible, it may be wise to limit fluid or consider implementing other monitoring techniques.

There are certain clinical situations in which assessing IVC size and collapsibility may be confusing or misleading. In patients with right heart failure, the IVC may be large and poorly collapsible despite intravascular volume depletion. Therefore, it is worthwhile to reiterate that ultrasound measurement of IVC indices is not perfect and should not be used in isolation, but in combination with the clinical exam and ultrasound assessment of cardiac function.

IVC Distensibility to Predict Fluid Responsiveness in Mechanically Ventilated Patients

In mechanically ventilated patients, the changes in IVC diameter during the respiratory cycle are opposite of the changes during spontaneous breathing. The IVC does not collapse but distends during insufflation, as venous return decreases and the volume of extrathoracic venous blood increases.[82] Also, variations in IVC diameter are much smaller during mechanical ventilation than with spontaneous breathing. However, if the magnitude of distention is carefully measured using M-mode ultrasound, it can be used to accurately predict fluid responsiveness.

Using IVC measurements at different times throughout the respiratory cycle, one study calculated the distensibility index, which reflects the increase in IVC diameter with mechanical insufflation. Distensibility index

$(dIVC) = IVCmax - IVCmin/IVCmin \times 100\%$. The dIVC was measured before and after a 7 mL/kg volume expansion by a plasma expander. Cardiac index (CI) was also calculated from aortic Doppler measurements before and after volume expansion, and fluid responsiveness was defined as an increase in CI. The study found that dIVC >18% was an accurate predictor of fluid responsiveness (sensitivity 90%, specificity 90%) and baseline CVP was a poor predictor of fluid responsiveness. Another study calculated distensibility index as $dIVC = IVCmax - IVCmin / IVCmean$ and found that dIVC >12% was an accurate predictor of fluid responsiveness (positive predictive value 93%, negative predictive value 92%).[82]

Measuring IVC distensibility to predict fluid responsiveness has several limitations. It is only reliable with mechanically ventilated patients who are perfectly synchronized to the ventilator (or paralyzed). The patient must be receiving a tidal volume of at least 8–10 mL/kg with positive pressure ventilation. Also, the patient must be in sinus rhythm and cannot have significant right-sided heart failure.

Respiratory Variation in Stroke Volume, Aortic Flow Velocity, and Arterial Peak Velocity to Predict Fluid Responsiveness in Mechanically Ventilated Patients

Intermittent positive pressure ventilation induces cyclic changes in left ventricular stroke volume, resulting in maximum stroke volume during mechanical insufflation and minimum stroke volume during exhalation.[281] The magnitude of respiratory changes in stroke volume is an indicator of biventricular preload dependence and a strong predictor of fluid responsiveness.[233,238,239,281] Respiratory variation in aortic flow velocity and pulse pressure accurately reflects the magnitude of stroke volume variation, so measurement of these indices can also reliably predict fluid responsiveness.[233,254,256,282] Transthoracic ultrasound or TEE can be used to measure stroke volume variation and aortic flow velocity variation.[83,100,283–285] In addition, point-of-care ultrasound can be used to measure peripheral artery peak velocity variation.[286,287]

There are some important limitations to using respiratory variations in stroke volume and aortic flow velocity to predict fluid responsiveness. The patient must be mechanically ventilated and perfectly synchronized with the ventilator (or paralyzed). They must be receiving positive pressure ventilation with a tidal volume of at least 8–10 mL/kg.[288,289] Finally, analysis of respiratory changes in stroke volume is not possible in patients with cardiac arrhythmias, so patients must be in sinus rhythm.[281]

Changes in Stroke Volume with Passive Leg Raising for Prediction of Fluid Responsiveness in Spontaneously Breathing and Mechanically Ventilated Patients

Passive leg raising allows reliable prediction of fluid responsiveness regardless of ventilation mode or cardiac rhythm.[290-293] Passive straight leg raising essentially employs an endogenous fluid challenge by effectively increasing central blood volume and filling pressures.[291] Several studies show that echocardiographic measurement of stroke volume before and after passive straight leg raising enables reliable prediction of fluid responsiveness (Figure 6-7).[100,102,294-296] A meta-analysis by Cavallaro et al. found that patients who had an increase in stroke volume (or cardiac output) of ≥18% with passive leg raising were fluid responsive, with a sensitivity

of 89% and a sensitivity of 91%.[290] In addition, point-of-care ultrasound can be used to measure changes in peripheral artery peak velocity with passive straight leg raising.[297]

Assessment of the Left Ventricle to Estimate Volume Status and Predict Fluid Responsiveness

Hyperdynamic left ventricular function is often seen in hypotensive patients and is generally considered an indicator of hypovolemia. Bedside cardiac ultrasound with a subjective assessment of hyperdynamic cardiac function and left ventricular systolic collapse has been found to be a better indicator of hypovolemia than CVP.[261] The presence of a hyperdynamic left ventricle in patients with nontraumatic undifferentiated hypotension

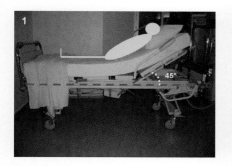
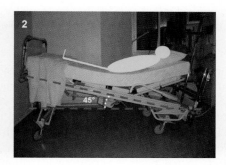
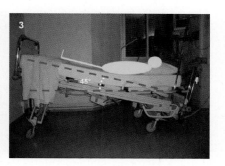

A

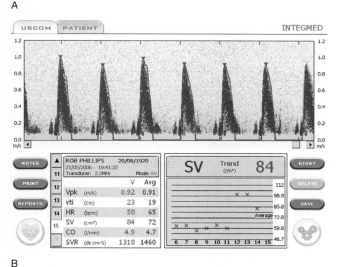

B

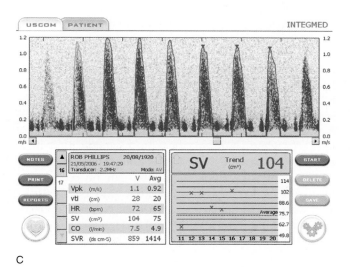

C

Figure 6-7. (A) The passive leg raising maneuver in three steps: Step 1, at baseline the patient is laying in a semirecumbent position, the trunk of the patient at 45° up to the horizontal; Step 2, the entire bed is pivoted to obtain a head down tilt at 45°; and Step 3, the head of the bed is adjusted to obtain a strictly horizontal trunk. Stroke volume is measured with an ultrasonic cardiac output monitor (USCOM, Sydney, Australia) before (B) and after (C) the passive leg raising maneuver and shows a 21% increase in stroke volume (from 84 to 104) after leg raising, which accurately predicts fluid responsiveness.[290,296] A standard ultrasound machine with a sector transducer and spectral Doppler can also be used to measure stroke volume (or aortic blood velocity) before and after passive leg raising. (A: Reproduced with permission from Levitov A, Mayo P, Slonim A. Critical care ultrasonography. New York, NY: McGraw-Hill, 2009. B,C: Reproduced with permission from Rob Phillips, Uscom, Ltd. http://www.uscom.com.au)

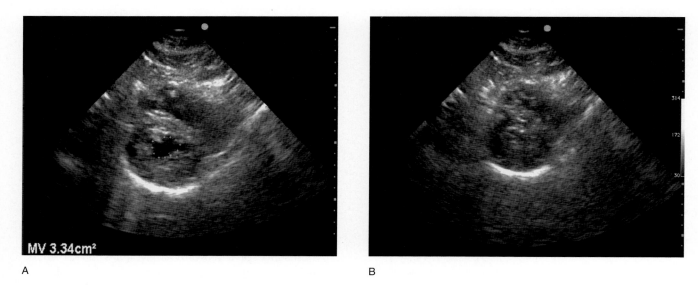

MV 3.34cm²

A   B

Figure 6-8. Severe hypovolemia, parasternal short-axis view. (A) Small LV cross-sectional area (<10 cm²) in diastole, and complete obliteration of the left ventricular chamber in systole (B).

has been demonstrated to be highly specific for sepsis as the etiology of shock.[33] A hyperdynamic left ventricle has been defined as "near or complete obliteration of the left ventricular cavity," meaning that the endocardial surfaces of the septum and posterior wall come in close contact with each other.[73] The presence of tachycardia is not a factor in making this assessment. Visual evaluation of hypercontractile left ventricular performance predicts volume responsiveness after cardiac arrest with 71–100% sensitivity.[87]

Left ventricular volume and end-diastolic area correlate with preload and can be assessed to help guide fluid therapy.[298] Left ventricular end-diastolic area is a reliable indicator of significant hypovolemia.[299–302] Subjective evaluation of left ventricular volume by assessing the size of the left ventricular cavity in the short- and long-axis views is often adequate to guide fluid therapy at the extremes of cardiac filling and function.[79] Also, significant volume depletion can be recognized by assessing left ventricular volume and end-diastolic area with a single measurement of left ventricular cross-sectional area. This is measured by tracing the endocardial border at end-diastole on a short-axis view at the level of the midpapillary muscles. A left ventricular cross-sectional area value of <10 cm² generally indicates hypovolemia (Figure 6-8A).[79,189] Also, a subjective but reliable indicator of hypovolemia is the "kissing papillary muscle sign," found to be 100% sensitive for detecting hypovolemia but only 30% specific for predicting volume responsiveness.[303] It is important to note that the finding of a large left ventricular area or volume should be interpreted with caution because it does not necessarily indicate adequate filling pressure (preload) in hypotensive patients with left ventricular dysfunction.

Complete systolic obliteration of the left ventricular cross-sectional area is an accurate predictor of severe hypovolemia (Figure 6-8B).[79] This is an important finding because it may be associated with dynamic left ventricular outflow obstruction. This can occur in elderly patients with concentric left ventricular hypertrophy, or in patients with apical myocardial infarction or Takotsubo cardiomyopathy. These patients are at risk for developing a dynamic outflow obstruction when they are exposed to dehydration, reduced afterload, and catecholamine stimulation.[104,304–309] This can be difficult to diagnose without cardiac ultrasound because filling pressures (CVP and PAP) may be elevated despite significant hypovolemia, and patients may quickly deteriorate if pressors are increased and fluid is withheld.

Quantitative Versus Qualitative Assessment of Hemodynamic and Volume Status

Although there are many measurements that can be obtained to determine volume status, filling status, and cardiac function, it is clear that clinicians can often use visual estimation to evaluate hemodynamic status. It has been found that measurements and subjective assessments were essentially equivalent when comparing serial qualitative and quantitative assessments of IVC collapsibility and left ventricular systolic function during early resuscitation in hypotensive ED patients.[73]

UNEXPLAINED HYPOTENSION

One of the most useful applications of point-of-care ultrasound is the assessment of patients with unexplained hypotension. Unexplained hypotension is a common presentation in the ED and other critical care settings. The etiology of shock is often difficult to determine due to lack of patient history, confusing symptoms, and unclear physical exam findings. These patients often need early aggressive therapy, even before the diagnosis is determined. The use of point-of-care ultrasound in these patients allows clinicians to quickly assess for conditions that may have similar clinical presentations but very different management strategies.[51] In this capacity, the ultrasound findings help clinicians narrow the differential diagnosis by identifying cardiac findings consistent with broad classifications of shock. In addition, other applications of point-of-care ultrasound (beyond the cardiac exam) can be used to further delineate the etiology of shock.[49,74]

Hypotension resulting from cardiac tamponade, massive PE, severe left ventricular dysfunction, or significant hypovolemia is usually readily apparent on bedside echocardiography.[5,38,44,49,52,56−58,61,92,127,246,248] Clinicians using focused cardiac ultrasound to differentiate shock states must realize that patients may have more than one abnormality or that they may have an acute illness superimposed on a chronic cardiac condition. As with all echocardiographic findings, clinical correlation is required, but gross cardiac abnormalities are clinically relevant in the setting of hypotension.

Ultrasound detection of a pericardial effusion that is large enough to cause hypotension is relatively straightforward.[55,108,139] Ultrasound's sensitivity for detecting a clinically important pericardial effusion is nearly 100%. When a pericardial effusion is detected in the setting of hypotension, the question is whether the effusion is causing cardiac tamponade.[46,149] The diagnosis of cardiac tamponade and the decision to perform pericardiocentesis are based on a combination of symptoms, physical exam findings, and ultrasound findings (see the section "Pericardial Effusion and Tamponade").

Bedside echocardiography is essential for rapidly making the diagnosis of massive PE.[26,32,39,135] Patients who are in shock due to PE, by definition, have a massive PE.[159,166,171,310−313] These patients have a very high mortality and clearly benefit from rapid diagnosis and aggressive medical or surgical therapy.[11,159,166,169,171,310−314] The echocardiographic findings are usually straightforward in cases of massive PE and include massive right ventricular dilatation and right-sided heart failure with a small, vigorously contracting left ventricle.[11,38,135,315] Underlying diseases, such as emphysema, cause chronic right-sided heart strain, making the diagnosis of acute cor pulmonale difficult and unreliable (see the section "Massive Pulmonary Embolism").[162] In unclear cases, further evaluation with CT may be necessary; however, when the diagnosis of massive PE is clear, aggressive management should not be delayed.[165]

Cardiogenic shock is common and occurs in 5–8% of patients hospitalized for ST elevation myocardial infarction. Most patients with cardiogenic shock present with moderate or severe left ventricular systolic dysfunction.[176,316,317] Isolated diastolic dysfunction can cause symptoms of heart failure, but most patients with cardiogenic shock have overt left ventricular systolic dysfunction that can be easily recognized by bedside echocardiography. Standard 2D point-of-care echocardiography can be used to quickly assess left ventricular systolic function (also see the section "Assessment of Left Ventricular Structure and Function"). Many studies have shown that simple visual estimation of left ventricular ejection fraction is a reliable method of determining left ventricular systolic function.[111,177−179] Furthermore, several studies have demonstrated that emergency physicians can use visual estimation to accurately assess left ventricular ejection fraction.[44,52,73,90,101,180−182]

The key to achieving a good outcome includes rapid diagnosis and prompt initiation of therapy to maintain blood pressure and cardiac output. Inotropes are used initially, followed by emergency cardiac catheterization and an intra-aortic balloon pump.[316,318] It is important to realize that left ventricular systolic dysfunction can also result from a variety of other etiologies like sepsis, metabolic disturbances, stress cardiomyopathy, or the endpoint of any shock state.[110,319−323] Early recognition and aggressive management of shock caused by left ventricular dysfunction are the key to improving mortality.[13,117,130,324] Patients with cardiogenic shock have a good prognosis if abnormalities are rapidly diagnosed and aggressively treated.

Some cardiogenic shock patients have a left ventricular outflow obstruction, which can be seen in hypertrophic cardiomyopathy, stress/takotsubo cardiomyopathy, or apical myocardial infarction with hyperkinesis of the remaining myocardium.[317] Acute treatment includes volume resuscitation and an intra-aortic balloon pump as needed. Inotropic agents will exacerbate obstruction and may cause rapid deterioration and death. Pure α−agonists may be used to increase afterload and reduce obstruction.[317]

Mechanical complications of myocardial infarction cause 12% of cases of cardiogenic shock.[317] These complications include rupture of the intraventricular septum, free wall, or papillary muscles. Bedside echocardiography can quickly identify most of these abnormalities.[56,325] The diagnosis of acute mitral regurgitation requires the use of color flow Doppler and more advanced skill. Acute mitral regurgitation can be caused by papillary muscle/chordae rupture, which is more common with inferior wall myocardial infarction, or left ventricular dilation with expansion of the mitral apparatus. Patients with suspected papillary/chordae rupture should have an urgent surgical consultation.

Hypovolemia is a common finding in hypotensive patients. Point-of-care ultrasound exam of the left ventricle and the IVC can be used to rapidly diagnose hypovolemia. Acute hemorrhage and sepsis are the most common causes of hypovolemia, and early aggressive fluid therapy is the initial management, regardless of the underlying etiology. While initial fluid resuscitation is ongoing, further ultrasound evaluation can help determine the etiology of hemorrhagic shock (see Chapter 5 "Trauma," Chapter 9 "Abdominal Aortic Aneurysm," and Chapter 8 "Critical Care"). In patients with septic shock, ongoing fluid requirements can be determined by serial measurements of fluid responsiveness (also see the section "Volume Status and Fluid Responsiveness").

Hyperdynamic left ventricular function is often seen in hypotensive patients and is generally considered an indicator of hypovolemia. Bedside cardiac ultrasound with a subjective assessment of hyperdynamic cardiac function and left ventricular systolic collapse has been found to be a better indicator of hypovolemia than CVP or IVC size or collapsibility.[76,79] In a study using bedside echocardiography to evaluate left ventricular function of ED patients with atraumatic, unexplained hypotension, it was demonstrated that the presence of a hyperdynamic left ventricle was highly specific for sepsis as the etiology of shock.[33]

Remember that the cardiac exam is only one part of a more comprehensive approach to using point-of-care ultrasound for shock.[1,2,49,53,55–57,61,74] (see Chapter 8, "Critical Care").

EMERGENCY CARDIAC PACING

Transcutaneous cardiac pacing is a common treatment for hemodynamically unstable bradycardias. Application and use of external pacing devices is straightforward, but assessment of mechanical ventricular capture during pacing can be confusing. If the pacing unit is used for electrocardiographic monitoring, then a pacing filter may allow correct assessment of electrical capture. Even with a filter, pacer spikes can drown out the native QRS complexes and give a false impression that there is electrical capture when there is none. An alternative means of assessing the capture is to feel the patients pulse and confirm that pulses correspond to pacer output. However, this can also be difficult especially if pacing causes significant skeletal muscle contractions.[24] The use of bedside echocardiography to assess pacemaker capture is straightforward.[4] One study showed that determination of mechanical cardiac capture by physicians at the bedside was both reliable and reproducible.[326]

Bedside echocardiography can also be used to help guide placement of a temporary transvenous pacing catheter. Emergency physicians have used ultrasound guidance to place pacing catheters into the apex of the right ventricle and confirm ventricular mechanical capture with excellent success.[4]

VALVULAR ABNORMALITIES

Only severe valvular abnormalities are of interest during a point-of-care cardiac ultrasound exam. Evaluation of the valves generally requires more advanced skill. This is a conundrum, because valvular abnormalities cannot be overlooked. Significant valvular abnormality may be the primary cause of acute hemodynamic compromise, and the ability to detect these abnormalities in a timely manner may be lifesaving. Fortunately, some valvular abnormalities can be detected with 2D inspection and a rudimentary color flow Doppler examination.

Mitral regurgitation, also known as mitral insufficiency, is a common disorder. Chronic mitral regurgitation can be caused by mitral valve prolapse, rheumatic disease, infective endocarditis, or congenital abnormalities. Acute mitral regurgitation is caused by rupture of chordae tendineae or papillary muscles as the result of a myocardial infarction or infective endocarditis.[327] Ischemic rupture is most likely to result from an inferior wall myocardial infarction with involvement of the right coronary artery. Acute mitral valve insufficiency causes dyspnea, pulmonary edema, and cardiogenic shock. Rupture of the entire papillary muscle usually results in acute severe mitral regurgitation and cardiogenic shock.[328] This process should be suspected in patients presenting with new onset severe pulmonary edema. Rapid diagnosis and emergency surgery are the key to survival for these patients.

Both leaflets of the mitral valve are usually clearly visualized on parasternal long-axis and apical four-chamber views. Normal valve leaflets should appear thin, produce uniform echoes, and be unrestricted in their motion. Thickened, immobile valve leaflets are often associated with regurgitation. Rupture of one of the mitral valve leaflets will usually result in a clearly visible flail leaflet if the entire papillary muscle is ruptured. Color flow Doppler is the key to detecting regurgitation and the easiest way to determine the severity of regurgitation. Mitral regurgitation is severe if the regurgitant jet area fills >40% of the left atrial area (Figure 6-9).[329]

Aortic regurgitation is an acute process in about 20% of cases and most commonly caused by infective endocarditis or proximal aortic dissection. In acute aortic valve incompetence, left ventricular failure develops rapidly and mortality from pulmonary edema and cardiac arrest is high, even with intensive medical therapy. The key to survival for these patients is rapid recognition of their condition and emergency surgery. Characteristic physical findings, including a murmur, are unreliable in the most severe cases. Cardiac ultrasound is indispensable in identifying the presence and severity of valvular

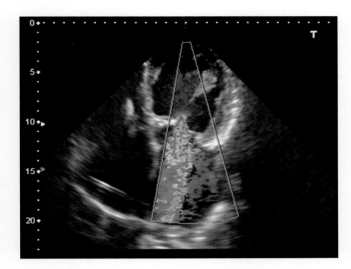

Figure 6-9. Color flow Doppler demonstrating severe mitral regurgitation. Apical view of the left ventricle and left atrium shows a turbulent jet filling the entire left atrial chamber.

regurgitation.[330] Patients with chronic aortic regurgitation are more likely to have obvious abnormalities, such as thickened and immobile leaflets or left ventricular enlargement. Those with acute regurgitation may have a normal-sized left ventricle and thin valve leaflets on 2D imaging. The aortic valve is usually well visualized on the parasternal long-axis view. Normal valve leaflets should appear thin, produce uniform echoes, and be unrestricted in their motion. During diastole the cusps coapt in the center of the aortic root and during systole they snap open and lie parallel to the aortic wall. Screening for aortic regurgitation requires utilization of color flow Doppler. Subjective visualization of a large regurgitant jet may be enough evidence to prompt further investigation. Measurement of the maximal proximal jet width and its ratio to the LVOT diameter is the best screening test for significant aortic regurgitation. A ratio of ≥65% is diagnostic of severe aortic regurgitation.[329]

Aortic stenosis can cause angina, syncope, and eventually heart failure. Sudden death from dysrhythmias occurs in 25% of such patients. Patients who present with congestive heart failure should be treated with oxygen and diuretics, but nitrates are not well tolerated in patients with severe aortic stenosis as decreasing preload may result in significant hypotension.[331] Aortic stenosis is most commonly caused by calcific changes to a congenital bicuspid valve, calcific stenosis of a trileaflet valve, or rheumatic valve disease. In the United States, roughly 50% of aortic stenosis cases are caused by bicuspid aortic valves and the other 50% by calcific stenosis. Rheumatic aortic stenosis is uncommon in the developed world, but common elsewhere. Rheumatic disease almost always affects the mitral valve first, so patients with rheumatic aortic stenosis will likely also have mitral stenosis.

Evidence of aortic stenosis may be apparent from gross inspection of valvular calcification and movements by 2D imaging. Gross inspection of the aortic valve is best done in the parasternal long- and short-axis views. Normal valve leaflets should appear thin, produce uniform echoes, and be unrestricted in their motion. During diastole the cusps coapt in the center of the aortic root and during systole they snap open and lie parallel to the aortic wall. Most patients with aortic stenosis have significant calcifications and thickening of the aortic valve leaflets, restricted mobility, and reduced leaflet separation, which may be easy to identify with 2D imaging. The finding of thickened leaflets alone is not diagnostic of aortic stenosis because 25% of adults over 65 years of age have aortic sclerosis (irregular valve thickening without left ventricular outflow obstruction). Measuring aortic stenosis severity requires continuous wave (CW) Doppler measurements. The simplest measurement of aortic stenosis severity is maximum jet velocity. Maximum jet velocity increases as stenosis severity increases; a velocity of >4 m/s is diagnostic of severe aortic stenosis.[332] Other measurements, such as mean transaortic gradient and calculation of valve area using the continuity equation, can also be employed. In addition, severe aortic stenosis usually causes concentric LVH and diffuse left ventricular wall thickening without chamber enlargement.

Significant mitral stenosis is nearly always caused by rheumatic disease.[333] This is uncommon in the United States, but developing countries have a high prevalence of rheumatic heart disease. Since the mitral valve is straightforward to visualize in the parasternal and apical views, significant mitral stenosis is usually obvious. Gross inspection of mitral valve opening can usually be seen best in the parasternal long-axis view. The valve opens widely with passive left ventricular filling and again with atrial contraction during diastole. This may be difficult to appreciate when the heart rate is very high, so it is important to slow or freeze images. The mitral valve may not open widely when the left ventricular function is extremely compromised. This is due to poor flow rather than stenosis. The severity of mitral stenosis can be determined by measuring the mitral valve area (MVA) by direct planimetry in the parasternal short-axis view. Normal MVA is 4–6 cm^2 and significant or symptomatic mitral stenosis occurs when MVA is <1.5 cm^2.[332]

Right-sided valvular abnormalities are less likely to cause acute decompensation and are less likely to be isolated problems. Most adults have some mild tricuspid regurgitation, which allows measurement of pressure gradients and estimation of right ventricle pressure during routine echocardiographic exams. Significant tricuspid regurgitation is usually due to right ventricular and tricuspid annular dilation due to pulmonary hypertension or right ventricular dysfunction. It may also be caused by endocarditis, carcinoid heart disease, rheumatic disease, or Ebstein's anomaly.[329] Tricuspid stenosis is uncommon and often associated with mitral stenosis when caused by rheumatic disease. It may also be caused by carcinoid syndrome (accompanied by significant tricuspid regurgitation), endocarditis, pacemaker-induced adhesions, or lupus. Tricuspid stenosis can be diagnosed by looking for valve thickening, restricted mobility with diastolic doming, reduced leaflet separation, and right atrial enlargement.[332]

The pulmonary valve is the most difficult to visualize by ultrasound, so it is more practical to look for accompanying abnormalities such as right ventricular enlargement and hypertrophy. Pulmonary stenosis is almost always congenital, so it is unlikely to be a new or isolated problem. Pulmonary regurgitation is most often seen in patients with pulmonary hypertension, which is often associated with dilation of the pulmonary artery, right ventricle, right atrium, and hepatic veins.[329]

AORTIC DISSECTION

Aortic dissection occurs when the intima is violated, allowing blood to enter the media and dissect between the intimal and adventitial layers. Common sites for tear include the ascending aorta and the region of the ligamentum arteriosum. The Stanford classification categorizes aortic dissection as type A, which involves the ascending aorta, and type B, which involves only the descending aorta.

Aortic dissection and intramural hematoma may be detected by transthoracic echocardiography on parasternal long-axis and suprasternal views. A linear echogenic flap, indicative of aortic dissection, may be seen across the aortic lumen anywhere along its length. In the parasternal long-axis view, the aortic root (proximal ascending aorta) is usually well visualized, but only a small section of the descending aorta is visualized (in cross section) posterior to the heart. The aortic arch can be visualized using the suprasternal view in most patients, but image quality depends on body habitus and operator experience.[334-337] A dissection that extends below the diaphragm may be detected with abdominal sonography. Transthoracic ultrasound is very useful if an abnormality is seen, but not sensitive for detecting thoracic aortic dissection, so it should not be used to rule out this diagnosis.

TEE provides much better resolution and visualization of aortic dissection than transthoracic echocardiography and can be used to rule out this diagnosis. Spiral CT, TEE, and magnetic resonance imaging (MRI) have been demonstrated to have comparable sensitivity, and

specificity, with accuracy rates approaching 100%.[334-337] One study found that all three modalities approach 100% sensitivity; the specificities for spiral CT, TEE, and MRI were 100%, 94%, and 94%, respectively.[338]

Important issues to address with aortic dissection include (1) presence of pericardial effusion as a sign of imminent mortality without surgical intervention, (2) presence of ascending aorta involvement without pericardial involvement, (3) evidence of isolated descending aorta involvement, (4) location of the entry site, and (5) evidence of involvement of major branch vessels.[334-337]

MYOCARDIAL ISCHEMIA AND INFARCTION

The diagnosis of acute myocardial ischemia can sometimes be made by echocardiographic findings of wall motion abnormalities. Myocardial function is immediately affected by ischemia and may precede ECG changes. Studies have demonstrated that the recognition of regional wall motion abnormalities by echocardiography in patients with acute chest pain is a sensitive predictor for Q-wave myocardial infarction. In experienced hands, the sensitivity for detecting a regional wall motion abnormality in acute myocardial infarction is high, but it may be hard to differentiate between new and old wall motion abnormalities without reviewing prior echocardiograms.[339,340] The myocardium is usually thinner at the site of an old wall motion abnormality, but this finding may be subtle, especially when the endocardium is difficult to visualize. Inability to obtain high-quality images and clearly visualize the endocardial border significantly decreases the accuracy of ultrasound for detecting wall motion abnormalities.

Clinicians using bedside echocardiography to identify wall motion abnormalities should be aware that left bundle branch block and a history of cardiac surgery can result in abnormal septal wall motion.[341-343] Patients with a left bundle branch block have a characteristic systolic rotating or twisting appearance in the parasternal short-axis view. In addition, patients with right ventricle cardiac pacing often have chronic regional wall motion changes that may be confused with acute abnormalities.[344,345]

Resting echocardiography in patients with acute chest pain is not sufficiently sensitive for exclusion of cardiac ischemia.[346,347] In the ED, however, the combination of resting echocardiography and cardiac enzyme serum markers may be a promising combination for the stratification of patients at risk of complications within the hospital and on discharge.[348] The identification of echocardiographic abnormalities may expedite admission for stable patients who are being evaluated in an ED.

Echocardiography plays an important role in the noninvasive evaluation of patients with known myocardial infarction, including evaluation of its complications such as left ventricular systolic dysfunction, development of ventricular septal defects, left ventricular rupture, and mitral regurgitation.[325] One study of ED patients reported six cases of myocardial rupture with hemopericardium from acute myocardial infarction with early ventricular rupture. As four of these patients met the criteria for emergency thrombolytic therapy, the emergency management was significantly changed by these findings on the focused echocardiogram.[56] Chronic complications such as pericarditis, pericardial effusion, left ventricular aneurysm, and left ventricular thrombus may also be evaluated by echocardiography.

► ANATOMIC CONSIDERATIONS

HEART

The heart is a hollow muscular organ, placed between the lungs, and enclosed within the pericardium. It is divided by a septum into two halves, right and left, each half being further subdivided into two cavities, the atrium and the ventricle. Blood flows from the right atrium into the right ventricle through the tricuspid valve. From the right ventricle, unoxygenated blood is carried to the lungs through the pulmonary artery. Blood flows from the left atrium into the left ventricle through the mitral valve. From the left ventricle, oxygenated blood is distributed to the body through the aorta. The outflow tract through the aortic valve into the proximal aorta starts anteriorly and curves posteriorly into the posterior mediastinum next to the esophagus. The aorta is divided into the ascending aorta, the aortic arch, and the descending aorta. The ascending aorta is approximately 5 cm in length; the only branches of the ascending aorta are the coronary arteries. The aortic arch has three branches: the innominate artery, the left common carotid artery, and the left subclavian artery.

The pericardium is composed of the parietal and visceral layers, which normally appose each other without any significant fluid accumulation. The pericardium attaches to the superior left atrium and envelops the proximal aspects of the great vessels.

THORACIC CAVITY

The thoracic cavity provides both windows and impediments to the accurate sonographic view of the heart. The heart has very few sonographic windows since ribs, the sternum, and the lungs surround it. Common windows include the parasternal, apical, subcostal, and suprasternal views. The left parasternal interspace allows for small

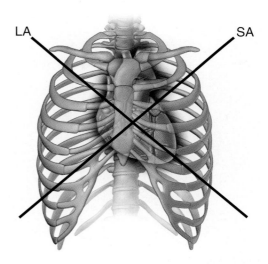

Figure 6-10. Orientation of the long (LA) and short (SA) cardiac axes relative to the torso.

sonographic windows into the mediastinum. The superior aspect of the abdomen also allows for soft-tissue windows via the left lobe of the liver. The heart can shift closer to the chest wall in the left decubitus position.

CARDIAC AXES AND SCANNING WINDOWS

The transducer position for all standard cardiac images is obtained relative to the long and short axis of the heart itself, not the torso. In general, the long axis of the heart is from the right shoulder to the left hip and the short axis is from the left shoulder to right hip (Figure 6-10), but cardiac axes can vary significantly in relation to the torso, depending on body habitus and age.

To obtain the standard transthoracic cardiac views, it is important to understand the three main cardiac axes (long, short, and four-chamber) and three main cardiac windows (subcostal, parasternal, and apical) (Figures 6-11–6-13).

► GETTING STARTED

Novice operators should understand that they can begin using point-of-care cardiac ultrasound for basic applications (pericardial effusion and gross cardiac function) after undergoing fundamental training. Clinically useful information can be obtained by providers with just a few hours of training concentrated on one or two cardiac ultrasound views (subcostal four-chamber and parasternal long axis). Novice operators should not be overwhelmed by the large amount of detail described in this chapter,

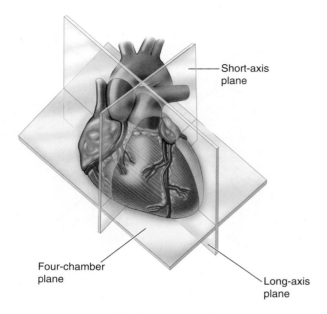

Figure 6-11. Cardiac axes.

which is intended for intermediate and advanced users, and as reference material. It is important to understand that most emergency providers use point-of-care cardiac ultrasound very effectively with 2D imaging, visual estimation, and very few specific measurements. Table 6-5 lists basic goals of point-of-care cardiac ultrasound.

Clinicians learning ultrasound may find transthoracic echocardiography difficult to learn initially because

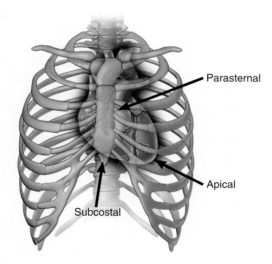

Figure 6-12. Cardiac ultrasound windows. Four-chamber views can be obtained from the subcostal and apical windows, short-axis views can be obtained from the parasternal or subcostal windows, and long-axis views can be obtained from the parasternal or apical windows.

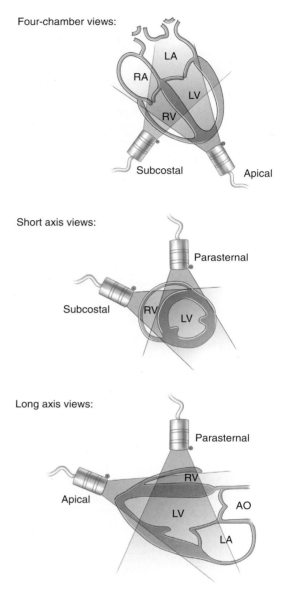

Figure 6-13. Standard transthoracic cardiac ultrasound views. These drawings demonstrate the position and orientation of the transducer relative to the heart.

of the complex anatomy of the heart and difficulty obtaining standard images due to the surrounding air-filled lungs. It is important to note that the long axis of the heart lies diagonal to the long axis of the torso (Figure 6-10). The long axis of the heart is more horizontal in short obese patients and more vertical in tall thin patients. Standard images of the heart are usually obtained from three anatomic locations on and below the chest wall: the subcostal window, the parasternal window, and the apical window. The heart lies higher in the chest cavity in younger patients, obese patients and those who are

► TABLE 6-5. **BASIC GOALS OF POINT-OF-CARE CARDIAC ULTRASOUND**

Identifying moderate or large pericardial effusions (subcostal view).

Identifying gross cardiac activity or cardiac standstill (subcostal or parasternal views)

Assessing relative and gross chamber sizes (apical four-chamber view)

Assessing the ejection fraction by 2D visual estimation (subcostal, parasternal, or apical views)

Measuring E-point septal separation to estimate the ejection fraction (parasternal long-axis view)

Evaluating gross valvular motion (parasternal long and short views)

Assessing volume status by IVC size and collapsibility (subcostal sagittal view)

supine. It lies lower in the chest cavity in elderly patients, thin patients and those who are sitting upright. The apex is found more medially in normal young patients and more laterally in patients with heart disease. Parasternal and apical images may be very difficult to obtain in patients with hyperexpanded lungs.

While most echocardiographers prefer to scan from the patient's left side, many clinicians scan from the patient's right. Cardiac presets should be selected if available on the machine. Patient positioning and ability to cooperate with inspiratory and expiratory maneuvers are critical to obtaining good images. The subcostal views are best obtained in the supine position, the parasternal views may be acquired in the supine or left lateral decubitus positions, and the apical views are usually best obtained in the left lateral decubitus position. Windows through intercostal spaces can be improved by positioning the patient's left hand behind their head, which may slightly widen the window. Nearly any change in patient position may improve cardiac windows and the ability to obtain good images. Subcostal cardiac images are often better when the patient takes a deep breath, and parasternal and apical views are often better when the patient exhales.

Having proper equipment and equipment settings is critical to obtaining good images. Using a phased array cardiac transducer is better than a curvilinear transducer for echocardiography. The phased array transducer allows imaging between the ribs and is especially important for the parasternal short-axis and all apical views. For transthoracic echocardiographic studies, a transducer with a median frequency of about 3.5 MHz (2.5–5.0 MHz) should be used. Most modern ultrasound machines allow operators to use presets for each particular type of examination. Using cardiac presets will produce the best results. Also, modern machines give the operator the ability to change the frequency range of the ultrasound transducer and activate tissue harmonics with the touch of a button. Testing different frequency ranges and activating tissue harmonics during each examination allows the operator to optimize images.

Overall gain and time-gain compensation are also simple to adjust and can be used to optimize each image. Ideal equipment settings produce images in which the edges of anatomic structures are sharply demarcated and the lumen of the cardiac chambers appear black, not grey.

There are several potential windows and views for echocardiography that will be described in detail below. From a practical standpoint, for clinical decision making in emergency and critical care medicine, often a single window and one or two views will provide the information needed for patient management. It is important, however, for clinicians to learn how to obtain images from all three standard anatomic locations (not just the subcostal window) because in any given patient one window may produce excellent images while the others are less optimal. Every patient has unique anatomy and no one anatomic location allows adequate imaging in all patients.

► TECHNIQUE AND NORMAL ULTRASOUND FINDINGS

For cardiac ultrasound the orientation marker (right/left indicator) on the monitor is usually oriented to the right side of the image, which is the opposite of the orientation for abdominal and pelvic imaging. This can be set-up automatically with a cardiac preset or changed manually. Table 6-6 provides a comparison of imaging techniques when using a cardiac preset versus an abdominal/pelvic preset. Regardless of the orientation of the indicator on the monitor, the key is to orient the transducer so as to produce the standard images pictured in this chapter. This facilitates recognition of normal cardiac anatomy and function as well as pathologic findings for the clinician and for any others who may review the images.

TRANSTHORACIC CARDIAC VIEWS

Subcostal Four-Chamber View

The subcostal views are often the most useful views for point-of-care cardiac ultrasound (Video 6-1 Cardiac Subcostal). Scanning from the subcostal window does not interfere in resuscitative measures such as thoracostomy, CPR, subclavian line insertion, or endotracheal intubation. It is easily learned, repeated, and performed as part of both the cardiac and trauma ultrasound evaluations.

▶ TABLE 6-6. **TRANSTHORACIC TRANSDUCER ORIENTATION ON THE SUPINE PATIENT**

Ultrasound Preset	Echocardiography	Abdomen/Pelvis
Machine/probe location	To the patient's left	To the patient's right
Monitor indicator	Right side of the image	Left side of the image
Subcostal	Probe marker directed to the patient's left flank	Probe marker directed to the patient's right flank
Apical four-chamber	Probe marker directed to the left side	Probe marker directed to the right side
	Probe aimed to right shoulder	Probe aimed to right shoulder
Parasternal long	Probe marker directed to the patient's right shoulder (10 o'clock)	Probe marker directed to the patient's left hip (4 o'clock)
Parasternal short	Probe marker directed to the patient's left shoulder (2 o'clock)	Probe marker directed to the patient's right hip (8 o'clock)

Perform the subcostal views at the subxiphoid position of the abdomen (Figure 6-14A). Hold the transducer at a 15° angle to the chest wall and aim the transducer marker toward the patient's left flank (using a cardiac preset). Angle the transducer up or down depending on the depth of the chest cavity to obtain images of the beating heart. Adjust the depth to visualize the atria at the bottom of the monitor screen. Initial poor-quality images may be improved upon by using an appropriate amount of ultrasound gel, using a shallow angle to the chest wall, moving the transducer to the right to use the left lobe of the liver as a window, and moving off

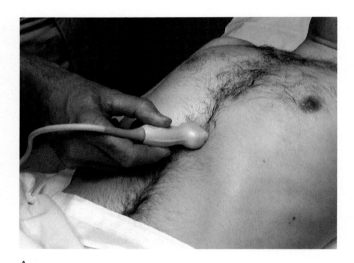

A

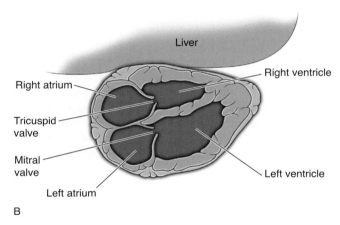

B

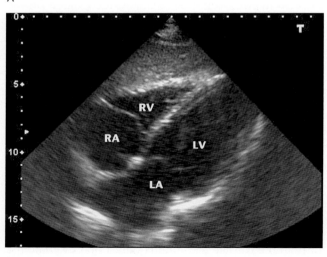

C

Figure 6-14. Transducer position for subcostal four-chamber view (A). Relevant anatomy (B). Subcostal four-chamber normal ultrasound (C). RA = right atrium, RV = right ventricle, LA = left atrium, LV = left ventricle. (C: Courtesy of Hennepin County Medical Center)

the xiphoid and over to the lower intercostal spaces to image the barrel-chested patient with a larger anterior–posterior diameter.

The subcostal four-chamber view should be seen primarily as a diagonal view of the ventricles, atria, pericardium, and the left lobe of the liver (Figures 6-14B,C). If the transducer is angled less acutely and into the upper abdomen from the subxiphoid position, the left lobe of the liver, IVC, and the hepatic veins will be visualized.

Subcostal Short-Axis View

The subcostal short axis view can be achieved by rotating the ultrasound transducer 90° counterclockwise from the four-chamber view (Figure 6-15). Images will resemble parasternal short axis images and they may provide virtually all of the same information (Figure 6-15). This view is especially useful in patients with COPD because hyperinflation of the lungs moves the heart into the subcostal region and makes parasternal and apical views difficult to obtain.

Subcostal Sagittal View of the IVC

The proximal IVC is found in the subcostal midline sagittal view as it courses posterior to the liver and into the right atrium. It is usually measured about 3–4 cm distal to its junction with the atrium or 2-cm distal to the entry of the hepatic veins (Video 6-2 Cardiac IVC).[37,276,349] The anterior–posterior diameter can be measured in the sagittal or transverse plane at any location between the hepatic vein and the left renal vein.[37,70,271,350]

The transducer is placed over the liver in the midline and aligned with the sagittal plane of the body. Emergency physicians usually align the transducer marker toward the patient's feet (using a cardiac preset) (Figure 6-16A). This will place the atrium/diaphragm on the left side of the screen as is the standard for abdominal longitudinal imaging. Cardiologists orient this image with the transducer marker pointing cephalad and the atrium/diaphragm on the right side of the screen. Either orientation is acceptable and provides identical information. The midline sagittal view provides visualization of the heart, the left lobe of the liver, the IVC, and hepatic

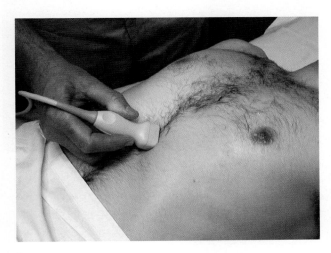

A

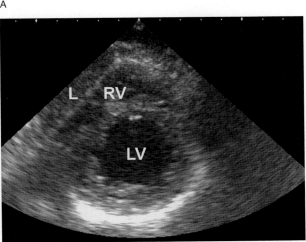

C

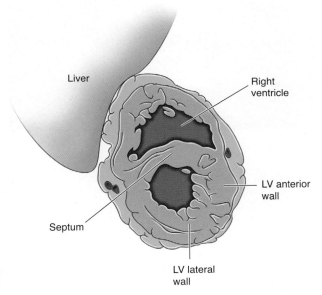

B

Figure 6-15. Transducer position for subcostal short-axis view (A). Relevant anatomy (B). Subcostal short-axis normal ultrasound (C). L = liver, RV = right ventricle, LV = left ventricle. (C: Courtesy of James Mateer, MD).

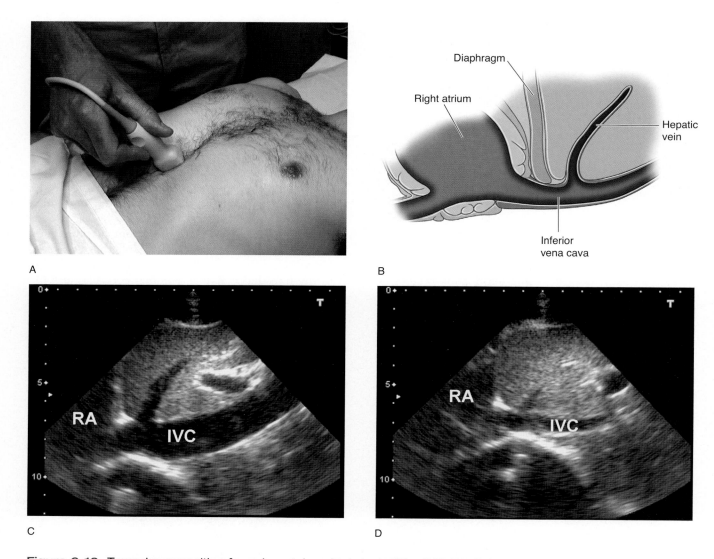

Figure 6-16. Transducer position for subcostal sagittal view of the IVC (A). Relevant anatomy (B). Proximal IVC during expiration (C) and inspiration (D). IVC = inferior vena cava, RA = right atrium. (C,D: Courtesy of Hennepin County Medical Center.)

veins (Figure 6-16B). This view allows evaluation of the proximal IVC during expiration and inspiration (Figure 6-16C,D). The anterior–posterior diameter of the proximal IVC usually measures about 1.5–2.0 cm during expiration and collapses with inspiration. Collapse of >50% during inspiration is consistent with normal (low) right sided filling pressure.

Although many studies use M-mode to accurately measure IVC size and the magnitude of variations, it should be noted that there is no evidence that it is superior to 2D imaging. Two-dimensional imaging is probably better because it is easier to locate the proper site for measurement in a 2D longitudinal view. In addition, transverse imaging of the IVC is also acceptable, but again it is more difficult to locate the best site for measurement in the transverse plane.

Parasternal Long-Axis View

The parasternal long-axis view is obtained by aligning the ultrasound plane with the long axis of the left ventricle (Figure 6-10 (Video 6-3 Cardiac Parasternal Long Axis). Place the transducer perpendicular to the chest wall at the 3rd or 4th intercostal space immediately to the left of the sternum with the transducer indicator directed toward the right shoulder (using a cardiac preset) (Figure 6-17A). The following structures can be visualized from anterior to posterior on the monitor: right ventricular free wall, right ventricular cavity, intraventricular septum (IVS), left ventricular cavity, and the posterior left ventricular free wall (Figure 6-17B). On the right side of the image the aortic and mitral valves and the proximal aorta and left atrium are usually well visualized. In

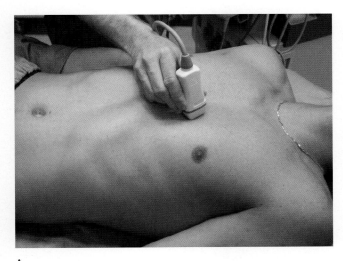

A

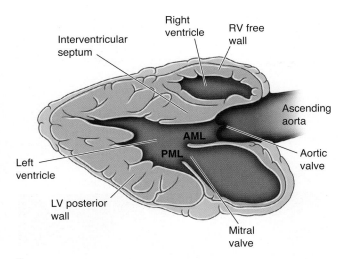

B

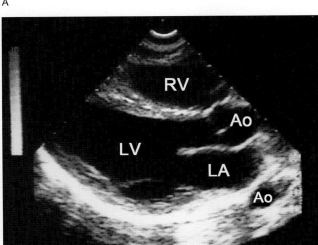

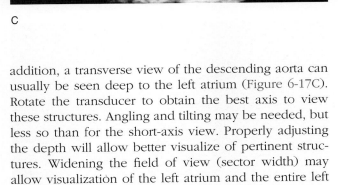

C

Figure 6-17. Transducer position for parasternal long-axis view (A). Note: May require left lateral decubitus position. Parasternal long-axis diagram (B). Parasternal long-axis normal ultrasound (C). RV = right ventricle, Ao - aorta, LV = left ventricle, LA = left atrium.

addition, a transverse view of the descending aorta can usually be seen deep to the left atrium (Figure 6-17C). Rotate the transducer to obtain the best axis to view these structures. Angling and tilting may be needed, but less so than for the short-axis view. Properly adjusting the depth will allow better visualize of pertinent structures. Widening the field of view (sector width) may allow visualization of the left atrium and the entire left ventricle simultaneously.

Parasternal Short-Axis View

The imaging plane for the parasternal short-axis view is oriented from the left shoulder to the right hip (Figure 6-10), and should be obtained in the left 3rd or 4th intercostal space just left of the sternum (Figure 6-18A). If the parasternal long-axis view has already been visualized, obtain the parasternal short-axis views by rotating the transducer marker 90° clockwise toward the left shoulder (using a cardiac preset)

(Video 6-4 Cardiac Parasternal Short Axis). With the transducer in this position, several different short-axis views can be obtained by tilting the transducer from the apex to the base (Figure 6-18B). Obtain parasternal short-axis views at the base of the heart, the level of the mitral valve (Figures 6-19A,B), the level of the papillary muscles, and at the apex. The short-axis view at the level of the papillary muscles is an important view because it allows identification of the different walls of the left ventricle (Figures 6-20A,B and 6-78). An ideal short-axis view at the base of the heart (Figures 6-21A,B) visualizes the left atrium, right atrium, tricuspid valve, right ventricle, and pulmonary valve encircling the aortic valve which is seen in cross section in the middle of the image (see the section "Valvular Abnomalities").

Apical Four-Chamber View

The apical four-chamber view is a coronal view of the heart that visualizes all four chambers in one plane

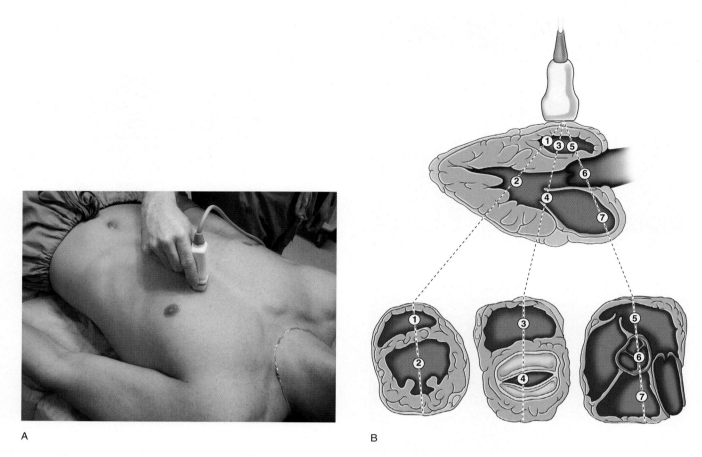

A

B

Figure 6-18. Transducer position for parasternal short-axis view (A). Note: May require left lateral decubitus position. Diagram of short-axis views from apex to base (B).

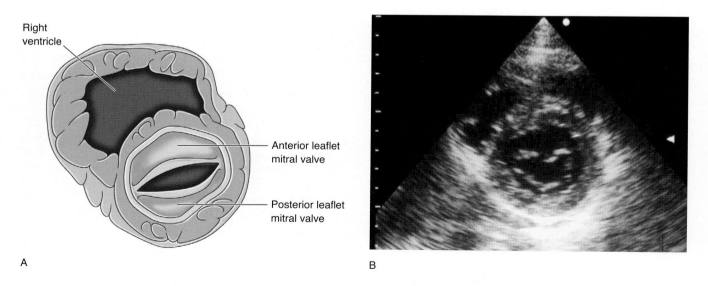

A

B

Figure 6-19. Parasternal short-axis diagram at mitral valve (A). Parasternal short-axis normal ultrasound at mitral valve (B).

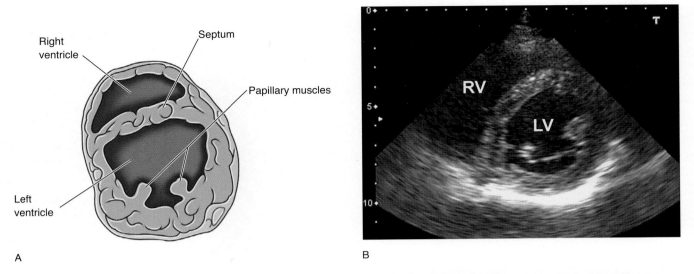

A

B

Figure 6-20. Parasternal short-axis diagram at papillary muscles (A). Parasternal short-axis normal ultrasound at papillary muscles (B). RV = right ventricle, LV = left ventricle. (B: Courtesy of Hennepin County Medical Center)

(Video 6-5 Cardiac Apical Four-Chamber). Other apical views include the apical five-chamber view, the apical two-chamber view, and the apical long-axis (three-chamber) view. The apical four-chamber view is the starting point from which all other apical views can be found. Start by placing the transducer at the point of maximal impulse (PMI) on the left lateral chest wall, generally in the 5th intercostal space or lower, and aim the transducer marker toward the left posterior axilla,

when using a cardiac preset (Figure 6-22A). Whenever possible, place the patient in the left lateral decubitus position to reduce lung artifact and to bring the heart closer to the chest wall. Some rotation may be needed to allow all four chambers to be visualized. The left ventricle should appear long and bullet shaped in proper apical views. The ventricle may appear short and round ("foreshortened") with cephalad or medial misplacement of the transducer on the chest wall. On the four-chamber

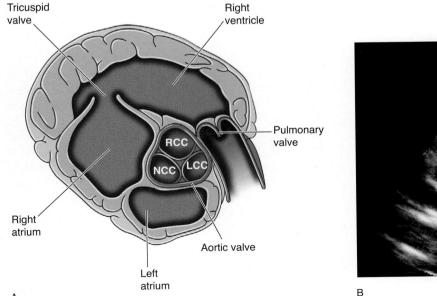

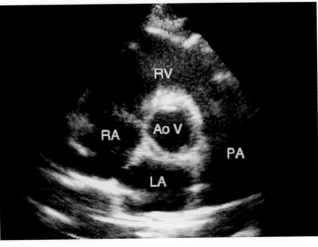

A

B

Figure 6-21. Parasternal short-axis diagram at aortic valve (A). Parasternal short-axis normal ultrasound at aortic valve (B). NCC= noncoronary cusp, RCC= right coronary cusp, LCC = left coronary cusp, RV = right ventricle, RA = right atrium, LA = left atrium, PA = pulmonary artery, Ao V = aortic valve.

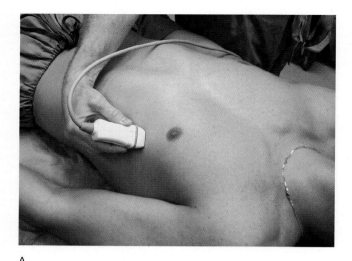

A

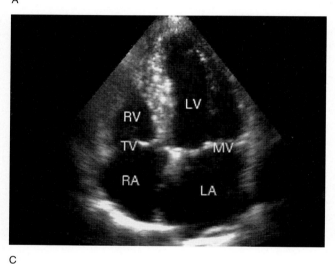

C

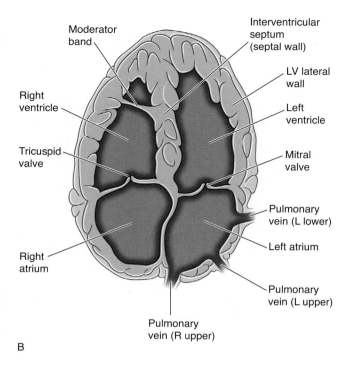

B

Figure 6-22. Transducer position for apical four-chamber view (A). Note: May require left lateral decubitus position with left arm elevated. Apical four-chamber diagram (B). Apical four-chamber normal ultrasound (C). RV = right ventricle, LV = left ventricle, MV = mitral valve, LA = left atrium, RA = right atrium, TV = tricuspid valve.

view, the right ventricle with its lateral wall, the IVS (septal wall), the left ventricle with its apex and lateral wall, the two atria, the interatrial septum, and the pulmonary veins will be visualized (Figure 6-22B,C). This view is advantageous for assessing left ventricular function as well as relative chamber sizes.

Doppler studies are often obtained with apical views because blood flow is parallel to the ultrasound beam (moving directly toward or away from the transducer) when the transducer is at the apex. When the image sector is swept anteriorly from the four-chamber view, the left ventricular outflow and aortic valve come into view (five-chamber).

Apical Five-Chamber View

The transducer position and orientation for the apical five-chamber view is nearly identical to the position and orientation for the apical four-chamber view. Beginning from the apical four-chamber view, the transducer is tilted or swept slightly anterior, to allow visualization of the LVOT (proximal aorta and aortic valve), which is the "5th" chamber (Figure 6-23A,B).

This view allows good visualization of the aortic valve and the LVOT in a vertical orientation, which is ideal for measuring blood flow. This is the primary view used for measuring Doppler flow across the LVOT and for calculation of stroke volume and cardiac output. It is also a good view for clinicians who may be confused about right-left orientation when obtaining the apical four-chamber view. When the mitral and aortic valves are both visualized simultaneously, there will be no doubt about which chamber is the left ventricle. Since the aortic valve is anterior to the mitral valve, the difference between the apical four-chamber and apical five-chamber views is just a slight anterior tilting of the transducer. The aortic valve and LVOT will appear in the center of the image between the mitral and tricuspid

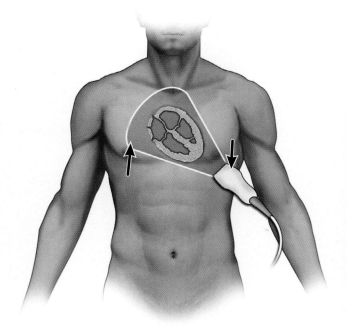

A

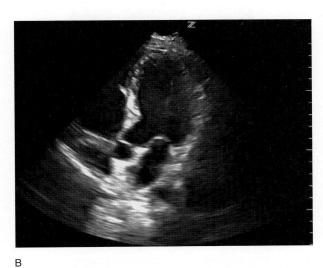

B

Figure 6-23. (A) Transducer movement (anterior tilt, no rotation) to get from the apical four-chamber view to the apical five-chamber view. (B) Apical five-chamber normal ultrasound.

valves. As noted above, ensure that the transducer is truly at the apex and the left ventricle appears long and bullet-shaped. This will align the LVOT vertically, so that blood flow through the aortic valve is moving directly away from the transducer. This will optimize the accuracy of Doppler flow measurements, which are best when blood flow is directly toward or away from the transducer.

Apical Two-Chamber View

To obtain the apical two-chamber view, first obtain the apical four-chamber view and then rotate the transducer about 60° counterclockwise (Figure 6-24A–C).

This view allows visualization of the anterior and inferior walls of the left ventricle complementing the apical four-chamber view for assessing wall motion and function (Figure 6-24B,C). Further counterclockwise rotation of the transducer from the two-chamber view (additional 30°) will produce the apical long-axis (three-chamber) view.

Apical Long-Axis (Three-Chamber) View

The apical long-axis or three-chamber view is another apical variation that provides essentially the same view as the parasternal long-axis view, but from a different vantage point. First obtain the apical four-chamber view,

then rotate counterclockwise beyond the apical two-chamber view until the aortic valve is visualized on the right side of the image (Figures 6-24A and 6-25A–C). Like the apical five-chamber view, this view aligns the mitral valve and LVOT in a vertical orientation. In this position, blood flow in and out of the left ventricle is directly toward and away from the transducer, which is optimal for Doppler flow measurements. The apical long-axis view provides visualization of the same structures as the parasternal long-axis view, including the IVS and posterior wall, with better visualization of the apex.

Suprasternal View

The suprasternal view allows visualization of the aortic arch with its three main branches: the innominate artery, the left carotid artery, and the left subclavian artery. Place the transducer in the sternal notch with the transducer marker pointed toward the patient's left scapula (using a cardiac preset) and the transducer aimed as far anteriorly as possible (Figure 6-26). This view may detect an aortic aneurysm or dissection. The right pulmonary artery, in cross section, can be seen below the aortic arch. If the transducer is rotated 90° to visualize the aortic arch in cross section, the left pulmonary artery may be better visualized. Occasionally, the superior vena cava may be visualized lateral to the ascending aorta.

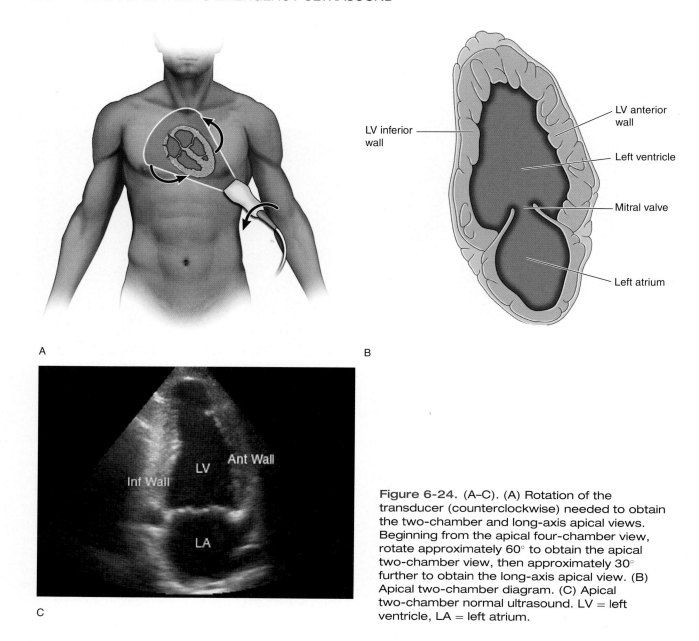

Figure 6-24. (A–C). (A) Rotation of the transducer (counterclockwise) needed to obtain the two-chamber and long-axis apical views. Beginning from the apical four-chamber view, rotate approximately 60° to obtain the apical two-chamber view, then approximately 30° further to obtain the long-axis apical view. (B) Apical two-chamber diagram. (C) Apical two-chamber normal ultrasound. LV = left ventricle, LA = left atrium.

► MEASUREMENTS

Most emergency providers use point-of-care cardiac ultrasound effectively without making any specific measurements, using just a visual estimation of cardiac structure and function, and most measurements are not considered part of the basic cardiac ultrasound examination (Table 6-5). Making 2D measurements or using M-mode or Doppler functions may be intimidating for novice operators. Some of the measurement techniques described below are simple to learn and may be used by novices, and some will only be useful for intermediate or advanced providers.

MEASUREMENTS OF LEFT VENTRICULAR STRUCTURE AND FUNCTION

There are several ways to measure left ventricular structure and function described in the following sections. These include visual estimation of ejection fraction and EPSS, 2D measurements of left ventricle chamber area/volume to calculate ejection fraction, M-mode measurements to calculate ejection fraction and left ventricle mass, and Doppler flow measurements to calculate stroke volume and cardiac output. Most ultrasound machines have software that can calculate these indices

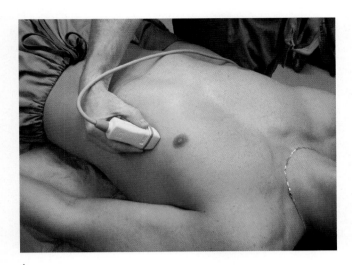

A

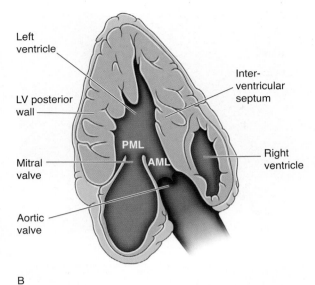

B

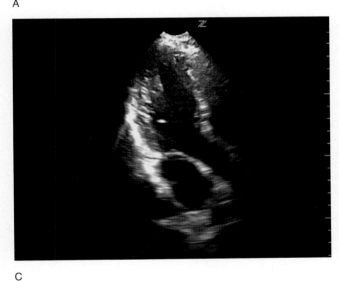

C

Figure 6-25. Transducer position for apical long-axis view (A). Apical long-axis diagram (B). Apical long-axis (three-chamber) normal ultrasound (C). PML = posterior mitral leaflet, AML = anterior mitral leaflet.

with a few simple measurements, but each calculation package is different, so it is important to learn the specifics of your machine's calculation software. Also, while it may be satisfying to calculate a value for ejection fraction, it has been shown that visual estimation of ejection fraction is as good or better than a calculated ejection fraction. Visual estimation is also easier and faster, so it is the most frequent method in clinical use today. Regardless, learning to measure cardiac structure and function is a useful exercise, to improve cardiac ultrasound skills and learn to obtain high-quality standard images. Measurements and visual estimation of ejection fraction will be inaccurate if the cardiac views are oblique, foreshortened, or otherwise of poor quality. Also, regional wall motion abnormalities, tachycardia, and bundle branch blocks can make it difficult to accurately estimate and measure ejection fraction.

Spectral Doppler measurements can be used to calculate stroke volume and cardiac output. It is impor-

tant to understand that these values provide a different type of information and do not necessarily correlate with ejection fraction. These parameters are rarely measured by emergency physicians, because a single measurement of stroke volume or cardiac output is rarely useful. Only serial or repeat measurements of these parameters, before and after a given treatment, are clinically useful. For example, measuring stroke volume before and after a fluid challenge, or with passive leg raising, can determine whether a patient has a positive hemodynamic effect with fluid resuscitation.

TWO-DIMENSIONAL MEASUREMENTS

Measure chamber dimensions and sizes at right angles to the long axis of the respective chamber. Measurement of chamber size, wall thickness, and the left ventricular function may be helpful. By measuring the left

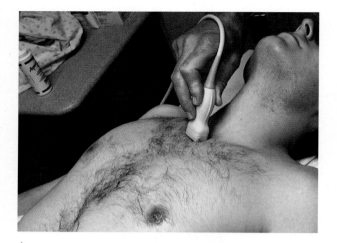

A

C

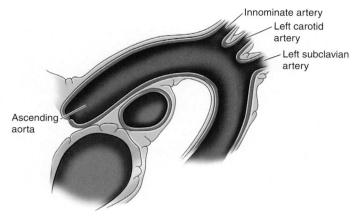

B

Figure 6-26. Transducer position for suprasternal view (A). From here, rotate the indicator towards the left scapula for a long axis view of the arch. Suprasternal diagram (B). Suprasternal normal ultrasound (C). The branch arteries may be closely approximated as in the diagram or spread apart for some patients as in the ultrasound example. Asc Ao = ascending aorta, Desc Ao = descending aorta.

ventricular dimensions in systole and diastole, one can calculate the ejection fraction manually or by using the ultrasound machine calculation package. Critical to the 2D measurement is the ability to visualize the endocardium and a cine memory in order to scroll to the correct point in the cardiac cycle for measurement. Table 6-7 lists abnormal cutoff values of common cardiac measurements.

Left Ventricular Diameter and Wall Thickness

Simple linear measurements of the left ventricle can be used to calculate left ventricular mass and ejection fraction (fractional shortening). These measurements are made in the mid-papillary region of the left ventricle, just beyond the tips of the mitral valve leaflets. Simply measuring the IVS, left ventricular internal diameter (LVID), and left ventricular posterior wall (LVPW) in diastole allows calculation of left ventricular mass and diagnosis of concentric or eccentric LVH (Figure 6-27, Table 6-8). Rapid measurements of chamber sizes can be made us-

ing 2D images. Simply freeze the 2D image, scroll back through the cine loop to end diastole, and make the appropriate measurements. A visual estimate comparing the chamber or wall to the image scale is often adequate, but calipers can also be used if visual estimation not adequate. The most accurate measurements are often made using M-mode images (see M-mode measurements in following section). If these measurements are made during both diastole and systole, the left ventricular ejection fraction (fractional shortening) can be calculated (see the section "M-Mode" for more details).

Left Ventricular Volumes and Ejection Fraction

Visual estimation is the most efficient method for estimating left ventricular ejection fraction. Simply obtain an apical four-chamber view (or any view for gross estimation) and answer the following question. Does the volume of blood ejected from the left ventricle appear to be >50–55% (normal), 30–50% (mild-to-moderate reduction in ejection fraction), or <25% (severely reduced

▶ TABLE 6-7. ABNORMAL CARDIAC ULTRASOUND MEASUREMENTS[189,265]

	Abnormal Values Female/Male
Left Ventricle	
Dimension/diastolic diameter, PLA view	>5.3 cm/>5.9 cm
Septal thickness, diastole PLA view	>1.2 cm*/>1.3 cm*
Posterior wall thickness, diastole PLA view	>1.2 cm*/>1.3 cm*
LV mass—from PLA linear dimensions	>190 g*/>260g*
LV mass—from PLA linear dimensions	>95 g/m²/>115 g/m²
E-point septal separation (EPSS)	>7 mm/>7 mm
Fractional shortening, PLA views	<25%/<25%
Ejection fraction, apical views are best	<55%/<55%
Left Atrium	
Dimension/diameter, PLA view	>4.0 cm/>4.0 cm
Area, apical four-chamber view	>20 cm/>20 cm²
Volume, apical four- and two-chamber views	>55 mL/>55 mL
Right Ventricle	
Free wall thickness, subcostal view	>0.5 cm/>0.5 cm
Mid-RV diameter, apical four-chamber view	>3.5 cm/>3.5 cm
Basal RV diameter, apical four-chamber view	>4.0 cm/>4.0 cm
Aorta	
Diameter—ascending aorta, PLA view	>3.5 cm/>3.5 cm

*These are moderate to severely abnormal values. LV mass/BSA is more accurate for diagnosing LVH.

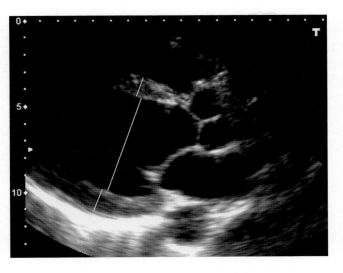

Figure 6-27. Linear measurements of the interventricular septum (IVS), left ventricular internal diameter (LVID), and left ventricular posterior wall (LVPW) in parasternal long-axis view. Use cine mode to adjust frame for diastole or systole as appropriate. These measurements can be used to calculate LV mass and LV ejection fraction (see the "M-Mode" section for details).

ejection fraction)? A rough estimate of the patient's left ventricular function can often guide the clinician to appropriate initial treatment, a precise number is not essential. Most quantitative measurements of left ventricular function are considered to be more advanced techniques and may not be appropriate or necessary for basic point-of-care cardiac ultrasound.

Quantitative measurements may be useful for ongoing treatment of critically ill patients and can be accomplished by measuring left ventricle chamber size by tracing the endocardial border in the apical four-chamber

▶ TABLE 6-8. FORMULAS FOR CARDIAC ULTRASOUND CALCULATIONS[189,265,332]

LV mass (g)	$= 0.8 \times \{1.04[(LVIDd + PWTd + SWTd)^3 - (LVIDd)^3]\} + 0.6$ g
Fractional shortening (%)*	$= (LVEDD - LVESD)/LVEDD \times 100$
Ejection fraction (%)	$= (LVEDV^2 - LVESV^2)/LVEDV^2 \times 100$
Stroke volume (mL)	$= CSA_{LVOT} \times VTI_{LVOT}$
Cardiac output (L/min)	$= SV \times HR/1000$
Cardiac index (L/min/m²)	$= CO/BSA$
Aortic valve area (cm²)	$= (VTI_{LVOT}/VTI_{AV}) \times CSA_{LVOT}$
Mitral valve area (cm²)	$= (VTI_{LVOT}/VTI_{MV}) \times CSA_{LVOT}$
Right ventricular systolic pressure (mm Hg)	$= 4(V_{TR})^2 + RAP$

LVIDd = left ventricular internal diameter in diastole, PWTd = posterior wall thickness in diastole, SWTd = septal wall thickness in diastole, LVEDD = left ventricular end-diastolic dimension, LVESD = left ventricular end-systolic dimension, LVEDV = left ventricular end-diastolic volume, LVESV = left ventricular end-systolic volume, CSA$_{LVOT}$ = cross-sectional area of the left ventricular outflow tract, VTI$_{LVOT}$ = velocity time integral measured in the left ventricular outflow tract, SV = stroke volume, HR = heart rate, CO = cardiac output, BSA = body surface area, VTI$_{AV}$ = velocity time integral measured in the aortic valve opening, VTI$_{MV}$ = velocity time integral measured in the mitral valve opening, V$_{TR}$ = peak velocity of tricuspid regurgitation (m/s), RAP = right atrial pressure (usually an estimate).
*Most modern ultrasound machines report ejection fraction based on measurement and calculation of fractional shortening.

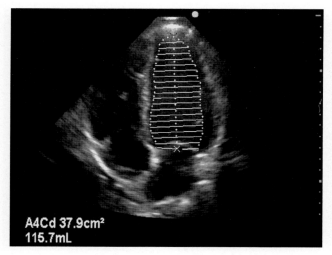
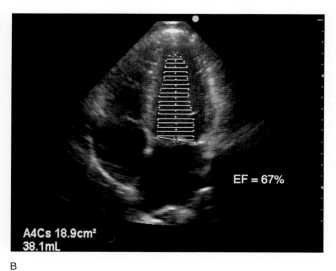

A4Cd 37.9cm²
115.7mL

A

A4Cs 18.9cm²
38.1mL

EF = 67%

B

Figure 6-28. Measurement of left ventricular volumes by the method of discs to calculate ejection fraction. The endocardial border is traced in diastole (A) and again in systole (B), and the computer calculates the ejection fraction. Only the apical four-chamber view is shown here, but the ejection fraction is more accurate if measurements are also made in the apical two-chamber view.

and apical two-chamber views. The left ventricular volumes are then calculated by the computer software, which fills the traced area with a stack of elliptical discs and calculates the volume based on that model (Figure 6-28A,B). Ejection fraction measurements are most accurate if the volumes are measured in both the apical four-chamber and apical two-chamber views, but most machines will display ejection fraction if just one view is obtained. It is important to obtain true apical views, so that the left ventricle is long and bullet shaped, not foreshortened or oblique, and a line drawn through the center of the long-axis of the ventricle intersects the center of the transducer. Utilization of this technique may be limited by time constraints and image quality. Even with good views it is often difficult to visualize the endocardial border, and contrast echocardiography significantly improves the accuracy and reproducibility of measuring left ventricular ejection fraction,[190,191] especially in obese patients and those with lung disease.[192]

Aortic Root and Left Atrial Diameter

Simple linear measurements of the aortic root and left atrial diameter (or dimension) are obtained from a parasternal long-axis view (Figure 6-29). The upper limit of normal of the aortic root is 3.5 cm and the upper limit of normal of the left atrium is 4.0 cm. A dilated aortic root can be associated with aortic aneurysm or dissection, but is usually just an age-related change. LAE can often be appreciated with just this single measurement, but a normal atrial diameter does not rule out LAE because the atrium often distends in other dimensions while the AP diameter remains normal.

Left Atrial Area and Volume

Left atrial size is most accurate if it is measured in both the apical four-chamber and apical two-chamber views. Measuring the left atrial volume is ideal but this may not be possible if it is not part of the ultrasound machines calculation package. An alternative is to simply trace the area of the left atrium (Figure 6-30A). The upper limit of normal for left atrial area is 20 cm². There are several methods for measuring left atrial volume. The biplane area-length measurement of volume involves tracing the atrial border and measuring the length perpendicular

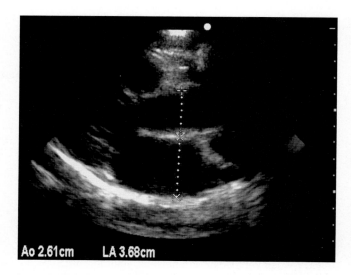

Ao 2.61cm   LA 3.68cm

Figure 6-29. Linear measurements of the aortic root (Ao) and the left atrial diameter (LA) in parasternal long-axis view. The atrium should be measured when it is largest. For 2D measurements, use cine mode to adjust frame for end systole.

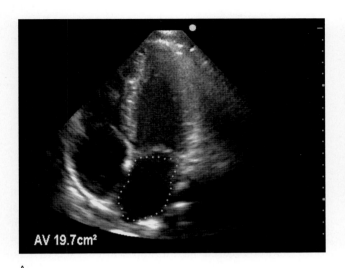

A

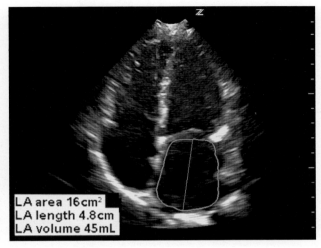

B

Figure 6-30. Measurement of left atrial area by a simple tracing of the atrial border (A) and measurement of left atrial volume by the biplane area-length method (B). The left atrium is measured when it is largest during systole. Measurement of the left atrium is more accurate if it is measured in both the apical four-chamber (shown) and apical two-chamber view.

from the center of the mitral annulus to the lower aspect of the atrium (Figure 6-30B).

Right Ventricular Dimensions

Right ventricular enlargement is often obvious and no measurements need to be made. The right ventricle is usually smaller than the left ventricle, so a rapid visual comparison of these two chambers in the apical four-chamber view is helpful. When the right ventricle becomes equal or larger in size than the left ventricle, it is easy to recognize right ventricular enlargement. In more subtle cases, it is useful to perform measurements of the right ventricle. Normal measurement of the mid-right ventricle diameter is <3.5 cm and normal measurement of the basal right ventricle diameter is <4 cm. Measurements significantly larger than normal are associated with cor pulmonale (Figure 6-31). Significantly elevated right-sided pressures often cause bowing of the IVS and significant tricuspid regurgitation, so it is useful to look for those findings if the right ventricle is enlarged.

Left Ventricular Outflow Tract

The LVOT diameter is commonly measured in the parasternal long-axis view at the level of the base of the valve leaflets (Figure 6-32). The computer then calculates the cross-sectional area, and this value is one of the variables in the equation for calculating stroke volume (see the section "Stroke Volume").

M-MODE

M-mode (motion mode) allows for a 1D tracing of structures over time. M-mode can record subtle changes

in motion of structures that typically move faster than human vision can perceive. Measurement of valve diameter, wall motion, wall thickness, and stroke volume is possible. There are several uses of M-mode tracing but the most common in point-of-care ultrasound is the tracing through the left ventricle for measurement of left ventricular size and function and to confirm the presence of a pericardial effusion.

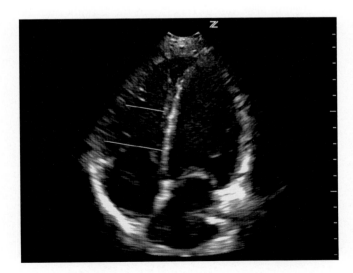

Figure 6-31. Measurements of the right ventricle (RV) in the apical four-chamber view. Measurements are made during diastole at the mid-portion and the base of the RV. Single measurements are generally positioned across the tips of the open tricuspid leaflets.

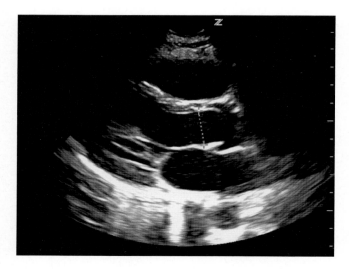

Figure 6-32. Measurement of the left ventricular outflow tract (LVOT). This measurement is performed in the parasternal long-axis view and the cursors are placed at the base of the aortic valve leaflets.

E-Point Septal Separation

An M-mode tracing at the mitral valve level in the parasternal long-axis view allows measurement of the right ventricular free wall, IVS, the mitral valve leaflets, the posterior left ventricular wall, and the pericardium. An M-mode tracing through the anterior leaflet of the mitral valve produces a double peak pattern (Figure 6-33A,B). The first peak is the E-point and is caused by passive filling of the left ventricle in early diastole. The second peak is the A-point and is caused by atrial contraction. This double peak pattern is evidence of sinus rhythm. The distance between the E-point and the IVS is EPSS. A large EPSS (in the absence of mitral stenosis) reflects left ventricular systolic dysfunction, left ventricular dilatation, or aortic regurgitation. Normal EPSS is ≤6 mm.[187] EPSS >7 mm indicates a ejection fraction of <50% and EPSS ≥13 mm indicates an ejection fraction of ≤35%.[186]

M-Mode Measurements of Left Ventricular Mass and Left Ventricular Function

Quantitative measurements of these parameters are generally considered more advanced techniques, and these measurements are not considered part of the basic point-of-care cardiac ultrasound exam (Table 6-5). However, understanding these concepts and how easy it is to make M-mode measurements will improve the providers understanding of how to visually assess 2D images in real time.

These measurements can be made in the parasternal long- or short-axis view (Figures 6-34A–D). The M-mode cursor is directed through the left ventricle at the level of the mid-papillary muscles. The measurements of the IVS, LVID, and LVPW are made using the calculation cursor. These simple measurements allow the calculation of left ventricular mass, diagnosis of concentric or eccentric LVH, and fractional shortening/ejection fraction (Figure 6-27, Tables 6-7 and 6-8). Note that determining left ventricular contractility using these measurements is technically called "fractional shortening," but most modern ultrasound machines report ejection fraction rather than fractional shortening when these measurements are made, because ejection fraction is a more familiar term and there is a linear correlation between ejection fraction and fractional shortening.

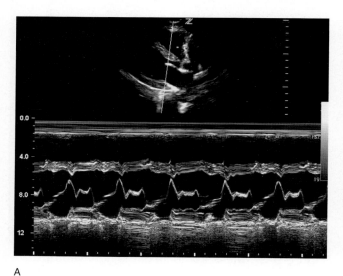

A

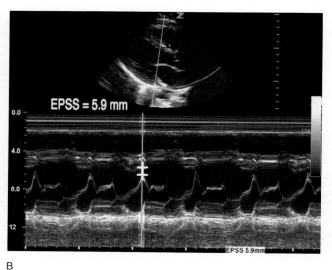

B

Figure 6-33. Normal E-point septal separation (EPSS) of M-mode at mitral leaflets from parasternal long-axis view. EPSS can be visually estimated (A), especially when there is good LV function, or it can be carefully measured (B). Increasing EPSS indicates worsening LV dysfunction.

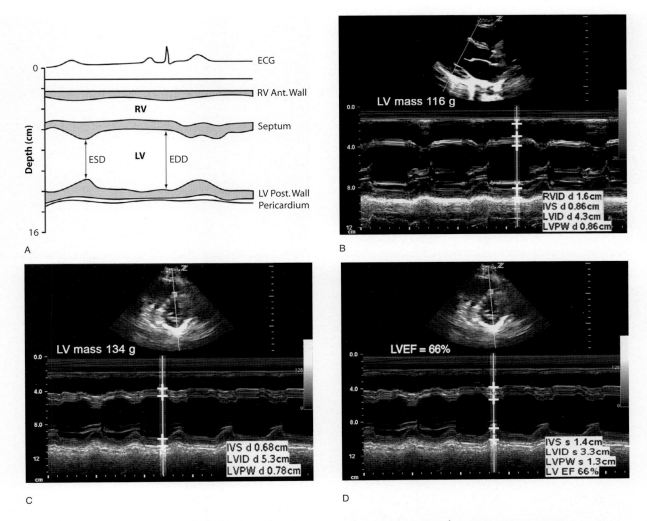

Figure 6-34. M-mode measurement of the left ventricle (LV). LV mass can be calculated by measuring the IVS, LVID, and LVPW in diastole (A–C). The LV ejection fraction can be calculated when these measurements are made during both diastole and systole (D). These measurements are usually made in the parasternal long-axis view just beyond the tips of the mitral valve leaflets (B), but can be made in the parasternal short-axis view at the mid-papillary level (C,D).

M-Mode Assessment of the IVC

M-mode assessment of the IVC allows for visual estimation and measurement of the diameter throughout the respiratory cycle. CVP can be estimated by measuring the diameter and inspiratory changes of the IVC in nonintubated patients (Table 6-4). If CVP is normal (<10 mm Hg), the IVC will collapse >50% with inspiration (Figure 6-35A,B). If CVP is elevated (>10 mm Hg), the IVC will be large (>2 cm) and will not collapse with inspiration (Figure 6-35C).

MEASUREMENTS OF VOLUME STATUS AND FLUID RESPONSIVENESS

There are several methods for determining volume status and fluid responsiveness described in the following sec-

tions. The traditional method is to measure the size and collapsibility of the IVC (Table 6-4); however, estimating fluid needs based on IVC indices alone may be oversimplified and can lead to clinical mistakes. Although IVC measurements cannot accurately measure CVP values, they can be used to effectively estimate whether CVP is very low or very high. For example, when the IVC is small (IVCe <1 cm) and collapses with inspiration, it is a good indication that the patient is volume depleted (also see the section "Volume Depletion and Fluid Responsiveness").

From a practical standpoint, the initial size and respiratory variation in the IVC are not as helpful (except when at the extremes) as the changes that occur in these parameters in response to a fluid challenge. When a patient presents with undifferentiated hypotension, the initial treatment often involves a fluid challenge. Serial monitoring of the IVC can help the clinician evaluate the

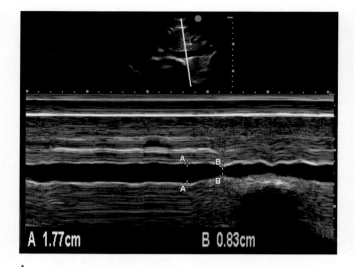

A

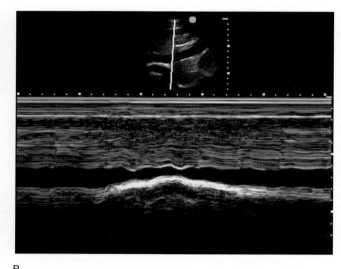

B

C

Figure 6-35. M-mode assessment of the IVC, from subcostal long-axis view. The size and dynamics of the IVC can be carefully measured (A) or visually estimated (B,C). The IVC normally collapses >50% with inspiration or sniffing (A, B), but has no inspiratory collapse when central venous pressure is elevated (C).

effect of this treatment more accurately. In general, if the patient's hemodynamics improve and the IVC changes little on ultrasound, more fluid can be given. When IVC measurements indicate a significant or rapid increase in CVP, it may be best to limit fluid therapy. Changes in IVC caliber should also be correlated with the patient's left ventricular function and capacity to accept a volume challenge.

IVC measurements may be helpful for initial determination of volume status and fluid needs, but they are not very useful after initial resuscitation for the ongoing assessment of fluid requirements. In these patients, there is significant evidence that CVP does not correlate with fluid responsiveness. It should be understood that fluid responsiveness is different from CVP (see the section "Volume Status and Fluid Responsiveness"). It is best to use IVC measurements along with other parameters, like changes in stroke volume, which have been proven to predict fluid responsiveness. The only IVC measurement

that has been proven to predict fluid responsiveness is IVC distension with mechanical insufflation in intubated patients. In intubated patients, there is no inspiratory collapse, rather mechanical insufflation has the opposite effect (distension); this may be subtle and distension of the IVC by 18% is highly predictive of fluid responsiveness. Another way to predict fluid responsiveness in intubated patients is to measure the stroke volume (or peak flow velocity or VTI) variation caused by changes in intrathoracic pressure during mechanical ventilation. The best way to predict fluid responsiveness with cardiac ultrasound may be to measure the stroke volume (or peak flow velocity or VTI) before and after passive leg raising, because this technique can be used in both intubated and nonintubated patients. This gives the patient an endogenous fluid challenge by significantly increasing venous return and will increase the stroke volume by >15% in patients who are fluid responsive (Figure 6-7A,B,C). See the following section on spectral

Doppler measurement of stroke volume, and the section "Volume Depletion and Fluid Responsiveness" under Common and Emergent Abnormalities.

DOPPLER PRINCIPLES AND MEASUREMENTS

Doppler ultrasound imaging requires more advanced skill and is not generally considered part of the basic point-of-care cardiac ultrasound exam (Table 6-5); however, some application of Doppler imaging (like transmitral flow) have been shown to be useful in the hands of emergency care providers. Doppler ultrasound uses the "Doppler effect" to identify or quantitate movement. The Doppler effect (or Doppler shift), named after Austrian physicist Christian Doppler, is the change in frequency as the source of the sound signal moves relative to the receiver. Using this principle, Doppler ultrasound can be used to identify and quantify movement of blood or tissue. Doppler ultrasound is most sensitive and accurate when movement of blood or tissue is directly toward or away from the transducer. The sampling beam must be positioned as close as possible to the direction of flow, since angle-correction is generally not used for cardiac Doppler measurements. Movement of blood or tissue can be displayed using a color display or as a waveform on a spectral display.

COLOR DOPPLER

Color Doppler flow imaging is used to visualize blood flow, and blood of different velocities and direction is assigned different colors. By convention, red represents flow toward the transducer and blue represents flow away from the transducer (Figure 6-36). It should be noted that the red and blue colors do not necessarily signify arterial or venous flow or specific vessels. In addition, degrees of velocity are mapped as shades of red and blue. Shades of orange, green, or yellow may represent degrees of velocity, variance, or turbulence. Optimizing the color flow image is accomplished by using the highest possible velocity scale. Decreasing the size of the color box increases pulse repetition frequency and allows more accurate depiction of high-frequency flow without artifacts. Color Doppler is used mostly for determining the presence and severity of valve regurgitation. The length and width of the color jet are factors in determining the severity of valve regurgitation (see the section "Valvular Abnormalities").

SPECTRAL DOPPLER

Spectral Doppler is a type of ultrasound image display in which flow velocity and direction are represented on

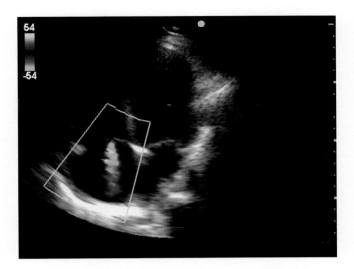

Figure 6-36. Apical view of color flow Doppler. This is an example of color Doppler identification of tricuspid regurgitation. The direction of the regurgitant jet is away from the transducer, so by convention it is blue in color.

the Y-axis and time is represented on the X-axis. Pulsed wave (PW) Doppler, CW Doppler, and tissue Doppler imaging (TDI) are displayed in this manner. PW Doppler is used to measure flow through the LVOT to calculate the left ventricular stroke volume and to document transmitral flow patterns to evaluate left ventricular diastolic function. CW Doppler is used to measure higher flow rates through stenotic or regurgitant valves, and is commonly used to measure tricuspid regurgitation to estimate right ventricular systolic pressure (RVSP) and to measure flow rates through stenotic lesions for valve area calculations. TDI is used to measure the movement of the mitral annulus during diastole, to assess left ventricular diastolic function.

Stroke Volume

Left ventricular stroke volume is determined by measuring the area of the LVOT and the Doppler flow through the LVOT. The cross-sectional area of the LVOT is calculated from a simple linear measurement (Figure 6-32). Blood flow through the LVOT is measured using pulsed Doppler, using the apical five-chamber or apical long-axis view (Figure 6-37A). The Doppler waveform is traced and the computer calculates the VTI (Figure 6-37B). The product of the VTI and the cross-sectional area of the LVOT is equal to the stroke volume (Table 6-8).

Vpeak (or Vmax) is the peak velocity of the pulsed Doppler blood flow and has a linear correlation with stroke volume. Visual estimation or measurements of changes in Vpeak, after passive leg raising, with respirations or after a fluid challenge, may be helpful in predicting fluid responsiveness.

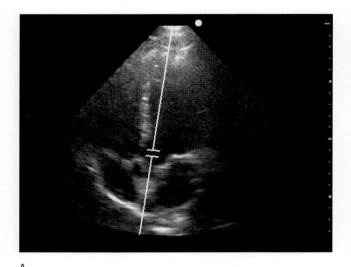
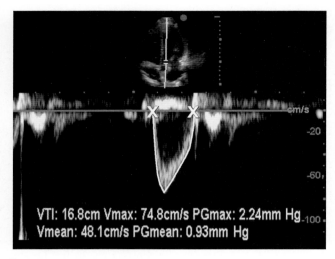

A

B

Figure 6-37. Pulsed Doppler flow through the left ventricular outflow tract (LVOT). (A) Positioning of the pulsed Doppler measuring gate into the LVOT in the apical five-chamber view. (B) Tracing of the pulsed Doppler waveform (white line between x's) allows the computer to calculate the velocity time integral (VTI).

Transmitral Flow

Transmitral Doppler flow is measured to determine left ventricular diastolic function. Pulsed Doppler is used in the apical four-chamber view, and the measuring gate is placed just inside the left ventricle beyond the tips of the mitral valve leaflets. Two distinct Doppler waveforms are created during diastole, corresponding with passive filling of the left ventricle and the atrial contraction. In a normal healthy heart, the majority of left ventricular filling occurs passively in early diastole (E-wave) and a small amount of filling occurs with atrial contraction (A-wave) (Figure 6-38A). The most important aspects of transmitral flow are the E/A pattern, the E/A ratio, and the measurement of the deceleration time of the E-wave (Figure 6-38B). The E/A ratio is normally 1–2 and the deceleration time is normally 160–240 ms (see the section "Diastolic Dysfunction" for abnormal filling patterns).

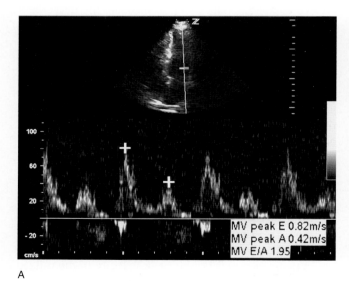
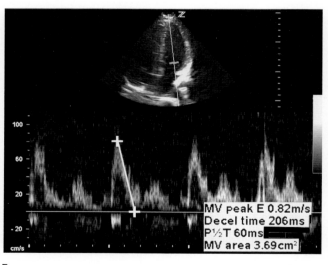

A

B

Figure 6-38. Normal transmitral Doppler flow pattern from apical views. (A) The majority of filling of the left ventricle occurs during early diastole, so the E-wave is more prominent than the A-wave. (B) The time interval from the peak of the E-wave to the baseline (deceleration time) is an important indicator of normal ventricular filling.

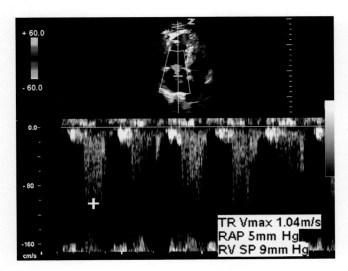

Figure 6-39. Measurement of the peak velocity of tricuspid regurgitation (TRV max) from apical view. RVSP is calculated (9 mm Hg) by the computer when the right atrial pressure is known or estimated (5 mm Hg).

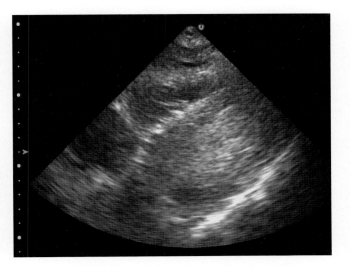

Figure 6-40. Cardiac arrest subcostal four-chamber view. Clotted blood in left ventricle is consistent with a complete lack of myocardial contractions.

Right Ventricular Systolic Pressure

Measurement of the peak velocity of tricuspid regurgitation is used to calculate RVSP. This is usually done using CW Doppler, but pulsed Doppler can also be used. The Doppler measuring gate is placed into the regurgitation jet using 2D and color Doppler flow guidance (Figure 6-39). The maximal velocity of regurgitant flow is measured (Vmax) and used to calculate RVSP from estimation of the right atrial pressure (RAP) (Table 6-8).

► COMMON AND EMERGENT ABNORMALITIES

CARDIAC ARREST

Asystole and true EMD are seen as a lack of myocardial contractions on ultrasound. Pooling of blood may be seen and echogenic clots may be formed under these conditions (Figure 6-40). A subjective assessment of the presence or absence of coordinated myocardial contractions (or kinetic wall motion) and an assessment of left ventricular function often change clinical management and are important prognostic indicators.[8,13,130] Movement of the valves can be seen just with positive pressure ventilation and should not be mistaken for spontaneous circulation in the absence of myocardial contractions.

CARDIAC TAMPONADE

Cardiac tamponade is not dependent on the amount of fluid in the pericardial sac but on the rate of fluid accumulation within the pericardial sac (Figure 6-2). Emergent echocardiographic findings of cardiac tamponade include a pericardial effusion, right atrial collapse during ventricular systole, right ventricular diastolic collapse (Figures 6-41 and 6-42), and lack of respiratory variation in the IVC and hepatic veins. Rarely, tamponade may present with isolated left atrial or left ventricular collapse in patients with loculated effusions or severe pulmonary hypertension.

PERICARDIAL EFFUSION

Pericardial effusion is typically characterized by an anechoic fluid collection between the parietal pericardium and the visceral pericardium (Figures 6-43A,B and 6-44). For all practical purposes, the visceral pericardium is not visualized by transthoracic echocardiography. However, the combined interface of the parietal and visceral pericardium is echogenic.

On transthoracic echocardiography, pericardial effusions may be judged as small or large. Small pericardial effusions are seen as an anechoic space <1 cm thick and are often localized, usually between the posterior pericardium and left ventricular epicardium. Large effusions are seen as an anechoic space >1.5 cm thick, and usually completely surround the heart. In patients with larger effusions, the heart may swing freely within the pericardial sac (Figure 6-45).

Pericardial volumes of up to 50 mL may be normal; however, pathologic fluid collections, if slow in

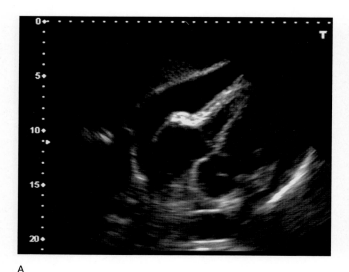

A

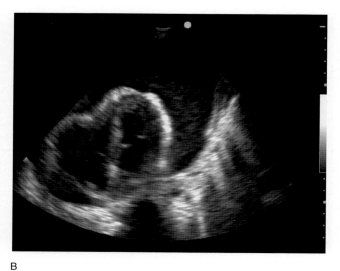

B

Figure 6-41. Cardiac tamponade. (A) Subcostal four-chamber view with a moderate pericardial effusion and right ventricular diastolic collapse. (B) Apical four-chamber view with a large echogenic effusion and right ventricular diastolic collapse.

progression, may accumulate hundreds of milliliters. Pericardial fluid is usually anechoic, but exudative effusions, such as pus, malignant effusions, and blood mixed with fibrin material, may be echogenic (Figure 6-46).

MASSIVE PULMONARY EMBOLISM

While direct visualization of a thrombus may occasionally be seen in the right heart, most echocardiographically detectable changes are indirect indices of right

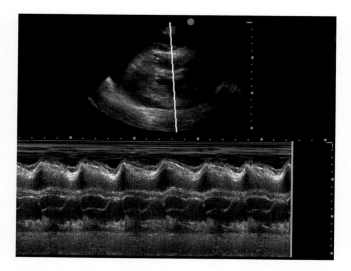

Figure 6-42. M-mode image demonstrating right ventricular diastolic collapse. In a parasternal long-axis view, the M-mode cursor is directed through the right ventricular free wall and the mitral valve.[46] The free wall of the right ventricle collapses toward the mitral valve as the valve opens during diastole.

heart strain caused by pumping against a fixed blood clot in the lung. These changes include right ventricular dilatation, right ventricular hypokinesis, tricuspid regurgitation, and abnormal septal motion. The normal right ventricular end-diastolic diameter measured in the apical four-chamber is ≤3.5 at the mid-right ventricle and ≤4.0 at the base of the ventricle (Figure 6-47). The normal right to left ventricle ratio is not consistently defined, but a ratio of 0.5–1.0 is generally considered normal and a ratio of >1.0 is seen with significant right ventricular enlargement.

With massive PE, the right ventricle will be significantly larger than the left ventricle and may be round in shape (Figures 6-3 and 6-48). McConnell's **sign**, described as diffuse hypokinesis of the right ventricular free wall with apical sparing, is a very specific but insensitive indicator of PE.[351] In addition to right-sided heart strain, a blood clot in the lung may cause decreased venous return to the left heart. This may result in decreased LVEDD as well as "paradoxical septal motion." The normal IVS relaxes outward (toward the right ventricle) in diastole. With increased right end-diastolic pressures and decreased left-sided pressures, abnormal motion of the septum in diastole may be visualized. While this septal deviation toward the left ventricle (also described as "septal flattening" or "**D-sign**") may also be observed in systole, its presence is more pronounced in diastole and is especially prominent in the acute phase of massive PE (Figure 6-49).

Tricuspid regurgitation may occur when pulmonary artery pressures exceed right ventricular end-diastolic (right atrial) pressures. Measurement of tricuspid regurgitation requires spectral Doppler velocity measurement and is usually obtained on the apical four-chamber view. This value is used to calculate the pressure gradient

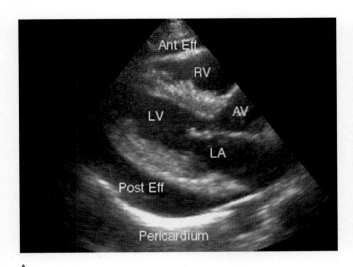

A

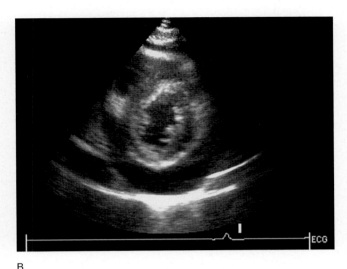

B

Figure 6-43. Pericardial effusion on parasternal long-axis view (A) and parasternal short-axis view (B). RV = right ventricle, LV = left ventricle, AV = aortic valve, LA = left atrium.

between the right atrium and right ventricle (Table 6-8). While many healthy persons have a trivial degree of tricuspid regurgitation, up to 90% of patients with PE will have measurable tricuspid regurgitation. Normal pulmonary artery systolic pressure is approximately 25 mm Hg in a healthy person, corresponding to a regurgitant jet of <2 m/s. Over 3 m/s would correspond to a pulmonary artery pressure of 46 mm Hg. Studies using cutoff values for diagnosis of PE typically cite velocities over 2.5–2.7 m/s as being elevated (Figure 6-50).

All of the indirect indicators of right-sided heart strain may occur in conditions other than PE. These conditions include right ventricular infarct, emphysema, and primary pulmonary hypertension. It is worthwhile to note that the acutely strained right-sided heart rarely has the muscle mass to elevate pulmonary artery pres-

sure into an extremely high range and values well over 40 mm Hg should suggest a chronic elevation. An increase in muscle mass on measurement of the right ventricular free wall may also indicate a more chronic etiology for right ventricular strain as opposed to a thin, acutely dilated right ventricle. The normal thickness of the right ventricular free wall is 2.4 ± 0.5 mm, and it is generally considered hypertrophied at measurements of 5 mm or greater.

LEFT VENTRICULAR SYSTOLIC DYSFUNCTION

Visual estimation is the best way to determine left ventricular function in the emergent setting. It is best to

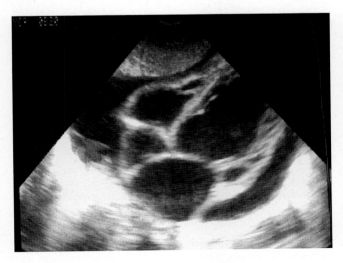

Figure 6-44. Chronic pericardial effusion (subcostal four-chamber view).

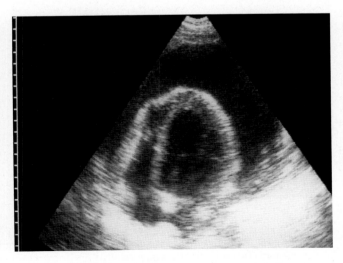

Figure 6-45. Large effusion (apical view). (Courtesy of James Mateer, MD)

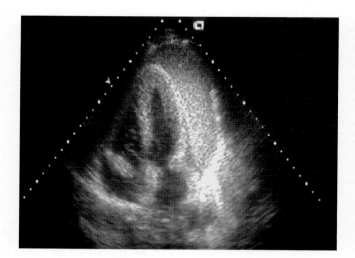

Figure 6-46. Exudative pericardial effusion (apical four-chamber view).

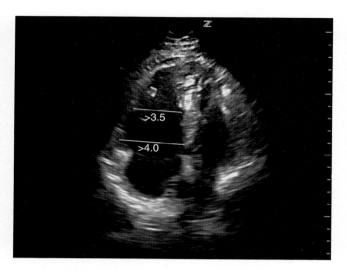

Figure 6-47. Right ventricular enlargement in a patient with a large pulmonary embolism, apical four-chamber view. The right ventricle is larger than the left ventricle and measurements of the diameter at the mid (4.5 cm) and basilar (6.6 cm) right ventricle are abnormally large.

visualize the left ventricle in multiple views (at least two), so that the function of the entire ventricle can be accurately assessed (Figure 6-51). Also, it is best to use a combination of findings to get the most accurate picture of overall cardiac function, including visual estimation of left ventricular function, EPSS, visual inspection of the valves, IVC size and collapsibility, pulmonary ultrasound findings, and simple measurements of systolic or diastolic function.

EPSS provides an objective measure of left ventricular function and is particularly important for those who are inexperienced with visual estimation of left ventricular function. Abnormally large EPSS is consistent with left ventricular dysfunction and increasing EPSS corre-

lates with worsening dysfunction (Figure 6-52). Normal EPSS is ≤6 mm.[187] EPSS >7 mm indicates a ejection fraction of <50% and EPSS ≥13 mm indicates an ejection fraction of ≤35%.[186]

Left ventricular dysfunction can also be measured and documented by measuring the change in left ventricular volume between diastole and systole (Figure 6-53). Volumes are calculated using the method of discs/modified Simpson's rule after tracing the endocardial border. Calculations are most accurate if measurements

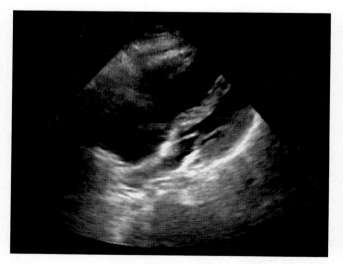

A

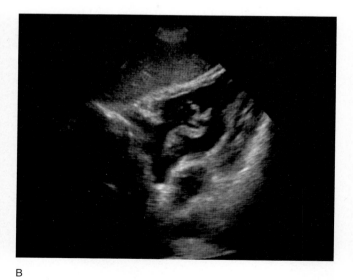

B

Figure 6-48. Massive pulmonary embolism. (A,B) Subcostal images demonstrating massive dilation of the right ventricle with bowing of the septum and an underfilled left ventricle. B shows a clot in transit passing through the tricuspid valve and into the right ventricle.

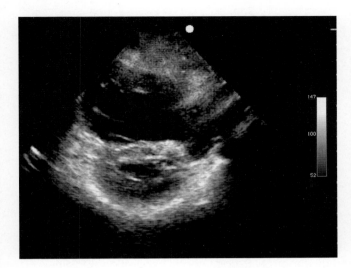

Figure 6-49. Massive pulmonary embolism with D-sign. Subcostal short-axis view showing a very large right ventricle (top) and collapsed left ventricle. The intraventricular septum is straight/bowed as a result of high right-sided pressure resulting in the classic "D-sign."

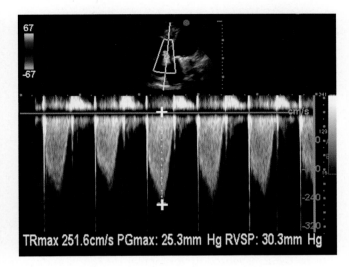

Figure 6-50. Determination of elevated right ventricular systolic pressure (RVSP) by measurement of the peak velocity of tricuspid regurgitation (TRmax). This patient has a RVSP of 30 mm Hg + RAP (right atrial pressure).

are performed in both apical four-chamber and two-chamber views.

LEFT VENTRICULAR DIASTOLIC DYSFUNCTION

Half of all patients with clinical heart failure have isolated diastolic dysfunction with normal left ventricular systolic function. Older patients with hypertension and LVH tend to have diastolic dysfunction. Also, diastolic dysfunction is the most common cause of LAE. Therefore, looking for LVH and LAE is part of assessing for diastolic dysfunction (see the sections "Left Ventricular Hypertrophy" and "Left Atrial Enlargement" for more details). Doppler imaging of left ventricular filling (referred to as transmitral flow or mitral inflow) and TDI of the mitral annulus are widely used to identify and determine the severity of diastolic dysfunction, and both techniques can be used by emergency physicians (Figure 6-54).[45,48]

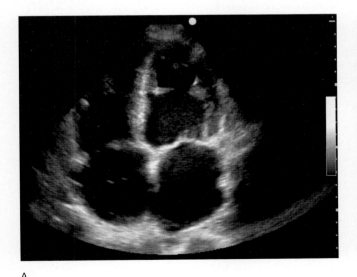

A

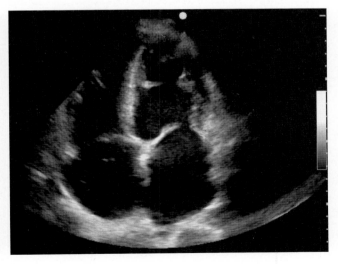

B

Figure 6-51. Severe left ventricular systolic dysfunction. Visual estimation of left ventricular function with an apical four-chamber view. This is an example of a patient with an ejection fraction of <10%, so there is minimal change in the LV area/volume between systole (A) and diastole (B).

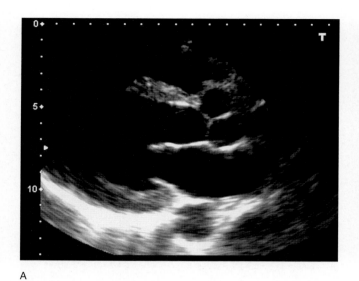

A

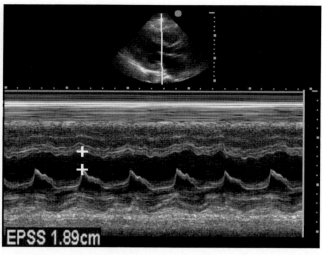

B

Figure 6-52. Severe left ventricular dysfunction determined by abnormal E-point septal separation (EPSS) parasternal long-axis view. EPSS can be visually estimated (A), especially if it is obviously abnormal; however, it is often measured and recorded with M-mode imaging (B).

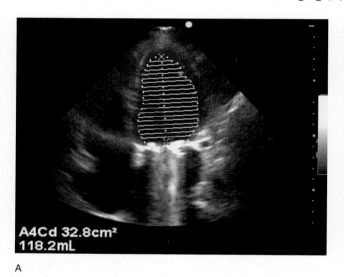

A

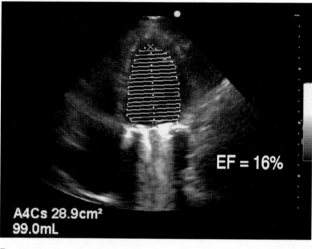

B

Figure 6-53. Apical views of severe LV dysfunction. This patient has an ejection fraction of 16%, which is calculated by the computer after the endocardial border is traced in diastole (A) and systole (B). The patient also has a prosthetic mitral valve with resultant image artifact shown in the left atrium.

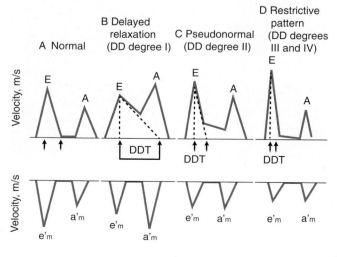

Figure 6-54. Left ventricular filling patterns. Transmitral Doppler flow (top) and mitral annular tissue Doppler (bottom) patterns associated with normal and progressively worsening diastolic function. From *Fontes-Carvalho R and Leite-Moreira A.* Heart Failure with Preserved Ejection Fraction: Fighting Misconceptions for a New Approach. *Arq Bras cardiol* 96:504, 2012.

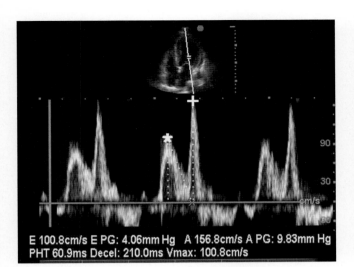

E 100.8cm/s E PG: 4.06mm Hg   A 156.8cm/s A PG: 9.83mm Hg
PHT 60.9ms Decel: 210.0ms Vmax: 100.8cm/s

A

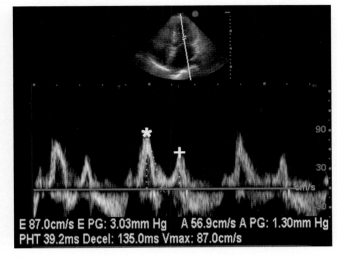

E 87.0cm/s E PG: 3.03mm Hg   A 56.9cm/s A PG: 1.30mm Hg
PHT 39.2ms Decel: 135.0ms Vmax: 87.0cm/s

B

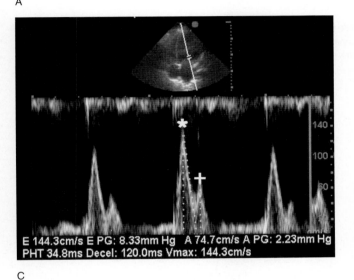

E 144.3cm/s E PG: 8.33mm Hg   A 74.7cm/s A PG: 2.23mm Hg
PHT 34.8ms Decel: 120.0ms Vmax: 144.3cm/s

C

Figure 6-55. Diastolic dysfunction with abnormal transmitral Doppler flow patterns. Impaired relaxation with reversal of normal E/A pattern (A). Pseudonormal E/A pattern with a short deceleration time = 135 m/s (B). Severe diastolic dysfunction with a restrictive pattern, E/A ratio >2, and a very short deceleration time = 120 ms (C).

Transmitral flow is measured by pulsed Doppler in the apical four-chamber or apical two-chamber view. The measuring gate is placed just inside the left ventricle at the tips of the mitral valve leaflets. There are two components to ventricular filling during diastole; early passive diastolic filling (E-wave) and late diastolic filling caused by the atrial contraction (A-wave). In a normal heart, without diastolic dysfunction, most of the ventricular filling occurs during early diastole, so E is larger than A, with an E/A ratio of 1–2 (Figure 6-38A). With early diastolic dysfunction (impaired relaxation), there is a reversal of the characteristic E/A pattern and E is smaller than A (Figure 6-55A). Also, impaired relaxation may cause prolongation (>240 ms) of the deceleration time of the E-wave (Figure 6-54). With worsening diastolic dysfunction, the E/A ratio reverses again, with E larger than A, which is referred to as "pseudonormalization"

(Figure 6-55B). A pseudonormal E/A pattern may be differentiated from a normal E/A pattern by measurement of an abnormally short deceleration time (<160 ms) or by measurement of decreased movement of the mitral annulus (using TDI) during early diastole (see below). Severe diastolic dysfunction is characterized by a restrictive filling pattern, with an E-wave much taller than the A-wave (E/A ratio >2) and a very short deceleration time (Figure 6-55C).

Movement of the mitral annulus is measured by obtaining an apical four-chamber view and placing the TDI gate over the septal portion of the mitral annulus. With normal left ventricular filling, the mitral annulus moves rapidly downward at a velocity of >8 cm/s and this movement is easily measured by TDI and referred to as e' (Figure 6-54). An e' of < 8 cm/s is diagnostic of diastolic dysfunction (Figure 6-56).

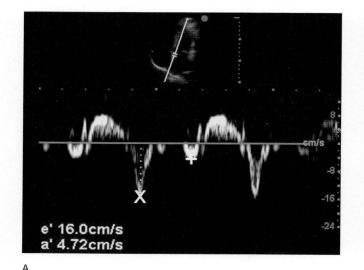

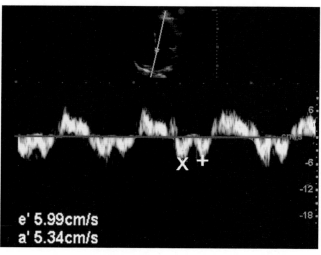

A

B

Figure 6-56. Normal (A) and abnormal (B) tissue Doppler imaging (TDI) of the septal portion of the mitral annulus. Early diastolic filling causes rapid downward movement of the mitral annulus (e' = 16 cm/s) in a normal heart (A). Decreased movement of the annulus (e' <8 cm/s) is diagnostic of diastolic dysfunction (B).

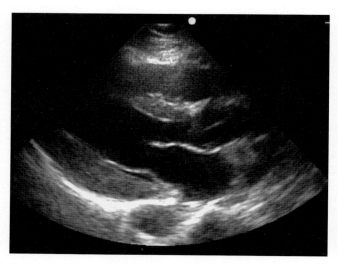

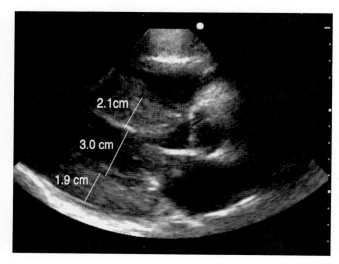

A

B

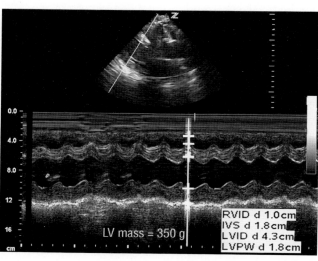

C

Figure 6-57. Left ventricular hypertrophy (LVH) parasternal long-axis views. LVH can be identified by visual estimation (A) or simple 2D measurements of the IVS, LVID and LVPW (B), but M-mode measurements (C) are classically used to make the diagnosis.

LEFT VENTRICULAR HYPERTROPHY

LVH may be concentric or eccentric. Patients with concentric hypertrophy have thick left ventricular walls and patients with eccentric hypertrophy have a large LVID. In patients with very thick left ventricle walls (Figure 6-57A), or a very large LVID, the diagnosis may be obvious without measurements. Measurements of left ventricular wall thickness >12 mm or LVID >5.3 cm in females or >5.9 cm in males (in diastole) are findings consistent with LVH (Figure 6-57B and Table 6-7). The most common way to make the diagnosis of LVH is to measure the left ventricular mass (using the area-length or the truncated-ellipse method) and divide it by the body mass index; however, this is somewhat cumbersome and requires the proper calculation software. A simpler way of identifying and classifying LVH is to use a nomogram (Figure 6-58). Measurements of the

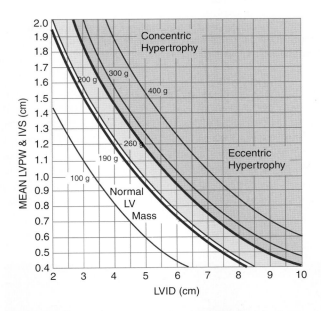

Figure 6-58. Nomogram for determination of left ventricular mass.[229] End-diastolic M-mode measurements are used, and the mean of the intraventricular septum (IVS) and left ventricular posterior wall (LVPW) thickness is found on the vertical axis and is followed to where it intersects with the left ventricular internal chamber diameter (LVID) on the horizontal axis. Coordinates in the gray zone are consistent with left ventricular hypertrophy (LVH), using cutoffs of 190 g for adult females and 260 g for adult males, which is consistent with moderate LVH.[189] Coordinates in the upper portion of the gray zone are consistent with concentric hypertrophy and those in the lower portion of the gray zone are consistent with eccentric hypertrophy. From Woythaler JN, Singer SL, Kwan OL, et al. Accuracy of echocardiography versus electrocardiography in detecting left ventricular hypertrophy: Comparison with postmortem mass measurements. *JACC* 2:305, 1983.

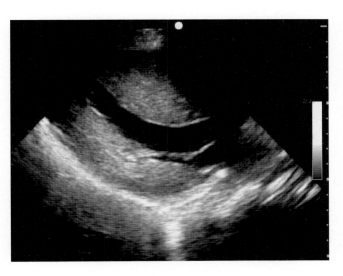

Figure 6-59. Hypertrophic cardiomyopathy, nonobstructive type, parasternal long-axis view. Hypertrophic cardiomyopathy is the leading cause of sudden cardiac death in preadolescent and adolescent children. This is an example of severe diffuse hypertrophy in a 12-year-old girl, which did not cause obstruction or a murmur, but she is still at high risk of arrhythmogenic sudden death.

IVS, LVID, and LVPW are made during diastole using M-mode (Figure 6-57C) and applied to the nomogram (Figure 6-58).

Hypertrophic cardiomyopathy is the leading cause of sudden cardiac death in preadolescent and adolescent children. This entity can be separated into obstructive and nonobstructive types (Figures 6-59 and 6-60).

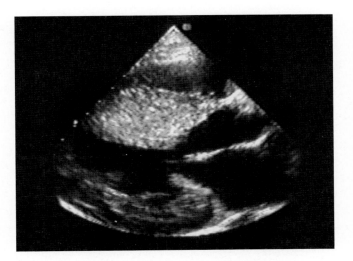

Figure 6-60. Hypertrophic cardiomyopathy, obstructive type, with asymmetric septal hypertrophy. The key finding is that the intraventricular septum is more than twice as thick as the posterior wall. This patient is at risk of obstruction of the left ventricular outflow tract during systole and at risk of arrhythmogenic sudden death.

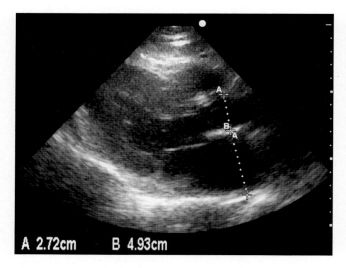

Figure 6-61. Left atrial enlargement (LAE). The LA diameter (dimension), measured in the parasternal long-axis view, is 4.93 cm. An LA diameter >4.0 cm is consistent with LAE.

Patients with asymmetric septal hypertrophy (obstructive type) are at risk of dynamic obstruction of the LVOT. However, patients with or without asymmetric septal hypertrophy are at high risk of arrhythmogenic sudden death.

LEFT ATRIAL ENLARGEMENT

LAE is a significant abnormality that is associated with high left ventricular filling pressure and often caused by

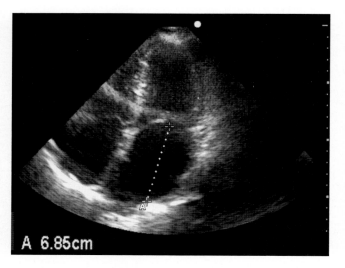

Figure 6-62. Left atrial enlargement. The left atrium is significantly larger than the left ventricle in the apical four-chamber view, so the diagnosis of LAE can be made by visual estimation. In addition, the major axis of the left atrium is >6 cm, which is consistent with LAE.

diastolic dysfunction or mitral regurgitation. The easiest way to document LAE is to measure the left atrial diameter (dimension) in the parasternal long-axis view during systole (when it is largest). Left atrial diameter >4.0 cm is consistent with LAE (Figure 6-61). The most accurate way to diagnose LAE is to measure the volume using both apical four-chamber and apical two-chamber views (Figure 6-30), but severe LAE may be obvious (Figure 6-62).

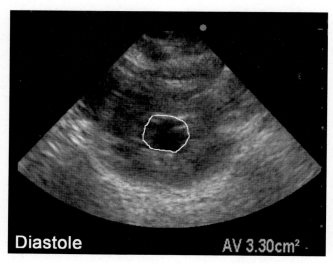

A

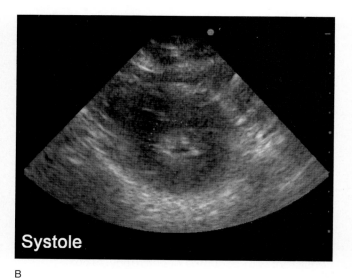

B

Figure 6-63. Short-axis views of hyperdynamic heart in a patient with significant volume depletion. (A) Measurement of a small left ventricular end-diastolic area (3.3 cm^2). (B) Nearly complete obliteration of the left ventricle during systole.

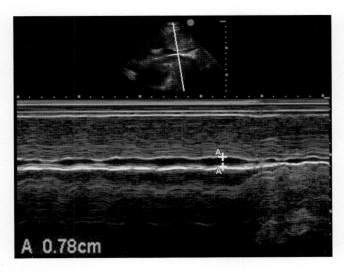

Figure 6-64. Small IVC. M-mode of the IVC in a patient with significant volume depletion. The largest diameter of the IVC during the respiratory cycle is <10 mm (0.78 cm), which is consistent with volume depletion.

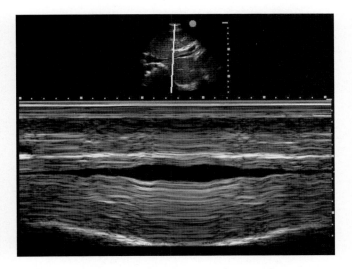

Figure 6-65. IVC distensibility. M-mode of the IVC in a mechanically ventilated patient. Distension of the IVC of >18% during insufflation predicts fluid responsiveness.

VOLUME DEPLETION AND FLUID RESPONSIVENESS

Signs of significant volume depletion on cardiac ultrasound are a hyperdynamic left ventricle with a small left ventricular end-diastolic area (<10 cm^2) and/or complete obliteration of the left ventricle during systole (Figure 6-63). A small IVC that measures <10 mm in diameter at its largest during the respiratory cycle (during expiration in spontaneously breathing patients and during insufflation in ventilated patients) is also consistent with significant volume depletion (Figure 6-64).

It is important to understand the concept of fluid responsiveness and why predicting fluid responsiveness is different from estimating CVP. The definition of fluid responsiveness is a positive hemodynamic response (increase in stroke volume of ≥15%) with a fluid bolus of 500 mL of crystalloid. The importance of differentiating between fluid responsiveness and CVP is based on the recognition that excess fluid can be harmful and that only about half of patients with septic shock have a positive hemodynamic response to a fluid bolus. In addition, CVP has been proven to be a poor predictor of fluid responsiveness. Parameters that have been shown to be good predictors of fluid responsiveness are an increase in the diameter (distensibility) of the IVC of >18% with insufflation in mechanically ventilated patients, stroke volume variation of >12% with the respiratory cycle in mechanically ventilated patients, and an increase in stroke volume of >15% with passive leg raising in both ventilated and spontaneously breathing patients (Figures 6-65, 6-66 and 6-7).

VALVULAR ABNORMALITIES

Patients with valvular abnormalities may be asymptomatic with incidental abnormal findings, symptomatic from acute decompensation from a chronic valve abnormality, or hemodynamically unstable from an acute severe valvular abnormality (usually acute regurgitation). A severe acute valve abnormality may be difficult to

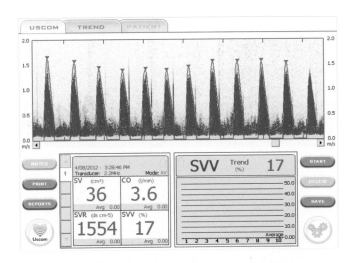

Figure 6-66. Stroke volume variation (SVV). This image demonstrates the measurement of the SVV with the USCOM device, which uses a nonimaging pencil transducer with continuous wave Doppler to measure flow in the left ventricular outflow tract. SVV of >12% with mechanical ventilations predicts fluid responsiveness. (Reproduced with permission from Rob Phillips, Uscom, Ltd. http://www.uscom.com.au)

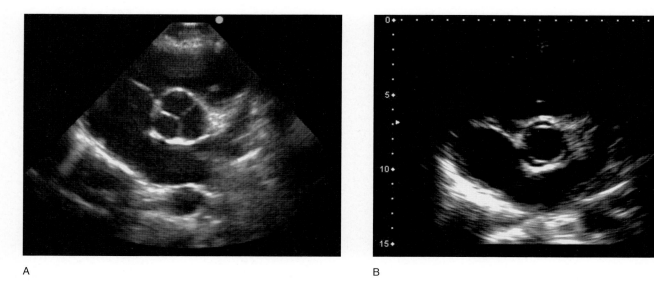

A   B

Figure 6-67. Aortic valve in the parasternal short-axis view. (A) Normal appearance in the closed position ("Mercedes Benz sign"). Bicuspid valves may have similar appearance when closed. (B) Visualization in the opened position rules out a bicuspid aortic valve and aortic stenosis.

recognize because the heart may look grossly normal or just hyperdynamic. Acute mitral regurgitation may result from rupture of a chorda tendinea or papillary muscle and acute aortic regurgitation may be associated with proximal aortic dissection. Chronic severe valvular abnormalities are often associated with significant cardiac dysfunction and chamber enlargement, so it is prudent to consider assessing valvular function in patients with these findings.

Valvular Stenosis

The initial evaluation for valvular stenosis can be accomplished using visual estimation. If good-quality images are obtained, valve opening can be well visualized and significant mitral and aortic stenosis can be ruled out very quickly.

Ruling out aortic stenosis may be straightforward if good 2D images of the aortic valve are obtained. Two cusps of the aortic valve (right coronary cusp and noncoronary cusp) are usually well visualized on the parasternal long-axis view, and a widely opened valve is easy to recognize (Figure 6-32). In the parasternal short-axis view, all three cusps of the aortic valve may be visualized in both the opened and closed position (Figure 6-67). It is important to visualize the valve in the opened position when trying to rule out a bicuspid valve because bicuspid aortic valves often have fusion of the right and left coronary cusps with a raphe replacing the inferior commissure, so the valve may look normal in the closed position (Figure 6-67A). Stenotic valves usually have significant thickening and calcifica-

tion, so a grossly abnormal valve should increase suspicion for stenosis. However, significant aortic thickening and calcific changes are present in about 25% of elderly patients, and the incidence of aortic stenosis is only a few percent, so most patients with these findings do not have aortic stenosis.

Calculation of the aortic valve area is usually accomplished with CW Doppler measurements at the level of the valve orifice and at the level of the LVOT. These measurements are placed into the continuity equation and the valve area is calculated (Table 6-8). An aortic valve area of 1.0–1.5 cm^2 is consistent with mild aortic stenosis, an area of 0.75–1.0 cm^2 is consistent with moderate stenosis, and an area <0.75 cm^2 is consistent with severe stenosis.

Potentially easier methods for determining significant aortic stenosis are to measure the maximal aortic jet velocity with CW Doppler or the maximal aortic cusp separation using M-mode imaging. Maximal jet velocity is the single highest velocity jet of flow that can be measured in the aortic valve region from any window using CW Doppler. A maximum jet velocity of 3–4 m/s is consistent with mild aortic stenosis and a maximal jet velocity >4 m/s is diagnostic of severe aortic stenosis.[332] Assessment of the aortic valve area by measurement of the maximal aortic cusp separation requires a good-quality parasternal long-axis view with the open valve cusps and proximal aorta aligned horizontally on the ultrasound image. Place the M-mode cursor through the aortic valve cusps. Normal aortic valve cusps are in close proximity to the walls of the proximal aorta when the valve is open and meet in the middle of the aorta when the valve is closed, giving a distinct M-mode

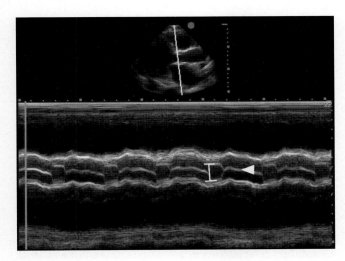

Figure 6-68. M-mode tracing of the aortic valve. The M-mode cursor is directed through the aortic valve cusps in the parasternal long-axis view and demonstrates the valve in the opened (measured) and closed (arrowhead) position. Measurement of the maximal aortic cusp separation estimates the aortic valve area.

pattern (Figure 6-68). Maximal aortic cusp separation >15 mm is normal, 12–15 mm is consistent with mild aortic stenosis, and <8 is consistent with severe aortic stenosis.[352]

Visual estimation to assess for mitral stenosis is usually straightforward. The mitral valve is often best visualized in the parasternal long-axis view and a widely opened valve is easy to recognize (Figure 6-69A). In addition, the area of the mitral valve orifice can eas-

ily be measured by 2D planimetry. To measure the valve with planimetry, a parasternal short-axis view is obtained and the mitral valve is traced at the point of maximal opening, at the level of the tips of the mitral valve (Figure 6-69B). Normal MVA is 4–6 cm^2, a valve area 1.0–1.5 cm^2 is consistent with moderate stenosis, and an area <1.0 cm^2 is considered severe stenosis. It is important to realize that decreased left ventricular function causes decreased mitral valve opening, which is why EPSS is useful (Figure 6-52A). Therefore, providers must differentiate mitral stenosis from severe left ventricular dysfunction by assessing the ventricle and the appearance of the valve during diastole. A stenotic mitral valve has a distinctive appearance with ballooning and a "hockey stick" shaped anterior leaflet during diastole (see Figure 6-90B).

Several genetic valvular anomalies may be easy to recognize with visual inspection of valve location and movement, and by recognition of abnormal chamber sizes (Figure 6-70).

Valvular Regurgitation

Color Doppler is the primary initial ultrasound test for valvular regurgitation. The angle of interrogation and the scale are the two most important factors when screening for regurgitant flow with color Doppler imaging. The color scale is optimal when it is adjusted to the highest possible velocity that still allows visualization of the regurgitation jet. Decreasing the size of the sampling box will allow the scale to be increased. The mitral valve is best evaluated in the apical four-chamber view or the parasternal long-axis view, the aortic valve is best evaluated in the parasternal long-axis view, the tricuspid valve

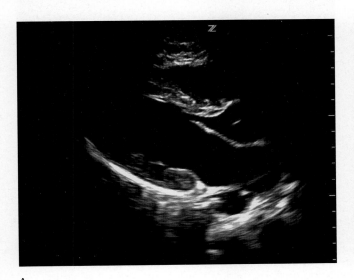

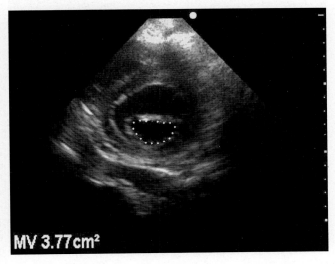

A

B

Figure 6-69. Normal mitral valve with obviously good opening in the parasternal long-axis view (A). Planimetry of the mitral valve in the parasternal short-axis view (B) with a valve area of 3.77 cm^2, which is consistent with minimal/mild mitral stenosis.

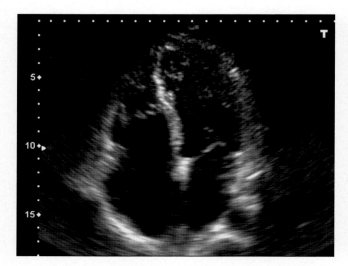

Figure 6-70. Ebstein's anomaly. Significant apical displacement of the tricuspid valve is noted on an apical four-chamber view. This congenital anomaly results in tricuspid stenosis and regurgitation and often requires surgical repair.

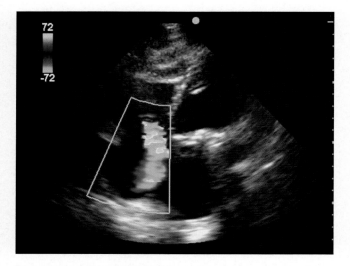

Figure 6-72. Moderate/severe tricuspid regurgitation. In the apical four-chamber view, color Doppler across the tricuspid valve reveals an eccentric jet with a wide vena contracta (neck) that extends to the opposite wall of the atria.

can be evaluated in the apical four-chamber view or the parasternal short-axis view, and the pulmonary valve can be evaluated in the parasternal short-axis view.

Color Doppler can also be used to judge the severity of valve regurgitation. Normal so-called "physiologic" regurgitation (with a short thin regurgitant jet) is com-

monly seen in the mitral and tricuspid valves in normal healthy individuals, and is clinically insignificant. Moderate or severe mitral and tricuspid regurgitation is consistent with a large regurgitant jet area (a long, wide jet). Regurgitant jets that occupy >40% of the atrial area and/or extend to the opposite wall of the atria are considered severe (Figures 6-71 and 6-72). Aortic

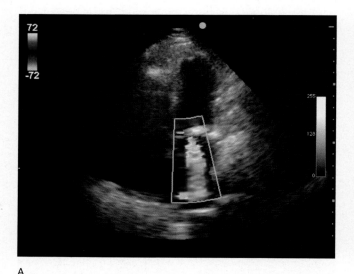

A   B

Figure 6-71. Mitral regurgitation. Apical four-chamber views demonstrating free (A) and eccentric (B) regurgitant jets. (A) A free jet occurs centrally and is easier to quantify as mild or severe, because it is clearly visualized in the center of the atria. (B) Eccentric jets are typically seen with flail leaflets or leaflet prolapse and are directed into the wall of the receiving chamber. Eccentric jets appear smaller in area than free jets, even when the regurgitant orifice area is the same, so their hemodynamic significance may be misjudged.

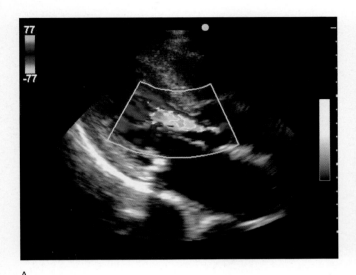

A

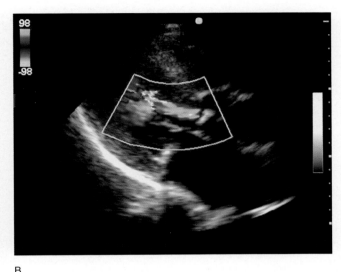

B

Figure 6-73. Severe aortic regurgitation in parasternal long-axis views. These images are from the same patient and demonstrate the importance of adjusting the color Doppler scale to the highest possible velocity. When the scale is set at –77 to 77 the regurgitant jet is a mixture of colors due to high velocity flow aliasing (A). When the color scale is adjusted upward, the blue regurgitant jet is more representative of the magnitude and direction of the flow (B). In this patient, the regurgitant jet occupies almost the entire width of the left ventricular outflow tract (>65%).

regurgitation is rare in normal healthy individuals. Aortic regurgitation is best seen in the parasternal long-axis view. The severity of aortic regurgitation is based on the regurgitant jet height (width) and the ratio of the jet height to the height (width) of the LVOT. Regurgitant jets that occupy >65% of the height of the LVOT are considered severe (Figure 6-73).

PLACEMENT OF EMERGENCY CARDIAC PACEMAKER

Please see Chapter 8 "Critical Care" for discussion.

MYOCARDIAL ISCHEMIA

Abnormal wall motion and abnormal ventricular emptying or relaxation characterizes left ventricular dysfunction. Ultrasound findings of acute left ventricular ischemia or infarction typically include wall motion abnormalities, usually regional in the distribution of a coronary artery or its branch, but without evidence of chronic thinning or scarring of the wall (Figure 6-74). Wall motion is graded as hypokinesis (reduced ventricular wall thickening and motion), akinesis (absent wall thickening and motion), and dyskinesia (paradoxical motion of the wall—outward movement of the wall during systole).[92,102] Ultrasound findings of chronic left ventricular in-

farction include a dilated left ventricle, global wall motion abnormalities with thinning of the ventricular wall (<7 mm or 30% less than the adjacent normal wall), and increased echogenicity of the segment due to fibrotic changes (Figure 6-75A,B).

Assessment of wall thickening requires ultrasound visualization of the myocardium and endocardium, which can be significantly limited for the typical emergency or critically ill patient. Contrast echocardiography provides a much better assessment of global and regional wall motion and has been proven to be very useful for assessing regional wall motion in ED patients with chest pain and potential acute coronary syndrome.[353–355] Wall motion may be characterized by

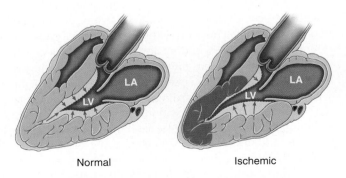

Normal   Ischemic

Figure 6-74. Wall motion abnormality.

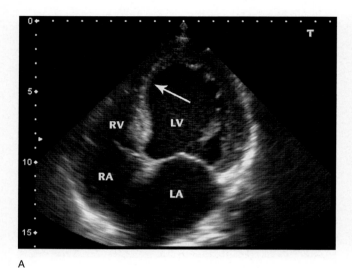
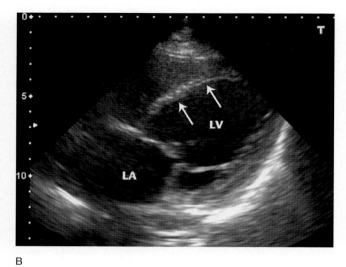

A

B

Figure 6-75. Chronic left ventricular infarction. Apical four-chamber view (A) demonstrates thinning and increased echogenicity of the apical septum (arrow) with increased size of LV and LA chambers. Subcostal four-chamber view (B) shows chronic thinning of the entire septum (arrows). RV = right ventricle, RA = right atrium, LV = left ventricle, LA = left atrium. (Courtesy of Hennepin County Medical Center)

gross ventricular wall dysfunction or segmental wall motion defects that usually follow the distribution of coronary vasculature (Figures 6-76 and 6-77). Multiple views of the left ventricle and a knowledge of the coronary vascular anatomy are required if the goal is to determine the region affected and correlate findings with the ECG (Figure 6-78A–D). In addition to improving visualization of the endocardial border and the myocardium, infusion of IV contrast also allows for assessment of regional myocardial perfusion, which provides significant additional information and value in the evaluation of patients presenting to the ED with chest pain.[354]

PROXIMAL AORTIC DISSECTION

Patients with a proximal thoracic aortic dissection often have a dilated aortic root (>3.5 cm), which is easily visualized on the parasternal long-axis view. An intimal flap can sometimes be seen within the dilated aortic root (Figure 6-79). The descending aorta may also be seen on the parasternal long-axis view in cross section posterior to the mitral valve. The arch of the aorta may be seen with transthoracic echocardiography using a suprasternal window. A dissection within the aortic arch or descending thoracic aorta may be seen in this view (Figure 6-80). In addition to the linear flap, aortic dissection is characterized on echocardiography as having two lumens, true and false, with different flow patterns. This may be best demonstrated using transesophageal views.

► COMMON VARIANTS AND SELECTED ABNORMALITIES

ASCENDING AORTIC ANEURYSM

Dilation of the ascending aorta over 1.5 times the normal segment may reflect an aneurysmal change (Figure 6-81). A true aneurysm of the ascending aorta involves all layers of the vessel wall. A false aneurysm, or pseudoaneurysm, involves a penetration of the intima and media layers only. Most thoracic aneurysms are fusiform but may be saccular. Concomitant aortic dissection may occur as well.

On echocardiography, the aorta is usually measured at several locations: aortic annulus, aortic leaflet tips, ascending aorta, aortic arch, and descending aorta. Note the length and levels of dilatation. As with the abdominal aorta, if the thoracic aorta diameter is measured at 5–6 cm, then obtain cardiothoracic surgery consultation.

The role of transthoracic echocardiography is limited as the aortic arch and descending aorta cannot be fully visualized because of the depth of the aorta in many views. There is also difficulty in viewing the endothelium and poor windows due to intervening bone and air. TEE, CT, and MRI are similar in accuracy for the detection and evaluation of aortic aneurysm and should be ordered if further evaluation is needed beyond transthoracic echocardiography.

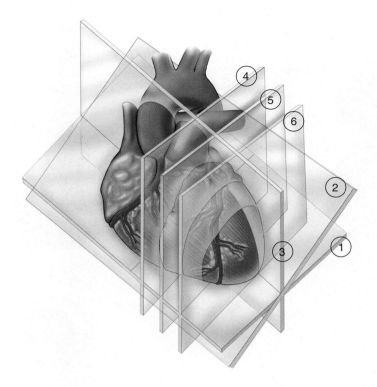

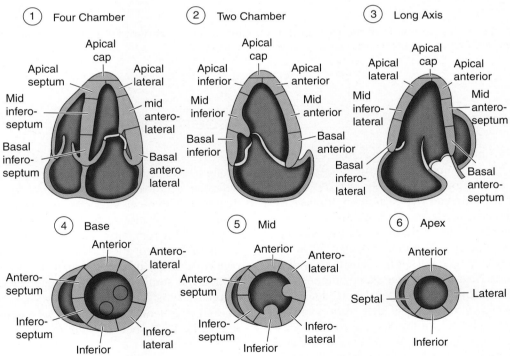

Figure 6-76. Left ventricular wall segments visualized on various cardiac ultrasound views.

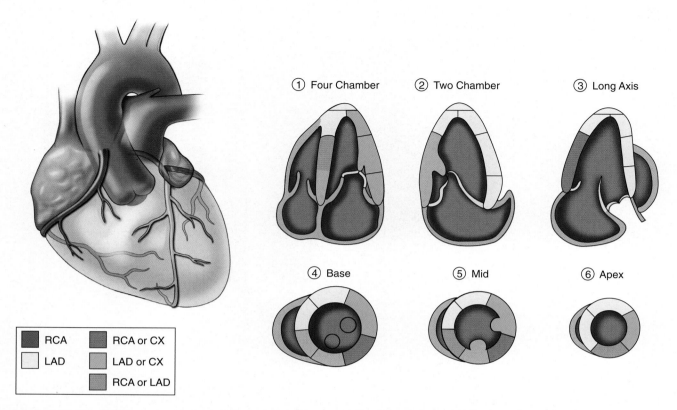

Figure 6-77. Coronary perfusion of the myocardium based on wall segments visualized in various cardiac ultrasound views. Coronary distribution varies between patients.

THROMBUS

While a thrombus may develop in any cardiac chamber, those with low pressure and low flow are at greater risk of developing a thrombus. A thrombus may be hyperechoic, isoechoic, and even hypoechoic in appearance (Figure 6-82). It is usually laminated with the layers paralleling the chamber wall. A thrombus is typically homogeneous with irregular borders, and may fill in the apex of a ventricle or attach itself to a chamber wall or valves of the atria. Near-field or time-gain compensation may have to be adjusted to visualize suspected areas.

Higher-frequency transducers that utilize cardiac scanning windows close to the cardiac chamber in question provide the best imaging. While transesophageal transducers are required for thrombus detection in atria, transthoracic scanning is adequate for thrombus detection within the ventricles in many cases. If color Doppler is available, the swirling vortices of flow may indicate the presence of a thrombus. Normal structures, such as the left atrial appendages, right atrial Chiari network, and right ventricular moderator bands must be distinguished from thrombus.

VEGETATIONS

Findings of irregularities on valvular surfaces should prompt further investigation and consultation for more definitive diagnosis (Figures 6-83 and 6-84). Vegetations may be echogenic or isoechoic and have an irregular appearance. Vegetations may be seen on any valve leaflet or part of the apparatus. Laminated or pedunculated attachments to the leaflet of the valve should prompt suspicion. In general, vegetations do not restrict valvular motion but some valve leaflets may not coapt together correctly. Typical appearance of normal valves includes smooth echogenic leaflets. Refer all suspected cases for TEE and cardiology consultation.

MYXOMA

Myxomas, which are uncommon benign fibrous tumors, are usually attached to a septal wall. Myxomas are usually echogenic, globular, and smooth. They are pedunculated with a stalk on one wall that may or may not be

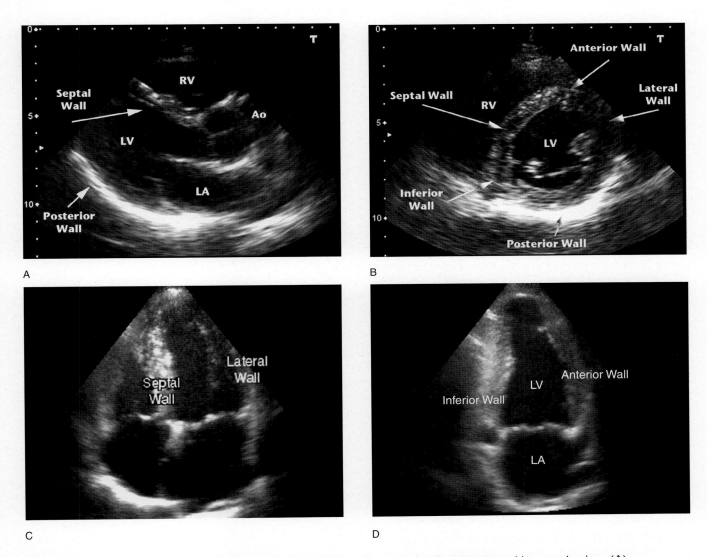

Figure 6-78. Corresponding ultrasound images of LV wall segments in parasternal long-axis view (A), parasternal short-axis view (B), apical four-chamber view (C), and apical two-chamber view (D). RV = right ventricle, LV = left ventricle, Ao = aorta, LA = left atrium.

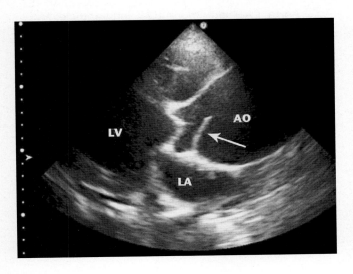

Figure 6-79. Proximal aortic dissection. Parasternal long-axis view shows dilated aortic root and proximal flap (arrow). Ao = aorta, LV = left ventricle, LA = left atrium. (Courtesy of Hennepin County Medical Center)

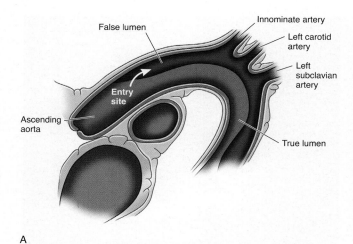

A

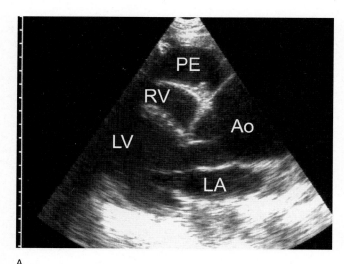

A

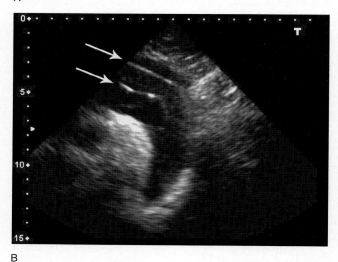

B

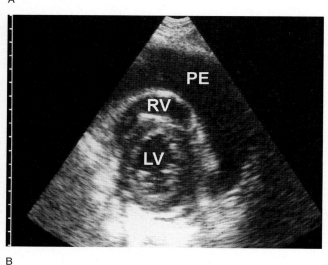

B

Figure 6-80. Type A aortic dissection diagram (A). Suprasternal ultrasound view of the aortic arch (B). The imaging plane crosses the intimal flap in two locations (arrows). (B: Courtesy of Hennepin County Medical Center)

Figure 6-81. Aortic aneurysm. Parasternal long-axis view shows a 6-cm aneurysm in the ascending aorta (A). Pericardial fluid collected anteriorly. The enlarged aorta may be pushing the LV against the posterior pericardial sac. This is best seen on the parasternal short-axis view (B). No intimal flap was found on TEE. Ao = Aorta, LA = left atrium, LV = left ventricle, RV = right ventricle, PE = pericardial effusion. (Courtesy of James Mateer, MD)

visualized. They are usually attached to an atrial wall, most often the left atrium (Figure 6-85A,B).

▶ PITFALLS

1. **Contraindications.** No contraindications exist to transthoracic echocardiography unless its use is interfering with lifesaving procedures and treatments.
2. **Inability to obtain adequate views.** Some patients cannot be imaged well by transthoracic echocardiography. These include patients with subcutaneous emphysema, pneumopericardium, large anterior–posterior girth, and chest wall deformities. Suggestions for improving image acquisition include maintaining transducer contact with the chest wall; use of an adequate amount of conduction gel; use of adjacent cardiac windows; and angling, rotating, and tilting the transducer, as necessary. The patient may be turned in the left lateral decubitus position to bring the heart closer to the anterior chest wall.

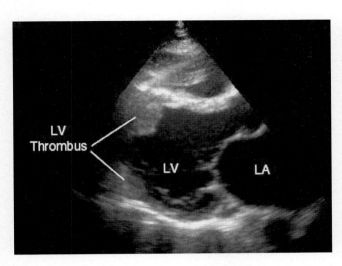

Figure 6-82. A left ventricular thrombus is located near the apex (parasternal long-axis view). LV = left ventricle, LA = left atrium.

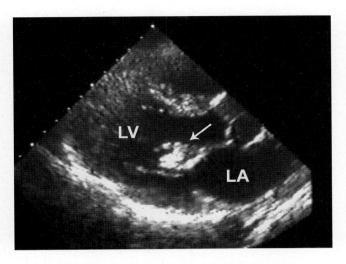

Figure 6-84. Endocarditis. Parasternal long-axis view with echogenic mobile vegetations on the mitral valve leaflets (arrow). LV = left ventricle, LA = left atrium. (Courtesy of Gulfcoast Ultrasound)

a. The subcostal window is a mainstay of the emergency cardiac ultrasound examination during resuscitation of a critically ill patient. Suggestions for improving image acquisition for this view include ensuring the transducer is at a shallow angle to the plane of the body (15° in general) and moving the transducer to the patient's right in the subcostal space instead of the more intuitive left side. This helps to avoid the air-filled stomach and uses the left lobe of the liver as a soft-tissue window. Also, asking the patient to take a deep

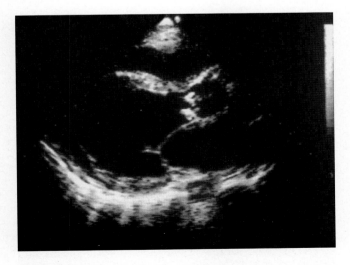

Figure 6-83. Endocarditis. Parasternal long-axis view reveals echogenic mobile vegetations on the aortic valve leaflets. (Courtesy of Gulfcoast Ultrasound)

inspiration or, if the patient is intubated, providing a large tidal volume will help push the heart toward the subcostal space.

b. The parasternal view is often limited by retrosternal air or altered anatomy. Moving the transducer to the left, and then up and down along the anterior–posterior axis may help with obtaining an improved view.

c. The apical view may be improved by changing the angle and aiming the transducer toward the head or right elbow instead of the right shoulder.

3. **Reversed orientation.** Proper imaging requires knowledge of the orientation of the transducer. Reversed orientation may lead the clinician to mistake ventricular enlargement for normal and vice versa. For example, a dilated right ventricle is an important clue for massive PE, but may be falsely identified as normal if a normal left ventricle is viewed on the reversed side of the monitor screen. When ventricle sizes are similar, the right ventricle can be identified on apical four-chamber view by recognizing that the tricuspid valve is positioned closer to the apex than the mitral valve. Another simple technique for confirming proper orientation with the apical four-chamber view is to tilt the transducer anteriorly to visualize the aortic outflow tract, thus obtaining the apical five-chamber view (Figure 6-86).

4. **Fluid versus blood clot or fat.** Fluid (serous pericardial fluid, or defibrinated blood) will

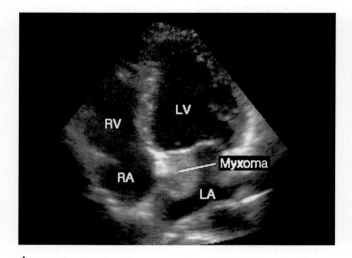

A

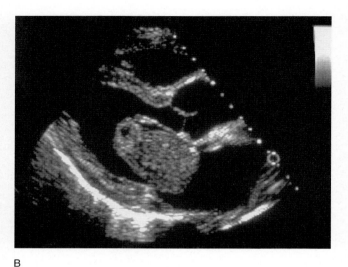

B

Figure 6-85. Left atrial myxoma shown on apical four-chamber view (A). Left atrial myxoma shown on a parasternal long-axis view in a different patient (B). The mass was mobile and prolapsing into the LV on the real-time exam. (Courtesy of Gulfcoast Ultrasound)

appear anechoic. However, a blood clot may be echogenic initially (Figure 6-87). The borders of clot usually have a thin anechoic stripe. Viewing other windows may assist with identifying free fluid in other aspects of the pericardium. Fat is commonly located in the anterior precordial space. In some patients, this appears hypoechoic and can be mistaken for fluid or hematoma. Clues to identification are mildly echoic septations characteristic of fat

and the lack of any dependent pooling of fluid within the posterior pericardial space.

5. **Gain issues.** Gain should be adjusted to allow the posterior aspect of the heart to have the highest time-gain compensation. Cardiac chambers should be anechoic and cardiac structures should be echogenic.

6. **Depth.** Adjust depth to visualize posterior to the cardiac structure in question. Place the focus, if adjustable, at the structure of interest. Too much magnification can alter proper interpretation and too shallow depth can minimize

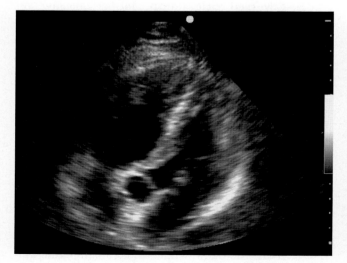

Figure 6-86. Apical five-chamber view in a patient with an enlarged right ventricle. Visualization of the left ventricular outflow tract confirms proper right left orientation.

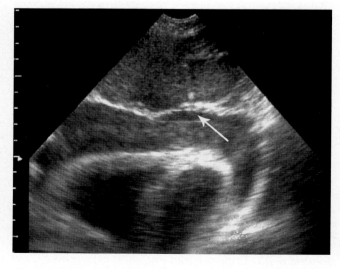

Figure 6-87. Hemopericardium. Echogenic clotted blood with a thin stripe of liquid blood (arrow) is shown in this subcostal view.

pathologic findings. The clinician might miss a large pericardial effusion if the depth is not adequate to capture the entire heart and the large fluid stripe between the right ventricular wall and diaphragm in the subcostal view is mistaken for the right ventricle.

7. **Dynamic range.** Many machines used for point-of-care ultrasound are preset for abdominal applications; this includes the dynamic range setting. In cardiac ultrasound, the image is more black and white. The dynamic range should be lower than the settings used in abdominal or pelvic imaging.

► CASE STUDIES

CASE 1

Patient Presentation

A 64-year-old woman presented to the ED by ambulance in severe respiratory distress. A nebulized albuterol treatment was in progress. She told paramedics that her shortness of breath had become progressively worse over the last several hours. She denied chest pain and any history of cardiac or pulmonary disease. The paramedics communicated that her respiratory distress was worsening.

On physical examination, her respiratory rate was 50–60 breaths per minute and she was using all accessory muscles. She could only speak in two- or three-word sentences due to her dyspnea. Her blood pressure was 161/101 mm Hg, heart rate 136 beats per minute, and oxygen saturation 94% despite receiving 100% supplemental oxygen by nonrebreather mask. Her temperature was normal. Auscultation of her chest revealed diffuse expiratory wheezes, decreased aeration, and a prolonged expiratory phase. There were no crackles appreciated. CV examination revealed tachycardia without murmurs and strong, equal peripheral pulses. Neck examination was without any noticeable jugular venous distention. Lower extremity edema was absent. The remainder of her examination was unremarkable.

Management Course

Two minutes after arrival, a bedside echocardiogram was performed and interpreted by the emergency physician. Notable findings were a dilated left ventricle with obvious severe left ventricular failure and a relatively small right ventricle (Figure 6-88A). The nebulization treatment was stopped and she was given high-flow oxygen and sublingual nitroglycerin. The patient received an IV bolus of furosemide and an IV nitroglycerin infusion was started. By the time her portable chest radiograph was available for viewing (Figure 6-88B) about 15 minutes after arrival, the patient's clinical condition had markedly improved. The chest radiograph confirmed the diagnosis of acute pulmonary edema. An ECG showed sinus tachycardia with nonspecific changes. She was admitted to the cardiac ICU and eventually diagnosed with severe diffuse ischemic cardiomyopathy.

Commentary

Bedside echocardiography was an important tool in the evaluation of this patient's undifferentiated respiratory

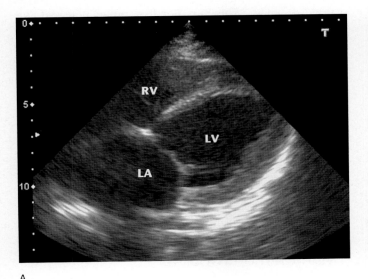

A

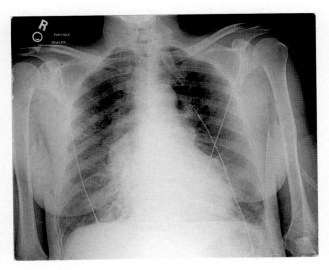

B

Figure 6-88. Case 1: Subcostal four-chamber ultrasound view (A). Portable chest radiograph (B). (Courtesy of Hennepin County Medical Center)

distress. The course of treatment delivered to this critically ill patient in the ED was significantly altered by the information provided by bedside echocardiography. Even though the patient could not tolerate lying flat, subcostal transducer positioning provided adequate visualization of her left ventricular dysfunction. This vital piece of information would not have been detectable by any other diagnostic modality within 2 minutes of the patient's arrival.

CASE 2

Patient Presentation

A 52-year-old man presented to the ED with vague, non-radiating chest pain over the previous 2–3 hours, gradual in onset over about 30 minutes. The patient had not experienced any significant shortness of breath, nausea, or palpitations. He acknowledged a history of inconsistently controlled hypertension over the past 20 years and a 40 pack-year history of smoking cigarettes.

On physical examination, blood pressure was noted at 182/100 mm Hg, heart rate 87 beats per minute, respiratory rate 15 breaths per minute, and oxygen saturation 98% on room air. The patient was afebrile. Head, neck, pulmonary, abdominal, and back examinations were unremarkable. CV examination revealed normal heart sounds without murmurs. Normal and equal peripheral pulses were palpable in the upper and lower extremities.

Management Course

The patient was given an aspirin and sublingual nitroglycerin without improvement. Morphine sulfate provided some relief. His ECG showed normal sinus rhythm and nonspecific ST changes. Chest radiograph was negative for pneumothorax and showed a normal appearing mediastinum. Laboratory studies, including the initial cardiac enzyme, were unremarkable. The patient was considered to have nonspecific but concerning chest pain and plans were made for observation unit admission, serial cardiac enzymes, cardiac monitoring, and further cardiac workup. As part of a routine chest pain evaluation, the emergency physician performed bedside echocardiography and noted a dilated aortic root with a diameter of 4.2 cm (Figure 6-89). Contrast-enhanced CT of the thoracic aorta confirmed suspicions of a proximal aortic dissection. CV surgery was emergently consulted and a timely repair was performed without incident.

Commentary

Case 2 exemplifies the utility of routine bedside echocardiography by emergency physicians during the evaluation of nonspecific chest pain. This patient's aortic dis-

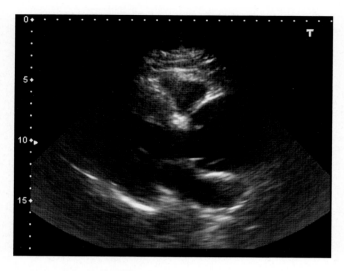

Figure 6-89. Case 2: Parasternal long-axis ultrasound view.

section may have caused a myocardial infarction, aortic valve failure, cardiac tamponade, or death had it not been identified in the ED. Patients with aortic dissection often present without classic symptoms or physical findings. Bedside echocardiography performed by emergency physicians can provide essential information to help expedite disposition and treatment.

CASE 3

Patient Presentation

A 30-year-old pregnant woman, 31-weeks gestational age, presented to the ED with 1 day of severe shortness of breath. This was her first pregnancy and she had regular prenatal care and an uncomplicated course. She was a recent immigrant from East Africa and reported no significant past medical history. She had mild swelling of her ankles, which was unchanged during the past few months. On physical examination, blood pressure was 105/60 mm Hg, heart rate 96 beats per minute, respiratory rate 20 breaths per minute, temperature 97°F, and oxygen saturation 97% on room air. The patient was in no distress. Abdominal exam revealed a gravid uterus consistent with the stated gestational age. Pulmonary exam revealed diffuse wheezes. There was no murmur appreciated on the initial cardiac examination. There was no appreciable jugular venous distension and minimal ankle edema.

Management Course

Initially she was thought to have reactive airway disease and given a nebulized albuterol treatment without improvement. There was concern for PE given the patient's

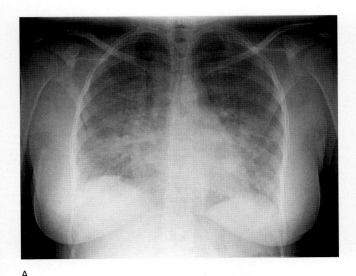

A

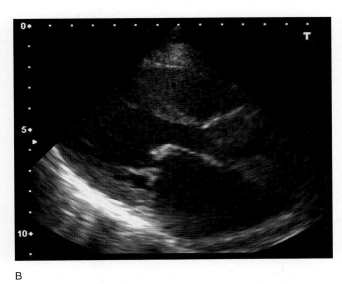

B

Figure 6-90. Case 3: Portable chest radiograph (A). Parasternal long-axis ultrasound view (B). The distinctive "hockey stick" shape of the anterior mitral leaflet is consistent with mitral stenosis.

severe symptoms and gestational status. ECG showed a normal sinus rhythm at 95 beats per minute with a small R wave in lead V_1. Cardiac enzymes were in the normal range, but the patient's chest radiograph showed pulmonary edema (Figure 6-90A). The tentative diagnosis was peripartum cardiomyopathy. Bedside echocardiography was performed by the emergency physician and showed normal left ventricular size and function, significant LAE, and obvious severe mitral stenosis (Figure 6-90B). Even after the diagnosis was established, a murmur could not be appreciated by several staff physicians. The patient was admitted to the intensive care unit (ICU) and had a cesarean section delivery the next day.

Commentary

This case shows the utility of point-of-care cardiac ultrasound for patients with undifferentiated shortness of breath and to determine the underlying etiology in patients with pulmonary edema. This patient had no past medical history, but emigrated from east Africa, where rheumatic valve disease is common. Also, she was in the third trimester of pregnancy and patients with significant mitral stenosis often experience hemodynamic deterioration during the third trimester or during labor and delivery. Additional displacement of blood volume into the systemic circulation during contractions makes labor particularly hazardous; therefore the patient had optimal medical management and early delivery via cesarean section. As is common in emergent settings, no murmur could be appreciated because the patient was in significant distress and had a rapid respiratory rate with

expiratory wheezes. This case demonstrates the significant limitations of the stethoscope and other parts of the physical exam, and highlights the utility of point-of-care cardiac ultrasound in patients with severe valve disease.

► ACKNOWLEDGMENTS

The authors thank Ben Dolan, MD and Sanjay Vasudeva, MD for their contributions to this chapter.

REFERENCES

1. Jehle D, et al.: Emergency department sonography by emergency physicians. *Am J Emerg Med* 7:605, 1989.
2. Mayron R, Gaudio FE, Plummer D, Asinger R, Elsperger J: Echocardiography performed by emergency physicians: Impact on diagnosis and therapy. *Ann Emerg Med* 17:150, 1988.
3. Plummer D: Principles of emergency ultrasound and echocardiography. *Ann Emerg Med* 18:1291, 1989.
4. Aguilera PA, Durham BA, Riley DA: Emergency transvenous cardiac pacing placement using ultrasound guidance. *Ann Emerg Med* 36:224, 2000.
5. Azim A, Rao PB, Srivastav P, Singh P: Cardiac tamponade mimicking septic shock diagnosed by early echocardiography. *J Emerg Trauma Shock* 3:306, 2010.
6. Blaivas M: Incidence of pericardial effusion in patients presenting to the emergency department with unexplained dyspnea. *Acad Emerg Med* 8:1143, 2001.
7. Blaivas M: Transesophageal echocardiography during cardiopulmonary arrest in the emergency department. *Resuscitation* 78:135, 2008.

8. Blaivas M, Fox JC: Outcome in cardiac arrest patients found to have cardiac standstill on the bedside emergency department echocardiogram. *Acad Emerg Med* 8:616, 2001.

9. Blehar DJ, Dickman E, Gaspari R: Identification of congestive heart failure via respiratory variation of inferior vena cava diameter. *Am J Emerg Med* 27:71, 2009.

10. Bocka JJ, Overton DT, Hauser A: Electromechanical dissociation in human beings: An echocardiographic evaluation. *Ann Emerg Med* 17:450, 1988.

11. Borloz MP, Frohna WJ, Phillips CA, Antonis MS: Emergency department focused bedside echocardiography in massive pulmonary embolism. *J Emerg Med* 41:658, 2011.

12. Bottiger BW, et al.: Efficacy and safety of thrombolytic therapy after initially unsuccessful cardiopulmonary resuscitation: A prospective clinical trial. *Lancet* 357:1583, 2001.

13. Breitkreutz R, et al.: Focused echocardiographic evaluation in life support and peri-resuscitation of emergency patients: A prospective trial. *Resuscitation* 81:1527, 2010.

14. Breitkreutz R, Walcher F, Seeger FH: Focused echocardiographic evaluation in resuscitation management: Concept of an advanced life support-conformed algorithm. *Crit Care Med* 35:S150, 2007.

15. Brunette DD: Twelve years of emergency medicine at Hennepin County Medical Center. Changing critical care experience. *Minn Med* 82:42, 1999.

16. Byrne MW, Czuczman AD, Hwang JQ: Images in emergency medicine. Elderly female with syncope. Venous thromboembolism in transit. *Ann Emerg Med* 58:105, 2011.

17. Chen L, Hsiao A, Langhan M, Riera A, Santucci KA: Use of bedside ultrasound to assess degree of dehydration in children with gastroenteritis. *Acad Emerg Med* 17:1042, 2010.

18. Cheng AB, Levine DA, Tsung JW, Phoon CK: Emergency physician diagnosis of pediatric infective endocarditis by point-of-care echocardiography. *Am J Emerg Med* 30:386.e1–e3, 2012.

19. Davis DP, Campbell CJ, Poste JC, Ma G: The association between operator confidence and accuracy of ultrasonography performed by novice emergency physicians. *J Emerg Med* 29:259, 2005.

20. Doniger SJ: Bedside emergency cardiac ultrasound in children. *J Emerg Trauma Shock* 3:282, 2010.

21. Doostan DK, Steffenson SL, Snoey ER: Cerebral and coronary air embolism: An intradepartmental suicide attempt. *J Emerg Med* 25:29, 2003.

22. Durham B: Emergency medicine physicians saving time with ultrasound. *Am J Emerg Med* 14:309, 1996.

23. Elavunkal J, Bright L, Stone MB: Emergency ultrasound identification of loculated pericardial effusion: The importance of multiple cardiac views. *Acad Emerg Med* 18:e29, 2011.

24. Ettin D, Cook T: Using ultrasound to determine external pacer capture. *J Emerg Med* 17:1007, 1999.

25. Fields JM, et al.: The interrater reliability of inferior vena cava ultrasound by bedside clinician sonographers in emergency department patients. *Acad Emerg Med* 18:98, 2011.

26. Frazee BW, Snoey ER: Diagnostic role of ED ultrasound in deep venous thrombosis and pulmonary embolism. *Am J Emerg Med* 17:271, 1999.

27. Hart D, Budhram G, Reardon R, Clinton J: Bedside echocardiography in the management of a thoracic stab wound with early pericardial tamponade. *Acad Emerg Med* 15:1322, 2008.

28. Hayhurst C, et al.: An evaluation of echo in life support (ELS): Is it feasible? What does it add? *Emerg Med J* 28:119, 2011.

29. Heller MB: Emergency ultrasound: echoes of the future. *Ann Emerg Med* 23:1353, 1994.

30. Heller MB, Verdile VP: Ultrasonography in emergency medicine. *Emerg Med Clin North Am* 10:27, 1992.

31. Hellmann DB, et al.: The rate at which residents learn to use hand-held echocardiography at the bedside. *Am J Med* 118:1010, 2005.

32. Johnson ME, Furlong R, Schrank K: Diagnostic use of emergency department echocardiogram in massive pulmonary emboli. *Ann Emerg Med* 21:760, 1992.

33. Jones AE, Craddock PA, Tayal VS, Kline JA: Diagnostic accuracy of left ventricular function for identifying sepsis among emergency department patients with nontraumatic symptomatic undifferentiated hypotension. *Shock* 24:513, 2005.

34. Jones AE, Tayal VS, Kline JA: Focused training of emergency medicine residents in goal-directed echocardiography: A prospective study. *Acad Emerg Med* 10:1054, 2003.

35. Jones AE, Tayal VS, Sullivan DM, Kline JA: Randomized, controlled trial of immediate versus delayed goal-directed ultrasound to identify the cause of nontraumatic hypotension in emergency department patients. *Crit Care Med* 32:1703, 2004.

36. Kosiak W, Swieton D, Piskunowicz M: Sonographic inferior vena cava/aorta diameter index, a new approach to the body fluid status assessment in children and young adults in emergency ultrasound–preliminary study. *Am J Emerg Med* 26:320, 2008.

37. Lyon M, Blaivas M, Brannam L: Sonographic measurement of the inferior vena cava as a marker of blood loss. *Am J Emerg Med* 23:45, 2005.

38. MacCarthy P, Worrall A, McCarthy G, Davies J: The use of transthoracic echocardiography to guide thrombolytic therapy during cardiac arrest due to massive pulmonary embolism. *Emerg Med J* 19:178, 2002.

39. Madan A, Schwartz C: Echocardiographic visualization of acute pulmonary embolus and thrombolysis in the ED. *Am J Emerg Med* 22:294, 2004.

40. Mandavia DP, Hoffner RJ, Mahaney K, Henderson SO: Bedside echocardiography by emergency physicians. *Ann Emerg Med* 38:377, 2001.

41. Mazurek B, Jehle D, Martin M: Emergency department echocardiography in the diagnosis and therapy of cardiac tamponade. *J Emerg Med* 9:27, 1991.

42. Miller JB, et al.: Inferior vena cava assessment in the bedside diagnosis of acute heart failure. *Am J Emerg Med* 30:778–83, 2012.

43. Moore CL, Copel JA: Point-of-care ultrasonography. *N Engl J Med* 364:749, 2011.

44. Moore CL, et al.: Determination of left ventricular function by emergency physician echocardiography of hypotensive patients. *Acad Emerg Med* 9:186, 2002.

45. Moore CL, et al.: Tissue Doppler of early mitral filling correlates with simulated volume loss in healthy subjects. *Acad Emerg Med* 17:1162, 2010.

46. Nagdev A, Stone MB: Point-of-care ultrasound evaluation of pericardial effusions: Does this patient have cardiac tamponade? *Resuscitation* 82:671, 2011.

47. Nagdev AD, Merchant RC, Tirado-Gonzalez A, Sisson CA, Murphy MC: Emergency department bedside ultrasonographic measurement of the caval index for noninvasive determination of low central venous pressure. *Ann Emerg Med* 55:290, 2010.

48. Nazerian P, et al.: Diagnostic accuracy of emergency Doppler echocardiography for identification of acute left ventricular heart failure in patients with acute dyspnea: Comparison with Boston criteria and N-terminal prohormone brain natriuretic peptide. *Acad Emerg Med* 17:18, 2010.

49. Perera P, Mailhot T, Riley D, Mandavia D: The RUSH exam: Rapid Ultrasound in SHock in the evaluation of the critically Ill. *Emerg Med Clin North Am* 28:29, 2010.

50. Perkins AM, Liteplo A, Noble VE: Ultrasound diagnosis of type a aortic dissection. *J Emerg Med* 38:490, 2010.

51. Pershad J, Chin T: Early detection of cardiac disease masquerading as acute bronchospasm: The role of bedside limited echocardiography by the emergency physician. *Pediatr Emerg Care* 19:E1, 2003.

52. Pershad J, et al.: Bedside limited echocardiography by the emergency physician is accurate during evaluation of the critically ill patient. *Pediatrics* 114:e667, 2004.

53. Plummer D: Diagnostic ultrasonography in the emergency department. *Ann Emerg Med* 22:592, 1993.

54. Plummer D: Whose turf is it, anyway? Diagnostic ultrasonography in the emergency department. *Acad Emerg Med* 7:186, 2000.

55. Plummer D, Brunette D, Asinger R, Ruiz E: Emergency department echocardiography improves outcome in penetrating cardiac injury. *Ann Emerg Med* 21:709, 1992.

56. Plummer D, Dick C, Ruiz E, Clinton J, Brunette D: Emergency department two-dimensional echocardiography in the diagnosis of nontraumatic cardiac rupture. *Ann Emerg Med* 23:1333, 1994.

57. Plummer D, et al.: Ultrasound in HEMS: Its role in differentiating shock states. *Air Med J* 22:33, 2003.

58. Randazzo MR, Snoey ER, Levitt MA, Binder K: Accuracy of emergency physician assessment of left ventricular ejection fraction and central venous pressure using echocardiography. *Acad Emerg Med* 10:973, 2003.

59. Riley DC, Cordi HP: Emergency department diagnosis of mitral stenosis and left atrial thrombus using bedside ultrasonography. *Acad Emerg Med* 17:e30, 2010.

60. Riley DC, Rezvankhoo K, Yi DH: Emergency department diagnosis of submassive pulmonary embolism using bedside ultrasonography. *Acad Emerg Med* 17:e78, 2010.

61. Rose JS, Bair AE, Mandavia D, Kinser DJ: The UHP ultrasound protocol: A novel ultrasound approach to the empiric evaluation of the undifferentiated hypotensive patient. *Am J Emerg Med* 19:299, 2001.

62. Salen P, et al.: Does the presence or absence of sonographically identified cardiac activity predict resuscitation outcomes of cardiac arrest patients? *Am J Emerg Med* 23:459, 2005.

63. Salen P, et al.: Can cardiac sonography and capnography be used independently and in combination to predict resuscitation outcomes? *Acad Emerg Med* 8:610, 2001.

64. Schefold JC, et al.: Inferior vena cava diameter correlates with invasive hemodynamic measures in mechanically ventilated intensive care unit patients with sepsis. *J Emerg Med* 38:632, 2010.

65. Schiavone WA, et al.: The use of echocardiography in the emergency management of nonpenetrating traumatic cardiac rupture. *Ann Emerg Med* 20:1248, 1991.

66. Scott Bomann J, Osborne M: Emergency physician diagnosis of an atrial septal defect: The bedside bubble study. *Acad Emerg Med* 17:e28, 2010.

67. Secko MA, Lazar JM, Salciccioli LA, Stone MB: Can junior emergency physicians use E-point septal separation to accurately estimate left ventricular function in acutely dyspneic patients? *Acad Emerg Med* 18:1223, 2011.

68. Shafer JS, Treaster MR, Fitzmaurice SC, Liao MM: Emergency bedside ultrasound diagnosis of traumatic cardiac tamponade—A case of blunt cardiac rupture. *Acad Emerg Med* 15:873, 2008.

69. Turturro MA: Emergency echocardiography. *Emerg Med Clin North Am* 10:47, 1992.

70. Wallace DJ, Allison M, Stone MB: Inferior vena cava percentage collapse during respiration is affected by the sampling location: An ultrasound study in healthy volunteers. *Acad Emerg Med* 17:96, 2010.

71. Wang HK, et al.: Cardiac ultrasound helps for differentiating the causes of acute dyspnea with available B-type natriuretic peptide tests. *Am J Emerg Med* 28:987, 2010.

72. Weekes AJ, Quirke DP: Emergency echocardiography. *Emerg Med Clin North Am* 29:759, 2011.

73. Weekes AJ, et al.: Comparison of serial qualitative and quantitative assessments of caval index and left ventricular systolic function during early fluid resuscitation of hypotensive emergency department patients. *Acad Emerg Med* 18:912, 2011.

74. American College of Emergency Physicians. Emergency ultrasound guidelines. *Ann Emerg Med* 53:550, 2009.

75. Labovitz AJ, et al.: Focused cardiac ultrasound in the emergent setting: A consensus statement of the American Society of Echocardiography and American College of Emergency Physicians. *J Am Soc Echocardiogr* 23:1225, 2010.

76. Beaulieu Y: Bedside echocardiography in the assessment of the critically ill. *Crit Care Med* 35:S235, 2007.

77. Beaulieu Y: Specific skill set and goals of focused echocardiography for critical care clinicians. *Crit Care Med* 35:S144, 2007.

78. Beaulieu Y, Marik PE: Bedside ultrasonography in the ICU: Part 2. *Chest* 128:1766, 2005.

79. Beaulieu Y, Marik PE: Bedside ultrasonography in the ICU: Part 1. *Chest* 128:881, 2005.

80. Canty DJ, Royse CF: Audit of anaesthetist-performed echocardiography on perioperative management decisions for non-cardiac surgery. *Br J Anaesth* 103:352, 2009.

81. Cowie B: Focused cardiovascular ultrasound performed by anesthesiologists in the perioperative period: Feasible and alters patient management. *J Cardiothorac Vasc Anesth* 23:450, 2009.

82. Feissel M, Michard F, Faller JP, Teboul JL: The respiratory variation in inferior vena cava diameter as a guide to fluid therapy. *Intensive Care Med* 30:1834, 2004.

83. Feissel M, et al.: Respiratory changes in aortic blood velocity as an indicator of fluid responsiveness in ventilated patients with septic shock. *Chest* 119:867, 2001.

84. Ferrada P, et al.: Limited transthoracic echocardiogram: So easy any trauma attending can do it. *J Trauma* 71:1327, 2011.

85. Ferrada P, et al.: Qualitative assessment of the inferior vena cava: Useful tool for the evaluation of fluid status in critically ill patients. *Am Surg* 78:468, 2012.

86. Ferrada P, Murthi S, Anand RJ, Bochicchio GV, Scalea T: Transthoracic focused rapid echocardiographic examination: Real-time evaluation of fluid status in critically ill trauma patients. *J Trauma* 70:56, 2011.

87. Gruenewald M, et al.: Visual evaluation of left ventricular performance predicts volume responsiveness early after resuscitation from cardiac arrest. *Resuscitation* 82:1553, 2011.

88. Guiotto G, et al.: Inferior vena cava collapsibility to guide fluid removal in slow continuous ultrafiltration: A pilot study. *Intensive Care Med* 36:692, 2010.

89. Gunst M, et al.: Accuracy of cardiac function and volume status estimates using the bedside echocardiographic assessment in trauma/critical care. *J Trauma* 65:509, 2008.

90. Gunst M, et al.: Bedside echocardiographic assessment for trauma/critical care: The BEAT exam. *J Am Coll Surg* 207:e1, 2008.

91. Jensen MB, Sloth E, Larsen KM, Schmidt MB: Transthoracic echocardiography for cardiopulmonary monitoring in intensive care. *Eur J Anaesthesiol* 21:700, 2004.

92. Joseph MX, Disney PJ, Da Costa R, Hutchison SJ: Transthoracic echocardiography to identify or exclude cardiac cause of shock. *Chest* 126:1592, 2004.

93. Kaplan A, Mayo PH: Echocardiography performed by the pulmonary/critical care medicine physician. *Chest* 135:529, 2009.

94. Kimura BJ, Amundson SA, Shaw DJ: Hospitalist use of hand-carried ultrasound: Preparing for battle. *J Hosp Med* 5:163, 2010.

95. Kimura BJ, Bocchicchio M, Willis CL, Demaria AN: Screening cardiac ultrasonographic examination in patients with suspected cardiac disease in the emergency department. *Am Heart J* 142:324, 2001.

96. Kirkpatrick JN, et al.: Effectiveness of echocardiographic imaging by nurses to identify left ventricular systolic dysfunction in high-risk patients. *Am J Cardiol* 95:1271, 2005.

97. Kirkpatrick JN, Ghani SN, Spencer KT: Hand carried echocardiography screening for LV systolic dysfunction in a pulmonary function laboratory. *Eur J Echocardiogr* 9:381, 2008.

98. Kobal SL, Atar S, Siegel RJ: Hand-carried ultrasound improves the bedside cardiovascular examination. *Chest* 126:693, 2004.

99. Kobal SL, et al.: Making an impossible mission possible. *Chest* 125:293, 2004.

100. Lamia B, et al.: Echocardiographic prediction of volume responsiveness in critically ill patients with spontaneously breathing activity. *Intensive Care Med* 33:1125, 2007.

101. Melamed R, Sprenkle MD, Ulstad VK, Herzog CA, Leatherman JW: Assessment of left ventricular function by intensivists using hand-held echocardiography. *Chest* 135:1416, 2009.

102. Monnet X, et al.: Passive leg raising predicts fluid responsiveness in the critically ill. *Crit Care Med* 34:1402, 2006.

103. Niendorff DF, et al.: Rapid cardiac ultrasound of inpatients suffering PEA arrest performed by nonexpert sonographers. *Resuscitation* 67:81, 2005.

104. Poelaert JI, Trouerbach J, De Buyzere M, Everaert J, Colardyn FA: Evaluation of transesophageal echocardiography as a diagnostic and therapeutic aid in a critical care setting. *Chest* 107:774, 1995.

105. Reuter DA, et al.: Stroke volume variations for assessment of cardiac responsiveness to volume loading in mechanically ventilated patients after cardiac surgery. *Intensive Care Med* 28:392, 2002.

106. Reuter DA, et al.: Usefulness of left ventricular stroke volume variation to assess fluid responsiveness in patients with reduced cardiac function. *Crit Care Med* 31:1399, 2003.

107. Rex S, et al.: Prediction of fluid responsiveness in patients during cardiac surgery. *Br J Anaesth* 93:782, 2004.

108. Rozycki GS, et al.: The role of ultrasound in patients with possible penetrating cardiac wounds: A prospective multicenter study. *J Trauma* 46:543, 1999.

109. Ruiz-Bailen M, et al.: Echocardiographic observations during in-hospital cardiopulmonary resuscitation. *Resuscitation* 71:264, 2006.

110. Vieillard-Baron A, et al.: Actual incidence of global left ventricular hypokinesia in adult septic shock. *Crit Care Med* 36:1701, 2008.

111. Vieillard-Baron A, Charron C, Chergui K, Peyrouset O, Jardin F: Bedside echocardiographic evaluation of hemodynamics in sepsis: Is a qualitative evaluation sufficient? *Intensive Care Med* 32:1547, 2006.

112. Vieillard-Baron A, et al.: Acute cor pulmonale in massive pulmonary embolism: incidence, echocardiographic pattern, clinical implications and recovery rate. *Intensive Care Med* 27:1481, 2001.

113. Vieillard-Baron A, Slama M, Cholley B, Janvier G, Vignon P: Echocardiography in the intensive care unit: From evolution to revolution? *Intensive Care Med* 34:243, 2008.

114. Vignon P, et al.: Diagnostic ability of hand-held echocardiography in ventilated critically ill patients. *Crit Care* 7:R84, 2003.

115. Vignon P, et al.: Focused training for goal-oriented handheld echocardiography performed by noncardiologist residents in the intensive care unit. *Intensive Care Med* 33:1795, 2007.

116. Heller K, Joing S, Dolan B, Reardon R: Emergency echocardiography. *Acad Emerg Med* 14:1157, 2007.

117. Neumar RW, et al.: Part 8: adult advanced cardiovascular life support: 2010 American Heart Association Guidelines for Cardiopulmonary Resuscitation and Emergency Cardiovascular Care. *Circulation* 122:S729, 2010.

118. Baker DW, Bahler RC, Finkelhor RS, Lauer MS: Screening for left ventricular systolic dysfunction among patients with risk factors for heart failure. *Am Heart J* 146:736, 2003.

119. Redfield MM, et al.: Burden of systolic and diastolic ventricular dysfunction in the community: Appreciating the scope of the heart failure epidemic. *JAMA* 289:194, 2003.

120. Berryman C: Electromechanical dissociation with directly measurable arterial blood pressure (Abstract). *Ann Emerg Med* 15:1986.

121. Lapostolles F, Le Toumelin P, Agostinucci JM, Catineau J, Adnet F: Basic cardiac life support providers checking the carotid pulse: Performance, degree of conviction, and influencing factors. *Acad Emerg Med* 11:878, 2004.

122. Tsung JW, Blaivas M: Feasibility of correlating the pulse check with focused point-of-care echocardiography during pediatric cardiac arrest: A case series. *Resuscitation* 77:264, 2008.

123. Deakin CD, Low JL: Accuracy of the advanced trauma life support guidelines for predicting systolic blood pressure using carotid, femoral, and radial pulses: observational study. *BMJ* 321:673, 2000.

124. Berg RA, et al.: Part 5: Adult basic life support: 2010 American Heart Association Guidelines for Cardiopulmonary Resuscitation and Emergency Cardiovascular Care. *Circulation* 122:S685, 2010.

125. Aichinger G, et al.: Cardiac movement identified on prehospital echocardiography predicts outcome in cardiac arrest patients. *Prehosp Emerg Care* 16:251–5, 2012.

126. Hendrickson RG, Dean AJ, Costantino TG: A novel use of ultrasound in pulseless electrical activity: The diagnosis of an acute abdominal aortic aneurysm rupture. *J Emerg Med* 21:141, 2001.

127. Tayal VS, Kline JA: Emergency echocardiography to detect pericardial effusion in patients in PEA and near-PEA states. *Resuscitation* 59:315, 2003.

128. Varriale P, Maldonado JM: Echocardiographic observations during in hospital cardiopulmonary resuscitation. *Crit Care Med* 25:1717, 1997.

129. Hernandez C, et al.: C.A.U.S.E: Cardiac arrest ultra-sound exam—A better approach to managing patients in primary non-arrhythmogenic cardiac arrest. *Resuscitation* 76:198, 2008.

130. Prosen G, Krizmaric M, Zavrsnik J, Grmec S: Impact of modified treatment in echocardiographically confirmed pseudo-pulseless electrical activity in out-of-hospital cardiac arrest patients with constant end-tidal carbon dioxide pressure during compression pauses. *J Int Med Res* 38:1458, 2010.

131. Kaul S, et al.: Value of two-dimensional echocardiography for determining the basis of hemodynamic compromise in critically ill patients: A prospective study. *J Am Soc Echocardiogr* 7:598, 1994.

132. Kurkciyan I, et al.: Pulmonary embolism as a cause of cardiac arrest: Presentation and outcome. *Arch Intern Med* 160:1529, 2000.

133. Silfvast T: Cause of death in unsuccessful prehospital resuscitation. *J Intern Med* 229:331, 1991.

134. Bottiger BW, Bohrer H, Bach A, Motsch J, Martin E: Bolus injection of thrombolytic agents during cardiopulmonary resuscitation for massive pulmonary embolism. *Resuscitation* 28:45, 1994.

135. Karavidas A, et al.: Emergency bedside echocardiography as a tool for early detection and clinical decision making in cases of suspected pulmonary embolism—A case report. *Angiology* 51:1021, 2000.

136. Hwang SO, et al.: Compression of the left ventricular outflow tract during cardiopulmonary resuscitation. *Acad Emerg Med* 16:928, 2009.

137. Alsaileek AA, et al.: Predictive value of normal left atrial volume in stress echocardiography. *J Am Coll Cardiol* 47:1024, 2006.

138. Moscati R, Reardon R: Clinical application of the FAST exam. In: Jehle D, Heller M, eds. *Ultrasonography in Trauma: The FAST Exam*. Dallas: American College of Emergency Physicians, 2003:39.

139. Thourani VH, et al.: Penetrating cardiac trauma at an urban trauma center: A 22-year perspective. *Am Surg* 65:811, 1999.

140. Cooper JP, Oliver RM, Currie P, Walker JM, Swanton RH: How do the clinical findings in patients with pericardial effusions influence the success of aspiration? *Br Heart J* 73:351, 1995.

141. Le Winter M, Samar K: Pericardial disease. In: Braunwald, E. ed. *Braunwauld's Heart Disease* Philadelphia, PA: Elsevier, 2005:1757.

142. Spodick DH: Acute cardiac tamponade. *N Engl J Med* 349:684, 2003.

143. Tsang TS, et al.: Clinical and echocardiographic characteristics of significant pericardial effusions following cardiothoracic surgery and outcomes of echo-guided pericardiocentesis for management: Mayo Clinic experience, 1979-1998. *Chest* 116:322, 1999.

144. Tsang TS, Oh JK, Seward JB: Diagnosis and management of cardiac tamponade in the era of echocardiography. *Clin Cardiol* 22:446, 1999.

145. Spodick DH: Pathophysiology of cardiac tamponade. *Chest* 113:1372, 1998.

146. Tsang TS, et al.: Consecutive 1127 therapeutic echocardiographically guided pericardiocenteses: Clinical profile, practice patterns, and outcomes spanning 21 years. *Mayo Clin Proc* 77:429, 2002.

147. Feldman J: Cardiac ultrasound in the ED. *Ann Emerg Med* 18:230, 1989.

148. Tsang TS, Freeman WK, Sinak LJ, Seward JB: Echocardiographically guided pericardiocentesis: Evolution and state-of-the-art technique. *Mayo Clin Proc* 73:647, 1998.

149. Roy CL, Minor MA, Brookhart MA, Choudhry NK: Does this patient with a pericardial effusion have cardiac tamponade? *JAMA* 297:1810, 2007.

150. Fowler NO: Cardiac tamponade. A clinical or an echocardiographic diagnosis? *Circulation* 87:1738, 1993.

151. Beckman MG, Hooper WC, Critchley SE, Ortel TL: Venous thromboembolism: A public health concern. *Am J Prev Med* 38:S495, 2010.

152. CDC website. Deep Vein Thrombosis/Pulmonary Embolism Data & Statistics. http://www.cdc.gov/ncbddd/dvt/data.html, accessed April, 2013.

153. Meyer G: Thrombolytic therapy for pulmonary embolism. *J Mal Vasc* 36 suppl 1:S33, 2011.

154. Konstantinides S: Thrombolysis in submassive pulmonary embolism? Yes. *J Thromb Haemost* 1:1127, 2003.

155. Konstantinides S: Should thrombolytic therapy be used in patients with pulmonary embolism? *Am J Cardiovasc Drugs* 4:69, 2004.

156. Konstantinides S: Pulmonary embolism: Impact of right ventricular dysfunction. *Curr Opin Cardiol* 20:496, 2005.

157. Konstantinides S: Diagnosis and therapy of pulmonary embolism. *Vasa* 35:135, 2006.

158. Konstantinides S, Geibel A, Heusel G, Heinrich F, Kasper W: Heparin plus alteplase compared with heparin alone in patients with submassive pulmonary embolism. *N Engl J Med* 347:1143, 2002.

159. Konstantinides S, Geibel A, Kasper W: Submassive and massive pulmonary embolism: A target for thrombolytic therapy? *Thromb Haemost* 82 (1):104, 1999.

160. Konstantinides S, Hasenfuss G: Acute cor pulmonale in pulmonary embolism. An important prognostic factor and a critical parameter for the choice of a therapeutic strategy. *Internist (Berl)* 45:1155, 2004.

161. Konstantinides S, et al.: Comparison of alteplase versus heparin for resolution of major pulmonary embolism. *Am J Cardiol* 82:966, 1998.

162. Jackson RE, Rudoni RR, Hauser AM, Pascual RG, Hussey ME: Prospective evaluation of two-dimensional transthoracic echocardiography in emergency department patients with suspected pulmonary embolism. *Acad Emerg Med* 7:994, 2000.

163. Carvalho EM, Macedo FI, Panos AL, Ricci M, Salerno TA: Pulmonary embolectomy: Recommendation for early surgical intervention. *J Card Surg* 25:261, 2010.

164. Piazza G, Goldhaber SZ: Fibrinolysis for acute pulmonary embolism. *Vasc Med* 15:419, 2010.

165. Kearon C, et al.: Antithrombotic therapy for venous thromboembolic disease: American College of Chest Physicians Evidence-Based Clinical Practice Guidelines (8th Edition). *Chest* 133:454S, 2008.

166. Jerjes-Sanchez C, et al.: Streptokinase and heparin versus heparin alone in massive pulmonary embolism: A randomized controlled trial. *J Thromb Thrombolysis* 2:227, 1995.

167. Wan S, Quinlan DJ, Agnelli G, Eikelboom JW: Thrombolysis compared with heparin for the initial treatment of pulmonary embolism: A meta-analysis of the randomized controlled trials. *Circulation* 110:744, 2004.

168. Aklog L, Williams CS, Byrne JG, Goldhaber SZ: Acute pulmonary embolectomy: A contemporary approach. *Circulation* 105:1416, 2002.

169. Leacche M, et al.: Modern surgical treatment of massive pulmonary embolism: Results in 47 consecutive patients after rapid diagnosis and aggressive surgical approach. *J Thorac Cardiovasc Surg* 129:1018, 2005.

170. Sareyyupoglu B, et al.: A more aggressive approach to emergency embolectomy for acute pulmonary embolism. *Mayo Clin Proc* 85:785, 2010.

171. Vohra HA, et al.: Early and late clinical outcomes of pulmonary embolectomy for acute massive pulmonary embolism. *Ann Thorac Surg* 90:1747, 2010.

172. Miniati M, et al.: Value of transthoracic echocardiography in the diagnosis of pulmonary embolism: Results of a prospective study in unselected patients. *Am J Med* 110:528, 2001.

173. Roy PM, et al.: Systematic review and meta-analysis of strategies for the diagnosis of suspected pulmonary embolism. *BMJ* 331:259, 2005.

174. Armstrong WF: Echocardiography. In: Braunwald E ed. *Braunwald's Heart Disease* Philadelphia, PA: Elsevier, 2005:187.

175. Kontos MC, Arrowood JA, Paulsen WH, Nixon JV: Early echocardiography can predict cardiac events in emergency department patients with chest pain. *Ann Emerg Med* 31:550, 1998.

176. Picard MH, et al.: Echocardiographic predictors of survival and response to early revascularization in cardiogenic shock. *Circulation* 107:279, 2003.

177. Amico AF, et al.: Superiority of visual versus computerized echocardiographic estimation of radionuclide left ventricular ejection fraction. *Am Heart J* 118:1259, 1989.

178. Mueller X, Stauffer, JC, Jaussi A, Goy JJ, Kappenberger L: Subjective visual echocardiographic estimate of left ventricular ejection fraction as an alternative to conventional echocardiographic methods: comparison with contrast angiography. *Clin Cardiol* 14:898, 1991.

179. Rich S, et al.: Determination of left ventricular ejection fraction by visual estimation during real-time two-dimensional echocardiography. *Am Heart J* 104:603, 1982.

180. Alexander JH, et al.: Feasibility of point-of-care echocardiography by internal medicine house staff. *Am Heart J* 147:476, 2004.

181. Manasia AR, et al.: Feasibility and potential clinical utility of goal-directed transthoracic echocardiography performed by noncardiologist intensivists using a small hand-carried device (SonoHeart) in critically ill patients. *J Cardiothorac Vasc Anesth* 19:155, 2005.

182. Mark DG, et al.: Hand-carried echocardiography for assessment of left ventricular filling and ejection fraction in the surgical intensive care unit. *J Crit Care* 24:470.e1–e7, 2009.

183. Kimura BJ, et al.: Value of a cardiovascular limited ultrasound examination using a hand-carried ultrasound device on clinical management in an outpatient medical clinic. *Am J Cardiol* 100:321, 2007.

184. Lehmann KG, Johnson AD, Goldberger AL: Mitral valve E point-septal separation as an index of left ventricular function with valvular heart disease. *Chest* 83:102, 1983.

185. Silverstein JR, Laffely NH, Rifkin RD: Quantitative estimation of left ventricular ejection fraction from mitral valve E-point to septal separation and comparison to magnetic resonance imaging. *Am J Cardiol* 97:137, 2006.

186. Ahmadpour H, et al.: Mitral E point septal separation: A reliable index of left ventricular performance in coronary artery disease. *Am Heart J* 106:21, 1983.

187. Lew W, Henning H, Schelbert H, Karliner JS: Assessment of mitral valve E point-septal separation as an index of left ventricular performance in patients with acute and previous myocardial infarction. *Am J Cardiol* 41:836, 1978.

188. Cheitlin MD, et al.: ACC/AHA/ASE 2003 guideline update for the clinical application of echocardiography: summary article: A report of the American College of Cardiology/American Heart Association Task Force on Practice Guidelines (ACC/AHA/ASE Committee to Update the 1997 Guidelines for the Clinical Application of Echocardiography). *Circulation* 108:1146, 2003.

189. Lang RM, et al.: Recommendations for chamber quantification: A report from the American Society of Echocardiography's Guidelines and Standards Committee and

the Chamber Quantification Writing Group, developed in conjunction with the European Association of Echocardiography, a branch of the European Society of Cardiology. *J Am Soc Echocardiogr* 18:1440, 2005.

190. Malm S, Frigstad S, Sagberg E, Larsson H, Skjaerpe T: Accurate and reproducible measurement of left ventricular volume and ejection fraction by contrast echocardiography: A comparison with magnetic resonance imaging. *J Am Coll Cardiol* 44:1030, 2004.

191. Reilly JP, et al.: Contrast echocardiography clarifies uninterpretable wall motion in intensive care unit patients. *J Am Coll Cardiol* 35:485, 2000.

192. Mulvagh SL, et al.: Contrast echocardiography: Current and future applications. *J Am Soc Echocardiogr* 13:331, 2000.

193. Carabello BA: Evolution of the study of left ventricular function: Everything old is new again. *Circulation* 105:2701, 2002.

194. Nagueh SF, et al.: Recommendations for the evaluation of left ventricular diastolic function by echocardiography. *J Am Soc Echocardiogr* 22:107, 2009.

195. Nishimura RA, Tajik AJ: Evaluation of diastolic filling of left ventricle in health and disease: Doppler echocardiography is the clinician's Rosetta Stone. *J Am Coll Cardiol* 30:8, 1997.

196. Dokainish H et al.: Optimal noninvasive assessment of left ventricular filling pressures: A comparison of tissue Doppler echocardiography and B-type natriuretic peptide in patients with pulmonary artery catheters. *Circulation* 109:2432, 2004.

197. Matyal R, Skubas NJ, Shernan SK, Mahmood F: Perioperative assessment of diastolic dysfunction. *Anesth Analg* 113:449, 2011.

198. Paulus WJ, et al.: How to diagnose diastolic heart failure: A consensus statement on the diagnosis of heart failure with normal left ventricular ejection fraction by the Heart Failure and Echocardiography Associations of the European Society of Cardiology. *Eur Heart J* 28:2539, 2007.

199. Zile MR, Brutsaert DL: New concepts in diastolic dysfunction and diastolic heart failure: Part I: Diagnosis, prognosis, and measurements of diastolic function. *Circulation* 105:1387, 2002.

200. Nguyen VT, Ho JE, Ho CY, Givertz MM, Stevenson LW: Handheld echocardiography offers rapid assessment of clinical volume status. *Am Heart J* 156:537, 2008.

201. Dokainish H, et al.: New, simple echocardiographic indexes for the estimation of filling pressure in patients with cardiac disease and preserved left ventricular ejection fraction. *Echocardiography* 27:946, 2010.

202. Kurtoglu N, Akdemir R, Yuce M, Basaran Y, Dindar I: Left ventricular inflow normal or pseudonormal. A new echocardiographic method: Diastolic change of left atrial diameter. *Echocardiography* 17:653, 2000.

203. Khoo CW, Krishnamoorthy S, Lim HS, Lip GY: Assessment of left atrial volume: A focus on echocardiographic methods and clinical implications. *Clin Res Cardiol* 100:97, 2011.

204. Moller JE, et al.: Left atrial volume: A powerful predictor of survival after acute myocardial infarction. *Circulation* 107:2207, 2003.

205. Ristow B, Ali S, Whooley MA, Schiller NB: Usefulness of left atrial volume index to predict heart failure hospitalization and mortality in ambulatory patients with coronary heart disease and comparison to left ventricular ejection fraction (from the Heart and Soul Study). *Am J Cardiol* 102:70, 2008.

206. Valocik G, Mitro P, Druzbacka L, Valocikova I: Left atrial volume as a predictor of heart function. *Bratisl Lek Listy* 110:146, 2009.

207. Abhayaratna WP, et al.: Left atrial size: physiologic determinants and clinical applications. *J Am Coll Cardiol* 47:2357, 2006.

208. Lim TK, Ashrafian H, Dwivedi G, Collinson PO, Senior R: Increased left atrial volume index is an independent predictor of raised serum natriuretic peptide in patients with suspected heart failure but normal left ventricular ejection fraction: Implication for diagnosis of diastolic heart failure. *Eur J Heart Fail* 8:38, 2006.

209. Pritchett AM, et al.: Diastolic dysfunction and left atrial volume: a population-based study. *J Am Coll Cardiol* 45:87, 2005.

210. Rossi A, Vassanelli C: Left atrium: No longer neglected. *Ital Heart J* 6:881, 2005.

211. Benjamin EJ, D'Agostino RB, Belanger AJ, Wolf PA, Levy D: Left atrial size and the risk of stroke and death. The Framingham Heart Study. *Circulation* 92:835, 1995.

212. Kimura BJ, Blanchard DG, Willis CL, DeMaria AN: Limited cardiac ultrasound examination for cost-effective echocardiographic referral. *J Am Soc Echocardiogr* 15:640, 2002.

213. Kimura BJ, Kedar E, Weiss DE, Wahlstrom CL, Agan DL: A bedside ultrasound sign of cardiac disease: The left atrium-to-aorta diastolic diameter ratio. *Am J Emerg Med* 28:203, 2010.

214. Lipczynska M, Szymanski P, Klisiewicz A, Hoffman P: Hand-carried echocardiography in heart failure and heart failure risk population: A community based prospective study. *J Am Soc Echocardiogr* 24:125, 2011.

215. Lucas BP, et al.: Diagnostic accuracy of hospitalist-performed hand-carried ultrasound echocardiography after a brief training program. *J Hosp Med* 4:340, 2009.

216. Quinones MA, et al.: Echocardiographic predictors of clinical outcome in patients with left ventricular dysfunction enrolled in the SOLVD registry and trials: Significance of left ventricular hypertrophy. Studies of Left Ventricular Dysfunction. *J Am Coll Cardiol* 35:1237, 2000.

217. Senior R, Galasko G, Hickman M, Jeetley P, Lahiri A: Community screening for left ventricular hypertrophy in patients with hypertension using hand-held echocardiography. *J Am Soc Echocardiogr* 17:56, 2004.

218. Trambaiolo P, et al.: A hand-carried cardiac ultrasound device in the outpatient cardiology clinic reduces the need for standard echocardiography. *Heart* 93:470, 2007.

219. Vourvouri EC, et al.: Experience with an ultrasound stethoscope. *J Am Soc Echocardiogr* 15:80, 2002.

220. Tsang TS, et al.: Prediction of cardiovascular outcomes with left atrial size: Is volume superior to area or diameter? *J Am Coll Cardiol* 47:1018, 2006.

221. Casale PN, et al.: Value of echocardiographic measurement of left ventricular mass in predicting cardiovascular morbid events in hypertensive men. *Ann Intern Med* 105:173, 1986.

222. Haider AW, Larson, MG, Benjamin EJ, Levy D: Increased left ventricular mass and hypertrophy are associated with increased risk for sudden death. *J Am Coll Cardiol* 32:1454, 1998.

223. Levy D, Garrison RJ, Savage DD, Kannel WB, Castelli WP: Left ventricular mass and incidence of coronary heart disease in an elderly cohort. The Framingham Heart Study. *Ann Intern Med* 110:101, 1989.

224. Vakili BA, Okin PM, Devereux RB: Prognostic implications of left ventricular hypertrophy. *Am Heart J* 141:334, 2001.

225. Devereux RB: Is the electrocardiogram still useful for detection of left ventricular hypertrophy? *Circulation* 81:1144, 1990.

226. Levy D et al.: Determinants of sensitivity and specificity of electrocardiographic criteria for left ventricular hypertrophy. *Circulation* 81:815, 1990.

227. Grossman W, Jones D, McLaurin LP: Wall stress and patterns of hypertrophy in the human left ventricle. *J Clin Invest* 56:56, 1975.

228. Vourvouri EC, et al.: Left ventricular hypertrophy screening using a hand-held ultrasound device. *Eur Heart J* 23:1516, 2002.

229. Woythaler JN, et al.: Accuracy of echocardiography versus electrocardiography in detecting left ventricular hypertrophy: comparison with postmortem mass measurements. *J Am Coll Cardiol* 2:305, 1983.

230. Rivers E, et al.: Early goal-directed therapy in the treatment of severe sepsis and septic shock. *N Engl J Med* 345:1368, 2001.

231. Boyd JH, Forbes J, Nakada TA, Walley KR, Russell JA: Fluid resuscitation in septic shock: A positive fluid balance and elevated central venous pressure are associated with increased mortality. *Crit Care Med* 39:259, 2011.

232. Durairaj L, Schmidt GA: Fluid therapy in resuscitated sepsis: Less is more. *Chest* 133:252, 2008.

233. Michard F, Teboul JL: Predicting fluid responsiveness in ICU patients: A critical analysis of the evidence. *Chest* 121:2000, 2002.

234. Murphy CV, et al.: The importance of fluid management in acute lung injury secondary to septic shock. *Chest* 136:102, 2009.

235. Rosenberg AL, Dechert RE, Park PK, Bartlett RH: Review of a large clinical series: Association of cumulative fluid balance on outcome in acute lung injury: A retrospective review of the ARDSnet tidal volume study cohort. *J Intensive Care Med* 24:35, 2009.

236. Wiedemann HP, et al.: Comparison of two fluid-management strategies in acute lung injury. *N Engl J Med* 354:2564, 2006.

237. Marik PE: Surviving sepsis: Going beyond the guidelines. *Ann Intensive Care* 1:17, 2011.

238. Marik PE, Monnet X, Teboul JL: Hemodynamic parameters to guide fluid therapy. *Ann Intensive Care* 1:1, 2011.

239. Charron C, Caille V, Jardin F, Vieillard-Baron A: Echocardiographic measurement of fluid responsiveness. *Curr Opin Crit Care* 12:249, 2006.

240. Levitov A, Marik P.E: Echocardiographic assessment of preload responsiveness in critically ill patients. *Cardiol Res Pract* 2012:819696, 2012.

241. Marik PE: Techniques for assessment of intravascular volume in critically ill patients. *J Intensive Care Med* 24:329, 2009.

242. Akilli B, Bayir A, Kara F, Ak A, Cander B: Inferior vena cava diameter as a marker of early hemorrhagic shock: A comparative study. *Ulus Travma Acil Cerrahi Derg* 16:113, 2010.

243. Chen L, Kim Y, Santucci KA: Use of ultrasound measurement of the inferior vena cava diameter as an objective tool in the assessment of children with clinical dehydration. *Acad Emerg Med* 14:841, 2007.

244. Goonewardena SN, et al.: Comparison of hand-carried ultrasound assessment of the inferior vena cava and N-terminal pro-brain natriuretic peptide for predicting readmission after hospitalization for acute decompensated heart failure. *JACC Cardiovasc Imaging* 1:595, 2008.

245. Hirayama S, Ando Y, Sudo Y, Asano Y: Improvement of cardiac function by dry weight optimization based on interdialysis inferior vena caval diameter. *ASAIO J* 48:320, 2002.

246. Sefidbakht S, Assadsangabi R, Abbasi HR, Nabavizadeh A: Sonographic measurement of the inferior vena cava as a predictor of shock in trauma patients. *Emerg Radiol* 14:181, 2007.

247. Tetsuka T, Ando Y, Ono S, Asano Y: Change in inferior vena caval diameter detected by ultrasonography during and after hemodialysis. *ASAIO J* 41:105, 1995.

248. Yanagawa Y, Nishi K, Sakamoto T, Okada Y: Early diagnosis of hypovolemic shock by sonographic measurement of inferior vena cava in trauma patients. *J Trauma* 58:825, 2005.

249. Yanagawa Y, Sakamoto T, Okada Y: Hypovolemic shock evaluated by sonographic measurement of the inferior vena cava during resuscitation in trauma patients. *J Trauma* 63:1245, 2007.

250. Yanagiba S, Ando Y, Kusano E, Asano Y: Utility of the inferior vena cava diameter as a marker of dry weight in nonoliguric hemodialyzed patients. *ASAIO J* 47:528, 2001.

251. Dellinger RP, et al.: Surviving Sepsis Campaign: international guidelines for management of severe sepsis and septic shock: 2008. *Intensive Care Med* 34:17, 2008.

252. Calvin JE, Driedger AA, Sibbald WJ: The hemodynamic effect of rapid fluid infusion in critically ill patients. *Surgery* 90:61, 1981.

253. Diebel L, et al.: End-diastolic volume versus pulmonary artery wedge pressure in evaluating cardiac preload in trauma patients. *J Trauma* 37:950, 1994.

254. Kramer A, Zygun D, Hawes H, Easton P, Ferland A: Pulse pressure variation predicts fluid responsiveness following coronary artery bypass surgery. *Chest* 126:1563, 2004.

255. Marik PE, Baram M, Vahid B: Does central venous pressure predict fluid responsiveness? A systematic review of the literature and the tale of seven mares. *Chest* 134:172, 2008.

256. Michard F, et al.: Relation between respiratory changes in arterial pulse pressure and fluid responsiveness in septic patients with acute circulatory failure. *Am J Respir Crit Care Med* 162:134, 2000.

257. Osman D, et al.: Cardiac filling pressures are not appropriate to predict hemodynamic response to volume challenge. *Crit Care Med* 35:64, 2007.

258. Reuse C, Vincent JL, Pinsky MR: Measurements of right ventricular volumes during fluid challenge. *Chest* 98:1450, 1990.

259. Schneider AJ, et al.: Biventricular performance during volume loading in patients with early septic shock, with emphasis on the right ventricle: A combined hemodynamic and radionuclide study. *Am Heart J* 116:103, 1988.

260. Tavernier B, Makhotine O, Lebuffe G, Dupont J, Scherpereel P: Systolic pressure variation as a guide to fluid therapy in patients with sepsis-induced hypotension. *Anesthesiology* 89:1313, 1998.

261. Carr BG, et al.: Intensivist bedside ultrasound (INBU) for volume assessment in the intensive care unit: A pilot study. *J Trauma* 63:495, 2007.

262. Brennan JM, et al.: Reappraisal of the use of inferior vena cava for estimating right atrial pressure. *J Am Soc Echocardiogr* 20:857, 2007.

263. Kircher BJ, Himelman RB, Schiller NB: Noninvasive estimation of right atrial pressure from the inspiratory collapse of the inferior vena cava. *Am J Cardiol* 66:493, 1990.

264. Kaplan A: Echocardiographic diagnosis and monitoring of the right ventricular function. In: Levitov A, Mayo PH, Slonim AD, eds. *Critical Care Ultrasonography.* New York, NY: McGraw Hill, 2009.

265. Rudski LG, et al.: Guidelines for the echocardiographic assessment of the right heart in adults: A report from the American Society of Echocardiography endorsed by the European Association of Echocardiography, a registered branch of the European Society of Cardiology, and the Canadian Society of Echocardiography. *J Am Soc Echocardiogr* 23:685, 2010.

266. Brennan JM, et al.: A comparison by medicine residents of physical examination versus hand-carried ultrasound for estimation of right atrial pressure. *Am J Cardiol* 99:1614, 2007.

267. Brennan JM, et al.: Handcarried ultrasound measurement of the inferior vena cava for assessment of intravascular volume status in the outpatient hemodialysis clinic. *Clin J Am Soc Nephrol* 1:749, 2006.

268. Goldberger JJ, Himelman RB, Wolfe CL, Schiller NB: Right ventricular infarction: Recognition and assessment of its hemodynamic significance by two-dimensional echocardiography. *J Am Soc Echocardiogr* 4:140, 1991.

269. Himelman RB, Kircher B, Rockey DC, Schiller NB: Inferior vena cava plethora with blunted respiratory response: A sensitive echocardiographic sign of cardiac tamponade. *J Am Coll Cardiol* 12:1470, 1988.

270. Mintz GS, Kotler MN, Parry WR, Iskandrian AS, Kane SA: Reat-time inferior vena caval ultrasonography: Normal and abnormal findings and its use in assessing right-heart function. *Circulation* 64:1018, 1981.

271. Moreno FL, et al.: Evaluation of size and dynamics of the inferior vena cava as an index of right-sided cardiac function. *Am J Cardiol* 53:579, 1984.

272. Nagueh SF, Kopelen HA, Zoghbi WA: Relation of mean right atrial pressure to echocardiographic and Doppler parameters of right atrial and right ventricular function. *Circulation* 93:1160, 1996.

273. Nakao S, Come PC, McKay RG, Ransil BJ: Effects of positional changes on inferior vena caval size and dynamics and correlations with right-sided cardiac pressure. *Am J Cardiol* 59:125, 1987.

274. Ommen SR, Nishimura RA, Hurrell DG, Klarich KW: Assessment of right atrial pressure with 2-dimensional and Doppler echocardiography: A simultaneous catheterization and echocardiographic study. *Mayo Clin Proc* 75:24, 2000.

275. Pepi M, et al.: A new formula for echo-Doppler estimation of right ventricular systolic pressure. *J Am Soc Echocardiogr* 7:20, 1994.

276. Simonson JS, Schiller NB: Sonospirometry: A new method for noninvasive estimation of mean right atrial pressure based on two-dimensional echographic measurements of the inferior vena cava during measured inspiration. *J Am Coll Cardiol* 11:557, 1988.

277. Stawicki SP, et al.: Intensivist use of hand-carried ultrasonography to measure IVC collapsibility in estimating intravascular volume status: Correlations with CVP. *J Am Coll Surg* 209:55, 2009.

278. Blair JE, et al.: Usefulness of hand-carried ultrasound to predict elevated left ventricular filling pressure. *Am J Cardiol* 103:246, 2009.

279. Jue J, Chung W, Schiller NB: Does inferior vena cava size predict right atrial pressures in patients receiving mechanical ventilation? *J Am Soc Echocardiogr* 5:613, 1992.

280. Ando Y, Yanagiba S, Asano Y: The inferior vena cava diameter as a marker of dry weight in chronic hemodialyzed patients. *Artif Organs* 19:1237, 1995.

281. Michard F, Teboul JL: Using heart-lung interactions to assess fluid responsiveness during mechanical ventilation. *Crit Care* 4:282, 2000.

282. Marik PE, Cavallazzi R, Vasu T, Hirani A: Dynamic changes in arterial waveform derived variables and fluid responsiveness in mechanically ventilated patients: A systematic review of the literature. *Crit Care Med* 37:2642, 2009.

283. Biais M, et al.: A comparison of stroke volume variation measured by Vigileo/FloTrac system and aortic Doppler echocardiography. *Anesth Analg* 109:466, 2009.

284. Durand P, Chevret L, Essouri S, Haas V, Devictor D: Respiratory variations in aortic blood flow predict fluid responsiveness in ventilated children. *Intensive Care Med* 34:888, 2008.

285. Pereira de Souza Neto E, et al.: Predicting fluid responsiveness in mechanically ventilated children under general anaesthesia using dynamic parameters and transthoracic echocardiography. *Br J Anaesth* 106:856, 2011.

286. Brennan JM, et al.: Radial artery pulse pressure variation correlates with brachial artery peak velocity variation in ventilated subjects when measured by internal medicine residents using hand-carried ultrasound devices. *Chest* 131:1301, 2007.

287. Monge Garcia MI, Gil Cano A, Diaz Monrove JC: Brachial artery peak velocity variation to predict fluid responsiveness in mechanically ventilated patients. *Crit Care* 13:R142, 2009.

288. De Backer D, Heenen S, Piagnerelli M, Koch M, Vincent JL: Pulse pressure variations to predict fluid responsiveness: Influence of tidal volume. *Intensive Care Med* 31:517, 2005.

289. Reuter DA, et al.: Influence of tidal volume on left ventricular stroke volume variation measured by pulse contour analysis in mechanically ventilated patients. *Intensive Care Med* 29:476, 2003.

290. Cavallaro F, et al.: Diagnostic accuracy of passive leg raising for prediction of fluid responsiveness in adults: Systematic review and meta-analysis of clinical studies. *Intensive Care Med* 36:1475, 2010.

291. Monnet X, Teboul JL: Passive leg raising. *Intensive Care Med* 34:659, 2008.

292. Teboul JL, Monnet X: Prediction of volume responsiveness in critically ill patients with spontaneous breathing activity. *Curr Opin Crit Care* 14:334, 2008.

293. Teboul JL, Monnet X: Detecting volume responsiveness and unresponsiveness in intensive care unit patients: Two different problems, only one solution. *Crit Care* 13:175, 2009.

294. Biais M, et al.: Changes in stroke volume induced by passive leg raising in spontaneously breathing patients: Comparison between echocardiography and Vigileo/FloTrac device. *Crit Care* 13:R195, 2009.

295. Maizel J, et al.: Diagnosis of central hypovolemia by using passive leg raising. *Intensive Care Med* 33:1133, 2007.

296. Thiel SW, Kollef MH, Isakow W: Non-invasive stroke volume measurement and passive leg raising predict volume responsiveness in medical ICU patients: An observational cohort study. *Crit Care* 13:R111, 2009.

297. Preau S, Saulnier F, Dewavrin F, Durocher A, Chagnon JL: Passive leg raising is predictive of fluid responsiveness in spontaneously breathing patients with severe sepsis or acute pancreatitis. *Crit Care Med* 38:819, 2010.

298. Swenson JD, Harkin C, Pace NL, Astle K, Bailey P: Transesophageal echocardiography: An objective tool in defining maximum ventricular response to intravenous fluid therapy. *Anesth Analg* 83:1149, 1996.

299. Brown JM: Use of echocardiography for hemodynamic monitoring. *Crit Care Med* 30:1361, 2002.

300. Dalibon N, Schlumberger S, Saada M, Fischler M, Riou B: Haemodynamic assessment of hypovolaemia under general anaesthesia in pigs submitted to graded haemorrhage and retransfusion. *Br J Anaesth* 82:97, 1999.

301. Cheung AT, Savino JS, Weiss SJ, Aukburg SJ, Berlin JA: Echocardiographic and hemodynamic indexes of left ventricular preload in patients with normal and abnormal ventricular function. *Anesthesiology* 81:376, 1994.

302. Reich DL, Konstadt SN, Nejat M, Abrams HP, Bucek J: Intraoperative transesophageal echocardiography for the detection of cardiac preload changes induced by transfusion and phlebotomy in pediatric patients. *Anesthesiology* 79:10, 1993.

303. Leung JM, Levine EH: Left ventricular end-systolic cavity obliteration as an estimate of intraoperative hypovolemia. *Anesthesiology* 81:1102, 1994.

304. Blazer D, Kotler MN, Parry WR, Wertheimer J, Nakhjavan FK: Noninvasive evaluation of mid-left ventricular obstruction by two-dimensional and Doppler echocardiography and color flow Doppler echocardiography. *Am Heart J* 114:1162, 1987.

305. Chenzbraun A, Pinto FJ, Schnittger I: Transesophageal echocardiography in the intensive care unit: Impact on diagnosis and decision-making. *Clin Cardiol* 17:438, 1994.

306. Haley JH, Sinak LJ, Tajik AJ, Ommen SR, Oh JK: Dynamic left ventricular outflow tract obstruction in acute coronary syndromes: An important cause of new systolic murmur and cardiogenic shock. *Mayo Clin Proc* 74:901, 1999.

307. Joffe II, et al.: Role of echocardiography in perioperative management of patients undergoing open heart surgery. *Am Heart J* 131:162, 1996.

308. Madu EC, Brown R, Geraci SA: Dynamic left ventricular outflow tract obstruction in critically ill patients: Role of transesophageal echocardiography in therapeutic decision making. *Cardiology* 88:292, 1997.

309. Mintz GS, Kotler MN, Segal BL, Parry WR: Systolic anterior motion of the mitral valve in the absence of asymmetric septal hypertrophy. *Circulation* 57:256, 1978.

310. Kucher N, Goldhaber SZ: Management of massive pulmonary embolism. *Circulation* 112:e28, 2005.

311. Kucher N, Rossi E, De Rosa M, Goldhaber SZ: Massive pulmonary embolism. *Circulation* 113:577, 2006.

312. Mehta N, Baron BJ, Stone MB: Successful thrombolysis of massive pulmonary embolism. *Acad Emerg Med* 18:e27, 2011.

313. Sadeghi A, et al.: Acute massive pulmonary embolism: role of the cardiac surgeon. *Tex Heart Inst J* 32:430, 2005.

314. Tayama, E, et al.: Treatment of acute massive/submassive pulmonary embolism. *Circ J* 66:479, 2002.

315. Grifoni S, et al.: Utility of an integrated clinical, echocardiographic, and venous ultrasonographic approach for triage of patients with suspected pulmonary embolism. *Am J Cardiol* 82:1230, 1998.

316. Hollenberg SM, Kavinsky CJ, Parrillo JE: Cardiogenic shock. *Ann Intern Med* 131:47, 1999.

317. Reynolds HR, Hochman JS: Cardiogenic shock: Current concepts and improving outcomes. *Circulation* 117:686, 2008.

318. Overgaard CB, Dzavik V: Inotropes and vasopressors: Review of physiology and clinical use in cardiovascular disease. *Circulation* 118:1047, 2008.

319. Forsythe SM, Schmidt GA: Sodium bicarbonate for the treatment of lactic acidosis. *Chest* 117:260, 2000.

320. Hurley K, Baggs D: Hypocalcemic cardiac failure in the emergency department. *J Emerg Med* 28:155, 2005.

321. Orchard CH, Kentish JC: Effects of changes of pH on the contractile function of cardiac muscle. *Am J Physiol* 258:C967, 1990.

322. Sharkey SW, Lesser JR, Maron BJ: Cardiology Patient Page. Takotsubo (stress) cardiomyopathy. *Circulation* 124:e460, 2011.

323. Sharkey SW, et al.: Natural history and expansive clinical profile of stress (tako-tsubo) cardiomyopathy. *J Am Coll Cardiol* 55:333, 2010.

324. Hick JL, Smith SW, Lynch MT: Metabolic acidosis in restraint-associated cardiac arrest: a case series. *Acad Emerg Med* 6:239, 1999.

325. Reardon MJ, et al.: Ischemic left ventricular free wall rupture: Prediction, diagnosis, and treatment. *Ann Thorac Surg* 64:1509, 1997.

326. Holger JS, Minnigan HJ, Lamon RP, Gornick CC: The utility of ultrasound to determine ventricular capture in external cardiac pacing. *Am J Emerg Med* 19:134, 2001.

327. Bonow R: Valvular heart disease. In: Braunwald E, ed.

Braunwald's Heart Disease Philadelphia, PA: Elsevier; 2005:1553.

328. Feigenbaum H, Armstrong WF, Ryan T: Mitral valve disease. In: Feigenbaum H, Armstrong WF, Ryan T, eds. *Feigenbaum's Echocardiography*. Philadelphia, PA: Lippincott Williams & Wilkins, 2005:306.

329. Zoghbi WA, et al.: Recommendations for evaluation of the severity of native valvular regurgitation with two-dimensional and Doppler echocardiography. *J Am Soc Echocardiogr* 16:777, 2003.

330. Bonow RO, et al.: ACC/AHA 2006 guidelines for the management of patients with valvular heart disease: A report of the American College of Cardiology/American Heart Association Task Force on Practice Guidelines (writing Committee to Revise the 1998 guidelines for the management of patients with valvular heart disease) developed in collaboration with the Society of Cardiovascular Anesthesiologists endorsed by the Society for Cardiovascular Angiography and Interventions and the Society of Thoracic Surgeons. *J Am Coll Cardiol* 48:e1, 2006.

331. Cline D: Valvular emergencies. In: Tintinalli JE, ed. *Emergency Medicine: A Comprehensive Study Guide*. New York, NY: McGraw Hill; 2003:373.

332. Baumgartner H, et al.: Echocardiographic assessment of valve stenosis: EAE/ASE recommendations for clinical practice. *J Am Soc Echocardiogr* 22:1, 2009.

333. Olson LJ, Subramanian R, Ackermann DM, Orszulak TA, Edwards WD: Surgical pathology of the mitral valve: A study of 712 cases spanning 21 years. *Mayo Clin Proc* 62:22, 1987.

334. DeSanctis RW, Doroghazi RM, Austen WG, Buckley MJ: Aortic dissection. *N Engl J Med* 317:1060, 1987.

335. Dmowski AT, Carey MJ: Aortic dissection. *Am J Emerg Med* 17:372, 1999.

336. Flachskampf, FA, Daniel, WG: Aortic dissection. *Cardiol Clin* 18:807, 2000.

337. Pretre R, Von Segesser LK: Aortic dissection. *Lancet* 349:1461, 1997.

338. Sommer T, et al.: Aortic dissection: A comparative study of diagnosis with spiral CT, multiplanar transesophageal echocardiography, and MR imaging. *Radiology* 199:347, 1996.

339. Horowitz RS, et al.: Immediate diagnosis of acute myocardial infarction by two-dimensional echocardiography. *Circulation* 65:323, 1982.

340. Sabia P, et al.: Value of regional wall motion abnormality in the emergency room diagnosis of acute myocardial infarction. A prospective study using two-dimensional echocardiography. *Circulation* 84:185, 1991.

341. Dillon JC, Chang S, Feigenbaum H: Echocardiographic manifestations of left bundle branch block. *Circulation* 49:876, 1974.

342. McDonald IG: Echocardiographic demonstration of abnormal motion of the intraventricular septum in left bundle branch block. *Circulation* 48:272, 1973.

343. Reynolds HR, et al.: Paradoxical septal motion after cardiac surgery: A review of 3,292 cases. *Clin Cardiol* 30:621, 2007.

344. Tse HF, et al.: Functional abnormalities in patients with permanent right ventricular pacing: The effect of sites of electrical stimulation. *J Am Coll Cardiol* 40:1451, 2002.

345. Xiao HB, Brecker SJ, Gibson DG: Differing effects of right ventricular pacing and left bundle branch block on left ventricular function. *Br Heart J* 69:166, 1993.

346. Levitt MA, et al.: Combined cardiac marker approach with adjunct two-dimensional echocardiography to diagnose acute myocardial infarction in the emergency department. *Ann Emerg Med* 27:1, 1996.

347. Muttreja MR, Mohler ER, 3rd: Clinical use of ischemic markers and echocardiography in the emergency department. *Echocardiography* 16:187, 1999.

348. Mohler ER, 3rd, et al.: Clinical utility of troponin T levels and echocardiography in the emergency department. *Am Heart J* 135:253, 1998.

349. Natori H, Tamaki S, Kira S: Ultrasonographic evaluation of ventilatory effect on inferior vena caval configuration. *Am Rev Respir Dis* 120:421, 1979.

350. Kimura BJ, et al.: The effect of breathing manner on inferior vena caval diameter. *Eur J Echocardiogr* 12:120, 2011.

351. Lodato JA, Ward RP, Lang RM: Echocardiographic predictors of pulmonary embolism in patients referred for helical CT. *Echocardiography* 25:584, 2008.

352. Godley RW, et al.: Reliability of two-dimensional echocardiography in assessing the severity of valvular aortic stenosis. *Chest* 79:657, 1981.

353. Kaul S, et al.: Incremental value of cardiac imaging in patients presenting to the emergency department with chest pain and without ST-segment elevation: a multicenter study. *Am Heart J* 148:129, 2004.

354. Rinkevich D, et al.: Regional left ventricular perfusion and function in patients presenting to the emergency department with chest pain and no ST-segment elevation. *Eur Heart J* 26:1606, 2005.

355. Senior R, Ashrafian H: Detecting acute coronary syndrome in the emergency department: the answer is in seeing the heart: Why look further? *Eur Heart J* 26:1573, 2005.

CHAPTER 7

Pulmonary

Fernando R. Silva and Lisa D. Mills

The lungs have traditionally been considered a barrier to ultrasound imaging because large changes in acoustic impedance result in ultrasound reflection and the acoustic impedance of air is extremely low compared with anatomic tissues. It was not until 1986 that the diagnosis of pneumothorax with ultrasound was reported in veterinary medicine.[1] In 1995, Lichtenstein published his landmark paper describing the most fundamental element of pulmonary ultrasound, the lung sliding sign.[2]

Lichtenstein opened the door for a large body of research based on the analysis of artifacts generated by the nearly complete reflection of the ultrasound beam when it encounters the interface between soft tissue and aerated parenchyma of the lung. What was initially seen as "noise" became useful information. The tissues and interfaces reflect the sound waves exhibiting notably different kinds of "noise" artifacts in several normal and pathologic conditions.

In 2011, the International Liaison Committee for the International Consensus Conference on Lung Ultrasound (ICC-LUS) critically evaluated the literature regarding point-of-care lung ultrasound. Over 300 publications were reviewed. From this, a consensus statement was written.[3] Overwhelmingly, the recommendations support the use of ultrasound to evaluate the lungs in critically ill and injured patients.[4–6]

▶ CLINICAL CONSIDERATIONS

The chest radiograph historically is one of the most iconic elements of the practice of medicine. It is un-

derstandable that many physicians resist ultrasound for lung pathology given the ingrained role of radiography. The advantages of lung ultrasound, however, outweigh the challenges of learning a new practice.

Sonography has many advantages over plain films and cross-sectional imaging. It is highly portable allowing its use in situations of limited resources as well as austere conditions. Ultrasound is feasible at the bedside and improves interaction during clinical interview increasing patient satisfaction.[7] Furthermore, the pulmonary applications of ultrasound consistently present levels of accuracy superior to plain films and comparable to CT scans, without exposing the patient to radiation.[8–10]

Point-of-care ultrasound provides an immediate diagnostic answer without the delays of media processing, transport, and consultative interpretation. This is particularly important in the critically ill.

Ultrasound plays a critical role for diagnosing lung pathology, including pneumothorax, hemothorax, interstitial syndromes, pneumonia, pulmonary edema, and contusion.[3] Point-of-care ultrasound provides the clinician with immediate, accurate data regarding lung pathology.

▶ CLINICAL INDICATIONS

Pulmonary ultrasound should be considered a first-line diagnostic modality for critically ill patients.[3] Point-of-care ultrasound, particularly lung ultrasound, is widely referred to as "the new stethoscope."

Clinical scenarios for performing lung ultrasound include

- Evaluation of acute dyspnea
- Airway management
- Pneumothorax
- Alveolar-interstitial syndromes: cardiogenic pulmonary edema, acute respiratory distress syndrome (ARDS), pulmonary contusion, and other interstitial syndromes
- Consolidations: pneumonia, atelectasis, other nonpneumonic consolidations
- Neonatal applications
- Pleural effusions

EVALUATION OF ACUTE DYSPNEA

Critical ultrasound achieves its prime role in the hands of the emergency and critical care physicians when dealing with unstable patients by providing immediate diagnostic answers, allowing for immediate therapeutic decisions. A number of ultrasound-guided protocols for diagnosis of undifferentiated shock rely heavily on chest ultrasound for the assessment of pneumothorax, pulmonary congestion, and pulmonary embolism.[4,11–17] Lichtenstein published the BLUE (bedside lung ultrasound in emergency) protocol[18] in 2008, which is primarily based on point-of-care lung ultrasound. This algorithm is a technically simple approach for the statistically accurate diagnosis of severe dyspnea in a selected population of intensive care patients. A similar approach was used in an ED population.[19] A high concordance between ultrasound and chest radiography was reported, and it questioned whether point-of-care ultrasound could replace standard chest radiography for evaluation of acute dyspnea in the ED. According to the evidence-based recommendations from the ICC-LUS, sonography should be considered a primary imaging modality for the diagnosis of acute dyspnea.[3]

AIRWAY MANAGEMENT

Sonography has a promising role in invasive airway management, especially with ultrasound-guided cricothyrotomy and percutaneous tracheostomy. Emergency physicians can use ultrasound to reliably identify the cricothyroid membrane,[20] but the clinical use is still to be investigated. Sonography assists with confirmation of endotracheal tube placement. Advantages over the traditional methods include detection of main stem intubation[21–23] and freedom from the false-negative results presented by end-tidal CO_2 detectors in hypoperfusion states.[24] These applications will be discussed

in detail in Chapter 8, "Critical Care," and Chapter 22, "Additional Ultrasound-Guided Procedures."

PNEUMOTHORAX

The most widely used application of lung ultrasound in the ED is the evaluation for pneumothorax in trauma. There is extensive literature supporting the superiority of ultrasound over plain films in this role.[25–37] This technique is discussed in Chapter 5, "Trauma," and Chapter 8, "Critical Care."

ALVEOLAR-INTERSTITIAL SYNDROMES

Cardiogenic Pulmonary Edema

One of the most exciting applications of lung ultrasound is cardiogenic pulmonary edema. Acutely dyspneic patients present diagnostic dilemmas due to the overlap and frequent coexistence of pathology as well as the time-dependent need for diagnosis and intervention. Acutely decompensated heart failure (ADHF) presents with the classic acutely dyspneic patient. Traditional ancillary testing, such as chest radiograph and labs, provides only moderate increase in our diagnostic accuracy and invokes tremendous delay in diagnosis.[38–40]

Sonography is a powerful tool to differentiate ADHF from other clinical entities,[4,41–46] and has been shown to provide quantitative information about the degree of pulmonary edema.[46–48]

ADHF presents a very typical finding on the ultrasound examination, called the B-pattern.[49] This pattern is based on the finding of multiple B-lines throughout the entire pulmonary surface. B-lines are the artifact found in the alveolar-interstitial syndromes and are generated when there is alveolar flooding and/or thickening of the interstitium by extravascular lung water or inflammatory products. In an ICU population, 100% of patients with ADHF had diffuse B-lines on exam, while 92% of COPD exacerbations did not.[50]

In a study of dialysis patients, a linear correlation was found between removed fluid and decrease in the quantity of B-lines.[48] The study confirmed previous findings that B-lines are present earlier than the clinical symptom of dyspnea is perceived by the patients.[47] The appearance of B-lines prior to physiologic dysfunction was also found in high-altitude pulmonary edema[51] and ARDS.[52]

B-lines (previously called "comet tails") are defined as discrete "laser-like vertical hyperechoic reverberation artifacts that arise from the pleural line, extend to the bottom of the screen without fading, and move

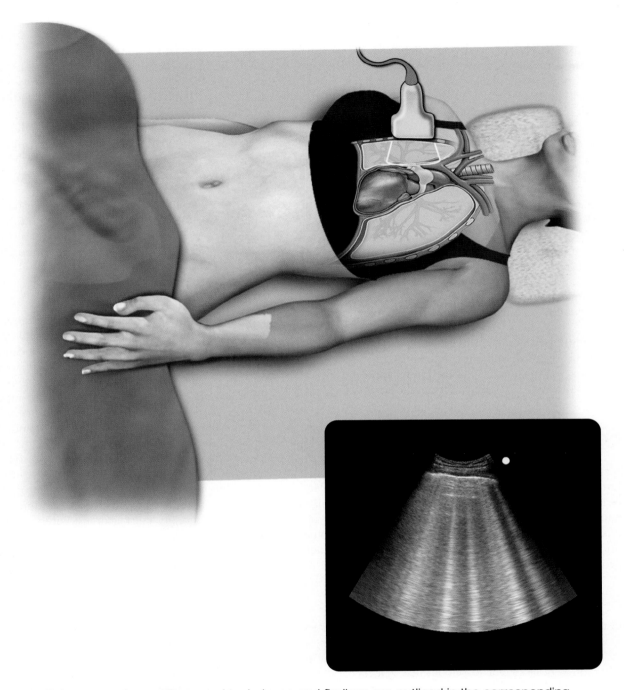

Figure 7-1. Pulmonary edema. Ultrasound techniques and findings are outlined in the corresponding sections of this chapter.

synchronously with lung sliding."[3] (Figure 7-1). The diagnosis of ADHF can usually be made within seconds in a patient with a consistent history.[39]

Often, scanning one focal area on the anterior chest at each hemithorax in a dyspneic patient is enough to assess for pulmonary congestion.[18] Even in cases where the clinical history is not immediately conducive to the diagnosis of ADHF, lung ultrasound still is recom-

mended as a first-line diagnostic tool, together with the traditional methods.[3]

ARDS and Other Interstitial Syndromes

ARDS can be clinically indistinguishable from ADHF, and there are several other diseases that mimic its clinical and radiologic appearance.[53] ARDS is still a diagnosis of exclusion, and the first step is excluding cardiogenic pulmonary edema.[54] BNP levels are a widely available test, but unfortunately are useful only if below 100 pg/mL, when they are suggestive of a noncardiogenic process. Levels above 100 pg/mL cannot confirm heart failure nor exclude ARDS.[55,56]

All interstitial syndromes that involve the subpleural parenchyma present a similar finding on lung ultrasound (B-line pattern). However, the findings of pleural line abnormalities (irregular, thickened, fragmented), anterior subpleural consolidations, presence of spared areas, reduction or absence of lung sliding, and nonhomogenous distribution of B-lines distinguish ARDS from ADHF.[3]

One review suggested that ultrasound could completely replace plain films and even CT scan for the diagnosis and monitoring of patients with ARDS and its usual complications, such as effusion and pneumothorax.[57] The same group reported successful use of ultrasound for guidance of alveolar recruitment maneuvers in ARDS.[58]

Pulmonary ultrasound has been shown to be useful in the diagnosis of other interstitial processes, like pulmonary contusion,[59-61] acute chest syndrome,[62] pulmonary fibrosis,[63-65] and viral pneumonitis.[66]

CONSOLIDATIONS

Several disease processes cause consolidation of the lung parenchyma. These include pneumonia, atelectasis, infarction (pulmonary embolism), and malignancy. Lung consolidation has a very characteristic ultrasound appearance; however, there are also some findings that allow differentiation between consolidative processes.[3,18,67]

Pneumonia

Clinical signs[68] and symptoms of pneumonia have a sensitivity of less than 50% compared with chest radiograph.[69] Although chest radiography is the most common way to diagnose pneumonia,[70] it has a sensitivity under 75%[71-74] compared with CT. Although CT is extremely sensitive for the diagnosis of pneumonia, it is not appropriate for routine use.[70] The literature supports using ultrasound for the diagnosis of pneumonia, with a reported sensitivity between 89% and 97% and a specificity between 95% and 98%.[3,8,9,75-81] In addition to improved sensitivity, point-of-care ultrasound allows

clinicians to perform serial exams in order to look for disease progression or ensure resolution of pneumonia without additional radiographic exams.[8-10]

Pulmonary consolidations that extend to the pleura are generally well visualized with ultrasound. One study showed that the consolidation reached the pleura in 98.5% of critically ill patients with CT-proven lung consolidations.[82] Limited data suggest that the sensitivity of lung ultrasound for the diagnosis of pneumonia in the ED may be better than the ICU setting,[75,82] possibly due to fewer limitations with patient mobility, dressings, tubes, etc.

The idea of imaging the entire pulmonary surface for consolidations may seem daunting to a time-pressed emergency physician; however, this examination may be successfully completed in less than 5 minutes.[75,77]

Nonpneumonic Subpleural Consolidations

Sonographic findings can reliably differentiate other causes of lung consolidation, particularly when providers use a combination of clinical and ultrasound findings to make a diagnosis.[4,24,61] Ultrasound findings that help define different types of consolidation are shape, boundaries, the presence and morphology of internal echoes (bronchograms), adjacent artifacts, and vascularity.[3,9,67,80-84] In addition, contrast agents are very useful for the evaluation of lung consolidations because different disease processes demonstrate remarkably different patterns of vascular morphology.

Pulmonary embolism is the most controversial topic in the lung ultrasound literature. Findings compatible with pulmonary embolism are wildly dichotomous. The literature espouses both a normal lung exam and pulmonary infarctions as findings consistent with pulmonary embolism. In the literature originating from critical care populations, the key finding in pulmonary embolism is a normal lung examination in the setting of DVT.[18] In contrast, other studies on nonacute and critically ill patients show that the vast majority presented with ultrasound findings compatible with pulmonary infarctions.[67,85,86] In this population, the overall accuracy of the examination was also increased if DVT was found. Our interpretation of this difference in the literature is that critical patients with massive or submassive pulmonary embolisms may have fewer but larger emboli, located more centrally in the vasculature, and with shorter time to examination. The noncritical patients may have a larger number of smaller emboli, with longer time before examination allowing for the complete development of the parenchymal inflammatory process and peripheral infarctions. Furthermore, unstable patients have had most of their examinations limited to the anterior chest, while most emboli are posterior.[87-89]

NEONATAL APPLICATIONS

Pulmonary ultrasound is revolutionary for the evaluation of respiratory distress in the neonatal population. It is remarkably accurate and negates radiation exposure in this sensitive group.[90,91] The cartilaginous ribcage and the small size of the lungs of a newborn allow for better evaluation and a complete exam.

Lung ultrasound was found to be useful for the diagnosis of transient tachypnea of the newborn.[92] In a mixed population of 132 infants with normal lungs or multiple interstitial diseases [transient tachypnea of the newborn, neonatal respiratory distress syndrome (NRDS), alveolar hemorrhage, pneumonia, atelectasis], a sensitivity and specificity of 100% compared with chest radiography were found.

Another study of 40 premature infants with radiographic signs of NRDS found ultrasound to be 100% sensitive and 100% specific,[93] suggesting that it could replace chest radiography, similar to what has been shown in adults with ARDS.[94,95]

PLEURAL EFFUSIONS

Ultrasound has a well-established role for the diagnosis and treatment of pleural effusions.[96] In addition to the intrinsic advantages of sonography over other methods, it is far more sensitive than plain films[97] and allows for differentiation of physiologic effusions,[98] and exudative and transudative processes.[99] In addition, ultrasound can differentiate effusion from pleural thickening,[100] estimate effusion volume in sitting or supine patients,[101] and drastically increase the safety[102] and success rates[103] of thoracentesis. Ultrasound-guided thoracentesis is covered in Chapter 22, "Additional Ultrasound-Guided Procedures."

▶ ANATOMIC CONSIDERATIONS

The subunits of the right and left lungs are called segments. The right lung is comprised of 10 segments: 3 in the right upper lobe (apical, anterior and medial), 2 in the right middle lobe (medial and lateral), and 5 in the right lower lobe (superior, medial, anterior, lateral, and posterior). The left lung comprises 8 segments: 4 in the left upper lobe (apicoposterior, anterior, superior lingula, and inferior lingula) and 4 in the left lower lobe (superior, anteromedial, lateral, and posterior). The lungs are covered by the visceral pleura, which is contiguous with the parietal pleura as it reflects from the lateral surfaces of the mediastinum.

Ultrasound of the lungs depends on findings generated by sonographic reflection from the lung and pleura. The lungs have a very large surface area, not all of which is accessible to ultrasound. Paravertebral regions and areas under the shoulders are not visible. Individual patient characteristics may limit the examination. Most pulmonary disease processes present with primary or secondary sonographic signs. They often involve a large portion of the pulmonary surface and/or accumulation of fluid in dependent regions. The combination of primary and secondary findings increases the sensitivity of pulmonary ultrasound.

In a group of 260 critically ill dyspneic patients, the correct diagnosis was reported in 53% of the patients by using a limited ultrasound exam that concentrated mostly on the anterior chest wall.[88] All examinations were performed in less than 3 minutes. The patient who presents with undifferentiated dyspnea will likely be in a semirecumbent or sitting position. The examination of a single spot[104] on each side of the anterior chest will likely provide the diagnostic answer because ADHF usually demonstrates diffuse B-lines bilaterally. However, routinely including an exam of the lateral chest may significantly increase sensitivity.[105]

▶ GETTING STARTED

BASIC PRINCIPLES OF LUNG ULTRASOUND

Pulmonary ultrasound is different from other sonographic examinations in that artifacts are good. Most lung ultrasound findings are based on the analysis of the artifacts, not of anatomical images. When encountering the interface of soft tissue and air at the level of the pleural line, the ultrasound beam is almost completely reflected back to the transducer. Think of air for ultrasound as a mirror is for light. This will help with the understanding of how both normal and pathologic pulmonary artifacts are generated.

MACHINES, TRANSDUCERS, AND SETTINGS

Less image processing is better since the goal in lung ultrasound is analysis of artifacts. Disable advanced filters, particularly tissue harmonics and spatial compounding. These capabilities were developed to eliminate the artifacts that decrease image quality for anatomical images.

These artifacts, however, are essential for pulmonary sonography.

Many contemporary machines do not have a factory preset for lung imaging. Nevertheless, disabling filters usually allows adequate imaging of the normal and pathologic lung artifacts.

If creation of a lung-specific preset is desirable, several settings have been found to be useful. Begin with a value of zero for the setting "persistence" and a high-contrast gray scale map. The other adjustments should favor achieving high frame-per-second rates, like the cardiac presets, because of the constant movement intrinsic to the pulmonary artifacts.

In spite of the enthusiastic recommendation of some authors for specific transducers or machines, there is no consensus among the experts.[3] Simple gray scale-only machines and microconvex 5 MHz transducers were traditionally recommended, but successful and comparable studies have been performed with virtually all common transducer arrays and machines. More superficial structures (e.g., pleura and chest wall) are better examined with high-frequency linear transducers to image anatomic detail. Deeper ultrasound-conducting structures (e.g., pleural effusions and consolidations) are better identified with lower frequency curvilinear or phased array transducers.

Our general recommendation considers clinical setting and goals of the examination. In the complete initial assessment involving an unstable or acutely ill patient, where multiple clinical questions exist, ideally the same transducer should be used for the entire examination. In this scenario, use phased array or curvilinear transducers. Examples of this include the acutely dyspneic patient, the critically injured patient, and the undifferentiated hypotensive patient; this helps avoid delays when switching transducers. To evaluate a focal process in a nonemergent fashion, such as detailed analysis of a subpleural consolidation, linear transducers afford superior resolution. An example would be differentiation of a metastatic lesion from a pulmonary infarct.

▶ TECHNIQUE AND NORMAL ULTRASOUND FINDINGS

LUNG SLIDING SIGN

The interface of the parietal and visceral pleura is the first element to consider when performing a pulmonary ultrasound exam. It is the initial reference for all normal and pathologic findings. The *lung sliding sign* is visible as a hyperechoic horizontal line at the pleural level, immediately deep to the ribs, which presents to-and-fro movement with ventilation. It is generated by the reflection of the ultrasound beam off the air contained in the aerated parenchyma, and the movement represents the visceral pleura sliding against the parietal pleura (See Video 7-1: Thoracic Normal).

Correctly locate the level of the pleural line when assessing lung sliding. Start the lung exam with a vertical transducer orientation in order to visualize at least two ribs as reference points so that the position of the pleural line can be identified with certainty as it extends between them (Figure 7-2).

Once the pleural line is identified, change the transducer orientation to remove the ribs from view and scan a larger length of pulmonary surface through the intercostal space.

When a pneumothorax is suspected, begin the exam on the anterior portion of the chest with the patient

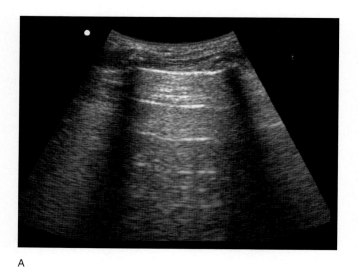

A

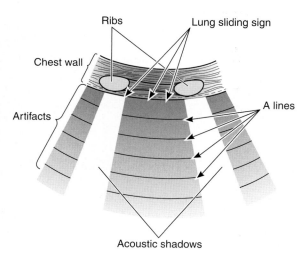

B

Figure 7-2. Normal lung. (A) Longitudinal intercostal scan. (B) Schematic representation of the same sonographic image.

in a supine position (See Video 7-2: Thoracic Abnormal). Free air will accumulate in the least dependent region of the chest cavity. If the initial exam shows lung sliding, then no further scanning is needed. If lung sliding is absent, then a pneumothorax is most likely present, but a more detailed exam can confirm the diagnosis. In this case, move the transducer laterally to find the spot where the lung loses contact from the chest wall—the lung point[33]—which clinches the diagnosis.

M-MODE SIGNS

The spherical shape of the alveoli gives the normal pleural interface a "rough" sonographic aspect by reflecting the ultrasound waves in multiple directions and causes the artifact below to present a "sparkling" pattern. The examination of normal lung in M-mode generates a pattern called the "seashore sign" (Figure 7-3A). This is not seen in the presence of a pneumothorax since the ul-

trasound beam is reflected off the smooth layer of air contained within the parietal pleura; hence, lung sliding sign is absent and the artifact is static. M-mode generates the linear pattern called the "stratosphere sign" (Figure 7-3B), which suggests the presence of a pneumothorax.

A-LINES

When the ultrasound beam reaches the pleural line, it is reflected almost entirely by the air in the alveoli or by a layer of free air. This causes a reverberation of the ultrasound waves within the thickness of the chest wall and the machine produces this image an infinite number of times. The image generated is expressed as the artifact below the pleural line as multiple horizontal lines (repetitions of the pleural line) separated by the distance equivalent to the thickness of the chest wall. These are called A-lines. They are seen whenever there is aerated parenchyma (e.g., normal lung, central pulmonary

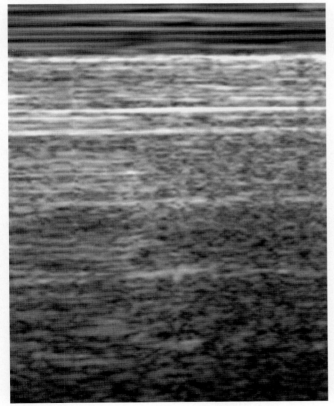

A

B

Figure 7-3. M-mode signs. (A) The seashore sign: note the two distinct patterns. The more superficial linear pattern is the tracing of the chest wall, devoid of any movement (the "waves"), and the deeper grainy pattern generated by the tracing of the sparkling artifact during normal pleural movement (the "sandy beach"). (B) The stratosphere sign: only horizontal lines are traced, recording the complete absence of movement on the screen. Both the chest wall and the artifact are static.

Increasing

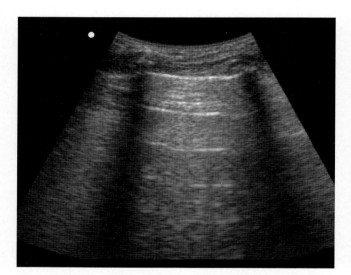
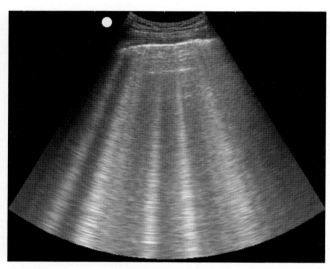

Normal

Edema

Figure 7-4. Progression of the artifacts in lung ultrasound according to increase in fluid/air ratio.

embolism, and COPD) or free air (pneumothorax). A-lines are more easily generated by free air than by aerated parenchyma. A-lines are usually present in images of normal lungs and are usually absent in the setting of interstitial syndromes, consolidations, or effusions.

► COMMON AND EMERGENT ABNORMALITIES

Understanding how lung ultrasound artifacts are generated makes it easier to appreciate how normal and pathologic images relate to specific disease processes. There is a predictable progression in the pattern of artifacts as the water/air ratio increases (Figure 7-4).[37]

Free air and aerated parenchyma reflect the ultrasound beam almost completely, while free fluid and soft tissue conduct the ultrasound beam almost completely, but certain lung diseases have a range of "in-between" conditions where there can be increased extravascular water content with engorgement of interalveolar/interlobular septa and alveolar flooding. They generate the artifact called B-lines. These artifacts are generated at the alveolar level, when the ultrasound

beam hits a layer of fluid or soft tissue surrounded by air, causing a reverberation of the beam within the soft tissue of thickened septa or flooded alveoli sandwiched between aerated alveoli. The machine interprets this reverberation as infinite repetitions of a tiny surface, stacking them up on the screen generating a vertical hyperechoic line. This phenomenon was demonstrated experimentally.[106]

To avoid confusion with other similar artifacts,[34] B-lines fulfill the following criteria[3]: laser-like hyperechoic lines, arise from the pleural line, move synchronously with the lung sliding, and extend to the bottom of the screen without fading.

A few (<3) isolated B-lines can be present in normal subjects, usually at the inferior lateral and posterior regions (Figure 7-5).

ALVEOLAR-INTERSTITIAL SYNDROMES

Cardiogenic Pulmonary Edema

The investigation of pulmonary edema, particularly in ADHF, is quite straightforward: the presence of diffuse

Fluid/Air Ratio

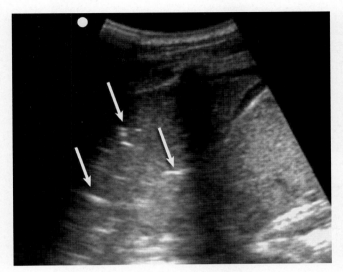

Consolidation

Effusion

Figure 7-4. (Continued)

B-lines bilaterally confirms this diagnosis. In most cases, a very limited scan of the anterior wall bilaterally is enough,[18] but a slightly more extensive exam, including the lateral walls, significantly increases sensitivity.[105] This is the method recommended by a consensus of experts.[3] For this exam, each hemithorax is divided into four regions—anterior superior, anterior inferior, lateral superior, and lateral inferior—limited by the parasternal, anterior axillary, and posterior axillary lines (Figure 7-6). A positive exam is defined as two or more positive regions bilaterally. A positive region is defined by the presence of three or more simultaneous B-lines seen in a single intercostal view.

Some experts endorse a more complete 28-point exam (Figure 7-7), acknowledging that this is not practical for routine use in the acute setting, but may be appropriate when accurate comparisons are needed (research or office follow-ups).[107]

Acute Respiratory Distress Syndrome

As opposed to ADHF, where the pattern of interstitial involvement is relatively homogenous, ARDS tends to present an irregular distribution, with patchy infiltrates and spared areas. The appearance of ARDS (and difference from ADHF) is usually straightforward on ultrasound examination, with areas of B-lines abutting areas of normal lung.

In addition to the irregular distribution pattern, ARDS has other findings. It can present as an irregular, thickened, and fragmented pleural line; small subpleural consolidations (Figure 7-8); and absence or reduction of lung sliding[3] due to decreased pulmonary compliance. As discussed above, the analysis of lung ultrasound is based on the lung sliding sign. However, in the absence of pulmonary expansion there will be no sliding with respirations, but it is still possible to identify the pleural line by identifying the lung pulse sign.[108] When there is pleural contact (no pneumothorax), but no lung expansion, the visceral pleura will show a tiny cyclic movement inflicted by the cardiac movement inside the chest. This has the appearance of a "shaking" at level of the pleural line, very similar to the lung sliding, but with a lower amplitude of movement.

Also, in ARDS, the B-lines are farther apart from each other when compared with the B-lines seen in ADHF, averaging 7 mm and 3 mm, respectively.[50] This

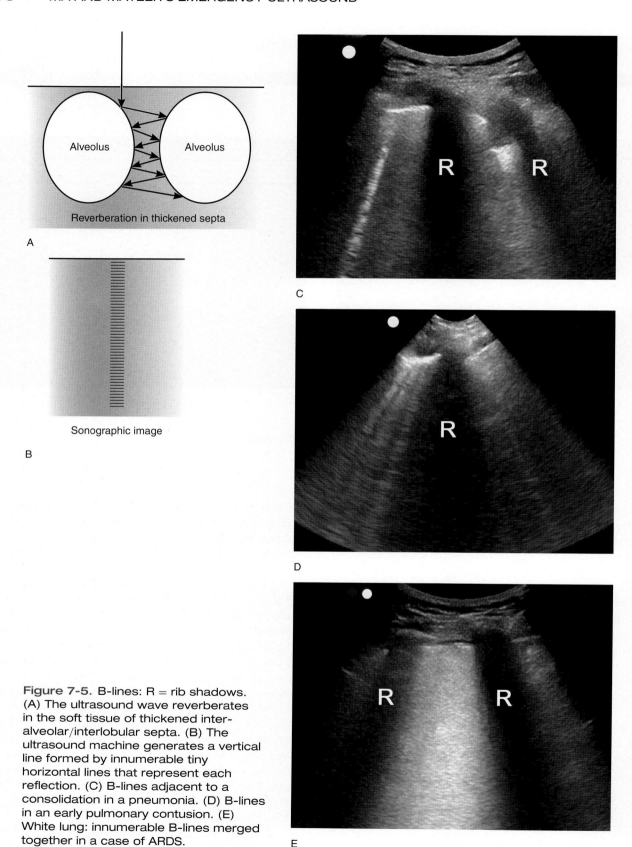

Figure 7-5. B-lines: R = rib shadows. (A) The ultrasound wave reverberates in the soft tissue of thickened inter-alveolar/interlobular septa. (B) The ultrasound machine generates a vertical line formed by innumerable tiny horizontal lines that represent each reflection. (C) B-lines adjacent to a consolidation in a pneumonia. (D) B-lines in an early pulmonary contusion. (E) White lung: innumerable B-lines merged together in a case of ARDS.

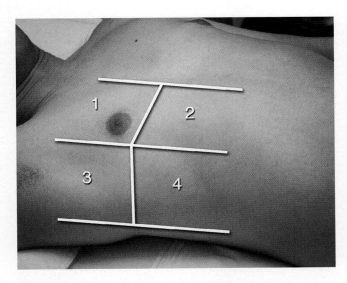

Figure 7-6. Eight-region exam for assessment of cardiogenic pulmonary edema. Two or more positive regions *bilaterally* define a positive exam.

makes sense when the histopathology of these diseases is considered: ARDS is an inflammatory process that starts in the cell-rich interlobular septa,[109] while the extravascular lung water seen in ADHF simultaneously engorges septa (interlobular and interalveolar) and floods peripheral alveoli.[107]

Pulmonary Contusion

Pulmonary contusion is a focal process since it is a direct bruise to the lung parenchyma.[110] The mecha-

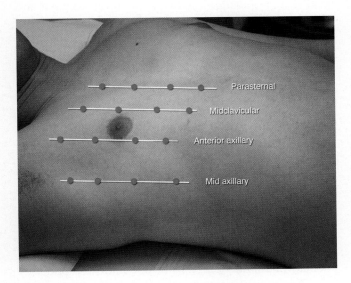

Figure 7-7. 28-Point exam. The points are at the intersections of the second to fifth intercostal spaces with the parasternal, midclavicular, anterior axillary, and midaxillary lines. The fifth intercostal space on the left is omitted to avoid the heart.

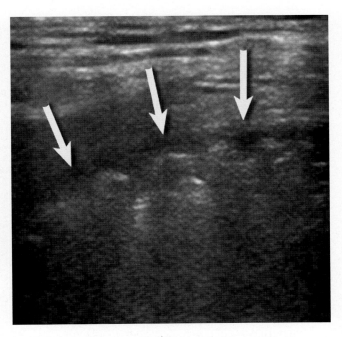

Figure 7-8. Detail of the pleural line changes in ARDS: irregular, thickened, and fragmented.

nism of injury, external signs of trauma, and the location of pain may all suggest the region of lung injury. The initial trauma causes alveolar disruption and interstitial edema, generating B-lines on ultrasound.[60] These abnormalities are obvious on ultrasound, but are missed by chest radiography.[111] Later in the course, the alveolar bleeding completely displaces the air from the affected parenchyma, forming the typical hepatization of the pulmonary tissue,[112] visible on ultrasound as subpleural consolidations.[113] At this point, the contusion may be visible on chest radiography.

Transient Tachypnea of the Newborn

Transient tachypnea of the newborn is considered a benign process secondary to the delayed clearance of fetal alveolar fluid.[114] As in all interstitial syndromes, transient tachypnea of the newborn will present with B-lines, but in a specific configuration: they are very dense in the lower regions of the lung, changing to barely present in the upper regions. This abrupt point of transition was called double lung point in the original paper by Copetti (not to be confused with the pneumothorax-specific lung point).

The B-lines in the lower regions are so dense that the sonographic appearance is of a white lung, meaning very prominent alveolar-interstitial syndrome.

The sonographic confirmation of transient tachypnea of the newborn can be very reassuring when caring for a tachypneic neonate after an unexpected ED delivery, and urgent transfer to a NICU-capable center can possibly be avoided.

Neonatal Respiratory Distress Syndrome

NRDS has very similar sonographic appearance to ARDS, but with generally more prominent findings. The combination of sonographic white lung (very densely distributed B-lines), pleural abnormalities (small subpleural consolidations, thickening, irregularity, and coarse appearance), and absence of spared areas is diagnostic.[93]

CONSOLIDATION

A more extensive examination might be required since consolidations are usually focal processes, especially when there is not an element of history that suggests a specific region (e.g., pleuritic chest pain). One study analyzed patients with pneumonia in the ED. It added posterior chest ultrasound to the eight areas described in Figure 7-6, and showed that this exam could always be completed in less than 5 minutes.[75]

The differential diagnosis of consolidations is usually apparent from the clinical history; nevertheless, there are several sonographic signs that allow differentiation[3]:

- quality of the deep margins of the consolidation
- presence of comet-tail artifacts at the far field margin
- presence of air bronchograms
- presence of fluid bronchograms
- vascular pattern within the consolidation

PNEUMONIA

Focal processes like pneumonia may require a somewhat more extensive examination if the examiner wishes to directly visualize the consolidation itself. However, narrowing the exam to a particular area (e.g., pleuritic pain on one side) may be helpful. Additionally, a pneumonia is surrounded by a regional interstitial process.[115] Because of regional impact of the disease, in the correct clinical setting, the finding of unilateral B-lines is strongly suggestive of pneumonia even if a consolidation is not seen.[18]

The vast majority of pneumonias reach the visceral pleura[82]; therefore, without an overlying layer of air the ultrasound beam can penetrate the hepatized parenchyma generating a soft tissue-like image (Figure 7-9). Pneumonia is particularly well visualized in the initial phases of the process and presents with certain sonomorphologic characteristics listed in Table 7-1.[37,67,83,115,116]

Air-filled bronchi and bronchioles are seen as hyperechoic tubular structures within the liver-like consolidation (Figure 7-10). Lentil-shaped echoes are

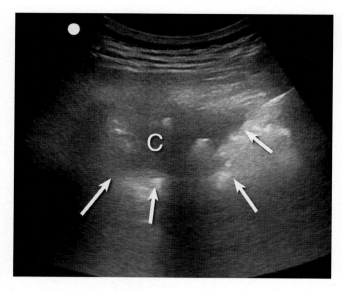

Figure 7-9. Pneumonia. Note the irregular limits (arrows) of the consolidation (C). The pleural line is not visible because there is no alveolar air to generate the lung sliding sign.

bronchi/bronchioles seen in cross section. Larger bronchi are seen within the consolidation in their normal branched distribution. Fluid mixed with the air inside these structures moves centrifugally with the inspiration, and this sign is called the dynamic air bronchogram. It is considered 100% specific for pneumonia.[83] A study[75] in the ED setting found it in 97% of the consolidations in a selected group with clinically suspected pneumonia, compared with 61% reported in a previous publication in an ICU population. Dynamic air bronchograms are the key feature in the differentiation of pneumonia and atelectasis, where the bronchograms will be static.

Superficial fluid alveologram refers to a small subpleural section completely devoid of bronchograms,[9] representing complete distal alveolar flooding.

Fluid bronchogram is the sonographic visualization of fluid contained in bronchi within the consolidations[117] (Figure 7-10A). They assume clinical importance because they suggest a postobstructive origin of the pneumonia (e.g., foreign body aspiration and expansive lesions) and bronchoscopy may be prudent.[37,67] Fluid bronchograms are hypoechoic/anechoic tubular structures seen within the consolidation. They can be differentiated from vessels by the higher echogenicity of the walls and absence of detectable Doppler signal.[116]

As opposed to expansive lesions (cancer) and ischemia (pulmonary embolism), pneumonia is primarily a fluid process that gradually occupies the airspace. In addition to the inflammatory process, the transition between flooded and nonflooded airspaces is gradual. This causes the typical irregular limits of pneumonic consolidations (the "shred sign"[18]), as well as comet-tail artifacts

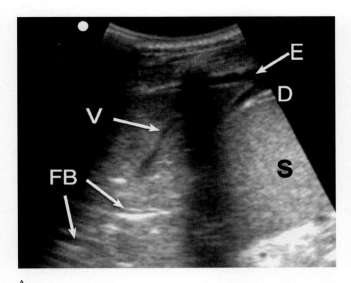

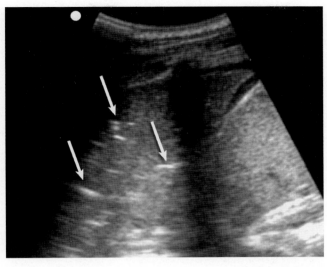

A

B

Figure 7-10. (A) Left lower lobe pneumonia at the lateral costophrenic recess. Fluid bronchograms (FB) can be seen. They have much more echogenic walls than vessels (V) and do not present flow with Doppler exam. A tiny pleural effusion (E) is seen above the diaphragm (D) overlying the spleen (S). (B) Dynamic air bronchograms. In another image of the same consolidation, movement of secretions could be seen within the air bronchograms (arrows) in real time.

arising from its deep margins and B-lines surrounding the consolidation (Figure 7-9). In addition, it has been shown that in patients with high clinical suspicion for pneumonia the finding of unilateral interstitial syndrome (multiple B-lines) is enough to make the diagnosis, even if a consolidation is not seen.[18,75]

ATELECTASIS

Atelectasis can be classified according to the causative mechanism: obstructive or compressive. Obstructive— or *absorption*—atelectasis is secondary to a proximal blockage of the airway and the distal air is absorbed, causing the collapse of the airspaces. This atelectasis is of particular importance because it quite often is radiographically similar to pneumonia.[118] There are, however, sonographic differences. By definition, obstructive

▶ **TABLE 7-1. SONOMORPHOLOGIC CHARACTERISTICS OF PNEUMONIA**

Dynamic air bronchograms
Lentil-shaped air bronchograms
Fluid alveologram
Fluid bronchogram
Irregular margins
Regional interstitial syndrome
Comet-tail artifacts arising from the deep margins
Normal anatomic distribution of the bronchial and vascular structures

atelectasis occurs after there is airway blockage; hence, there will be no pressure changes within the distal airway. The air bronchograms in atelectasis will always be static, without sonographically detectable movement of secretions or bubbles within the bronchi.[83] Also, when air is absorbed from the airspaces, there is massive loss of parenchymal volume. This causes structural collapse toward the pulmonary hilum, resulting in a more parallel relationship between the bronchi, as opposed to the normal branching pattern seen in pneumonia. This phenomenon is much more expressive in the pediatric population, but can also be seen in adults.[37]

In the very proximal airway obstructions (e.g., main stem intubations), there will not be any pulmonary ventilation and this will eventually lead to complete pulmonary atelectasis. In these cases, the lung sliding sign will also be replaced by the lung pulse sign,[108] independently of the degree of parenchyma aeration, allowing ultrasound to be an excellent resource for the detection of correct tube placement.[21–24]

Compressive atelectasis (Figure 7-11) is secondary to extrinsic compression of the peripheral pulmonary tissue, usually seen in pleural effusions. The space-occupying fluid crushes the peripheral lung, expressing the air out of that region. There is normal variation in the air pressure with ventilation since there is no proximal airway obstruction. This may cause intermittent alveolar recruitment at the interface between atelectatic and aerated tissue, a phenomenon that can easily be seen with ultrasound, allowing its differentiation from pneumonia. In addition, the use of contrast agents and Doppler

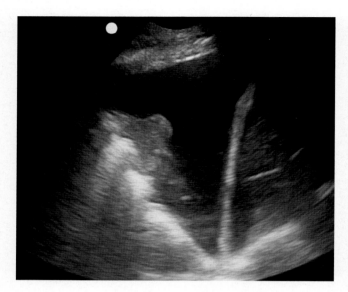

Figure 7-11. Compressive atelectasis in a patient with pleural effusion in renal failure. The reduction in parenchymal volume in atelectasis becomes obvious when compared with the pneumonia in Figure 7-9, at the same anatomic location.

vascular analysis may allow for accurate differentiation of atelectasis and other consolidations.[116]

PULMONARY EMBOLISM

Two different approaches exist for the sonographic diagnosis of pulmonary embolism. In the critical care and emergency medicine literature, findings of normal lung, presence of DVT, and presence of right heart strain confirm the diagnosis.[18] In the pulmonary and radiology literature, sonomorphologic findings of consolidations are key, including vascular Doppler and contrast-enhanced findings.[67,86,116,119] We recommend the former approach, but occasionally the emergency physician may need differentiation of a subpleural consolidation. Unlike pneumonia and atelectasis, ischemic subpleural consolidations (Figure 7-12) have the following characteristics:[86]

- Well delimited, usually small (average 1.4 × 1 cm) wedge-shaped, hypoechoic, or anechoic consolidations;
- Not surrounded by interstitial syndrome;
- Occasionally, one isolated air bronchogram can be seen at the center of the consolidation;
- A small contained perilesional effusion can occasionally be seen, secondary to the acute inflammatory process in the ischemic region under the visceral pleura. Being subpleural, this effusion is static, overlying the lesion, and moves with the ventilatory movement.

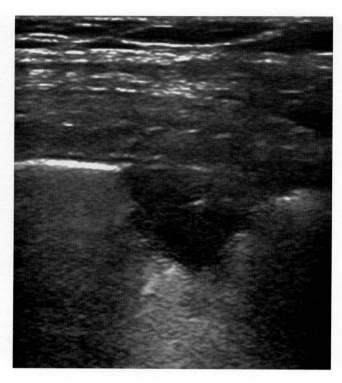

Figure 7-12. Typical subpleural consolidation in pulmonary embolism: triangular shaped with sharp edges, no surrounding interstitial syndrome, and a small central hyperechoic lenticular bronchogram.

EFFUSIONS

Pleural effusions are highly gravity dependent. Unless extremely loculated and organized, an effusion will flow to the most dependent regions of the pleural cavity. Therefore, initially assess the posterior costophrenic recess in a sitting patient. In supine position, such as an immobilized trauma patient, place the transducer at the most posterior spot reachable by the transducer without rotating the patient, which would only displace the fluid away from the transducer. The traditional transhepatic/transplenic approach of the FAST exam can also be used.

Large and moderate effusions are usually quite obvious, but small echogenic effusions can be harder to differentiate from pleural thickening using B-mode only. Ventilatory movements cause free fluid to shift, which can be detected with color Doppler, allowing accurate differentiation.[120]

The sinusoid sign is also specific for effusions (Figure 7-13). The ventilatory movements cause the lung to come closer to the chest wall in inspiration and to move away in expiration. This cyclic movement can be detected as a typical sinusoid tracing in M-mode.

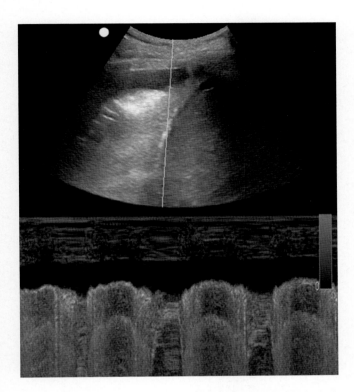

Figure 7-13. The sinusoid sign in pleural effusion.

TRANSUDATE VS. EXUDATE

Pleural effusions can be divided into four categories based on sonographic appearance: anechoic, complex nonseptated, complex septated, and homogenously echogenic. Transudates are always anechoic and hemothoraces are homogenously echogenic. Unfortunately, inflammatory exudates can present as any of these categories; therefore, thoracentesis is still needed when the clinical presentation is not clear and the differentiation is necessary. Ultrasound should be used for guidance of thoracentesis when it is indicated, and should also be used to determine when it is contraindicated. Plain films can be deceiving in estimating the size and position of an effusion. In general, a thoracentesis is recommended only when a pleural fluid collection is at least 15 mm thick.[121]

VOLUME ESTIMATION

Estimation of the volume of a pleural effusion is generally classified as small, moderate, or large. Multiple techniques for measuring volume have been reported,[101] usually with margins of error around 25%; this is far superior to estimating the volume with a chest radiograph.[122] The most straightforward technique on supine patients is to measure the largest thickness of

the effusion at the lateral wall (D) and use the following formula: D (mm) × 47.6 − 837 = volume (mL).

DIAGNOSIS OF DYSPNEA

In 2008, Lichtenstein proposed the BLUE protocol as a straightforward method to diagnose the cause of dyspnea in critically ill patients. It is based on the analysis of three spots on each hemithorax: one anterior, one anterolateral and caudal, and one posterolateral and caudal (Figure 7-14), as well as lower extremity venous analysis for DVT. A brief cardiac analysis is not part of the protocol, but is recommended.

Each anterior point will be analyzed for presence or absence of lung sliding, presence of A-lines or B-lines, and presence of consolidations.

The posterolateral point may then be analyzed for the presence of PLAPS, or posterior/lateral alveolar/pleural syndrome, which is a combination of effusion and/or consolidation limited to the posterolateral regions.

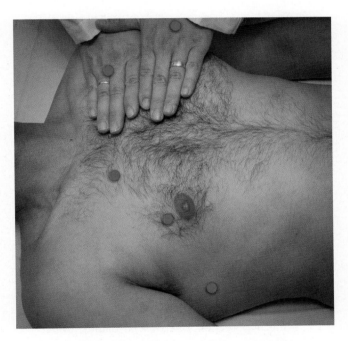

Figure 7-14. The BLUE points can be found by placing two hands on the patient's chest, side by side, with the little finger of the upper hand aligned with the lower limit of the clavicle and index fingers side by side and the fingertips over the midline. The little finger of the lower hand should then be parallel to the diaphragmatic line. The first point is between the bases of the ring and middle finger of the upper hand. The second point is at the center of the palm of the lower hand. The third point (PLAPS point) is at the intersection of a straight line traced under the little finger of the lower hand and the midaxillary line.

The combination of the findings will determine one of the following profiles:

A profile: Lung sliding present, A-lines predominant. This profile rules out pneumothorax and should prompt a search for DVT. If DVT is present, this suggests a diagnosis of pulmonary embolism. If DVT is absent, then begin a search for PLAPS. If PLAPS is present, it suggests a diagnosis of pneumonia.

A' profile: Lung sliding absent, A-lines predominant. This profile suggests a pneumothorax is present. This profile may also be present in cases of markedly decreased or absent lung sliding, such as in advanced COPD or posttherapeutic pleurodesis. It should prompt a search for a lung point (100% specific).[3]

B profile: Lung sliding present, anterior B-lines predominant bilaterally. This profile suggests pulmonary edema.

B' profile: Lung sliding absent, anterior B-lines predominant. This profile suggests extensive pneumonia, with markedly decreased pulmonary compliance. ARDS should also be considered.

A/B profile: B-lines predominant on one side, A-lines on the other side. This profile suggests a diagnosis of pneumonia.

C profile: anterior consolidations. This profile suggests a diagnosis of pneumonia.

Normal profile: A profile without PLAPS. This profile suggests a diagnosis of COPD or asthma.

▶ PITFALLS

1. **Identification of the pleural line.** Always use the ribs to initially identify the pleural line, and only then appreciate the presence or absence of lung sliding at that level. The misidentification of fascia and muscle planes within the chest wall for lung sliding sign could be disastrous. A typical example would be a muscular trauma patient, with dyspnea secondary to a pneumothorax. This patient would likely present with exaggerated ventilatory movement secondary to dyspnea and the chest wall muscles may slide on each other, generating a moving hyperechoic line (fascial planes) above the ribs.

2. **Subcutaneous emphysema.** The sonographic appearance of subcutaneous emphysema can mimic B-lines arising from the pleural line. The air trapped in the subcutaneous tissue can generate hyperechoic vertical artifacts, but these do not move with the ventilation and do not arise from the pleural line. Ribs are usually not visible, as they are obscured by the artifact. These lines have been called W-lines (when arising from multiple levels) or E-lines (when arising

from the same plane).[34] Once again, the correct identification of the pleural line as the first step of the exam cannot be emphasized enough, particularly in trauma. In most cases, if the patient can tolerate this maneuver, applying more pressure with the transducer will force the free air out of the scanning plane, allowing for visualization of the pleural line.

3. **Pulmonary embolism.** Normal lungs on the ultrasound exam are the hallmark of a large pulmonary embolism. Therefore, when evaluating the lungs in a dyspneic patient, the clinician should not be deterred by a normal ultrasound exam, and should proceed to evaluate for DVT. The finding of pulmonary infarction adds weight to the diagnosis of pulmonary embolus.

4. **BLUE protocol for dyspnea.** The BLUE protocol was designed based on a population of ICU patients with profound dysfunction. Its utility for stable patients was not studied. Its use in noncritical patients is currently discouraged.

▶ CASE STUDIES

CASE 1

Patient Presentation

A 65-year-old-man presented to the ED by ambulance in respiratory distress with an oxygen saturation of 86%. The patient was unable to speak in full sentences. The paramedics gleaned that the patient had increasing shortness of breath for several days. He acutely worsened this evening. The patient and his family were not able to provide a past medical history. The patient's medications included furosemide, albuterol, and metoprolol. On physical examination, his blood pressure was 185/78 mm Hg, pulse 115 beats per minute, respirations 25 per minute, and temperature 37.0°C. His lung exam revealed poor aeration in all fields. Lower extremities had pitting edema of the feet bilaterally.

Management Course

The patient was placed on noninvasive positive pressure ventilation with 100% oxygen with an in-line albuterol and ipratropium nebulized treatment. IV methylprednisolone and furosemide were ordered. A stat portable chest radiograph was ordered. A point-of-care lung ultrasound examination revealed diffuse B-lines throughout the bilateral lung fields and a small pleural effusion on the right. The portable chest radiograph showed poor inspiratory effort with vascular congestion and concern for pulmonary edema. The patient's BiPAP inspiratory effort was increased to maximize displacement of interstitial fluid. The nebulized treatments were stopped to promote slowing of the heart rate. Within 30 minutes, the patient's respiratory status was markedly improved. BiPAP was discontinued and oxygen was decreased to a nasal cannula.

Commentary

In this case, point-of-care lung ultrasound rapidly narrowed the differential diagnosis and allowed early treatment of ADHF. The chest radiograph was suggestive, but not diagnostic due to the inability of the patient to comply with a breath-hold. The patient was immediately maximized on appropriate therapy and noncontributory therapies were discontinued. Pulmonary ultrasound is rapid and accurate in the evaluation of the acutely dyspneic patient.

CASE 2

Patient Presentation

A 20-year-old man presented to the ED by ambulance in respiratory distress with an oxygen saturation of 86% on 15 L of oxygen via a non-rebreather mask. The patient was unable to speak full sentences. The paramedics reported that the patient had asthma. He experienced coughing and wheezing for the past week, which became worse today. On physical examination, his blood pressure was 130/78 mm Hg, pulse 125 beats per minute, respirations 30 per minute, and temperature 37.0°C. The lung exam revealed decreased air movement throughout with diffuse expiratory wheezes.

Management Course

The patient was placed on maximal oxygen with an albuterol and ipratropium nebulized treatment. IV methylprednisolone was administered. Point-of-care lung ultrasound examination identified the pleural line in the second intercostal space. The pleural line on the right exhibited lung sliding. The pleural line on the left was identified, and lung sliding was not found. The transducer was moved laterally and a lung point was detected (Figure 7-15). The differential diagnosis was expanded from acute asthma exacerbation to include pneumothorax. Since the patient remained hypoxic and in respiratory distress, the decision was made to perform tube thoracostomy in the left chest. There was a large rush of air and the patient's respiratory status improved markedly.

Commentary

Lung ultrasound played a critical role in the early evaluation and rapid management of this patient in respiratory distress. The unexpected finding of a pneumothorax on ultrasound directed clinical management. Any delays for

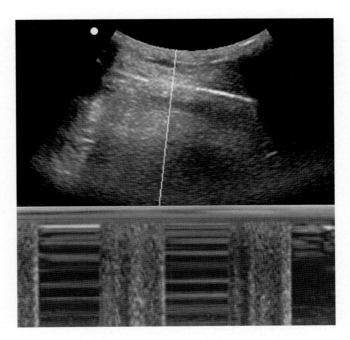

Figure 7-15. The lung point sign, a very specific indicator of pneumothorax. In a live video, lung sliding is seen only on one side of the screen, and the point of transition moves with ventilation. M-mode records alternation of stratosphere and seashore signs.

traditional imaging tests may have resulted in an unnecessary intubation for a condition that was immediately reversible. The timeliness of point-of-care pulmonary ultrasound facilitates the diagnosis and treatment of critically ill patients.

CASE 3

Patient Presentation

A 9-month-old, full-term, healthy female infant was brought to the ED by her mother. The patient had a cough, rhinorrhea, and fever for 2 days. She was experiencing more difficulty breathing today. Her mother reported that she could hear wheezing. On physical examination, her blood pressure was 80/60 mm Hg, pulse 130 beats per minute, respirations 40 per minute, temperature 38.0°C, and oxygen saturation 96%. She was a tachypneic infant in mild respiratory distress with intercostal retractions. There were diffuse expiratory wheezes on auscultation of the lungs. It was RSV season so the clinician had a stronger suspicion for RSV than lobar pneumonia.

Management Course

The patient had minimal improvement after a treatment of nebulized albuterol was administered. The clinician performed a point-of-care pulmonary ultrasound exam and did not identify consolidative processes. Occasional B-lines were seen. Subsequently, the patient received nebulized racemic epinephrine with significant improvement. Tachypnea did not recur. A rapid RSV came back positive. Given the entire clinical picture, the clinician opted to not order a chest radiograph. The patient was discharged with a diagnosis of RSV bronchiolitis. Return precautions and close follow-up were instituted.

Commentary

Pulmonary ultrasound findings are best used in combination with other diagnostic information to help providers support or refute their clinical impression. In this case, the RSV test, clinical improvement, and the ultrasound findings all contributed to the care of this infant.

REFERENCES

1. Rantanen NW: Diseases of the thorax. *Vet Clin North Am Equine Pract* 2(1):49–66, 1986.
2. Lichtenstein DA, Menu Y: A bedside ultrasound sign ruling out pneumothorax in the critically ill. Lung sliding. *Chest* 108(5):1345–1348, 1995.
3. Volpicelli G, Elbarbary M, Blaivas M, et al.: International evidence-based recommendations for point-of-care lung ultrasound. *Intensive Care Med* 38(4):577–591, 2012.
4. Neesse A, Jerrentrup A, Hoffmann S, et al.: Prehospital chest emergency sonography trial in Germany. *Eur J Emerg Med* 19(3):161–166, 2011.
5. Ma OJ, Norvell JG, Subramanian S: Ultrasound applications in mass casualties and extreme environments. *Crit Care Med* 35(5 suppl):S275–S279, 2007.
6. Hamilton DR, Sargsyan AE, Kirkpatrick AW, et al.: Sonographic detection of pneumothorax and hemothorax in microgravity. *Aviat Space Environ Med* 75(3):272–277, 2004.
7. Lindelius A, Törngren S, Nilsson L, Pettersson H, Adami J: Randomized clinical trial of bedside ultrasound among patients with abdominal pain in the emergency department: Impact on patient satisfaction and health care consumption. *Scand J Trauma Resusc Emerg Med* 17:60, 2009.
8. Bouhemad B, Liu Z-H, Arbelot C, et al.: Ultrasound assessment of antibiotic-induced pulmonary reaeration in ventilator-associated pneumonia. *Crit Care Med* 38(1):84–92, 2010.
9. Reissig A, Kroegel C: Sonographic diagnosis and follow-up of pneumonia: A prospective study. *Respiration* 74(5):537–547, 2007.
10. Peris A, Tutino L, Zagli G, et al.: The use of point-of-care bedside lung ultrasound significantly reduces the number of radiographs and computed tomography scans in critically ill patients. *Anesth Analg* 111(3):687–692, 2010.
11. Kirkpatrick AW, Sirois M, Laupland KB, et al.: Hand-held thoracic sonography for detecting post-traumatic pneumothoraces: The Extended Focused Assessment with Sonography for Trauma (EFAST). *J Trauma* 57(2):288–295, 2004.
12. Jones AE, Tayal VS, Sullivan DM, Kline JA: Randomized, controlled trial of immediate versus delayed goal-directed ultrasound to identify the cause of nontraumatic hypotension in emergency department patients. *Crit Care Med* 32(8):1703–1708, 2004.
13. Lanctôt J-F, Valois M, Beaulieu Y: EGLS: echo-guided life support. *Crit Ultrasound J* 3:123–129, 2011.
14. Perera P, Mailhot T, Riley D, Mandavia D: The RUSH Exam: Rapid Ultrasound in SHock in the evaluation of the critically ill. *Emerg Med Clin North Am* 28(1):29–56, 2010
15. Atkinson PRT, McAuley DJ, Kendall RJ, et al.: Abdominal and cardiac evaluation with sonography in shock (ACES): An approach by emergency physicians for the use of ultrasound in patients with undifferentiated hypotension. *Emerg Med J* 26(2):87–91, 2009.
16. Cibinel GA, Casoli G, Elia F, et al.: Diagnostic accuracy and reproducibility of pleural and lung ultrasound in discriminating cardiogenic causes of acute dyspnea in the emergency department. *Intern Emerg Med* 7(1):65–70, 2012.
17. Copetti R, Copetti P, Reissig A: Clinical integrated ultrasound of the thorax including causes of shock in nontraumatic critically ill patients. A practical approach. *Ultrasound Med Biol* 38(3):349–359, 2012.
18. Lichtenstein DA, Mezière GA: Relevance of lung ultrasound in the diagnosis of acute respiratory failure: The BLUE protocol. *Chest* 134(1):117–125, 2008.
19. Zanobetti M, Poggioni C, Pini R: Can chest ultrasonography replace standard chest radiography for evaluation of acute dyspnea in the ED? *Chest* 139(5):1140–1147, 2011.
20. Nicholls SE, Sweeney TW, Ferre RM, Strout TD: Bedside sonography by emergency physicians for the rapid identification of landmarks relevant to cricothyrotomy. *Am J Emerg Med* 26(8):852–856, 2008.
21. Blaivas M, Tsung JW: Point-of-care sonographic detection of left endobronchial main stem intubation and obstruction versus endotracheal intubation. *J Ultrasound Med* 27(5):785–789, 2008.
22. Weaver B, Lyon M, Blaivas M: Confirmation of endotracheal tube placement after intubation using the ultrasound sliding lung sign. *Acad Emerg Med* 13(3):239–244, 2006.
23. Chun R, Kirkpatrick AW, Sirois M, et al.: Where's the tube? Evaluation of hand-held ultrasound in confirming endotracheal tube placement. *Prehosp Disaster Med* 19(4):366–369, 2004.
24. Galicinao J, Bush AJ, Godambe SA: Use of bedside ultrasonography for endotracheal tube placement in pediatric patients: A feasibility study. *Pediatrics* 120(6):1297–1303, 2007.
25. Reissig A, Kroegel C: Accuracy of transthoracic sonography in excluding post-interventional pneumothorax and hydropneumothorax. Comparison to chest radiography. *Eur J Radiol* 53(3):463–470, 2005.
26. Weinecke K, Galanski M, Peters PE, Hansen J: Pneumothorax: evaluation by ultrasound–preliminary results. *J Thorac Imaging* 2(2):76–78, 1987.

27. Dulchavsky SA, Schwarz KL, Kirkpatrick AW, et al.: Prospective evaluation of thoracic ultrasound in the detection of pneumothorax. *J Trauma* 50(2):201–205, 2001.

28. Zhang M, Liu Z-H, Yang J-X, et al.: Rapid detection of pneumothorax by ultrasonography in patients with multiple trauma. *Crit Care* 10(4):R112, 2006.

29. Wilkerson RG, Stone MB: Sensitivity of bedside ultrasound and supine anteroposterior chest radiographs for the identification of pneumothorax after blunt trauma. *Acad Emerg Med* 17(1):11–17, 2010.

30. Silva F: Shirt fold mimicking pneumothorax on chest radiograph: Accurate diagnosis by ultrasound. *Intern Emerg Med* 2(3):236–238, 2007.

31. Kirkpatrick AW, Ng AK, Dulchavsky SA, et al.: Sonographic diagnosis of a pneumothorax inapparent on plain radiography: confirmation by computed tomography. *J Trauma* 50(4):750–752, 2001.

32. Knudtson JL, Dort JM, Helmer SD, Smith RS: Surgeon-performed ultrasound for pneumothorax in the trauma suite. *J Trauma* 56(3):527–530, 2004.

33. Lichtenstein D, Mezière G, Biderman P, Gepner A: The "lung point": An ultrasound sign specific to pneumothorax. *Intensive Care Med* 26(10):1434–1440, 2000.

34. Lichtenstein DA, Mezière G, Lascols N, et al.: Ultrasound diagnosis of occult pneumothorax. *Crit Care Med* 33(6):1231–1238, 2005.

35. Lichtenstein D, Mezière G: Ultrasound probably has a bright future in the diagnosis of pneumothorax. *J Trauma* 52(3):607, 2002.

36. Liu DM, Forkheim K, Rowan K, Mawson JB, Kirkpatrick A, Nicolaou S: Utilization of ultrasound for the detection of pneumothorax in the neonatal special-care nursery. *Pediatr Radiol* 33(12):880–883, 2003.

37. Soldati G, Copetti R: *Ecografia Toracica.* 1st ed. Casagranda I, ed. Torino, Italy: C. G. Edizioni Medico Scientifiche S.r.l, 2006.

38. Remes J, Miettinen H, Reunanen A, Pyörälä K: Validity of clinical diagnosis of heart failure in primary health care. *Eur Heart J* 12(3):315–321, 1991.

39. Wong GC, Ayas NT: Clinical approaches to the diagnosis of acute heart failure. *Curr Opin Cardiol* 22(3):207–213, 2007.

40. Wang CS, FitzGerald JM, Schulzer M, Mak E, Ayas NT: Does this dyspneic patient in the emergency department have congestive heart failure? *JAMA.* 294(15):1944–1956, 2005.

41. Lichtenstein D, Mezière G: A lung ultrasound sign allowing bedside distinction between pulmonary edema and COPD: The comet-tail artifact. *Intensive Care Med* 24(12):1331–1334, 1998.

42. Copetti R, Soldati G, Copetti P: Chest sonography: A useful tool to differentiate acute cardiogenic pulmonary edema from acute respiratory distress syndrome. *Cardiovasc Ultrasound* 6:16, 2008.

43. Soldati G, Gargani L, Silva FR: Acute heart failure: New diagnostic perspectives for the emergency physician. *Intern Emerg Med* 3(1):37–41, 2008.

44. Rempell JS, Noble VE: Using lung ultrasound to differentiate patients in acute dyspnea in the prehospital emergency setting. *Crit Care* 15(3):161, 2011.

45. Volpicelli G, Mussa A, Garofalo G, et al.: Bedside lung ultrasound in the assessment of alveolar-interstitial syndrome. *Am J Emerg Med* 24(6):689–696, 2006.

46. Picano E, Frassi F, Agricola E, Gligorova S, Gargani L, Mottola G: Ultrasound lung comets: A clinically useful sign of extravascular lung water. *J Am Soc Echocardiogr* 19(3):356–363, 2006.

47. Agricola E, Bove T, Oppizzi M, et al.: "Ultrasound comet-tail images": A marker of pulmonary edema: a comparative study with wedge pressure and extravascular lung water. *Chest* 127(5):1690–1695, 2005.

48. Noble VE, Murray AF, Capp R, Sylvia-Reardon MH, Steele DJR, Liteplo A: Ultrasound assessment for extravascular lung water in patients undergoing hemodialysis. Time course for resolution. *Chest* 135(6):1433–1439, 2009.

49. Lichtenstein D: Lung ultrasound in acute respiratory failure an introduction to the BLUE-protocol. *Minerva Anestesiol* 75(5):313–317, 2009.

50. Lichtenstein D, Mezière G, Biderman P, Gepner A, Barré O: The comet-tail artifact. An ultrasound sign of alveolar-interstitial syndrome. *Am J Respir Crit Care Med* 156(5):1640–1646, 1997.

51. Fagenholz PJ, Gutman JA, Murray AF, Noble VE, Thomas SH, Harris NS: Chest ultrasonography for the diagnosis and monitoring of high-altitude pulmonary edema. *Chest* 131(4):1013–1018, 2007.

52. Gargani L, Lionetti V, Di Cristofano C, Bevilacqua G, Recchia FA, Picano E: Early detection of acute lung injury uncoupled to hypoxemia in pigs using ultrasound lung comets. *Crit Care Med* 35(12):2769–2774, 2007.

53. Schwarz MI, Albert RK: "Imitators" of the ARDS: Implications for diagnosis and treatment. *Chest* 125(4):1530–1535, 2004.

54. Hansen-Flaschen J, Siegel M: *Acute Respiratory Distress Syndrome: Definition, Clinical Features and Diagnosis.* 19th ed. Basow D, ed. Waltham, MA: UpToDate, 2012.

55. Rudiger A, Gasser S, Fischler M, Hornemann T, Eckardstein von A, Maggiorini M: Comparable increase of B-type natriuretic peptide and amino-terminal pro-B-type natriuretic peptide levels in patients with severe sepsis, septic shock, and acute heart failure. *Crit Care Med* 34(8):2140–2144, 2006.

56. Levitt JE, Vinayak AG, Gehlbach BK, et al.: Diagnostic utility of B-type natriuretic peptide in critically ill patients with pulmonary edema: A prospective cohort study. *Crit Care* 12(1):R3, 2008.

57. Arbelot C, Ferrari F, Bouhemad B, Rouby J-J: Lung ultrasound in acute respiratory distress syndrome and acute lung injury. *Curr Opin Crit Care* 14(1):70–74, 2008.

58. Bouhemad B, Brisson H, Le-Guen M, Arbelot C, Lu Q, Rouby JJ: Bedside ultrasound assessment of positive end-expiratory pressure-induced lung recruitment. *Am J Respir Crit Care Med* 183(3):341–347, 2011.

59. Wüstner A, Gehmacher O, Hämmerle S, Schenkenbach C, Häfele H, Mathis G: Ultrasound diagnosis in blunt thoracic trauma. *Ultraschall Med* 26(4):285–290, 2005.

60. Soldati G, Testa A, Silva FR, Carbone L, Portale G, Silveri NG: Chest ultrasonography in lung contusion. *Chest* 130(2):533–538, 2006.

61. Stone MB, Secko MA: Bedside ultrasound diagnosis of pulmonary contusion. *Pediatr Emerg Care* 25(12):854–855, 2009.

62. Stone MB: Acute chest syndrome diagnosed by lung sonography. *Am J Emerg Med* 27(4):516.e5–e6, 2009.

63. Doveri M, Frassi F, Consensi A, et al.: Ultrasound lung comets: New echographic sign of lung interstitial fibrosis in systemic sclerosis. *Reumatismo* 60(3):180–184, 2008.

64. Sperandeo M, Varriale A, Sperandeo G, et al.: Transthoracic ultrasound in the evaluation of pulmonary fibrosis: Our experience. *Ultrasound Med Biol* 35(5):723–729, 2009.

65. Delle Sedie A, Doveri M, Frassi F, et al.: Ultrasound lung comets in systemic sclerosis: A useful tool to detect lung interstitial fibrosis. *Clin Exp Rheumatol* 28(5 suppl 62):S54, 2010.

66. Volpicelli G, Frascisco MF: Sonographic detection of radio-occult interstitial lung involvement in measles pneumonitis. *Am J Emerg Med* 27(1):128.e1–3, 2009.

67. Reissig A, Görg C, Mathis G: Transthoracic sonography in the diagnosis of pulmonary diseases: A systematic approach. *Ultraschall Med* 30(5):438–454; quiz 455–456, 2009.

68. Wipf JE, Lipsky BA, Hirschmann JV, et al.: Diagnosing pneumonia by physical examination: Relevant or relic? *Arch Intern Med* 159(10):1082–1087, 1999.

69. Metlay JP, Fine MJ: Testing strategies in the initial management of patients with community-acquired pneumonia. *Ann Intern Med* 138(2):109–118, 2003.

70. Mandell LA, Wunderink RG, Anzueto A, et al.: Infectious Diseases Society of America/American Thoracic Society consensus guidelines on the management of community-acquired pneumonia in adults. *Clin. Infect. Dis* S27–S72, 2007.

71. Wilkins TR, Wilkins RL: Clinical and radiographic evidence of pneumonia. *Radiol Technol* 77(2):106–110, 2005.

72. Hagaman JT, Rouan GW, Shipley RT, Panos RJ: Admission chest radiograph lacks sensitivity in the diagnosis of community-acquired pneumonia. *Am J Med Sci* 337(4):236–240, 2009.

73. Syrjälä H, Broas M, Suramo I, Ojala A, Lähde S: High-resolution computed tomography for the diagnosis of community-acquired pneumonia. *Clin Infect Dis* 27(2):358–363, 1998.

74. Lynch T, Bialy L, Kellner JD, et al.: A systematic review on the diagnosis of pediatric bacterial pneumonia: When gold is bronze. *PLoS ONE* 5(8):e11989, 2010.

75. Cortellaro F, Colombo S, Coen D, Duca PG: Lung ultrasound is an accurate diagnostic tool for the diagnosis of pneumonia in the emergency department. *Emerg Med J* 29(1):19–23, 2012.

76. Sperandeo M, Carnevale V, Muscarella S, et al.: Clinical application of transthoracic ultrasonography in inpatients with pneumonia. *Eur J Clin Invest* 41(1):1–7, 2011.

77. Parlamento S, Copetti R, Di Bartolomeo S: Evaluation of lung ultrasound for the diagnosis of pneumonia in the ED. *Am J Emerg Med* 27(4):379–384, 2009.

78. Gibikote S, Verghese VP: Diagnosis of pneumonia in children: Ultrasound better than CXR? *Radiol Med* 113(7):1079–1080; author reply 1080–1081, 2008.

79. Copetti R, Cattarossi L: Ultrasound diagnosis of pneumonia in children. *Radiol Med* 113(2):190–198, 2008.

80. Lichtenstein D, Peyrouset O: Is lung ultrasound superior to CT? The example of a CT occult necrotizing pneumonia. *Intensive Care Med* 32(2):334–335, 2006.

81. Gehmacher O, Mathis G, Kopf A, Scheier M: Ultrasound imaging of pneumonia. *Ultrasound Med Biol* 21(9):1119–1122, 1995.

82. Lichtenstein DA, Lascols N, Mezière G, Gepner A: Ultrasound diagnosis of alveolar consolidation in the critically ill. *Intensive Care Med* 30(2):276–281, 2004.

83. Lichtenstein D, Mezière G, Seitz J: The dynamic air bronchogram. A lung ultrasound sign of alveolar consolidation ruling out atelectasis. *Chest* 135(6):1421–1425, 2009.

84. Lichtenstein DA: Ultrasound in the management of thoracic disease. *Crit Care Med* 35(5 suppl):S250–61, 2007.

85. Mathis G, Blank W, Reissig A, et al.: Thoracic ultrasound for diagnosing pulmonary embolism: A prospective multicenter study of 352 patients. *Chest* 128(3):1531–1538, 2005.

86. Reissig A, Heyne JP, Kroegel C: Sonography of lung and pleura in pulmonary embolism: Sonomorphologic characterization and comparison with spiral CT scanning. *Chest* 120(6):1977–1983, 2001.

87. Mathis G: Why look for artifacts alone when the original is visible? *Chest* 137(1):233–233, 2010.

88. Reissig A, Kroegel C: Relevance of subpleural consolidations in chest ultrasound. *Chest* 136(6):1706; author reply 1706–1707, 2009.

89. Mathis G: Sonographie bei Lungenembolie: drei Fliegen auf einen Streich. *Pneumologie* 60(10):600–606, 2006.

90. Brenner D, Elliston C, Hall E, Berdon W: Estimated risks of radiation-induced fatal cancer from pediatric CT. *AJR Am J Roentgenol* 176(2):289–296, 2001.

91. Linet MS, Slovis TL, Miller DL, et al.: Cancer risks associated with external radiation from diagnostic imaging procedures. *CA Cancer J Clin* 62:75–100, 2012.

92. Copetti R, Cattarossi L: The "double lung point": an ultrasound sign diagnostic of transient tachypnea of the newborn. *Neonatology* 91(3):203–209, 2007.

93. Copetti R, Cattarossi L, Macagno F, Violino M, Furlan R: Lung ultrasound in respiratory distress syndrome: A useful tool for early diagnosis. *Neonatology* 94(1):52–59, 2008.

94. Lichtenstein D, Goldstein I, Mourgeon E, Cluzel P, Grenier P, Rouby J-J: Comparative diagnostic performances of auscultation, chest radiography, and lung ultrasonography in acute respiratory distress syndrome. *Anesthesiology* 100(1):9–15, 2004.

95. Lichtenstein DA: Ultrasound examination of the lungs in the intensive care unit. *Pediatr Crit Care Med* 10(6):693–698, 2009.

96. Doelken P, Mayo P: *Thoracic Ultrasound: Indications, Advantages, and Technique.* 19th ed. Basow D, ed. Waltham, MA: UpToDate, 2012.

97. Xirouchaki N, Magkanas E, Vaporidi K, et al.: Lung ultrasound in critically ill patients: Comparison with bedside chest radiography. *Intensive Care Med* 37(9):1488–1493, 2011.

98. Kocijancic KV, Vidmar G, Kocijancic I: Sonographic evaluation of pleural fluid in a large group of adult healthy

individuals—end trial results. *Coll Antropol* 33(3):805–810, 2009.

99. Yang PC, Luh KT, Chang DB, Wu HD, Yu CJ, Kuo SH: Value of sonography in determining the nature of pleural effusion: Analysis of 320 cases. *AJR Am J Roentgenol* 159(1):29–33, 1992.

100. Koegelenberg C, Diacon A, Bolliger C: Transthoracic ultrasound for chest wall, pleura and the peripheral lung. In: Bolliger C, ed. *Clinical Chest Ultrasound*. 1st ed. Basel, Switzerland: Karger, 2009.

101. Reuss JP, Mathis G, eds. *Chest Sonography*. 3rd ed. Berlin, Germany: Springer, 2012.

102. Duncan DR, Morgenthaler TI, Ryu JH, Daniels CE: Reducing iatrogenic risk in thoracentesis: Establishing best practice via experiential training in a zero-risk environment. *Chest* 135(5):1315–1320, 2009.

103. Weingardt JP, Guico RR, Nemcek AA, Li YP, Chiu ST: Ultrasound findings following failed, clinically directed thoracenteses. *J Clin Ultrasound* 22(7):419–426, 1994.

104. Lichtenstein D: The BLUE-points: Three standardized points used in the BLUE-protocol for ultrasound assessment of the lung in acute respiratory failure. *Crit Ultrasound J* 3:109–110, 2011.

105. Volpicelli G, Noble V, Liteplo A, Cardinale L: Decreased sensitivity of lung ultrasound limited to the anterior chest in emergency department diagnosis of cardiogenic pulmonary edema: A retrospective analysis. *Crit Ultrasound J* 2(2), 2010.

106. Soldati G, Copetti R, Sher S: Sonographic interstitial syndrome: The sound of lung water. *J Ultrasound Med* 1;28(2):163–174, 2009.

107. Jambrik Z, Monti S, Coppola V, et al.: Usefulness of ultrasound lung comets as a nonradiologic sign of extravascular lung water. *Am J Cardiol* 93(10):1265–1270, 2004.

108. Lichtenstein DA, Lascols N, Prin S, Mezière G: The "lung pulse": An early ultrasound sign of complete atelectasis. *Intensive Care Med* 29(12):2187–2192, 2003.

109. Matthay MA, Zimmerman GA: Acute lung injury and the acute respiratory distress syndrome: Four decades of inquiry into pathogenesis and rational management. *Am J Respir Cell Mol Biol* 33(4):319–327, 2005.

110. Eckstein M, Henderson S: Thoracic trauma. In: Marx J, Hockberger R, Walls R, eds. *Rosen's Emergency Medicine*. 7th ed. Philadelphia, PA: Mosby Elsevier, 2010.

111. Miller LA: Chest wall, lung, and pleural space trauma. *Radiol Clin North Am* 44(2):213–224, viii, 2006.

112. Allen GS, Coates NE: Pulmonary contusion: A collective review. *Am Surg* 62(11):895–900, 1996.

113. Silva F: *Thoracic Ultrasound in Lung Contusion*. Macedo Neto A, ed. Porto Alegre: Universidade Federal do Rio Grande do Sul, 2006:90.

114. Avery ME, Gatewood OB, Brumley G: Transient tachypnea of newborn. Possible delayed resorption of fluid at birth. *Am J Dis Child* 111(4):380–385, 1966.

115. Volpicelli G, Silva F, Radeos M: Real-time lung ultrasound for the diagnosis of alveolar consolidation and interstitial syndrome in the emergency department. *Eur J Emerg Med* 17(2):63–72, 2010.

116. Mathis G, Beckh S, Görg C: Lung consolidation. In: Mathis G, ed. *Chest Sonography*. 3rd ed. Berlin: Springer-Verlag, 2011.

117. Dorne HL: Differentiation of pulmonary parenchymal consolidation from pleural disease using the sonographic fluid bronchogram. *Radiology* 158(1):41–42, 1986.

118. Woodring JH, Reed JC: Types and mechanisms of pulmonary atelectasis. *J Thorac Imaging* 11(2):92–108, 1996.

119. Reissig A, Kroegel C: Transthoracic ultrasound of lung and pleura in the diagnosis of pulmonary embolism: A novel non-invasive bedside approach. *Respiration* 70(5):441–452, 2003.

120. Wu RG, Yuan A, Liaw YS, et al.: Image comparison of real-time gray-scale ultrasound and color Doppler ultrasound for use in diagnosis of minimal pleural effusion. *Am J Respir Crit Care Med* 150(2):510–514, 1994.

121. Lichtenstein D: *Pleural Effusion and Introduction to the Lung Ultrasound Technique. General Ultrasound in the Critically Ill*. 1st ed. Berlin: Springer-Verlag, 2005.

122. Eibenberger KL, Dock WI, Ammann ME, Dorffner R, Hörmann MF, Grabenwöger F: Quantification of pleural effusions: Sonography versus radiography. *Radiology* 191(3):681–684, 1994.

123. Tso P, Rodriguez A, Cooper C, et al.: Sonography in blunt abdominal trauma: A preliminary progress report. *J Trauma* 33(1):39–43, 1992.

124. Filly RA: Ultrasound: The stethoscope of the future. *Radiology* 167(2):400, 1988.

CHAPTER 8

Critical Care

Gavin R. Budhram, Robert F. Reardon, and David W. Plummer

The management of critically ill patients becomes more challenging when they are hemodynamically unstable or clinically deteriorating, and the underlying etiology of their condition is unclear. This often occurs shortly after arrival to the ED, but can also occur in other parts of the hospital hours or days after care has been established, with unexpected deterioration of a previously stable patient. In these situations, clinicians are often forced to make treatment decisions before diagnostic tests can be performed. A focused physical examination of the critical organ systems is often inaccurate or misleading. Point-of-care ultrasound can rapidly examine the same organ systems with a higher degree of accuracy.

Point-of-care ultrasound, performed and interpreted by the clinician, was introduced into emergency medicine in the 1980s. In many institutions, it is now the most commonly used diagnostic tool in the initial evaluation of critically ill patients (Figure 8-1). Clinicians using ultrasound can rapidly detect previously occult findings, such as the etiology of cardiac arrest or shock, causes of shortness of breath, sources of sepsis, and volume status and fluid responsiveness. In unstable patients, the ability to obtain this information immediately at the bedside can be lifesaving.

This chapter describes how to apply and integrate several different types of ultrasound exams for the diagnosis and management of critically ill patients. The details of how to perform each exam and most of the normal ultrasound findings are detailed in other chapters.

▶ CLINICAL CONSIDERATIONS

There are a wide variety of ultrasound applications that have great utility in the evaluation and management of critically ill patients. Many clinicians who manage critically ill patients do not appreciate the extent to which point-of-care ultrasound will improve their diagnostic ability and patient care. In the United States, emergency physicians tend to focus on abdominal, cardiac, and shock applications, while intensivists concentrate on cardiac function and hemodynamic parameters.[1] In Europe, clinicians tend to have a much better understanding of pulmonary ultrasound and use it extensively for the benefit of critically ill patients. Those with the most experience often advocate "whole body ultrasonography" in critically ill patients.[2]

▶ CLINICAL INDICATIONS

Critically ill patients often present with ill-defined disease entities. A variety of ultrasound applications can help clinicians make management decisions when dealing with common problems encountered in the care of critically ill patients.

- Cardiac arrest and near-arrest states
- Evaluation of undifferentiated hypotension
- Assessment of volume status and fluid requirements
- Assessment of shortness of breath or respiratory distress

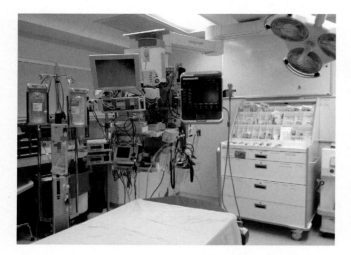

Figure 8-1. Ultrasound machine mounted on an articulating arm in an ED critical care bay. This assures that the machine is always available and ready to use.

- Evaluation of deep venous thrombosis (DVT)
- Evaluation of abdominal sources of shock or sepsis
- Critical ultrasound-guided procedures

CARDIAC ARREST AND NEAR-ARREST STATES

Critically ill patients are frequently hypotensive and it is occasionally difficult to palpate their pulses (See Chapter 6 Cardiac and Videos 6-1 to 6-5). Managing severe hypovolemia is a precarious situation as the line between hypotension and cardiac arrest is blurred. Assessment of pulses and blood pressure is unreliable in unstable or near-arrest patients. It has been demonstrated that rescuers misjudged pulselessness in 22% of pediatric "cardiac arrest" patients, which led them to withhold cardiac compression in 14% of cases when they were needed and perform compressions in 36% of cases when they were not needed.[3] Another study disproved the long-held belief that carotid, femoral, and radial pulses correspond to certain blood pressure measurements, finding instead that there is wide variation and little correlation between pulse palpation and blood pressure.[4] Noninvasive blood pressure measurement is equally unreliable in the near-arrest state. A study of 15 resuscitated cardiac arrest patients showed that 33% had unrecordable cuff blood pressures but adequate mean arterial pressures when measured directly.[5] In addition, 27% had a cuff blood pressure approaching normal yet a very poor cardiac output. Therefore, without invasive blood pressure monitoring and cardiac ultrasound, clinicians may be flying blind in near-arrest situations,

TABLE 8-1. TREATABLE CAUSES OF CARDIAC ARREST FROM THE 2010 AHA ADVANCED CARDIAC LIFE SUPPORT GUIDELINES

H's	T's
Hypoxia	Toxins
Hypovolemia	Tamponade (cardiac)
Hydrogen ion (acidosis)	Tension pneumothorax
Hypo-/hyperkalemia	Thrombosis, pulmonary
Hypothermia	Thrombosis, coronary

Reprinted with permission from Neumar RW, et al.: Part 8: adult advanced cardiovascular life support: 2010 American Heart Association Guidelines for Cardiopulmonary Resuscitation and Emergency Cardiovascular Care. *Circulation* 122:S729, 2010.

often unsure whether to do chest compressions, give fluid or pressors, or perform other therapeutic interventions. Clinicians who use cardiac ultrasound extensively in these situations often see patients with a normal or hyperdynamic heart but no pulses on physical exam. Also, some patients may show a "normal" automatic blood pressure cuff displayed while cardiac ultrasound shows no activity.

Data support the utility of point-of-care ultrasound in patients with cardiac arrest or near-arrest situations. It is clear that decreased time to diagnosis and therapeutic interventions in these patients results in improved patient outcomes.[6,7] The key is to rapidly diagnose and treat reversible conditions. In patients with pulseless electrical activity (PEA), ACLS guidelines suggest searching for the "5 H's and 5T's" (Table 8-1).[8]

Cardiac function cannot be directly observed without ultrasound. Consequently, potentially treatable causes of cardiac arrest or near-arrest, such as tamponade, pulmonary embolism (PE), severe hypovolemia, and cardiogenic shock, may go undetected. For example, autopsy studies show that PE is often unrecognized clinically when it is the cause of cardiac arrest.[9–11] The utility of ultrasound has been demonstrated in identifying reversible causes of cardiac arrest.[12–18] One study showed that 12% of cardiac arrest patients had a therapeutic intervention as a direct result of an ultrasound exam.[14] Another study showed that 86% of patients with presumed electromechanical dissociation actually had myocardial contractions on cardiac ultrasound.[19] The largest report of ultrasound use for cardiac arrest and near-arrest states analyzed 200 patients and demonstrated that ultrasound findings changed management in 78% of cases.[13] Also, they found that 35% of patients who were initially thought to be in asystole had cardiac wall motion on ultrasound. Severe bradycardia and subclinical ventricular fibrillation (VF) can both masquerade as asystole. In a study of 18 patients with in-hospital cardiac arrest and initial rhythm of asystole, the

▶ **TABLE 8-2. ULTRASOUND-GUIDED MANAGEMENT OF UNSTABLE PATIENTS: ULTRASOUND ABNORMALITIES AND SPECIFIC TREATMENTS IN CARDIAC ARREST OR NEAR-ARREST SITUATIONS**

Abnormality	Treatment
Severe hypovolemia	Fluid
Severe left ventricular dysfunction	Pressor/inotrope (low-dose bolus in near arrest)[22] or balloon pump
Cardiac tamponade	Pericardiocentesis or thoracotomy
Massive pulmonary embolism	Thrombolytic agent or embolectomy
Bradyarrhythmia	Inotrope (low-dose bolus in near-arrest)[22] or emergency pacing
Fine ventricular fibrillation	Defibrillation

investigators identified four patients who actually had severe bradyarrhythmia and responded to fluids and inotropic support.[18] Also, an echocardiographic assessment for subclinical VF is essential in cardiac arrest. It has long been recognized that the amplitude of VF is dependent on several factors: duration of VF, size and position of electrodes, skin resistance, body habitus, ventricular hypertrophy, and lead gain.[20,21] The amplitude of VF may be so low as to appear asystolic on the cardiac monitor. Therefore, it is recommended that the asystole on the cardiac monitor be sonographically confirmed with direct observation of cardiac standstill at the bedside. If fine fibrillations are seen instead, defibrillation should be performed (Table 8-2).

Withholding chest compressions in pulseless patients is controversial, but investigators of one study modified the advanced life support algorithm based on cardiac ultrasound findings and held compressions briefly in patients who had visible cardiac contractility.[15] In patients with PEA who had cardiac activity by ultrasound, they held compressions while rapidly administering 20 IU of vasopressin. Fifteen of sixteen patients (94%) had return of spontaneous circulation and eight (50%) had a good neurologic outcome. This study provided evidence to support the notion that all pulseless patients may not need chest compressions.

EVALUATION OF UNDIFFERENTIATED HYPOTENSION

Point-of-care ultrasound is a powerful tool that can help clinicians determine the etiology of shock. Shock is traditionally classified into one of the five categories: hypovolemic, cardiogenic, distributive, obstructive, and neurogenic. Ultrasound provides objective, visual, and recordable evidence to help classify shock. The initial ultrasound exam usually concentrates on the heart, lungs, and inferior vena cava (IVC). Cardiogenic shock is suspected with sonographic findings of a poorly contractile left ventricle, distended IVC, and B-lines on thoracic scan. Obstructive shock is indicated by a distended IVC, lack of B-lines, and a hyperdynamic left ventricle. Right ventricular distention suggesting PE or large pericardial effusion may further elucidate the cause of obstructive shock. Finally, a collapsed IVC coupled with a hyperdynamic poorly filled left ventricle and lack of B-lines indicates hypovolemic or distributive shock (see Table 8-3).

In addition, ultrasound examination of the pleural spaces, intraperitoneal space, aorta, deep veins, and the urologic and biliary systems may be useful for identifying hemorrhage, infection, or obstruction. The RUSH (Rapid Ultrasound in SHock) exam is an algorithmic approach to categorization of shock based on a similar concept of "whole body" ultrasound (Table 8-4).[23] The benefits of a comprehensive approach to point-of-care ultrasound for shock in order to quickly narrow the differential diagnosis and focus initial management have been demonstrated.[6,24]

In critically ill patients, cardiac ultrasound starts with a visual assessment of the overall cardiac function and relative chamber sizes. Severe abnormalities, such as hypovolemia, tamponade, and massive PE, are usually recognized with visual inspection and do not require specific measurements (Figure 8-2).

▶ **TABLE 8-3. SUMMARY OF IMPORTANT CARDIAC AND THORACIC ULTRASOUND FINDINGS IN SHOCK**

Type of Shock	Inferior Vena Cava	Cardiac Ultrasound	Thoracic Ultrasound
Hypovolemic	Collapsed	Hyperdynamic	No B-lines
Cardiogenic	Distended	Hypodynamic	B-lines
Distributive	Collapsed	Hyperdynamic	No B-lines
Obstructive	Distended	Hyperdynamic	No B-lines

▶ **TABLE 8-4.** **THE RUSH (RAPID ULTRASOUND IN SHOCK) PROTOCOL. AN ALGORITHM BASED ON THE CONCEPT OF WHOLE BODY ULTRASOUND. RUSH INCLUDES ULTRASOUND OF THE HEART (PUMP), THE INFERIOR VENA CAVA, CHEST AND ABDOMEN (TANK), AND THE AORTA AND DEEP EXTREMITY VEINS (PIPES)**

RUSH Evaluation	Hypovolemic Shock	Cardiogenic Shock	Obstructive Shock	Distributive Shock
Pump	Hypercontractile heart Small chamber size	Hypercontractile heart Dilated heart	Hypercontractile heart Pericardial effusion Cardiac tamponade RV strain Cardiac thrombus	Hypercontractile heart (early sepsis) Hypercontractile heart (late sepsis)
Tank	Flat IVC Flat jugular veins Peritoneal fluid (fluid loss) Pleural fluid (fluid loss)	Distended IVC Distended jugular veins Lung rockets (pulmonary edema) Pleural fluid Peritoneal fluid (ascites)	Distended IVC Distended jugular veins Absent lung sliding (pneumothorax)	Normal or small IVC (early sepsis) Peritoneal fluid (sepsis source) Pleural fluid (sepsis source)
Pipes	Abdominal aneurysm Aortic dissection	Normal	DVT	Normal

Abbreviations: DVT, deep venous thrombosis, IVC, inferior vena cava; RV, right ventricle.
Reprinted with permission from Perera P, Mailhot T, Riley D, Mandavia D: The RUSH exam: Rapid Ultrasound in SHock in the evaluation of the critically Ill. *Emerg Med Clin North Am* 28:29, 2010.

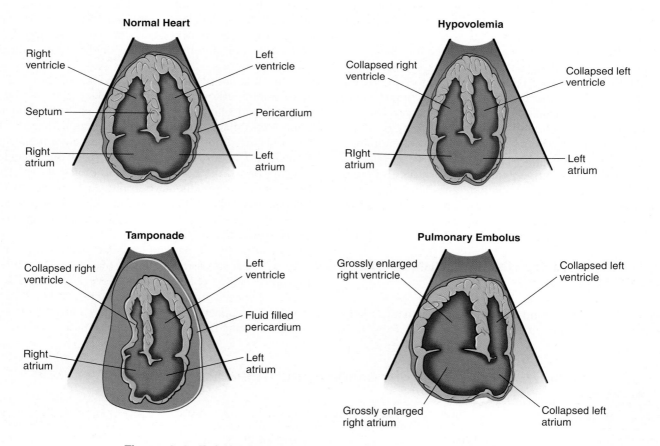

Figure 8-2. Relative cardiac chamber size in different shock states.

There are several ways to measure left ventricular function with echocardiography, but a qualitative visual estimation of global left ventricular function is best in critical situations because it is faster and just as accurate as doing measurements.[25-27] Also, it has been clearly shown that emergency physicians and intensivists can accurately estimate left ventricular function using point-of-care ultrasound.[28,29] Visual estimation is used to classify global left ventricular contractility into three groups: poor, normal, or hyperdynamic. This determination, though deceptively simple, is profoundly useful in critically ill patients, and with practice, noncardiologists are able to make this estimation with sufficient accuracy.

Poor left ventricular contractility suggests a cardiogenic etiology in patients with shock. Clinicians should remember, however, that all decompensated shock states will eventually result in decreased left ventricular performance, so it is prudent to keep a broad differential and search for other potential sources of shock when indicated. Regardless, it is critical to know whether diminished cardiac function is at least contributory to the shock state. Transthoracic echocardiography has been demonstrated to be 100% sensitive and 95% specific for identifying cardiogenic shock.[30]

By contrast, a hyperdynamic, vigorously contracting left ventricle suggests a physiologic compensation for hypovolemic, distributive, or obstructive shock. Time constraints may limit quantifiable echocardiographic measurements, but gross estimations of left ventricular contractility, E-point septal separation (EPSS), left ventricular and right ventricular filling, and IVC indices may be quickly obtained (see Chapter 6, "Cardiac," for cardiac measurements). A small, poorly filled and vigorously beating heart coupled with a narrow, collapsed IVC will usually be evident in patients with severe hypovolemia. In severe cases, complete obliteration of the left ventricular cavity in systole will be seen.

A hyperdynamic left ventricle with increased ejection fraction may develop without tachycardia and may be a warning of fluid loss and pending decompensation. These findings should prompt the physician to rapidly seek etiologies of shock that may be reversible if discovered and treated. This may occur in the setting of trauma, hemorrhage, sepsis, diabetic ketoacidosis, hyperosmolar nonketotic coma, or a host of other clinical scenarios. Clinicians should be mindful of preexisting heart failure, use of beta-blockers or calcium channel blockers, or later stages of shock associated with metabolic decompensation that may prevent a compensatory hyperdynamic state. The left ventricle may also be small and hyperdynamic in shock caused by PE or cardiac tamponade. In hypovolemic and distributive shock, poor left ventricular filling is due to central volume depletion. In obstructive shock, this may be due to a large PE resulting in a right ventricular outflow obstruction preventing left heart filling.[31]

Cardiac tamponade is a clinical and sonographic diagnosis.[32-37] Be aware that physical examination findings of tamponade are inconsistent; Beck's triad is not usually present; and pulsus paradoxus may be absent in patients with preexisting left ventricular dysfunction, atrial septal defect, regional tamponade, and positive pressure ventilation.[33,38] The combination of shock (without another clear source) and a moderate or large pericardial effusion is an indication for emergent pericardiocentesis. Since ultrasound-guided pericardiocentesis is a safe procedure, delaying it while trying to obtain more specific ultrasound findings is generally not prudent. Volume resuscitation may be a temporizing measure but once tamponade is diagnosed the effusion should be removed as soon as possible. Patients with simple fluid are candidates for ultrasound-guided pericardiocentesis; those with penetrating trauma or pericardial clot are usually best served with an emergent thoracotomy.[39] Also, it is generally not acceptable to use the landmark (or "blind") technique for pericardiocentesis if ultrasound guidance is available.[40-43]

It is common to see sonographic signs of impending tamponade in patients who are normotensive. Sonographically, the first sign of tamponade is collapse of the right atrial free wall during systole (Figure 8-3). As pericardial pressure increases, impaired filling of the right ventricle will also be evident, as well as collapse of the right ventricular free wall during diastole. These changes may be difficult to appreciate in real-time B-mode (2D) imaging but will be more apparent if the video is frozen and rolled backward slowly. A distended IVC that does not collapse with inspiration is also a sensitive sign of current or impending tamponade.[44]

PE is often a difficult diagnosis to make clinically, especially if the patient cannot give history of shortness of breath or chest pain. There are no pathognomonic signs on physical exam, and leg swelling is only clinically evident in about 4% of cases. The diagnosis is clinically missed in up to 84% of cases when it is the cause of cardiac arrest.[45] Point-of-care ultrasound is invaluable in the early detection of massive PE and obstructive shock. Classic echocardiographic findings of a massive PE are a thin-walled, dilated, and hypokinetic right ventricle, with bowing of the septum into the left ventricle (Figure 8-2). Patients with chronic pulmonary hypertension may also have a large, poorly-functioning right ventricle, but it will have a thick free wall (see Chapter 6, "Cardiac"). Several studies have demonstrated that ultrasound findings of acute right heart strain have only moderate sensitivity (41–66%) but excellent specificity (87–91%) for the diagnosis of massive PE.[46-50] McConnell's sign, described as diffuse hypokinesis of the right ventricular free wall with apical sparing, is a very specific indicator of PE and may help differentiate acute from chronic right heart strain.[50] Another sonographic

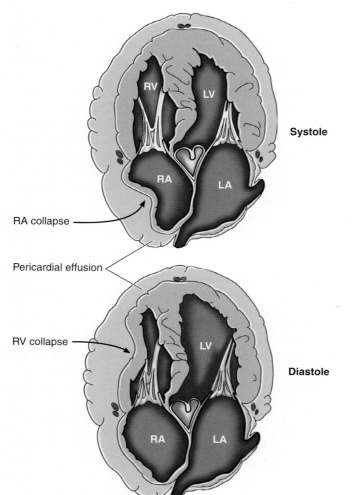

Figure 8-3. Physiology of cardiac tamponade.

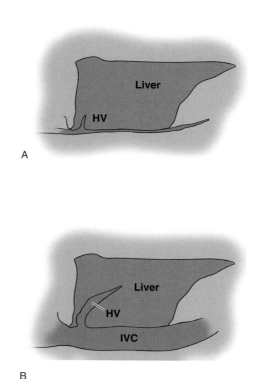

Figure 8-4. Drawing of the IVC at the extremes of volume status. (A) Small collapsing IVC. (B) Distended IVC and hepatic vein with no respiratory collapse.

sign of pulmonary artery obstruction is a distended IVC that does not collapse with inspiration.

Patients with sonographic signs of acute right heart strain consistently have a massive clot load and severe pulmonary artery obstruction.[51,52] These patients have a high mortality rate, so they may be candidates for surgical embolectomy or thrombolytic therapy.[47,53–56] Patients who are in shock (systolic BP <90 mm Hg) and have sonographic signs of massive PE are definitely candidates for thrombolytic therapy.[57] Several studies have demonstrated improved patient outcomes with thrombolytics in this scenario.[58]

ASSESSMENT OF VOLUME STATUS AND FLUID REQUIREMENTS

Physical examination findings and vital signs are notoriously inaccurate for estimating volume status and fluid needs. Sonographic assessment of the size and collapsibility of the IVC is widely used as an indicator of volume status and fluid needs. A small IVC (<1 cm) that completely collapses with inspiration is a reliable indicator of low central venous pressure and a good indicator of hypovolemic or distributive shock (Figure 8-4A). A large IVC (>2 cm) with no inspiratory collapse during forcible inspiration or sniffing is a good indicator of a high central venous pressure and a good predictor of heart failure (Figure 8-4B). This will also be seen with obstructive shock due to a massive PE and in cardiac tamponade. Be aware that patients with chronic pulmonary hypertension will have a large fixed IVC regardless of their hydration status. At the extremes and in intubated or chronically ill patients, IVC measurements are often confusing and they may not be good indicators of fluid requirements. Also, IVC measurements should not be used in isolation but rather in unison with other clinical and ultrasound findings.

Sonographic assessment of the heart is critical to determine volume status and the need for fluid resuscitation. Point-of-care cardiac ultrasound with a subjective assessment of hyperdynamic cardiac function and left ventricular end-systolic collapse has been found to be a better indicator of hypovolemia than central venous pressure or IVC size or collapsibility.[59] One study

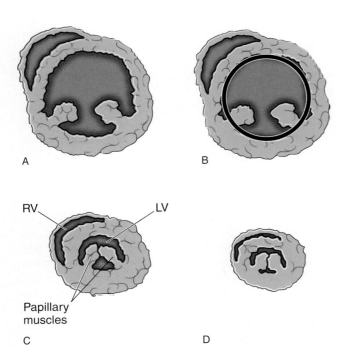

A

B

RV   LV

Papillary
muscles

C   D

Figure 8-5. Left ventricular area. (A) Short-axis cardiac view at the level of the papillary muscles. (B) Measurement of the left ventricular end-diastolic area (LVEDA). (C) Significantly decreased end-systolic area with "kissing papillary muscles." (D) Systolic obliteration of cavity of the left ventricle. LVEDA <10 cm², kissing papillary muscles, and systolic obliteration of the left ventricle are all indicators of significant volume depletion. The parasternal long axis, apical four-chamber, and subcostal views are also helpful for identifying hyperdynamic left ventricular function.

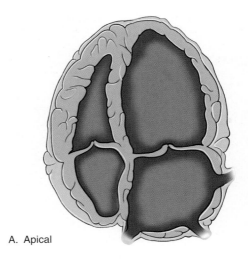

A. Apical

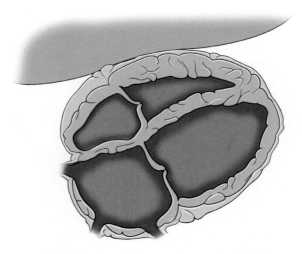

B. Subcostal

C. Parasternal

Figure 8-6. Anatomic changes associated with chronic left ventricular dysfunction A: 4-chamber view, B: Subcostal view, C: Parasternal long axis. The left ventricle and left atrium are significantly dilated. These are very common findings in patients with chronic heart disease. Patients with these findings have chronically elevated filling pressures and it is often difficult to determine their fluid requirements.

demonstrated that visual evaluation of hyperdynamic left ventricular function predicted volume responsiveness with a sensitivity of 71–100%.[60] Hyperdynamic left ventricular function is defined as the endocardium of the opposing ventricular walls coming in close proximity or touching during systole (Figure 8-5). Be aware that the opposite finding, a large, poorly-functioning left ventricle, does not necessarily mean that the patient is overloaded with fluid (Figure 8-6). Even patients with severe left ventricular dysfunction sometimes need fluid resuscitation. Patients with chronic left ventricle failure (systolic or diastolic) have chronically elevated left ventricular filling pressure and may deteriorate rapidly if they become hypovolemic, but they are also at risk of volume overload. Fluid management decisions in these patients are difficult, and it is best to measure indices that have been proven to predict fluid responsiveness (see Chapter 6, "Cardiac"). A simple way to estimate fluid status is to do a pulmonary ultrasound exam to help differentiate patients with signs of pulmonary edema from those who may need fluid resuscitation.

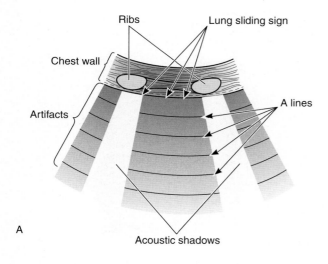

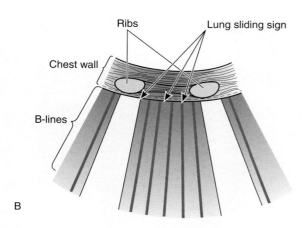

Figure 8-7. Pulmonary ultrasound to evaluate for extravascular lung water. (A) Normal "dry lung" has a prominent A-line pattern. (B) Prominent B-line pattern is consistent with "wet lung" (alveolar-interstitial syndrome: pulmonary edema or ARDS).

Pulmonary ultrasound is one of the best ways to determine volume status, especially for recognizing fluid overload (Figure 8-7). The finding of diffuse and bilateral B-lines is extremely sensitive for the diagnosis of pulmonary edema and extravascular lung water (which is associated with increased pulmonary wedge pressure and left ventricular systolic and diastolic dysfunction).[61-65] One study found a direct linear correlation between an increased number of B-lines and increased intravascular volume as measured by invasive techniques (pulmonary capillary wedge pressure and extravascular lung water by pulse contour cardiac output).[66] Another study found that the number of B-lines decreased in real time as intravascular fluid volume decreased during hemodialysis.[67] Lung ultrasound is more sensitive for detecting early pulmonary edema than chest radiography or the clinical symptom of dyspnea.[63,66,67]

Prominent B-lines can also be seen in ARDS, but the distribution will be patchy rather than diffuse (see Chapter 7, "Pulmonary").

Although a rapid sonographic assessment of the IVC, heart, and lungs provides a good initial estimate of volume status, this information does not necessarily predict fluid responsiveness. When determining fluid requirements, it is important to understand the concept of fluid responsiveness and how it differs from central venous pressure or filling pressures. Historically, central venous or filling pressures were measured and used to make decisions about fluid resuscitation. However, significant evidence shows that these parameters are poor predictors of fluid responsiveness.[68,69] Fluid responsiveness is defined as an increase in cardiac output with a fluid challenge. Measuring parameters that predict fluid responsiveness is ultimately the best way to make decisions about the need for fluid resuscitation (see section "Volume Status and Fluid Responsiveness" in Chapter 6, "Cardiac").

ASSESSMENT OF SHORTNESS OF BREATH OR RESPIRATORY DISTRESS

In patients with respiratory distress of unknown etiology, it is important to initiate treatment as quickly as possible. Chest radiography is the traditional initial imaging choice, but awaiting results would often cause an unacceptable delay in initiation of treatment. One study showed high concordance between chest ultrasound and chest radiography in patients presenting with acute dyspnea.[70] In addition, ultrasound results were available much more quickly than radiography results. The authors suggested that chest ultrasound could replace the standard chest radiograph in this setting (See Videos 7-1 and 7-2).

Pneumothorax

Missed pneumothorax is a common cause of morbidity and mortality.[71] For patients who are rapidly deteriorating, there is good evidence that ultrasound is better than chest radiography for diagnosing pneumothorax. One study found that the sensitivity of ultrasound for detecting pneumothoraces was 98% compared with 75% for radiography.[72] Several studies have shown that the negative predictive value of ultrasound for ruling out a pneumothorax is 100%.[72-78] Most importantly, ultrasound is much quicker than chest radiography. One study showed that chest ultrasound was performed in an average of 2 minutes, while chest radiography took

20 minutes.[78] A single sagittal window through the upper lung fields is dependable, but sensitivity is increased by scanning several areas along the anterior and lateral chest. In the presence of a pneumothorax, the clinician will appreciate an absence of lung sliding and comet-tail artifact at the pleural interface. This may be accentuated by obtaining an M-mode tracing at this level. It is important to remember that several other clinical scenarios may cause an absence of lung sliding, including pulmonary blebs, adhesions, and atelectasis.[79,80] In addition, the same concept that is used to rule out or diagnose a pneumothorax, the presence or absence of the *lung sliding sign* can be used to diagnose or rule out a main stem or esophageal intubation.[81,82]

Detection of Main Stem Intubation

When critically ill patients are intubated, it is important to assess the position of the endotracheal tube. Auscultation of breath sounds is inaccurate for detecting both esophageal intubation and main stem intubation.[83–85] Therefore, waveform capnography is the gold standard for detecting esophageal intubation, and chest radiography is the gold standard for determining endotracheal tube depth and diagnosing main stem intubation. However, the use of chest radiography usually causes a delay in the diagnosis of main stem intubation. This delay may be avoided by looking for the lung sliding sign immediately before and after intubation. The presence of bilateral lung sliding after intubation is an accurate indicator of good endotracheal tube position.[81,82,86,87] Unilateral lack of lung sliding may indicate a main stem intubation and the endotracheal tube depth should be checked.[81,87] If lack of sliding is thought to be the result of a main stem intubation, the endotracheal tube can be pulled back as the operator watches for the return lung sliding in real time.

Pulmonary Edema

Pulmonary edema is a common problem in critically ill patients. However, "classic" diagnostic characteristics such as rales, jugular venous distention, and interstitial edema on chest radiograph are absent in more than 50% of patients who present with dyspnea from acute congestive heart failure.[88,89] Pulmonary edema is very straightforward to recognize on chest ultrasound. It causes thickened subpleural intralobular septa that result in long vertical hyperechoic lines (B-lines) emanating from the pleural interface (Figure 8-7B).[90] B-lines are very sensitive for pulmonary edema.[63,67,91] Some B-lines are present at the lung bases in 27% of patients without pulmonary edema, but are a very sensitive indicator of pulmonary edema when prominent in the upper lung fields.[64]

Multiple B-lines visualized in the upper lung fields are very specific for pulmonary edema, and very accurate for discriminating pulmonary edema from chronic obstructive pulmonary disease (COPD) in patients with acute dyspnea and severe respiratory distress.[63,92] B-lines precede the development of radiographic findings of pulmonary edema and correlate well with pro-BNP levels.[91] Also, they resolve as fluid is removed from the body during hemodialysis.[67] In the hypotensive patient, B-lines are 94% sensitive and 84% specific for a cardiac etiology.[93]

Pleural Effusions

Ultrasound is extremely sensitive (96.2%) and specific (100%) for the diagnosis of fluid in the hemithoraces, detecting as little as 20 mL.[94,95] Pleural effusions may be present in a wide variety of pathologies including trauma, congestive heart failure, malignancy, renal failure, and pneumonia. In the setting of chest trauma and hypotension, a pleural effusion may signal hypovolemic shock due to a hemothorax. In a patient with poor cardiac function and B-lines, pleural effusions are consistent with a diagnosis of heart failure. A pleural effusion in a patient with pleuritic chest pain may increase suspicion for a PE. The clinician should interpret the finding of pleural effusion in the context of other clinical and sonographic information.

Pericardial Effusions

It is well known that patients with a pericardial effusion often present with nonspecific symptoms or with a primary complaint of dyspnea.[37,38] One study evaluated the use of point-of-care echocardiography on 103 ED patients with unexplained dyspnea and found that 14 had pericardial effusions. Four patients had large effusions requiring pericardiocentesis and three had moderate-sized effusions that were treated conservatively. It was recommended that ED patients with unexplained dyspnea be evaluated for a pericardial effusion.[96]

EVALUATION OF DEEP VENOUS THROMBOSIS

Ultrasound of the peripheral venous system has become the modality of choice for the diagnosis of DVT (See Video 17-1). Multiple studies have shown that clinicians can accurately detect DVTs using a modified compression technique, with a sensitivity ranging from 98% to 100% compared with a comprehensive duplex exam performed in a vascular lab (Figure 8-8).[96–98] In the management of critically ill patients, this exam is most useful when an acute PE is suspected.[99] In one study of 383 patients with known PE who underwent compression ultrasound, a lower extremity DVT was found in

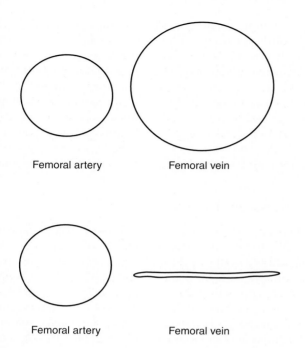

Figure 8-8. Simple compression test for DVT. The vast majority of DVTs are located in either the proximal femoral vein or at the popliteal vein. Locating and compressing the veins in these locations is an accurate way to rapidly evaluate for DVT. This is an example of normal complete compression of the femoral vein, which rules out DVT at this location.

289 (76%).[100] Signs or symptoms of DVT were present in only 31%.

Point-of-care ultrasound may be useful in the ICU setting when surveying for the development of hospital-acquired DVTs because the true prevalence of acute DVTs in the ICU setting is unknown and may be as high as 60% depending on the patient population, detection methods, and the application of surveillance programs.[101–103] Upper extremity sonography is important for patients with prolonged internal jugular, subclavian, basilic, or brachial catheters.

EVALUATION OF ABDOMINAL SOURCES OF SHOCK OR SEPSIS

Abdominal ultrasound is often overlooked by critical care practitioners, but it is very useful for identifying several specific life-threatening causes of shock and sepsis.

Ruptured Abdominal Aortic Aneurysm

Patients with ruptured abdominal aortic aneurysm (AAA) are initially misdiagnosed in 30–60% of cases.[104,105] This is an avoidable problem, because point-of-care ultrasound is nearly 100% accurate for the diagnosis of aortic aneurysm (See Video 9-1).[106,107] In addition, ruptured AAA is a relatively common cause of cardiac arrest.[108] Although some physicians argue that cardiac arrest resulting from ruptured AAA presents a miniscule chance of survival and operative intervention is a waste of resources, this is not well supported in the literature. One study demonstrated 28% (11 of 39) survival in patients with ruptured AAA presenting as cardiac arrest.[108]

Intra-Abdominal Free Fluid

The utility of the FAST exam is well described and accepted in the trauma literature, primarily because of the ease of detecting intraperitoneal fluid. It is highly sensitive for intra-abdominal hemorrhage in hypotensive trauma patients (See Videos 5-1 to 5-6).[109] Several studies report the ability of the FAST exam to detect intraperitoneal fluid collections from 250 to 620 mL, with overall sensitivity of 79% and specificity of 99%.[109–112] It is a small cognitive leap for most physicians to use the same exam for other nontraumatic abdominal catastrophes that present with intra-abdominal fluid collections. In unstable pregnant women, a positive FAST exam coupled with lack of intrauterine pregnancy is extremely sensitive for ectopic pregnancy and mandates immediate operative intervention. Abdominal free fluid is estimated to be present in 26% of patients with intestinal ischemia due to superior mesenteric artery occlusion.[113]

Cholecystitis

In elderly patients with sepsis and hypotension but without a clear infectious source, sonography of the gallbladder is recommended (See Videos 10-1 and 10-2). In cases of abdominal sepsis in the elderly, approximately 25% are due to acute cholecystitis and cholangitis.[114] Diagnosis is delayed in as much as 33% of these patients due to lack of physical exam findings.[115,116] A point-of-care ultrasound of the gallbladder may elucidate the etiology of undifferentiated septic shock, especially in the elderly patient unable to provide a history. Acute acalculous cholecystitis, although infrequent as an overall cause of cholecystitis, is seen more frequently in the ICU setting postoperatively or as a consequence of sepsis, trauma, or major burns. The sonographic evaluation of acalculous cholecystitis involves the same findings as calculous cholecystitis: a thickened gallbladder wall with pericholecystic fluid. An enlarged gallbladder, exceeding 9 cm longitudinally and 5 cm transversely is another typical feature. Although gallstones are absent, sludge should be present in the lumen of the gallbladder. Murphy's sign may be unreliable or absent, likely due to ICU sedation and pain control.

One study evaluated the routine use of gallbladder ultrasound in 53 intubated ICU patients and found three septic patients with acalculous cholecystitis in whom surgical intervention was performed and judged to be lifesaving.[117]

Hollow Viscus Perforation

An intraperitoneal air collection may be so large that underlying structures are obscured by dirty shadows. Smaller amounts of fluid may be detectable as bright reverberation artifact arising from the inner wall of the peritoneum. These reverberation artifacts, caused by air adjacent to the peritoneal wall, will be displaced with gentle pressure.[118] These findings are usually best detected in the right upper quadrant between the anterior abdominal wall and the liver where there is no intervening bowel.[119] Using these methods, ultrasound has been demonstrated to be 86% sensitive and 99% specific for detecting pneumoperitoneum. In contrast, abdominal plain films are reported to be 50–60% sensitive for intraperitoneal free air.[120–123]

Urosepsis

Complications of pyelonephritis, including abscess formation and emphysematous pyelonephritis, are commonly missed causes of sepsis, especially in the elderly population. Only 15–25% of perinephric or intrarenal abscesses were diagnosed at the time of admission.[124–126] The clinician should be rigorous in the bedside renal ultrasound evaluation of patients with sepsis with presumed pyelonephritis as a source (See Videos 12-1 and 12-2). Patients with diabetes, renal stones, immunosuppression, and renal failure are especially at risk.

Source control is an important part of early goal-directed therapy, and is known to decrease mortality in patients with sepsis.[127] The early identification of abscess or emphysematous pyelonephritis can expedite surgical intervention, either by percutaneous drainage or open nephrectomy. Ultrasound has been shown to be an effective initial tool for the detection of retroperitoneal abscess.[128] A renal abscess is typically a solitary, round hypoechoic mass with posterior acoustic enhancement, typically containing internal septations or mobile debris. Emphysematous pyelonephritis is a rare but deadly infection, occurring more commonly in diabetic or immunocompromised patients. Gas formation by bacteria in the kidneys causes dirty shadowing on ultrasound. This finding should prompt CT scanning; early emergent surgical consultation and intervention may be lifesaving for these patients.

Acute Renal Failure

Etiologies of acute renal failure are often divided into pre-renal, intrinsic, and post-renal causes. Most causes of intrinsic renal failure do not cause any sonographic abnormality, though occasionally the clinician may detect the absence of a kidney, or small, atrophic, hyperechoic kidneys. These suggest a more chronic nature of the renal failure.

Ultrasound is extremely useful in the diagnosis of postobstructive renal failure. Although only accounting for 5% of all causes of renal failure, obstructive renal failure is the most imminently reversible and most amenable to ultrasound investigation. In the presence of bilateral hydronephrosis, the clinician should assess for bladder outlet obstruction. This will usually include an ultrasound exam of the bladder for masses, clot (possibly around a urinary catheter), or prostatic hypertrophy. Bilateral hydronephrosis in patients with acute renal failure requires emergency decompression of the kidneys.

CRITICAL ULTRASOUND-GUIDED PROCEDURES

Ultrasound guidance of procedures allows clinicians to improve their success with procedures that are not routinely performed, such as pericardiocentesis and transvenous pacemaker placement. In addition, ultrasound guidance allows increased speed and accuracy, and decreased complications, with procedures that are routinely performed such as placement of a central line, paracentesis, and thoracocentesis (see Chapter 21, "Vascular Access," and Chapter 22, "Additional Ultrasound-Guided Procedures").[129]

Troubleshooting and Ensuring Proper Placement of Central Venous Catheters

Ultrasound guidance has replaced the landmark technique as the standard of care in placing central venous catheters, with a reduction in failed attempts and complications (see Chapter 21, "Vascular Access").[129] However, the risk of carotid artery puncture or cannulation is present even when proper technique is followed.[130] Also, malposition of a catheter into an aberrant location, outside of the central circulation, occurs in 2–50% of procedures depending on the site of venous puncture.[131] In addition to ultrasound guidance of the needle puncture and direct observation of the catheter inside the vein at the puncture site, there are two other ultrasound techniques that can be used to ensure that the tip of the catheter is in the proper venous location.

Cardiac Bubble Test

Performing a cardiac bubble test is an effective method to assure venous catheter placement and rule out arterial catheter placement.[132] This test involves observing the heart while the catheter is flushed with 10 mL of normal saline. Any cardiac view that shows the right atrium or right ventricle is sufficient.

Visualization of the Guidewire in the IVC

Another method to assure proper central venous catheter placement is to visualize the guidewire inside of the IVC during the procedure. Visualization of the guidewire within the IVC proves that the wire is in a vein (not an artery) and also assures that the catheter will end up in the central venous circulation as it is placed over the guidewire. This technique can confirm venous placement of the wire before the dilator is inserted, so it assures that an arterial puncture will not be dilated and cannulated. Some providers argue that overinsertion of the guidewire is dangerous and will cause cardiac sustained arrhythmias, but this practice has been studied and found to be safe.[133] Guidewires are straightforward to visualize because their irregular surface reflects ultrasound and any view of the IVC will suffice, although a longitudinal view is usually more visually pleasing.

Ultrasound-Guided Pericardiocentesis

Ultrasound guidance for pericardiocentesis is the preferred technique, as it is safer and more effective than the traditional technique.[42] The traditional technique is essentially "blind" and has a high rate of procedural failure and major complications.[40] Ultrasound-guided pericardiocentesis has been reported to have a success rate of 97% and a major complication rate of 1.2%.[41] The location of needle placement through the chest wall should allow for the shortest distance between the skin surface and cardiac effusion.[41–43] Aim the needle toward the largest, most accessible part of the effusion, with the needle trajectory such that the risk of cardiac puncture is minimized.

Ultrasound-Guided Placement of Transvenous Pacer

Ultrasound-guided placement of a transvenous pacing catheter enables more accurate placement than the traditional approach of observing electrical waveforms. When compared against fluoroscopy, sonographic guidance allows shorter time to pacing with a lower incidence of complications and a lower incidence of pacemaker malfunction during pacing.[134]

Confirmation of IV position of a central venous catheter may be achieved with the rapid instillation of 10 mL of agitated normal saline while observing the heart for bubbles moving through the right ventricle.[132] Confirmation of both IV position and proper placement toward the central circulation can be achieved

by visualization of the guidewire in the IVC during the procedure.

Ultrasound-Guided Cricothyroidotomy or Tracheostomy

Emergency cricothyroidotomy is a relatively rare procedure. Recent studies report cricothyroidotomy rates of only 0.4–1.2%.[121,122] Complication rates are high, ranging from 9% to 40%, with the most frequent being misplacement of the tracheal tube through the thyrohyoid membrane.[135,136] Percutaneous tracheostomy is commonly performed in the critical care setting; early complications occur in about 11% of patients.[137] Late complications, including tracheal stenosis from inappropriately high placement and erosion into mediastinal vessels from inappropriately low placement, occur in approximately 17% of patients.[138]

Both cricothyroidotomy and percutaneous tracheostomy techniques rely on palpation of the neck to identify anatomic landmarks. However, anterior neck anatomy is often difficult to palpate. Sonographic assessment of relevant anatomy and guidance of percutaneous needle puncture has been described.[139–142] The thyroid and cricoid cartilage, the cricothyroid membrane, and tracheal rings are identified on a sagittal ultrasound window. Point of needle entry may be quickly marked for static ultrasound guidance before the procedure. The mean time to visualization of the cricothyroid membrane has been reported to be 24 seconds and did not vary significantly with patient body habitus.[141] Ultrasound guidance increases success of tracheostomy placement.[140,142]

▶ GETTING STARTED

Ideally, all clinicians who care for critically ill patients should have significant experience with point-of-care cardiac, pulmonary, abdominal, and vascular ultrasonography. Clinicians who are relative ultrasound novices should concentrate on a handful of applications to get started. The pulmonary exam to assess for pneumothorax, basic cardiac exam to assess for gross function and a pericardial effusion, and ultrasound-guided peripheral and central venous access are ideal starting points.

When using ultrasound in critical care situations, it is important not to interfere with other more important diagnostic tests or patient management. Like the focused physical exam, point-of-care ultrasound should be brief and performed simultaneously with other diagnostic tests and ongoing care.

▶ COMMON ABNORMAL ULTRASOUND FINDINGS IN CRITICALLY ILL PATIENTS

This section demonstrates actual findings from the use of point-of-care ultrasound in critically ill patients. The reader is encouraged to review other chapters within this book for more specific information on interpretation of abnormal ultrasound findings.

CARDIAC ARREST AND NEAR-ARREST STATES

Cardiac imaging may be challenging in critically ill patients. Adequate windows often require the patient to be in the left-lateral decubitus position with the left arm elevated, but this is difficult to accomplish in such scenarios. In these cases, the clinician may choose other windows or settle for suboptimal or nonstandard images. Patients with long-standing obstructive pulmonary disease often have difficult cardiac visualization due to hyperinflation of the lungs and only the subcostal window allows reasonable cardiac images. Sonography during cardiac arrest is difficult because it requires the ability to obtain and interpret technically adequate images quickly; this is possible and extremely useful in clinical practice.[143,144] In this situation, cardiac ultrasound should be done quickly and concurrently with the 5-second pause for pulse and rhythm check. The subcostal four-chamber view is usually the "go to" view in car-

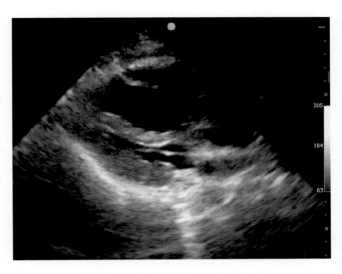

Figure 8-9. Cardiac arrest from massive PE, parasternal long-axis view. The right ventricle (top) is massively dilated and compressing the left ventricle.

diac arrest, and the parasternal long-axis position is an excellent alternative when the subcostal view is inadequate.

The objective is to rapidly identify any potentially treatable causes for cardiac arrest and/or profound shock (see Tables 8-1 and 8-2). Common findings are outlined in the following case examples (Figures 8-9 through 8-13).

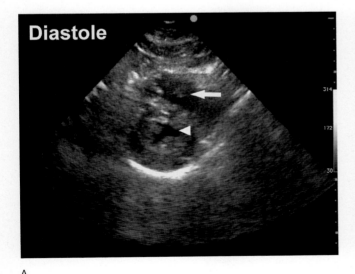

A

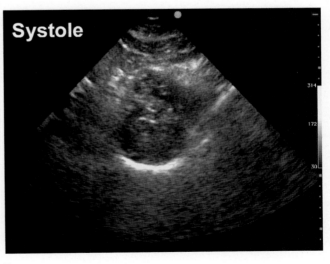

B

Figure 8-10. Underfilled hyperdynamic heart, parasternal short-axis views. (A) The left ventricular chamber is very small at the end of diastole (arrowhead) and the right ventricular chamber is barely visible (arrow). (B) The left ventricle and right ventricle are completely obliterated during systole, an accurate indicator of severe volume depletion. This patient presented in PEA from a ruptured abdominal aortic aneurysm.

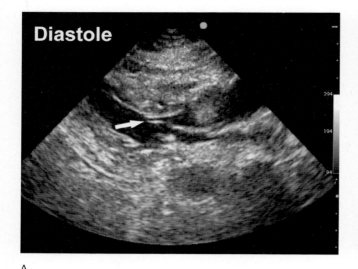
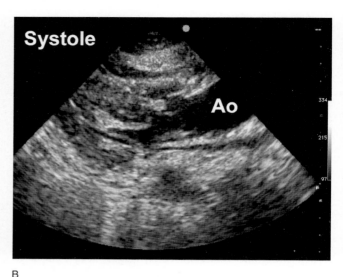

A   B

Figure 8-11. Underfilled hyperdynamic heart, parasternal long-axis views. The anterior leaflet of the mitral valve (arrow) touches the intraventricular septum during diastole (A) and the septum and posterior left ventricular walls touch during systole (B). The right ventricle is very small during diastole and systole. The left ventricular outflow track and aorta (Ao) are the only fluid-filled areas visible during systole. This patient presented in PEA from severe septic shock and responded to aggressive volume resuscitation.

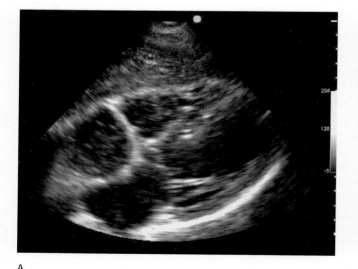
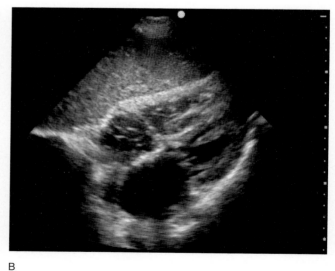

A   B

Figure 8-12. (A, B) Cardiac arrest, subcostal four-chamber views. These patients had primary cardiac events and presented in PEA with extremely poor left ventricular function. All four-chambers are filled and well visualized, but there is minimal contractility.

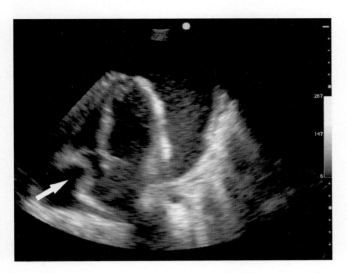

Figure 8-13. Cardiac arrest from tamponade, apical four-chamber view. This patient was getting chest compressions until a massive echogenic pericardial effusion was identified. Note collapsing right atrium (arrow). Pericardiocentesis was quickly performed by inserting an 18-gauge needle adjacent to the ultrasound transducer.

UNIDIFFERENTIATED HYPOTENSION

Assessment of the left ventricular filling and function is the first step to evaluating patients with undifferentiated shock. The most straightforward technique is visual esti-

mation of left ventricular size and systolic function (Figures 8-14–8-18). Visual estimation of the IVC size and dynamics as well as pulmonary ultrasound to diagnose or rule out pulmonary edema adds supporting information.

VOLUME STATUS AND FLUID REQUIREMENTS

A small IVC is a reliable indicator of low central venous pressure and volume depletion. Normal patients may have an IVC that collapses completely with inhalation or sniffing, but an IVC that remains small (<1 cm) throughout the respiratory cycle is a sign of significant volume loss (Figures 8-19 and 8-20). A dilated (>2 cm) and fixed (no change with respirations) IVC and dilated hepatic veins are consistent with an elevated central venous pressure; however, these findings do not necessarily mean that a patient is acutely volume overloaded because patients with preexisting heart disease or pulmonary hypertension will have these findings at baseline (Figures 8-21). Therefore, it should be understood that IVC size and collapsibility provide some basic information about volume status, especially at the extremes, but they are not good indicators of the need for fluid in most patients. Using a combination of IVC, cardiac, and pulmonary findings is much more accurate. A small hyperdynamic left ventricle is a reliable indicator of volume depletion. Measuring the left ventricular end-diastolic area (LVEDA) by simply tracing the endocardial

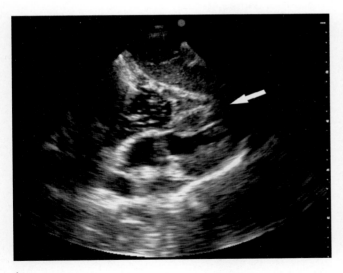

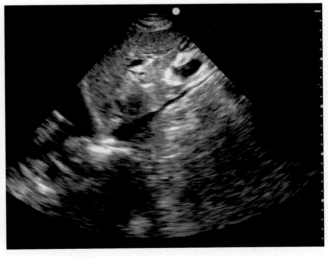

A   B

Figure 8-14. Septic shock. (A) Subcostal four-chamber cardiac view with position of interventricular septum indicated (arrow). Left ventricular and right ventricular chambers are ≤2 cm in diameter. (B) Long-axis view of the IVC. The findings of a small hyperdynamic heart and completely collapsed IVC are consistent with hypovolemic or distributive shock. The provider should consider looking for an abdominal aortic aneurysm or abdominal sources of hemorrhage or sepsis. This patient had urosepsis and acute renal failure. Also visible is a significant left pleural effusion above the diaphragm (B).

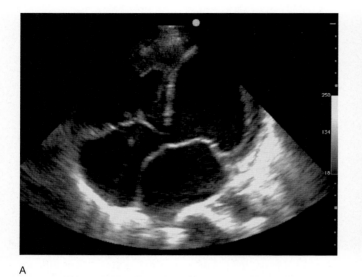

A

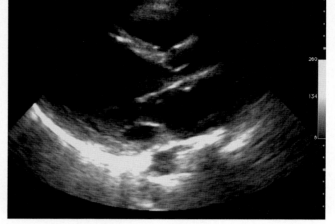

B

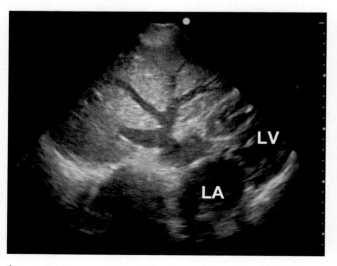

C

Figure 8-15. Acutely decompensated heart failure and cardiogenic shock, apical four-chamber (A), and parasternal long-axis (B) views. Obvious changes associated with chronic heart disease, including biatrial and biventricular enlargement. These findings suggest that shock could be cardiogenic in etiology. Supporting evidence can be obtained by assessing the lungs and other body regions looking for other possible causes of shock. This patient was found to have a normal abdominal aorta and diffuse bilateral B-lines on pulmonary ultrasound, consistent with pulmonary edema from heart failure. The static lung image (C) demonstrates multiple diffuse B-lines emanating from the entire pleural surface (more obvious during real-time exam). Using a curved or phased array transducer, these lines can be seen to radiate to the full depth of the image. (Image C Courtesy of James Mateer, MD)

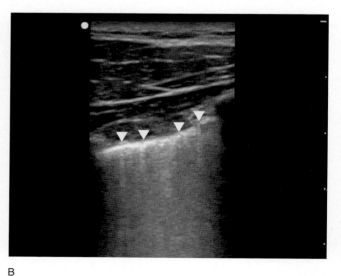

A

B

Figure 8-16. Cardiogenic shock. (A) Subcostal four-chamber view angled toward the midline. LA enlargement is noted, and dilated hepatic veins are seen with spontaneous echo contrast noted on real-time exam. These are all signs of poor forward flow and cardiogenic shock. (B) High-frequency linear array image of the pleura. The finding of a diffuse bilateral B-line pattern on lung ultrasound is diagnostic for pulmonary edema. The origins of the B-lines are indicated (arrowheads) and were obvious on real-time exam. LA = left atrial, LV = left ventricle.

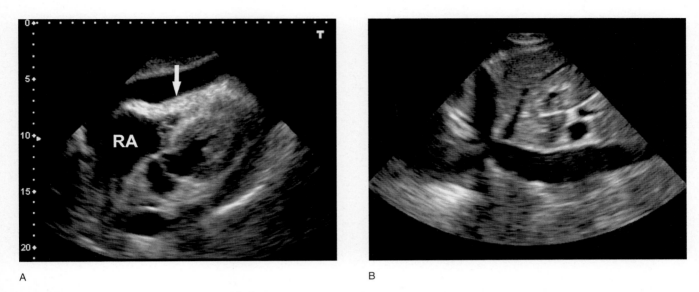

A

B

Figure 8-17. Cardiac tamponade. The classic ultrasound finding of tamponade is early-diastolic collapse of the right ventricle. (A). Subcostal four-chamber view with right atrium visible, but right ventricular chamber is completely collapsed (arrow). A moderate-to-large pericardial effusion is surrounding the heart. A dilated fixed IVC (B) is supportive evidence of the hemodynamic significance of the pericardial effusion. RA = right atrium.

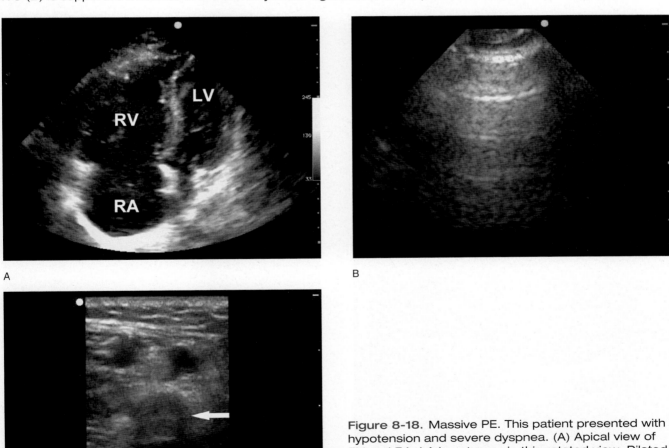

A

B

C

Figure 8-18. Massive PE. This patient presented with hypotension and severe dyspnea. (A) Apical view of RV and RA. LA is not seen in this rotated view. Dilated and poorly functioning right ventricle noted on real-time views. (B) Intact lung sliding and A-line pattern on lung ultrasound (phased array transducer) rule out pneumothorax and pulmonary edema. (C) Right popliteal vein is noncompressible and contains echogenic clot (arrow). RV= right ventricle, RA = right atrium, LV = left ventricle.

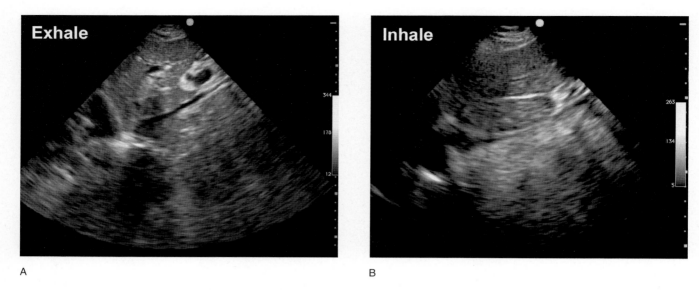

Figure 8-19. Low-volume IVC. Longitudinal view of the IVC during exhalation (A) and inhalation (B). Note narrow initial diameter (< 1 cm) and complete collapse with inhalation.

border in a short-axis view at the mid-papillary muscle level provides some objective evidence to allow recognition of an underfilled left ventricle (Figure 8-22A). A hyperdynamic ventricle is one in which the opposing endocardial surfaces make contact or are in close proximity during systole (Figure 8-22B and C). Pulmonary ultrasound can be used to differentiate "dry lungs" from "wet lungs" (see next section), which provides valuable additional information. Ultrasound is very sensitive for identifying early pulmonary edema or ARDS, so patients

with "dry lungs" are unlikely to be harmed by a fluid challenge. Therefore, in unstable patients, who are often at the extremes of hypovolemia or fluid overload, the combination of IVC indices, cardiac filling and function, and pulmonary ultrasound findings provides a good estimate of fluid status. When these findings are unclear or indeterminate, it is best to measure specific indices that are known to predict fluid responsiveness (see section "Volume Status and Fluid Responsiveness" in Chapter 6, "Cardiac").

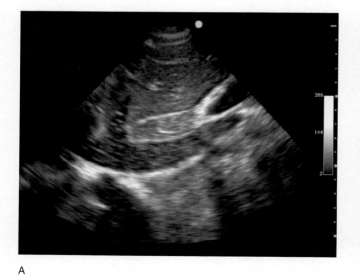

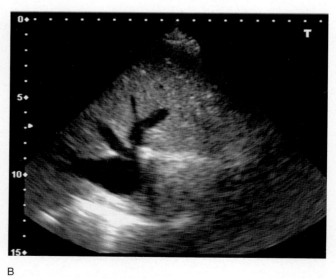

Figure 8-20. High-volume IVC. Longitudinal view of the IVC (A) shows a large diameter (≥2 cm) and spontaneous contrast. There was no change with respirations on real-time views. Also note dilated hepatic veins branching anteriorly. Corresponding transverse view of the IVC (B).

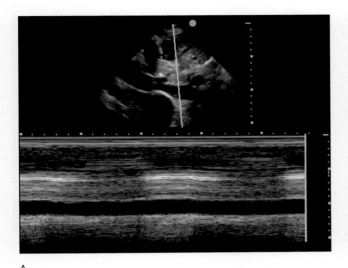

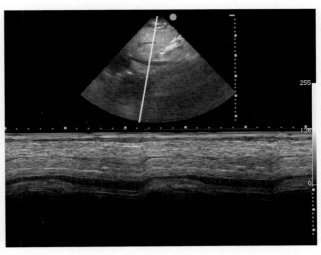

A

B

Figure 8-21. M-mode ultrasound of the IVC. A dilated fixed IVC (A) is consistent with an elevated central venous pressure and has the appearance of a straight column with a diameter >2 cm. A small collapsing IVC (B) is consistent with a low central venous pressure and has the appearance of a ribbon that changes diameter from <1 cm during expiration to 0 cm during inspiration.

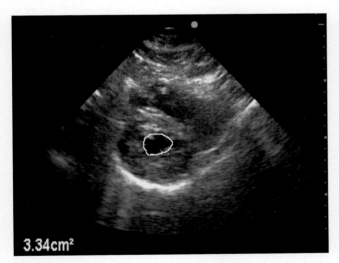

3.34cm²

A

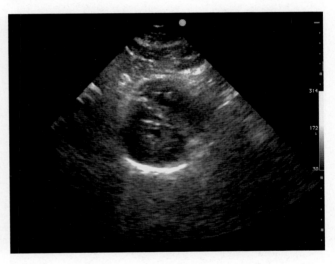

B

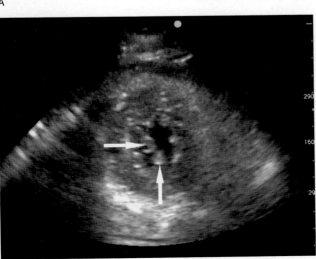

C

Figure 8-22. Small hyperdynamic heart, parasternal short-axis views. Small left ventricular end-diastolic area (<10 cm²) is consistent with significant volume depletion (A). Complete systolic obliteration of the left ventricle (B) and "kissing papillary muscles" (arrows) (C) are also specific signs of severe volume depletion.

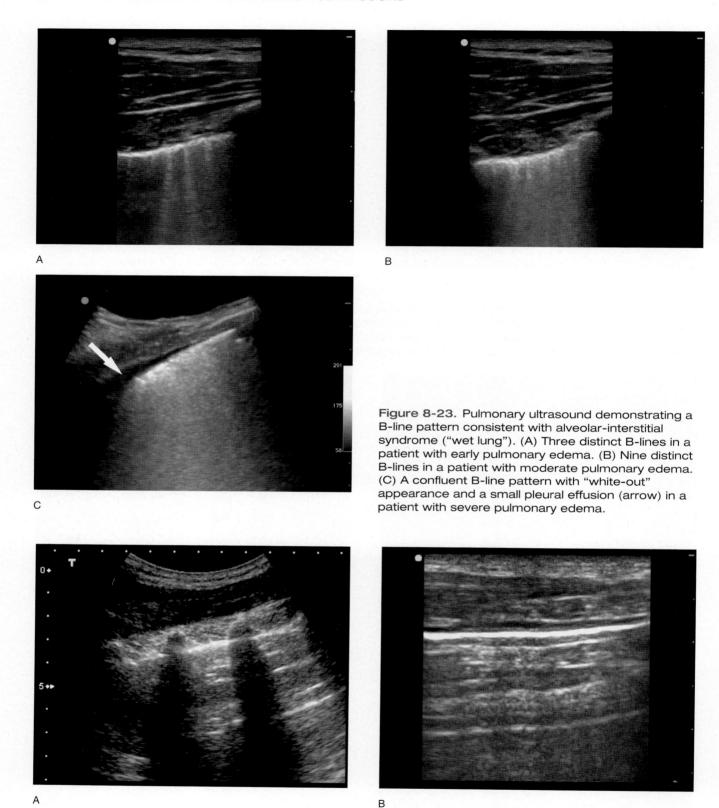

A

B

C

Figure 8-23. Pulmonary ultrasound demonstrating a B-line pattern consistent with alveolar-interstitial syndrome ("wet lung"). (A) Three distinct B-lines in a patient with early pulmonary edema. (B) Nine distinct B-lines in a patient with moderate pulmonary edema. (C) A confluent B-line pattern with "white-out" appearance and a small pleural effusion (arrow) in a patient with severe pulmonary edema.

A

B

Figure 8-24. Pulmonary ultrasound demonstrating an A-line pattern consistent with normal lung ("dry lung"). This is the appearance of normal lung. Bright horizontal lines of reverberation (A-lines) repeat at intervals equal to the distance from skin to pleura. This finding essentially rules out the diagnosis of pulmonary edema, but it may also be seen in patients with a pneumothorax (see below), COPD, or PE. (A) Sagittal view with curved array transducer includes multiple rib shadows that help determine the location of the pleural surface. (B) Intercostal view with linear array transducer without rib shadows allows better visualization of the A-line pattern.

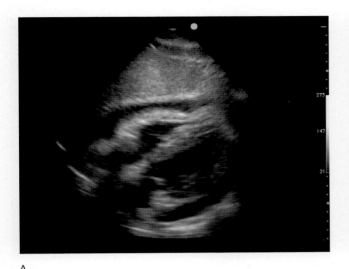
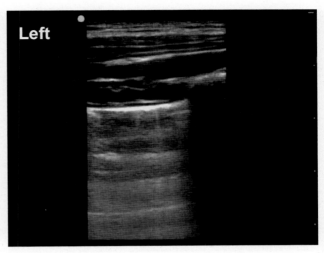

A   B

Figure 8-25. Pericardial effusion in a dyspneic patient. Dyspnea is a common symptom in patients with pericardial effusions and cardiac tamponade. Early-diastolic collapse of the right ventricular free wall (A) is the classic ultrasound sign of tamponade. An A-line pattern on ultrasound of the lungs (B) rules out pulmonary edema as the cause of dyspnea and supports the diagnosis of early tamponade.

SHORTNESS OF BREATH AND RESPIRATORY DISTRESS

Pulmonary ultrasound allows an accurate assessment of "wet lungs" versus "dry lungs" (Figure 8-7). A B-line pattern on pulmonary ultrasound indicates alveolar-interstitial syndrome ("wet lung"). Pulmonary edema and ARDS are the most common causes of a B-line pattern. If the B-line pattern is diffuse throughout both lungs, then pulmonary edema is the diagnosis (Figure 8-23). ARDS will cause patchy B-lines with areas of sparing that have a normal A-line appearance

(see Chapter 7, "Pulmonary"). The severity of pulmonary edema can be determined by the number of B-lines on each image (Figure 8-23). B-lines are very sensitive for detecting early pulmonary edema, so a diffuse A-line pattern essentially rules out pulmonary edema (Figure 8-24). Simply differentiating wet lungs from dry lungs in patients who are short of breath, in shock, or have unclear volume status has great clinical utility. In addition, point-of-care ultrasound can be used to accurately identify other causes of shortness of breath, such as pneumothorax, pleural effusion, lung consolidation, or pericardial effusion (Figures 8-25–8-27).

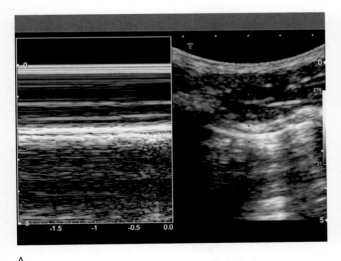
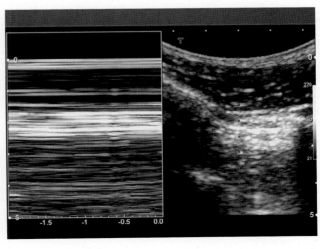

A   B

Figure 8-26. M-mode ultrasound of the lung. The normal "seashore sign" (A) confirms lung sliding and rules out a pneumothorax at this location on the chest wall. The "stratosphere sign" (B) is seen when there is no lung sliding, which is consistent with a pneumothorax or lack of lung ventilation. Lack of lung sliding on the left side after endotracheal intubation may be secondary to right main stem intubation.

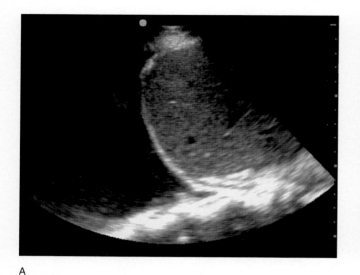

A

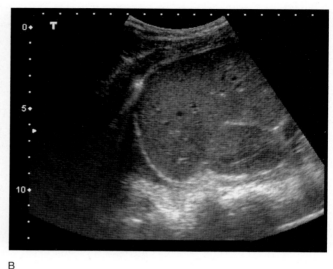

B

C

Figure 8-27. Pleural effusion and lung consolidation, right intercostal oblique view. A large pleural effusion (A) can be the primary cause of dyspnea. A small effusion (B) is unlikely to cause dyspnea, but may be a clue to the diagnosis of pulmonary edema, PE, or pneumonia. Pneumonia (C) often causes a localized hepatization of the lung (arrow), which allows good visualization of the lung parenchyma with ultrasound.

DEEP VENOUS THROMBOSIS

Screening all critically ill patients for DVT is not unreasonable. Multiple studies show that the rate of DVT in critically ill patients is very high, especially those with clinical signs of PE and those with central venous catheters.[100–103] Two-point simple compression ultrasound of the femoral and popliteal regions (see Chapter 17, "Deep Venous Thrombosis") has been proven to be extremely accurate compared with more comprehensive DVT studies, and visualization of clot around IV catheters is relatively straightforward (Figure 8-28).[97,98,145]

ABDOMINAL SOURCES OF SHOCK AND SEPSIS

The concept of evaluating the abdomen as a source of shock and sepsis is well described, yet this portion of the body is often overlooked in critically ill patients as clinicians concentrate on cardiac and pulmonary exams that are perceived to be more important. As with the physical exam, an incomplete evaluation may miss critical findings that can make a major difference in patient care and outcome (Figures 8-29–8-33). It is no surprise that critical care providers who have the greatest experience with point-of-care ultrasound support the concept of "whole body ultrasonography in the critically ill."[2]

CRITICAL ULTRASOUND-GUIDED PROCEDURES

Many procedures that were previously performed using landmark (blind) techniques have a higher success rate and are safer when performed with ultrasound

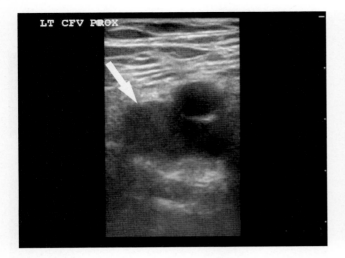

A

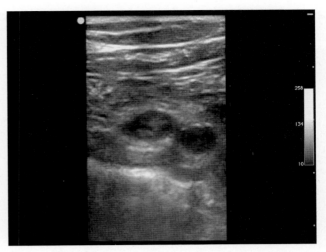

B

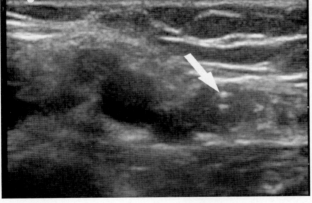

C

Figure 8-28. Deep venous thrombosis in three different patients who all presented with severe dyspnea and were eventually diagnosed with PE. (A) Left common femoral vein (arrow) does not compress and echogenic clot is visible within the vessel. (B) Clot in the popliteal vein. The vein is to the left of the artery; it does not compress with firm pressure and contains visible echogenic clot. (C) Clot in the basilic vein surrounding a PICC line. The vessel on the left is the brachial vein and the one on the right is the basilic vein. The wall of the catheter (arrow) creates two small bright artifacts in the center of the basilic vein and the vein should collapse down around the catheter with compression. This image is with compression, the vessel does not compress, and contains echogenic material around the PICC catheter.

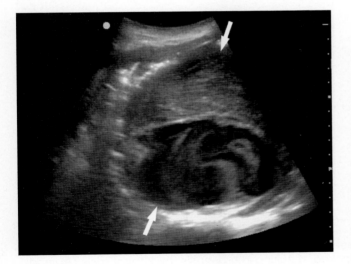

Figure 8-29. Abdominal aortic aneurysm, transverse view. This patient presented with shock and altered mental status. He was noted to be hypovolemic with a hyperdynamic heart and small IVC. This aneurysm (measuring 10 cm in diameter) had ruptured. Spontaneous echo contrast, caused by slow blood flow, gives the appearance of flames flickering within the lumen. Note large mural thrombus anteriorly. Arrows indicate outer walls of the aneurysm.

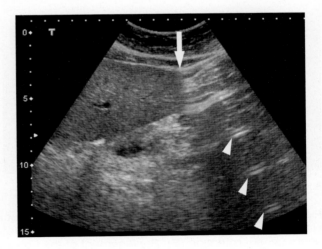

Figure 8-30. Hollow viscus perforation with abdominal free air. There is a transition point at the center/right of the image (arrow) where the liver parenchyma is abruptly replaced by an A-line pattern (arrowheads), beginning at the level of the posterior abdominal wall. With firm pressure the liver was visualized and without firm pressure the A-pattern obscured the liver completely.

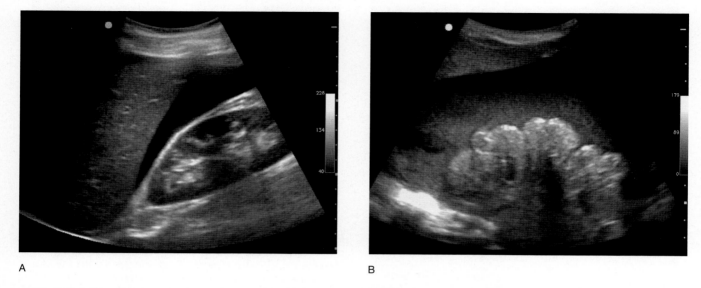

Figure 8-31. Intraperitoneal fluid. Both images show a large amount of free intraperitoneal fluid. (A) Anechoic fluid in Morison's pouch. Hemorrhage and ascites often have a similar appearance. (B) Complex intraperitoneal fluid surrounding the echogenic bowel wall in a patient with bacterial peritonitis. Consider performing an ultrasound-guided diagnostic needle aspiration in order to characterize the fluid or obtain a culture.

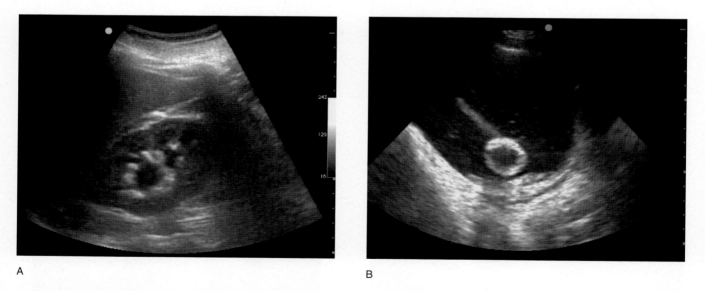

Figure 8-32. Urosepsis and obstruction. This patient presented with urosepsis, shock, and acute renal failure. He had a chronic indwelling Foley catheter, which was blocked, resulting in urosepsis, hydronephrosis (A), and acute urinary retention (B). Replacement of the Foley catheter allowed a liter of purulent urine to drain from the bladder. The hydronephrosis subsequently resolved.

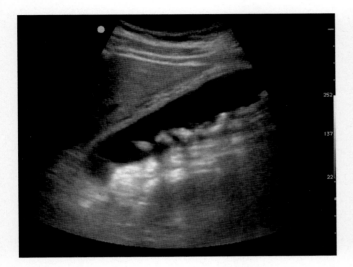

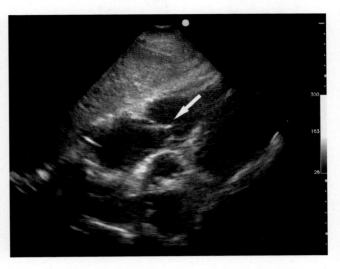

Figure 8-33. Cholecystitis. Longitudinal view of the gallbladder. This gallbladder is large and contains multiple echogenic gallstones. There is also wall thickening and pericholecystic fluid, which are specific ultrasound findings associated with cholecystitis. The sonographic Murphy's sign may be absent in patients who have shock and altered mental status.

Figure 8-34. Placement of an ultrasound-guided emergency transvenous pacing catheter—subcostal four-chamber view. The catheter (arrow) is visualized in real time as it passes through the tricuspid valve and into the right ventricle.

guidance (Figures 8-34–8-37). In addition, point-of-care ultrasound can be used to diagnose significant complications caused by invasive procedures, including pneumothorax, main stem intubation, and pericardial effusion.

▶ PITFALLS

1. **Poor quality images or nonstandard views.** This is a common problem because there are many uncontrollable factors during the performance of point-of-care ultrasound for critically ill patients. Patient positioning and cooperation is almost never optimal. Time constraints are

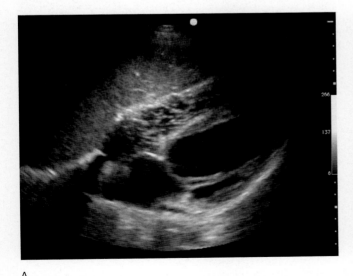

A

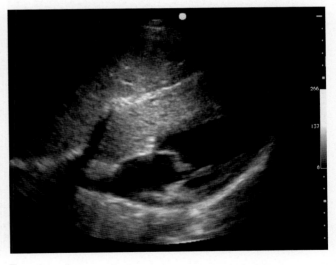

B

Figure 8-35. Cardiac bubble test to confirm IV location of central venous catheters—subcostal four-chamber view. Ten mL of sterile saline is rapidly injected into the catheter. Bubbles immediately begin to appear in the right ventricle (A), and then the right side of the heart becomes completely opacified (B).

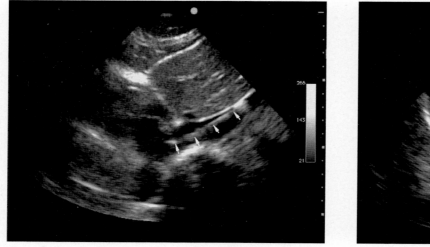

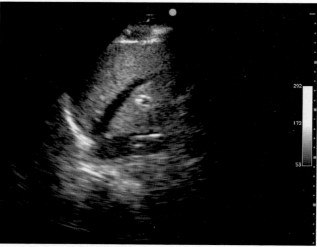

A

B

Figure 8-36. Visualization of guidewire in the IVC to predict proper placement of central venous catheters—longitudinal view of IVC in upper abdomen. This technique helps assure that the guidewire is in a vein and that the tip of the catheter will ultimately reside within the central venous circulation. (A) The guidewire is clearly visualized (arrows) inside the IVC after insertion from the right internal jugular vein (B). In a separate case, the J-shaped tip of the guidewire is clearly visualized inside the IVC after insertion from the left femoral vein.

significant and images may need to be obtained within just a few seconds. Finally, important ergonomic factors like placement of the ultrasound machines and operator comfort, which are carefully choreographed in more controlled settings, are not usually considered in the critical care setting. Operators should try to optimize conditions and images, but also learn to deal with poor quality images and avoid making important diagnostic decisions if proper images cannot be obtained.

2. **Operator inexperience.** Since point-of-care ultrasound is a relatively new technology in many critical care settings, lack of operator

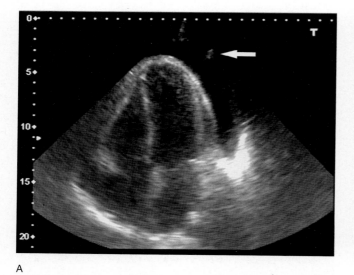

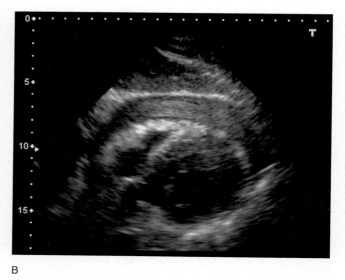

A

B

Figure 8-37. Significant pericardial fluid. Apical (A) and subcostal four-chamber views (B): Pericardiocentesis (A) in a patient with a large pericardial effusion and tamponade. The tip of the needle is entering the effusion at about the 2 o'clock position (arrow). A catheter was placed using the Seldinger technique after a bubble test confirmed the location of the needle tip inside the effusion. A total of 500 mL of straw-colored fluid was removed. (B) Tamponade from a pericardial clot secondary to an acute myocardial infarction and ventricular free wall rupture. This is not a good candidate for a pericardiocentesis and needs a thoracotomy.

experience is a significant factor. It is best for inexperienced operators to understand which ultrasound exams can be learned rapidly and which require intensive practice and experience. For example, pulmonary ultrasound for visualization of the sliding lung sign can be quickly learned and used in practice almost immediately, whereas the cardiac ultrasound exam is more complex and requires more hands-on training. Inexperienced operators should avoid making important clinical decisions based on their ultrasound findings until they have a basic level of experience.

3. **Prolonged ultrasound examination.** Novice operators tend to spend too much time on the cardiac ultrasound during pulse checks. In order to maintain cerebral and tissue perfusion, it is imperative that interruptions in chest compressions be kept to a minimum. Recording a short video clip that can be reviewed once chest compressions have resumed may be helpful. If the clinician is unable to obtain an adequate view of the heart during the pulse check, compressions should resume immediately. It may be helpful to attempt a parasternal long-axis window during the next pulse check.

4. **Preexisting heart failure.** Patients with preexisting heart failure or on beta-blockers or calcium channel blockers may not be able to mount an appropriate compensatory inotropic or chronotropic response in distributive or hypovolemic shock. This will confuse the sonographic evaluation of hypotension so the clinician should be aware of these elements of the medical history.

5. **Preexisting pulmonary hypertension.** Patients with long-standing pulmonary hypertension from pulmonary fibrosis, sleep apnea, or other chronic conditions resulting in chronic cor pulmonale may have long-standing right ventricular dilatation. Although the right ventricular free wall will usually display compensatory hypertrophy, be wary of these elements of the medical history to avoid erroneous diagnosis of PE.

► CASE STUDIES

CASE 1

Patient Presentation

A 72-year-old man presented to the ED from a nursing home for altered mental status and hypotension. He had a history of dementia and hypertension, but no signif-

icant cardiac history. Further history was unobtainable. He was awake but incoherent and diaphoretic. On physical examination, his blood pressure was 80/40 mm Hg, pulse 160 beats per minute, respirations 20 breaths per minute, and temperature 37.5°C. He had flat neck veins, clear lungs, and an irregular heart rate.

Management Course

The patient was placed on a cardiac monitor, IV access was established, and a fluid bolus was initiated. An EKG was performed, which revealed rapid atrial fibrillation. The ED physician performed a sonographic evaluation, which revealed IVC collapse (Figure 8-38A) and the heart to be hyperdynamic with poor left ventricular filling (Figure 8-38B). Pulmonary ultrasound revealed a diffuse A-line pattern (Figure 8-38C), essentially ruling out pulmonary edema. Rapid fluid resuscitation was performed and serial ultrasound exams showed improvement in left ventricular filling. The patient spontaneously converted to normal sinus rhythm 30 minutes after arrival and his blood pressure improved to 112/70 mm Hg. Abdominal ultrasound revealed no intraperitoneal fluid and a normal aorta; it also revealed a markedly abnormal gallbladder with multiple gallstones, gallbladder wall edema, and pericholecystic fluid (Figure 8-38D). A surgical consult was obtained for acute cholecystitis and the patient was given broad-spectrum antibiotics for suspected biliary sepsis.

Commentary

This case represents a common clinical scenario of a patient with new onset atrial fibrillation and hypotension. Using ultrasound, the clinician was able to quickly determine that the patient was hypovolemic and not fluid overloaded. Fluid resuscitation and finding the primary etiology of the hypovolemia (cholecystitis and early sepsis) were the keys to managing this patient.

CASE 2

Patient Presentation

A 43-year-old obese woman presented to the ED with chest pain and near syncope. The symptoms occurred while she was in her bathroom and EMS was called for a complaint of "weakness." She reported to paramedics that she was recently discharged from the hospital after being evaluated for chest pain and was told that she may have a "heart condition." On physical examination, the patient was awake, alert, and agitated. Her blood pressure was difficult to obtain because of morbid obesity, pulse 120 beats per minute, respirations 24 breaths per minute, temperature 37.0°C, and oxygen saturation 90%

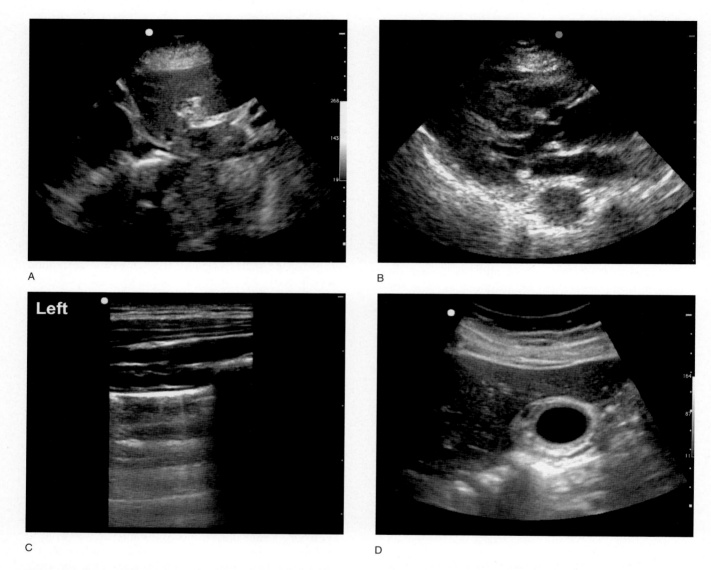

Figure 8-38. Small collapsing IVC is consistent with volume depletion. (A). Hyperdynamic heart that is nearly completely collapsed during systole (parasternal long-axis view) (B). A-line pattern on pulmonary exam (C) essentially rules out pulmonary edema. Abdominal ultrasound with classic signs of cholecystitis: (D) gallbladder wall thickening and pericholecystic fluid.

on 2 L of oxygen by nasal cannula. She was pale and slightly diaphoretic. She had clear breath sounds bilaterally; heart sounds were difficult to auscultate; and the abdomen was obese, soft, and nontender. There were no signs of leg swelling or tenderness.

Management Course

Immediately after arrival to the ED, point-of-care ultrasound was performed during the primary survey. A subcostal four-chamber cardiac view revealed hyperdynamic left ventricular function and an enlarged, thinwalled, hypodynamic right ventricle, with no pericardial effusion (Figure 8-39A). Pulmonary ultrasound revealed

a diffuse A-line pattern, consistent with "dry lungs." A radial arterial line was established and revealed a blood pressure of 80/50 mm Hg. While the arterial line was being placed, venous ultrasound of the lower extremities was performed and revealed a right popliteal DVT (Figure 8-39B). The patient was administered 150 mg of TPA IV approximately 15 minutes after arrival and prior to admission to the ICU.

Commentary

This case represents a good example of a massive PE causing acute right heart strain and shock. The differential diagnosis of chest pain and weakness was broad.

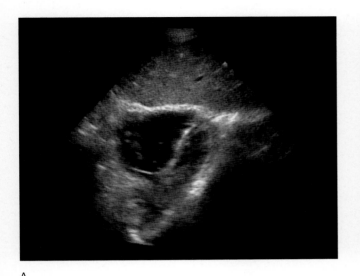

A

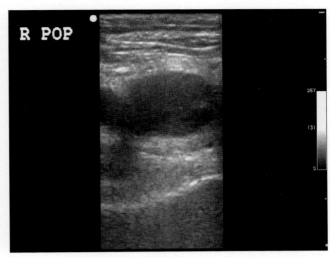

B

Figure 8-39. Massive PE and DVT. Subcostal view shows a large thin-walled right ventricle and small underfilled left ventricle (A). Transverse view of the popliteal region reveals a dilated popliteal vein that does not compress with firm pressure (B). There is also a echogenic clot visible inside the vein.

The emergency physician approached this case as undifferentiated hypotension. The determination of a hyperdynamic left ventricle ruled out a cardiogenic etiology and indicated an attempt to compensate for systemic hypoperfusion. The triad of an enlarged, thin-walled, hypokinetic right ventricle strongly suggested acute right ventricular outflow obstruction (cor pulmonale). In the setting of obesity with recent hospitalization, this was interpreted as indirect evidence of a massive PE. The physician rapidly acquired sufficient clinical information to initiate therapy very early after arrival. Traditionally, this patient would have been subjected to diagnostic studies like EKG, chest radiograph, and CT pulmonary angiogram before the initiation of proper therapy.

CASE 3

Patient Presentation

A 19-year-old man sustained a single stab wound to the epigastric region during a domestic dispute. The patient was intoxicated and combative at the scene. En route to the hospital, he lost consciousness, had no palpable pulse, and required positive pressure ventilation. The prehospital cardiac monitor revealed a narrow complex tachycardia.

Management Course

In anticipation of the patient's arrival, preparations were made for bilateral needle thoracostomies and an ED thoracotomy. On arrival, the patient was unresponsive, un-dergoing face mask ventilation, and chest compressions. Chest compressions were interrupted for a pulse check. Although no pulse was demonstrated, the cardiac ultrasound revealed a small hyperdynamic heart with no pericardial effusion (Figure 8-40A and B). Pulmonary ultrasound revealed a normal sliding lung sign bilaterally and abdominal ultrasound revealed a large amount of fluid in Morison's pouch (Figure 8-40C). Chest compressions were withheld while aggressive volume resuscitation was delivered through three large-bore peripheral IV lines. Within 2 minutes, the patient's volume status improved markedly, as indicated by serial ultrasound exams, which showed better filling of the cardiac chambers and the IVC. The patient's heart rate, which was initially 160 beats per minute, decreased to 120 beats per minute before a carotid pulse could be palpated. The patient underwent rapid sequence intubation and was transported emergently to the operating room for laparotomy without further diagnostic imaging.

Commentary

This case represents an example of a patient who presented with PEA caused by volume depletion. This illustrates how point-of-care ultrasound can be used to rapidly evaluate cardiac function, rule out a pneumothorax, and locate the source of hemorrhage. Performing blind needle thoracostomies or an ED thoracotomy would not have been beneficial to this patient. Withholding chest compressions from a pulseless patient is controversial, but compressing an underfilled hyperdynamic heart makes no sense and compressions may interfere with placement of lines,

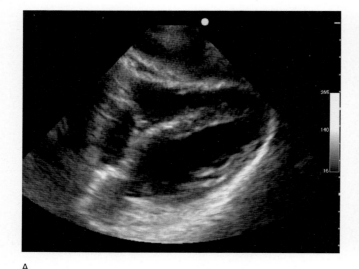

A

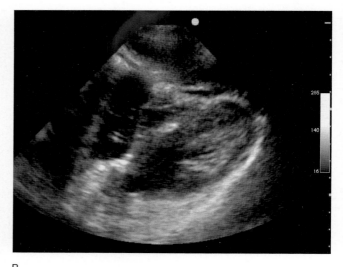

B

C

Figure 8-40. Hyperdynamic heart (subcostal views) and large intraperitoneal-free fluid. Note the poorly filled right ventricle during diastole (A) and complete emptying of the left ventricle during systole (B). A large hemoperitoneum with a thick anechoic stripe is present in Morison's pouch (C).

aggressive volume resuscitation, airway management, and emergent transport to the operating room.

REFERENCES

1. Levitov A, Mayo PH, Slonim AD: *Critical Care Ultrasonography*. New York, NY: McGraw Hill, 2009.
2. Lichtenstein DA: *Whole Body Ultrasonography in the Critically Ill*. Heidelberg: Springer, 2010.
3. Tibballs J, Russell P: Reliability of pulse palpation by healthcare personnel to diagnose paediatric cardiac arrest. *Resuscitation* 80:61, 2009.
4. Deakin CD, Low JL: Accuracy of the advanced trauma life support guidelines for predicting systolic blood pressure using carotid, femoral, and radial pulses: observational study. *BMJ* 321:673, 2000.
5. Ryan BP, Redmond AD, Edwards JD: When to stop resuscitation—The significance of cuff blood pressure. *Arch Emerg Med* 8:177, 1991.
6. Jones AE, Tayal VS, Sullivan DM, Kline JA: Randomized, controlled trial of immediate versus delayed goal-directed ultrasound to identify the cause of nontraumatic hypotension in emergency department patients. *Crit Care Med* 32:1703, 2004.
7. Mullie A, Van Hoeyweghen R, Quets A: Influence of time intervals on outcome of CPR. The Cerebral Resuscitation Study Group. *Resuscitation* 17(suppl):S23, 1989.
8. Neumar RW, et al.: Part 8: adult advanced cardiovascular life support: 2010 American Heart Association Guidelines for Cardiopulmonary Resuscitation and Emergency Cardiovascular Care. *Circulation* 122:S729, 2010.
9. McKelvie PA: Autopsy evidence of pulmonary thromboembolism. *Med J Aust* 160:127, 1994.
10. Combes A, et al.: Clinical and autopsy diagnoses in the intensive care unit: A prospective study. *Arch Intern Med* 164:389, 2004.

11. Perkins GD, McAuley DF, Davies S, Gao F: Discrepancies between clinical and postmortem diagnoses in critically ill patients: An observational study. *Crit Care* 7:R129, 2003.

12. Blaivas M, Fox JC: Outcome in cardiac arrest patients found to have cardiac standstill on the bedside emergency department echocardiogram. *Acad Emerg Med* 8:616, 2001.

13. Breitkreutz R, et al.: Focused echocardiographic evaluation in life support and peri-resuscitation of emergency patients: A prospective trial. *Resuscitation* 81:1527, 2010.

14. Hayhurst C, et al.: An evaluation of echo in life support (ELS): Is it feasible? What does it add? *Emerg Med J* 28:119, 2011.

15. Prosen G, Krizmaric M, Zavrsnik J, Grmec S: Impact of modified treatment in echocardiographically confirmed pseudo-pulseless electrical activity in out-of-hospital cardiac arrest patients with constant end-tidal carbon dioxide pressure during compression pauses. *J Int Med Res* 38:1458, 2010.

16. Salen P, et al.: Does the presence or absence of sonographically identified cardiac activity predict resuscitation outcomes of cardiac arrest patients? *Am J Emerg Med* 23:459, 2005.

17. Salen P, et al.: Can cardiac sonography and capnography be used independently and in combination to predict resuscitation outcomes? *Acad Emerg Med* 8:610, 2001.

18. Varriale P, Maldonado JM: Echocardiographic observations during in hospital cardiopulmonary resuscitation. *Crit Care Med* 25:1717, 1997.

19. Bocka JJ, Overton DT, Hauser A: Electromechanical dissociation in human beings: An echocardiographic evaluation. *Ann Emerg Med* 17:450, 1988.

20. Callaway CW, Menegazzi JJ: Waveform analysis of ventricular fibrillation to predict defibrillation. *Curr Opin Crit Care* 11:192, 2005.

21. Endoh H, et al.: Prompt prediction of successful defibrillation from 1-s ventricular fibrillation waveform in patients with out-of-hospital sudden cardiac arrest *J Anesth* 25:34, 2011.

22. Weingart S: Push-Dose Pressors. In: *EMCrit Blog*. Vol. 6. 2012.

23. Perera P, Mailhot T, Riley D, Mandavia D: The RUSH exam: Rapid Ultrasound in SHock in the evaluation of the critically Ill. *Emerg Med Clin North Am* 28:29, 2010.

24. Rose JS, Bair AE, Mandavia D, Kinser DJ: The UHP ultrasound protocol: A novel ultrasound approach to the empiric evaluation of the undifferentiated hypotensive patient. *Am J Emerg Med* 19:299, 2001.

25. Amico AF, et al.: Superiority of visual versus computerized echocardiographic estimation of radionuclide left ventricular ejection fraction. *Am Heart J* 118:1259, 1989.

26. Stamm RB, Carabello BA, Mayers DL, Martin RP: Two-dimensional echocardiographic measurement of left ventricular ejection fraction: Prospective analysis of what constitutes an adequate determination. *Am Heart J* 104:136, 1982.

27. Mueller X, Stauffer JC, Jaussi A, Goy JJ, Kappenberger L: Subjective visual echocardiographic estimate of left ventricular ejection fraction as an alternative to conventional echocardiographic methods: Comparison with contrast angiography. *Clin Cardiol* 14:898, 1991.

28. Melamed R, Sprenkle MD, Ulstad VK, Herzog CA, Leatherman JW: Assessment of left ventricular function by intensivists using hand-held echocardiography. *Chest* 135:1416, 2009.

29. Moore CL, et al.: Determination of left ventricular function by emergency physician echocardiography of hypotensive patients. *Acad Emerg Med* 9:186, 2002.

30. Joseph MX, Disney PJ, Da Costa R, Hutchison SJ: Transthoracic echocardiography to identify or exclude cardiac cause of shock. *Chest* 126:1592, 2004.

31. MacCarthy P, Worrall A, McCarthy G, Davies J: The use of transthoracic echocardiography to guide thrombolytic therapy during cardiac arrest due to massive pulmonary embolism. *Emerg Med J* 19:178, 2002.

32. Azim A, Rao PB, Srivastav P, Singh P: Cardiac tamponade mimicking septic shock diagnosed by early echocardiography. *J Emerg Trauma Shock* 3:306, 2010.

33. Fowler NO: Cardiac tamponade. A clinical or an echocardiographic diagnosis? *Circulation* 87:1738, 1993.

34. Levine MJ, Lorell BH, Diver DJ, Come PC: Implications of echocardiographically assisted diagnosis of pericardial tamponade in contemporary medical patients: Detection before hemodynamic embarrassment. *J Am Coll Cardiol* 17:59, 1991.

35. Nagdev A, Stone MB: Point-of-care ultrasound evaluation of pericardial effusions: Does this patient have cardiac tamponade? *Resuscitation* 82:671, 2011.

36. Roy CL, Minor MA, Brookhart MA, Choudhry NK: Does this patient with a pericardial effusion have cardiac tamponade? *JAMA* 297:1810, 2007.

37. Spodick DH: Acute cardiac tamponade. *N Engl J Med* 349:684, 2003.

38. Tsang TS, et al.: Clinical and echocardiographic characteristics of significant pericardial effusions following cardiothoracic surgery and outcomes of echo-guided pericardiocentesis for management: Mayo Clinic experience, 1979-1998. *Chest* 116:322, 1999.

39. Hart D, Budhram G, Reardon R, Clinton J: Bedside echocardiography in the management of a thoracic stab wound with early pericardial tamponade. *Acad Emerg Med* 15:1322, 2008.

40. Fagan SM, Chan KL: Pericardiocentesis: Blind no more! *Chest* 116:275, 1999.

41. Tsang TS, et al.: Consecutive 1127 therapeutic echocardiographically guided pericardiocenteses: Clinical profile, practice patterns, and outcomes spanning 21 years. *Mayo Clin Proc* 77:429, 2002.

42. Tsang TS, Freeman WK, Sinak LJ, Seward JB: Echocardiographically guided pericardiocentesis: Evolution and state-of-the-art technique. *Mayo Clin Proc* 73:647, 1998.

43. Tsang TS, Oh JK, Seward JB: Diagnosis and management of cardiac tamponade in the era of echocardiography. *Clin Cardiol* 22:446, 1999.

44. Himelman RB, Kircher B, Rockey DC, Schiller NB: Inferior vena cava plethora with blunted respiratory response: A sensitive echocardiographic sign of cardiac tamponade. *J Am Coll Cardiol* 12:1470, 1988.

45. Karwinski B, Svendsen E: Comparison of clinical and postmortem diagnosis of pulmonary embolism. *J Clin Pathol* 42:135, 1989.

46. Grifoni S, et al.: Utility of an integrated clinical, echocardiographic, and venous ultrasonographic approach for triage of patients with suspected pulmonary embolism. *Am J Cardiol* 82:1230, 1998.

47. Carvalho EM, Macedo FI, Panos AL, Ricci M, Salerno TA: Pulmonary embolectomy: Recommendation for early surgical intervention. *J Card Surg* 25:261, 2010.

48. Miniati M, et al.: Value of transthoracic echocardiography in the diagnosis of pulmonary embolism: Results of a prospective study in unselected patients. *Am J Med* 110:528, 2001.

49. Vieillard-Baron A, et al.: Acute cor pulmonale in massive pulmonary embolism: Incidence, echocardiographic pattern, clinical implications and recovery rate. *Intensive Care Med* 27:1481, 2001.

50. Lodato JA, Ward RP, Lang RM: Echocardiographic predictors of pulmonary embolism in patients referred for helical CT. *Echocardiography* 25:584, 2008.

51. Kjaergaard J, Schaadt BK, Lund JO, Hassager C: Quantification of right ventricular function in acute pulmonary embolism: Relation to extent of pulmonary perfusion defects. *Eur J Echocardiogr* 9:641, 2008.

52. Ribeiro A, Juhlin-Dannfelt A, Brodin LA, Holmgren A, Jorfeldt L: Pulmonary embolism: relation between the degree of right ventricle overload and the extent of perfusion defects. *Am Heart J* 135:868, 1998.

53. Leacche M, et al.: Modern surgical treatment of massive pulmonary embolism: Results in 47 consecutive patients after rapid diagnosis and aggressive surgical approach. *J Thorac Cardiovasc Surg* 129:1018, 2005.

54. Sareyyupoglu B, et al.: A more aggressive approach to emergency embolectomy for acute pulmonary embolism. *Mayo Clin Proc* 85:785, 2010.

55. Tayama E, et al.: Treatment of acute massive/submassive pulmonary embolism. *Circ J* 66:479, 2002.

56. Vohra HA, et al.: Early and late clinical outcomes of pulmonary embolectomy for acute massive pulmonary embolism. *Ann Thorac Surg* 90:1747, 2010.

57. Fesmire FM, et al.: Critical issues in the evaluation and management of adult patients presenting to the emergency department with suspected pulmonary embolism. *Ann Emerg Med* 57:628, 2011.

58. Bottiger BW, et al.: Efficacy and safety of thrombolytic therapy after initially unsuccessful cardiopulmonary resuscitation: A prospective clinical trial. *Lancet* 357:1583, 2001.

59. Carr BG, et al.: Intensivist bedside ultrasound (INBU) for volume assessment in the intensive care unit: A pilot study. *J Trauma* 63:495, 2007.

60. Gruenewald M, et al.: Visual evaluation of left ventricular performance predicts volume responsiveness early after resuscitation from cardiac arrest. *Resuscitation* 82:1553, 2011.

61. Agricola E, et al.: Assessment of stress-induced pulmonary interstitial edema by chest ultrasound during exercise echocardiography and its correlation with left ventricular function. *J Am Soc Echocardiogr* 19:457, 2006.

62. Lichtenstein D: Lung ultrasound in acute respiratory failure: An introduction to the BLUE-protocol. *Minerva Anestesiol* 75:313, 2009.

63. Lichtenstein D, Meziere G: A lung ultrasound sign allowing bedside distinction between pulmonary edema and COPD: The comet-tail artifact. *Intensive Care Med* 24:1331, 1998.

64. Lichtenstein D, Meziere G, Biderman P, Gepner A, Barre O: The comet-tail artifact. An ultrasound sign of alveolar-interstitial syndrome. *Am J Respir Crit Care Med* 156:1640, 1997.

65. Picano E, et al.: Ultrasound lung comets: A clinically useful sign of extravascular lung water. *J Am Soc Echocardiogr* 19:356, 2006.

66. Agricola E, et al.: "Ultrasound comet-tail images": A marker of pulmonary edema: A comparative study with wedge pressure and extravascular lung water. *Chest* 127:1690, 2005.

67. Noble VE, et al.: Ultrasound assessment for extravascular lung water in patients undergoing hemodialysis. Time course for resolution. *Chest* 135:1433, 2009.

68. Marik PE, Baram M, Vahid B: Does central venous pressure predict fluid responsiveness? A systematic review of the literature and the tale of seven mares. *Chest* 134:172, 2008.

69. Osman D, et al.: Cardiac filling pressures are not appropriate to predict hemodynamic response to volume challenge. *Crit Care Med* 35:64, 2007.

70. Zanobetti M, Poggioni C, Pini R: Can chest ultrasonography replace standard chest radiography for evaluation of acute dyspnea in the ED? *Chest* 139:1140, 2011.

71. Lockey D, Crewdson K, Davies G: Traumatic cardiac arrest: Who are the survivors? *Ann Emerg Med* 48:240, 2006.

72. Blaivas M, Lyon M, Duggal S: A prospective comparison of supine chest radiography and bedside ultrasound for the diagnosis of traumatic pneumothorax. *Acad Emerg Med* 12:844, 2005.

73. Dulchavsky SA, et al.: Prospective evaluation of thoracic ultrasound in the detection of pneumothorax. *J Trauma* 50:201, 2001.

74. Garofalo G, Busso M, Perotto F, De Pascale A, Fava C: Ultrasound diagnosis of pneumothorax. *Radiol Med* 111:516, 2006.

75. Knudtson JL, Dort JM, Helmer SD, Smith RS: Surgeon-performed ultrasound for pneumothorax in the trauma suite. *J Trauma* 56:527, 2004.

76. Sartori S, et al.: Accuracy of transthoracic sonography in detection of pneumothorax after sonographically guided lung biopsy: Prospective comparison with chest radiography. *AJR Am J Roentgenol* 188:37, 2007.

77. Soldati G, et al.: Occult traumatic pneumothorax: Diagnostic accuracy of lung ultrasonography in the emergency department. *Chest* 133:204, 2008.

78. Zhang M, et al.: Rapid detection of pneumothorax by ultrasonography in patients with multiple trauma. *Crit Care* 10:R112, 2006.

79. Lichtenstein DA, Meziere GA: Relevance of lung ultrasound in the diagnosis of acute respiratory failure: The BLUE protocol. *Chest* 134:117, 2008.

80. Slater A, Goodwin M, Anderson KE, Gleeson FV: COPD can mimic the appearance of pneumothorax on thoracic ultrasound. *Chest* 129:545, 2006.

81. Blaivas M, Tsung JW: Point-of-care sonographic detection of left endobronchial main stem intubation and

obstruction versus endotracheal intubation. *J Ultrasound Med* 27:785, 2008.

82. Pfeiffer P, Rudolph SS, Borglum J, Isbye DL: Temporal comparison of ultrasound vs. auscultation and capnography in verification of endotracheal tube placement. *Acta Anaesthesiol Scand* 55:1190, 2011.

83. Knapp S, et al.: The assessment of four different methods to verify tracheal tube placement in the critical care setting. *Anesth Analg* 88:766, 1999.

84. Grmec S: Comparison of three different methods to confirm tracheal tube placement in emergency intubation. *Intensive Care Med* 28:701, 2002.

85. Rudraraju P, Eisen LA: Confirmation of endotracheal tube position: A narrative review. *J Intensive Care Med* 24:283, 2009.

86. Chun R, et al.: Where's the tube? Evaluation of hand-held ultrasound in confirming endotracheal tube placement. *Prehosp Disaster Med* 19:366, 2004.

87. Weaver B, Lyon M, Blaivas M: Confirmation of endotracheal tube placement after intubation using the ultrasound sliding lung sign. *Acad Emerg Med* 13:239, 2006.

88. Januzzi JL, Jr, et al.: The N-terminal pro-BNP investigation of dyspnea in the emergency department (PRIDE) study. *Am J Cardiol* 95:948, 2005.

89. Stevenson LW, Perloff JK: The limited reliability of physical signs for estimating hemodynamics in chronic heart failure. *JAMA* 261:884, 1989.

90. Lichtenstein D: Introduction to lung ultrasound. In: Lichtenstein D, ed. *Whole Body Ultrasonography in the Critically Ill.* Heidelberg: Springer, 2010.

91. Manson WC, Bonz JW, Carmody K, Osborne M, Moore CL: Identification of sonographic B-lines with linear transducer predicts elevated B-type natriuretic peptide level. *West J Emerg Med* 12:102, 2011.

92. Volpicelli G, et al.: Bedside lung ultrasound in the assessment of alveolar-interstitial syndrome. *Am J Emerg Med* 24:689, 2006.

93. Cibinel GA, et al.: Diagnostic accuracy and reproducibility of pleural and lung ultrasound in discriminating cardiogenic causes of acute dyspnea in the emergency department. *Intern Emerg Med* 7:65, 2012.

94. Barry BN, Mallick A, Bodenham AR, Vucevic M: Lack of agreement between bioimpedance and continuous thermodilution measurement of cardiac output in intensive care unit patients. *Crit Care* 1:71, 1997.

95. Rothlin MA, et al.: Ultrasound in blunt abdominal and thoracic trauma. *J Trauma* 34:488, 1993.

96. Blaivas M: Incidence of pericardial effusion in patients presenting to the emergency department with unexplained dyspnea. *Acad Emerg Med* 8:1143, 2001.

97. Lensing AW, et al.: Detection of deep-vein thrombosis by real-time B-mode ultrasonography. *N Engl J Med* 320:342, 1989.

98. Poppiti R, Papanicolaou G, Perese S, Weaver FA: Limited B-mode venous imaging versus complete color-flow duplex venous scanning for detection of proximal deep venous thrombosis. *J Vasc Surg* 22:553, 1995.

99. Barrellier MT, Lezin B, Monsallier JM: [Isolated iliac deep venous thrombosis. Study of 48 cases seen in 7 years among 18,297 echo-Doppler evaluations of the lower limbs]. *J Mal Vasc* 26:290, 2001.

100. Pomero F, et al.: Venous lower-limb evaluation in patients with acute pulmonary embolism. *South Med J* 104:405, 2011.

101. Burns GA, Cohn SM, Frumento RJ, Degutis LC, Hammers L: Prospective ultrasound evaluation of venous thrombosis in high-risk trauma patients. *J Trauma* 35:405, 1993.

102. Harris LM, et al.: Screening for asymptomatic deep vein thrombosis in surgical intensive care patients. *J Vasc Surg* 26:764, 1997.

103. Marik PE, Andrews L, Maini B: The incidence of deep venous thrombosis in ICU patients. *Chest* 111:661, 1997.

104. Marston WA, Ahlquist R, Johnson G Jr, Meyer AA: Misdiagnosis of ruptured abdominal aortic aneurysms. *J Vasc Surg* 16:17, 1992.

105. Akkersdijk GJ, van Bockel JH: Ruptured abdominal aortic aneurysm: Initial misdiagnosis and the effect on treatment. *Eur J Surg* 164:29, 1998.

106. Lanoix R, Leak LV, Gaeta T, Gernsheimer JR: A preliminary evaluation of emergency ultrasound in the setting of an emergency medicine training program. *Am J Emerg Med* 18:41, 2000.

107. Kuhn M, Bonnin RL, Davey MJ, Rowland JL, Langlois SL: Emergency department ultrasound scanning for abdominal aortic aneurysm: Accessible, accurate, and advantageous. *Ann Emerg Med* 36:219, 2000.

108. Gloviczki P, et al.: Ruptured abdominal aortic aneurysms: Repair should not be denied. *J Vasc Surg* 15:851, 1992.

109. Jehle D, Stiller G, Wagner D: Sensitivity in detecting free intraperitoneal fluid with the pelvic views of the FAST exam. *Am J Emerg Med* 21:476, 2003.

110. Stengel D, Bauwens K, Rademacher G, Mutze S, Ekkernkamp A: Association between compliance with methodological standards of diagnostic research and reported test accuracy: Meta-analysis of focused assessment of US for trauma. *Radiology* 236:102, 2005.

111. Gracias VH, et al.: Defining the learning curve for the Focused Abdominal Sonogram for Trauma (FAST) examination: implications for credentialing. *Am Surg* 67:364, 2001.

112. Branney SW, et al.: Quantitative sensitivity of ultrasound in detecting free intraperitoneal fluid. *J Trauma* 39:375, 1995.

113. Grassi R, et al.: [Twenty-six consecutive patients with acute superior mesenteric infarction. Comparison of conventional radiology, ultrasonography, and computerized tomography]. *Radiol Med* 93:699, 1997.

114. Nee PA, Rivers EP: The end of the line for the Surviving Sepsis Campaign, but not for early goal-directed therapy. *Emerg Med J* 28:3, 2011.

115. Morrow DJ, Thompson J, Wilson SE: Acute cholecystitis in the elderly: A surgical emergency. *Arch Surg* 113:1149, 1978.

116. Adedeji OA, McAdam WA: Murphy's sign, acute cholecystitis and elderly people. *J R Coll Surg Edinb* 41:88, 1996.

117. Myrianthefs P, et al.: Is routine ultrasound examination of the gallbladder justified in critical care patients? *Crit Care Res Pract* 2012:565617, 2012.

118. Karahan OI, Kurt A, Yikilmaz A, Kahriman G: New method for the detection of intraperitoneal free air by sonography: Scissors maneuver. *J Clin Ultrasound* 32:381, 2004.

119. Hefny AF, Abu-Zidan FM: Sonographic diagnosis of intraperitoneal free air. *J Emerg Trauma Shock* 4:511, 2011.

120. Grassi R, Di Mizio R, Pinto A, Romano L, Rotondo A: Serial plain abdominal film findings in the assessment of acute abdomen: Spastic ileus, hypotonic ileus, mechanical ileus and paralytic ileus. *Radiol Med* 108:56, 2004.

121. Levitan RM, Rosenblatt B, Meiner EM, Reilly PM, Hollander JE: Alternating day emergency medicine and anesthesia resident responsibility for management of the trauma airway: A study of laryngoscopy performance and intubation success. *Ann Emerg Med* 43:48, 2004.

122. Sakles JC, Laurin EG, Rantapaa AA, Panacek EA: Airway management in the emergency department: A one-year study of 610 tracheal intubations. *Ann Emerg Med* 31:325, 1998.

123. Tayal VS, Kline JA: Emergency echocardiography to detect pericardial effusion in patients in PEA and near-PEA states. *Resuscitation* 59:315, 2003.

124. Salvatierra O Jr, Bucklew WB, Morrow JW: Perinephric abscess: A report of 71 cases. *J Urol* 98:296, 1967.

125. Thorley JD, Jones SR, Sanford JP: Perinephric abscess. *Medicine (Baltimore)* 53:441, 1974.

126. Anderson KA, McAninch JW: Renal abscesses: Classification and review of 40 cases. *Urology* 16:333, 1980.

127. Rivers E, et al.: Early goal-directed therapy in the treatment of severe sepsis and septic shock. *N Engl J Med* 345:1368, 2001.

128. Chern CH, et al.: Psoas abscess: Making an early diagnosis in the ED. *Am J Emerg Med* 15:83, 1997.

129. Leung J, Duffy M, Finckh A: Real-time ultrasonographically-guided internal jugular vein catheterization in the emergency department increases success rates and reduces complications: A randomized, prospective study. *Ann Emerg Med* 48:540, 2006.

130. Blaivas M: Video analysis of accidental arterial cannulation with dynamic ultrasound guidance for central venous access. *J Ultrasound Med* 28:1239, 2009.

131. Dunbar RD, Mitchell R, Lavine M: Aberrant locations of central venous catheters. *Lancet* 1:711, 1981.

132. Prekker ME, Chang R, Cole JB, Reardon R: Rapid confirmation of central venous catheter placement using an ultrasonographic "Bubble Test". *Acad Emerg Med* 17:e85, 2010.

133. Sunder-Plassmann G, Muhm M, Drum W: Placement of central venous catheters by overinsertion of guide wires: Low complication rate in 1527 central venous access devices. *Nephrol Dial Transplant* 11:911, 1996.

134. Pinneri F, et al.: Echocardiography-guided versus fluoroscopy-guided temporary pacing in the emergency setting: An observational study. *J Cardiovasc Med* 14:242, 2013.

135. Bair AE, Panacek EA, Wisner DH, Bales R, Sakles JC: Cricothyrotomy: A 5-year experience at one institution. *J Emerg Med* 24:151, 2003.

136. McGill J, Clinton JE, Ruiz E: Cricothyrotomy in the emergency department. *Ann Emerg Med* 11:361, 1982.

137. Petros S, Engelmann L: Percutaneous dilatational tracheostomy in a medical ICU. *Intensive Care Med* 23:630, 1997.

138. van Heurn LW, Theunissen PH, Ramsay G, Brink PR: Pathologic changes of the trachea after percutaneous dilatational tracheotomy. *Chest* 109:1466, 1996.

139. Hatfield A, Bodenham A: Portable ultrasonic scanning of the anterior neck before percutaneous dilatational tracheostomy. *Anaesthesia* 54:660, 1999.

140. Kleine-Brueggeney M, et al.: Ultrasound-guided percutaneous tracheal puncture: A computer-tomographic controlled study in cadavers. *Br J Anaesth* 106:738, 2011.

141. Nicholls SE, Sweeney TW, Ferre RM, Strout TD: Bedside sonography by emergency physicians for the rapid identification of landmarks relevant to cricothyrotomy. *Am J Emerg Med* 26:852, 2008.

142. Sustic A, Kovac D, Zgaljardic Z, Zupan Z, Krstulovic B: Ultrasound-guided percutaneous dilatational tracheostomy: A safe method to avoid cranial misplacement of the tracheostomy tube. *Intensive Care Med* 26:1379, 2000.

143. Breitkreutz R, Walcher F, Seeger FH: Focused echocardiographic evaluation in resuscitation management: Concept of an advanced life support-conformed algorithm. *Crit Care Med* 35:S150, 2007.

144. Hernandez C, et al.: C.A.U.S.E.: Cardiac arrest ultra-sound exam—A better approach to managing patients in primary non-arrhythmogenic cardiac arrest. *Resuscitation* 76:198, 2008.

145. Crisp JG, Lovato LM, Jang TB: Compression ultrasonography of the lower extremity with portable vascular ultrasonography can accurately detect deep venous thrombosis in the emergency department. *Ann Emerg Med* 56:601, 2010.

CHAPTER 9

Abdominal Aortic Aneurysm

Robert F. Reardon, Michelle E. Clinton, Frank Madore, and Thomas P. Cook

Aneurysm of the abdominal aorta is a relatively common disease in patients over 50 years of age.[1-3] Rupture of an abdominal aortic aneurysm (AAA) has a high mortality and causes as many as 30,000 deaths per year in the United States, which is more than AIDS or prostate cancer.[4] It is one of the least-known killers in American society.[4]

More than 100 years ago, William Osler said, "There is no disease more conducive to clinical humility than aneurysm of the aorta." This remains true today, as the diagnosis of ruptured AAA continues to confound clinicians. Misdiagnosis of ruptured AAA is common because many patients have not had a previously asymptomatic AAA formally diagnosed; they also may present with nonspecific complaints and have normal vital signs.[5-7] Mortality due to AAA is decreased if the diagnosis is made prior to rupture or if the diagnosis is made rapidly after rupture of AAA.[8-13]

The availability of point-of-care ultrasound in the ED has allowed emergency physicians to change their approach to patients at risk for a ruptured AAA. A screening point-of-care ultrasound examination can now be obtained on patients over 50 years of age who present with pain in the abdomen, back, flank, or groin, and on those who present with dizziness, syncope, unexplained hypotension, or cardiac arrest.[2,14] This practice is analogous to the immediate acquisition of an ECG for all patients with possible myocardial infarction. In this capacity, ultrasound clearly can save lives, making this application one of the indisputable benefits of emergency point-of-care ultrasound.[8,9,13,15]

► CLINICAL CONSIDERATIONS

AAA occurs in 2–5% of the population over 50 years of age and about 10% of men over 65 years of age who have risk factors for vascular disease.[16-22] The prevalence is even higher in patients with first-degree relatives who have an AAA and those with peripheral vascular disease.[4,23] AAA is about four times more prevalent in men than in women.[24-26] The prevalence has been steadily rising in both men and women over the past several decades, so despite advances in diagnostic imaging and surgical techniques there has been essentially no change in the number of patients presenting with ruptured AAA.[27-31]

The risk of AAA rupture is directly related to the largest diameter of the aneurysm and increases dramatically in those >5 cm. Estimates of rupture risk are as follows: <2% per year for aneurysms <4 cm, 1–5% per year for those 4–5 cm, 3–15% per year for those 5–6 cm, 10–20% per year for those 6–7 cm, and 20–50% per year for those >7 cm.[32-37] Other factors such as continued smoking, uncontrolled hypertension, and emphysema increase the risk of rupture.[38,39] Also, women have a higher risk for rupture than men with the same-size aneurysm.[32,40-42] Current guidelines for elective treatment of AAA suggest operative repair of aneurysms 5.5 cm or larger in the "average" patient.[43] Of course, each patient's situation is unique and requires an analysis of the risks and benefits prior to elective surgery.[4]

Most patients with an AAA are asymptomatic until rupture occurs. The overall mortality for ruptured AAA is roughly 80%. About 60% die prior to receiving any medical care and 40–50% of those who have emergent operative repair die.[18,44–49] Rapid diagnosis and early surgical management have been shown to decrease mortality.[10–13] Unfortunately, 30–60% of patients with a ruptured AAA may be initially misdiagnosed.[6,44,50,51] Delayed or misdiagnosis occurs because the symptoms may mimic other common conditions such as renal colic, musculoskeletal back pain, diverticulitis, GI hemorrhage, sepsis, or acute coronary syndrome. Patients do not usually know that they have an aneurysm, and many have normal vital signs and initially appear well.[6,18,47,51–53]

Emergency physicians routinely manage a large number of patients over 50 years of age who have symptoms that could be consistent with a ruptured AAA. Most of these patients do not have a ruptured AAA, but those who do must be diagnosed rapidly. Even when an aneurysm is suspected, physical examination findings are not reliable for excluding or confirming the diagnosis.[6,18,47,51–55] Therefore, clinicians need an accurate diagnostic screening test that can be effectively used on a large number of patients. The diagnostic test must be rapid and easy to obtain so that clinicians will have a low threshold for using it. The only diagnostic test that fits this description is point-of-care ultrasound performed by the clinician who is already caring for the patient.[50] Laboratory tests are unhelpful and plain radiographs are unreliable; the two essentially have no place in the diagnostic evaluation for an acute AAA. Computed tomography (CT) is very accurate for detecting AAA but it exposes patients to ionizing radiation, is very expensive, and is not practical in unstable patients. The use of point-of-care ultrasound performed by clinicians has been extensively studied and is nearly 100% accurate for detecting or excluding AAA.[5,7,56–59]

In 1989, the first report on the use of point-of-care ultrasound by emergency physicians to rapidly diagnose ruptured AAA was published.[60] Two prospective studies reported that emergency physicians with limited training could diagnose AAA with sensitivity and specificity approaching 100%.[57,61] In 2000, a study analyzed 68 patients over 50 years of age presenting to an ED with symptoms worrisome for a ruptured AAA.[56] Point-of-care ultrasound was performed by emergency physicians who had attended a 3-day point-of-care ultrasound training course but had no prior experience performing or interpreting sonograms. They detected 26 AAAs and had 100% sensitivity and 100% specificity. They concluded that relatively inexperienced providers can perform aortic ultrasound examinations accurately. In 2003, a prospective study analyzed 114 patients presenting to an ED with symptoms suggestive of ruptured AAA.[7] Point-of-care ultrasound examinations were performed by emergency physicians and senior emergency

medicine residents. The investigators diagnosed AAA in 29 patients, had 100% sensitivity, and 98% specificity compared with confirmatory testing, and concluded that emergency physicians could use point-of-care ultrasound to diagnose or exclude AAA. A 2005 study evaluated 238 patients who presented to an ED with symptoms concerning for ruptured AAA.[5] Ultrasound examinations were performed by senior emergency medicine residents who had been trained following guidelines of the American College of Emergency Physicians.[62] They found 36 ruptured AAAs and had 100% sensitivity for making the diagnosis, although their measurements were not perfect. They correctly measured aneurysm diameter in 34 of 36 patients and incorrectly measured 2 aneurysms, but recognized that the aorta was abnormal, leading to the correct diagnosis in those cases. The investigators concluded that appropriately trained emergency medicine residents can accurately determine the presence of AAA.

A 1998 study conducted by Plummer and colleagues dramatically demonstrated the need for emergency point-of-care ultrasound.[13] They reviewed the medical records of 50 consecutive patients presenting to their ED with a ruptured AAA. Twenty-five patients who had an immediate point-of-care ultrasound examination had an average time to diagnosis of 5.4 minutes and a median time to disposition for operative intervention of 12 minutes. Twenty-five patients who did not receive an immediate point-of-care ultrasound examination had an average time to diagnosis of 83 minutes and a median time to disposition for operative intervention of 90 minutes. Their most important finding was that those patients who received an early point-of-care ultrasound examination had a 40% mortality compared with a 72% mortality for those patients who did not receive a point-of-care ultrasound examination.

Although ultrasound is operator dependent and the quality of the examination may be influenced by the expertise of the clinician as well as patient body habitus, point-of-care aortic ultrasound can achieve 100% accuracy with brief training.[56,63–66] There is not much inter-observer variability, even in inexperienced hands, though more experienced clinicians tend to be more accurate.[64,67] Training in point-of-care ultrasound of the abdominal aorta to evaluate for AAA is now a standard part of the core point-of-care ultrasound curriculum across all US emergency medicine residency programs.[68]

▶ CLINICAL INDICATIONS

The main indication for point-of-care aortic ultrasound examination is to rapidly identify patients with an AAA (Figure 9-1). Patients with signs or symptoms that could be attributable to a ruptured AAA should

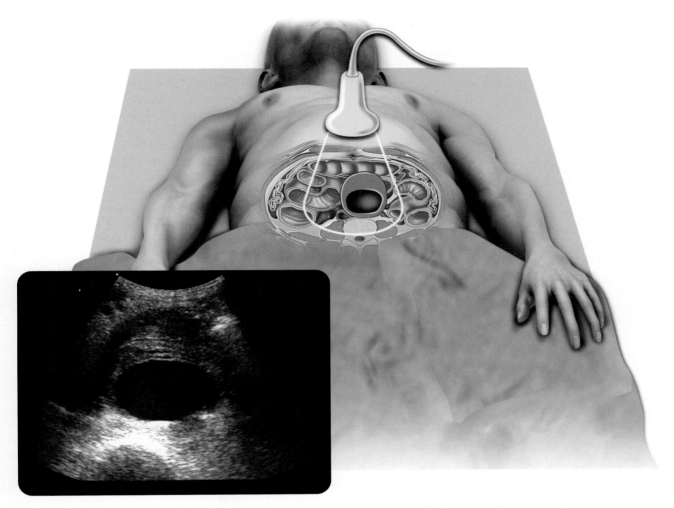

Figure 9-1. Abdominal aortic aneurysm. Ultrasound techniques and findings are outlined in the corresponding sections of this chapter.

undergo an immediate point-of-care ultrasound examination. Patients with a ruptured AAA have widely varying presentations. Reasonable indications for bedside aortic ultrasound examination include all patients over 50 years of age with the following signs or symptoms:

- The classic presentation of ruptured AAA
- Any pain consistent with ruptured AAA
- Unexplained hypotension, dizziness, or syncope
- Cardiac arrest

It is certainly preferable to diagnose AAA prior to rupture since early recognition and repair carries a much lower mortality. In 2005, the US Preventive Services Task Force published recommendations that endorsed the one-time screening for AAA by ultrasonography in men aged 65–75 who had any history of tobacco use. It has been demonstrated that screening for AAA and sur-

gical repair of large AAAs (5.5 cm or more) in men aged 65–75 with a history of tobacco use (current or former smokers) lead to decreased AAA-specific mortality.[8]

CLASSIC PRESENTATION OF RUPTURED AAA

The "classic" presentation of a ruptured AAA is the triad of abdominal, back, or flank pain; a palpable abdominal mass; and hypotension. This "classic" presentation is found in <25% of cases.[6,47,50,51,53] Pain is the most consistent part of the triad and is present in >80% of those seeking medical attention.[6,51,53] Palpation of an abdominal mass on physical examination is an unreliable finding. One study reported that a palpable mass was noted in only 18% of 329 patients presenting with a ruptured AAA.[53] In addition, many thin patients with an apparent pulsatile abdominal mass have a normal abdominal aorta.[54] Finally, hypotension is not universally present with ruptured AAA. Most aneurysms rupture into the retroperitoneum, resulting in a transient tamponade effect; thus, 30–50% of patients have a normal blood pressure at the time of presentation with ruptured AAA.[6,18,51–53,69]

PAIN CONSISTENT WITH RUPTURED AAA

Pain is the most common reason for patients with a ruptured AAA to seek medical care. Most patients complain of pain in the abdomen, back, or flank. Studies have found that about 80% of ruptured AAA patients have abdominal pain, about 60% have back or flank pain, and 22% have groin pain at the time of presentation.[6,51] In another study of 329 cases of ruptured AAA, it was found that 49% had abdominal pain and 36% had back pain at the time of presentation.[53] Clinicians should be aware that patients often present with referred pain to the scrotum, buttocks, thighs, shoulders, chest, or other locations.[2] Many patients with ruptured AAA are misdiagnosed with renal colic, diverticulitis, or musculoskeletal pain.[50] When patients present with nonspecific pain and stable vital signs, it is common to miss or delay the diagnosis. In these difficult patients, it is imperative to rapidly diagnose a ruptured AAA because those who develop hypotension prior to surgery have a higher mortality.[10,13,18,70] No patient with a known or suspected AAA rupture should be considered stable regardless of initial vital signs.[52]

UNEXPLAINED HYPOTENSION, DIZZINESS, OR SYNCOPE

Hypotension is present in 50% or more of patients presenting with ruptured AAA.[6,18,51–53,69] Altered mental status secondary to hypotension can make it difficult to obtain a history of abdominal, back, or flank pain. Therefore, patients may present with unexplained hypotension and no other clues of a ruptured AAA. Many of these patients are misdiagnosed with GI hemorrhage, sepsis, or myocardial infarction.[6,50,51,53] Both hypotension and altered mental status prior to surgery are independent predictors of mortality from a ruptured AAA.[18,70,71] Multiple protocols for screening ED patients who present with undifferentiated hypotension have been developed.[72] One study used an empiric ultrasound examination to screen for pericardial effusion, free intraperitoneal fluid, and AAA. Another study

used a similar approach that included additional ultrasound windows to evaluate the inferior vena cava (IVC), perisplenic region, and pelvis.[73] Both studies pointed out that empiric abdominal ultrasonography is especially valuable when clinical history is limited or unknown and suggested that it should be a routine part of evaluation of patients with unexplained hypotension.

Relative hypotension, orthostatic hypotension, dizziness, or syncope may be precursors to overt hypotension and are indications for ultrasound examination of the abdominal aorta. Relative hypotension occurs in patients with baseline hypertension who have a decrease in blood pressure level but still have values that are within the "normal" range. These patients may present with altered mental status, vague weakness, dizziness, or syncope. A study that reviewed the records of 23 patients with a ruptured AAA found that 61% were initially misdiagnosed.[51] Only 13% of patients had overt hypotension (systolic blood pressure <90 mm Hg) but 26% had syncope and 48% had an initial systolic blood pressure <110 mm Hg or orthostatic hypotension.

CARDIAC ARREST

Cardiac arrest is a fairly common presentation in patients with ruptured AAA.[18] Clinicians should recognize that patients with pulseless electrical activity may be in a state of severe hypotension that could possibly be reversible if the cause is rapidly identified and aggressively treated.[74] A case report described a patient with pulseless electrical activity in whom emergency physicians used point-of-care ultrasound to immediately identify mechanical cardiac activity despite lack of pulses.[75] This finding led to aggressive resuscitation and a search for potential hemorrhage. They then used point-of-care ultrasound to detect a large AAA, allowing the patient to proceed directly to the operating room for surgical repair. They concluded that patients presenting with pulseless electrical activity who are found to have mechanical cardiac activity should have immediate ultrasound imaging of their aorta. Multiple approaches to rapid ultrasound exam of the pulseless electrical activity arrest victim have been described. If hypovolemia is suggested by decreased cardiac chamber volume and increased IVC collapsibility, the aorta should be promptly assessed to evaluate for possible AAA rupture.[76–79]

Some physicians argue that patients who have sustained cardiac arrest from a ruptured AAA have a miniscule chance of survival and that surgical repair is a waste of resources, but this view is not supported by data.[70] One study found that preoperative cardiac arrest occurred in 24% of patients with ruptured AAA, but 28% of those survived operative repair.[18]

SCREENING FOR AAA IN HIGH-RISK ASYMPTOMATIC PATIENTS

Ultrasound screening for AAA and its impact on mortality have been extensively studied.[16,80−84] A 2005 evidence-based systematic review of population-based screening for AAA concluded that selective screening for AAA significantly improves AAA-related mortality. When the study extrapolated the findings to the entire US population of men aged 65–74 years, it estimated that 11,392 AAA deaths could be prevented over a 5-year period.[9] A 2007 Cochrane review of four randomized controlled trials involving 127,891 men and 9342 women found significant decrease in mortality from AAA in men who were screened, but not for women. Only one of the analyzed trials included women, leading to the conclusion that there is insufficient evidence to determine the benefit of AAA screening in women.[85]

A study analyzing the cost-effectiveness of a "quick-screen" program for AAA found that the cost-effectiveness ratio (cost per life saved) was lower than the cost of breast cancer screening. A study evaluating the efficacy and cost of a large-scale screening effort in men between the ages of 65 and 75 years who had smoked at least 100 cigarettes in their lifetime found that AAA was diagnosed in 5.1% of screened patients. The cost of the exam per patient was $53.[86] Properly trained emergency physicians can perform limited AAA screening examinations with 100% sensitivity.[7,56] The rapidity and accuracy of an ED screening exam was reported to have an average time of 141 seconds and a mean size discrepancy of 3.9 mm between the ED exam and comprehensive imaging.[87] Other trainees, such as internal medicine and surgery residents, can learn to perform accurate AAA screening examinations with little training.[88,89]

The Society for Vascular Surgery, the American Association of Vascular Surgery, and the Society for Vascular Medicine and Biology endorse screening of the following patient groups (based on a review of six prospective randomized trials):[4,16,25,80,82,84,90−92]

1. all men aged 60–85 years;
2. women aged 60–85 years with CV risk factors;
3. men and women older than 50 years with a family history of AAA.

They also recommended that patients found to have an AAA 3–4 cm in diameter have an annual follow-up ultrasound examination, those with an AAA 4–4.5 cm have a follow-up examination every 6 months, and those with an AAA >4.5 cm be referred to a vascular surgeon. While these guidelines are widely accepted and adhered to in the United States, a systematic review of seven national or international guidelines for AAA screening published in 2012 found consensus only in screening men over the age of 65 for AAA and in referring patients with AAAs >5.5 cm for surgical repair.[93]

▶ ANATOMICAL CONSIDERATIONS

The abdominal aorta is entirely a retroperitoneal structure. It begins at the aortic hiatus of the diaphragm at approximately the 12th thoracic vertebrae and courses anterior to the spine before bifurcating into the common iliac arteries. The IVC courses to the right of the abdominal aorta and may be confused for the abdominal aorta by inexperienced operators. The psoas muscle and kidney are posterior–lateral to the abdominal aorta on the left side. The left lobe of the liver is located anterior to the proximal abdominal aorta and acts as the primary acoustic window for this area of the vessel. More caudal, the aorta is posterior to the transverse colon, the pancreas, and proximal duodenum. The distal duodenum crosses over the abdominal aorta distal to the superior mesenteric artery (SMA). Other areas of the small bowel lie anterior to the abdominal aorta as it courses distally to its bifurcation at approximately the 2nd lumbar vertebrae (or umbilicus). Components of the GI system may contain air that can block visualization of the abdominal aorta and its branches.

The abdominal aorta is 10–20 cm in length in adults with a maximum external diameter that is normally <3.0 cm (2.1 cm for men over 55 years and 1.8 cm for women over 55 years). It tapers to approximately 1.5 cm at the bifurcation, but it can be <1.0 cm in diameter in smaller adults. The first large branch of the abdominal aorta is the celiac trunk (Figure 9-2). It comes off the anterior wall of the abdominal aorta approximately 1–2 cm below the level of the diaphragm and courses anteriorly for 1–2 cm before splitting into the common hepatic and splenic arteries. The splenic artery courses to the left and follows the superior border of the pancreas before entering the spleen. The common hepatic artery courses to the right and supplies blood to the liver, stomach, pancreas, and duodenum. The SMA arises from the anterior wall of the aorta approximately 1–2 cm distal from the celiac trunk and courses caudally to supply blood to the small bowel. Both renal arteries come off the lateral wall of the abdominal aorta, just distal to the SMA; the right renal artery courses under the IVC. The paired gonadal arteries (testicular and ovarian) come off the anterior wall distal to the renal vessels. The inferior mesenteric artery comes off the anterior wall 2–3 cm proximal to the iliac bifurcation and supplies blood to the lower GI tract. Both the gonadal vessels and inferior mesenteric artery are usually difficult to visualize by ultrasound and rarely contribute to evaluation and management of the patient.

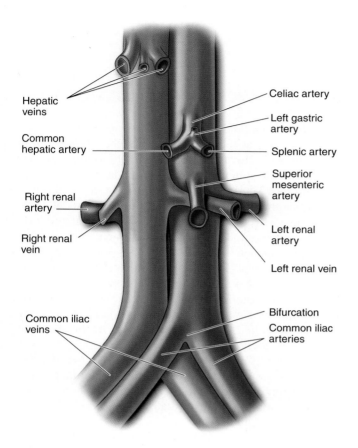

Figure 9-2. Branches of the abdominal aorta and inferior vena cava.

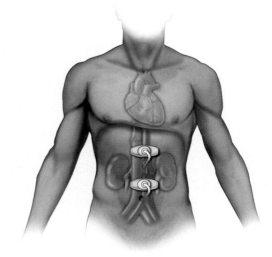

Figure 9-3. Ultrasound transducer positions for imaging the abdominal aorta. The length of the aorta can be imaged using sweeping views from these transducer positions. This can avoid potential interference from gas in the transverse colon.

▶ GETTING STARTED

The bedside scenario when performing an ultrasound examination of the aorta can vary from a calm physician's office to a resuscitation bay crowded with medical personnel working together to provide simultaneous components of patient care. There are a variety of protocols that clinicians may adopt to complete an examination; however, an abbreviated examination of the aorta is usually easy to complete in <1 or 2 minutes. Ideally, evaluate the entire length of the abdominal aorta from the diaphragm to the bifurcation in both the longitudinal and transverse planes.

Examine most patients in the supine position; however, place the patient into the right or left decubital positions if excessive bowel gas is present. Bowel gas is the most common cause for inability to view the abdominal aorta; by placing the patient in either decubitus position, bowel gas may be displaced from the aorta.

Since there are no ribs or other bony structures overlying the abdominal aorta, a variety of transducers can be used for the examination, ranging from curvilinear transducers with large footprints to small phased array transducers typically designed for echocardiography. Most examiners use abdominal "presets" for the examination. Focal zones and frequency may need to be augmented to accommodate the patient's body habitus.

Situate the machine at the patient's right side. Place a liberal amount of gel in the area from the xiphoid process to the umbilicus. By convention, scan the abdominal aorta in the longitudinal (sagittal) plane by pointing the transducer marker dot toward the patient's head and in the transverse (axial) plane by pointing the transducer marker dot toward the patient's right side. The vast majority of imaging of the abdominal aorta is performed on the anterior surface along the patient's midline (Figure 9-3). The critical portion of the abdominal aorta examination (just above the bifurcation) is accomplished in the transverse orientation with the transducer indicator pointed toward the patient's right side.

A curved array transducer is typically used to examine the aorta. Base frequency selection on body habitus to achieve the best balance of resolution and penetration. An average-sized adult is usually scanned at approximately 3.5 MHz. Select a lower frequency for greater penetration in patients with a large body habitus. Scan smaller or thinner adults at resolutions as high as 5 MHz. Standard two-dimensional gray scale imaging is adequate; additional features such as color Doppler and power Doppler are not required but can facilitate differentiation of the abdominal aorta from other structures. Select a sufficient depth at the beginning of the examination until the abdominal aorta is identified. Upon visualizing the aorta, adjust the depth, focal zone, and frequency to optimize the image.

Although not required for all examinations of the abdominal aorta, identification of landmark structures including arterial branches, venous structures, and other abdominal organs can ensure that an adequate segment of the aorta has been imaged. Visualization of this entire length of abdominal aorta is required to exclude AAA. Should its diameter be adequately visualized and appear normal over this length, then a ruptured AAA can be confidently excluded.

There are two primary obstacles to obtaining adequate images of the abdominal aorta: bowel gas and obesity. Bowel gas may require the examiner to move the transducer slightly to either side of the midline to acquire views. Another option is to apply gentle, continuous pressure in order to compress the bowel with the transducer and move bowel gas away from the area of interest. This may require 1–2 minutes of continuous pressure on the abdominal wall with the transducer.

Strategies to overcome obesity include using firm pressure to decrease the distance from the skin–transducer interface to the target organ and rolling the patient in a left lateral decubitus position to swing the pannus away from the midline. Firm pressure on the transducer will allow visualization of the aorta in nearly all patients. Iatrogenic rupture of an AAA by firm pressure during physical examination or an ultrasound examination has not been reported.[52]

► TECHNIQUE AND NORMAL ULTRASOUND FINDINGS

If time permits for a complete examination of the abdominal aorta, initially place the transducer just caudal to the xiphoid process (Figures 9-4 and 9-5; Video 9-1: Aorta). In the transverse plane, an excellent point of reference is the spine. It appears as a posteriorly oriented concave structure that is highly reflective (hyperechoic) and casts a shadow. The abdominal aorta is easily found immediately anterior and slightly to the left of the spine. It is pulsatile and round to ovular in shape. This usually makes it easy to differentiate from the IVC, which is thin-walled, varies in size with respiration, and is often flattened by minimal pressure from the transducer. This view also provides an opportunity to angle the transducer beam into the frontal plane (i.e., toward the head) in order to acquire a subcostal view of the heart. Superficial to the most proximal abdominal aorta will be the subcutaneous tissue and left lobe of the liver. The left lobe of the liver acts as the acoustic window for imaging the proximal portion of the abdominal aorta (See Video 9-1: Abdominal Aorta).

As the transducer is moved more caudal, branches of the abdominal aorta come into view starting with the celiac trunk and then the SMA. The latter is in close proximity to several other vascular structures in the transverse plane (Figure 9-6A). The left renal vein courses under the SMA and over the abdominal aorta joining the IVC. The splenic vein crosses over the SMA along the body of the pancreas before joining the superior mesenteric vein to create the portal vein in the liver. One or both renal arteries and veins may be seen just inferior to the take-off of the SMA coursing posterior and lateral to the kidneys. When the renal arteries are not visible, involvement of an aneurysm with these branch vessels can be

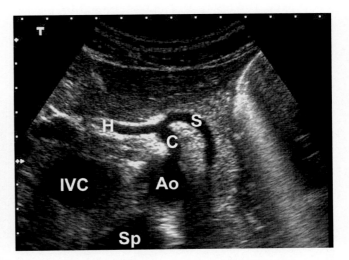

Figure 9-5. Transverse view of the upper aorta (at the level of the celiac trunk). By using a large convex transducer in a thin patient, the relative positions of the anatomical landmarks can be visualized. The liver serves as an acoustic window to the structures below. The aorta and IVC are immediately above the spine. H = hepatic artery, S = splenic artery, C = celiac artery, IVC = inferior vena cava, Ao = aorta, Sp = spine.

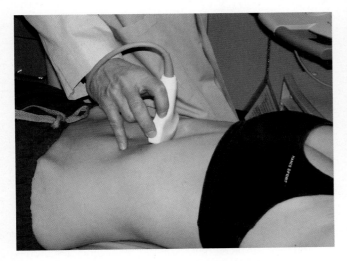

Figure 9-4. Initial transducer position for complete imaging of the abdominal aorta–transverse with indicator to the patient's right.

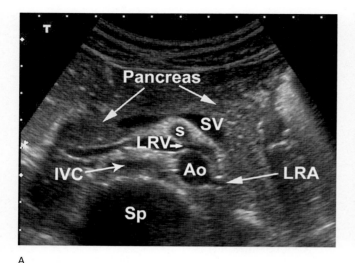

A

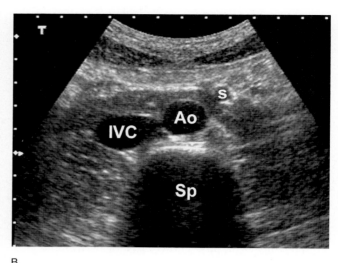

B

Figure 9-6. (A) Transverse view of the middle portion of the abdominal aorta (at a level just below the branching point for the SMA). LRV = left renal vein, s = superior mesenteric artery (SMA), SV = splenic vein, IVC = inferior vena cava, Ao = aorta, LRA = left renal artery, Sp = spine. (B) Transverse view of the distal abdominal aorta (at a level above the bifurcation). IVC = inferior vena cava, Ao = aorta, s = superior mesenteric vein (or artery). Sp = spine.

predicted on the basis of proximity to the SMA. The renal arteries are likely to be involved if the aneurysm is within 2 cm of the branching point for the SMA.

Since the distal abdominal aorta is the most common location of an AAA, clinicians may opt to examine the distal aorta first in the hemodynamically unstable patient. The distal aorta is best viewed by placing the transducer just superior to the umbilicus in the transverse plane (Figure 9-3). However, there is much to be said for starting in the epigastric region every time and

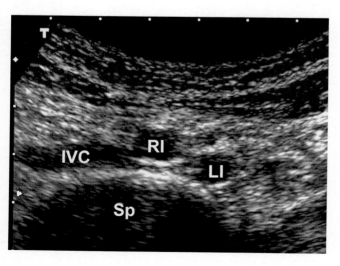

Figure 9-7. Transverse view of the bifurcation of the abdominal aorta. IVC = inferior vena cava, RI = right iliac artery, LI = left iliac artery, Sp = spine.

taking the additional seconds to orient to the anatomy before moving distally. The distal transverse view often visualizes only the abdominal aorta and posterior spine as the IVC may be collapsed because of compression from the transducer (Figure 9-6B). Anterior–posterior (AP) diameter from outer wall to outer wall in transverse section provides the most accurate measurement of the diameter of the abdominal aorta. In contrast, measurement of the longitudinal dimension may cause a "cylinder tangent" error (described in Pitfalls section). If a careful measurement is required, then use the freeze frame option on the ultrasound machine along with the caliper measurement software. In some patients, the bifurcation of the aorta can be seen, and iliac arteries followed to exclude iliac artery aneurysm if suspected (Figure 9-7).

In the longitudinal plane at the xiphoid process (Figures 9-8 and 9-9), angle the transducer from left to right to image the proximal IVC and the aorta. Some clinicians utilize a "sniff" test to help with differentiation of these structures as well. By having the patient quickly sniff, a sudden drop in thoracic pressure is created that pulls blood from the IVC into the thorax and causes the IVC to collapse. In addition, the IVC is often seen directly entering the right atrium of the heart (Figure 9-10), while the abdominal aorta will demonstrate the celiac trunk and SMA exiting from its anterior surface. The splenic vein and left renal vein may be seen in their short axes above and below the SMA, respectively, and the left renal vein may be seen coursing under the IVC. When rotating the

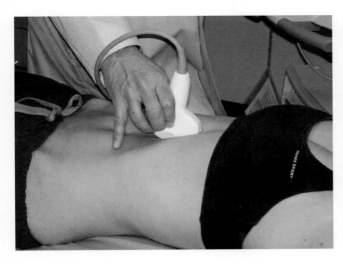

Figure 9-8. Transducer position for longitudinal views of the aorta—indicator is cephalad.

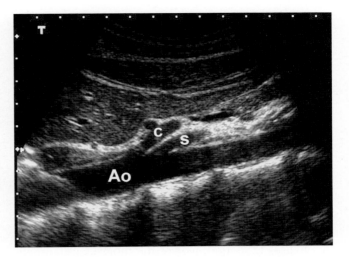

Figure 9-9. Longitudinal view of the abdominal aorta. The celiac artery (C) is the first vessel to branch off the aorta. The superior mesenteric artery (S) is immediately below the celiac artery and courses parallel to the aorta (Ao).

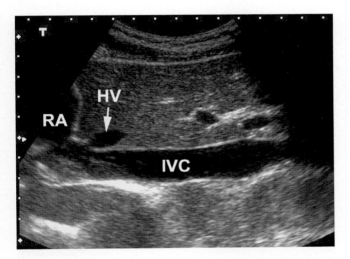

Figure 9-10. Longitudinal view of the inferior vena cava (IVC). RA = right atrium, HV = hepatic vein.

transducer from a transverse to longitudinal view of the aorta, avoid inadvertently sliding the transducer over the IVC. In some patients, the IVC may appear pulsatile due to cardiac motion.

A final option for ultrasound imaging of the aorta is the coronal view. Place the transducer in the right anterior axillary line and, using the hepatic acoustic window, scan the aorta in the coronal plane. Initiate the examination with the image display at maximum depth. This will yield an image with the IVC toward the top of the screen and the aorta lying deeper (Figures 9-11 and 9-12).

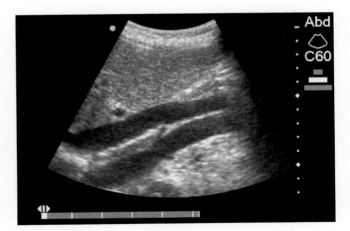

Figure 9-12. Coronal view of the aorta. The IVC is above the aorta in this right coronal view. Both renal arteries are seen branching off the aorta at a 45° angle (forming an arrowhead appearance in the mid aorta). The renal arteries are not routinely visualized in this view. (Courtesy of James Mateer, MD)

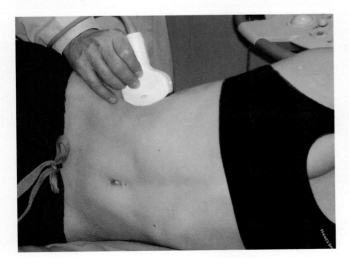

Figure 9-11. Transducer position for coronal views of the aorta—indicator is cephalad.

▶ COMMON ABNORMALITIES

ABDOMINAL AORTIC ANEURYSM

The primary abnormality is aneurysmal enlargement of the abdominal aorta. This is most frequently seen in the transverse view as an aorta >3.0 cm in diameter (Figure 9-13). Aneurysmal dilation is usually fusiform, resulting in a uniform concentric enlargement of the circumference (Figure 9-14). Localized outpouching of a segment of the aortic wall results in the more unusual saccular aneurysm formation (Figure 9-15). Aneurysmal dilatation is most often confined to the infrarenal aorta and usually terminates proximal to the bifurcation. Contiguous thoracoabdominal aneurysm occurs in a minority of cases (2%) and involves the thoracic aorta in addition to the abdominal aorta, including the segment involving the celiac, superior mesenteric, and renal arteries. The iliac arteries are involved in some patients with AAA (Figure 9-16A), and occasionally, iliac artery aneurysms occur in an isolated fashion. More than 90% of AAAs occur in the distal abdominal aorta, inferior to the renal arteries. An AAA may rarely be detected only in the proximal abdominal aorta (Figure 9-16B). Rupture most commonly occurs into the left retroperitoneum. Less commonly, intraperitoneal rupture can occur.[94] Ultrasonography is inadequate to demonstrate the presence of extraluminal retroperitoneal blood associated with rupture, which is found with a sensitivity <5%.[95] However, in the appropriate clinical setting, a large AAA should be considered ruptured until proven otherwise.[52,96]

INTRALUMINAL THROMBUS

With increasing diameter, the laminar flow rate decreases at the periphery, resulting in blood stagnation and thrombus formation. This intraluminal thrombus is well visualized on ultrasound and is more common anteriorly

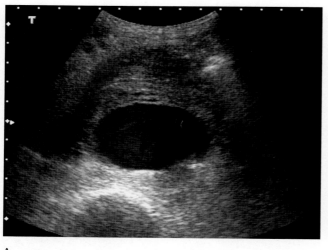

A

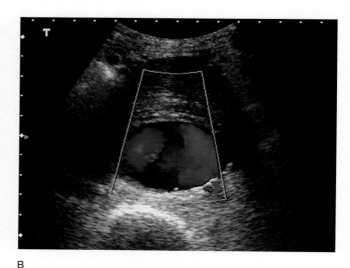

B

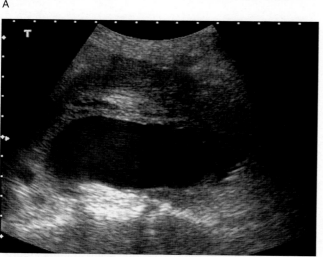

C

Figure 9-13. AAA. This fusiform aneurysm demonstrates a thickened wall secondary to mural thrombus. Transverse view (A). Color Doppler confirms this is a vascular structure (B). Longitudinal view (C).

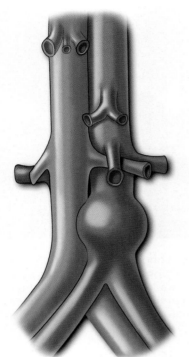

Figure 9-14. Fusiform aneurysm.

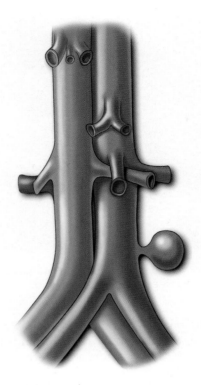

Figure 9-15. Saccular aneurysm (uncommon).

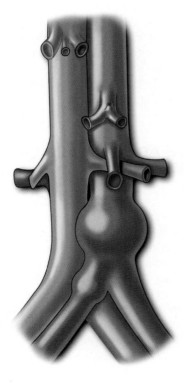

A

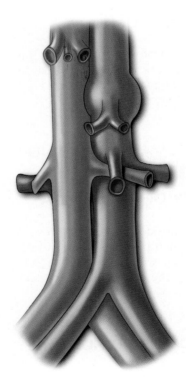

B

Figure 9-16. (A) Iliac artery aneurysm. A fusiform AAA with extension into the right common iliac artery is illustrated. (B) Isolated proximal AAA (uncommon).

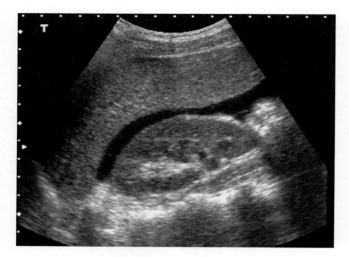

Figure 9-17. Coronal view of the right kidney demonstrates free intraperitoneal fluid.

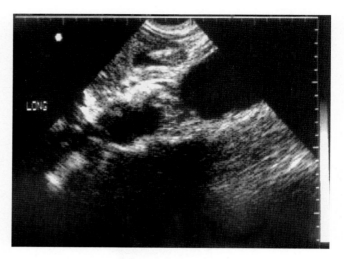

Figure 9-18. Longitudinal view of an AAA. The normal distal tapering of the aorta is reversed. The echogenic area within the aorta is not a clot, but is the sidewall of the vessel due to tortuosity. (Courtesy of James Mateer, MD)

and laterally but may be circumferential (Figure 9-13). Thrombus is found in both ruptured and unruptured AAAs. It is not an indication of rupture or dissection, and is not a false lumen. Complete occlusion of the abdominal aorta has also been described and has been successfully diagnosed with point-of-care ultrasound.[97]

HEMOPERITONEUM

Rupture into the peritoneal cavity may present with acute hemoperitoneum that may be visualized with the right intercostal oblique window of the FAST examination (Figure 9-17) or other windows.

► COMMON VARIANTS AND OTHER ABNORMALITIES

TORTUOSITY OF THE AORTA

Variations in the position and size of vessels are common. The aorta often becomes tortuous with age. This can cause difficulty with following the course of the vessel and finding the correct plane for transverse and longitudinal views (Figure 9-18).

CONTAINED AORTIC RUPTURE

A contained rupture of an AAA is not commonly diagnosed with ultrasound. When present, it may be seen as a hypoechoic mixed density area (from contained hemorrhage and hematoma) surrounding the aorta (Figure 9-19).

HYDRONEPHROSIS

A large AAA can cause secondary complications by compressing surrounding structures. Compression of the left ureter can lead to hydronephrosis and eventually to a perinephric urinoma from calyceal rupture (Figure 9-20). Hydronephrosis is, of course, a much more common finding in patients being imaged for suspected ureterolithiasis. Thus, the finding of hydronephrosis in a patient with AAA risk factors and flank pain should not reassure the clinician that the cause is an obstructing ureteral stone.

ACUTE ABDOMINAL AORTIC DISSECTION

This disease entity may be confused with ruptured AAA and can occur with or without a coexisting aneurysm. Only 2%–4% of patients with an aortic dissection experience it in the abdominal aorta. The presenting symptoms are similar to those seen in ruptured AAA but may mimic other disease entities such as pancreatitis.[98] Occasionally, clinicians will encounter mild aortic dilation caused by an aortic dissection and mistakenly diagnose an early AAA thought to be too small for rupture. Care should thus be taken to examine for a flap in the lumen (Figure 9-21). Utilizing color Doppler will occasionally show flow in only one portion of the abdominal aorta in transverse orientation. Even if the flap cannot be well visualized, a finding of mild aortic dilatation in the correct clinical scenario should raise the suspicion for an abdominal aortic dissection.

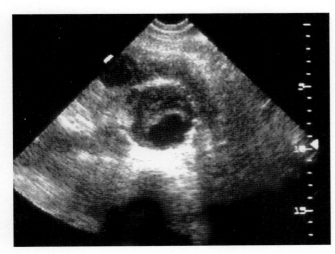

A

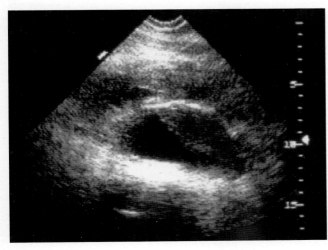

B

Figure 9-19. Contained rupture of an AAA: Transverse view reveals an AAA with mural thrombus (A). Wrapping around the anterior aorta is a hypoechoic mixed density area (from contained hemorrhage and hematoma). Longitudinal view of the same patient (B). (Courtesy of James Mateer, MD)

AORTOVENOUS FISTULA

Formation of an arteriovenous fistula occurs when an AAA ruptures into an adjacent vein; the left renal vein or the IVC is most often involved. Because these aneurysms are usually large (11–13 cm on average), a pulsatile mass can often be palpated on physical examination. The presenting symptoms are similar to those seen in AAA rupture. An ultrasound examination demonstrating a large AAA, along with a CT scan documenting a retroaortic left renal vein and an IVP showing absence of left renal filling, may help confirm the diagnosis.

ISOLATED ILIAC ARTERY ANEURYSM

Iliac artery aneurysms are present in up to 20% of AAAs but are found in the absence of AAA in 2–7% of cases. Thus, include careful examination of the bifurcation of the abdominal aorta (found posterior to the umbilicus) as well as the proximal iliac arteries in every bedside aorta ultrasound exam. The normal diameter of the iliac arteries is about 1 cm. Aneurysms measure >1.5 cm and elective repair is generally considered at 3.5 cm.[99]

ENDOLEAK

In a patient with a previously grafted AAA, abdominal pain may occur from expansion of the aneurysm sac due to leakage of blood through or around the endoluminal graft. The ability to detect endoleak by ultrasound is limited, but if comparison images are available, an expanding aneurysm sac post-repair should prompt further investigation by CT. If no comparison images are available, an endoleak may be definitively diagnosed by demonstrating flow out of the graft by color Doppler.[94]

► PITFALLS

1. **Contraindication.** The only absolute contraindication to performing this ultrasound examination of the abdominal aorta is if it delays clearly indicated, immediate surgical intervention.
2. **Overreliance on examination.** The finding of an enlarged aorta alone is not sufficient to diagnose rupture of the abdominal aorta. There are no reliable ultrasound findings of retroperitoneal hematoma associated with the most common form of AAA rupture. However, the finding of AAA (especially with a diameter >5 cm) accompanied by other clinical manifestations, such as acute hemodynamic compromise, strongly suggests the diagnosis of AAA rupture. Correlate the location of the aneurysm with the SMA origin and recognize that if dilation is within 2 cm inferior to the SMA, the renal arteries are likely to be involved. When hemodynamically stable, patients with contained rupture may be diagnosed by definitive imaging prior to surgical intervention.
3. **Patient factors limiting imaging.** Obesity and bowel gas always render ultrasound imaging more difficult. Failure to determine the involvement of the major branches of the aorta makes operative planning more difficult for the surgeon. When bowel gas or other technical factors

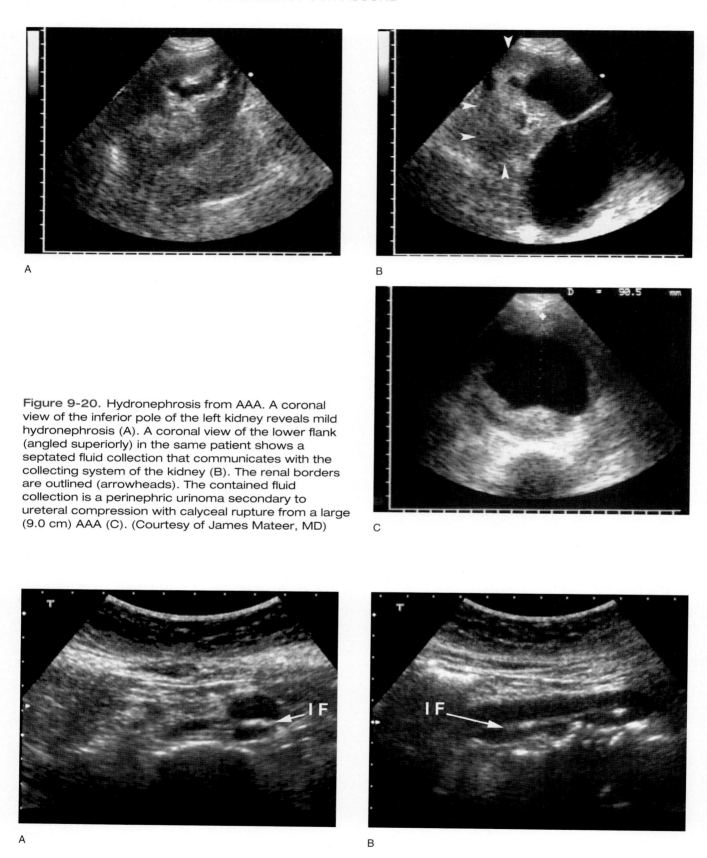

Figure 9-20. Hydronephrosis from AAA. A coronal view of the inferior pole of the left kidney reveals mild hydronephrosis (A). A coronal view of the lower flank (angled superiorly) in the same patient shows a septated fluid collection that communicates with the collecting system of the kidney (B). The renal borders are outlined (arrowheads). The contained fluid collection is a perinephric urinoma secondary to ureteral compression with calyceal rupture from a large (9.0 cm) AAA (C). (Courtesy of James Mateer, MD)

Figure 9-21. Acute abdominal aortic dissection. Transverse (A) and longitudinal views (B) showing intimal flap (IF).

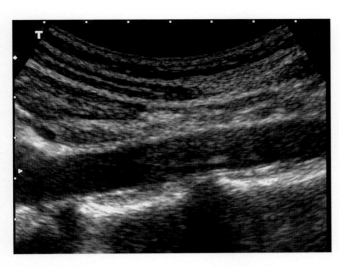

Figure 9-22. Long-axis view of the distal aorta. Obtain a transverse view to avoid confusing the IVC and aorta.

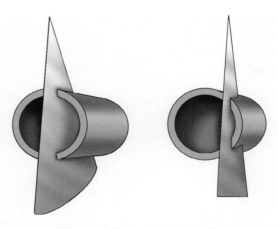

Figure 9-24. The cylinder tangent effect. A longitudinal beam slice through the center of the vessel will show the maximum diameter, while an off center slice will show a reduced diameter.

prevent a complete systematic real-time scan through all tissue planes, identify and document these limitations. Such limitations may mandate further evaluation by alternative methods, as clinically indicated.[100]

4. **Errors in imaging.** Two common errors in imaging must be avoided. First, the physician must take care not to inadvertently sweep the plane of the beam into a right parasagittal plane, which may result in a long-axis view of the IVC. The IVC here is thin walled and easily compressed, and can be mistaken for the abdominal aorta. The examiner can avoid this error by visualizing the aorta and IVC in the transverse plane

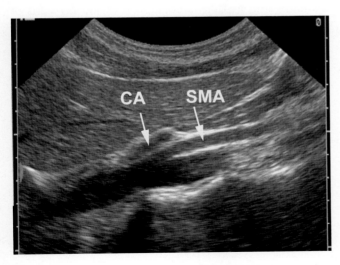

Figure 9-23. Long-axis view of the aorta. The upper abdominal aorta shows characteristic thick echogenic walls and anterior branching vessels. CA, celiac artery; SMA, superior mesenteric artery.

(Figure 9-22), or when in longitudinal plane by visualizing the celiac trunk and SMA at the proximal abdominal aorta (Figure 9-23). The second error may result from the "cylinder tangent" effect (Figure 9-24). Limited window accessibility may result in a situation in which the plane of the beam enters the cylinder of the aorta at a tangent and displays an incorrect AP diameter. This is not an artifact error but an operator error. Measure the aorta in both sagittal and transverse planes to avoid this error.

5. **A small aneurysm does not preclude rupture.** A patient with symptoms and signs consistent with acute AAA and an aortic diameter >3.0 cm should have this diagnosis (or alternative vascular catastrophes) fully investigated.

6. **Large paraaortic nodes may be confused for AAA.** Large paraaortic nodes usually occur anterior to the aorta, but may be posterior, displacing the aorta away from the vertebral body. They can be distinguished by an irregular nodular shape, which is identifiable in real time. If color flow Doppler is utilized, the nodes will not demonstrate luminal flow.

▶ CASE STUDIES

CASE 1

Patient Presentation

A 65-year-old man presented to the ED after a witnessed syncopal episode. Upon awaking in the morning, the patient complained of feeling weak and constipated. The patient had a history of well-controlled hypertension.

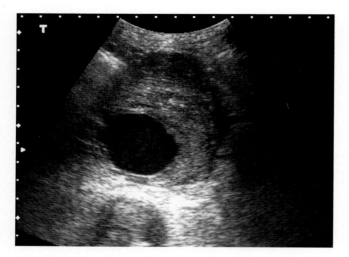

Figure 9-25. Case 1. AAA 7.2 cm. Transverse view.

On physical examination, the patient was awake, alert, and oriented. His blood pressure was 110/50 mm Hg, pulse 100 beats per minute, respirations 18 per minute, and temperature 98.9°F. He appeared pale and slightly diaphoretic. His lungs were clear to auscultation, neck veins flat, and abdomen soft and nontender with no peripheral edema. The remainder of his physical examination was unremarkable.

Management Course

On arrival, two large-bore IVs were established in the upper extremities, while the primary examination was simultaneously performed. As part of his secondary survey, a rapid cardiac view by the subcostal window revealed a hyperdynamic heart. Repositioning of the transducer immediately revealed an enlarged abdominal aorta with an AP diameter of 7.2 cm (Figure 9-25). There was no free intraperitoneal fluid. Surgical consultation was initiated.

Reassessment revealed a decline in blood pressure to 80/50 mm Hg. No other diagnostic maneuvers were employed and the patient was transported directly to the operating room for exploratory laparotomy. Operative findings included a ruptured 7.4 cm AAA that was successfully grafted.

Commentary

Case 1 is an example of a patient presenting to the ED with hemodynamic alteration from a ruptured AAA. This type of syncope followed by near-normalization of vital signs with subsequent decline in perfusion parameters is one of the most common presentations for ruptured AAA. This patient exemplifies an hemodynamically unstable profile that requires limited diagnostic evaluation and rapid surgical intervention. It is impor-

tant to note that the same ultrasound examination was used to demonstrate marked global hyperkinesis of the heart, essentially excluding left ventricular failure as a cause of gradual hemodynamic decline. This was done before performing either an ECG or a chest radiograph.

CASE 2

Patient Presentation

A 74-year-old man presented to the ED at 2 AM, complaining of left "hernia" pain. The patient said that he had been diagnosed with a left inguinal hernia more than 10 years earlier, and he had decided against surgical repair, because it did not cause him pain. He said that he began having left groin pain last night after supper and it had gradually worsened. He denied any other medical history.

On physical examination, the patient was awake and alert and was in no distress. His blood pressure was 160/80 mm Hg, pulse rate 85 beats per minute, respirations 20 per minute, and temperature 99.0°F. He had a left inguinal hernia that was moderately tender to palpation. The hernia sac was firm and protruded into his scrotum about 3–4 cm and could not be reduced on examination. His abdomen was mildly obese and nontender. The remainder of his examination was unremarkable.

Management Course

An IV line was established and the patient was given fentanyl 50 micrograms IV with good relief of his pain. A second attempt to reduce the hernia was unsuccessful. Basic laboratory tests, including a urinalysis, were unremarkable and a plain radiograph revealed no signs of bowel obstruction. The on-call surgeon was consulted because the patient was thought to have an incarcerated inguinal hernia. While awaiting surgical consultation, the patient became diaphoretic and dizzy, his blood pressure dropped to 100/60 mm Hg, and he began complaining of left flank pain. A point-of-care ultrasound examination was performed in the ED and he was noted to have an 8-cm AAA (Figure 9-26). The surgeon was called again and informed of the new information. The patient had an additional large-bore IV placed and was aggressively resuscitated and taken to the operating room within 20 minutes. Despite these efforts, he died on the operating table.

Commentary

This case demonstrated a complex presentation of a ruptured AAA. The patient's long-standing inguinal hernia convinced both the patient and the emergency physician that the etiology of his pain was the hernia. It is common

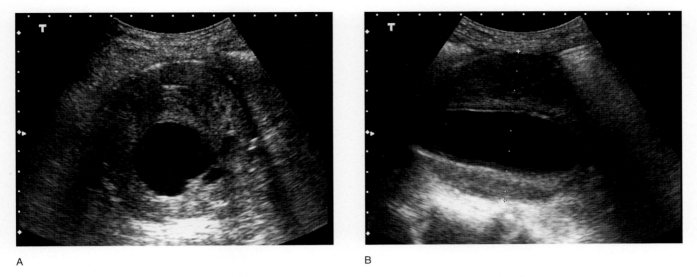

A   B

Figure 9-26. Case 2. AAA 8 cm. Transverse (A) and longitudinal (B) views.

to delay or miss the diagnosis of ruptured AAA because referred pain to the groin, back, or flank is thought to be caused by another disease process. In this case, the physician did not initially consider the diagnosis of ruptured AAA because of the patient's atypical symptoms and normal vital signs.

CASE 3

Patient Presentation

An emergency physician was giving his 62-year-old father a tour of his ED. While showing off for his father, he performed a bedside abdominal aortic ultrasound ex-

amination on his father and was surprised to discover a 4.2-cm AAA (Figure 9-27). His father had a history of smoking, but was asymptomatic and had no other medical history or risk factors.

Management Course

The AAA was monitored every 6 months with serial ultrasound examinations. Two years after it was initially discovered, the AAA measured 5.2 cm in AP diameter. The patient was referred to a surgeon who advised that he delay elective repair until the AAA became 5.5 cm. The patient saw another surgeon for a second opinion and was advised to have the AAA repaired as soon as possible. The second surgeon also recommended

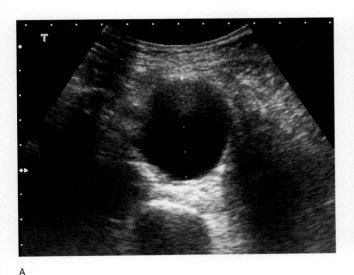
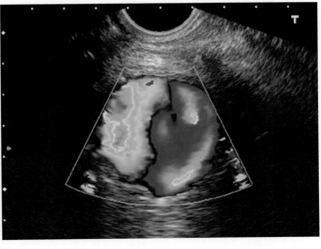

A   B

Figure 9-27. Case 3. AAA 4.2 cm. Transverse (A) and color Doppler transverse views (B).

having an open repair rather than an angiographic stent because he was otherwise healthy and a good surgical candidate. The patient had an open repair and placement of a Gortex graft without complications and had an uneventful recovery. He was able to play golf just a few months later and continues to be asymptomatic.

Commentary

This case demonstrated the importance of screening asymptomatic patients who are at risk for AAA. Men over 60 years of age who have ever smoked are at higher risk for AAA (up to 10%). There are over 50,000 elective AAA repairs per year in the United States, with a very low surgical mortality rate. Conversely, the mortality rate after AAA rupture is 80%.

► ACKNOWLEDGMENT

The authors would like to thank Ben Dolan, MD, and Scott Joing, MD, for their contributions to this chapter. The authors additionally thank Dave Plummer, MD, for his contributions to this chapter in previous editions.

REFERENCES

1. Collin J, Araujo L, Walton J, Lindsell D: Oxford screening programme for abdominal aortic aneurysm in men aged 65 to 74 years. *Lancet* 2:613–615, 1988.

2. Phelan MP, Emerman CL: Focused aortic ultrasound to evaluate the prevalence of abdominal aortic aneurysm in ED patients with high-risk symptoms. *Am J Emerg Med* 24:227–229, 2006.

3. Scott RA, Ashton HA, Kay DN: Routine ultrasound screening in management of abdominal aortic aneurysm. *Br Med J (Clin Res Ed)* 296:1709–1710, 1988.

4. Kent KC, Zwolak RM, Jaff MR, et al.: Screening for abdominal aortic aneurysm: a consensus statement. *J Vasc Surg* 39:267–269, 2004.

5. Costantino TG, Bruno EC, Handly N, Dean AJ: Accuracy of emergency medicine ultrasound in the evaluation of abdominal aortic aneurysm. *J Emerg Med* 29:455–460, 2005.

6. Marston WA, Ahlquist R, Johnson G, Jr., Meyer AA: Misdiagnosis of ruptured abdominal aortic aneurysms. *J Vasc Surg* 16:17–22, 1992.

7. Tayal VS, Graf CD, Gibbs MA: Prospective study of accuracy and outcome of emergency ultrasound for abdominal aortic aneurysm over two years. *Acad Emerg Med: Official Journal of the Society for Academic Emergency Medicine* 10:867–871, 2003.

8. US Preventive Services Task Force. Screening for abdominal aortic aneurysm: Recommendation statement. *Ann Intern Med.* 142:198–202, 2005.

9. Fleming C, Whitlock EP, Beil TL, Lederle FA: Screening for abdominal aortic aneurysm: A best-evidence systematic review for the U.S. Preventive Services Task Force. *Ann Intern Med* 142:203–211, 2005.

10. Hans SS, Huang RR: Results of 101 ruptured abdominal aortic aneurysm repairs from a single surgical practice. *Arch Surg* 138:898–901, 2003.

11. Harris LM, Faggioli GL, Fiedler R, Curl GR, Ricotta JJ: Ruptured abdominal aortic aneurysms: factors affecting mortality rates. *J Vasc Surg* 14:812–818; discussion 9–20, 1991.

12. Hoffman M, Avellone JC, Plecha FR, et al.: Operation for ruptured abdominal aortic aneurysms: A community-wide experience. *Surgery* 91:597–602, 1982.

13. Plummer D, Clinton J, Matthew B: Emergency department ultrasound improves time to diagnosis and survival of abdominal aortic aneurysm. *Acad Emerg Med: Official Journal of the Society for Academic Emergency Medicine* 5:417, 1998.

14. ACOEP: Clinical policy: Critical issues for the initial evaluation and management of patients presenting with a chief complaint of nontraumatic acute abdominal pain. *Ann Emerg Med* 36:406–415, 2000.

15. Miller J, Miller J: Small ruptured abdominal aneurysm diagnosed by emergency physician ultrasound. *Am J Emerg Med* 17:174–175, 1999.

16. Ashton HA, Buxton MJ, Day NE, et al.: The Multicentre Aneurysm Screening Study (MASS) into the effect of abdominal aortic aneurysm screening on mortality in men: A randomised controlled trial. *Lancet* 360:1531–1539, 2002.

17. Boll AP, Verbeek AL, van de Lisdonk EH, van der Vliet JA: High prevalence of abdominal aortic aneurysm in a primary care screening programme. *Br J Surg* 85:1090–1094, 1998.

18. Gloviczki P, Pairolero PC, Mucha P, Jr., et al.: Ruptured abdominal aortic aneurysms: repair should not be denied. *J Vasc Surg* 15:851–857; discussion 7–9, 1992.

19. Lederle FA. Ultrasonographic screening for abdominal aortic aneurysms. *Ann Intern Med* 139:516–522, 2003.

20. Lederle FA, Johnson GR, Wilson SE, et al.: The aneurysm detection and management study screening program: Validation cohort and final results. Aneurysm detection and management veterans affairs cooperative study investigators. *Arch Intern Med* 160:1425–1430, 2000.

21. Smith FC, Grimshaw GM, Paterson IS, Shearman CP, Hamer JD: Ultrasonographic screening for abdominal aortic aneurysm in an urban community. *Br J Surg* 80:1406–1409, 1993.

22. Vohra R, Reid D, Groome J, Abdool-Carrim AT, Pollock JG: Long-term survival in patients undergoing resection of abdominal aortic aneurysm. *Ann Vasc Surg* 4:460–465, 1990.

23. Webster MW, Ferrell RE, St Jean PL, Majumder PP, Fogel SR, Steed DL: Ultrasound screening of first-degree relatives of patients with an abdominal aortic aneurysm. *J Vasc Surg* 13:9–13; discussion 13–4, 1991.

24. Lederle FA, Johnson GR, Wilson SE: Abdominal aortic aneurysm in women. *J Vasc Surg* 34:122–126, 2001.

25. Scott RA, Bridgewater SG, Ashton HA: Randomized clinical trial of screening for abdominal aortic aneurysm in women. *Br J Surg* 89:283–285, 2002.

26. Singh K, Bonaa KH, Jacobsen BK, Bjork L, Solberg S: Prevalence of and risk factors for abdominal aortic aneurysms in a population-based study: The Tromsø Study. *Am J Epidemiol* 154:236–244, 2001.

27. Acosta S, Ogren M, Bengtsson H, Bergqvist D, Lindblad B, Zdanowski Z: Increasing incidence of ruptured abdominal aortic aneurysm: A population-based study. *J Vasc Surg* 44:237–243, 2006.

28. Best VA, Price JF, Fowkes FG: Persistent increase in the incidence of abdominal aortic aneurysm in Scotland, 1981–2000. *Br J Surg* 90:1510–1515, 2003.

29. Bickerstaff LK, Hollier LH, Van Peenen HJ, Melton LJ, 3rd, Pairolero PC, Cherry KJ: Abdominal aortic aneurysms: The changing natural history. *J Vasc Surg* 1:6–12, 1984.

30. Heller JA, Weinberg A, Arons R, et al.: Two decades of abdominal aortic aneurysm repair: Have we made any progress? *J Vasc Surg* 32:1091–1100, 2000.

31. Melton LJ, 3rd, Bickerstaff LK, Hollier LH, et al.: Changing incidence of abdominal aortic aneurysms: A population-based study. *Am J Epidemiol* 120:379–386, 1984.

32. Brown LC, Powell JT: Risk factors for aneurysm rupture in patients kept under ultrasound surveillance. UK Small Aneurysm Trial Participants. *Ann Surg* 230:289–296; discussion 96–97, 1999.

33. Jones A, Cahill D, Gardham R: Outcome in patients with a large abdominal aortic aneurysm considered unfit for surgery. *Br J Surg* 85:1382–1384, 1998.

34. Lederle FA, Johnson GR, Wilson SE, et al.: Rupture rate of large abdominal aortic aneurysms in patients refusing or unfit for elective repair. *JAMA* 287:2968–2972, 2002.

35. Nevitt MP, Ballard DJ, Hallett JW Jr: Prognosis of abdominal aortic aneurysms. A population-based study. *New Eng J Med* 321:1009–14, 1989.

36. Reed WW, Hallett JW Jr, Damiano MA, Ballard DJ: Learning from the last ultrasound. A population-based study of patients with abdominal aortic aneurysm. *Arch Intern Med* 157:2064–2068, 1997.

37. Scott RA, Tisi PV, Ashton HA, Allen DR: Abdominal aortic aneurysm rupture rates: A 7-year follow-up of the entire abdominal aortic aneurysm population detected by screening. *J Vasc Surg* 28:124–128, 1998.

38. Cronenwett JL, Sargent SK, Wall MH, et al: Variables that affect the expansion rate and outcome of small abdominal aortic aneurysms. *J Vasc Surg* 11:260–268; discussion 8–9, 1990.

39. Strachan DP: Predictors of death from aortic aneurysm among middle-aged men: The Whitehall study. *Br J Surg* 78:401–404, 1991.

40. Brown PM, Sobolev B, Zelt DT: Selective management of abdominal aortic aneurysms smaller than 5.0 cm in a prospective sizing program with gender-specific analysis. *J Vasc Surg* 38:762–765, 2003.

41. Evans SM, Adam DJ, Bradbury AW: The influence of gender on outcome after ruptured abdominal aortic aneurysm. *J Vasc Surg* 32:258–262, 2000.

42. Powell JT, Brown LC: The natural history of abdominal aortic aneurysms and their risk of rupture. *Acta Chirurgica Belgica* 101:11–16, 2001.

43. Brewster DC, Cronenwett JL, Hallett JW, Jr, Johnston KW, Krupski WC, Matsumura JS: Guidelines for the treatment of abdominal aortic aneurysms. Report of a subcommittee of the Joint Council of the American Association for Vascular Surgery and Society for Vascular Surgery. *J Vasc Surg* 37:1106–1117, 2003.

44. Akkersdijk GJ, van Bockel JH: Ruptured abdominal aortic aneurysm: Initial misdiagnosis and the effect on treatment. *Eur J Surg Acta Chirurgica* 164:29–34, 1998.

45. Bown MJ, Sutton AJ, Bell PR, Sayers RD: A meta-analysis of 50 years of ruptured abdominal aortic aneurysm repair. *Br J Surg* 89:714–730, 2002.

46. Ingoldby CJ, Wujanto R, Mitchell JE: Impact of vascular surgery on community mortality from ruptured aortic aneurysms. *Br J Surg* 73:551–553, 1986.

47. Kiell CS, Ernst CB: Advances in management of abdominal aortic aneurysm. *Adv Surg* 26:73–98, 1993.

48. Magee TR, Galland RB, Collin J, et al.: A prospective survey of patients presenting with abdominal aortic aneurysm. *Eur J Vasc Endovasc Surg: Official Journal of the European Society for Vascular Surgery* 13:403–406, 1997.

49. Tambyraja AL, Murie JA, Chalmers RT: Outcome and survival of patients aged 65 years and younger after abdominal aortic aneurysm rupture. *World J Surg* 29:1245–1247, 2005.

50. Colucciello S, Dasley W, Decker W, et al.: Clinical policy: Critical issues for the initial evaluation and management of patients presenting with a chief complaint of nontraumatic acute abdominal pain. *Ann Emerg Med* 36:406–415, 2000.

51. Lederle FA, Parenti CM, Chute EP: Ruptured abdominal aortic aneurysm: The internist as diagnostician. *Am J Med* 96:163–167, 1994.

52. Bessen H: Abdominal aortic aneurysm. In: Marx J, ed. *Rosen's Emergency Medicine: Concept's and Clinical Practice.* 6th ed. Philadelphia, PA: Mosby Elsevier, 2006:1330–1341.

53. Rose J, Civil I, Koelmeyer T, Haydock D, Adams D: Ruptured abdominal aortic aneurysms: Clinical presentation in Auckland 1993–1997. *ANZ J Surg* 71:341–344, 2001.

54. Fink HA, Lederle FA, Roth CS, Bowles CA, Nelson DB, Haas MA: The accuracy of physical examination to detect abdominal aortic aneurysm. *Arch Intern Med* 160:833–836, 2000.

55. Lederle FA, Simel DL: The rational clinical examination. Does this patient have abdominal aortic aneurysm? *JAMA* 281:77–82, 1999.

56. Kuhn M, Bonnin RL, Davey MJ, Rowland JL, Langlois SL: Emergency department ultrasound scanning for abdominal aortic aneurysm: accessible, accurate, and advantageous. *Ann Emer Med* 36:219–223, 2000.

57. Lanoix R, Leak LV, Gaeta T, Gernsheimer JR: A preliminary evaluation of emergency ultrasound in the setting of an emergency medicine training program. *Am J Emer Med* 18:41–45, 2000.

58. Lee TY, Korn P, Heller JA, et al.: The cost-effectiveness of a "quick-screen" program for abdominal aortic aneurysms. *Surgery* 132:399–407, 2002.

59. Salen P, Melanson S, Buro D: ED screening to identify abdominal aortic aneurysms in asymptomatic geriatric patients. *Am J Emerg Med* 21:133–135, 2003.

60. Jehle D, Davis E, Evans T, et al.: Emergency department sonography by emergency physicians. *Am J Emerg Med* 7:605–611, 1989.

61. Schlager D, Lazzareschi G, Whitten D, Sanders AB: A prospective study of ultrasonography in the ED by emergency physicians. *Am J Emerg Med* 12:185–189, 1994.

62. American College of Emergency Physicians. ACEP emergency ultrasound guidelines-2001. *Ann Emer Med* 38:470–481, 2001.

63. Beales LWS, Evans, J, West R, Scott D: Reproducibility of ultrasound measurement of the abdominal aorta. *Br J Surg* 98(11):1517–1525, 2011.

64. Heegaard W, Hildebrandt D, Spear D, Chason K, Nelson B, Ho J: Prehospital ultrasound by paramedics: Results of field trial. *Acad Emerg Med: Official Journal of the Society for Academic Emergency Medicine* 17:624–630, 2010.

65. LaRoy LL, Cormier PJ, Matalon TA, Patel SK, Turner DA, Silver B: Imaging of abdominal aortic aneurysms. *AJR* 152:785–792, 1989.

66. Wong I, Jayatilleke T, Kendall, R, Atkinson P: Feasibility of a focused ultrasound training programme for medical undergraduate students. *Clin Teach* 8(1):3–7, 2011.

67. Hoffman B, Bessman E, Um P, Ding R, McCarthy ML: Successful sonographic visualisation of the abdominal aorta differs significantly among a diverse group of credentialed emergency department providers. *Emerg Med J* 28(6):472–476, 2010.

68. Akhtar S, Theodoro D, Gaspari R, et al.: Resident training in emergency ultrasound: Consensus recommendations from the 2008 council of emergency medicine residency directors conference. *Acad Emerg Med: Official Journal of the Society for Academic Emergency Medicine* 16:S32–S36, 2009.

69. Ernst CB: Abdominal aortic aneurysm. *New Eng J Med* 328:1167–1172, 1993.

70. Kniemeyer HW, Kessler T, Reber PU, Ris HB, Hakki H, Widmer MK: Treatment of ruptured abdominal aortic aneurysm, a permanent challenge or a waste of resources? Prediction of outcome using a multi-organ-dysfunction score. *Eur J Vasc Endovasc Surg: Official Journal of the European Society for Vascular Surgery* 19:190–196, 2000.

71. Shackleton CR, Schechter MT, Bianco R, Hildebrand HD: Preoperative predictors of mortality risk in ruptured abdominal aortic aneurysm. *J Vasc Surg*: Official publication of the Society for Vascular Surgery [and] International Society for Cardiovascular Surgery, North American Chapter 6:583–589, 1987.

72. Rose JS, Bair AE, Mandavia D, Kinser DJ: The UHP ultrasound protocol: A novel ultrasound approach to the empiric evaluation of the undifferentiated hypotensive patient. *Am J Emerg Med* 19:299–302, 2001.

73. Atkinson PR, McAuley DJ, Kendall RJ, et al.: Abdominal and Cardiac Evaluation with Sonography in Shock (ACES): An approach by emergency physicians for the use of ultrasound in patients with undifferentiated hypotension. *J Emerg Med* 26:87–91, 2009.

74. Neumar RW, Otto CW, Link MS, et al.: Part 8: Adult advanced cardiovascular life support: 2010 American Heart Association Guidelines for Cardiopulmonary Resuscitation and Emergency Cardiovascular Care. *Circulation* 122:S729, 2010.

75. Hendrickson RG, Dean AJ, Costantino TG: A novel use of ultrasound in pulseless electrical activity: The diagnosis of an acute abdominal aortic aneurysm rupture. *J Emerg Med* 21:141–144, 2001.

76. Hernandez C, Shuler K, Hannan H, Sonyika C, Likourezos A, Marshall J: C.A.U.S.E.: Cardiac arrest ultra-sound examination: a better approach to managing patients in primary non-arrhythmogenic cardiac arrest. *Resuscitation* 76:198–206, 2008.

77. Perera P, Mailhot T, Riley D, Mandavia D: The RUSH exam: Rapid Ultrasound in SHock in the evaluation of the critically Ill. *Emerg Med Clin North Am* 28:29–56, vii, 2010.

78. Volpicelli G: Usefulness of emergency ultrasound in non-traumatic cardiac arrest. *Am J Emerg Med* 29:216–223, 2011.

79. Labovitz AJ, Noble VE, Bierig M, et al.: Focused cardiac ultrasound in the emergent setting: A consensus statement of the American Society of Echocardiography and American College of Emergency Physicians. *J Am Soc Echocardiogr: Official Publication of the American Society of Echocardiography* 23:1225–1230, 2010.

80. Lawrence-Brown MM, Norman PE, Jamrozik K, et al.: Initial results of ultrasound screening for aneurysm of the abdominal aorta in Western Australia: Relevance for endoluminal treatment of aneurysm disease. *Cardiovasc Surg* 9:234–940, 2001.

81. Lederle FA, Johnson GR, Wilson SE, et al.: Prevalence and associations of abdominal aortic aneurysm detected through screening. Aneurysm Detection and Management (ADAM) Veterans Affairs Cooperative Study Group. *Ann Inter Med* 126:441–449, 1997.

82. Lindholt JS, Juul S, Fasting H, Henneberg EW: Hospital costs and benefits of screening for abdominal aortic aneurysms. Results from a randomised population screening trial. *Eur J Vasc Endovasc Surg: Official Journal of the European Society for Vascular Surgery* 23:55–60, 2002.

83. Norman PE, Jamrozik K, Lawrence-Brown MM, et al.: Population based randomised controlled trial on impact of screening on mortality from abdominal aortic aneurysm. *BMJ* 329:1259, 2004.

84. Scott RA, Wilson NM, Ashton HA, Kay DN: Influence of screening on the incidence of ruptured abdominal aortic aneurysm: 5-year results of a randomized controlled study. *Br J Surg* 82:1066–1170, 1995.

85. Cosford PA, Leng GC: Screening for abdominal aortic aneurysm. *Cochrane Database Syst Rev* 18(2):CD002945, 2007.

86. Lee ES, Pickett E, Hedayati N, Dawson DL, Pevec WC: Implementation of an aortic screening program in clinical practice: Implications for the Screen For Abdominal Aortic Aneurysms Very Efficiently (SAAAVE) Act. *J Vasc Surg*: Official publication of the Society for Vascular Surgery [and] International Society for Cardiovascular Surgery, North American Chapter 49:1107–1111, 2009.

87. Moore CL, Holliday RS, Hwang JQ, Osborne MR: Screening for abdominal aortic aneurysm in asymptomatic at-risk patients using emergency ultrasound. *Am J Emerg Med* 26:883–887, 2008.

88. Bailey RP, Ault M, Greengold NL, Rosendahl T, Cossman D: Ultrasonography performed by primary care residents for abdominal aortic aneurysm screening. *J Gen Intern Med* 16:845–849, 2001.

89. Lin PH, Bush RL, McCoy SA, et al.: A prospective study of a hand-held ultrasound device in abdominal aortic aneurysm evaluation. *Am J Surg* 186:455–459, 2003.

90. Heather BP, Poskitt KR, Earnshaw JJ, Whyman M, Shaw E: Population screening reduces mortality rate from aortic aneurysm in men. *Br J Surg* 87:750–753, 2000.

91. Irvine CD, Shaw E, Poskitt KR, Whyman MR, Earnshaw JJ, Heather BP: A comparison of the mortality rate after elective repair of aortic aneurysms detected either by screening or incidentally. *Eur J Vasc Endovas Surg: Official Journal of the European Society for Vascular Surgery* 20:374–378, 2000.

92. Wilmink TB, Quick CR, Hubbard CS, Day NE: The influence of screening on the incidence of ruptured abdominal aortic aneurysms. *J Vasc Surg: Official publication of the Society for Vascular Surgery [and] International Society for Cardiovascular Surgery, North American Chapter* 30:203–208, 1999.

93. Ferket BS, Grootenboer N, Colkesen EB, et al.: Systematic review of guidelines on abdominal aortic aneurysm screening. *J Vasc Surg: Official publication of the Society for Vascular Surgery [and] International Society for Cardiovascular Surgery, North American Chapter,* 2011.

94. Bhatt S, Dogra VS: Catastrophes of abdominal aorta: Sonographic evaluation. *Ultrasound Clin* 3(1):83–91, 2008.

95. Shuman WP, Hastrup W Jr, Kohler TR, et al.: Suspected leaking abdominal aortic aneurysm: Use of sonography in the emergency room. *Radiology* 168:117–119, 1988.

96. Chandler JJ: The Einstein sign: The clinical picture of acute cholecystitis caused by ruptured abdominal aortic aneurysm. *New Eng J Med* 310:1538, 1984.

97. Zaremba J, NJ. Ultrasound diagnosis of acute thrombosis of an abdominal aortic aneurysm: A case report. *J Emerg Med* 42:437–439, 2012.

98. Kaban J, Raio C: Emergency department diagnosis of aortic dissection by bedside transabdominal ultrasound. *Acad Emerg Med* 16:809–810, 2009.

99. Uberoi RDT, Vivek S, Morgan R, Belli A: Standard of practice for the interventional management of isolated iliac artery aneurysms. *Cardiovasc Intervent Radiol* 34:3–13, 2011.

100. Kendall JL, Bahner DP, Blaivas M, et al.: Emergency ultrasound imaging criteria compendium. American College of Emergency Physicians. *Ann Emerg Med* 48:487–510, 2006.

CHAPTER 10

Hepatobiliary

Resa E. Lewiss and Daniel L. Theodoro

Abdominal pain is consistently one of the top reasons that patients present to the ED.[1] In 2009, 668970 ED visits resulted in a diagnosis of gallbladder or bile duct pathology. Overall, 39% of these cases required admission and 80% were diagnosed with acute gallbladder and bile duct-related conditions such as cholecystitis. When the emergency physician diagnosed gallstones without acute inflammatory conditions, 88% of cases were discharged from the ED.[2] Consequently, emergency physicians who can effectively perform point-of-care ultrasound have the potential to efficiently impact the care of patients with right upper quadrant abdominal pain.

► CLINICAL CONSIDERATIONS

The primary tools in the evaluation of acute hepatobiliary disease are ultrasound, hepatobiliary iminodiacetic acid scintigraphy (commonly referred to as HIDA scan or cholescintigraphy), computed tomography (CT), and endoscopic retrograde cholangiopancreatography (ERCP). Prior to the late 1980s and early 1990s, several imaging modalities were in use to diagnose hepatobiliary disease, such as oral and IV cholangiography. These methods were time consuming, required the ingestion or injection of potentially harmful contrast agents, and exposed the patient to radiation.[3] Ultrasound largely replaced these imaging modalities in the 1990s. Ultrasound can be performed rapidly at the bedside and does not expose the patient to ionizing radiation. Ultrasound also has the highest sensitivity for detecting the presence of gallstones, while HIDA has a reportedly higher sensitivity for detecting the presence of acute cholecystitis.[4] Data derived solely from ED patients, however, suggest that point-of-care ultrasound of the gallbladder may prove as accurate for the detection of acute cholecystitis as HIDA.[5,6] HIDA has very limited utility for the detection of acute cholecystitis when the point-of-care ultrasound examination is normal.[7] Although CT is limited by its inability to detect 25% of gallstones, CT may play a greater role when other causes of abdominal pain are being considered.[8,9] ERCP is time consuming and resource heavy, and its complications include iatrogenic pancreatitis, perforation, and even death.

► CLINICAL INDICATIONS

Indications for clinicians to perform point-of-care hepatobiliary ultrasound include the evaluation of

- Biliary colic
- Acute cholecystitis
- Jaundice and biliary duct dilatation
- Sepsis
- Ascites
- Hepatic abnormalities

BILIARY COLIC

In the United States, more patients undergo cholecystectomies (both elective and emergent) than appendectomies. Emergency physicians expect to see biliary pathology in up to a third of all patients with abdominal pain, making the differentiation of acute and subacute pathology important.[10,11] The classic presentation of biliary colic portrays an obese woman of childbearing age with recurrent colicky pain in the right upper quadrant shortly after the consumption of a fatty meal. While gallstones are more prevalent in young, multiparous women than in young men, the effect of gender disappears with advancing age.[12] In older patients, the pain does not wax and wane after meals but is constant and occurs mostly at night at predictable times, lasting for an average of 1–5 hours.[13] Prospective data on the prevalence of gallstones and cholecystitis in the pediatric and adolescent population has not been reported. One study suggests that these patients do not have a classic presentation, are often misdiagnosed, and have a delay in diagnosis due to a low suspicion on the part of pediatric providers.[14] Retrospective data on gallstones in this population note that the cause is often due to hemolytic anemia, long-term IV antibiotic therapy, or idiopathic in nature.[15]

Physiologic studies conducted on patients while they were undergoing cholecystectomy concluded that a majority of patients with cholelithiasis experience epigastric discomfort or dyspepsia with mechanical stimulation of the gallbladder. Symptoms may not migrate to the right upper quadrant until the inflamed gallbladder irritates the peritoneum.[16–18] Patients with biliary disease may also complain of right flank pain, scapular pain, or chest pain.[19]

Since the differential diagnosis for the patient with upper abdominal pain is extensive, point-of-care ultrasound of the gallbladder can reduce the number of diagnoses the clinician must consider.[20] Patients with isolated epigastric pain may not routinely get a biliary ultrasound exam, especially if their pain resolves. However, one study showed that one-third of patients with isolated epigastric pain had gallstones, and one-third of the patients with gallstones had cholecystitis.[21] Many patients who present to the ED with biliary disease have ongoing pain, and in these patients point-of-care ultrasound can expedite the diagnosis, and focus the clinician's effort and use of resources.[10,22] An algorithmic approach to the patient presenting with suspected biliary colic is outlined in Figure 10-1.

Several studies demonstrate that emergency physicians with adequate experience acquire and interpret ultrasound images with skill similar to traditional imaging providers, especially in the detection of gallstones.[7,15,23,24] In the hands of emergency physicians, the sensitivity and specificity for detecting gallstones (86–96% and 88–97%, respectively) resembled the pooled sensitivities and specificities in data gathered from imaging specialists (84% and 99%, respectively). On average, emergency providers take 10 minutes to conduct a focused ultrasound examination of the gallbladder. This expedient and accurate information has been shown to effectively decrease ED length of stay

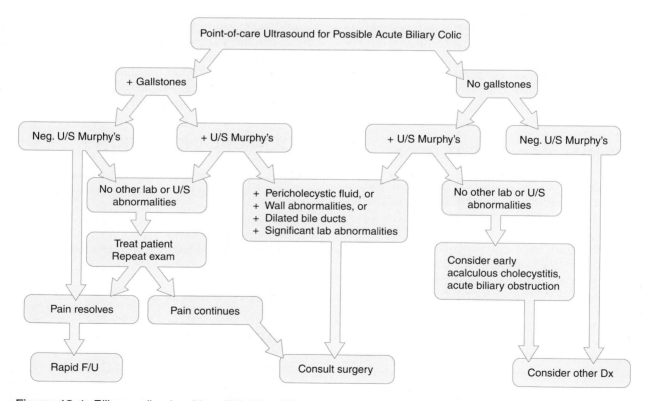

Figure 10-1. Biliary colic algorithm. This flow diagram outlines some of the decision points to consider for patient disposition based on clinical parameters and ultrasound findings. (Courtesy of James Mateer, MD)

and influence provider's probabilistic judgments especially when diagnosing diseases that are not readily apparent by the clinical presentation.[10,25]

Providers must use caution, however, when interpreting the findings of gallstones in a patient with atypical symptoms. Cholelithiasis is a prevalent disease and a majority of patients are asymptomatic. Although it may be convenient to attribute a patient's symptoms to biliary disease, the astute clinician will always remember that biliary colic remains a clinical diagnosis and not a sonographic diagnosis.

ACUTE CHOLECYSTITIS

Classically, the patient presenting with right upper quadrant abdominal pain, fever, and a leukocytosis on laboratory examination raises the concern for a diagnosis of acute cholecystitis. In the ED, however, these findings are not present in a majority of patients. The lack of clinical sensitivity makes the definitive diagnosis of acute cholecystitis dependent on imaging studies (Figure 10-2).[26,27]

In general, ultrasound has a 94% sensitivity and 84% specificity for making the diagnosis of cholecystitis.[4] One study showed that point-of-care ultrasound performed by emergency physicians had a 91% sensitivity and a 66% specificity for making the diagnosis; however, most of the providers using ultrasound in this study had no structured training. Ninety-five percent to ninety-nine percent of patients with acute cholecystitis have gallstones.[28] The sonographic Murphy's sign (pain elicited by pressing over the fundus of the gallbladder with an ultrasound transducer) may be present in

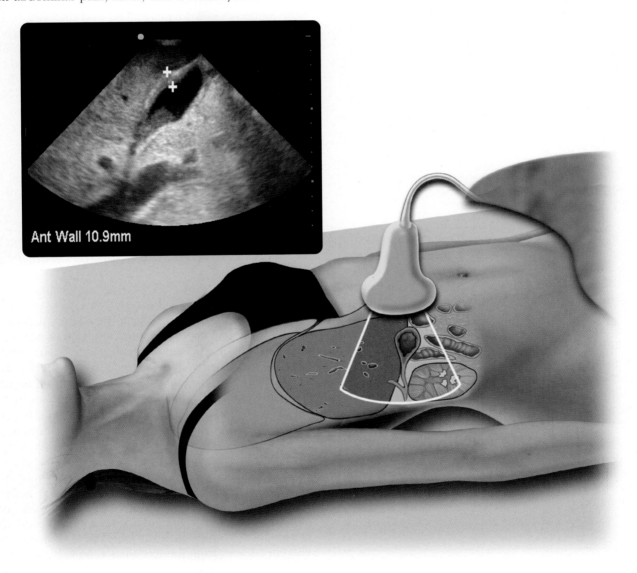

Figure 10-2. Acute cholecystitis. Ultrasound techniques and findings are outlined in the corresponding sections of this chapter.

98.8% of cases, but is not by itself specific for cholecystitis. In a pooled sample of emergency biliary ultrasound studies, the sensitivity of the sonographic Murphy's sign for cholecystitis was 75% when an emergency physician performed the test but only 45% when performed by the department of radiology.[11,24–29] Nevertheless, the sonographic Murphy's sign helps localize the source of the abdominal pain. When focal tenderness is present, along with an ultrasound study demonstrating gallstones, the patient likely has at least a diagnosis of biliary colic (Figure 10-1). Although no single ultrasound finding predicts cholecystitis with sufficient accuracy for definitive diagnosis, multiple studies have shown that a combination of positive findings increases the accuracy of ultrasound for this diagnosis. One prospective study reported a positive predictive value of 92%, for the combination of gallstones and a sonographic Murphy's sign, whereas a combination of gallstones and gallbladder wall thickening had a positive predictive value of 95% for the diagnosis of acute cholecystitis.[28]

In general, the emergency physician can rely on the presence of gallstones and a thickened gallbladder wall in conjunction with the clinical presentation and laboratory findings to identify cases with a high probability of acute cholecystitis. Gallstones are the most common obstruction causing acute cholecystitis, but other causes such as sludge or tumor may be visualized.

JAUNDICE AND BILIARY DUCT DILATATION

When a patient presents to the ED with jaundice, the emergency physician must elucidate the cause as a physical obstruction of the biliary tree or as another disease process. Ultrasound is useful for detecting dilatation of intrahepatic ducts or the common hepatic and bile ducts.[30] Once an obstructive process is detected, the next concern is whether the patient is presenting with clinical signs of cholangitis (fever, leukocytosis), which may precipitate the need for urgent ductal decompression (by surgery, ERCP, or transhepatic stenting). Ultrasound is less sensitive at defining the exact etiology of obstruction, which may include a common bile duct stone, pancreatic head tumor, ampullary carcinoma, or bile duct compression from another cancer.[31] While ultrasound may detect dilated ducts and the presence of gallstones, other modalities such as CT and ERCP may be needed to determine the ultimate diagnosis and direct treatment.

SEPSIS

Patients who present to the ED with severe sepsis benefit from early goal-directed therapy.[32] Identifying and treating the source of sepsis remains a core component that significantly contributes to the success of the protocol. Identifying the source of sepsis is challenging, especially in the elderly population.[33] It has been reported that acute cholecystitis and acute cholangitis are responsible for 25% of intra-abdominal sepsis.[34] Point-of-care ultrasound may offer prompt and accurate diagnosis in these cases.[35]

ASCITES

Detection of peritoneal fluid by physical examination is notoriously insensitive. Although the finding of a "fluid wave" has been described and is classically taught, the accuracy of this sign is low. In the emergency and acute care settings, determining whether a patient has ascites may influence initial management and disposition. For example, in a patient with abdominal pain and/or a fever with abdominal ascites, the clinician must consider bacterial peritonitis as a potential cause. Ultrasound can also be used to assess for ascites in patients with an unknown cause of abdominal distention.

HEPATIC ABNORMALITIES

Several hepatic abnormalities have a characteristic ultrasound appearance, such as cirrhosis, metastatic liver disease, liver mass, liver abscess, or hepatomegaly.[36]

▶ ANATOMICAL CONSIDERATIONS

The predominant organ in the right upper quadrant of the abdomen is the liver, bordered superiorly by the diaphragm and coronary/triangular ligament confluence, inferomedially by the duodenum and head of pancreas, and inferiorly by the gallbladder, hepatic flexure of the ascending colon, and superior pole of right kidney. The gastric fundus is located posterolateral to the left hepatic lobe. The liver is divided into right and left lobes by the major lobar fissure, which contains the middle hepatic vein and extends from the gallbladder fossa anteriorly to the inferior vena cava posteriorly. The right lobe is divided into anteromedial and posterolateral segments by the right hepatic vein, and the left lobe is divided into anterior and posterior segments by the left hepatic vein. After draining the liver of venous blood, all hepatic veins converge at the inferior vena cava posteriorly, just inferior to the atriocaval junction. The main portal vein courses from the intestinal venous drainage arcades, through the lesser omentum to the hepatic hilum, where it bifurcates into right and left branches and enters the liver (Figure 10-3A).

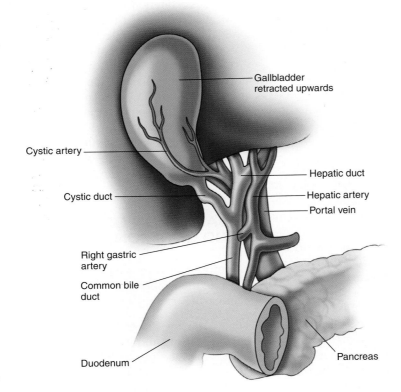

Figure 10-3. (A) Surgical anatomy of the liver. (Redrawn from Feliciano et al. *Trauma*. 3rd ed. New York, NY: Appleton & Lange/McGraw-Hill, 1996:489.) (B) Normal anatomy. The diagram depicts the relationships in the porta hepatis. The triangle of Calot is bordered by the edge of the liver, the cystic duct, and the hepatic duct. (Redrawn from Schwartz et al. *Principles of Surgery*. 6th ed. New York, NY: McGraw-Hill, 1994:1368.)

The hepatic artery courses toward the hepatic hilum in the lesser omentum, occupying a position anterior to the main portal vein. At the hilum, the hepatic artery divides into right and left branches and enters the liver parenchyma (Figure 10-3B).

The biliary system begins with the intrahepatic right and left hepatic ducts, which course toward the hilum, uniting to form the extrahepatic common hepatic duct. After exiting the hilum, the common hepatic duct is joined by the cystic duct (from the gallbladder) to form the common bile duct, which courses anterior to the main portal vein, and usually to the right of the hepatic artery in the lesser omentum before entering the duodenum (Figure 10-3B). It is important to remember the anatomical relationships of the hepatic artery, common bile duct, and main portal vein. They traverse the lesser omentum in the region of the hepatic hilum to form the main portal triad. Within the liver, branches of the main portal vein, proper hepatic artery, and biliary tree follow parallel pathways of distribution to the liver parenchyma in bundles known as lesser portal triads. Hepatic venous tributaries do not follow this system.

The gallbladder is divided into the fundus, body, and neck. The body of the gallbladder is contiguous with the inferior surface of the liver and narrows at the neck. The neck often contains spiral valves known as spiral valves of Heister that are occasionally misdiagnosed as impacted stones. The neck is continuous with the cystic duct, which empties into the common hepatic duct to create the common bile duct.

▶ GETTING STARTED

Patient positioning and respiratory maneuvers play an important role in the hepatobiliary ultrasound examination. The gallbladder is not a fixed organ in the right upper quadrant.

When the patient's gallbladder lies inferior to the lower rib cage, the patient can be scanned in the recumbent position. The right lower rib cage overlies the gallbladder and may interfere with direct visualization of the gallbladder. The patient may then be asked to take and hold a deep breath. This maneuver shifts the liver and gallbladder inferiorly, so it can be visualized below the costal margin. When the gallbladder cannot be well visualized in the recumbent position, moving the patient to the left lateral decubitus position may significantly improve visualization (Figure 10-4A). In this position, the liver and gallbladder move with gravity toward the patients left, contacting the anterior abdominal wall and providing a better "acoustic window" below the costal margin. Rarely, the patient must roll past the left lateral decubitus position to a nearly prone position in order to allow good visualization of the gallbladder. It may also be helpful to scan patients in the upright position,

especially when good images cannot be obtained in the supine or left lateral decubitus positions.

Adjusting the depth, focus point(s), and gain optimizes most sonographic images. Adjust the depth so that the gallbladder fills at least two-third of the screen. Direct the focus point(s) at the structures of interest.[37] Do not set the gain too high or low because image quality may be distorted. Tissue harmonic imaging may help identify smaller stones that are typically difficult to visualize.[38]

▶ TECHNIQUE AND NORMAL ULTRASOUND FINDINGS

The goal of point-of-care ultrasound is to answer focused questions that facilitate the diagnostic, therapeutic, or procedural workup of the patient. A low- to medium-frequency (2–5 MHz) curvilinear ultrasound transducer will suffice for most ultrasound examinations of the gallbladder. A phased array transducer can be helpful when there is no option but to image between ribs. Less commonly, a linear transducer for a very anterior gallbladder in a thin patient may be required. (See Video 10-1: Hepatobiliary Normal)

Initially, position the transducer sagittally (transducer indicator toward the patient's head) just inferior to the right costal margin to help locate the gallbladder. Color flow Doppler can be used to confirm that the cystic structure is not a vessel. Since there is great variability in anatomy, transducer position can vary widely from patient to patient. After localizing the gallbladder, orient the transducer to obtain standard images in the long- and short-axis view of the gallbladder.

EVALUATION OF THE GALLBLADDER AND COMMON BILE DUCT

Components necessary to complete the focused evaluation of the gallbladder in cases of suspected biliary colic and acute cholecystitis are as follows:

1. View the gallbladder in two orthogonal planes (long and short axis).
2. Trace the gallbladder from the fundus to the neck, carefully examining for small stones impacted in the neck.
3. Measure the anterior gallbladder wall at its clearest point, which is usually in the mid-portion of the ultrasound image. If focal wall thickening is encountered, make several measurements, one of which includes the focally thickened area.
4. Measure the common bile duct and trace it as far medially as possible.
5. Assess the gallbladder for pericholecystic fluid.

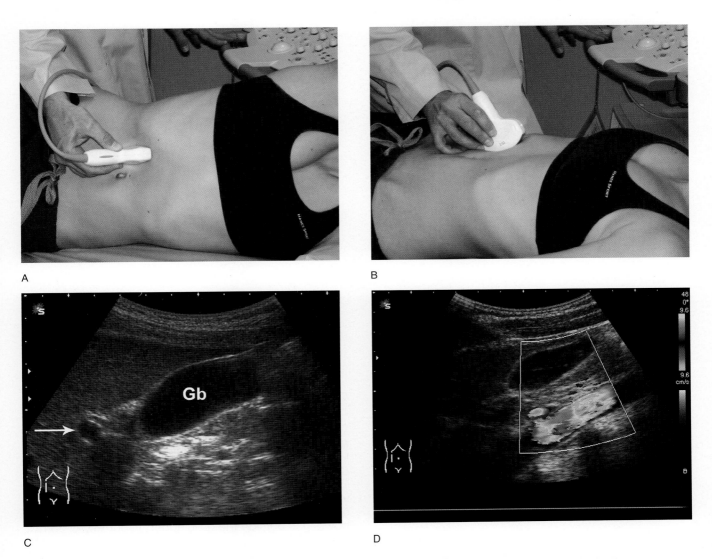

Figure 10-4. Longitudinal views of the gallbladder. Initial transducer position with patient in lateral decubitus (A) and supine positions (B). Gallbladder imaging is often facilitated with a deep inspiratory hold. Transducer is angled cephalad under the rib margins. Corresponding ultrasound image (C) with main portal vein indicated (arrow). Color Doppler may assist in delineating large vascular structures (D). Gb, gallbladder. (Courtesy of James Mateer, MD)

6. Assess for tenderness (sonographic Murphy's sign) by applying ultrasound-guided pressure directly on the gallbladder.
7. The gallbladder size is less relevant, although it may have clinical implications when it is especially enlarged.

Begin with a sagittal orientation to locate the gallbladder (Figure 10-4B). Place the transducer under the right costal margin at about the mid-clavicular line with the transducer marker directed toward the patient's head, then sweep the right upper quadrant until an image of the gallbladder is obtained (Figure 10-4C). Ask the patient to take and hold a deep breath. Color and power Doppler aid in distinguishing large vascular structures.

The gallbladder should have no Doppler signal and is typically the most anterior cystic structure in the right upper quadrant (Figure 10-4D). Additionally, identify the main portal vein to help identify the gallbladder. Typically, the main portal vein connects to the gallbladder via the main lobar fissure. Locating the main portal vein and following the main lobar fissure to the gallbladder is a good way to locate the gallbladder when it is collapsed or in an odd position.

Obtain a sagittal view of the gallbladder by rotating or sweeping the transducer to align it with the long-axis view of the gallbladder. Examine the gallbladder neck and consider having the patient take and hold a deep breath, to help identify the main portal triad adjacent to the neck of the gallbladder. One of the most difficult

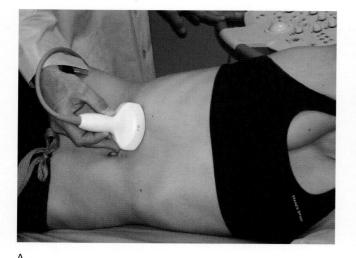

A

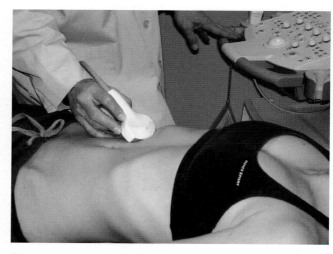

B

C

Figure 10-5. Transverse views of the gallbladder. Initial transducer position with patient in lateral decubitus (A) and supine positions (B). Note the deep inspiration used and cephalad angulation of the transducer to view under rib margins. Corresponding ultrasound image (C). Shadowing is from adjacent bowel gas outside the gallbladder. (Courtesy of James Mateer, MD)

skills for the novice operator is the technique of moving between long-axis views and short-axis views. To change planes, move the transducer slowly and keep some element of the gallbladder in view. This is the time to adjust the patient's position or perform respiratory maneuvers if the gallbladder is not well visualized. Obtain short-axis views after long-axis views, by rotating the transducer about 90° counterclockwise, with the transducer marker toward the patients right (Figure 10-5). Visualizing the gallbladder from multiple views helps to differentiate normal anatomy and artifacts from abnormal findings. If imaging remains difficult after patient positioning and deep inspiratory efforts, consider imaging the gallbladder from intercostal views (Figure 10-6). Intercostal views may be obtained with the patient in the supine or lateral decubitus position. These are helpful when the gallbladder is positioned under the ribs and/or the patient is unable to take a deep breath. Many emergency providers like using intercostal views because the position of the transducer is similar to that used when

visualizing Morison's pouch during the FAST exam. A phased array transducer with a narrow "footprint" may be particularly helpful for intercostal imaging.

It is not clear how much training is required to gain competency in emergency gallbladder ultrasound. One report suggests that novice operators who perform and interpret at least 25 gallbladder ultrasound exams demonstrate excellent proficiency in detecting gallstones.[39]

Gallbladder ultrasound images should be examined and assessed for the presence of gallstones, for the determination of wall thickness, and for the presence of pericholecystic fluid. An accurate measurement of wall thickness is made on the anterior wall that is perpendicular to the imaging plane (>3 mm is considered abnormally thick). If gallstones are detected, change the patient's position (roll to the left lateral decubitus or prone position) to document that they are mobile.

Visualization of the portal vein in the sagittal plane aids in identifying the main portal triad (Figure 10-7A).

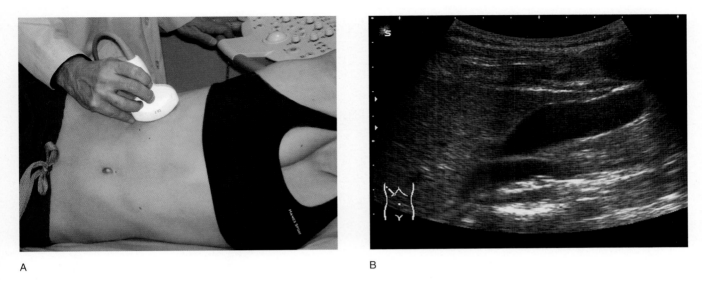

Figure 10-6. Intercostal views of the gallbladder. Initial transducer position with patient in lateral decubitus (A). Initial imaging plane is aligned parallel to the ribs. Corresponding ultrasound image (B). A small segment of the portal vein is seen below the neck of the gallbladder. (Courtesy of James Mateer, MD)

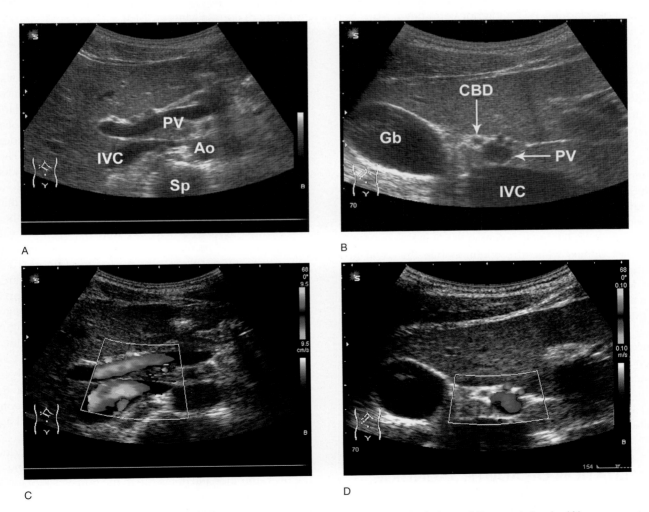

Figure 10-7. Portal vein and normal common bile duct. Longitudinal view of the portal vein (A). Transverse view of the portal vein (B). Corresponding color Doppler images (C,D). Patient has a duplicated hepatic artery. IVC = inferior vena cava, PV = portal vein, Ao = aorta, Sp = spine, Gb = gallbladder, CBD = common bile duct. (Courtesy of James Mateer, MD)

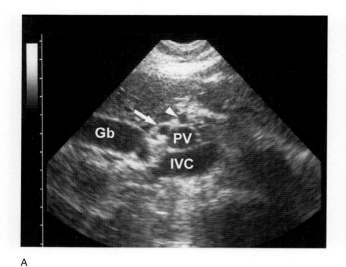

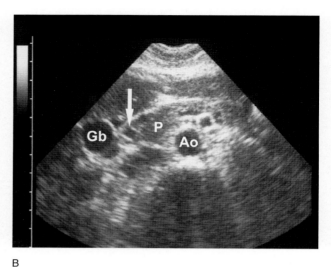

Figure 10-8. (A) Short-axis view of the PV, with the associated common bile duct (anterior/lateral) (arrow) and hepatic artery (anterior/medial) (arrowhead). The relative positions of the Gb and IVC are noted. (B) Transverse view of the upper abdomen. The position of the common bile duct (arrow) near its termination by the pancreatic head (P) is noted along with the relative positions of the Gb and Ao. PV = portal vein, Gb = gallbladder, IVC = inferior vena cava, Ao = aorta. (Courtesy of James Mateer, MD)

The portal vein will have bright echogenic walls compared with the hepatic veins. It can usually be visualized coursing toward the porta hepatis. The main portal triad is made up of the main portal vein, hepatic artery, and the common bile duct. By rotating the transducer 90° (counterclockwise) from a sagittal orientation, a transverse image of the portal vein with the associated common bile duct (anterior/lateral) and hepatic artery (anterior/medial) may be visualized (Figure 10-7B). This is referred to as the "Mickey Mouse sign." Use color or power Doppler to identify vascular structures. The portal vein and hepatic artery will demonstrate color Doppler signals while the common bile duct will not (Figure 10-7C,D). Measure the common bile duct at the level of the porta hepatis from inner wall to inner wall, which is normally <6–7 mm.[40–42,43] (C) Tissue harmonic imaging may help delineate the common bile duct. However, tissue harmonics increase the apparent thickness of walls and must be used with caution. Common bile duct dilatation is an indirect indication of obstruction. The site of common bile duct obstruction from stones is often near its termination close to the pancreatic head and is difficult to visualize in most patients (Figure 10-8).

EVALUATION OF ACUTE JAUNDICE AND BILIARY OBSTRUCTION

Evaluating the bile ducts may reveal important information when biliary obstruction is the suspected cause of

jaundice. The initial step of this examination is to locate the main portal triad, which can be accomplished in two ways. The first method uses the portal vein as a landmark, as described above. The second method involves tracing more peripheral branches of the portal venous system as they course centrally toward the hilum. Their echogenic walls and their normal enlargement can identify portal venous branches as they course centrally toward the hilum to join the main portal vein in the main portal triad. They are clearly distinguished from the hepatic venous system, which has thin hypoechoic walls and vessels that increase in diameter as they converge toward the inferior vena cava posteriorly (Figure 10-9). In the absence of biliary disease the bile ducts are rarely visible within the hepatic parenchyma. Color Doppler helps differentiate between the portal veins and biliary ducts by demonstrating flow within the veins (Figure 10-7). Once the main portal triad has been identified, examination and measurement of the common duct are performed. The duct is usually normal if the transverse diameter, in millimeters, is less than one tenth of the patient's age. However, after cholecystectomy, the common bile duct may normally range up to 1 cm in all age groups.

The most convenient method for intrahepatic duct evaluation involves transverse imaging of the left lobe of the liver. Intrahepatic ducts run in the transverse plane in this location, allowing longitudinal images of the ducts to be obtained by orienting the ultrasound beam axis transversely. Longitudinal imaging of the ducts allows easier detection and evaluation of abnormalities in the

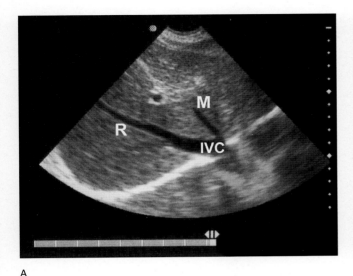

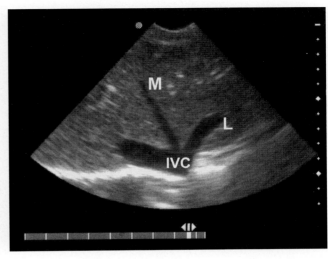

A

B

Figure 10-9. (A) Transverse view of the upper portion of the liver. The hepatic venous system, with its thin, hypoechoic walls and enlargement as it converges on the IVC posteriorly is noted. The right hepatic vein (R) and a portion of the middle hepatic vein (M) are seen in this view. (B) Transverse/oblique view of the upper liver demonstrating the junction of the IVC with the middle hepatic vein (M) and the left hepatic vein (L). IVC = inferior vena cava. (Courtesy of James Mateer, MD)

intrahepatic system. While it was once thought that any visualization of the intrahepatic ducts was abnormal, this may not be the case with modern equipment and the greatly improved resolution it delivers.

▶ COMMON AND EMERGENT ABNORMALITIES

ACUTE CHOLELITHIASIS AND CHOLECYSTITIS

Gallstones typically appear as hyperechogenic foci with acoustic shadowing posteriorly. They can range in size but the majority will be >5 mm in diameter (Figures 10-10, 10-11, 10-12) (Video 10-2: Hepatobiliary Abnormal).[44] The shadow is produced by ultrasound waves that are strongly reflected off of the gallstone. Shadowing may not be present if the gallstone diameter is <2 mm depending on the transducer being used and its frequency and resolution. Gallstones will layer in the most dependent region of the gallbladder. If stones do not respond to a change in the patient's position, then they may be impacted in the gallbladder neck. Calcified polyps are rare, but may have a similar appearance. Nonshadowing stones may be difficult to distinguish from echogenic nonshadowing polyps or cholesterol collections (Figure 10-13).

Complications of gallstones include acute cholecystitis, gallbladder empyema, chronic cholecystitis, cholangitis, and gallstone pancreatitis. Acute cholecystitis is as-

sociated with a particularly high morbidity and mortality rate when progression to gangrenous or hemorrhagic cholecystitis occurs. When organisms that produce gas are involved, emphysematous changes in the gallbladder wall may be seen. In cases of hemorrhagic cholecystitis, internal echoes caused by bleeding represent sloughing of the gallbladder mucosa. The wall of the gallbladder will be enlarged and have a striated appearance in these cases (Figure 10-14).[45]

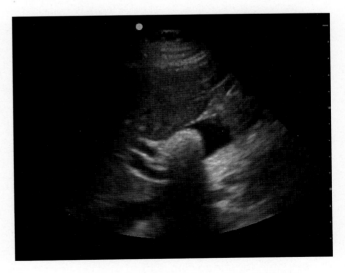

Figure 10-10. Longitudinal view of the gallbladder demonstrating a large solitary stone with prominent posterior acoustic shadowing.

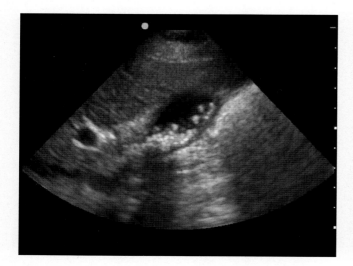

Figure 10-11. Longitudinal view of the gallbladder demonstrating multiple small stones. There is prominent posterior acoustic shadowing toward the neck of the gallbladder that contrasts with the acoustic enhancement artifact noted toward the fundus. The portal triad is visible on the left side of the image.

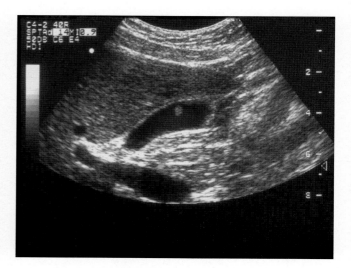

Figure 10-13. Longitudinal view of the gallbladder with solitary small polyp attached to the anterior wall. There was no shadowing and no movement with patient positioning. (Courtesy of Gulfcoast Ultrasound)

In patients with cholelithiasis and the appropriate clinical presentation, sonographic findings consistent with cholecystitis may include one or more of the following: wall thickness >3 mm (Figure 10-15), pericholecystic fluid, and the presence of a sonographic Murphy's sign. Ninety-two percent of patients with chole-

cystitis will have a thickened gallbladder wall >3 mm. However, gallbladder wall thickening can occur in a variety of conditions such as pancreatitis, ascites, and alcoholic hepatitis. Although sensitive for acute cholecystitis, gallbladder wall thickening cannot be considered pathognomonic.[20,46,47] Measurements between 3 and 5 mm are recognized as being abnormal but lack

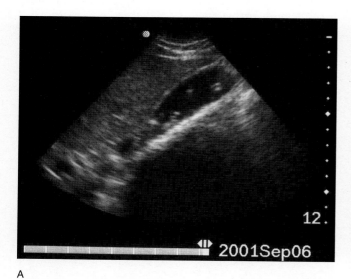

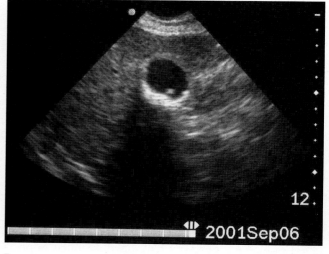

A   B

Figure 10-12. (A) Longitudinal view of the gallbladder shows multiple polyps suspended inside the wall. The dense posterior shadowing is from multiple tiny stones (sand-like) layering along the posterior wall of the gallbladder. This is best appreciated in the transverse view. (B) Transverse view. The posterior layering of the sand-like stones and the source of the shadowing is best appreciated in this view. (Courtesy of James Mateer, MD)

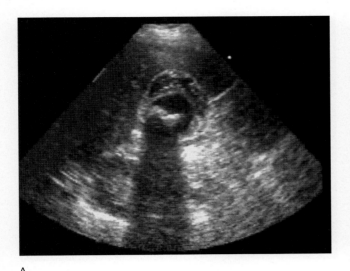

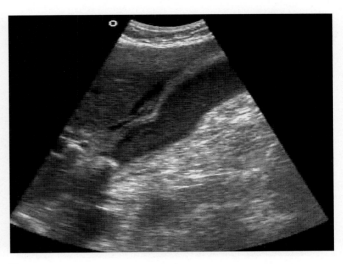

A   B

Figure 10-14. (A) Transverse view of the gallbladder shows marked thickening of the anterior wall and associated edema separating the layers of the wall. Cholelithiasis with shadowing is obvious. This patient was diagnosed with acute cholecystitis. (B) Hemorrhagic cholecystitis. Internal echoes caused by bleeding from sloughing of the gallbladder mucosa. The wall of the gallbladder is thickened and may have a striated appearance. Note the shadowing stone lodged in the gallbladder neck.

diagnostic certainty. A contracted gallbladder, commonly occurring in the postprandial patient, may be difficult to detect, and may demonstrate a nonpathologically thickened wall (Figure 10-16). Other causes of a thickened gallbladder wall include renal failure, HIV disease, congestive heart failure, and hypoalbuminemic states. In addition, nearly all patients with ascites will have a thickened gallbladder wall.

In the case of a gallstone lodged at the level of the cystic duct, the diameter of the gallbladder increases and may measure >5 cm in the transverse plane.[48]

The sonographic Murphy's sign is present when the point of maximal tenderness elicited by pressure from the ultrasound transducer occurs over the sonographically identified gallbladder. If clinically applicable, use the transducer to "palpate" the gallbladder in an attempt

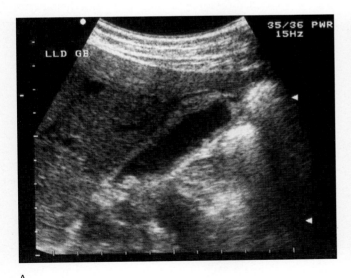

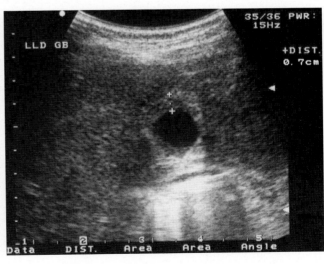

A   B

Figure 10-15. (A) Longitudinal view of a gallbladder with abnormal thickening of the wall. The bright echoes and shadowing below the gallbladder are from gas within the colon. (B) Transverse view. Wall thickness measures 7 mm. This patient was diagnosed with chronic cholecystitis. (Courtesy of Lori Sens, Gulfcoast Ultrasound)

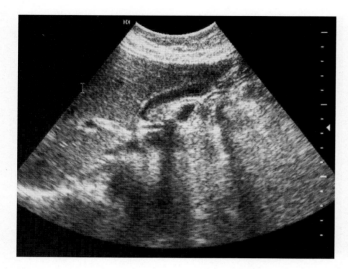

Figure 10-16. Contracted gallbladder. Can be difficult to detect, and may demonstrate a nonpathologically thickened wall.

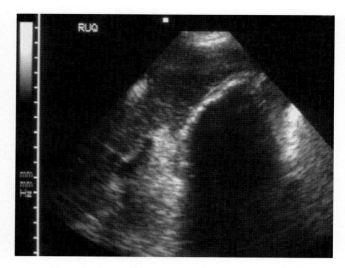

Figure 10-17. The WES sign. Note the superficial echogenic line arising from the near wall of the gallbladder, an intervening anechoic stripe generated from bile when present, and a posterior brightly echogenic line representing stone material, followed by a prominent posterior acoustic shadow. WES = wall echo shadow. (Courtesy of James Mateer, MD)

to elicit this sign. Administering opioid analgesia for patients in pain will not mask this clinical sign.[49] Furthermore, transducer pressure not directly over the gallbladder should elicit much less or no pain. Pericholecystic fluid is a less common finding, but when present it is quite specific for cholecystitis.[50]

The wall echo shadow (WES) sign occurs when the gallbladder is contracted around many gallstones with most of the bile emptied. The WES sign consists of an anterior echogenic line arising from the near wall of the gallbladder, an intervening anechoic stripe generated from bile when present, and a posterior brightly echogenic line representing stone material followed by a prominent posterior acoustic shadow (Figure 10-17).

Chronic cholecystitis is caused by chronic inflammation and subsequent fibrosis of the gallbladder with the presence of gallstones. Progressive loss of function of the gallbladder develops. A nonfunctional and calcified gallbladder is also called a porcelain gallbladder. Patients with chronic cholecystitis or porcelain gallbladder are predisposed to gallbladder cancer.

A patient with ascending cholangitis classically presents with jaundice, fever, and right upper quadrant pain. A common bile duct stone often causes obstruction. With the interruption of flow from the liver to the intestine, dilation of bile ducts with bacterial overgrowth results.

In 2% of cases, cholecystitis may be diagnosed in the absence of gallstones (acalculous cholecystitis). Typically, such patients are chronically debilitated, diabetic, immunocompromised, on hyperalimentation therapy, or recovering from a recent traumatic injury. This diagnosis is most commonly made in intensive care unit patients.[20]

BILIARY OBSTRUCTION AND JAUNDICE

Interpret isolated extrahepatic biliary duct dilatation in the context of the clinical presentation. Extrahepatic ductal dilatation should prompt evaluation of the intrahepatic ducts, duct wall thickening, presence of sludge, stones, a mass, and the presence of external compression. Ductal dilatation may be normal in elderly patients and those who have undergone cholecystectomy.[43]

A dilated extrahepatic bile duct will appear as an enlarged anechoic tubular structure (with echogenic walls) in the main portal triad, anterior to and following the course of the main portal vein. This is referred to as the parallel channel sign (Figure 10-18). Dilatation of the extrahepatic ducts implies obstruction of the common bile duct. The common hepatic duct is commonly labeled as the common bile duct on ultrasound images, although it is technically not the common bile duct (Figures 10-18 and 10-19). Common causes of extrahepatic obstruction include choledocholithiasis pancreatic masses and strictures (Figure 10-19). Left untreated, an extrahepatic obstruction will eventually also lead to dilatation of the intrahepatic ducts. Dilated intrahepatic ducts appear as anechoic tubules with echogenic walls coursing through the hepatic parenchyma. Morphologically, they are described as "antler signs" (Figure 10-20). Dilatation of the intrahepatic ducts alone suggests an obstructive process within the common hepatic duct or more proximally. Causes of primary intrahepatic

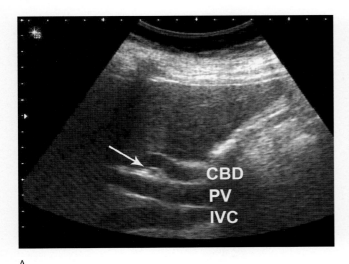

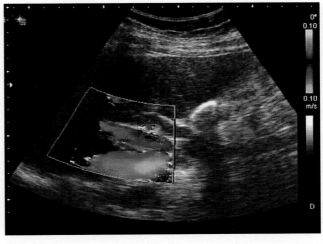

A

B

Figure 10-18. Dilated CBD (A) above the portal vein with the hepatic artery (arrow) between the two ("olive sandwich" appearance). Including the IVC below, three tubular structures are also known as the "parallel channel sign." Color Doppler (B) distinguishes structures with flow (portal vein and hepatic artery) from those without flow (dilated CBD). CBD = common bile duct, PV = portal vein, IVC = inferior vena cava.

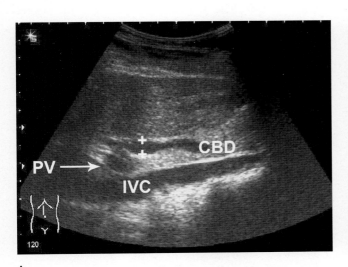

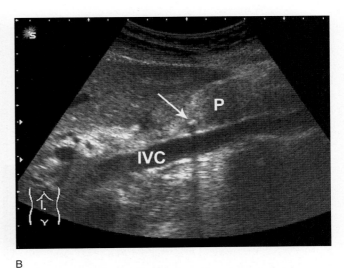

A

B

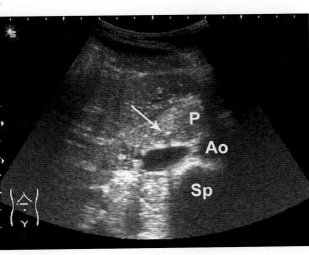

C

Figure 10-19. Choledocholithiasis. The CBD of a patient with biliary colic s/p cholecystectomy measures 8 mm (cursors) (A). Longitudinal view (B) shows pancreas above IVC with a 4-mm stone (arrow) lodged in the distal CBD. Transverse view (C) confirms. CBD = common bile duct, PV = portal vein, IVC = inferior vena cava, P = pancreas, Ao = aorta, Sp = spine. (Courtesy of James Mateer, MD)

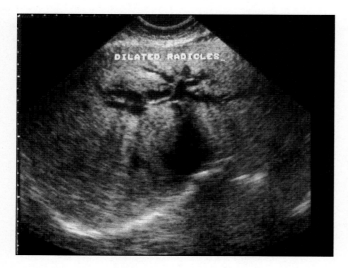

Figure 10-20. Antler signs. Transverse view of the liver. Dilated intrahepatic ducts appear as irregular anechoic tubules coursing through the hepatic parenchyma. (Courtesy of Gulfcoast Ultrasound)

stones.[51] The definitive etiology is often determined by other modalities such as CT, MRI, or ERCP.

Common causes of nonobstructive jaundice are hepatitis and cirrhosis. Sonographically, hepatitis usually appears as a relatively decreased parenchymal echogenicity secondary to the increased fluid content of the tissue.[52] The diaphragm and portal vessel walls are not involved in the edema, and remain brightly echogenic. Their relative "accentuated brightness" is the classic finding associated with acute hepatitis but this ultrasound finding is often not obvious. As inflammation becomes more chronic, and cirrhosis develops, the liver size decreases, parenchymal echogenicity and surface irregularity increase, and intrahepatic anatomy becomes distorted (Figure 10-22).[53]

ASCITES

In patients presenting with abdominal distention, ultrasound can quickly differentiate a patient with dilated gas-filled loops of bowel from a patient with ascites (Figure 10-22). The ultrasound technique for detecting ascites is similar to that used in the FAST examination (see Chapter 5, "Trauma"). Carefully note the sonographic characteristics of any visualized intraperitoneal fluid. Large free floating echogenic particles may indicate clotted blood, while multiple small free floating particles may indicate spilled abdominal contents and/or peritonitis (Figure 10-23A). Most frequently the fluid is

obstruction may include inflammatory conditions intrahepatic masses, or biliary duct cancer (Figure 10-21). Although ultrasound is sensitive in detecting ductal dilation, it may be less accurate for detecting the underlying cause of the obstruction. For example, ultrasound has a sensitivity of 15–55% for detecting common duct

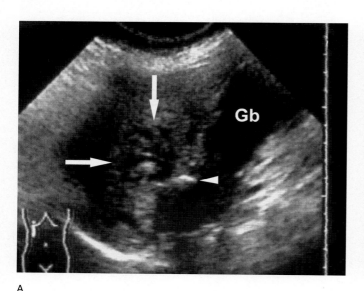

A

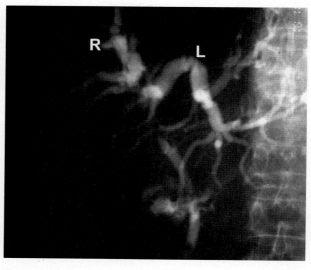

B

Figure 10-21. (A) Mirizzi syndrome. Longitudinal view of the Gb reveals massive enlargement (hydrops) and evidence of dilated intrahepatic ducts (arrows). At laparotomy, a large stone was found in the gallbladder neck area (arrowhead) with surrounding inflammation resulting in common hepatic duct obstruction. This is an unusual cause of intrahepatic obstruction. (B) ERCP radiograph of the same patient demonstrates dilatation of the right (R) and left (L) hepatic ducts. Gb = gallbladder. (Courtesy of James Mateer, MD)

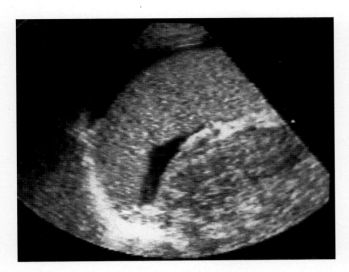

Figure 10-22. Cirrhosis of the liver. This oblique view of the right lobe demonstrates the findings of contracted size, increased echogenicity, and irregular texture of the liver. There is surrounding echo-free ascites.

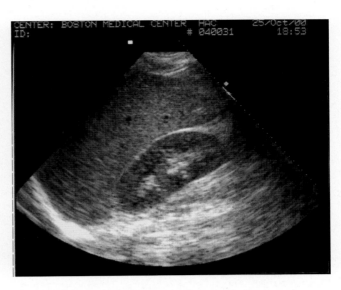

Figure 10-24. Longitudinal view of the liver and kidney shows possible hepatomegaly. The liver parenchyma of the right lobe extends to or beyond the inferior pole of the right kidney.

homogeneously anechoic (Figure 10-23B). It is difficult to discern the etiology of ascites by ultrasound.[54] The incidence of complications during paracentesis is about 3%.[55] Ultrasound guidance decreases the risk of complications and increases the success of fluid collection for diagnostic analysis.[56] Paracentesis is performed successfully in 95% of cases when using point-of-care ultrasound guidance.[57]

HEPATOMEGALY AND SPLENOMEGALY

Ultrasound is an ideal bedside tool for detection of hepatomegaly. If the parenchyma of the right lobe of the liver extends to or beyond the inferior pole of the right kidney, hepatic enlargement is probable (Figure 10-24). Alternatively, obtain a longitudinal scan at the mid-hepatic line, and measure the liver from

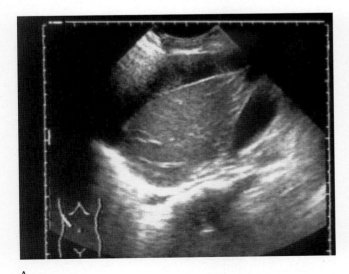

A

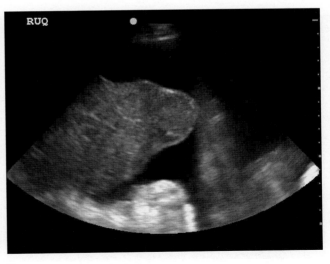

B

Figure 10-23. Coronal view of the right lobe of the liver and gallbladder shows echogenic ascites fluid with strand-like projections on the liver surface (A). The patient was diagnosed with bacterial peritonitis. RUQ view of the liver edge demonstrates homogeneously anechoic ("clear") ascites fluid (B). (Courtesy of James Mateer, MD)

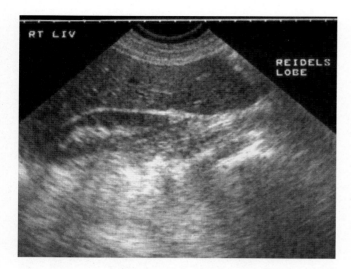

Figure 10-25. Riedel's lobe. Longitudinal view of the abdomen at the anterior axillary line, centered over the kidney. A projection of normal hepatic tissue extends from the right lobe inferiorly toward the iliac crest. (Courtesy of Lori Sens, Gulfcoast Ultrasound)

the dome (diaphragm) to the inferior margin. Enlargement is considered to be a measurement >12.8 cm.[28] Riedel's lobe of the liver is a thin projection of otherwise normal hepatic tissue extending from the right lobe inferiorly toward the iliac crest (Figure 10-25). If not recognized, this could be mistaken for hepatomegaly.

Since enlargement of the left lobe of the liver and splenomegaly can be confused on physical examination, complete the ultrasound evaluation for possible hepatomegaly with long-axis views of the spleen. Splenomegaly is confirmed when the length measured in long-axis exceeds 12–14 cm (Figure 10-26).

► COMMON VARIANTS AND SELECTED ABNORMALITIES

BILIARY SLUDGE

Biliary sludge may be detected as a dependent layer of variable nonshadowing echogenicity in the gallbladder (Figure 10-27). Typically, this is an aggregate of biliary mucous with bile salts, which over time form stones. Sludge and stones may be visualized together and both can cause symptoms of biliary colic. Sludge is frequently detected in states associated with biliary stasis, such as limited oral intake.[58] Tumefactive sludge is nonlayering, thickened, polypoid sludge that can be mistaken for a gallbladder wall tumor (Figure 10-28).

SEPTATIONS

A number of common variants may be noted with respect to point-of-care ultrasound of the gallbladder. Gallbladder wall mucosal indentations may produce septations of the lumen, which can be mistaken for gallstones. A distinguishing factor is that shadowing does not usually occur (Figure 10-29). Folds of the gallbladder fundus may produce a Phrygian cap (Figure 10-30). Agenesis of the gallbladder has an incidence of <0.05%. Consider an intrahepatic gallbladder, secondary to embryologically abnormal migration of the gallbladder bud,

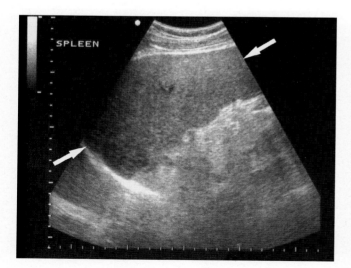

Figure 10-26. Long-axis view of the spleen measures >17 cm. Calipers should be placed on the longest length from the diaphragm to the spleen tip (arrows). (Courtesy of Lori Sens, Gulfcoast Ultrasound)

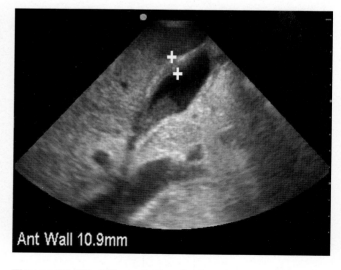

Figure 10-27. Biliary sludge is demonstrated as a dependent layer of nonshadowing mid-level echoes in this long-axis view of the gallbladder. Abnormal wall thickening is also noted in this example.

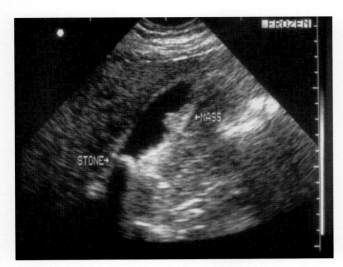

Figure 10-28. Tumefactive sludge. Dense polypoid sludge can be mistaken for a gallbladder wall tumor (<MASS). The patient also has a stone impacted in the gallbladder neck (STONE>). (Courtesy of James Mateer, MD)

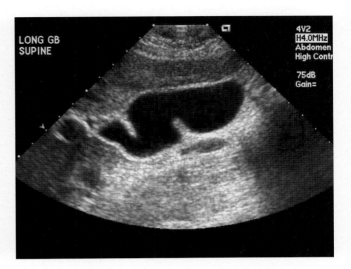

Figure 10-29. Longitudinal view of the gallbladder demonstrates nonshadowing mucosal folds on the mid-posterior wall and the anterior neck areas. (Courtesy of James Mateer, MD)

if the gallbladder is not found in its typical location. A duplicated gallbladder occurs with an incidence of 0.02%.

LIVER ABNORMALITIES

Simple hepatic cysts are often an incidental finding. Their features include sharp margins, no internal echoes, and increased "through transmission" (Figure 10-31).[59]

Hepatic abscesses, although an uncommon finding, are worthy of mention. Sonographic features include thickened, poorly defined walls surrounding fluid of variable echogenicity, which is dependent on the nature of the internal pus (Figure 10-32).[60]

Intrinsic and metastatic tumors of the liver produce variable sonographic patterns, depending on the histology (benign or malignant), secondary tumor necrosis, and/or hemorrhage.[61] Metastatic lesions can exhibit smooth, well-defined, or irregular borders, and can have increased or decreased echogenicity relative

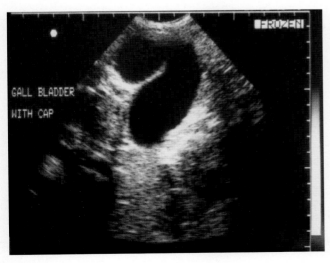

A   B

Figure 10-30. (A) Phrygian cap. Longitudinal view demonstrates a folded gallbladder at the fundus. (B) Transverse views of the same patient create the illusion of a double gallbladder in this plane. (Courtesy of James Mateer, MD)

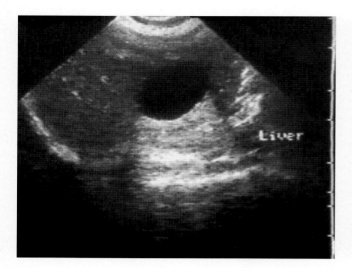

Figure 10-31. Liver cyst. Sharp margins, no internal echoes, and increased "through transmission" are demonstrated in this simple cyst of the right lobe of the liver. (Courtesy of Gulfcoast Ultrasound)

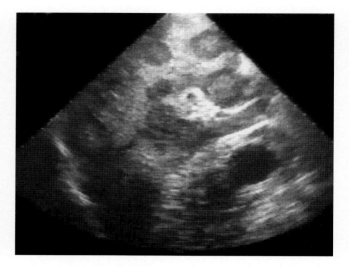

Figure 10-33. Metastatic tumors. Longitudinal view of the right lobe shows numerous target lesions. A cyst is also present within the lower pole of the kidney. (Courtesy of Gulfcoast Ultrasound)

to the surrounding hepatic tissue. Common sources of metastatic lesions include colon, breast, and pancreas (Figure 10-33).[62] Necrosis produces areas of decreased echogenicity, whereas hemorrhage can create foci of increased or decreased echogenicity depending on the age and degeneration of blood. Common benign tumors include hemangiomas, with well-defined margins and a hyperechoic appearance, and hepatic adenomas, with well-defined margins and variable echogenicity (Figures 10-34 and 10-35).

▶ PITFALLS

1. **Misidentifying the gallbladder.** Both the inferior vena cava and the duodenum can be mistaken for the gallbladder. This pitfall can be avoided by ensuring the main lobar fissure is visualized connecting the gallbladder to the main portal triad. Additionally, the gallbladder is typically the most anterior cystic structure in the right upper quadrant of the abdomen and will not demonstrate Doppler color flow. Bowel can

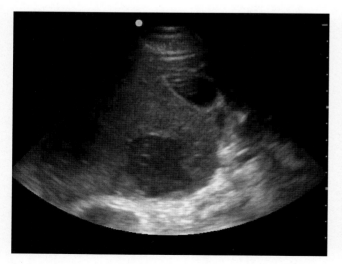

A

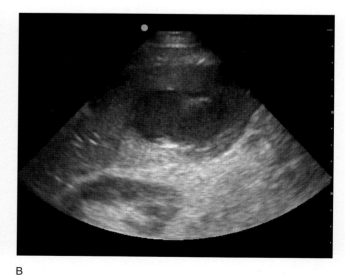

B

Figure 10-32. Liver abscess. A transverse view of the right lobe shows a large irregular hypoechoic mass below the gallbladder (A). On longitudinal view, the complex mass demonstrates mid-level echoes and posterior acoustic enhancement (which confirms the fluid density nature of the mass) (B).

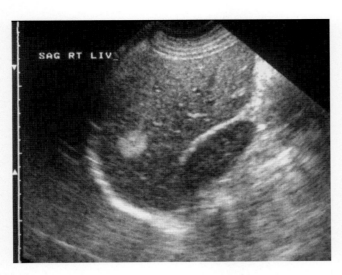

Figure 10-34. Hemangioma. Longitudinal view of the right lobe of the liver demonstrates the typical appearance. (Courtesy of Gulfcoast Ultrasound)

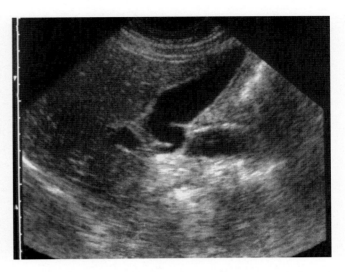

Figure 10-36. Hartman's pouch. Long-axis view of the gallbladder neck (Hartman's pouch) demonstrates the spiral valves of Heister. (Courtesy of Gulfcoast Ultrasound)

easily mimic the gallbladder, especially if it contains both fluid and solids. Differentiation occurs by visualizing a segment of bowel, which typically shows peristaltic movement.

2. **Inadequate visualization of the gallbladder and biliary system.** Intestinal gas can interfere with focused emergency imaging of the gallbladder and biliary system. Try alternating the patient's position (e.g., left lateral decubitus, upright, or prone). If time permits, have the patient drink water since this may encourage gas to move.

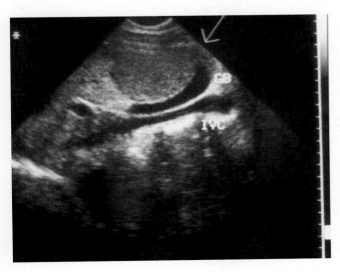

Figure 10-35. Hepatic adenoma. A hypoechoic mass (arrow) is seen compressing the gallbladder in this long-axis view. (Courtesy of Gulfcoast Ultrasound)

3. **Confusion with shadowing.** A common error after detecting shadowing is making the diagnosis of a small gallstone impacted in the gallbladder neck without actually visualizing a gallstone. Causes of shadowing in the region of the gallbladder neck include the spiral valves of Heister (Figure 10-36), fat in the porta, duodenal gas, and edge artifacts from the gallbladder wall/fluid interface. Bowel loops filled with echogenic material posterior to the gallbladder are a frequent mimic. Any potential stone should actually be contained within the gallbladder lumen. When a solitary gallstone is lodged in the neck of the gallbladder, however, it can be easily missed (Figure 10-37). A persistent clean shadow behind a rounded bright echo that is present from several viewing angles should be identified. Tissue harmonics may be exceedingly useful in detecting such small stones due to improved contrast resolution. A stone-filled gallbladder containing little or no bile may be confusing because of dense shadowing in the area that must be differentiated from shadowing caused by bowel gas (Figure 10-38).

4. **Misdiagnosing cholelithiasis and cholecystitis.** Cholesterol polyps and mucosal folds can be mistaken for gallstones. Gallstones can be missed when they are small or when the entire gallbladder is not visualized because of intestinal gas or large mucosal folds. A thickened gallbladder wall is a nonspecific finding, and may be consistent with cholecystitis, hepatitis,

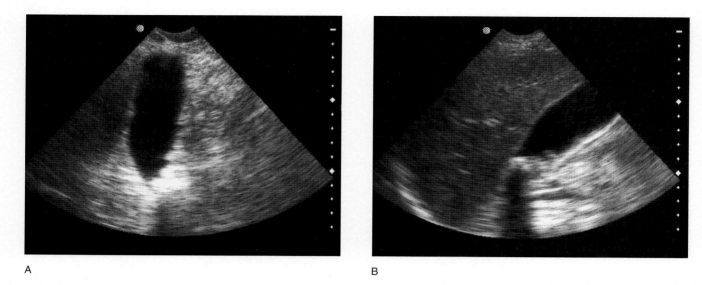

A   B

Figure 10-37. (A) Longitudinal view with the transducer positioned at the tip of the gallbladder. Cholelithiasis is not obvious. (B) Intercostal oblique view of the same patient. Impacted stone in the gallbladder neck and prominent shadowing are more obvious in this view. (Courtesy of James Mateer, MD)

ascites, hypoalbuminemia, and systemic volume overload states (Figure 10-39). The entire clinical picture should always be considered.

5. **Misdiagnosing dilated intrahepatic ducts.** Intrahepatic branches of the portal vein may be mistaken for dilated intrahepatic ducts as both have echogenic walls and become larger near the hepatic hilum. Color or power Doppler can differentiate the vascular structures as bile ducts do not demonstrate flow.

6. **Misdiagnosing ascites.** On ultrasound, ascites can be confused with hemoperitoneum, and vice versa. This can occur between simple transudative ascites and fresh blood (both typically anechoic) and between complex exudative fluid and partially clotted blood (varying degrees of echogenicity). Clinical correlation, along with fluid sampling, should be used to make the correct diagnosis. Also, patients with ascites almost always have gallbladder wall thickening,

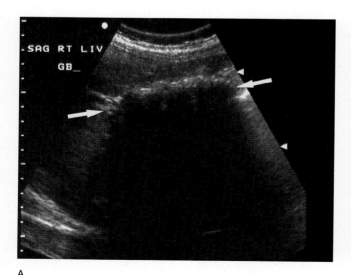

A

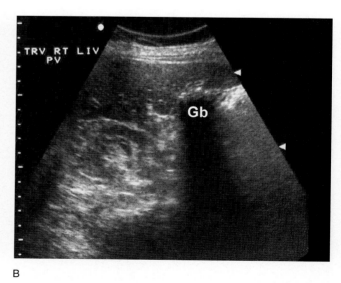

B

Figure 10-38. (A) Packed gallbladder. Longitudinal view of the Gb (arrows) shows dense shadowing from a collapsed Gb filled with stones. (B) Transverse views of the same patient clarify that the shadowing emanates from the Gb fossa. Gb = gallbladder. (Courtesy of Lori Sens, Gulfcoast Ultrasound)

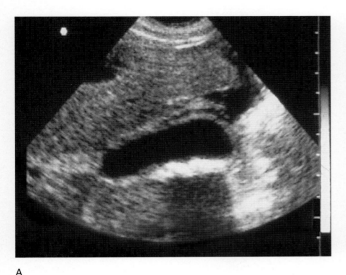

A

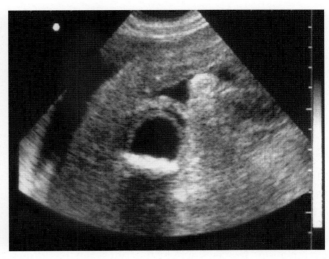

B

Figure 10-39. (A) Long-axis view of the gallbladder shows typical ultrasound signs of cholecystitis: stones, a thickened wall, and pericholecystic fluid. (B) Transverse views of the same patient demonstrate ascites as the cause for wall thickening. The patient did not have cholecystitis on further clinical evaluation. (Courtesy of James Mateer, MD)

whereas those with hemoperitoneum and other acute processes should have a normal thin gallbladder wall.

7. **Cystic duct stone.** Stones in the cystic duct may be difficult to identify as the gallbladder may appear free of stones. A stone lodged in the cystic duct can appear in a different plane from the gallbladder and may be mistaken, even by experienced operators, for bowel gas not associated with the gallbladder. Investigate any bright echogenic structure in the vicinity of the gallbladder, at least until peristalsis is seen.

8. **Common bile duct stones.** Common bile duct stones can be exceedingly difficult to identify, especially if they are not highly echogenic (Figure 10-19). Many common bile duct stones are not seen at all and the only abnormality is dilation of the duct. Complicating this further is the fact that the common bile duct may not be dilated with all stones, especially if there is only partial duct obstruction or the obstruction has occurred very recently.

9. **Misdiagnosis of biliary colic.** In the United States, at least 20% of women and 8% of men over 40 years of age have been found to have gallstones at autopsy. It is estimated that 20 million persons in the United States have gallstones, and the vast majority are asymptomatic.[63] When a patient presents with abdominal pain and is found to have gallstones on point-of-care ultrasound, exercise caution when attributing the symptoms to gallbladder disease. Make the diagnosis of biliary colic based on a combination of clinical and ultrasound findings.

▶ CASE STUDIES

CASE 1

Patient Presentation

A 55-year-old man presented to the ED complaining of abdominal swelling. He was known to the staff as he had had many prior visits due to alcohol intoxication and on this visit he seemed similarly intoxicated. Vital signs revealed a temperature of 37.8°C, blood pressure 130/80 mm Hg, pulse 105 beats per minute, and respiratory rate 18 breaths per minute. He appeared in no distress. There was no evidence of scleral icterus, the lungs were clear, and he did not exhibit costovertebral angle tenderness. There was gynecomastia, palmar erythema, and relative hairlessness on examination of his skin. The abdomen was large, soft, diffusely tender without guarding or rebound, and there were no pulsatile masses. There seemed to be a fluid wave. Stool was guaiac negative.

Management Course

A point-of-care glucose, urinalysis, ECG, and chest radiograph were normal. The WBC was 11,000/μL, hemoglobin 10.5, and platelets 155,000. A paracentesis tray was set at the bedside. Prior to performing the procedure, a point-of-care ultrasound examination of the right upper quadrant of the abdomen revealed a relatively small sized liver and no ascites. The paracentesis was deferred and the patient was frequently reassessed. When clinically sober, he denied abdominal symptoms and had normal vital signs. He improved and was discharged home with alcohol cessation counseling as well as referral to a detox program.

Commentary

This patient had a very typical presentation for alcoholic liver disease with liver cirrhosis and ascites. Before the regular availability of point-of-care ultrasound, a patient such as this may have undergone an unsuccessful paracentesis. Ascites may be difficult to detect on physical examination. In cases where the physician has a suspicion for ascites, point-of-care ultrasound provides a quick and efficient way to make the diagnosis. If ascites is present, ultrasound can identify a deep fluid pocket easily drained for diagnostic or therapeutic purposes. If no ascites is visible, then the physician should look for other sources of intra-abdominal disease.

CASE 2

Patient Presentation

An 88-year-old woman was brought to the ED by ambulance. When the family arrived, they noted she had become increasingly confused and somnolent over the past 2 days with generalized weakness. She was noted to have been sleeping a lot. At the bedside, the patient was observed to be completely unresponsive and tachypneic. Vital signs revealed a temperature of 39.1°C, blood pressure 78/52 mm Hg, pulse 128 beats per minute, respirations 28 breaths per minute, and pulse oximetry 98% on room air. The patient was jaundiced with minimal response to verbal and tactile stimuli. She moaned occasionally with her eyes closed. On lung auscultation, she had clear breath sounds, and on heart auscultation, she had a regular and tachycardic cardiac rhythm and her extremities were cool with slight mottling. Abdominal examination revealed questionable diffuse tenderness.

Management Course

The patient was intubated for airway protection and expectant management. IV fluids and vasopressors were initiated with good response in the patient's hemodynamic parameters. An ECG and portable chest radiograph were normal. Urinalysis was normal. Further laboratory data revealed a WBC of 14,000/μL, a normal lipase, a total bilirubin of 14 with a direct component of 9, and an ALT and AST that were twice normal in

value. A serum lactate was 5.8. A focused ultrasound examination revealed multiple small shadowing gallstones contained within the gallbladder, a thickened anterior gallbladder wall, and a common bile duct that measured 1.2 cm. A diagnosis of cholangitis was made. The patient underwent ERCP and sphincterotomy with removal of two gallstones from the common bile duct.

Commentary

Biliary pathology accounts for 25% of all suspected abdominal sepsis in the elderly. Point-of-care ultrasound can quickly identify a source of infection and expedite therapy. In addition, point-of-care ultrasound of the common bile duct can readily differentiate between obstructive and nonobstructive causes of jaundice and be used to direct either medical or surgical management.

CASE 3

Patient Presentation

A 35-year-old female presented to the ED with epigastric pain that began 2 hours before arrival after eating a fried egg sandwich with bacon. She had presented with similar symptoms 5 days prior and noted that the medication administered at that time relieved her pain. Upon review of the patient's ED note from the prior visit, it was noted that a diagnosis of gastritis was made without any documentation of testing or a point-of-care ultrasound. The patient noted that her pain was intermittent in nature associated with nausea and radiation to her right shoulder. Vital signs revealed a temperature of 37.3°C, blood pressure 110/74 mm Hg, pulse 105 beats per minute, and respirations 18 breaths per minute. The patient appeared in mild discomfort, but was nontoxic. There was no evidence of jaundice. Heart sounds and breath sounds were normal. Her abdomen was soft and mildly tender in the epigastric region and nontender in the right upper quadrant.

Management Course

IV antiemetic and pain medications were administered with good response. A point-of-care urinalysis was negative for both pregnancy and infection. Laboratory data also revealed a WBC of 10,000/μL, a normal lipase, bilirubin, ALT, and AST. A focused ultrasound examination revealed multiple small shadowing gallstones contained within the gallbladder and a thickened anterior gallbladder wall. No sonographic Murphy's sign, pericholecystic fluid, or dilated common bile duct was noted. A diagnosis of biliary colic was made. The patient's pain was relieved and she asked to go home. She was scheduled for an outpatient surgery clinic appointment.

Commentary

A second presentation to the ED with epigastric pain should raise the clinician's suspicion for a diagnosis other than gastritis. Patients with biliary colic and isolated epigastric pain are often initially misdiagnosed with gastritis or dyspepsia. This patient's history, constellation of symptoms, and ultrasound findings are consistent with a diagnosis of biliary colic.

REFERENCES

1. Summers SM, Scruggs W, Menchine MD, et al.: A prospective evaluation of emergency department bedside ultrasonography for the detection of acute cholecystitis. *Ann Emerg Med* 56:114–122, 2010.
2. Jang TB, Ruggeri W, Dyne P, Kaji AH: The learning curve of resident physicians using emergency ultrasonography for cholelithiasis and cholecystitis. *Acad Emerg Med* 17:1247–1252, 2010.
3. Matolo N, Stadainik R, McGahan J: Comparison of ultrasonography, computerized tomography, and radionuclide imaging in the diagnosis of acute and chronic cholecystitis. *Am J Surg* 144:676–681, 1982.
4. Shea JA, Berlin JA, Escarce JJ, et al.: Revised estimates of diagnostic test sensitivity and specificity in suspected biliary tract disease. 10.1001/archinte.154.22.2573. *Arch Intern Med* 154:2573–2581, 1994.
5. Justice AC, Covinsky KE, Berlin JA: Assessing the generalizability of prognostic information. *Ann Intern Med* 130:515–524, 1999.
6. Blaivas M: Utility of cholescintigraphy as an adjunct to emergency bedside ultrasonographic evaluation of cholecystitis. *Ann Emerg Med* 40:A 268, 2002.
7. Horrow M: Ultrasound of the extrahepatic bile duct. *Ultrasound Quarterly* 26:67–74, 2010.
8. Bennett GL, Balthazar EJ: Ultrasound and CT evaluation of emergent gallbladder pathology. *Radiol Clin North Am* 41:1203–1216, 2003.
9. Harvey RT, Miller WT Jr: Acute biliary disease: Initial CT and follow-up US versus initial US and follow-up CT. *Radiology* 213:831–836, 1999.
10. Bassler D, Snoey ER, Kim J: Goal-directed abdominal ultrasonography: Impact on real-time decision making in the emergency department. *J Emerg Med* 24:375–378, 2003.
11. DeFrances CP, MN: 2004 National hospital discharge survey. *In advance data from vital and health statistics.* Hyattsville, MD: National Center for Health Statistics, 2006.
12. Friedman GD: Natural history of asymptomatic and symptomatic gallstones. *Am J Surg* 165:399–404, 1993.
13. Traverso L: Clinical manifestations and the impact of gallstone disease. *Am J Surg* 163:405–409, 1993.
14. Tsung JW, Raio CC, Ramirez-Schrempp D, Blaivas M: Point-of-care ultrasound diagnosis of pediatric cholecystitis in the ED. *Am J Emerg Med* 28:338–342, 2010.
15. Testa A, Lauritano EC, Giannuzzi R, Pignataro G, Casagranda I, Silveri NG: The role of emergency ultrasound in the diagnosis of acute non-traumatic epigastric pain. *Intern Emerg Med* 5:401–401, 2010.
16. Zollinger R: Observations following distension of the gallbladder and common duct in man. *Proc Soc Exp Biol Med* 30:1260–1261, 1933.
17. Zollinger R: Localization of pain following faradic stimulation of the common bile duct. *Proc Soc Exp Biol Med* 35:267–268, 1936.
18. Gallbladder Survey Committee OC, ACS: 28621 cholecystectomies in Ohio. *Am J Surg* 119:714–717, 1970.
19. Diehl AK, Sugarek NJ, Todd KH: Clinical evaluation for gallstone disease: Usefulness of symptoms and signs in diagnosis. *Am J Med* 89:29–33, 1990.
20. Nelson BP, Senecal EL, Hong C, Ptak T, Thomas SH: Opioid analgesia and assessment of the sonographic Murphy sign. *J Emerg Med* 28:409–413, 2005.
21. Nazeer SR, Dewbre H, Miller AH: Ultrasound-assisted paracentesis performed by emergency physicians vs the traditional technique: A prospective, randomized study. *Am J Emerg Med* 23:363–367, 2005.
22. Jehle D, Davis E, Evans T, et al.: Emergency department sonography by emergency physicians. *Am J Emerg Med* 7:605–611, 1989.
23. Schlager D, Lazzareschi G, Whitten D, Sanders AB: A prospective study of ultrasonography in the ED by emergency physicians. *Am J Emerg Med* 12:185–189, 1994.
24. Kendall JL, Shimp RJ: Performance and interpretation of focused right upper quadrant ultrasound by emergency physicians. *J Emerg Med* 21:7–13, 2001.
25. Blaivas M, Harwood RA, Lambert MJ: Decreasing length of stay with emergency ultrasound examination of the gallbladder. *Acad Emerg Med* 6:1020–1023, 1999.
26. Trowbridge RL, Rutkowski NK, Shojania KG: Does this patient have acute cholecystitis? 10.1001/jama.289.1.80. *JAMA* 289:80–86, 2003.
27. Singer AJ, McCracken G, Henry MC, Thode J, Henry C, Cabahug CJ: Correlation among clinical, laboratory, and hepatobiliary scanning findings in patients with suspected acute cholecystitis. *Ann Emerg Med* 28:267–272, 1996.
28. Ralls P, Colletti P, Lapin S, et al.: Real-time sonography in suspected acute cholecystitis. Prospective evaluation of primary and secondary signs. *Radiology* 155:767–771, 1985.
29. Bree RL: Further observations on the usefulness of the sonographic Murphy sign in the evaluation of suspected acute cholecystitis. *J Clin Ultrasound* 23:169–172, 1995.
30. Abboud P, Malet P, Berlin J, et al.: Predictors of common bile duct stones prior to cholecystectomy: A meta-analysis. *Gastrointest Endosc* 44:450–457, 1996.
31. Haubek A, Pedersen J, Burcharth F, Gammelgaard J, Hancke S, Willumsen L: Dynamic sonography in the evaluation of jaundice. *Am J Roentgenol* 136:1071–1074, 1981.
32. Rivers E, Nguyen B, Havstad S, et al.: The early goal-directed therapy collaborative group: Early goal-directed therapy in the treatment of severe sepsis and septic shock. *N Engl J Med* 345:1368–1377, 2001.
33. Martin G, Mannino D, Moss M: The effect of age on the development and outcome of adult sepsis. *Crit Care Med* 34:15–21, 2006.
34. Podnos YD, Jimenez JC, Wilson SE: Intra-abdominal sepsis in elderly persons. *Clin Infect Dis* 35:62–68. Epub 2002 Jun 2007, 2002.

35. Cobden I, Venables CW, Lendrum R, James OFW: Gallstones presenting as mental and physical debility in the elderly. *Lancet* 323:1062–1064, 1984.

36. Gaspari RJ, Dickman E, Blehar D: Learning curve of bedside ultrasound of the gallbladder: *J Emerg Med* 37:51–56, 2009.

37. AIUM Official Statement: 3D Technology. November 12, 2005 [cited; Available from: http://www.aium.org/publications/statements/?statementSelected.asp?statement=23.

38. Choudhry S, Gorman B, Charboneau JW, et al.: Comparison of tissue harmonic imaging with conventional US in abdominal disease. *Radiographics* 20:1127–1135, 2000.

39. Spence SC, Teichgraeber D, Chandrasekhar C: Emergent right upper quadrant sonography. *J Ultrasound Med* 28(4):479–496, 2009.

40. Cooperberg P: High-resolution real-time ultrasound in the evaluation of the normal and obstructed biliary tract. *Radiology* 129:477–480, 1978.

41. Koenigsberg M, Wiener S, Walzer A: The accuracy of sonography in the differential diagnosis of obstructive jaundice: A comparison with cholangiography. *Radiology* 133:157–165, 1979.

42. Ortega D, Burns PN, Hope Simpson D, Wilson SR: Tissue harmonic imaging: Is it a benefit for bile duct sonography? *Am J Roentgenol* 176:653–659, 2001.

43. Scruggs W, Fox JC, Potts B, et al.: Accuracy of ED Bedside Ultrasound for Identification of gallstones: Retrospective analysis of 575 studies. *West J Emerg Med* 9:1–5, 2008.

44. Jensen K, Jorgensen T: Incidence of gallstones in a Danish population. *Gastroenterology* 100:790–794, 1991.

45. Teefey S, Baron R, Bigler S: Sonography of the gallbladder: Significance of striated (layered) thickening of the gallbladder wall. *Am J Roentgenol* 156:945–947, 1991.

46. Sanders RC: The significance of sonographic gallbladder wall thickening. *J Clin Ultrasound* 8:143–146, 1980.

47. Laing F, Federle M, Jeffrey R, Brown T: Ultrasonic evaluation of patients with acute right upper quadrant pain. *Radiology* 140:449–455, 1981.

48. Blaivas M, Adhikari S: Diagnostic utility of cholescintigraphy in emergency department patients with suspected acute cholecystitis: Comparison with bedside RUQ ultrasonography. *J Emerg Med* 33:47–52, 2007.

49. Miller AH, Pepe PE, Brockman CR, Delaney KA. ED ultrasound in hepatobiliary disease. *J Emerg Med* 30:69–74, 2006.

50. Elyaderani MK: Accuracy of cholecystosonography with pathologic correlation. *W V Med J* 80:111–115, 1984.

51. Laing FC, Jeffrey RB: Choledocholithiasis and cystic duct obstruction: difficult ultrasonographic diagnosis. *Radiology* 146:475–479, 1983.

52. Kurtz AB, Rubin CS, Cooper HS, et al.: Ultrasound findings in hepatitis. *Radiology* 136:717–723, 1980.

53. Taylor KJ, Gorelick FS, Rosenfield AT, et al.: Ultrasonography of alcoholic liver disease with histological correlation. *Radiology* 141:157–161, 1981.

54. Edell S, Gefter W: Ultrasonic differentiation of types of ascitic fluid. *Am J Roentgenol* 133:111–114, 1979.

55. Mallory A, Schaefer JW: Complications of diagnostic paracentesis in patients with liver disease. *JAMA* 239:628–630, 1978.

56. Blaivas M: Emergency diagnostic paracentesis to determine intraperitoneal fluid identity discovered on bedside ultrasound of unstable patients. *J Emerg Med* 29:461–465, 2005.

57. Wang HP, Chen SC: Upper abdominal ultrasound in the critically ill. *Crit CareMed* 35(5 suppl):S208–S215, 2007.

58. Angelico M, De Santis A, Capocaccia L: Biliary sludge: A critical update. *J Clin Gastroenterol* 12(6):656–662, 1990.

59. Weaver RM, Goldstein HM, Green B, et al.: Gray scale ultrasonographic evaluation of hepatic cystic disease. *Am J Roentgenol* 130:849–852, 1978.

60. Kuligowska E, Connors SK, Shapiro JH: Liver abscess: Sonography in diagnosis and treatment. *Am J Roentgenol* 138:253–257, 1982.

61. Green B, Bree RL, Goldstein HM, et al.: Gray scale ultrasound evaluation of hepatic neoplasms: Patterns and correlations. *Radiology* 124:203–208, 1977.

62. Viscomi G, Gonzalez R, Taylor K: Histopathological correlation of ultrasound appearances of liver metastases. *J Clin Gastroenterol* 3:395, 1981.

63. Johnston DE, Kaplan MM: Medical progress: Pathogenesis and treatment of gallstones. *N Engl J Med* 328:412–415, 1993.

64. National Hospital Ambulatory Medical Care Survey: 2008 Emergency Department Summary. Sponsored by the Center for Disease Control and Prevention.

65. Healthcare Cost and Utilization Project. *Agency for Healthcare Research and Quality*. Rockville, MD. http://hcupnet.ahrq.gov/

66. Adhikari S, Morrison D, Zeger W, Chandwani D, Krueger A. Utility of bedside biliary ultrasound in the evaluation of emergency department patients with isolated epigastric pain. *Ann Emerg Med* 54(3):S89, 2009.

CHAPTER 11

General Surgery Applications

Masaaki Ogata

Over the past three decades, abdominal sonography has become increasingly utilized as a diagnostic tool for surveying hepatobiliary, vascular, urologic, or GYN disorders. With progress in the resolution of scanning devices, it has also been used for the evaluation of various acute GI abnormalities. In the emergency setting, the focused assessment with sonography for trauma (FAST) examination has been widely performed by growing numbers of nonradiologist physicians, such as emergency physicians and surgeons, and accepted as a rapid and appropriate screening tool for trauma. In the same way, bedside abdominal sonography has been increasingly utilized for surveying the acute abdomen. The operator-dependent nature of ultrasonography, however, may limit the application of the examination in the emergency or acute care setting. In many hospitals, the difficulty in providing 24-hour ultrasonography service has been a major factor in preventing ultrasound from becoming a primary imaging modality. However, it is quite important to utilize the advantages of sonography to improve patient evaluation in the emergency or acute care setting.

This chapter discusses practical applications of sonography for the acute abdomen, especially for surgical emergencies associated with this presentation.

► CLINICAL CONSIDERATIONS

The evaluation of acute abdominal disorders begins with a careful history and physical examination. When re-

quired, the clinical findings may be supplemented by laboratory tests or conventional plain radiographs. Plain radiography may show some significant findings, such as pneumoperitoneum and bowel dilatation, but unsatisfactorily, it shows nonspecific findings in a significant number of patients. The development of high-resolution CT and ultrasonography has greatly facilitated the identification of pathology in many patients with an acute abdomen.

CT is an excellent imaging modality to evaluate not only intraperitoneal disorders but also retroperitoneal abnormalities. CT has a greater specificity than plain radiography. Multiple-detector CT (MDCT), which has taken the place of single-detector CT in recent years, shows three-dimensional, high-quality images of the viscera and presents detailed structures of acute abdominal abnormalities. Both plain radiography and CT are noninvasive, but are contraindicated in pregnant patients. The level of irradiation for CT may be more than a hundred times of that in plain radiography.

In contrast, sonography does not expose patients to ionizing radiation and is noninvasive, readily available, repeatable at the bedside, and less expensive than CT. It has been accepted as a useful imaging modality for hepatobiliary, CV, urologic, or GYN disorders. In addition, it has been demonstrated that sonography is applicable and accurate for acute GI disorders such as acute appendicitis, acute colonic diverticulitis, intussusception, and bowel obstruction. Abdominal sonography, however, has some disadvantages such as difficulty in visualizing abnormalities in patients who are obese or who have excessive bowel gas.

The operator-dependent nature of ultrasonography is one factor influencing the reliability of point-of-care ultrasound performed by nonradiologist physicians. Indeed, the clinical applications and results of point-of-care ultrasound are influenced by the clinical experience, skill, and interest of the clinician. In several European countries and Japan, however, point-of-care ultrasound performed by nonradiologist physicians has been accepted as a rapid and useful screening tool for evaluating the acute abdomen as well as for abdominal trauma. Physicians who are well trained to perform point-of-care ultrasound will significantly improve patient evaluation, initial treatment, selection of further diagnostic modalities, and timely consultation of surgeons or GI specialists.

Color and power Doppler imaging have been applied to a variety of GI disorders, vascular disorders, and various tumors in the abdomen. In addition, contrast-enhanced ultrasound has been used for differentiating ischemic intestinal disorders. These modalities may enable visualization of vascularity in the affected segment of the intestine. In the emergency setting, however, they have been of limited use because of the uncertain efficacy and the difficulties in application. At present, they are not essential to the diagnosis of inflammatory disorders, but are complementary to differentiating between inflammation and ischemia.

► CLINICAL INDICATIONS

In general, the clinical indications for performing a point-of-care ultrasound examination in this setting are

- Acute abdominal pain and peritonitis
- Intractable nausea and vomiting
- Abdominal distention or mass
- Unexplained shock or sepsis

All patients who have been diagnosed with an acute abdomen on the basis of clinical findings are candidates for the examination. Table 11-1 lists the common etiologies of an acute abdomen.

HEMORRHAGE

Active intraperitoneal or GI bleeding is a life-threatening etiology for which rapid diagnosis and treatment are required. If patients are hemodynamically unstable,

► **TABLE 11-1. COMMON ETIOLOGIES OF AN ACUTE ABDOMEN**

Hemorrhage
GI perforation
Bowel obstruction
Inflammatory disorder
Circulatory impairment

adequate resuscitation is the first priority. Rapid assessment for the approximate site of hemorrhage (intraperitoneal or GI) should be made on the basis of clinical findings. The use of sonography for patients with massive hematemesis is limited in the emergency setting because they should be referred for emergency endoscopy. Patients who are hemodynamically unstable without GI bleeding should be urgently examined for intraperitoneal hemorrhage. In this setting, abdominal sonography is very useful and reliable for the evaluation of intraperitoneal hemorrhage. It can be utilized during the resuscitation of the unstable patient in the emergency setting.

Intraperitoneal Hemorrhage

Rapid detection of free intraperitoneal fluid is essential since intraperitoneal hemorrhage may be severe enough to produce hypovolemic shock. For this purpose, the FAST examination is beneficial. As described in Chapter 5, "Trauma," sonography has been recognized as a rapid, sensitive, and specific diagnostic modality for detecting free intraperitoneal fluid.[1,2] Appropriately trained nonradiologist physicians, such as emergency physicians and surgeons, can accurately perform and interpret abdominal sonography for free intraperitoneal fluid. Plain radiographs are insensitive and inappropriate for the early recognition of intraperitoneal hemorrhage since radiographic signs for the accumulation of peritoneal fluid, such as widening of the paracolic gutter or a "dog's ear" appearance, require a large amount of peritoneal fluid. While CT is very useful for detecting intraperitoneal hemorrhage and retroperitoneal hematoma, it is inappropriate for hemodynamically unstable patients.

In making a decision for surgical exploration, it is important to detect the presence and the amount of intraperitoneal hemorrhage even if primary lesions are not identified. As abdominal sonography can be used to estimate not only the amount but also the rate of intraperitoneal hemorrhage through serial examinations, it will supplement clinical findings in evaluating whether the hemorrhage is active or not.

Common sites where free intraperitoneal fluid accumulates are Morison's pouch, the rectovesical pouch, the pouch of Douglas, and bilateral subphrenic spaces. A small amount of free intraperitoneal fluid may be seen only between bowel loops. A large amount of free intraperitoneal fluid can be seen above the bowels, located adjacent to the anterior peritoneum. On sonographic images, hemoperitoneum appears anechoic with coarse internal echoes as the blood is clotted. Bloody or purulent ascites or peritoneal fluid containing intestinal contents also may be shown as having similar images. It is not very difficult, however, to differentiate hemoperitoneum from ascites on the basis of a careful history and physical examination. If required, paracentesis (guided by ultrasound) can be applied for the definitive diagnosis of hemoperitoneum.

The pathology causing intraperitoneal hemorrhage can be evaluated with abdominal sonography. While CT remains the gold standard for detecting specific intraabdominal pathology, it is beneficial to utilize point-of-care ultrasound for this purpose, especially with unstable patients. Common causes of intraperitoneal hemorrhage are rupture of a hepatoma, abdominal aortic aneurysm, ectopic pregnancy, or ovarian lesion. Abdominal sonography can be performed as a rapid screening tool for detecting such specific lesions as hepatoma and abdominal aortic aneurysm. Early recognition of these etiologies is beneficial for selecting further imaging tests and strategizing on treatment options, such as immediate surgery or interventional radiology procedures. In young women who present with hypotensive shock and associated lower abdominal pain, disorders, such as rupture of an ectopic pregnancy or ovarian bleeding unrelated to pregnancy, should always be taken into consideration. Although transabdominal sonography may demonstrate only nonspecific findings, massive hemorrhage warrants immediate surgical intervention.

GI Hemorrhage

Patients with an upper GI hemorrhage generally present with varying degrees of hematemesis or melena. However, some may present with only complaints of epigastric pain or with unexplained shock. Primary causes of upper GI hemorrhage are listed in Table 11-2. Patients suspected of having massive GI hemorrhage should be referred for emergency endoscopy, which makes it possible to identify the bleeding source in up to 90% of cases of upper GI hemorrhage. Diagnostic modalities such as plain radiography, ultrasonography, CT, and GI contrast studies do not contribute to the diagnosis of acute GI hemorrhage. When appropriate, point-of-care ultrasound may be used to detect adjunct findings such as liver cirrhosis and splenomegaly. Abnormalities of the gastroduodenal wall occasionally may be shown with sonography in cases of gastric cancer, peptic ulcer, or acute gastric mucosal lesion.[3,4]

In cases of massive lower GI hemorrhage, direct endoscopic evaluation may be disturbed by a large amount of blood and stool in the colon. Furthermore, at times, the causes of lower GI hemorrhage originate in the small bowel. For these reasons, emergency angiography or scintigraphy is reserved for patients in whom

▶ **TABLE 11-2. PRIMARY CAUSES OF UPPER GI HEMORRHAGE**

Duodenal ulcer
Gastric ulcer
Hemorrhagic gastritis
Esophageal or gastric varices
Mallory–Weiss syndrome

colonoscopy is unsuccessful in locating the bleeding source. Abdominal sonography can be used as a screening tool to evaluate intra-abdominal abnormalities suggesting a bleeding source (e.g., colon cancer and ischemic colitis) and its adjunct findings (e.g., liver cirrhosis, bowel obstruction, or abscess formation).

GI PERFORATION

GI perforations are serious disorders requiring rapid diagnosis and treatment. Since they may be severe enough to produce septic or hypovolemic shock, rapid decision making for urgent laparotomy is crucially important. The initial diagnosis is generally made on the basis of clinical symptoms and signs of peritonitis and then supplemented by plain radiographs demonstrating pneumoperitoneum. Plain radiographs, however, may not always show pneumoperitoneum in cases of GI perforation, and are useless in detecting underlying etiologies. The incidence of pneumoperitoneum appreciated on conventional radiographs was reported 80–90% in cases of gastroduodenal perforation but only 20–30% and 30–50%, respectively, in cases of small bowel and large bowel perforation.[5,6] Moreover, in the elderly, signs of peritonitis on physical examination may be obscured and laboratory tests may show a normal WBC. These clinical and radiographic features may cloud the diagnosis of GI perforation in elderly patients. Consequently, any delay in making a decision for urgent laparotomy may lead to further deterioration in the clinical status of the patients, especially in cases of large bowel perforation. To avoid such delay in the diagnosis and treatment, conventional plain radiography should be supplemented with other diagnostic modalities, which include CT, sonography, contrast studies, or endoscopy. CT is very sensitive for demonstrating not only pneumoperitoneum but also ectopic gas in the retroperitoneal space. CT may demonstrate a very small pneumoperitoneum that is not appreciated on conventional plain radiography.[7]

Abdominal sonography is not as sensitive as plain radiography for demonstrating pneumoperitoneum. It may be valuable, however, in complementing plain radiographs by rapidly identifying pneumoperitoneum in the supine patient.[8–12] Subphrenic free air can be identified as an echogenic line with posterior reverberation artifacts on the ventral surface of the liver. It should be discriminated from gas in the GI lumen or the lung to avoid a false diagnosis. Hyperventilation may interfere with the examination for visualization of free air. Hepatodiaphragmatic interposition of the colon also may cause subphrenic gas echoes.

As for the underlying pathology, point-of-care ultrasound can be applied for the evaluation of specific lesions. It may detect a primary lesion, such as acute colonic diverticulitis, colon cancer, or an acute duodenal ulcer, and secondary abnormalities, such as free peritoneal fluid, a localized abscess, or paralytic ileus. Upper GI perforation is not very difficult to diagnose on the basis of clinical and radiographic findings. If required, emergency endoscopy can be adopted for identifying gastroduodenal lesions. Therefore, it is not essential to detect images of a peptic ulcer or gastric cancer by sonography or CT. As a screening tool available at bedside, however, abdominal sonography may occasionally demonstrate a gastroduodenal ulcer or gastric cancer as hypoechoic wall thickening.[3,4]

The strategies for treatment of a peptic ulcer, which is the leading cause of upper GI perforation, have been changed in recent years. Nonoperative treatments using antiulcerative agents have been successful in selected patients with a perforated duodenal ulcer. This new option in treating perforated peptic ulcers may influence the use of diagnostic modalities. A patient with a perforated duodenal ulcer can be a candidate for nonoperative treatments when signs of peritonitis are localized in the right upper quadrant. In this setting, consequently, pneumoperitoneum itself is not considered to be an absolute indication for immediate surgery. Serial examinations with sonography can be used as follow-up studies to evaluate the accumulation of peritoneal fluid or occurrence of any other abnormalities when nonoperative treatments are adopted for a perforated duodenal ulcer.

On sonographic images of GI perforation, free intraperitoneal fluid often contains gray level echoes inside an anechoic space in the pelvis or Morison's pouch, or adjacent to intestinal loops. The image is regarded as showing turbulent, purulent, or feculent peritoneal fluid. Gas echoes may be occasionally identified as echogenic spots inside an anechoic space. Although the nature of peritoneal fluid cannot be ascertained strictly on ultrasound, such sonographic images can be helpful in making a decision for surgical intervention when pneumoperitoneum is not identified.

BOWEL OBSTRUCTION

Bowel obstruction is a common etiology of acute abdomen. The clinical picture of a patient with bowel obstruction varies depending on location, form, etiology, and degree of the obstruction. Thus, strategies for treatment should be carefully determined on the basis of clinical findings, laboratory tests, and imaging methods. Generally, plain radiography is conventionally used as an initial imaging method when bowel obstruction is considered. It serves to confirm the distribution of gaseous dilated bowel and the approximate site of obstruction. However, it is widely known that plain radiography cannot reliably differentiate strangulation from simple obstruction and is useless to demonstrate causative lesions for bowel obstruction.[13,14]

For years, the application of sonography for bowel obstruction has been regarded as inappropriate and unreliable because of the significant artifact arising from GI gas. This misconception has prevented not only radiologists but also surgeons and emergency physicians from utilizing sonography for the evaluation of bowel obstruction. With progress in the resolution of scanning devices, however, abdominal sonography has become more popular for the evaluation of GI diseases.[15-17] Ultrasound's role in recognizing fluid-filled distended bowel was reported in the literature during the latter half of 1970s.[18,19] Fleischer and coworkers first introduced sonographic patterns of distended, fluid-filled bowel both in vivo and in vitro in 1979.[18] Since the latter half of 1980s, abdominal sonography has gained increasing popularity for the evaluation of bowel obstruction in Japan and Germany. Some studies have shown the usefulness of abdominal sonography for demonstrating a radiograph-negative small bowel obstruction, and for differentiating between a small bowel obstruction and a paralytic ileus.[20-23] In the 1990s, the use of sonography for the differentiation between strangulation and simple small bowel obstruction was reported.[24-26] Ogata and colleagues introduced the usefulness of sonography in identifying radiograph-negative large bowel obstruction, and Ogata and Mateer prospectively demonstrated that initial point-of-care ultrasound was as sensitive as, and more specific than, plain radiographs for the diagnosis of bowel obstruction in an ED setting.[27,28]

The pathophysiologic appearances of bowel obstruction are characterized primarily by the accumulation of fluid in the GI tract proximal to the obstruction.[29] Along with further progression of bowel obstruction, the bowel loops become distended with accumulated fluid in the lumen (Figure 11-1). In addition, the bowel wall may be thickened with interstitial edema, and free fluid may accumulate in the peritoneal cavity. Taking these features into consideration, abdominal sonography as well as CT may be appropriate and applicable to the diagnosis of bowel obstruction because it is superior to plain radiography in visualizing accumulated fluid. Furthermore, real-time sonography can provide a dynamic view of intestinal peristalsis, which is not recognized with CT. These advantages of real-time sonography have made a revolutionary progress in the diagnosis of bowel obstruction, especially in the early recognition of strangulated small bowel obstruction.

Strangulated small bowel obstruction involves compromise of blood supply to the strangulated loop of bowel and requires early surgical intervention. It is difficult to recognize the early stages of strangulation because of lack of reliable criteria.[13] Difficulty in making the early diagnosis of strangulation has resulted in a recommendation of early surgical intervention. While this strategy seems logical in reducing delays in surgical repair, it increases the number of surgical cases for nonstrangulated obstruction that could have been relieved

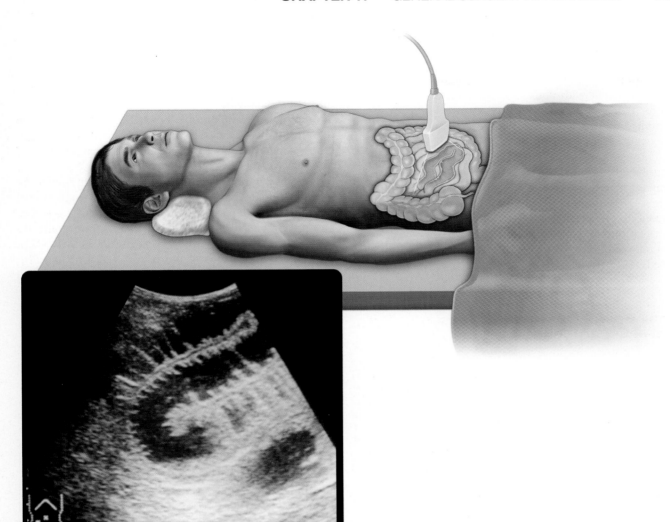

Figure 11-1. Fluid-filled dilated small bowel.

without operative therapy. However, in order to safely elect nonoperative treatment, the exclusion of strangulation is essential. Ogata and associates reported that abdominal sonography was useful in revealing the presence of strangulation that was not suspected by clinical judgment. Abdominal sonography was also useful for excluding the presence of strangulation in patients with simple obstruction who were clinically suspected of having strangulation.[24] According to their reports, the sensitivity and specificity of sonography for strangulation were 90% and 92%, respectively, in the study of 231 patients with small bowel obstruction by adhesions. The use of sonography to differentiate strangulation from simple obstruction may permit earlier operative intervention for strangulation and allow wider use of nonoperative management for simple small bowel obstruction.

When abdominal sonography is applied for the evaluation of bowel obstruction, it is clinically important to analyze the following points in each case:

1. To identify the evidence of mechanical bowel obstruction
2. To locate the level of obstruction
3. To differentiate strangulation from simple obstruction
4. To evaluate the etiology of bowel obstruction
5. To estimate the severity of bowel obstruction
6. To survey the whole abdomen for other abnormalities

Mechanical Bowel Obstruction Versus Ileus

The clinical manifestations of a mechanical bowel obstruction depend on the level of the obstruction (proximal or distal small bowel or large bowel) and the blood supply to the affected loop of bowel (simple or strangulated obstruction). The evidence of a mechanical bowel obstruction is confirmed by demonstrating a distinct point of transition between dilated proximal bowel and collapsed distal bowel with an imaging modality such as plain radiography, sonography, or CT. In contrast, the diagnosis of ileus is based on the absence of such a distinct point of transition along with a clinical presentation consistent with ileus. Abdominal sonography, as well as plain radiography and CT, can be used for the differentiation of a mechanical bowel obstruction versus an ileus.[20,28,30] In the early stage of ileus, slightly dilated small bowel loops (<25 mm wide in diameter) are often recognized on ultrasound. Gas echoes, which are more dominant than fluid collection inside the bowel, are featured in the sonographic images of ileus. Also, other abnormalities suggesting the primary etiology of ileus may be shown on ultrasound. In the advanced stage of ileus, real-time sonography may occasionally show fluid-filled dilated bowel loops without peristaltic activity.

Small Bowel Obstruction Versus Large Bowel Obstruction

Initially, abdominal sonography was used in suggesting the diagnosis of small bowel obstruction in patients with atypical plain radiographs, such as a "pseudotumor" appearance or a totally "gasless" abdomen, and also in demonstrating an intussusception in patients with an abdominal mass suspected of the entity. Real-time point-of-care ultrasound can be used as an initial imaging method for the evaluation of small bowel obstruction.[21,23,25] According to the report by Ogata and associates, GI gas interfered with ultrasound examinations in only 3 of 231 patients with small bowel obstruction by adhesions.[24]

As for patients clinically suspected of having a large bowel obstruction, plain radiographs are routinely used as the initial imaging modality as it serves to confirm the diagnosis and locate the obstruction in the majority of the cases. However, plain radiographs may show an isolated small bowel dilatation but no gaseous colonic dilatation in approximately 15% of patients with large bowel obstruction.[14,27] In such cases, it is difficult to differentiate a large bowel obstruction from a small bowel obstruction on plain radiographs alone. The use of sonography for the diagnosis of large bowel obstruction has not yet been fully evaluated because of the belief that accumulated gas in the colon interferes with the examination. Indeed, it is difficult to evaluate the gaseous distended colon with sonography. In cases of large bowel obstruction, however, abdominal sonography often reveals dilated colon filled with dense spot echoes, which seem to represent feculent, liquid contents including small bubbles of gas. In one study, abdominal sonography provided a diagnosis of large bowel obstruction in 33 of 39 patients with this condition, and proved useful in detecting radiograph-negative colonic dilatation that was occasionally seen in patients with large bowel obstruction proximal to the splenic flexure.[27]

Strangulation Versus Simple Obstruction

Adhesive bands most commonly cause strangulated small bowel obstruction. The strangulated closed loop may occasionally be shown as a "pseudotumor" appearance on plain radiographs. Sonography is effective in demonstrating the closed loop filled with fluid. Real-time sonography also can provide a dynamic view of peristalsis in the obstructed loops.

The sonographic criteria for simple small bowel obstruction include the presence of dilated small bowel proximal to collapsed small bowel or ascending colon, and the presence of peristaltic activity in the entire dilated proximal small bowel. The peristaltic activity is appreciated as peristalsis of the bowel wall or to-and-fro movements of spot echoes inside the fluid-filled dilated small bowel.

The criteria for early strangulation include (1) the presence of an akinetic dilated loop, (2) the presence of peristaltic activity in dilated small bowel proximal to the akinetic loop, and (3) rapid accumulation of intraperitoneal fluid after the onset of obstruction. An established strangulation is recognized by asymmetric wall thickening (>3 mm) with increased echogenicity in the akinetic loop, or a large amount of peritoneal fluid containing scattered spot echoes indicating bloody ascites.

The presence of intraperitoneal fluid is not specific for strangulation, but the quantitative evaluation of intraperitoneal fluid is helpful in differentiating strangulation from simple obstruction. The presence of an akinetic dilated loop is an ominous sign, but should be judged carefully with several minutes' observation or serial observations in order to avoid overlooking intermittent peristaltic activity. In some cases, when the obstruction becomes prolonged or anticholinergic drugs are administered, peristaltic activity may cease in dilated intestinal loops *without* circulatory impairment. In addition, peristaltic activity may occasionally be observed in a viable state of an early or partially strangulated loop.

Color or power Doppler imaging may demonstrate reduced blood flow within the strangulated loop in hemorrhagic necrosis, but does not surpass B-mode ultrasound in the early recognition of strangulated obstruction.

Specific Etiologies of Obstruction

Abdominal sonography offers the advantage of providing additional information about specific etiologies of obstruction that is not obtained with plain radiographs. Although adhesions obstructing the small bowel cannot be visualized, ultrasound can image the specific etiologies of small bowel obstruction, which are listed in Table 11-3. With the exception of intussusception and incarceration of external hernia, these specific etiologies are relatively rare but should be considered.

► **TABLE 11-3. ETIOLOGIES OF SMALL BOWEL OBSTRUCTION SEEN ON ULTRASOUND**

Cecal carcinoma
Intussusception
External hernias
Inflammatory bowel diseases
Small bowel tumors
Afferent loop obstruction following Billroth gastrectomy
Gallstone ileus

Intussusception is a common etiology of bowel obstruction in children but relatively rare in adults, accounting for only about 5% of all intussusception cases and 1–3% of adult patients with bowel obstruction. Unlike in children, the causative lesion can be identified in more than 80% of adult patients. The most common cause is a polypoid tumor of the small bowel. Ileocolic intussusception is the most common form (>70%), followed by enteroenteric and colocolic intussusception. Plain radiographs rarely define the intussusception as a mass of soft tissue density, and show no evidence of bowel obstruction in the acute stage. In contrast, abdominal sonography can present the characteristic appearances of intussusception. The cross-sectional image is well known as the "multiple concentric ring sign" or "target sign."[31,32] The multilaminar structure also can be demonstrated in the long-axis planes. It is very rare, however, to demonstrate the causative lesion itself (i.e., tumor or diverticulum) with sonography. The sonographic appearance of bowel obstruction may not yet be established when the diagnosis of intussusception is obtained.

Incarceration, which is a common complication of external hernias, produces a bowel obstruction and impairs the blood supply to the entrapped bowel segment. Among the common external hernias including external inguinal hernia, internal inguinal hernia, femoral hernia, and abdominal incisional hernia, incarceration occurs most frequently in cases of femoral hernia. The common hernia content is small bowel. The diagnosis is not difficult to make on the basis of a careful physical examination in most cases. If physical examination findings are equivocal, abdominal sonography can be used to demonstrate an incarcerated hernia, showing an entrapped bowel segment in the abdominal wall. However, incarcerated obturator hernia is a rare entity among the external hernias, and hardly noticed as a mass because it is located deep in the femoral region. It occurs occasionally in thin, elderly females, and is usually diagnosed as a small bowel obstruction by clinical symptoms, physical examination, and plain radiographs. Abdominal sonography can demonstrate an entrapped bowel segment medial to the femoral artery and vein, and posterior to the pectineus muscle in the femoral region. CT of the pelvis demonstrates an entrapped bowel segment between the pectineus muscle and the obturator externus (or internus) muscle.

As for the etiologies of large bowel obstruction, obstructing colon carcinoma, which is by far the most common cause of large bowel obstruction, may be detected as an irregular-shaped hypoechoic mass with echogenic core inside or a localized circular wall thickening. Intraluminal tumor obstructing the lumen may be occasionally demonstrated with sonography. Ogata and associates reported that sonography demonstrated the obstructing lesion in 14 of 35 patients with primary or metastatic colorectal carcinoma.[27] Even when the obstructing lesion is not visualized, detecting the associated lesions such as metastatic liver tumors would be useful in making the diagnosis. In volvulus of the sigmoid colon, however, sonography shows only vast gas echoes that spread beneath the abdominal wall because the twisted and obstructed colon loop is markedly distended with excessive gas. Plain radiography is diagnostic of this entity by presenting the classic "coffee bean" sign. In volvulus of the entire small bowel, a rare entity in the Western countries, sonography may show fluid-filled dilated loops with mural thickening and intraperitoneal fluid. Peristaltic activity dwindles as the intestinal infarction progresses.

INFLAMMATORY DISORDER

Various kinds of inflammatory disorders are included in the etiologies of acute abdomen. Abdominal sonography can be used for evaluating the site, extent, or severity of the inflammatory disorder by visualizing interstitial edema or hemorrhage, and peritoneal fluid. Segmental wall thickening of the bowel may be demonstrated in inflammatory GI disorders such as appendicitis, diverticulitis, infectious enterocolitis, ischemic colitis, or Crohn's disease.[17] Also, wall thickening of the gallbladder can show the severity of acute cholecystitis, and the echogenicity of the pancreas varies according to the degree of interstitial edema or hemorrhage in acute pancreatitis.

Color and power Doppler imaging can be used to evaluate vascularity in the affected segment of the intestine or the gallbladder and may present complementary findings in the diagnosis of inflammatory diseases. Without careful interpretation of B-mode sonograms, however, their utility would be of limited value.

Acute Appendicitis

Acute appendicitis is the most common cause of the acute abdomen in Western countries. The diagnosis is straightforward in most patients who present with typical clinical symptoms and signs. It is not uncommon, however, to face difficulties in making a diagnosis of appendicitis in patients who have an equivocal presentation.

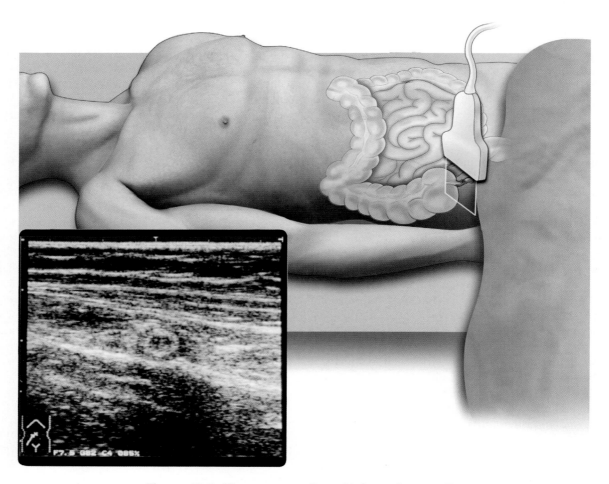

Figure 11-2. The cross-section of inflamed appendix.

Conventional radiographs present nonspecific findings, such as regional bowel dilatation, in most cases of acute appendicitis. The most specific finding on plain radiographs is the presence of a calcified appendicolith, which is noted in about 10% of adults with appendicitis.

However, abdominal sonography has been increasingly used for the diagnosis of acute appendicitis, and consequently, is considered to be useful for (1) direct visualization of the inflamed appendix (Figure 11-2), (2) assessment for the degree of inflammatory changes, (3) identification of abscess formation or free peritoneal fluid, (4) differentiation from other acute abdominal disorders, and (5) application to pregnant patients.

Since the first report that high-resolution ultrasound with a graded compression technique was successful in visualizing the abnormal appendix in a high percentage of cases, many physicians have adopted the technique and confirmed high diagnostic accuracy of the technique for acute appendicitis.[33-39] The sensitivity and specificity of graded compression sonography in expe-

rienced hands were reported to be 76–90% and 90–98%, respectively. In the United States, abdominal CT scan is commonly utilized for evaluating patients with possible appendicitis; its accuracy for confirming or ruling out appendicitis has been reported to be 93–98%.

The accuracy of sonography is operator dependent. Practically, inexperienced operators will face difficulties in obtaining a high accuracy rate in the diagnosis of acute appendicitis.[40,41] The most important reason for a false-negative study is overlooking the inflamed appendix. Dilated bowel loops due to an associated ileus may obscure the appendix. Optimal images may not be obtained because of the inability to achieve adequate compression of the right lower quadrant. This is caused by severe pain or marked obesity. False-negative studies may also occur in patients with retrocecal or perforated appendicitis. A false-positive diagnosis can be made if a normal appendix is mistaken for an inflamed one or if a terminal ileum is confused with an enlarged inflamed appendix. With adequate training and enough experience, however, nonradiologist physicians can obtain an acceptable accuracy rate in comparison with experienced operators.[42–45]

Sonography is more sensitive for the detection of an appendicolith than plain radiographs, and has been reported as detecting intraluminal fecaliths in up to 30% of cases.[46] In general, a normal appendix (about 6 mm or smaller) can rarely be visualized by graded compression sonography although some investigators have reported that in the majority of patients a normal appendix can be identified in experienced hands.[46,47]

Acute appendicitis may present in various stages at the time of diagnosis: catarrhal, phlegmonous, gangrenous, or perforated accompanying pericecal abscess or purulent peritonitis. Abdominal sonography can be used to evaluate the pathologic severity of acute appendicitis by delineating the layer structure of thickened appendiceal wall. In cases of catarrhal or phlegmonous appendicitis, a swollen appendix maintains the mural lamination. In contrast, focal loss of the layer structure is often observed in patients with gangrenous appendicitis. A pericecal abscess can be demonstrated as fluid collection with a thick, noncompressible wall. With a pericecal abscess secondary to perforated appendicitis, it may be quite difficult to identify the gangrenous appendix itself. Even if an inflamed appendix is not detected, identifying an abscess or free peritoneal fluid in the pelvis or the pericecal region can be valuable for surgeons to make a decision for urgent exploration. However, it is still controversial whether surgical intervention or conservative treatment with antibiotics should be adopted in the early stage of appendicitis. In general, sonographic findings should be correlated with both clinical and laboratory findings to determine an indication for surgery.

Acute appendicitis in pregnant women can be rather difficult to diagnose because of the deviated location of the appendix and equivocal presentation. Abdominal sonography can be applied for the evaluation of appendicitis in pregnant patients. In this setting, it is important to take the deviated location of the appendix into consideration.

Sonography is also useful for establishing an alternative diagnosis in patients examined with suspicion of appendicitis.[48] The spectrum of differential diagnoses includes mesenteric lymphadenitis (particularly in children), right-sided adnexal pathology in young women, enterocolitis, diverticulitis, Crohn's disease, cholecystitis, and colon cancer.

Acute Colonic Diverticulitis

The prevalence of colonic diverticulosis increases with age. Acute colonic diverticulitis is a relatively common etiology of the acute abdomen in elderly patients, although approximately 80–90% of all diverticula remain asymptomatic for life. The rectosigmoid colon is the most frequently involved segment in acute colonic diverticulitis. Diverticulitis in the ascending colon and cecum is less frequently involved, but seen in younger patients and frequently in the Asian countries. It is occasionally misdiagnosed as acute appendicitis since it is accompanied with the symptoms or signs similar to the entity.

Plain radiographs are of little value in obtaining direct findings of acute diverticulitis, but may demonstrate pneumoperitoneum or ileus in complicated cases. The use of contrast barium enema for demonstrating the extent of the disease is limited to the cases of clinically mild diverticulitis because it is hazardous in cases of possible colonic perforation. Water-soluble contrast enema is safe and available in complicated cases, although the quality of images is inferior to barium contrast enema.

Abdominal sonography can be applied for the initial evaluation of possible diverticulitis. Both the sensitivity and specificity of sonography for this etiology was reported more than 80% when the examination was performed by experienced operators.[49–52] Abdominal sonography may reveal additional findings such as pericolonic abscess or free intraperitoneal fluid in complicated cases. CT is better in demonstrating not only colonic diverticula but also extracolonic complications, including pericolonic or pelvic abscess, free perforation, or colovesical fistula.

Acute Pancreatitis

Acute pancreatitis is defined as an inflammation of the pancreas associated with typical abdominal complaints and elevated serum pancreatic enzymes, and may be classified according to the clinical picture, etiologic factors, or pathologic changes. The clinical course ranges from a mild, benign process to a severe, fulminant process that may lead to fatal outcomes. The two most common etiologic factors are alcoholism and biliary stone disease, although up to 10–30% of patients with acute pancreatitis may present without a history of either.

The pathologic forms are classified generally as edematous and necrotizing pancreatitis. Edematous pancreatitis is characterized by interstitial edema and mild pancreatic and peripancreatic inflammation, and accounts for 80–85% of cases. The mortality rate is less than 2%. Necrotizing pancreatitis is characterized by interstitial hemorrhage, fat necrosis, extensive extrapancreatic infiltration, and suppuration. Bacterial infection occurs in up to 40% of patients with necrotizing pancreatitis and is gradually manifested within several weeks after the onset of pancreatitis. On the whole, necrotizing pancreatitis is a far more severe form of acute pancreatitis that often requires hemodynamic support and mechanical ventilation, and leads to severe complications and mortality rates of 10–40%.[53,54] Although it is clinically important to distinguish patients with either edematous or necrotizing pancreatitis in terms of therapy and prognosis, it is rather difficult at the early stage of their clinical course. Quantitative assays of serum pancreatic enzymes may be useful for the diagnosis of acute pancreatitis, but the degree of the enzymes does not correlate with the severity of the disease. Plain radiographs may show nonspecific findings such as the "sentinel loop sign," "colon cut-off sign," or a generalized ileus, but are of little use in evaluating acute pancreatitis.

Direct imaging of the pancreas with CT or sonography may provide morphologic information to establish the diagnosis of pancreatitis and its complications.[54–56] In general, CT is clearly superior to ultrasound in demonstrating complex extrapancreatic involvement as well as contour irregularities or focal changes in the pancreas, and used as the gold standard imaging modality for acute pancreatitis and its complications. Contrast CT is recommended to discriminate necrotizing pancreatic tissues from other parts. It is also advantageous in locating fluid collections to specific anatomic compartments. Pancreatic abscess is often associated with extensive, ill-defined multicompartmental changes. However, it is difficult to distinguish pancreatic abscess from uninfected necrosis or fluid collections. CT-guided fine-needle aspiration can be used to make an early diagnosis of pancreatic abscess.

Ultrasound examinations are frequently disturbed by excessive GI gas caused by an accompanying ileus, especially in cases of severe pancreatitis. Therefore, the primary role of point-of-care ultrasound is to evaluate the biliary tree for gallstone disease as a remediable cause. Sonographic diagnosis of choledocholithiasis or significant dilatation of the common bile duct may obviate the need for invasive diagnostic procedures. The secondary role is to evaluate peripancreatic fluid collections or intraperitoneal fluid. Extrapancreatic fluid collections are most commonly detected in the superior recess of the lesser sac and the anterior pararenal space in cases of acute pancreatitis. Fluid collections are generally visualized as anechoic or hypoechoic images on ultrasound.

Acute peripancreatic fluid collections resolve with conservative therapy in 70–90% of the cases. The remaining fluid collections persist long enough (at least 6 weeks) to develop a fibrous wall, and then are called pancreatic pseudocysts. Pseudocysts may develop in association with chronic pancreatitis, or after pancreatic surgery or trauma. Uncomplicated small pseudocysts (smaller than 6 cm) may allow persistent observation, but larger pseudocysts should be drained by surgical, endoscopic, or percutaneous means to reduce the risk of complications, which include secondary infection, rupture, and hemorrhage.[53,54] Serial examinations with CT or sonography can document the gradual development of pseudocysts. The advantage of sonography is lower cost for follow-up studies. On sonographic images, pancreatic pseudocysts are generally visualized as cystic masses of various sizes, which are well defined

by adjacent organs and a visible capsule. However, small well-defined cystic masses should be examined with color Doppler scanning to exclude a pancreatic pseudoaneurysm, which may occasionally develop 2–3 weeks after the onset of severe pancreatitis.

Abdominal sonography can also be used for the initial survey of acute pancreatitis. The echogenicity of the pancreas generally decreases in acute pancreatitis as a result of interstitial edema. In some patients, however, the echogenicity is normal or increased. The echogenicity of the pancreas compared to the liver has been found to be increased in 16% and normal in 32% of patients with acute pancreatitis.[55] The variability may be caused by pancreatic hemorrhage, necrosis, or fat saponification. Enlargement of the pancreas is also variable in acute pancreatitis, and significant individual variations are recognized in pancreatic dimensions. Therefore, enlargement of the pancreas is of limited value for the diagnosis of acute pancreatitis. Echogenic pancreatic masses may suggest the progress of necrotizing pancreatitis, and should be confirmed with both contrast and noncontrast CT for the definitive diagnosis.

Acute Cholecystitis

Since acute cholecystitis may lead to serious complications such as sepsis, pericholecystic abscess, or bilious peritonitis secondary to gallbladder perforation, immediate surgery is often required. Therefore, it is critically important to make a rapid and accurate diagnosis of acute cholecystitis and to determine the indication for surgical intervention. Abdominal sonography is a rapid and reliable technique for establishing or excluding the diagnosis of acute cholecystitis, even though sonographic findings should be always correlated with clinical and laboratory findings (see also Chapter 10, "Hepatobiliary").

There are three important indirect signs to establish the diagnosis of acute cholecystitis.[57,58] Gallstones are the prime etiologic factor since approximately 90% of cases with acute cholecystitis develop as a complication of cholelithiasis. The identification of impacted stones in the gallbladder neck or cystic duct is highly specific for acute calculous cholecystitis, although sonography may be unable to detect a small impacted gallstone in a few cases of calculous cholecystitis. Biliary sludge along with the absence of gallstones in the expanded gallbladder can be identified in cases of acalculous cholecystitis. The most specific sign of acute cholecystitis is the "sonographic Murphy's sign," which corresponds to the spot of maximum tenderness directly over the gallbladder (Murphy's sign is elicited with focal tenderness over the gallbladder with inspiratory arrest). According to one study, 99% of patients with acute cholecystitis had calculi and a positive sonographic Murphy's sign.[58] In cases of acalculous cholecystitis, however, focal tenderness over the gallbladder may be difficult to obtain.

Thickening of the gallbladder wall to more than 3 mm is another sign for acute cholecystitis, although it is not specific as long as the wall maintains a distinct three-layer structure with a hypoechoic band surrounded by two hyperechoic lines. Irregular sonolucent layers in the gallbladder wall may be indicative of more advanced cholecystitis. The presence of asymmetric thickening of the gallbladder wall or intraluminal membranes parallel to the gallbladder wall may be identified in patients with acute gangrenous cholecystitis. Localized pericholecystic fluid collection may be caused by gallbladder perforation and abscess formation. The site of perforation may occasionally be visualized as a defect in the gallbladder wall. These sonographic findings can be indicative of the need for immediate surgery.

CIRCULATORY IMPAIRMENT

Ischemic bowel disease requires prompt treatment, either by surgical exploration or interventional radiology. It is challenging to demonstrate ischemia at the early stage of the disease entity. Consequently, delay in diagnosis may lead to intestinal necrosis in a significant number of patients with ischemic bowel disease.

In theED, acute mesenteric ischemia and ischemic colitis should always be considered in the elderly patient who presents with acute abdomen or unexplained shock. Acute mesenteric ischemia is caused mainly by embolism or thrombosis of the superior mesenteric artery (SMA). Nonocclusive mesenteric ischemia may develop secondary to hypoperfusion of the intestine in cases of serious illness, including heart failure, sepsis, or shock. Superior mesenteric vein thrombosis may develop secondary to abdominal surgery, trauma, acute pancreatitis, or coagulopathy.

Superior Mesenteric Artery Occlusion

Acute mesenteric artery occlusion is notoriously difficult to diagnose early in its clinical course, and subsequently often results in delayed surgical intervention in a number of cases. Patients present with sudden onset of abdominal pain, diarrhea, or vomiting. However, the symptoms are nonspecific and there may be a striking disparity between the severity of symptoms and the lack of direct physical findings. Progressive signs of shock may be apparent in the initial stage. Therefore, it is clinically important to suspect an SMA occlusion when elderly patients present with nonspecific abdominal symptoms. An SMA embolism may develop in cases of mitral valve disorders or atrial fibrillation. SMA thrombosis is related to atherosclerotic disorders.

Routine abdominal sonography does not provide specific findings in cases of an SMA occlusion. In the initial stage, fluid-filled dilatation of the small bowel is minimal. Peritoneal fluid and mural thickening in the small bowel without peristaltic activity are nonspecific, but suggest the possibility of acute mesenteric ischemia. Compared with strangulated small bowel obstruction, dilatation of the small bowel is not recognized as significant. In the advanced stages, a large amount of peritoneal fluid can be demonstrated. The application of color Doppler ultrasound is limited to detecting an occlusion of the main trunk of the SMA.[59] However, it is not so easy to confirm the etiology by examination because excessive GI gas caused by an accompanying ileus disturbs the examination. Segmental mesenteric arteries cannot be demonstrated with color Doppler ultrasound.

Contrast and noncontrast CT can demonstrate decreased enhancement in the vascular territories of the SMA, and may directly demonstrate an occluding thrombus within the SMA, pneumatosis of the bowel wall, or gas in the portal vein in conjunction with peritoneal fluid, bowel wall thickening, or dilatation of fluid-filled loops of the small bowel. When SMA occlusion is suspected, immediate angiography should be applied for the definite diagnosis or nonsurgical intervention.

Ischemic Colitis

Ischemic colitis is characterized by the abrupt onset of crampy abdominal pain and diarrhea that often contains blood. Since the clinical features are nonspecific and few symptoms may be present initially, it is especially important to consider this entity in elderly patients. Unlike small bowel ischemia, most cases of colonic ischemia are not associated with a visible arterial occlusion. The pathophysiology is believed to relate to decreased perfusion of the colon wall due to peripheral vasoconstriction (e.g., in cardiac failure), sepsis, or hypovolemia. Age-related atherosclerotic disease is a predisposing factor. The most common site of involvement is the distal colon within the vascular territory of the inferior mesenteric artery. The proximal colon to the splenic flexure area (the so-called "watershed zone") may be involved. The effects of ischemia range from reversible mucosal ischemia to transmural infarction. Most cases of ischemic colitis are resolved conservatively with medical treatment. Urgent laparotomy is required in complicated cases with gangrene or perforation of the affected colon.

While colonoscopy remains the primary method to evaluate patients with clinically suspected ischemic colitis, abdominal sonography can be used as an initial diagnostic method for the entity. In the acute phase, circumferential hypoechoic wall thickening is demonstrated in the affected segment of the colon. The laminar structure of the wall is visualized as less distinct on ultrasound exams using a high-frequency transducer. As routine sonography cannot reliably differentiate inflammatory changes from ischemic changes, color Doppler ultrasound should be applied for the differentiation.[60–62] Mural blood flow is diminished in the affected segment of ischemic colitis. Both routine sonography and color

Doppler scanning can be used for a follow-up study of ischemic colitis. In cases of reversible mucosal ischemia, wall thickening is gradually reduced and mural blood flow increases approximately in 1 week. In cases of transmural infarction, sonography may show rapid accumulation of peritoneal fluid. CT scan can be used for the same purpose and is more sensitive for complications such as perforation or abscess formation.

► ANATOMICAL CONSIDERATIONS

FREE INTRAPERITONEAL FLUID

The site of accumulation of intraperitoneal fluid is dependent on the position of the patient and the etiology that causes free fluid to accumulate. In the supine patient, intraperitoneal fluid in the pelvis or Morison's pouch is most easily detected by sonography.

STOMACH

The stomach can be identified by the subcostal or subxiphoid scanning. The gastric antrum is generally located posterocaudally to the left lobe of the liver. The cardia is identified posterior to the lateral segment of the liver. In the emergency setting, the proximal stomach is difficult to clearly delineate due to the significant artifact arising from gas in the stomach.

DUODENUM

The duodenal bulb is located medially to the gallbladder, posterior to the liver, and anterior to the pancreatic head. The inferior vena cava is another landmark located posterior to the duodenal C-loop.

SMALL BOWEL

Generally, the jejunum is located in the left upper and mid abdomen and the ileum is located in the right mid and lower abdomen. The small bowel cannot be traced continuously by sonography.

LARGE BOWEL

The ascending colon is easily demonstrated anterior to the right kidney in the right flank. The transverse colon can be identified caudally to the gastric antrum in a sagittal plane. The descending colon can be demonstrated anterior to the lower pole of the left kidney in the left flank. The sigmoid colon may be difficult to examine. The rectum can be demonstrated posterior to the uterus or prostate.

APPENDIX VERMIFORMIS

The psoas muscle and the external iliac artery and vein are important anatomic landmarks when searching for the appendix. The position of the appendix is highly variable. The most common position is caudal to the cecum and terminal ileum, followed by a retrocecal position. Other less common positions are deep within the pelvis, lateral to the cecum, and mesocecal.

PANCREAS

The pancreas is easily located by its vascular landmarks. In transverse planes, the pancreas lies posterocaudal to the left lobe of the liver and crosses over the aorta and the inferior vena cava. The splenic vein is a useful landmark for identifying the pancreas as it runs along the posterior surface of the pancreas. In sagittal planes, the pancreatic body is located posterior to the gastric antrum and the left lobe of the liver, and anterior to the splenic vein and the SMA. The pancreatic head lies anterior to the inferior vena cava and caudal to the portal vein. The pancreatic duct runs along the length of the gland, and is best imaged in the pancreatic body. The duct can be frequently visualized as a tubular structure with reflective walls with maximum diameter up to 2 mm. The anteroposterior diameters of the head and body are, in general, less than 3 cm and 2 cm, respectively. Wide normal variations are noted in pancreatic dimensions, and tend to decrease with age. The normal pancreas is homogeneous with the echogenicity greater than or equal to the adjacent liver.

► GETTING STARTED

In the emergency and acute medical care setting, a rapid, focused inspection and systematic survey of the entire abdomen are required for obtaining useful information. Among a number of factors that influence the accuracy of point-of-care ultrasound, the most critical is the clinician's experience, which includes not only the technique of scanning but also the knowledge of the clinical and pathologic findings in acute abdominal disorders.

Positioning of the patient during the point-of-care ultrasound examination is important for obtaining optimal images. Place the patient in the supine position. To avoid interference by gas echoes, place the patient in the semilateral, lateral, or semierect positions. Oblique or coronal planes are more frequently used than sagittal or transverse planes, especially in patients who have a bowel obstruction or ileus. Perform the standard examination using a sweeping motion with a convex transducer (3–5 MHz). Use a higher-frequency (>7 MHz) transducer for delineating the laminar structure of the appendix, GI wall, or specific lesions of the abdominal wall.

Focused assessment with sonography is recommended according to the purposes, situations, and various levels of examiners. Avoid an unnecessary, time-consuming examination for obtaining unfocused findings so as not to delay patient treatment. Inexperienced operators should begin with the survey for free intraperitoneal fluid, and then proceed to the focused assessment for gallstone-related disorders, hydronephrosis, abdominal aortic aneurysm, dilated small bowel, or large abdominal tumors. Intraperitoneal fluid is the first priority to evaluate in cases of acute abdomen as well as trauma, since the presence, amount, location, and internal echoes of accumulated intraperitoneal fluid are correlated with the etiology or severity of acute abdominal disorders.

► TECHNIQUE AND NORMAL ULTRASOUND FINDINGS

FOCUSED ASSESSMENT WITH SONOGRAPHY FOR THE ACUTE ABDOMEN

For cases of an acute abdomen, perform a rapid inspection for free intraperitoneal fluid in a manner similar to the FAST examination (see Chapter 5, "Trauma") (See Videos 5-1–5-6). Use the right intercostal and coronal views to examine for free intraperitoneal fluid in Morison's pouch and the right subphrenic space. From these views, the right kidney and the right lobe of the liver can be inspected briefly. Use the left intercostal and left coronal views to examine for free intraperitoneal fluid in the left subphrenic space and the splenorenal recess. From these views, the spleen and the left kidney

can be inspected briefly. Then, use the pelvic (sagittal and transverse) views to examine for free intraperitoneal fluid in the pelvis. From these views, the bladder and the prostate or uterus can be inspected briefly.

Next, perform a focused inspection for acute abdominal disorders in a systematic fashion. Determine the areas to be examined first according to the clinical findings, but survey the entire abdomen to exclude less suspicious disorders in the differential diagnosis. Subphrenic free air is best visualized on the ventral surface of the liver with right intercostal scanning. The patient may be placed in the semilateral position elevating the right flank.

SCANNING PROCEDURES FOR GASTRODUODENAL ABNORMALITIES

In scanning the epigastric region, demonstrate the gastric antrum anterior to the pancreatic body and posterocaudal to the left lobe of the liver (Figure 11-3). Visualize the proximal stomach posterior to the left lobe of the liver by using the liver as an acoustic window (Figure 11-4), although the examination is often disturbed by a significant artifact arising from gas in the stomach or the transverse colon. Identify the distended proximal stomach filled with liquid contents medially to the splenic hilum with left intercostal or coronal scanning.

Evaluate the five-layer structure of the gastric wall, which can be demonstrated with a high-frequency transducer, as closely corresponding to the histological layers (Figure 11-5):

1st layer: inner hyperechoic layer—superficial mucosal interface;

2nd layer: inner hypoechoic layer—mucosa;

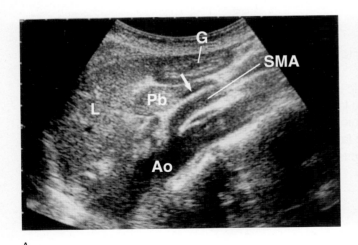

A

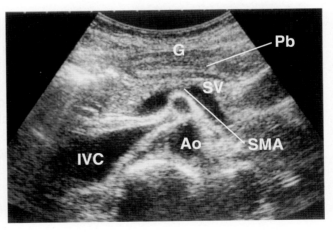

B

Figure 11-3. Gastric antrum. (A) In an epigastric sagittal plane, the cross section of gastric antrum is visualized anterior to the pancreatic body and caudal to the left lobe of the liver. The pancreatic body is located anterior and cephalad to the splenic vein (arrow) and the SMA. (B) In a transverse plane, the gastric antrum is demonstrated anterior to the pancreatic body. G = gastric antrum, L = left lobe of the liver, Pb = pancreatic body, Ao = aorta, IVC = inferior vena cava, SMA = superior mesenteric artery, SV = splenic vein.

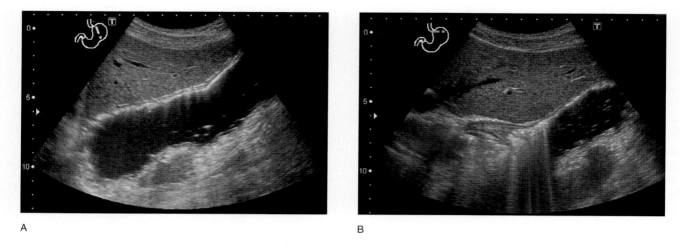

A   B

Figure 11-4. Proximal stomach. (A) The anterior wall of the gastric corpus filled with fluid is visualized in an epigastric plane using the left liver lobe as an acoustic window. (B) The cardia is visualized in an epigastric plane using the left liver lobe as an acoustic window.

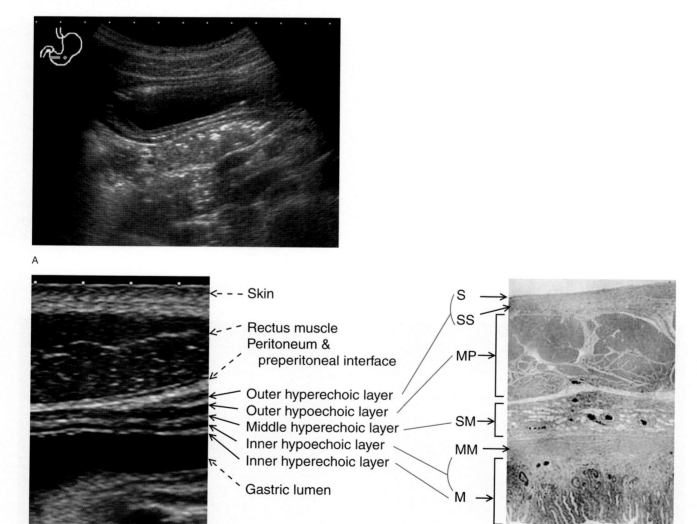

Figure 11-5. Sonographic layer structure of the normal gastric wall. (A) Five-layer structure of the gastric wall is demonstrated in a transverse scanning with a high-frequency transducer. (B) Comparison of the sonographic layer structure with the histological image of the gastric wall. M = mucosa, MM = muscularis mucosa, SM = submucosa, MP = muscularis propria, SS = subserosa, S = serosa.

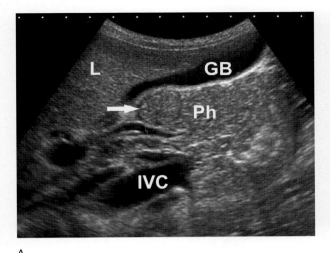

A

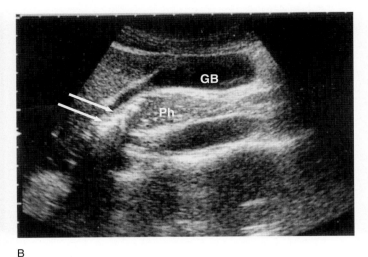

B

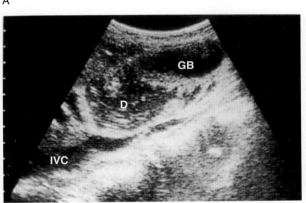

C

Figure 11-6. Duodenum. Longitudinal views. (A) A normal proximal duodenum (arrow) is visualized between the gallbladder and the pancreatic head. (B) The posterior wall of the duodenum is usually impossible to demonstrate because of the gas in the lumen. (C) A slightly dilated duodenal C-loop is visualized anterolateral to the inferior vena cava and posterior to the gallbladder. L = liver, D = duodenum, GB = gallbladder, Ph = pancreatic head, IVC = inferior vena cava.

3rd layer: middle hyperechoic layer—submucosa;

4th layer: outer hypoechoic layer—muscularis propria;

5th layer: outer hyperechoic layer—serosa and interface to the serosa.

The layer structure visualized on the sonograms depends on the resolution of scanning devices and undergoes changes corresponding to the pathologic changes in the stomach.

Visualize the duodenal bulb between the gallbladder and the gastric antrum. It is difficult to clearly visualize the duodenal C-loop except when it is dilated with accumulated fluid (Figure 11-6). It may be visualized anterior to the inferior vena cava in a coronal or oblique plane from the right anterior flank.

SCANNING PROCEDURES FOR BOWEL OBSTRUCTION

For cases of possible bowel obstruction, begin the examination by scanning the ascending colon and the hepatic flexure in the right flank. View the hepatic flexure at the ventral side of the right kidney, and then evaluate the longitudinal views of the ascending colon by positioning the transducer caudally in the mid- to posterior axillary line. A sequence of gas echoes separated with the haustra of the colon can be seen inside the hypoechoic wall (Figure 11-7). When a distended ascending colon is identified, scan the left flank to inspect the descending colon. Evaluate the approximate site of obstruction on the basis of whether or not the descending colon is distended. When an ascending colon is not distended, carefully examine the ileocecal region to guard against overlooking collapsed ileal loops or specific lesions. Then, survey the degree of dilatation, peristaltic activities, wall thickening, or specific lesions in the small bowel loops, and intraperitoneal fluid between the loops.

Sonographic images of the normal small bowel are generally recognized as a tubular structure with peristalsis (Figure 11-8A), but vary depending on the nature and volume of the intestinal contents. The Kerckring's folds (the valvulae conniventes) are typical of the small bowel and are best visualized in a fluid-filled dilated small bowel. They are not essential for the identification of the small bowel because they decrease in number and height from the proximal jejunum to the distal

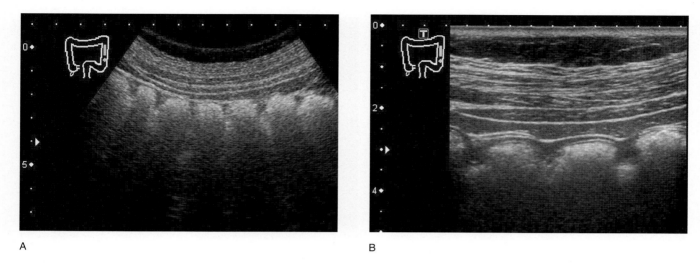

A   B

Figure 11-7. Normal colon. (A) A sequence of gas echoes separated with the haustra is shown inside the hypoechoic wall (3.5 MHz). (B) Five-layer structure is delineated in the colonic wall with a high-frequency transducer (6 MHz).

ileum. Peristaltic activity of the intestine can be visualized in real time as peristalsis of the bowel wall or to-and-fro movements of intestinal contents. Akinesis of the affected loop can be established with observation for several minutes or serial observations.

Wall thickness of the small bowel is less than 3 mm under normal conditions. It should not be measured at a contracted segment or a Kerckring's fold in order to prevent misinterpretation. Routine sonography with a

3.5 MHz transducer shows single or three-layer structure in the small bowel wall. Three-layer structure in the small bowel wall becomes clearer as the submucosa is more edematous. The layer structures of the bowel wall can be more clearly demonstrated with a high-frequency transducer when the bowel segment is located closely beneath the abdominal wall (Figure 11-8B). The layer structures of the small bowel wall are not the same as those of the gastric wall. Sonograms of the small bowel

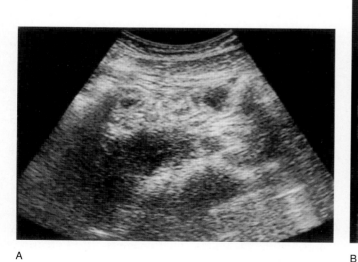

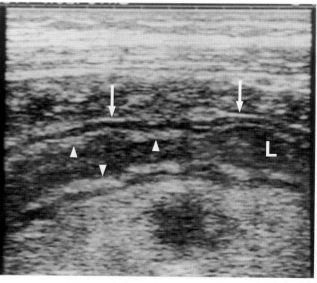

A   B

Figure 11-8. Normal small bowel loop. (A) No unified images of the small bowel are obtained with routine sonography using a 3.5 MHz transducer. (B) Wall structure of the small bowel is demonstrated with a high-frequency transducer. The lumen is bounded by the broad hyperechoic layer (arrowheads), and then surrounded by the hypoechoic muscular layer, which is bounded externally by the fine, hyperechoic reflection from the serosa (arrows). L = intestinal lumen.

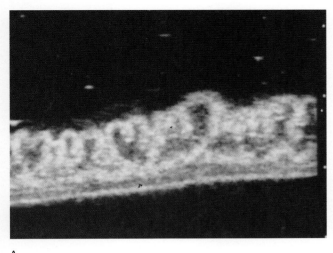

A

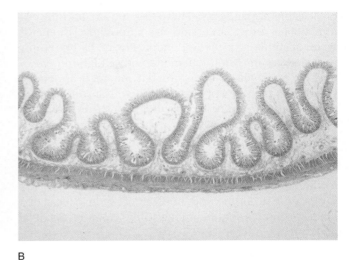

B

Figure 11-9. Sonographic layer structures in the small bowel wall with submucosal edema. Ultrasonogram of the small bowel wall in a water tank (A) clearly presents layer structures corresponding to the histological changes (B) in the wall.

wall in a water tank clearly show laminar structures corresponding to the histological layers (Figure 11-9):

1st layer: inner hyperechoic layer—superficial mucosal interface and mucosa

2nd layer: inner hypoechoic layer—submucosa (edematous submucosa)

3rd layer: middle hyperechoic layer—submucosa and interface to the muscularis propria

4th layer: outer hypoechoic layer—muscularis propria

5th layer: outer hyperechoic layer—subserosa and interface to the serosa

In normal conditions, however, it is difficult to discriminate the five layers on transabdominal sonograms.

SCANNING PROCEDURES FOR ACUTE APPENDICITIS

Survey the anatomic orientation in the right lower quadrant with a standard transducer (Figure 11-10) for cases

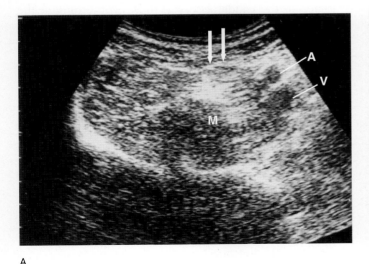

A

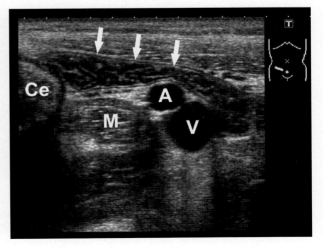

B

Figure 11-10. Transverse ultrasonogram of the right lower quadrant. The psoas muscle and external iliac artery and vein are important anatomic landmarks for the appendix. The terminal ileum (arrows) crosses over the psoas muscle to the cecum. (A) 3.5 MHz, (B) 7.5 MHz. M = psoas muscle, A = iliac artery, V = iliac vein, Ce = cecum.

of possible appendicitis. The psoas muscle and the external iliac artery and vein are important landmarks when searching for the appendix (Figure 11-10). Apply a graded compression technique with a high-frequency transducer when searching for an inflamed appendix. Gentle progressive application and withdrawal of pressure are important not to elicit peritoneal irritation for the patient. Express all overlying fluid or gas from normal bowel with graded compression to visualize the inflamed noncompressible appendix. The terminal ileum can be recognized as crossing over the psoas muscle to the cecum. Just caudal to this area is the cecal tip. To locate a tip of the appendix, carefully inspect with a graded compression technique to the point of maximal abdominal tenderness.

SCANNING PROCEDURES FOR ACUTE PANCREATITIS

For cases of possible pancreatitis, it may be difficult to obtain optimal sonographic images of the pancreas because of the significant artifacts arising from intestinal gas. To avoid such interference, place the patient in the semierect position to visualize the pancreatic head and body. In this position, gas in the stomach rises to the fundus, and the left lobe of the liver often provides an acoustic window for imaging the pancreas and the lesser sac. The standard planes are sagittal and transverse along the vascular landmarks (Figures 11-3 and 11-11). The tail of the pancreas can be best visualized with a coronal view in a right posterior oblique posi-

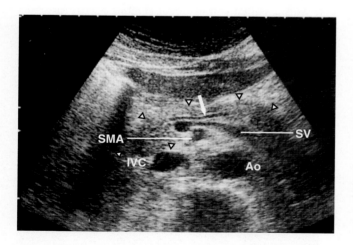

Figure 11-11. Normal pancreas. In a transverse plane, the pancreas (arrowheads) lies caudal to the left lobe of the liver and crosses over the aorta and the inferior vena cava. The splenic vein runs along the posterior surface of the pancreas. The pancreatic duct (arrow) is visualized as a tubular structure with reflective walls. Ao = aorta, IVC = inferior vena cava, SMA = superior mesenteric artery, SV = splenic vein.

tion. The spleen is used as an acoustic window in this position. The anterior pararenal space is best imaged through a coronal flank approach.

► COMMON ABNORMALITIES

FREE INTRAPERITONEAL FLUID

Free intraperitoneal fluid is delineated as an anechoic stripe with sharp edges (Figure 11-12). Intraperitoneal hemorrhage, bloody or purulent ascites, or intraperitoneal fluid containing intestinal contents may be shown as having gray level echoes inside.

RETROPERITONEAL HEMORRHAGE

Retroperitoneal hematoma is delineated as an anechoic or heterogenous hypoechoic space (Figure 11-13A). Common atraumatic causes of retroperitoneal hemorrhage are rupture of an abdominal aortic aneurysm or an iliac artery aneurysm (see Chapter 5, "Trauma," and Chapter 9, "Abdominal Aortic Aneurysm"). Pararenal hematoma is discriminated from intraperitoneal hemorrhage, as it is visualized as a fluid space between the kidney and the Gerota's fascia (Figure 11-13B).

PNEUMOPERITONEUM

Subphrenic free air can be identified as an echogenic line with posterior reverberation artifacts on the ventral surface of the liver, separated from gas echoes in the GI lumen at the caudal side and those in the lung at the cephalic side (Figure 11-14A and B).

Gas in an abscess or free intraperitoneal fluid may be occasionally recognized as echogenic spots inside the anechoic or hypoechoic fluid (Figure 11-14C).

SPECIFIC ETIOLOGIES OF GI PERFORATION

Duodenal ulcer, gastric ulcer, colonic diverticulitis, and GI cancer are specific etiologies for GI perforation. Gas echoes penetrating the GI wall may be visualized as direct evidence for perforation (Figure 11-15A and C). It is not easy, however, to visualize a perforated segment directly with ultrasound in cases of peritonitis due to a GI perforation. A gastroduodenal ulcer may be visualized as a deformity or disruption of the wall in the duodenal bulb or the stomach (Figure 11-15A and B).

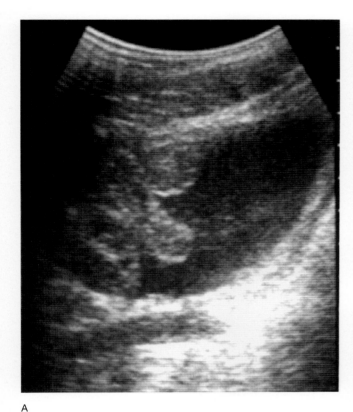

A

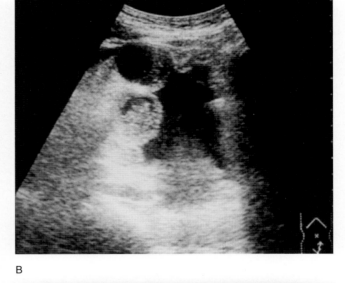

B

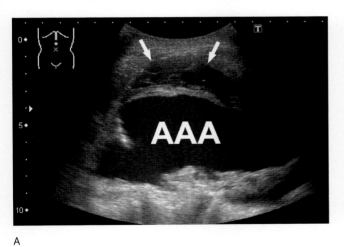

C

Figure 11-12. Free intraperitoneal fluid. (A) Free intraperitoneal fluid with internal echoes is demonstrated in pelvic space. The patient was diagnosed with intraperitoneal hemorrhage secondary to ovarian bleeding. (B) Bloody ascites secondary to strangulated small bowel obstruction is demonstrated as an anechoic space with fine internal echoes in the pouch of Douglas. (C) A large amount of ascites is shown in a case of peritoneal carcinomatosis.

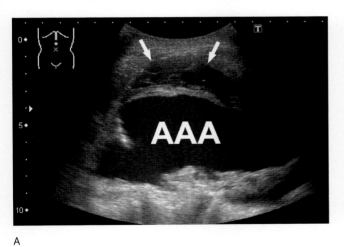

A

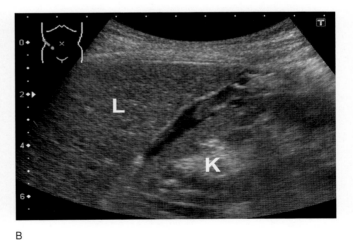

B

Figure 11-13. Retroperitoneal hemorrhage. (A) Retroperitoneal hematoma (arrows) is delineated anterior to a ruptured abdominal aortic aneurysm. (B) Right pararenal hematoma is delineated as a complex fluid collection containing both liquid and partially clotted blood. It is located between the right kidney and the Gerota's fascia (visualized as a echogenic line beneath the liver). AAA = abdominal aortic aneurysm, L = liver, K = kidney.

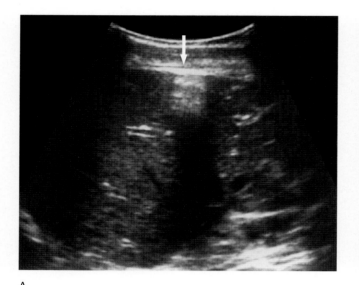

A

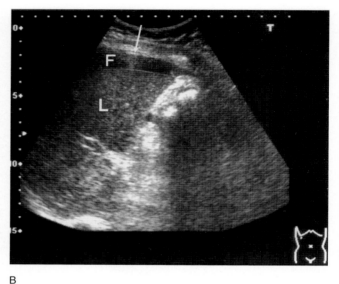

B

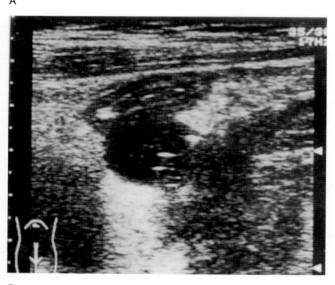

C

Figure 11-14. Pneumoperitoneum. (A) Subphrenic free air (arrow) is recognized at the ventral side of the liver in a case of perforated duodenal ulcer. (B) A small collection of free air (arrow) within the peritoneal fluid is recognized in the subphrenic space. (C) Gas in a paracolonic abscess is demonstrated as echogenic spots inside the hypoechoic fluid in a case of perforated colonic diverticulitis. F = fluid.

SMALL BOWEL OBSTRUCTION

In cases of small bowel obstruction, dilated small bowel proximal to collapsed small bowel or ascending colon can be identified (Figure 11-16). Dilated small bowel is usually visualized as fluid-filled dilated loops with the maximal diameter more than 25 mm (usually >30 mm) at the time of diagnosis of small bowel obstruction. In the early stage of distal small bowel obstruction, no dilated loops may be observed in the proximal jejunum.

The sonographic images of dilated loops vary depending on the degree of distention and the nature of intestinal contents (Figure 11-17). The well-known "keyboard sign" is not essential for the diagnosis of small

bowel obstruction. The sonographic appearance of Kerckring's folds varies depending on scanning planes and intestinal contents, and they are rarely visualized in the distal ileum. The intestinal wall of a dilated small bowel loop is usually visualized as having a hyperechoic single layer (standard transducer). When edematous, it may be visualized as having a three-layer (hypo-, hyper-, hypoechoic layer) structure.

In most cases of simple obstruction, the entire dilated proximal small bowel is visualized as having peristaltic activity (Figure 11-18). No intraperitoneal fluid is visualized in approximately half of the patients with simple small bowel obstruction by adhesions. A large amount of peritoneal fluid is seldom seen in cases of simple small bowel obstruction by adhesions, and when

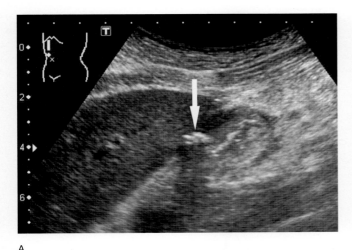

A

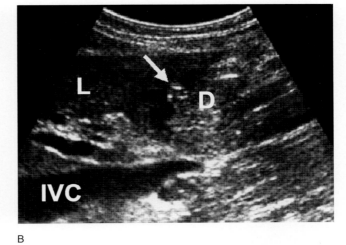

B

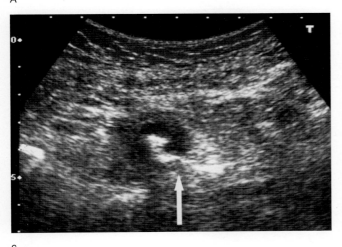

C

Figure 11-15. GI perforation. (A) Longitudinal epigastric view. A perforated duodenal ulcer is delineated as penetrating gas echoes (arrow) in the thickened wall of the duodenal bulb with echogenic lumen. (B) Longitudinal epigastric view. A perforated duodenal ulcer is delineated as a deformity of the duodenal bulb (arrow) posterior to the left liver lobe. (C) Perforation of a diverticulum in the sigmoid colon is delineated as penetrating gas echoes (arrow) in the thickened wall of the colon in the pelvic space. D = duodenal bulb, L = liver, IVC = inferior vena cava.

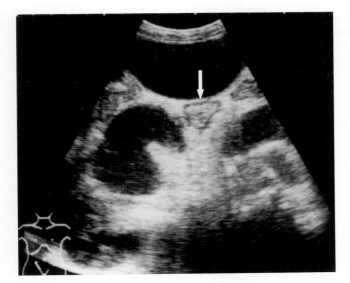

Figure 11-16. Mechanical small bowel obstruction. Both dilated small bowel and a collapsed one (arrow) are demonstrated in the right lower abdomen.

present, the following conditions should be considered: peritoneal carcinomatosis, liver cirrhosis, or circulatory impairment in the intestine.

STRANGULATED OBSTRUCTION

A strangulated loop is demonstrated as an akinetic dilated small bowel loop with real-time sonography (Figure 11-19). In contrast, peristaltic activity can be recognized in the dilated small bowel proximal to the akinetic loop. Intraperitoneal fluid can be demonstrated in most cases and rapidly accumulates after the onset of obstruction.

With an established strangulation, real-time sonography may demonstrate wall thickening with increased echogenicity and flattened folds within the akinetic loop, or a large amount of intraperitoneal fluid (Figure 11-20). Alternately, in cases of incomplete strangulation with viable tissue, the examination may reveal weak motion or submucosal edema in the intestinal wall of the strangulated loop (Figure 11-21).

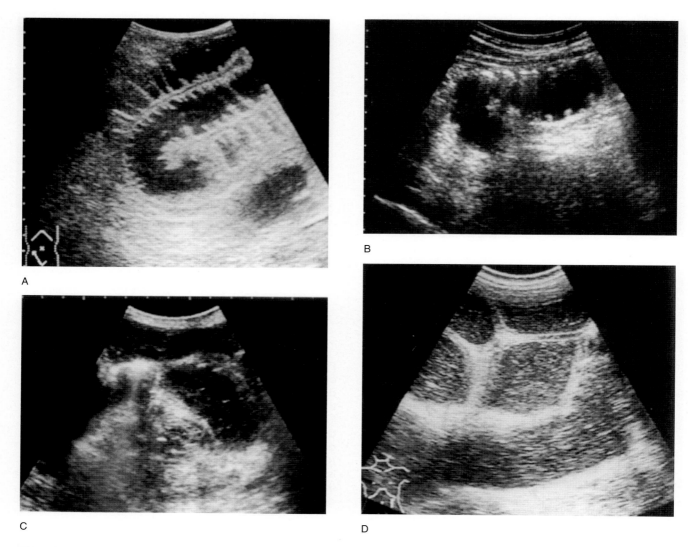

Figure 11-17. Varied sonographic images of dilated small bowel. (A) The "keyboard sign" is characteristic of fluid-filled dilated jejunum. (B) The sonographic image of small bubbles of gas entrapped between the Kerckring's folds inside dilated small bowel loops is similar to the "string of beads sign" on plain radiographs. (C) In mild or early stages of small bowel obstruction, gas echoes may be more dominant than anechoic fluid in the dilated loops. (D) Dilated small bowel may be filled with spot echoes when intestinal contents become more feculent.

LARGE BOWEL OBSTRUCTION

With large bowel obstruction, the dilated colon proximal to the obstruction is usually delineated as filled with dense spot echoes around the periphery of the abdomen (Figure 11-22A), whereas the dilated small bowel loops are located more centrally. Haustral indentations may be visualized as widely spaced in the dilated ascending colon. Real-time sonography can occasionally reveal to-and-fro movements of the intestinal contents through the ileocecal valve when the valve is incompetent (Figure 11-22B). With large bowel obstruction distal to the splenic flexure, however, sonography may show a dilated colon simply as wide gas echoes around the periphery of the abdomen (Figure 11-22C).

The criterion for large bowel obstruction is the presence of dilated colon proximal to normal or collapsed large bowel. Ascending colon and descending colon are the initial checkpoints for the sonographic evaluation of large bowel obstruction. The site of obstruction can be estimated on the basis of distribution of the dilated colon (>50 mm for the ascending colon). Clinically, it is unnecessary to strictly define the accurate site or cause of obstruction with sonography because water-soluble contrast enema or colonoscopy demonstrates the degree and level of obstruction and helps to clarify its cause.

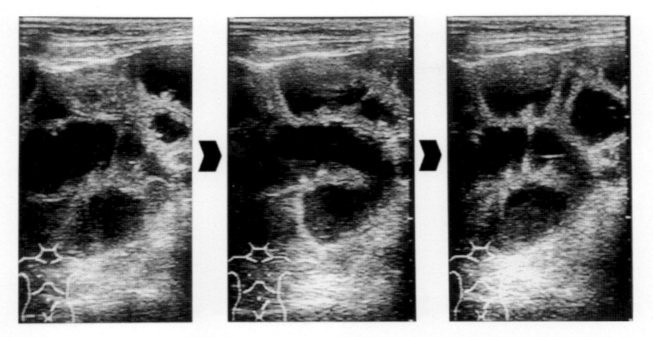

Figure 11-18. Simple small bowel obstruction. Selected images from real-time sonography reveal intermittently increased peristaltic activity of the entire dilated small bowel proximal to the obstruction.

SPECIFIC ETIOLOGIES OF BOWEL OBSTRUCTION

Intussusception

The cross-sectional image of intussusception is known as the "multiple concentric ring sign" or "target sign" (Figure 11-23A). Multilaminar structure may be demon-

strated with scanning along the long axis of the intussusception (Figure 11-23B).

Incarcerated Hernia

An incarcerated small bowel segment can be demonstrated as entrapped within the hernia sac in the

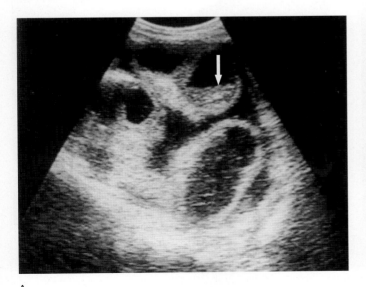

A

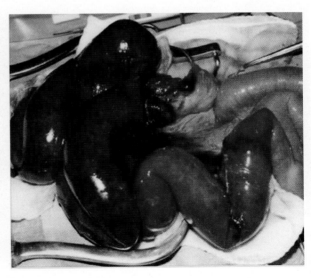

B

Figure 11-19. Strangulated small bowel obstruction. (A) Ultrasonogram (3.5 MHz). Real-time sonography reveals an akinetic dilated loop accompanied by a large amount of intraperitoneal fluid in the cul-de-sac. Inside the akinetic loop, spot echoes are demonstrated as deposited like sludge (arrow). (B) Operative picture. Laparotomy showed hemorrhagic necrosis of the affected small bowel.

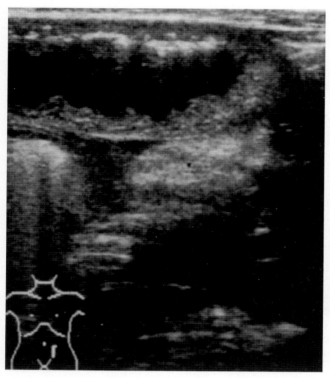

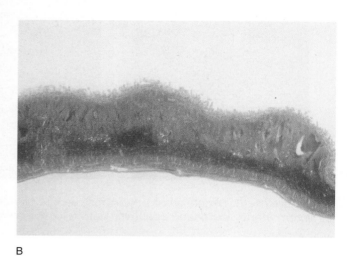

A

B

Figure 11-20. Strangulated small bowel obstruction. (A) In a case of established strangulation with hemorrhagic necrosis, wall thickening with increased echogenicity and flattened folds is visualized within the akinetic loop. The layer structure of the wall is delineated as an indistinct image with a high-frequency transducer (7.5 MHz). (B) Histology of the small bowel wall with hemorrhagic necrosis.

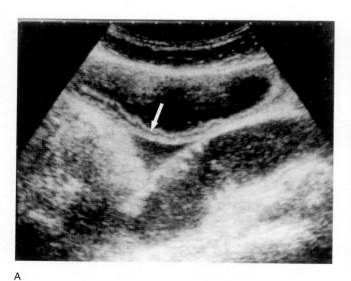

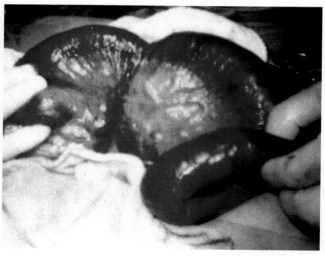

A

B

Figure 11-21. Strangulated small bowel obstruction. (A) Ultrasonogram (3.5 MHz). Submucosal edema caused by mild strangulation is demonstrated as a hypoechoic layer (arrow) of the wall. (B) Operative picture. The strangulated small bowel loop was still viable, although it had some hemorrhagic and edematous changes.

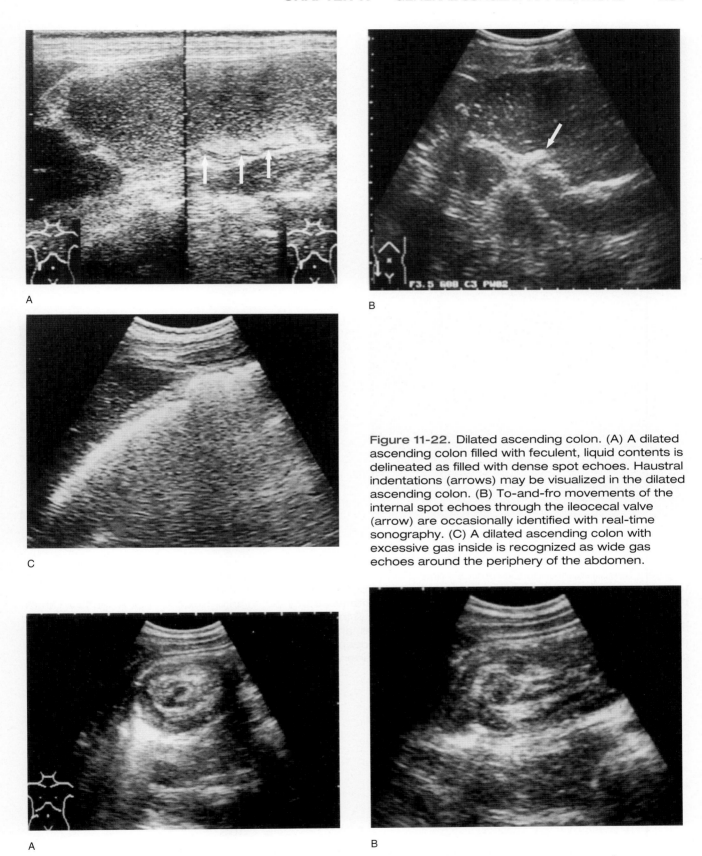

Figure 11-22. Dilated ascending colon. (A) A dilated ascending colon filled with feculent, liquid contents is delineated as filled with dense spot echoes. Haustral indentations (arrows) may be visualized in the dilated ascending colon. (B) To-and-fro movements of the internal spot echoes through the ileocecal valve (arrow) are occasionally identified with real-time sonography. (C) A dilated ascending colon with excessive gas inside is recognized as wide gas echoes around the periphery of the abdomen.

Figure 11-23. Ileocolic intussusception in an adult patient. (A) A cross-sectional image of intussusception is demonstrated as a "multiple concentric ring sign." (B) Multiple layer structure of intussusception in the long-axis plane is demonstrated.

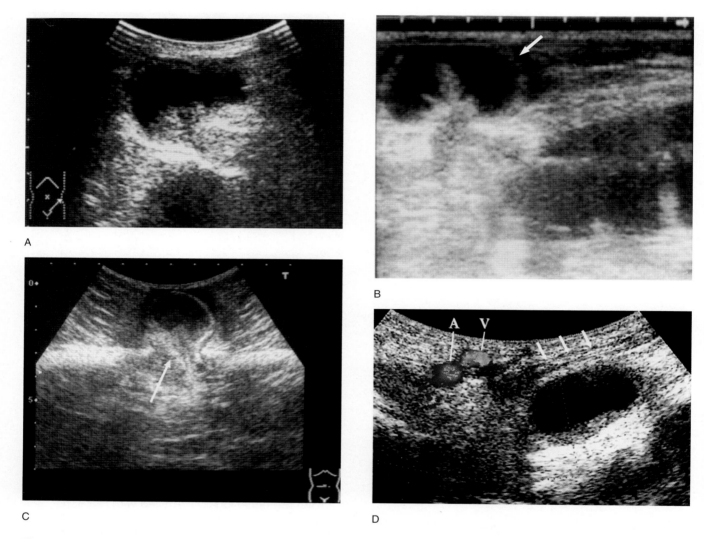

Figure 11-24. Incarcerated hernia. (A) An incarcerated femoral hernia is demonstrated as a small bowel segment herniated through the femoral canal. (B) In an incarcerated incisional hernia, a small bowel segment (arrow) is demonstrated as herniated through a small orifice in the abdominal wall. Dilated small bowel loops proximal to the incarceration are also shown in the peritoneal cavity. (C) In an umbilical hernia, a herniated small bowel segment is demonstrated within the fluid space in the hernia sac. The segment was softly strangulated at the hernia orifice (arrow) formed by defect of the fascia, and was easily reduced by manipulation in the case. (D) An incarcerated obturator hernia is demonstrated deep in the femoral region. It locates posterior to the pectineus muscle (arrows) and medial to the femoral artery and vein. A = femoral artery, V = femoral vein.

abdominal wall (Figure 11-24). An incarcerated obturator hernia is delineated posterior to the pectineus muscle in the femoral region. In contrast, an incarcerated femoral hernia is located in the subcutaneous space anterior to the muscle.

Afferent Loop Obstruction

Afferent loop obstruction after a Billroth's gastrojejunostomy may result from adhesions or recurrent carcinoma. Abdominal sonography can show a dilated duodenum and jejunum proximal to the anastomosis (Figure 11-25). The diagnosis of afferent loop obstruction can be made on the basis of the sonographic features and the clinical findings consistent with acute pancreatitis in patients with a prior history of a Billroth's gastrectomy.

Gallstone Ileus

Gallstone ileus is a rare complication of acute cholecystitis. The sonographic features diagnostic of gallstone ileus include pneumobilia, small bowel obstruction, and

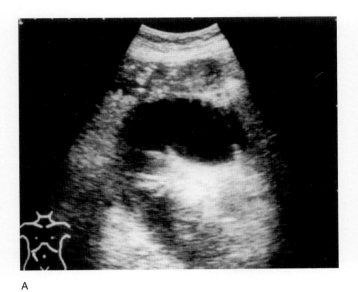

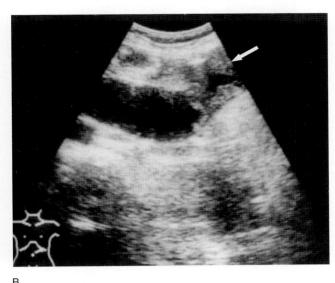

A   B

Figure 11-25. Afferent loop obstruction. (A) Dilated duodenal C-loop and (B) dilated jejunum proximal to the anastomosis are demonstrated in a case of recurrent carcinoma (arrow) at the site of anastomosis.

a large calculus (average diameter >3 cm) obstructing the small bowel (Figure 11-26A). The most common site of impaction is the ileocecal valve. Biliary-enteric fistula may be suggested by gas echoes inside the intra- or extrahepatic biliary tree (Figure 11-26B).

Small Bowel Tumor

It is rare for a small bowel tumor to cause a bowel obstruction. Malignant small bowel tumor, such as metastatic

carcinoma, malignant lymphoma, or leiomyosarcoma, may be occasionally identified by sonography (Figure 11-27).

Inflammatory Bowel Disease

Segmental wall thickening of the small bowel may be identified in cases of inflammatory bowel disease such as intestinal tuberculosis, Crohn's disease, or radiation enteritis (Figure 11-28).

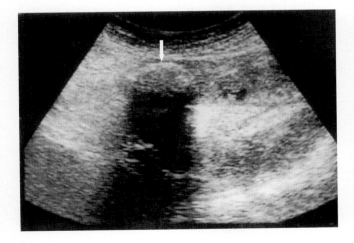

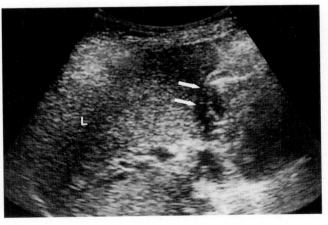

A   B

Figure 11-26. Gallstone ileus. (A) The impacted gallstone (arrow) obstructing the small bowel is directly visualized with a prominent acoustic shadow inside the dilated small bowel. (B) Gas echoes in the atrophic gallbladder (arrows) are recognized as showing the presence of a biliary-enteric fistula between the gallbladder and the duodenum (or less commonly the stomach, jejunum). L = liver.

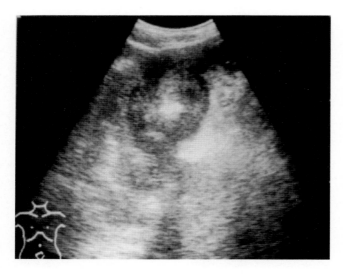

Figure 11-27. Small bowel tumor. A leiomyosarcoma causing a small bowel obstruction is recognized as an oval-shaped mass with a mosaic image.

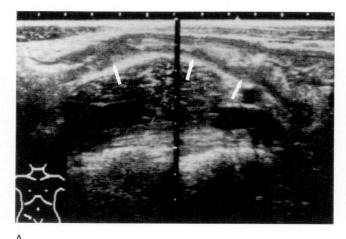

A

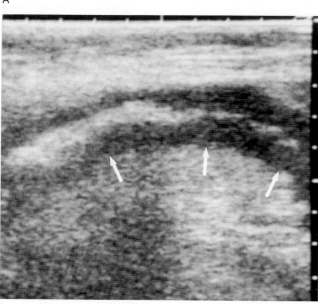

C

Colon Cancer

Colorectal cancer is by far the most common cause of large bowel obstruction, and may be detected as an irregular-shaped hypoechoic mass with echogenic core inside (Figure 11-29A) or a localized circular wall thickening (Figure 11-29B and C). Intraluminal tumor obstructing the lumen may occasionally be demonstrated (Figure 11-29D).

ILEUS

In the early stage of an ileus, slightly dilated small bowel loops (<25 mm wide in diameter) may be recognized on ultrasound. Gas echoes are more dominant than fluid collection inside the bowel (Figure 11-30).

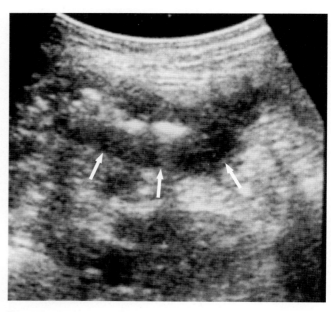

B

Figure 11-28. Inflammatory bowel diseases. A segmental wall thickening (arrows indicate posterior wall) of the small bowel is demonstrated in cases of (A) intestinal tuberculosis (7.5 MHz), (B) Crohn's disease (3.5 MHz), or (C) radiation enteritis (3.5 MHz).

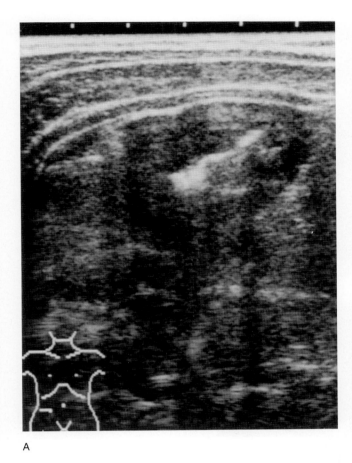

A

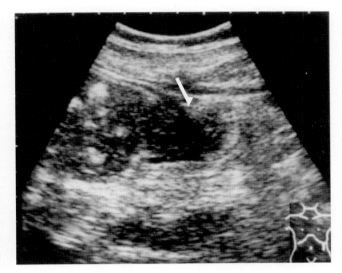

B

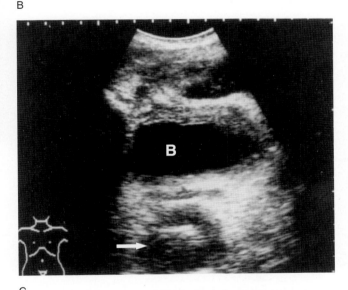

C

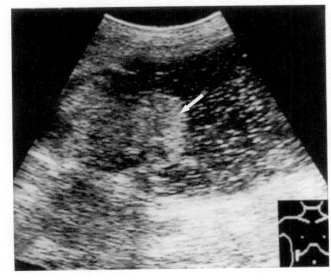

D

Figure 11-29. Colon carcinoma. (A) A colon cancer is often demonstrated as an irregular-shaped hypoechoic mass with an echogenic core inside, which is called the "pseudokidney sign" (7.5 MHz). (B) An obstructing colon cancer (arrow) is demonstrated as a circular wall thickening at the site of obstruction, where dilated colon filled with dense spot echoes is tapering (3.5 MHz). (C) Circular wall thickening of the rectum (arrow) is demonstrated in a case of recurrent gastric carcinoma (3.5 MHz). (D) Occasionally, a prominent tumor (arrow) obstructing the lumen may be demonstrated (3.5 MHz). B = urinary bladder.

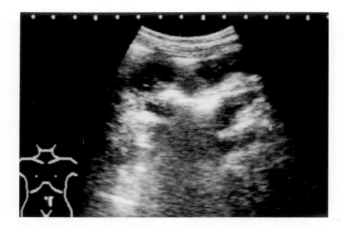

Figure 11-30. Ileus. Slightly dilated small bowel is demonstrated in a case of peritonitis secondary to perforated appendicitis.

ACUTE APPENDICITIS

Demonstration of a swollen, noncompressible appendix more than 6 mm in diameter is the prime sonographic criterion for the diagnosis of acute appendicitis. The typical appearance of an inflamed appendix is a tubular structure with one blind end. Maximal outer diameter ranges from 7 to 20 mm. In cases of catarrhal or phlegmonous appendicitis, a swollen appendix maintains the layer structure of the wall (Figure 11-31). In cases of gangrenous appendicitis, a progressive loss of mural lamination and organ contours can be demonstrated as a result of gangrene (Figure 11-32). Color Doppler

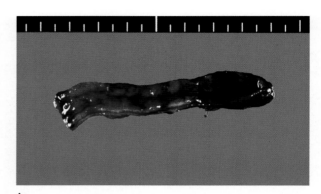

A

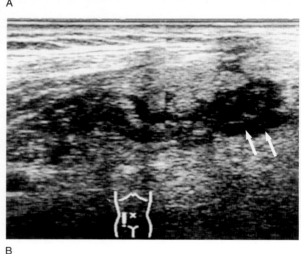

B

Figure 11-32. Acute appendicitis. Gangrenous tip in the appendix (A) is demonstrated as a focal loss of mural lamination (arrows) on the ultrasonogram (B).

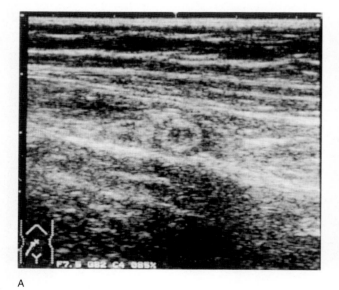

A

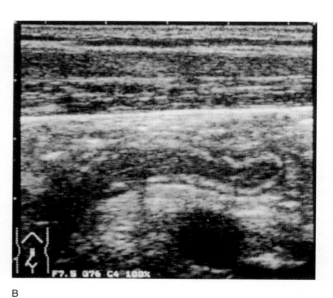

B

Figure 11-31. Acute appendicitis. A noncompressible, inflamed appendix is shown in (A) a cross-sectional view (7.5 MHz) and (B) a longitudinal section (7.5 MHz). Mural lamination of the swollen appendix is maintained in the early stages of acute appendicitis.

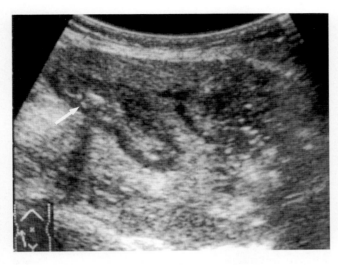

Figure 11-33. Acute appendicitis. An appendicolith (arrow) with acoustic shadowing is demonstrated (5 MHz).

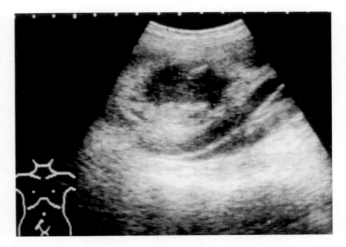

Figure 11-34. Pericecal abscess. A pericecal abscess secondary to perforated appendicitis is demonstrated as a hypoechoic fluid collection with a thick, noncompressible wall.

imaging is not essential for the disease, but may be supplementary to the sonographic differentiation between gangrene and phlegmon. Sonography may also demonstrate an appendicolith with acoustic shadowing (Figure 11-33). The presence of appendicolith is always indicative of acute appendicitis in patients with acute right lower quadrant abdominal pain. The appendix is aperistaltic, and infrequently contains gas in the lumen.

With progression of the inflammation, free intraperitoneal fluid may be demonstrated in the pelvis, and the inflamed appendix or pericecal abscess may be observed as surrounded by reflective fatty tissue that

represents the mesentery or omentum. A pericecal abscess can be demonstrated as fluid collection with a thick, noncompressible wall (Figure 11-34). Gas echoes may be visualized in the abscess (Figure 11-35). Atony of the terminal ileum may be seen as swelling of the cecal wall.

ACUTE COLONIC DIVERTICULITIS

On ultrasound, acute diverticulitis is shown as hypoechoic wall thickening (5–18 mm in thickness) of the

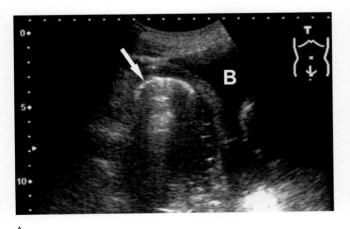

A

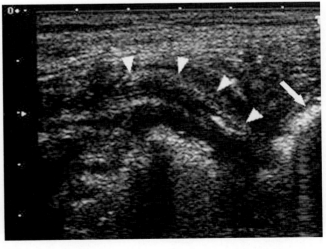

B

Figure 11-35. Acute perforated appendicitis with a pelvic abscess. (A) A fluid collection with gas echoes (arrow) is demonstrated in the pelvis. (B) The appendix (arrowheads) is recognized as a tubular structure with an echogenic fecalith inside, located adjacent to the pelvic abscess (arrow). In this case, perforated appendiceal tip is not detected. B = urinary bladder.

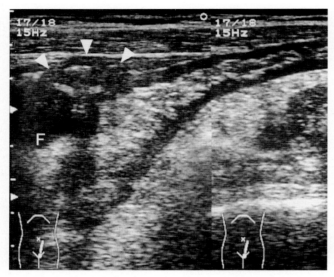

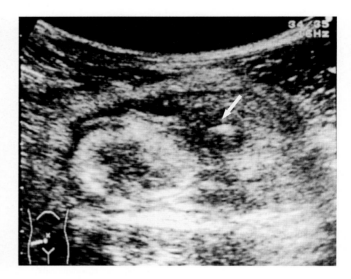

A   B

Figure 11-36. Acute colonic diverticulitis. (A) In a case of perforated diverticulitis of the sigmoid colon, a focal hypoechoic prominence (arrowheads) with gas echoes inside is visualized along the thickened intestinal wall. Paracolonic fluid collections also visualized adjacent to the hypoechoic lesion (7.5 MHz). (B) In a case of diverticulitis of the ascending colon, a solitary diverticulum (arrow) within the thickened wall is demonstrated at the maximum point of tenderness (7.5 MHz). F = fluid.

affected segment (Figure 11-36A). Graded compression over the site of tenderness is a simple method of localizing any inflammatory mass. Diverticulum may be demonstrated as a focal hypoechoic prominence with a hyperechoic fecalith or gas echoes inside, although it is not always identified in all cases of acute colonic diverticulitis (Figure 11-36B). Color Doppler imaging may show increased blood flow in the affected segment and the surrounding fatty tissue. Peridiverticular abscess or purulent intraperitoneal fluid may be recognized in cases of complicated diverticulitis (Figure 11-14C).

ACUTE PANCREATITIS/PANCREATIC PSEUDOCYST

Diffuse swelling of the pancreas is often recognized in cases of acute edematous pancreatitis. Decreased echogenicity of the pancreas represents interstitial edema (Figure 11-37). In cases of severe pancreatitis, peripancreatic fluid collections or echogenic pancreatic masses may be demonstrated (Figure 11-38A and B). Pancreatic pseudocysts are generally visualized as well-defined cystic masses in which sludge-like echoes may be identified (Figure 11-39).

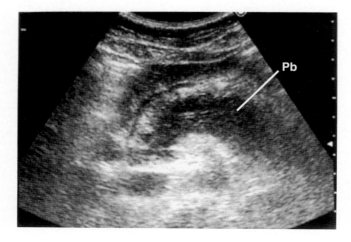

Figure 11-37. Acute edematous pancreatitis. Transverse view of the upper abdomen. Diffuse, homogeneous swelling of the pancreatic body (Pb) with decreased echogenicity is demonstrated in a case of acute edematous pancreatitis.

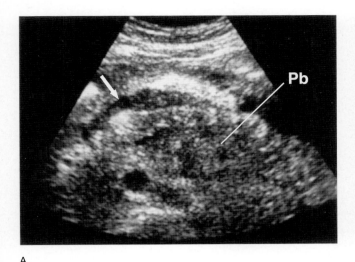
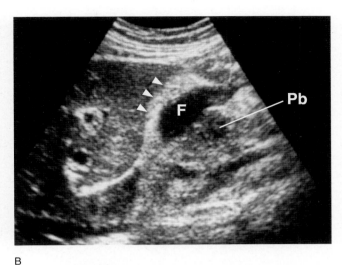

A

B

Figure 11-38. Acute necrotizing pancreatitis. (A) Transverse view of the upper abdomen. In a case of acute necrotizing pancreatitis, the pancreatic body is visualized as heterogenous mass with unclear border. Hypoechoic inflammatory exudate (arrow) is demonstrated anterior to the pancreatic body. (B) Peripancreatic fluid collection is demonstrated between the hypoechoic pancreatic body and reflective fatty tissue (arrows). Pb = pancreatic body, F = fluid collection.

ACUTE CHOLECYSTITIS

Irregular sonolucent layers in the gallbladder wall are indicative of acute cholecystitis (Figure 11-40A; Videos 10-1 and 10-2: Hepatobiliary). The presence of asymmetric thickening of the gallbladder wall or intra-luminal membranes parallel to the gallbladder wall can be identified in patients with acute gangrenous chole-cystitis. Pericholecystic fluid collection can be caused by gallbladder perforation or abscess formation (Figure 11-40B).

ACUTE MESENTERIC ISCHEMIA

Wall thickening of the small bowel associated with a significant amount of intraperitoneal fluid is nonspecific but suggestive of acute mesenteric ischemia as well as

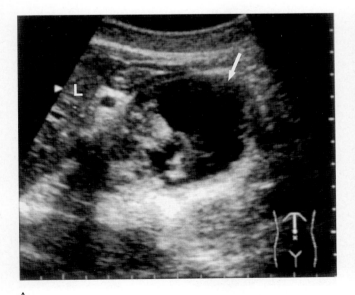
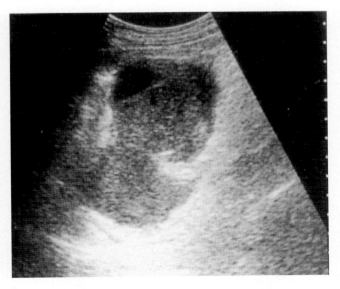

A

B

Figure 11-39. Pancreatic pseudocyst. (A) A well-defined cystic mass (arrow) is demonstrated posterior to the gastric antrum. (B) An irregular-shaped cystic mass filled with spot echoes is demonstrated medial to the splenic hilum in a case of infected pseudocyst. L = liver.

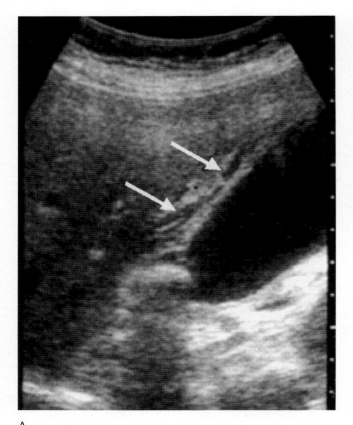

A

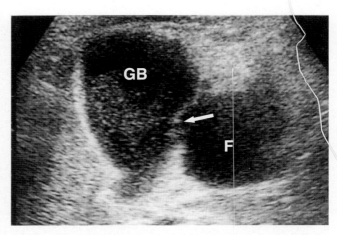

B

Figure 11-40. Acute cholecystitis. (A) Irregular sonolucent layers (arrows) in the swollen gallbladder wall are accompanied by an impacted stone in the gallbladder neck. (B) Pericholecystic fluid collection with a defect (arrow) in the gallbladder wall, which represents a gallbladder perforation, is directly visualized with sonography. GB = gallbladder, F = fluid collection.

peritonitis and peritoneal carcinomatosis (Figure 11-41). Color Doppler ultrasound can potentially be used to evaluate the blood flow through the main trunk of the SMA in a patient suspected of having an SMA occlusion (Figure 11-42). However, it is not easy to confirm the etiology by this examination because excessive GI gas caused by an accompanying ileus often disturbs the examination. Segmental mesenteric arteries cannot be demonstrated with color Doppler ultrasound, but segmental wall thickening of the small bowel may suggest the etiology (Figure 11-43).

ISCHEMIC COLITIS

In cases of ischemic colitis, hypoechoic wall thickening is often demonstrated in the affected segment especially from the splenic flexure to the rectosigmoid junction (Figures 11-44). The laminar structure of the wall becomes indistinct (Figures 11-45 and 11-46). Color or power Doppler ultrasound shows poor blood flow in the affected segment and demonstrates increased blood

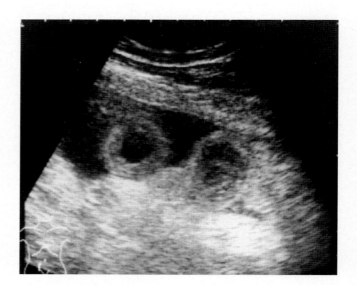

Figure 11-41. Acute mesenteric ischemia. Slightly dilated small bowel with wall thickening and intraperitoneal fluid are nonspecific but suggestive of acute mesenteric ischemia.

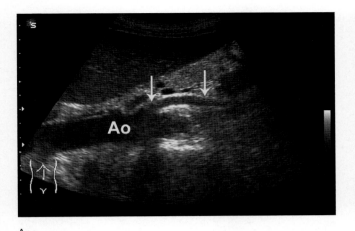

A

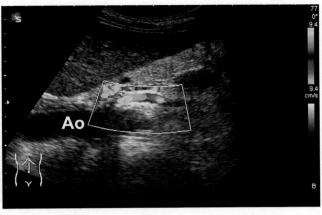

B

Figure 11-42. Application of color Doppler ultrasound technique for mesenteric ischemia. (A) Longitudinal view of the aorta and SMA (arrows). (B) A color Doppler ultrasound of the same area shows blood flow through the SMA on longitudinal view. Ao = aorta, SMA = superior mesenteric artery. (Courtesy of James Mateer, MD)

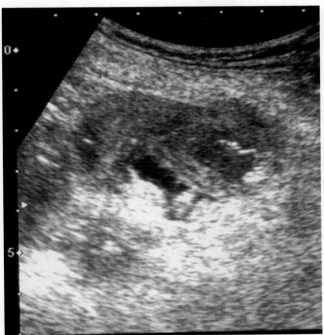

A

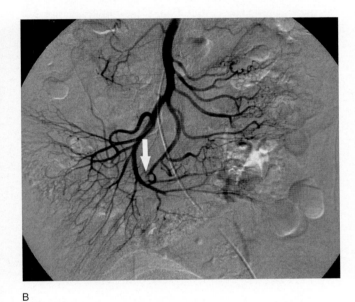

B

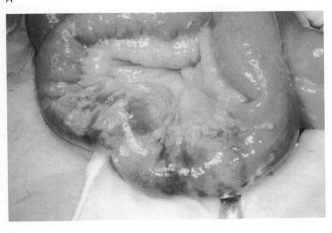

C

Figure 11-43. A case of acute segmental mesenteric ischemia. (A) Segmental wall thickening in the affected small bowel was detected with sonography. (B) An occlusion (arrow) in the branch of the superior mesenteric artery was demonstrated by selective angiography. (C) Laparotomy revealed a segmental ischemia of the small bowel.

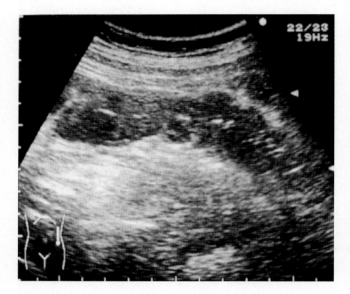

Figure 11-44. Ischemic colitis. Hypoechoic wall thickening is delineated in the descending colon (3.5 MHz).

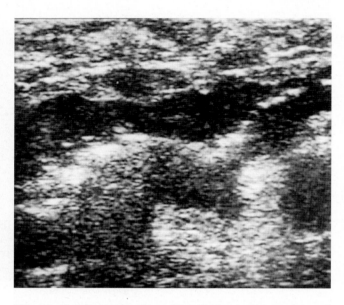

Figure 11-46. Ischemic colitis. An irregular contour of the wall of the affected segment with decreased echogenicity is visualized in the advanced stage of ischemic colitis (5 MHz).

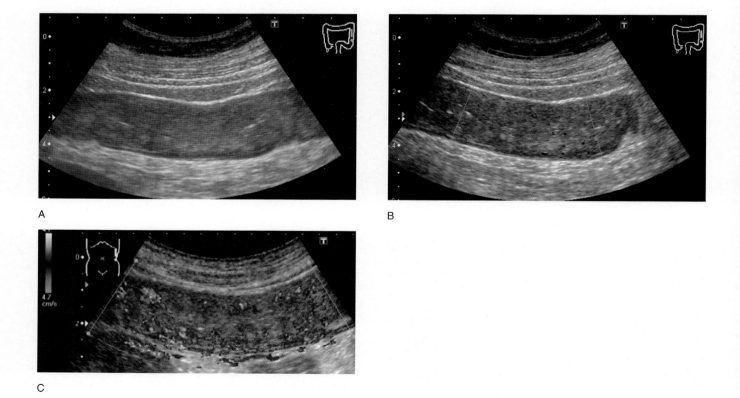

A

B

C

Figure 11-45. Ischemic colitis. (A) In the affected segment, the laminar structure of the wall is delineated as indistinct (5 MHz). (B) Color Doppler ultrasound demonstrates poor blood flow in the affected segment. (C) Color signals of the blood flow in the segment increased over several days, as the segment recovered from ischemia.

flow in approximately 1 week when the segment recovers from ischemia (Figure 11-45B and C).

► COMMON VARIANTS AND OTHER ABNORMALITIES

Common normal variants that may be erroneously identified as free intraperitoneal fluid are discussed in Chapter 5, "Trauma." Fluid in the stomach when examining the perisplenic views and fluid in a collapsed bladder or an ovarian cyst when examining the pelvic views may be erroneously identified as free intraperitoneal fluid. Also, premenopausal women can occasionally have a small amount of free fluid in the pouch of Douglas.

Collapsed small bowel can be visualized similarly to a swollen appendix vermiformis, leading to a false-positive diagnosis of acute appendicitis (Figure 11-47). Peristaltic activity is not observed in the appendix, while it should be recognized in the small bowel.

GASTRIC OUTLET OBSTRUCTION

Gastric outlet obstruction may be demonstrated with point-of-care ultrasound (Figure 11-48). It can be caused by gastric cancer, chronic duodenal ulcer, or pancreatic cancer. To confirm the diagnosis, endoscopy and con-

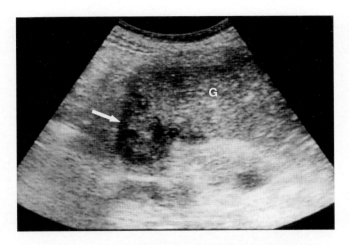

Figure 11-48. Gastric outlet obstruction. Distended stomach filled with spot echoes is demonstrated proximal to the circular, hypoechoic wall thickening (arrow) in the pylorus, which represents a gastric cancer. G = stomach.

trast studies are usually applied after decompression of the distended stomach.

TORSION OF THE PEDICLE OF OVARIAN TUMOR

Ovarian torsion rarely occurs in patients without ovarian tumors or enlarged cysts. The clinical symptoms and physical findings may be confused with appendicitis, salpingitis, or gastroenteritis. The sonographic findings may be nonspecific and demonstrate a complex or cystic-appearing mass accompanied by free fluid in the pouch of Douglas (Figure 11-49). With a hemorrhagic infarction, the ovarian tumor may be hyperechoic.

RECTUS SHEATH HEMATOMA

Acute or subacute hematoma in the rectus sheath, generally confined to the upper or lower quadrant, can occasionally be experienced without trauma in a patient who has bleeding diathesis after strenuous physical exertion. It is not always easy to differentiate rectus sheath hematoma from intra-abdominal pathology because most patients with the hematoma present with significant abdominal swelling and tenderness. Without suspicion of this pathologic entity, a nontherapeutic laparotomy might be performed for an acute abdomen when conservative treatment or percutaneous drainage is indicated. Abdominal sonography is useful in this clinical situation by demonstrating the hematoma within the abdominal wall (Figure 11-50).

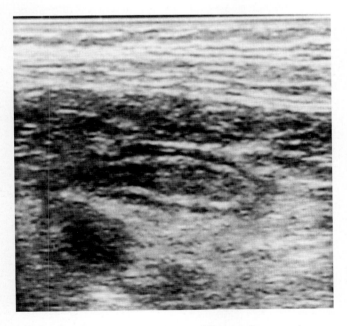

Figure 11-47. Normal collapsed ileum. A normal ileum may be misdiagnosed as a swollen appendix vermiformis (7.5 MHz). Peristaltic activity is recognized in the normal small bowel, while it is not observed in the appendix.

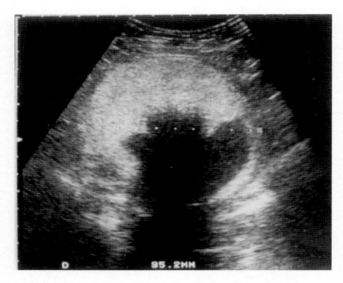

Figure 11-49. Torsion of the pedicle of an ovarian tumor. A solid and cystic tumor is demonstrated in the pouch of Douglas. The dense central shadowing suggests calcified components. The mixed components may represent a dermoid tumor. Significant tenderness on the tumor suggests possible torsion of the pedicle. Color Doppler may be helpful if available.

ACUTE ENTEROCOLITIS

Sonography has been increasingly applied for acute enterocolitis in recent years. Slightly dilated bowel loops with normal wall thickness and hyperperistalsis can be visualized in cases of mild enterocolitis. Mural thickening of the ileum or the colon may be identified in more severe cases (Figure 11-51A). Color Doppler imaging shows increased blood flow in the affected intestinal wall. The most affected segment depends on the etiologies of enterocolitis. Some pathologic microorganisms such as Campylobacter, Salmonella, and Yersinia may specifically infect the ileocecal region, which is known as infectious ileocecitis.[63] The terminal ileitis is often accompanied with enlarged mesenteric lymph nodes.

Anisakiasis, a parasitic infection of the GI tract, may present as acute abdomen within hours after ingestion of raw or undercooked seafood containing larvae of the nematode Anisakis simplex. It may occasionally lead to small bowel obstruction from segmental intestinal edema (Figure 11-51B).[64]

▶ PITFALLS

1. **Contraindication.** When a patient presents with an acute abdomen, there is no absolute contraindication to performing a point-of-care ultrasound examination. A rapid ultrasound examination can be applied even when the resuscitation efforts are performed on patients in shock.
2. **Overreliance on the point-of-care ultrasound examination.** A pitfall is the overreliance of an initial negative ultrasound

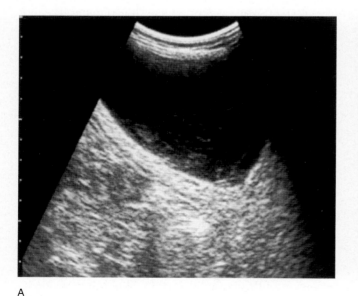

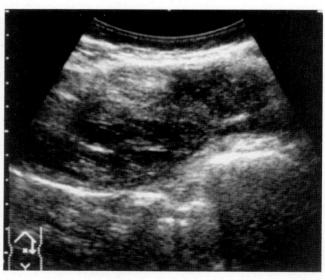

A   B

Figure 11-50. Rectus sheath hematoma. (A) Sonography shows a large hematoma as a circumscribed fluid collection within the abdominal wall. (B) In the early stage, a rectus sheath hematoma may be shown as a heterogeneous image.

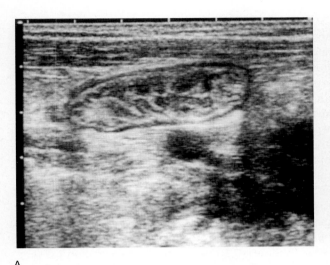

A

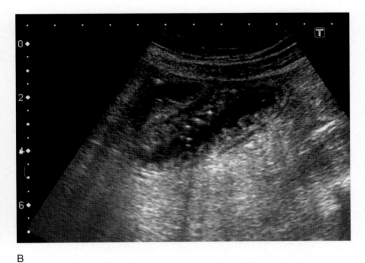

B

Figure 11-51. Infectious enterocolitis. (A) Mural thickening of the ileum is regarded as reflective of inflammatory changes in the intestinal wall (5 MHz). (B) Ultrasonogram (5 MHz) of intestinal anisakiasis. The affected small bowel is recognized as an edematous segment, which may cause a small bowel obstruction, accompanied by a small amount of intraperitoneal fluid.

examination in caring for patients with an acute abdomen. Each examination is a single data point in the overall clinical picture. As the clinical symptoms and findings change, perform serial ultrasound examinations to evaluate any changes of sonographic findings. If the ultrasound examination presents equivocal findings, utilize abdominal CT, other radiographic procedures using contrast media, or endoscopy for further evaluation.

3. **Limitations of the point-of-care ultrasound examination.** Limitations include difficulty in imaging patients who are morbidly obese or have an immense amount of GI gas. Various artifacts may interfere with the examination in obtaining optimal images. Also, it may be difficult to determine the nature of free intraperitoneal fluid. If clinically required, an ultrasound-guided paracentesis of the fluid can be applied to clarify the issue. Another limitation is that ultrasound is an operator-dependent examination for both obtaining and interpreting the images.

4. **Limitations associated with pregnancy.** In pregnant patients, the distortion of usual landmarks caused by the presence of a gravid uterus can complicate the identification of an inflamed appendix. Interpreting sonographic images of extrauterine vasculature may be difficult for inexperienced operators. Nonobstructive dilatation of the renal collecting system may occur after 6 weeks in a normal pregnancy.

5. **Technical difficulties with the point-of-care ultrasound examination.** Many clinicians do not have enough experience to confidently apply sonography for the diagnosis of GI disorders such as bowel obstruction, acute appendicitis, or acute diverticulitis. Significant tenderness, peritoneal irritability, or hyperventilation can interfere with the examination.

6. **Etiologies undetected by sonography.** Certain etiologies that can cause an acute abdomen may not be detected initially by the point-of-care ultrasound examination. These include perforation of a vesical bladder or GI tract, embolism of the SMA, colonic volvulus, and GI hemorrhage.

► CASE STUDIES

CASE 1

Patient Presentation

A 68-year-old man presented with complaints of intermittent epigastric pain, nausea, and vomiting. He felt the sudden onset of pain prior to dinner. The pain increased intermittently and was accompanied by emesis of bilious fluid. He had a bowel movement earlier in the day. He had a medical history of gastrectomy for gastric cancer and cholecystectomy for gallstone disease.

On physical examination, his blood pressure was 160/90 mm Hg, pulse 82 beats per minute, respirations 16 per minute, and temperature 37.1°C. His head, neck, pulmonary, and CV examinations were unremarkable. His abdomen was soft and flat but had moderate tenderness to palpation and rebound tenderness in the epigastric region. No muscle guarding was appreciated. On rectal examination, his stool was guaiac negative.

Management Course

Plain radiographs revealed dilated small bowel with multiple air–fluid levels. Laboratory tests revealed leukocytosis (WBC 10,300/μl). A point-of-care ultrasound revealed dilated loops of small bowel with peristaltic activity in the entire abdomen and collapsed loops localized in the right lower quadrant (Figure 11-52A). A small amount of peritoneal fluid was also identified between the dilated loops. No evidence of hepatobiliary disorders, splenomegaly, or pancreatitis was found.

The patient was admitted with the diagnosis of small bowel obstruction by adhesions and treated conservatively with nasogastric tube decompression and IV fluids. Although his symptoms were relieved after the nasogastric tube decompression, sonographic appearances of small bowel obstruction were slightly progressive. Three days after admission, a long intestinal tube was inserted for decompression of dilated small bowel and for a contrast study to confirm the site and degree of the obstruction. A small amount of water-soluble contrast medium was passed through the obstruction to the ascending colon, and thus the patient was suspected to have a partial obstruction on radiograph findings. At that time, laboratory tests showed only slight elevation of serum C-reactive protein (CRP) level (2.0 mg/dL). The WBC count was 7,100/μL. However, more than 1,000 mL of intestinal fluid were drained via the long intestinal tube in 24 hours. Reexamination with sonography revealed an aperistaltic, dilated loop with slight mural thickening in the right lower abdomen (Figure 11-52B),

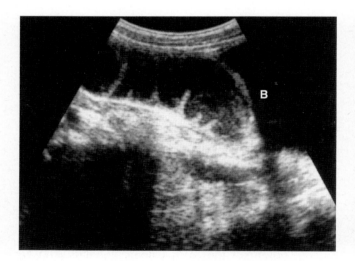

A

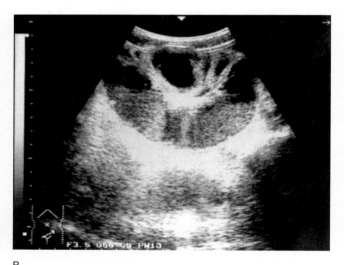

B

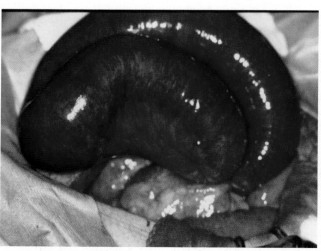

C

Figure 11-52. Sonograms of case 1. (A) An initial ultrasound examination revealed dilated loops of small bowel with peristaltic activity. (B) Reexamination with sonography revealed an akinetic, dilated loop with slight mural thickening and an increased amount of intraperitoneal fluid in the pelvis. Inside the akinetic loop, spot echoes are deposited like sludge. (C) Operative picture. The strangulated small bowel was still viable and relieved by adhesiolysis. B = bladder.

and increased amount of intraperitoneal fluid. Slowly progressing strangulated obstruction was suspected on sonographic images contrary to his minimal clinical and radiograph findings. He underwent an urgent laparotomy, which revealed a large amount of serobloody ascites and a congestive, hemorrhagic loop of bowel that was twisted and strangulated by an adhesive band (Figure 11-52C). The strangulated loop was still viable and relieved by adhesiolysis.

Commentary

Case 1 was an example of a patient who had a slowly progressing strangulated obstruction. The clinical picture of a strangulated obstruction varies by the severity of circulatory impairment, the length of strangulated loop, and the period after the onset. Diagnosis of strangulated small bowel obstruction is difficult preoperatively unless the patient presents with severe pain or peritoneal signs. In general, laboratory tests and plain radiographs are not diagnostic in the early stage of strangulation. Real-time sonography, however, can evaluate not only the morphologic changes but also the physiologic changes observed in bowel obstruction. An aperistaltic, dilated loop distal to the dilated loops with peristaltic activity is essential in the sonographic diagnosis of strangulated small bowel obstruction. The increase in the amount of intraperitoneal fluid, which is also diagnostic for strangulation, can be assessed by serial ultrasound examinations. In this particular case, the information provided by serial examinations was crucial in the decision process to proceed with an urgent laparotomy, and this prevented an enterectomy for hemorrhagic necrosis of the strangulated loop.

CASE 2

Patient Presentation

A 55-year-old man presented with a 5-day history of lower abdominal pain and watery diarrhea. He denied nausea and vomiting. He had a medical history of chronic hepatitis and cerebral infarction, and was a heavy smoker and heavy drinker.

On physical examination, his blood pressure was 145/84 mm Hg, pulse 110 beats per minute, and temperature 38.4°C. His head, neck, pulmonary, and CV examinations were unremarkable. The abdominal examination was soft, diffusely tender, and without peritoneal signs.

Management Course

An upright chest radiograph and abdominal radiographs showed no evidence of bowel obstruction or GI perfora-

tion. His laboratory tests showed an elevated serum CRP level (4.5 mg/dL) and leukocytosis (WBC 11,000/μL. A point-of-care ultrasound examination revealed no free intraperitoneal fluid but slightly thickened wall of the sigmoid colon (Figure 11-53A). Abdominal CT scan was negative for intraperitoneal and retroperitoneal pathology. The patient was treated conservatively with antibiotics and IV fluid therapy. Two days after the admission, he complained of having severe abdominal pain. A repeat point-of-care ultrasound revealed mural thickening of the sigmoid colon and turbulent intraperitoneal fluid, including gas echoes in the anterior pelvis (Figure 11-53B and C). He underwent an urgent laparotomy, which revealed feculent peritonitis due to perforative diverticulitis of the sigmoid colon.

Commentary

Case 2 had an initial negative ultrasound examination and CT scan. Reexamination with point-of-care ultrasound revealed turbulent-free intraperitoneal fluid and mural thickening of the sigmoid colon. These findings were suggestive of a sigmoid colon perforation due to acute diverticulitis, and thus, negated the need for a repeat CT scan while making a decision for surgical intervention. As abdominal ultrasound is available at the bedside, it should be repeated for a patient with an acute abdomen whose etiology is not yet defined.

CASE 3

Patient Presentation

A 26-year-old pregnant woman presented with complaints of right lower abdominal pain radiating to the right flank. She initially experienced epigastric pain accompanied by nausea and vomiting. She denied urinary retention, dysuria, hematuria, diarrhea, and constipation. She was 18 weeks pregnant and had no vaginal bleeding. She denied any significant medical history.

On physical examination, her vital signs were within normal limits. Her pulmonary and CV examinations were normal. The abdominal examination was soft but had significant peritoneal signs localized in the right lower quadrant laterally and superiorly deviated from McBurney's point. She also felt a severe pain on percussion in the costovertebral angle and right lumbar region. A gravid uterus, 3 cm below the umbilicus, was noted.

Management Course

Her urinalysis showed no RBCs or bacteria. Her laboratory tests demonstrated leukocytosis (WBC 12,000/μL) and elevated CRP level (10 mg/dL). A point-of-care ultrasound examination using a standard transducer

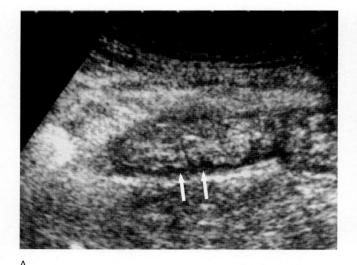

A

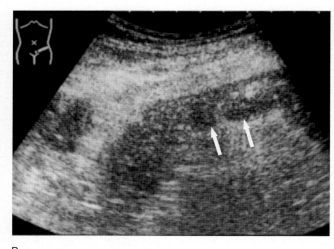

B

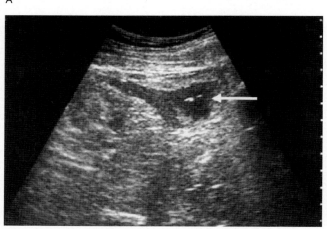

C

Figure 11-53. Sonograms of case 2. (A) No free peritoneal fluid but slightly thickened wall of the sigmoid colon (arrows) was revealed with an initial ultrasound examination. (B) Mural thickening of the sigmoid colon (arrows) was identified with reexamination. (C) Turbulent intraperitoneal fluid (arrow) including gas echoes was recognized in the anterior pelvis.

revealed a target figure of the appendix that was draped over by omental tissues (Figure 11-54A), dilated pyelocaliceal system in the right kidney (Figure 11-54B), and the fetus moving actively within the gravid uterus. There was no evidence of peritoneal fluid. The patient was suspected of having an acute appendicitis accompanied with acute hydronephrosis. For the purpose of differential diagnosis and treatment, the urologist performed a retrograde ureteral catheterization under cystoscopic procedures. No evidence of pyuria or apparent obstructive lesions was confirmed, and subsequently, the patient was suspected of having nonobstructive dilatation of the renal collecting system, which is occasionally recognized in pregnant women. The patient underwent an urgent laparotomy, which revealed an acute gangrenous appendicitis without abscess. An appendectomy was performed and her postoperative course was uneventful. The right hydronephrosis was slightly reduced but lasted throughout pregnancy.

Commentary

Case 3 was an example of a pregnant patient who presented with an acute abdomen. She had acute appendicitis with puzzling symptoms and signs. The sonographic findings were compatible with her complicated clinical findings. The diagnosis of acute appendicitis in pregnant patients can be more challenging even when they present with a typical clinical picture for the disease. Abdominal sonography should be utilized for pregnant women and can assist physicians with their management strategy.

Nonobstructive dilatation of the collecting system occurs in normal pregnancy onward after 6–10 weeks, with both hormonal factors and pressure of the gravid uterus on the ureters considered to be likely causes. The dilatation is marked more on the right than on the left and increases in severity throughout pregnancy. In this case, the retroperitoneal involvement of the inflammation from the appendicitis may have caused

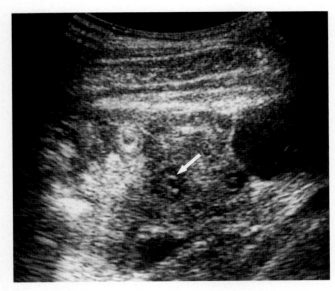

A

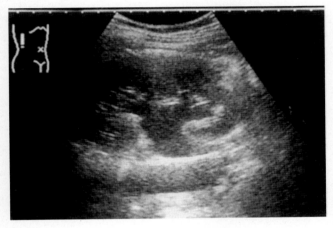

B

Figure 11-54. Sonograms of case 3. (A) A point-of-care ultrasound examination using a standard transducer revealed a target figure of the appendix (arrow), which was draped over by omental tissues, in the right lower flank. (B) A coronal view in the right upper flank showed moderately dilated pyelocaliceal system within the right kidney.

paresis of the ureter and, consequently, aggravated urinary retention.

► ACKNOWLEDGMENT

The author thanks the staff of the ultrasound section in the Kobe City Medical Center West Hospital and the Kobe City General Hospital, especially Mr. Toshiaki Fujimoto and Mr. Shuji Tamura, for their assistance in obtaining the images used in this chapter.

REFERENCES

1. Gore RM, Gore MD: Ascites and peritoneal fluid collections. In: Gore RM, Levine MS, eds. *Textbook of Gastrointestinal Radiology*, 2nd ed. Philadelphia, PA: WB Saunders, 2000:1969.
2. Jeffrey RB, McGahan JP: Gastrointestinal tract and peritoneal cavity. In: McGahan JP, Goldberg BB, eds. *Diagnostic Ultrasound—A Logical Approach*. Philadelphia, PA: Lippincott-Raven, 1998:511.
3. Lim JH, Lee DH, Ko YT: Sonographic detection of duodenal ulcer. *J Ultrasound Med* 11:91, 1992.
4. Garcia SJM: Direct sonographic signs of acute duodenal ulcer. *Abdom Imaging* 24:226, 1999.
5. Winek TG, Mosely HS, Grout G, et al.: Pneumoperitoneum and its association with ruptured abdominal viscus. *Arch Surg* 123:709, 1988.
6. Williams N, Everson NW: Radiological confirmation of intraperitoneal free gas. *Ann R Coll Surg Engl* 79:8, 1997.
7. Jeffrey RB, Federle MP, Wall S: Value of computed tomography in detecting occult gastrointestinal perforation. *J Comput Assist Tomogr* 7:825, 1983.
8. Meiser G, Meissner K: Clinical relevance of sonography in acute diagnosis of perforated gastroduodenal ulcers. *Langenbecks Arch Chir* 368:197, 1986.
9. Chanda D, Kedar RP, Malde HM: Sonographic detection of pneumoperitoneum: An experimental and clinical study. *Australas Radiol* 37:182, 1993.
10. Kainberger P, Zukriegel M, Sattlegger P, et al.: Ultrasound detection of pneumoperitoneum based on typical ultrasound morphology. *Ultraschall Med* 15:122, 1994.
11. Braccini G, Lamacchia M, Boraschi P, et al.: Ultrasound versus plain film in the detection of pneumoperitoneum. *Abdom Imaging* 21:404, 1996.
12. Grechenig W, Peicha G, Clement HG, et al.: Detection of pneumoperitoneum by ultrasound examination: An experimental and clinical study. *Injury* 30:173, 1999.
13. Corn I: Intestinal obstruction. In: Berk JE, ed. *Bockus Gastroenterology*, 4th ed., Vol. 3. Tokyo: WB Saunders, 1985: 2056.
14. Ziter FMH Jr, Markowitz SK: Radiologic diagnosis. In: Welch JP, ed. *Bowel Obstruction: Differential Diagnosis and Clinical Management*. Philadelphia, PA: WB Saunders, 96, 1990.
15. Stephanie R, Wilson MD: Ultrasonography of the hollow viscera. In: Gore RM, Levine MS, eds. *Textbook of Gastrointestinal Radiology*, 2nd ed. Philadelphia, PA: WB Saunders, 67, 2000.
16. Peck R: The small bowel. In: Meire H, Cosgrove D, Dewbury K, et al., eds. *Clinical Ultrasound* (Vol. 2, Abdominal and General Ultrasound). 2nd ed. New York, NY: Churchill Livingstone, 823, 1999.
17. O'Malley ME, Wilson SR: US of gastrointestinal tract abnormalities with CT correlation. *Radiographics* 23:59, 2003.
18. Fleischer AC, Dowling AD, Weinstein ML, et al.: Sonographic patterns of distended, fluid-filled bowel. *Radiology* 133:681, 1979.
19. Scheible W, Goldberger LE: Diagnosis of small bowel obstruction: The contribution of diagnostic ultrasound. *AJR* 133:685, 1979.

20. Meiser G, Meissner K: Ileus and intestinal obstruction: Ultrasonic findings as a guideline to therapy. *Hepatogastroenterology* 34:194, 1987.

21. Cho KC, Hoffman-Tretin JC, Alterman DD: Closed-loop obstruction of the small bowel: CT and sonographic appearance. *J Comput Assist Yomogr* 13:256, 1989.

22. Truong S, Arlt G, Pfingsten F, et al.: Importance of sonography in diagnosis of ileus. A retrospective study of 459 patients. *Chirurg* 63:634, 1992.

23. Schmutz GR, Benko A, Fournier L, et al.: Small bowel obstruction: Role and contribution of sonography. *Eur Radiol* 7:1054, 1997.

24. Ogata M, Imai S, Hosotani R, et al.: Abdominal ultrasonography for the diagnosis of strangulation in small bowel obstruction. *Br J Surg* 81:421, 1994.

25. Ogata M: Ultrasonographic findings in the intestinal wall with hemorrhagic necrosis caused by strangulation ileus. *Jpn J Med Ultrasonics* 17:19, 1990.

26. Czechowski J: Conventional radiography and ultrasonography in the diagnosis of small bowel obstruction and strangulation. *Acta Radiol* 37:186, 1996.

27. Ogata M, Imai S, Hosotani R, et al.: Abdominal sonography for the diagnosis of large bowel obstruction. *Jpn J Surg* 24:791, 1994.

28. Ogata M, Mateer JR, Condon RE: Prospective evaluation of abdominal sonography for the diagnosis of bowel obstruction. *Ann Surg* 223:237, 1996.

29. Russell JC, Welch JP: Pathophysiology of bowel obstruction. In: Welch JP, ed. *Bowel Obstruction: Differential Diagnosis and Clinical Management*. Philadelphia, PA: WB Saunders, 28, 1990.

30. Suri S, Gupta S, Sudhakar PJ, et al.: Comparative evaluation of plain films, ultrasound and CT in the diagnosis of intestinal obstruction. *Acta Radiol* 40:422, 1999.

31. Weissberg DL, Scheible W, Leopld GR: Ultrasonographic appearance of adult intussusception. *Radiology* 124:791, 1977.

32. Holt S, Samuel E: Multiple concentric ring sign in the ultrasonographic diagnosis of intussusception. *Gastrointest Radiol* 3:307, 1978.

33. Puylaert JBCM: Acute appendicitis: US evaluation using graded compression. *Radiology* 158:335, 1986.

34. Jeffrey RB, Laing FC, Lewis FR: Acute appendicitis: High-resolution real-time US findings. *Radiology* 163:11, 1987.

35. Jeffrey RB, Laing FC, Townsend RR: Acute appendicitis: Sonographic criteria based on 250 cases. *Radiology* 167:327, 1988.

36. Schwerk WB, Wichtrup B, Rothmund M, et al.: Ultrasonography in the diagnosis of acute appendicitis: A prospective study. *Gastroenterology* 97:630, 1989.

37. Douglas DD, Macpherson NE, Davidson PM, et al.: Randomised controlled trial of ultrasonography in diagnosis of acute appendicitis, incorporating the Alvarado score. *BMJ* 321:919, 2000.

38. Terasawa T, Blackmore CC, Bent S, et al.: Systematic review: Computed tomography and ultrasonography to detect acute appendicitis in adults and adolescents. *Ann Intern Med* 141:537, 2004.

39. Birnbaum BA, Wilson SR: Appendicitis at the Millenium. *Radiology* 215:337–348, 2000.

40. Skaane P, Schistad O, Amland PF, et al.: Routine ultrasonography in the diagnosis of acute appendicitis: A valuable tool in daily practice? *Am Surg* 63:937, 1997.

41. Pohl D, Golub R, Schwartz GE, et al.: Appendiceal ultrasonography performed by nonradiologists: Does it help in the diagnostic process? *J Ultrasound Med* 17:217, 1998.

42. Amgwerd M, Rothlin M, Candinas D, et al.: Ultrasound diagnosis of appendicitis by surgeons—A matter of experience? A prospective study. *Lagenbecks Arch Chir* 379:335, 1994.

43. Williams RJ, Windsor AC, Rosin RD, et al.: Ultrasound scanning of the acute abdomen by surgeons in training. *Ann R Coll Surg Engl* 76:228, 1994.

44. Zielke A, Hasse C, Sitter H, et al: Influence of ultrasound on clinical decision making in acute appendicitis: A prospective study. *Eur J Surg* 164:201, 1998.

45. Chen SC, Wan HP, Huang PM, et al: Accuracy of ED sonography in the diagnosis of acute appendicitis. *Am J Emrg Med* 18:449, 2000.

46. Puylaert JBCM, Rioux M, Oostayen JA: The appendix and small bowel. In: Meire H, Cosgrove D, Dewbury K, et al., eds. *Abdominal and General Ultrasound*, 2nd ed. New York, NY: Churchill Livingstone, 1999:841.

47. Simonovsky V: Sonographic detection of normal and abnormal appendix. *Clin Radiol* 54:533, 1999.

48. Van Breda Vriesman AC, Puylaert JBCM: Mimics of appendicitis: Alternative nonsurgical diagnoses with sonography and CT. *Am J Roentgenol* 187:1103–1112, 2006.

49. Wilson SR, Toi A: The value of sonography in the diagnosis of acute diverticulitis of the colon. *AJR* 154:1199–1202, 1990.

50. Schwerk WB, Schwarz S, Rothmund M: Sonography in acute colonic diverticulitis. A prospective study. *Dis Colon Rectum* 35:1077, 1992.

51. Zielke A, Hasse C, Kisker O, et al.: Prospective evaluation of ultrasonography in acute colonic diverticulitis. *Br J Surg* 84:385, 1997.

52. Pradel JA, Adell JF, Taourel P, et al.: Acute colonic diverticulitis: Prospective comparative evaluation with US and CT. *Radiology* 205:503–512, 1997.

53. Glazer G, Mann D: Acute pancreatitis. In: Monson J, Duthie G, O'Malley K, eds. *Surgical Emergencies*. Oxford, UK: Blackwell Science, 1999:134.

54. Balthazar EJ: Pancreatitis. In: Gore RM, Levine MS, eds. *Textbook of Gastrointestinal Radiology*, 2nd ed. Philadelphia, PA: WB Saunders, 2000:1767.

55. Jeffrey RB: The pancreas. In: Jeffrey RB, ed. *CT and Sonography of the Acute Abdomen*. New York, NY: Raven Press, 1989:111.

56. Cosgrove DO: The pancreas. In: Meire H, Cosgrove D, Dewbury K, et al., eds. *Clinical Ultrasound* (Vol. 1, abdominal and general ultrasound), 2nd ed. New York, NY: Churchill Livingstone, 1999:349.

57. Laing F: Ultrasonography of the acute abdomen. *Radiol Clin N Am* 30:389, 1992.

58. Ralls PW, Colletti PM, Lapin SA, et al.: Real-time sonography in suspected acute cholecystitis. *Radiology* 155:767, 1985.

59. Danse EM, Laterre PF, Van Beers BE, et al.: Early diagnosis of acute intestinal ischaemia: Contribution of colour Doppler sonography. *Acta Chir Belg* 97:173, 1997.

60. Ripolles T, Simo L, Martinez-Perez MJ, et al.: Sonographic findings in ischemic colitis in 58 patients. *AJR* 184:777–785, 2005.

61. Teefey SA, Roarke MC, Brink JA, et al.: Bowel wall thickening: Differentiation of inflammation from ischemia with color Doppler and duplex US. *Radiology* 198:547, 1996.

62. Danse EM, Van Beers BE, Jamart J, et al.: Prognosis of ischemic colitis: Comparison of color Doppler sonography with early clinical and laboratory findings. *AJR* 175: 1151–1154, 2000.

63. Puylaert JBCM, Van der Zant FM, Mutsaers JAEM: Infectious ileocecitis caused by Yersinia, Campylobacter, and Salmonella: Clinical, radiological and US findings. *Eur Radiol* 7:3–9, 1997.

64. Ido K, Yuasa H, Ide M, et al.: Sonographic diagnosis of small bowel anisakiasis. *J Clin Ultrasound* 26:125–130, 1998.

CHAPTER 12

Renal

Dina Seif and Stuart P. Swadron

The kidney and bladder are two of the most sonographically accessible organs. Both are easily recognizable to those who are new to ultrasound and thus the urinary tract can be a simple starting point for learning point-of-care sonography in the acute care setting.

The primary focus of renal ultrasonography in the emergency setting has been to determine the presence or absence of hydronephrosis.[1-4] As with other areas of point-of-care ultrasound, physicians using the modality for this specific goal have begun to explore new indications for imaging the urinary tract. Ultrasound determination of bladder volume and evaluation of bladder filling before catheterization are two such examples.[5-14] Another important consideration that has arisen with the focused use of renal ultrasound is the management of unexpected or incidental findings, such as masses and cysts.[15-18]

► CLINICAL CONSIDERATIONS

For many years, the standard imaging modality in cases of suspected renal colic was the intravenous pyelogram (IVP). Although IVP is more specific than ultrasound for the detection and characterization of a ureteral stone,[19-23] it has several disadvantages in the emergency and acute care settings, which include the use of iodinated contrast material and exposure to ionizing radiation. Noncontrast spiral CT and ultrasound have largely replaced IVP as the preferred imaging studies for patients presenting to the ED with renal colic.[24-26]

The sensitivity of CT scan in the detection of renal stone disease varies from 86% to 100%.[27-35] CT provides excellent visualization of the urinary tract and renal stones, and has a higher sensitivity for renal calculi compared with ultrasound.[36] However, CT remains less accessible, involves a considerable exposure to radiation, and does not need to be performed emergently in stable patients with uncomplicated clinical presentations. Many physicians are now using CT in place of both ultrasound and IVP because it allows visualization of the urinary tract as well as extraurinary structures such as the appendix and aorta. A retrospective analysis of ED visits from 1996 to 2007 found a 10-fold increase in the use of CT in patients with suspected renal stone disease.[37] However, there was no corresponding increase in the proportion of renal stone diagnoses or hospital admissions. Another study showed that in patients who had resolution of pain with analgesics, immediate imaging by CT in the ED did not lead to reduced morbidity when compared to imaging by CT 2–3 weeks later.[38] The widespread use of CT has raised concerns within the imaging community because of the large cumulative radiation dosage being delivered to patients. The successive and repetitive nature of renal colic virtually assures these patients (especially younger ones) a higher iatrogenic cancer risk and, thus, forms a logical argument for judicious use of CT in this population.[39,40]

Ultrasound, however, can be performed safely and quickly at the bedside with essentially no risks. It is the modality of choice for patients in whom radiation should be avoided such as children and pregnant women. While ultrasound does not give information about renal function, the presence of unilateral hydronephrosis or hydroureter in the setting of hematuria and acute flank pain is very sensitive for the presence of a ureteral stone. Studies comparing point-of-care ultrasound with CT for the detection of hydronephrosis have found sensitivities comparable to comprehensive ultrasonography performed in the radiology suite.[41–44]

The degree of hydronephrosis, in combination with the patient's history and response to analgesics, is helpful to determine the need for urgent consultation with a urologist. Studies have found a relationship between the degree of hydronephrosis on point-of-care ultrasound and ureteral stone size on CT.[45] In this respect, point-of-care ultrasound often provides sufficient information to efficiently guide the treatment and disposition of the patient. Although a patient with mild-to-moderate hydronephrosis can, with few exceptions, be managed on an outpatient basis, the presence of severe hydronephrosis should prompt further definition of the obstruction by CT and urgent consultation or close follow-up.

In the course of utilizing ultrasound of the urinary tract to detect obstruction, practitioners are identifying other abnormalities with increasing frequency. Some of these represent life- or kidney-threatening processes and may prompt timely definitive treatment. Ultrasound is especially sensitive for the presence of cysts and for distinguishing between solid and cystic masses.[46]

Since the differential diagnosis in patients with flank or abdominal pain involves other organs visualized well by point-of-care ultrasound, invaluable additional information may be available. Specifically, if no hydronephrosis is seen on ultrasound examination, the physician may proceed to visualize the gallbladder, common bile duct, and abdominal aorta.

In the setting of trauma, ultrasound is not the definitive imaging modality; however, it may be used to triage unstable patients in whom renal injury is suspected but who cannot undergo CT. An evolving application of ultrasound in trauma uses semiquantitative Doppler measurements to evaluate renal blood flow. The renal Doppler resistive index, a measurement of tissue resistance to perfusion caused by vasoconstriction, has been shown to predict occult hemorrhagic shock in normotensive polytrauma patients with high sensitivity and specificity.[47]

One of the major advantages of ultrasound is that it can be performed directly at the point of care, in conjunction with the physical examination and without having to move the patient to the radiology suite. Sonography in this fashion is being performed by urologists evaluating patients in the ED and is also helpful in remote or austere locations where other imaging may not exist.[48,49]

► CLINICAL INDICATIONS

Indications for ultrasound examination of the urinary tract in the emergency and acute care setting are as follows:

- Acute flank pain/suspected renal colic
- Acute urinary retention and bladder size estimation
- Acute renal failure
- Hematuria
- Acute pyelonephritis and renal abscess
- Possible renal mass
- Trauma

ACUTE FLANK PAIN/SUSPECTED RENAL COLIC

A focused point-of-care ultrasound examination of the kidneys is indicated for evaluation of the patient with suspected renal colic. Because of the prevalence of renal stone disease, this diagnosis is in the differential of all patients presenting with abdominal or flank pain. While ultrasonography is primarily utilized in patients presenting with flank pain and hematuria, its use also may be considered in the broader group of patients with undifferentiated abdominal pain and the absence of hematuria since renal stone disease may present in this fashion as well.

Studies have reported very high sensitivity of ultrasound for the detection of urolithiasis.[44,50] These studies employed specific protocols, including fasting and IV hydration prior to a comprehensive renal ultrasound that can last up to 30 minutes. Such conditions are not always possible in the ED; more importantly, the goal of emergency renal ultrasound is not to identify stones, but rather to detect hydronephrosis, an important consequence of obstructive uropathy (Figure 12-1). The ability to detect acute urinary obstruction is what makes ultrasound an invaluable tool in the emergency setting.[51] Sensitivity and specificity of point-of-care ultrasound for the detection of hydronephrosis range from 80% to 94% and 82% to 99%, respectively.[18,41,42,52,53] This is comparable to the sensitivities reported in the urology literature for point-of-care ultrasound[48] and in the radiology literature for traditional renal ultrasound.[43,50,54]

In patients who have no or mild hydronephrosis, a ureteral calculus larger than 5 mm is unlikely.[45] Patients who are dehydrated may fail to show the signs of hydronephrosis on ultrasound,[20,56] and it is for this reason that oral or IV hydration is recommended before obstructive hydronephrosis can be excluded. Conversely, a patient with a full bladder may have the appearance of bilateral hydronephrosis; if such a situation is

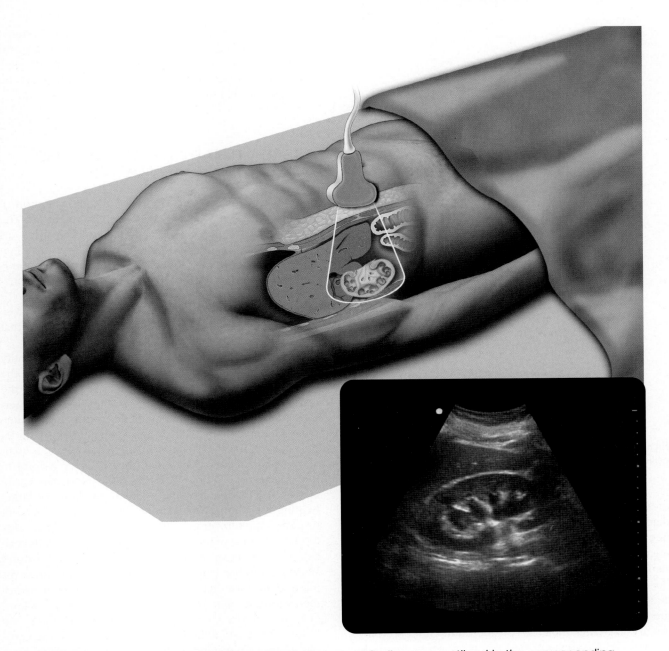

Figure 12-1. Hydronephrosis. Ultrasound techniques and findings are outlined in the corresponding sections of this chapter.

encountered, the ultrasound examination should be repeated after the patient voids.[56] Because of the variations in hydration and bladder volume, it is extremely important to obtain images of both kidneys (for comparison) and the bladder, and to correlate point-of-care ultrasound findings with the clinical picture.

The persistence of bilateral hydronephrosis may indicate bladder outlet obstruction and thus further study is indicated. With long-standing hydronephrosis, thinning of the medulla and cortex begins to occur.[46] The presence of right-sided hydronephrosis is a common finding in pregnancy and should not be confused for pathology.[57] Occasionally, the finding of calyceal rupture will be noted by the presence of perinephric fluid with mild-to-moderate hydronephrosis. The finding of urinary extravasation is a specific sign of severe acute urinary obstruction and should prompt urgent urologic consultation.

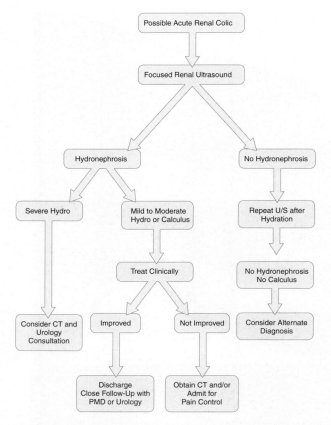

Figure 12-2. Algorithm for the evaluation of renal colic.

In a patient without hematuria and a negative point-of-care ultrasound examination for hydronephrosis, the diagnosis of renal colic becomes extremely unlikely; the negative predictive value of this combination is high.[41] If microscopic hematuria is present and no hydronephrosis is seen, the consideration of other diagnoses should be made even though the diagnosis of renal stone is still possible. Those diagnoses that are immediately life threatening, such as a ruptured abdominal aortic aneurysm (AAA), must be considered in either scenario. Once the clinician is satisfied that more serious pathologies are not present, the patient may be discharged for further workup as necessary on an outpatient basis, which may include CT, comprehensive renal ultrasound, or stone analysis, if collected. The presence of a solitary kidney, renal failure, or urinary tract infection may be indications for admission or further investigation, despite the absence of significant hydronephrosis, when the diagnosis of renal stones is still under consideration.

An algorithm for the evaluation of renal colic that incorporates the use of focused emergency ultrasonography is outlined in Figure 12-2. Some investigators have used a similar algorithm to safely discharge >50% of patients presenting to the ED with flank pain using only urinalysis, analgesia, and point-of-care ultrasound of the kidneys and aorta.[53]

An evolving technique in the evaluation of renal outflow obstruction involves the imaging of ureteral jets.[58,59] In the normal bladder, the intermittent ejection of urine into the bladder from the ureters can be visualized in real-time examination.

ACUTE URINARY RETENTION AND BLADDER SIZE ESTIMATION

Point-of-care ultrasound can assist in the evaluation of patients with symptoms of acute urinary retention. The placement of a urinary catheter for residual urine, as both a diagnostic and therapeutic procedure, has been the traditional approach when acute urinary retention is being considered. Although this approach does quantify the amount of urine retained, it is uncomfortable for patients and incurs a risk of infection. It is therefore preferable to avoid this procedure unless it is clear that urinary retention exists.

Ultrasound can immediately confirm and quantify the degree of obstruction and retention by imaging the urinary bladder and estimating its size. Many of the studies examining bladder volume have been performed by urologists in conjunction with urodynamic measurements.[5,7–12,59–67] In this setting, even small degrees of error may be unacceptable. By contrast, a qualitative estimate of bladder size may be very helpful in the emergency setting. Bedside ultrasound can easily classify the bladder volume as small, medium, or large, helping the clinician determine the need for emergent urinary catheterization. The presence of a large distended bladder mandates emergency urinary catheterization, whereas an empty or small bladder on ultrasound suggests another cause for the patient's symptoms. An intermediate size may require bladder volume measurements to determine the need for catheterization. Whenever the bladder is imaged in this fashion, examine the kidneys for bilateral hydronephrosis, a concerning complication of long-standing bladder outlet obstruction.

When quantitative data are necessary, as in the evaluation of patients with possible spinal cord compression or cauda equina syndrome, ultrasound can reliably estimate the postvoid residual urinary volume. Studies performed on postoperative patients have demonstrated that three-dimensional measurements correlate with volume measured by catheter drainage, which may obviate the need for this invasive procedure (Figure 12-3).[67]

Another indication for point-of-care ultrasound of the urinary tract is the assessment of bladder volume prior to urinary catheterization of children. Studies have demonstrated that confirming the existence of urine in the bladder prior to catheterization can successfully reduce or even eliminate unsuccessful procedures,[13,14] which are painful and often very traumatic.

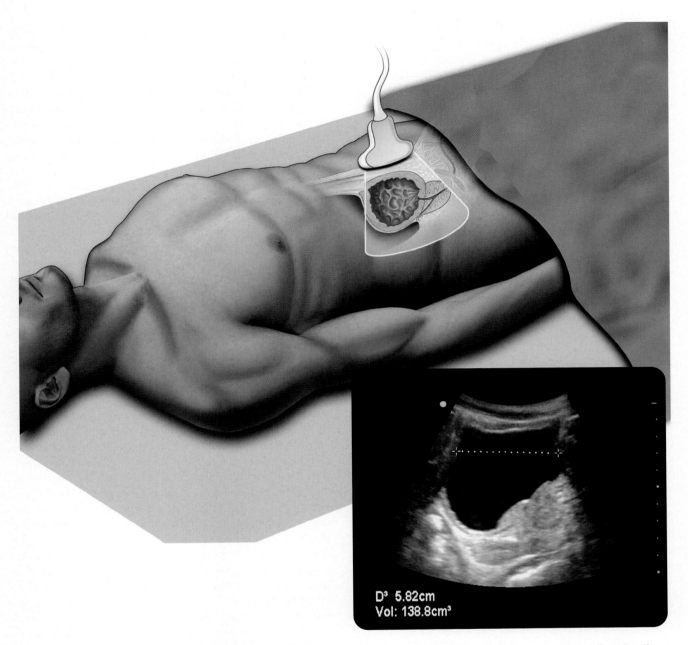

D³ 5.82cm
Vol: 138.8cm³

Figure 12-3. Urinary retention. Ultrasound techniques and findings are outlined in the corresponding sections of this chapter.

ACUTE RENAL FAILURE

Renal ultrasound can be a useful adjunct in the evaluation of acute renal failure. The clinical evaluation of acute renal failure begins with a determination of whether the cause is proximal to the kidneys ("pre-renal" failure), distal to the kidneys ("post-renal" failure), or intrinsic to the kidneys themselves ("renal" failure). Because post-renal causes such as obstruction of either ureteric or urethral outflow are readily reversible if identified in a timely fashion, these are most often considered first in the evaluation. Ultrasound is clearly an effec-

tive tool in the identification of post-renal obstruction, easily detecting bilateral hydronephrosis, and bladder distention. If only a solitary kidney is visualized and hydronephrosis is present, the need for acute decompression becomes particularly urgent. Moreover, prostatic enlargement, one of the most common causes of lower tract obstruction, can be identified on ultrasound.

After a post-renal cause has been excluded, renal ultrasound may provide still further diagnostic information. Although pre-renal causes of renal failure will not generally cause sonographic abnormalities, several causes of acute and acute-on-chronic intrinsic renal failure will manifest themselves on ultrasound examination. Small, atrophic, and hyperechoic kidneys suggest chronic pathologic processes such as hypertensive nephropathy and chronic glomerulonephritis. The finding of enlarged kidneys with multiple cysts distorting the renal architecture suggests polycystic kidney disease (PCKD) as the cause of renal failure. Unfortunately, many causes of acute renal failure that are intrinsic, such as acute glomerulonephritis and acute tubular necrosis, may have nonspecific or minimal sonographic findings. Furthermore, different clinical entities may have different sonographic manifestations at different stages in their presentation. For this reason, other clinical methods, such as volume status determination, response to fluid therapy, microscopic urinalysis, and measurement of the fractional excretion of sodium must be utilized to distinguish between pre-renal and intrinsic causes of renal failure and guide therapy. Renal biopsy, often necessary to establish a definitive diagnosis, may be facilitated by ultrasound guidance.

HEMATURIA

Hematuria occurs in a vast array of medical conditions. In the patient with renal colic, hematuria is a common finding. However, presence of red blood cells on urinalysis has been found to be nonspecific and may occur in life-threatening conditions such as AAA, ectopic pregnancy, and appendicitis. Patients with microscopic hematuria may benefit from a screening bedside renal ultrasound to rule out hydronephrosis, AAA, and any obvious bladder or renal mass. Initial evaluation of patients with gross hematuria should include a bedside renal ultrasound in addition to laboratory testing of hematocrit and renal function.

In the setting of blunt trauma, patients may have microscopic or gross hematuria. Hemodynamically stable patients with profound hematuria in the setting of trauma should undergo contrast-enhanced CT.

ACUTE PYELONEPHRITIS AND RENAL ABSCESS

Acute pyelonephritis, an extremely common emergency diagnosis, does not necessarily require imaging. In fact, the sonographic appearance of the kidney in acute pyelonephritis is most commonly normal.[51] However, in complex cases or those not responding to medical management, ultrasound may be helpful in ruling out complications of pyelonephritis that require surgical management. For example, the formation of a renal abscess may complicate pyelonephritis. Renal abscesses are typically solitary, round hypoechoic masses, often with internal septations or mobile debris, and a degree

of posterior acoustic enhancement.[51,57] Suspicious lesions identified in the course of the point-of-care ultrasound may prompt consultation with a urologist, a comprehensive sonographic study, and, in some cases, CT scanning to further characterize the lesion and formulate a surgical treatment plan.[68] Perinephric abscesses extend beyond the kidney and may be visualized on ultrasound, but are better evaluated with CT. This modality should be sought when lesions are seen to extend beyond the kidney on ultrasound.[51]

Emphysematous pyelonephritis, a rare but life-threatening infection, deserves special mention. Patients with this infection are most frequently diabetic or immunocompromised for other reasons. Because patients with emphysematous pyelonephritis may have toxic and nonspecific presentations, suggestive findings on point-of-care ultrasound may prompt surgical intervention (either percutaneous drainage or open nephrectomy) that would have otherwise been overlooked or unduly delayed.[69–71]

POSSIBLE RENAL MASSES

Renal masses are being seen with increasing frequency as a result of both emergency sonography and the incorporation of screening abdominal ultrasound into periodic health evaluations.[15,18,72–74] There is no question that the mortality and morbidity of malignancies detected in this incidental fashion are greatly reduced.[75–77] Although there is concern regarding the cost-effectiveness of routine use of ultrasound in the absence of specific symptomatology, a mechanism for the follow-up of abnormalities found in the emergency and acute care setting must be available. It cannot be overemphasized that the focused use of ultrasound to evaluate a patient for hydronephrosis is not a substitute for comprehensive sonography or other follow-up studies. Moreover, renal masses discovered on ultrasound almost always require further characterization with another modality, usually CT.[51] The majority of malignancies seen in the kidney are renal cell carcinoma (RCC).[16,74,78,79] These tumors are extremely variable in their sonographic appearance and may be isoechoic, hyperechoic, or hypoechoic relative to the adjacent parenchyma. It is also important to note that many of these tumors have a partially cystic presentation and may be mistaken for a simple benign cyst.[51]

Another common tumor seen in the kidney is angiomyolipoma (AML).[51,78] These tumors are mostly benign and may be treated conservatively.[80] Although they are usually well demarcated and brightly echogenic on ultrasound, there is a significant overlap in their sonographic appearance with that of echogenic RCC.[81] This serves to underscore the caution that is required in the interpretation of any mass found incidentally during ultrasound. Any such finding requires follow-up with a comprehensive ultrasound examination, a CT scan, or urologic consultation.

Other tumors that are commonly seen on ultrasound are lymphomas and metastatic malignancies, which commonly appear as irregular nodules, either single or multiple. These may also be diffuse, grossly disturbing the renal architecture or infiltrative, extending into the perirenal and surrounding structures.[51] Transitional cell carcinoma (TCC), which is more commonly found in the bladder and ureter than in the renal pelvis, is frequently not visible on renal ultrasound. This is because it is frequently symptomatic (with gross hematuria) before sufficient tumor mass can be seen in the renal pelvis. Its sonographic appearance is one of a hypoechoic mass within the highly echogenic renal sinus.[51]

Renal cysts are an extremely common finding on ultrasound. Although simple cysts are benign, malignancies may present with a cystic appearance.[82] For this reason, caution needs to be exercised before dismissing a lesion seen on sonography as a simple cyst.

PCKD can be recognized as an abundance of cysts of varying sizes that both enlarge and distort the regular renal architecture.[51,57,82] Ultrasound is the modality of choice to evaluate this inheritable disorder, which may present with hematuria, flank pain, hypertension, or renal failure. Cysts are frequently present in multiple organs in the body, and there is an association with cerebral aneurysms.[82] Urology or nephrology referral is indicated upon discovery of this disorder. Patients with chronic renal failure undergoing long-term dialysis also tend to develop multiple renal cysts. This disorder, known as acquired renal cystic disease (ARCD), is characterized by a huge increase in the incidence of renal malignancies, and for this reason regular surveillance of this condition is indicated.[51,82]

RENAL TRAUMA

The primary sonographic indicators of major renal trauma are subcapsular hematoma, perinephric hematoma, or calyceal dilation associated with internal echogenicity. These findings may be recognized on the initial trauma ultrasound screening examination or on subsequent examinations. Studies show that while standard B-mode sonography has high specificity for urologic trauma, the sensitivity is low and may miss significant injuries.[83-85] Therefore, hemodynamically stable patients with major trauma in whom injury of the renal pedicle is suspected are best evaluated with contrast-enhanced CT, which provides information about renal function and is considered the modality of choice.[83] If CT is not available, newer ultrasound techniques such as color Doppler or contrast ultrasound may provide much more information than standard B-mode sonography.[86-89]

Ultrasound may have a role in the follow-up and management of patients with identified parenchymal injury, such as hematomas and lacerations. These lesions are often well visualized by ultrasound and can be evaluated periodically to monitor their resolution.

► ANATOMICAL CONSIDERATIONS

COMPARTMENTS OF THE RETROPERITONEUM

Before describing the gross anatomy of the kidney, ureter, and bladder, it is first important to review where these structures lie within the abdominal cavity and their relation to surrounding structures.

The retroperitoneal cavity is divided into three distinct compartments (Figure 12-4), with the kidneys occupying the middle or perirenal compartment. The anterior compartment contains the duodenum, pancreas, descending colon, celiac trunk, and superior mesenteric vessels, as well as associated fat. The posterior compartment, which lies anterior to the quadratus lumborum and psoas muscles, simply contains fat. The anterior and posterior compartments are also referred to as the pararenal compartments.

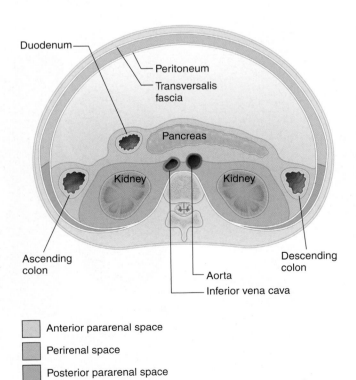

Figure 12-4. Anatomic compartments of the retroperitoneum.

The perirenal compartment is bounded by Gerota's fascia both anteriorly and posteriorly, although many authors refer to the posterior component of the renal fascia as Zuckerkandl's fascia. This fascia, which invests the kidneys, adrenal glands, renal hila, proximal collecting system and perinephric fat, merges laterally to form the lateroconal fascia that extends to the parietal peritoneum of the lateral paracolic gutter. This completes the separation of the anterior and posterior retroperitoneal compartments. Thus, the kidneys are surrounded by two distinct layers of fat: the perinephric fat, which lies immediately outside the true fibrous capsule of the kidney, bounded by Gerota's fascia, and the paranephric fat, which lies in the pararenal compartments outside of Gerota's fascia.

This compartmentalization of the retroperitoneum is important clinically as it serves to localize various pathologic processes. It also creates a barrier to the progression of various pathologic processes such as hemorrhage and infection. Collections of fluid in the anterior pararenal compartment, for example, are commonly related to pancreatitis or trauma, whereas collections of fluid in the posterior pararenal compartment are uncommon, usually representing spontaneous hemorrhage in patients with coagulopathy or related to trauma.

ANATOMIC RELATIONSHIPS OF THE URINARY SYSTEM

There is significant asymmetry in the position of the two kidneys within the abdominal cavity. The right kidney is bounded anteriorly by the liver, which serves as an excellent acoustic window for sonography. It is usually slightly larger and slightly inferior to the left kidney. The left kidney is bounded anteriorly by several structures, including the pancreas, stomach, spleen, and large and small bowel, making it somewhat more difficult to image, as only the spleen serves as an acoustic window of equal quality to the liver. Both kidneys have symmetrical relationships, with the diaphragms superiorly and the musculature of the retroperitoneum (psoas and quadratus) posteriorly. In the supine position, the superior pole of the left kidney is at the level of the 12th thoracic vertebrae and the inferior pole is at the level of the 3rd lumbar vertebrae. However, it is important to realize that the kidneys are mobile structures within the retroperitoneum, moving with changes in position and with phases of respiration. Figure 12-5 demonstrates the anatomical relationships of the two kidneys.

The renal hilum is the specific area of the sinus where the renal artery enters and the renal vein and

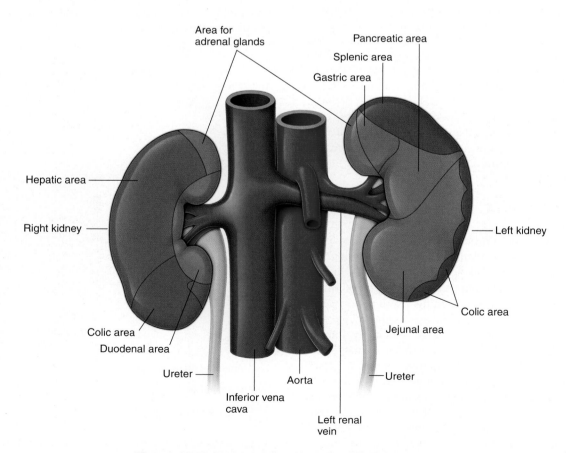

Figure 12-5. Anatomic relationship of the kidneys.

ureter exit the kidney on its medial concave surface. The ureters, which arise from the hila of each kidney, travel inferiorly toward the bladder in close relation to the psoas muscle, just anterior to the transverse process of the lumbar spine. As they enter the pelvis, they course medially to cross the iliac vessels and then laterally once again to parallel the margins of the bony pelvis before inserting posteriorly into the bladder.

The bladder, when empty, abuts the posterior aspect of the pubis. As it fills, it expands to fill more of the pelvis, displacing bowel loops into the abdomen. A distended bladder moves into the lower abdomen and gains relationships to the anterior abdominal wall.

RENAL ANATOMY

The kidneys are paired structures that lie obliquely with respect to every anatomic plane. They are situated so that their inferior poles are anterior and lateral to their superior poles. In addition, each hilum is directed obliquely in an anteromedial rather than simply medial orientation. The sonographic significance of this orientation is that the technique for imaging the kidneys must involve adjusting the transducer obliquely in each plane to match the anatomy.[56,90]

Each kidney is between 9 and 13 cm in its maximum longitudinal measurement, and they decrease in size with advanced age and chronic renal failure. The approximate width and depth of the kidneys is 5 cm and 3 cm, respectively. Each kidney is surrounded by a true fibrous capsule and can be divided into two parts (Figure 12-6), the renal parenchyma and the renal sinus. The renal parenchyma, which surrounds the sinus on all sides except at the hilum, is composed of the outer cortex, consisting of the filtration components of the nephrons, and the inner medulla, consisting of the reabsorptive components (loops of Henle). The cone-shaped medullary pyramids are oriented with their apices, or papillae, protruding inward toward the renal sinus. Thus, the functional unit of the kidney, or renal lobe, consists of a medullary pyramid and its surrounding cortex: urine being filtered by the cortex and then excreted through the papillae into the collecting system. There are between 8 and 18 such lobes in each kidney, bounded by interlobar arteries and veins. The arcuate

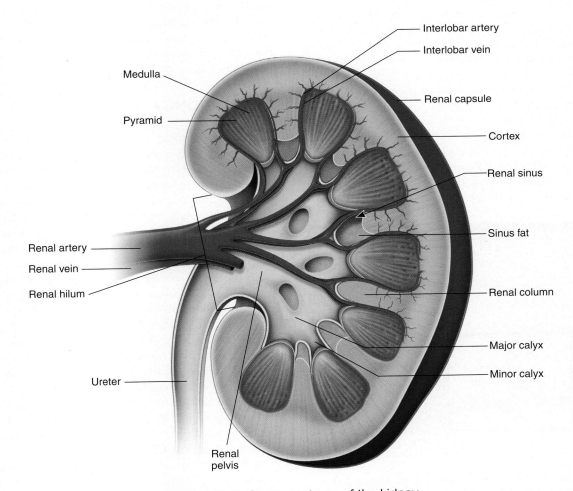

Figure 12-6. Gross anatomy of the kidney.

arteries, which branch from these interlobar arteries, are found at the base of the medullary pyramids and can serve as important landmarks in the interpretation of sonographic images.

The renal sinus, the central portion of the kidney, begins where the renal papillae empty their urine into the smallest subunit of the collecting system, the minor calyces. There are, therefore, between 8 and 18 minor calyces in each kidney corresponding to the pyramids. These minor calyces in turn coalesce into two to three major calyces. The major calyces merge with the renal pelvis, which is the dilated proximal end of the ureter as it joins the kidney. In addition to the collecting system, the renal sinus also contains the renal artery and vein, as well as fatty tissue, which is an extension of the perinephric fat bounded by Gerota's fascia.

► GETTING STARTED

Basic renal sonography can be performed with almost any machine suitable for point-of-care ultrasound. An ideal transducer is a phased array 3.5–5.0 MHz transducer, which has a small footprint and allows easier navigation through the ribs. A larger curved array transducer can be used, but rib shadows may be problematic and could obscure critical areas. Images from a curved array transducer will tend to have higher quality and resolution, and may show greater detail. A starting depth of 15 cm will suffice for most patients and can be adjusted as needed.

The right kidney is easily visualized given its proximity to the liver, which provides an excellent acoustic window (Figure 12-7). The right kidney can usually be imaged well with the patient in a supine position (as in obtaining Morison's pouch in the FAST examination), but the left kidney may be difficult to image given the

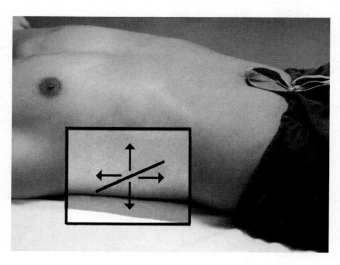

Figure 12-7. Transducer placement for imaging the right kidney. Central line represents the longitudinal axis of the kidney.

lack of a similar acoustic window on that side. Having the patient raise their arms often helps obtain a better window. It is reasonable to start with the patient in the supine position, then, if needed, to move the patient to the right lateral decubitus position (when clinically permissible), which allows the clinician to access the far posterior aspects of the left flank. Initially scan kidneys in the longitudinal plane, which is enhanced by orienting the beam of the transducer in the same plane as the ribs. Once the longitudinal plane has been well visualized, rotate the transducer 90° to obtain the transverse plane.

► TECHNIQUE AND NORMAL ULTRASOUND FINDINGS

While the kidneys are usually imaged using the 3.5 MHz transducer, a 5.0 MHz transducer may be used to yield greater anatomic detail in thin patients or in those patients with a transplanted kidney located in the pelvis. Obtain images of the affected and unaffected kidneys in both the longitudinal and transverse planes. As with other structures, carefully scan through the kidneys in both of these planes to image the entire parenchyma.[90] Identify both kidneys for comparison, and to rule out congenital or surgical absence. Include views of the bladder to assess total filling and identify possible abnormalities (See Video 12-1: Renal Normal).

RIGHT KIDNEY

Scan the right kidney with the patient supine from a position in the mid-axillary line at the right costal margin (Figure 12-8). With the transducer marker directed toward the patient's head, move the transducer inferiorly until the kidney comes into view. Alternatively, move the transducer anteromedially to use the anterior subcostal approach. Because of the kidney's oblique lie, rotate the transducer to obtain the image of the kidney in its maximal length. This is the longitudinal axis, and once the image is obtained, sweep the transducer anteriorly and posteriorly to scan the entire parenchyma. In many patients it will not be possible to view the entire kidney longitudinally in one window, and separate images are often required of the superior and inferior poles. It also may be necessary to obtain some of the images using intercostal windows or by having the patient inhale deeply and briefly hold their breath, which moves the kidneys inferiorly to a subcostal window. If clinically permissible, it may be useful to have the patient turn toward their left side or lay prone to scan from a subcostal approach.

To obtain the transverse plane images, rotate the transducer 90° from the longitudinal plane so that the transducer marker is toward the patient's right (Figure 12-9). Once in the transverse plane, sweep the

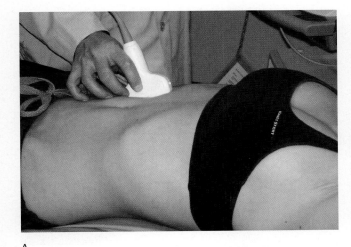

A

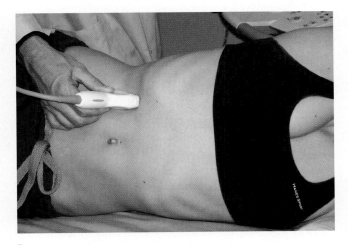

B

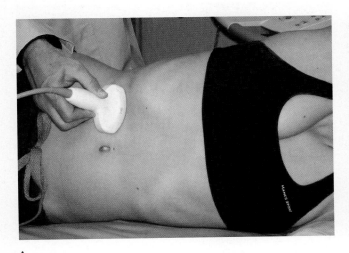

C

Figure 12-8. Longitudinal ultrasound view of the normal right kidney. Transducer position for supine patient (A), transducer position for patient in lateral decubitus (B), and corresponding ultrasound image (C). Model is holding a deep breath for improved kidney imaging. (Courtesy of James Mateer, MD)

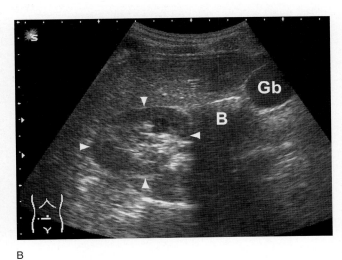

A

B

Figure 12-9. Transverse ultrasound view of the normal right kidney. Transducer position (A) and corresponding ultrasound image (B) with kidney border outlined (arrowheads). Gb = gallbladder, B = bowel with posterior shadowing. (Courtesy of James Mateer, MD)

transducer superiorly and inferiorly to locate the renal hilum, the superior pole, and the inferior pole. Color Doppler imaging is useful to demonstrate flow in the renal artery and vein at the level of the hilum as well as flow in the intrarenal vasculature.

LEFT KIDNEY/BLADDER

Unlike the right kidney, with a generous acoustic window provided by the liver, the clinician has to contend with interference from air in the stomach and intestine in order to obtain images of the left kidney. To obtain the longitudinal images of the left kidney, initially place the transducer in the left posterior axillary line at the costal margin with the transducer marker directed toward the patient's head, moving between the costal margin superiorly and the iliac crest inferiorly to find the kidney (Figure 12-10). As with the right kidney, find the longest

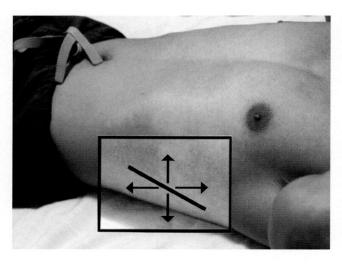

Figure 12-10. Transducer placement for imaging the left kidney. Central line represents the longitudinal axis of the kidney.

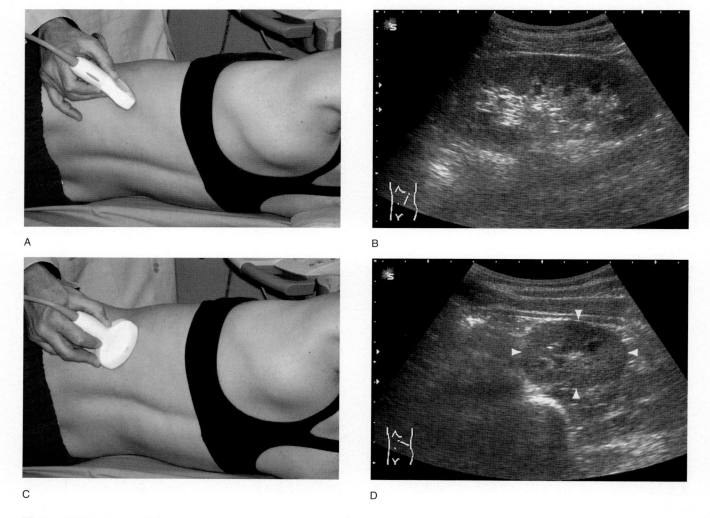

A

B

C

D

Figure 12-11. Normal left kidney. Longitudinal coronal transducer position (A) and long-axis ultrasound image of the kidney (B). Transverse coronal transducer position (C) and short-axis ultrasound image of the kidney (arrowheads) (D). (Courtesy of James Mateer, MD)

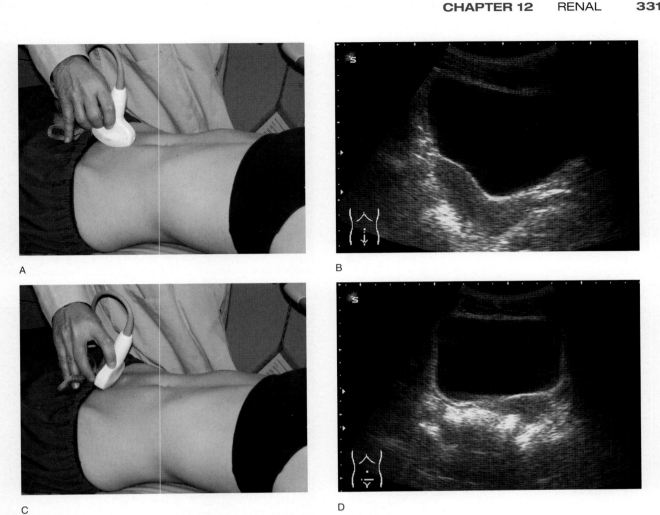

A

B

C

D

Figure 12-12. Normal filled urinary bladder— female model. Longitudinal transducer position (A) and long-axis ultrasound image of the bladder (B). Transverse transducer position (C) and short-axis ultrasound image of the bladder (D). (Courtesy of James Mateer, MD)

axis first before scanning the kidney throughout in this plane (Figure 12-11). To obtain transverse images of the left kidney, simply rotate the transducer 90° so that the transducer marker is toward the patient's right and scan throughout the superior and inferior poles. The renal hilum is often easily identified in the transverse view. If the left kidney is not easily visualized with the patient supine, use a more posterior approach by having the patient turn toward the examiner in the right lateral decubitus position.[56,90] The coronal view is particularly helpful for imaging the inferior pole of the left kidney, which is often obscured by overlying gas within the descending colon.

Scan the bladder with the transducer in the suprapubic position; a moderately filled bladder is optimal for imaging. If the bladder is not seen, aim the transducer inferiorly into the pelvis. Scan thoroughly in the sagittal plane (transducer marker toward the patient's head) and transverse plane (transducer marker toward the patient's right) (Figures 12-12,12-13).

SONOGRAPHIC APPEARANCE OF THE KIDNEY, URETER, AND BLADDER

Each kidney is well demarcated by a brightly echogenic fibrous capsule surrounded by a variable amount of perinephric fat. When compared to the liver, the normal renal parenchyma typically has a less echogenic appearance. Within the parenchyma, the outer cortex can often be distinguished from the medulla, which, because of its urine-filled tubules, forms a hypoechoic, saw-toothed ribbon deep to the margin of the cortex. Individual pyramids may or may not be visible as hypoechoic triangular structures within the medulla. The central area of the kidney is the renal sinus, which lies deep to the medulla, and appears highly echogenic because of its high fat content. The renal sinus contains the minor and major calyces that empty into the renal pelvis. In well-hydrated patients, anechoic pockets of urine may be seen within the calyces. When scanned in real time, the continuity of these pockets with the renal

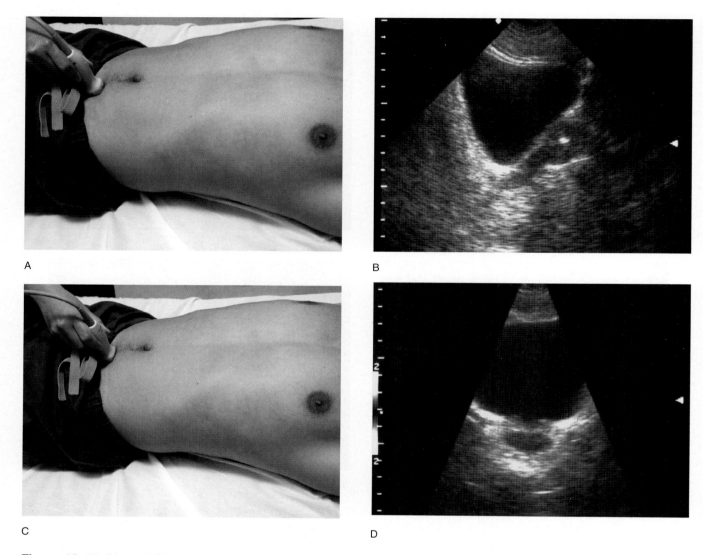

Figure 12-13. Normal filled urinary bladder—male model. Longitudinal transducer position (A) and long-axis ultrasound image of the bladder (B). Note prostate posteriorly that also contains a small central calcification. Transverse transducer position (C) and short-axis ultrasound image of the bladder (D).

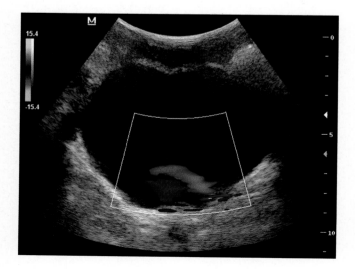

Figure 12-14. Ureteral jet—Color Doppler. Transverse view of the bladder reveals a normal, ureteral flow jet arising from the trigone area on the left. (Courtesy of James Mateer, MD)

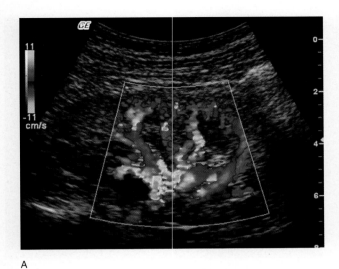

A

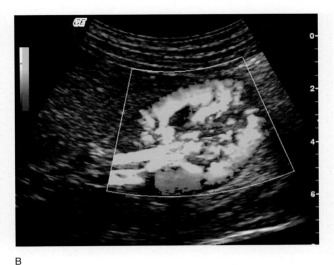

B

Figure 12-15. Color Doppler of right kidney—longitudinal views. Color flow Doppler may demonstrate directional flow in both the renal arteries and veins (A). Power Doppler imaging of the kidney may identify general tissue blood flow (B). (Reprinted with permission from GE Healthcare.)

pelvis can be demonstrated. Figures 12-8 and 12-9 show normal longitudinal and transverse ultrasound images of the right kidney. Although the normal ureter is not seen on ultrasound, a proximally distended ureter can often be visualized.

The shape and relationships of the bladder on ultrasound examination depend on its degree of filling (Figures 12-12, 12-13). With urine in the bladder, its wall appears as an echogenic line surrounding an anechoic cavity. The prostate gland may be recognized as a hyperechoic ovular mass at the bladder neck (Figure 12-13).

In patients with normal hydration and no ureteral obstruction, intermittent ureteral flow jets can be observed near the trigone area. These can be visualized with gray scale sonography but are more obvious using color Doppler techniques (Figure 12-14). As urine flows into a filled bladder, the ureteral jets appear as color signals that flow in an anteromedial direction and should cross the midline.[86]

The vascularity of the kidneys makes them amenable to Doppler imaging for confirmation of normal blood flow. The quality of these images will depend on patient factors, skill of the operator, and the sensitivity of the color Doppler imaging on the ultrasound machine. Color flow Doppler can be used to identify arterial versus venous flow (Figure 12-15A), while power Doppler is used primarily to demonstrate overall tissue flow (Figure 12-15B).

► COMMON ABNORMALITIES

OBSTRUCTIVE UROPATHY

The degree of hydronephrosis seen on ultrasound represents a continuum of urinary obstruction (See Video 12-2: Renal Abnormal). Anechoic areas can be seen within the echogenic renal sinus as urine distends the collecting system. Designations of mild, moderate, and severe hydronephrosis are commonly used (Figures 12-16 and 12-17);

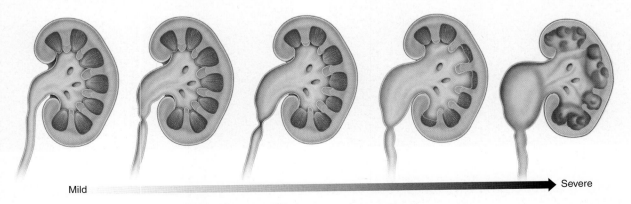

Mild   Severe

Figure 12-16. Grades of hydronephrosis.

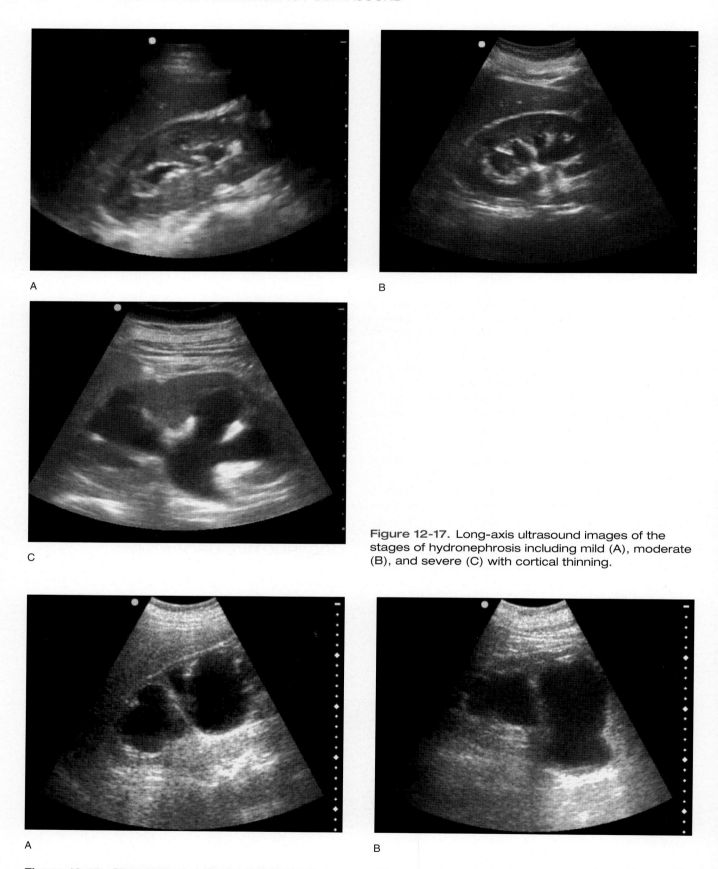

A

B

C

Figure 12-17. Long-axis ultrasound images of the stages of hydronephrosis including mild (A), moderate (B), and severe (C) with cortical thinning.

A

B

Figure 12-18. Chronic, severe hydronephrosis. Coronal views of the kidney show severe hydronephrosis and cortical atrophy (A). Another view of the same kidney demonstrates severe urinary distention of the renal pelvis (B). (Courtesy of James Mateer, MD)

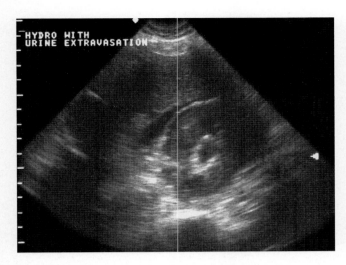

Figure 12-19. Hydronephrosis with acute calyceal rupture. Transverse view of right kidney (outlined by rib shadows) with hydronephrosis and urinary extravasation into the perirenal space.

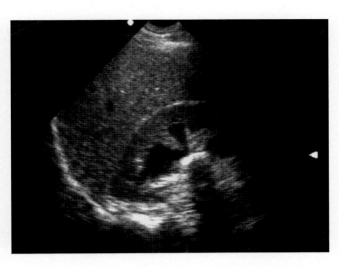

Figure 12-21. Longitudinal view of right kidney shows moderate hydronephrosis and a large stone within the renal pelvis.

however, this grading is quite subjective. Mild hydronephrosis appears as minimal separation of the renal sinus. Intrarenal vasculature can mimic mild hydronephrosis, but color Doppler demonstrating absent flow confirms the diagnosis of hydronephrosis. Moderate hydronephrosis causes greater separation of the renal sinus and extends into the calyces. The designation of severe hydronephrosis is generally reserved for kidneys with marked dilation of the collecting system that demonstrate some degree of parenchymal thinning. For those with chronic severe hydronephrosis, cortical atrophy will be more obvious (Figure 12-18). Occasionally,

high-grade obstruction with hydronephrosis can result in perinephric fluid signifying a ruptured calyx (Figure 12-19).

Renal stones can be seen within the kidney itself and, like gallstones, have a strongly echogenic appearance and cause acoustic shadowing (Figures 12-20, 12-21). Stones are rarely visualized in the mid-ureter, but may occasionally be identified at the ureteropelvic (Figure 12-22) or ureterovesical junctions (Figure 12-23), which are two common locations of obstruction. Stones may also be seen in the bladder.

A phenomenon known as "twinkling artifact" can be seen when color Doppler is applied to a highly

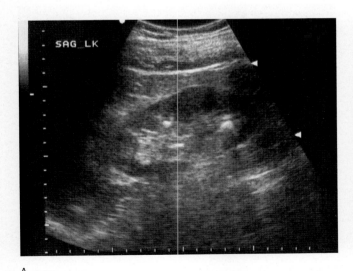

A

B

Figure 12-20. Longitudinal (A) and transverse (B) views of the left kidney show intrarenal stones (with posterior shadowing below the larger of the two stones). (Courtesy of Lori Sens, Gulfcoast Ultrasound)

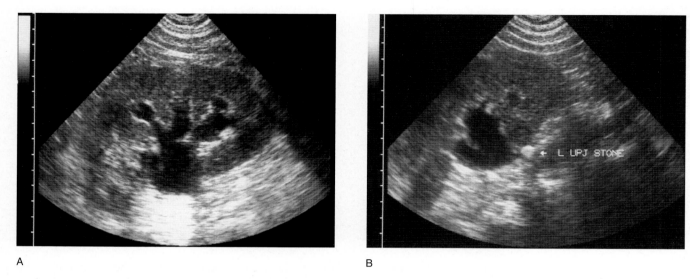

A   B

Figure 12-22. Ureteropelvic junction stone. Coronal view of the kidney (A) shows moderate hydronephrosis. A slightly different angle of the same kidney demonstrates a ureteropelvic junction stone with posterior shadowing (B) as the cause of the urinary obstruction. (Courtesy of James Mateer, MD)

reflective surface, such as a kidney stone. This may be particularly useful when a suspected stone appears indistinct and has poor posterior acoustic shadowing. In place of the stone shadow, an irregular erratic color signal may be seen.

In the presence of unilateral obstruction, ureteral jet flow to the ipsilateral side is slow, continuous, prolonged, diverted, decreased, or absent. Asymmetric or absent flow may suggest high-grade obstruction;[58] the sonographer should perform prolonged imaging to confirm the absence of flow.[91] Abnormalities in ureteral jets

are more likely to be seen in high-grade obstruction than low-grade obstruction. Thus, ultrasound imaging of ureteral jets can provide valuable information on urinary tract function.

In patients with indwelling urinary catheters who have flank or abdominal pain, point-of-care ultrasound is useful to evaluate malfunction of the catheter. A functioning catheter will appear as a spherical object representing the fluid-filled balloon within a decompressed bladder (Figure 12-24). An obstructed catheter

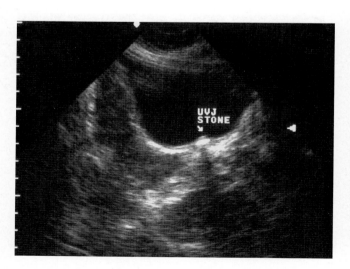

Figure 12-23. Ureterovesical junction stone. Ureteral stone shown at the ureterovesical junction through a transverse view of the bladder.

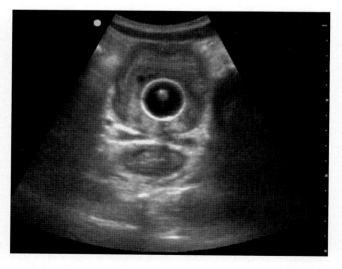

Figure 12-24. Urinary catheter balloon. Transverse view of decompressed bladder with urinary catheter balloon. Circumferential bladder wall thickening is seen, which was due to chronic cystitis.

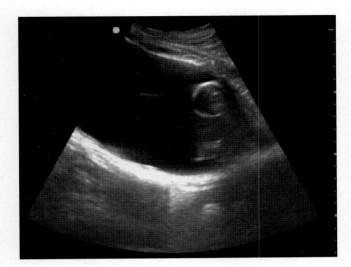

Figure 12-25. Obstructed urinary catheter. Longitudinal view of distended bladder secondary to obstructed urinary catheter. The spherical catheter balloon is easily visualized.

will demonstrate a full bladder (Figure 12-25) and, possibly, hydronephrosis. Ultrasound is also useful for real-time guidance of urinary bladder catheter balloon puncture in cases of balloon malfunction.

BLADDER VOLUME MEASUREMENT

This technique involves measuring the bladder in its maximal width, depth, and length to noninvasively esti-mate urinary volume. It has been used for >25 years and was first performed using B-mode imaging.[5,10] Scan the bladder in two planes in order to obtain three unique measurements. In the transverse plane, measure the diameter between the lateral walls to obtain the width. The height is the anteroposterior diameter, which can be obtained in the transverse or sagittal plane. The length is the craniocaudal diameter, which is obtained by measuring from the superior to inferior wall of the bladder in the sagittal plane. Most current machines contain automated calculators for volume measurement (Figure 12-26). As an alternate, the simple formula (L × W × H × 0.75) can be used to estimate bladder volume.[11] Because of the inherent variability of bladder shape and the variation in this shape with differing degrees of filling, bladder volume measurements obtained in this fashion may have an error rate between 15% and 35%.[5,9–12] This should, however, provide a reliable estimate of the postvoid residual in patients with neurogenic urinary retention. The normal postvoid residual urine volume is 100 mL or less, or 20% of the volume voided.[92]

Point-of-care ultrasound can be used to increase success rates of urethral catheterization in children by identifying the precatheterization volume.[14] The volume may be calculated as described above. Alternatively, using only two measurements, the bladder index volume can be calculated by the product of the anteroposterior and transverse bladder diameters. A calculated bladder index volume of 2.4 cm^2 corresponds to a bladder volume of 2 mL, the minimum volume necessary for accurate urinalysis. Therefore, catheterization should be deferred when the index is less than 2.4 cm^2.[13]

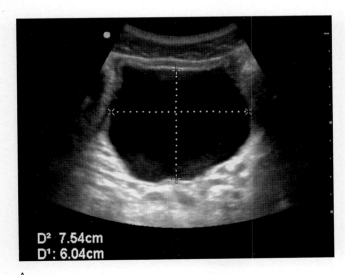

D² 7.54cm
D¹: 6.04cm

A

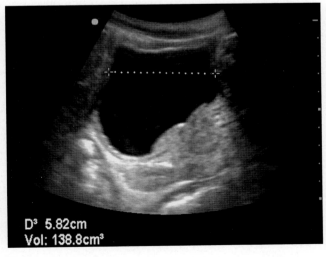

D³ 5.82cm
Vol: 138.8cm³

B

Figure 12-26. Transverse (A) and longitudinal (B) views of the bladder show the use of a software calculation program to determine bladder volume.

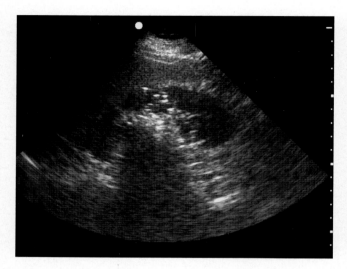

Figure 12-27. Emphysematous pyelonephritis. Longitudinal view of the kidney shows multiple hyperechoic foci with dirty shadowing that represents gas in the renal parenchyma (Courtesy of Thomas Mailhot, MD).

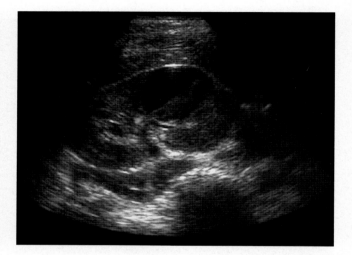

Figure 12-28. Longitudinal view of the kidney shows a large complex cyst in the mid portion of the cortex. The echogenic layer was persistent with transducer angle and position (not an artifact) and was documented as inflammatory debris from a renal abscess (Reproduced with permission from Charles Lanzieri, MD, University Hospitals of Cleveland.)

ACUTE PYELONEPHRITIS AND RENAL ABSCESS

The sonographic appearance of the kidney in acute pyelonephritis is most commonly normal, but cortical inflammation may appear as ill-defined hypoechogenicity. Ultrasound is more useful to evaluate abnormalities in complicated urinary tract infections such as emphysematous pyelonephritis and renal abscess. Emphysematous pyelonephritis is characterized by gas within the parenchyma due to infection by gas-forming bacteria. This appears as hyperechoic areas that distort the renal sinus and shadow posteriorly, often obscuring the deeper structures (Figure 12-27). These hyperechoic areas could potentially be confused with renal stone disease; however, the shadowing of gas is echogenic and "dirty," while calculi tend to cast "clean" shadows. In the setting of pyelonephritis, this finding should prompt further imaging and emergent surgical consultation.

Renal abscesses are typically solitary, round, hypoechoic masses, often with internal septations or mobile debris and a degree of posterior acoustic enhancement (Figure 12-28). When these rupture or extend into the perinephric space, complex fluid may be appreciated surrounding a portion of the kidney.

RENAL MASSES

The majority of malignancies seen in the kidney are RCC.[16,74,78] These tumors are extremely variable in their sonographic appearance and may be isoechoic, hy-perechoic, or hypoechoic to the adjacent parenchyma (Figure 12-29). Many of these tumors have a cystic presentation and may be mistaken for a simple benign cyst.[51]

Another common tumor seen in the kidney is AML.[80] Although they are usually well demarcated and brightly echoic on ultrasound, there is a significant overlap in their sonographic appearance with that of echogenic RCC.[81]

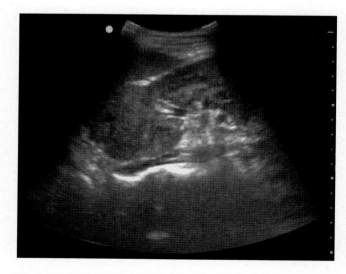

Figure 12-29. Renal cell carcinoma. Longitudinal view of the right kidney showing renal cell carcinoma with enlargement of the upper pole.

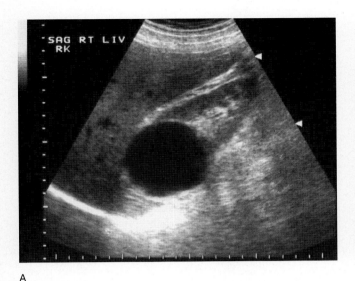

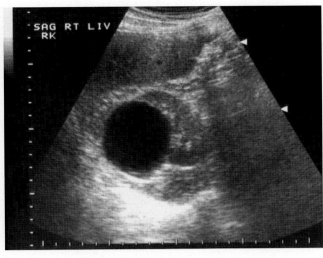

A

B

Figure 12-30. Renal cyst. Longitudinal (A) and transverse (B) views of the right kidney demonstrate the usual features of a simple cyst. (Courtesy of Lori Sens, Gulfcoast Ultrasound).

RENAL CYSTS

Renal cysts are an extremely common finding on ultrasound. A benign cyst must meet all of the following criteria:[51,56,57]

1. Smooth, round, or oval shaped
2. No internal echoes or solid elements
3. Well-defined interface between the cyst and the adjacent renal parenchyma in all planes and orientations
4. Posterior echo enhancement beyond the cyst

Figures 12-30 and 12-31 show the sonographic appearance of simple cysts.

RENAL TRAUMA

Ultrasound is not the definitive modality in the evaluation of renal trauma due to poor sensitivity. Sonography does, however, have high specificity for evidence of renal trauma.[85] The sonographic indicators of major renal trauma are subcapsular hematoma and perinephric hematoma (Figure 12-32). Calyceal dilation with internal echogenicity may also be seen. Ultrasound will not

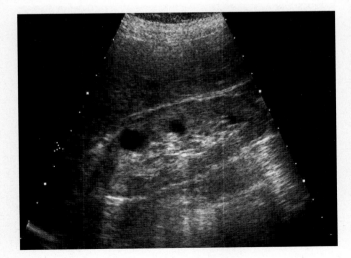

Figure 12-31. Longitudinal view of the right kidney with two small, simple appearing cysts within the middle and upper pole.

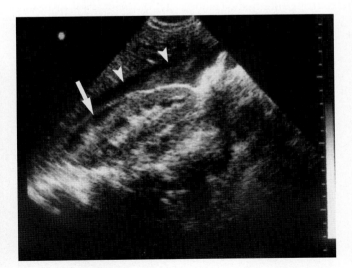

Figure 12-32. Renal trauma. Longitudinal view of the right upper quadrant shows fluid and clots in Morison's pouch (arrowheads) from hepatic injury and capsular elevation and a subcapsular hematoma of the kidney (arrow) related to blunt renal trauma. (Courtesy of James Mateer, MD)

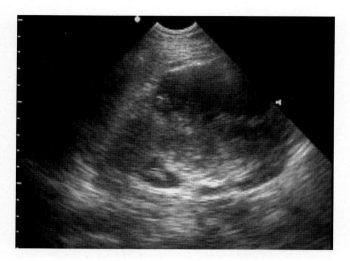

Figure 12-33. Longitudinal view of the kidney demonstrates a large complex subcapsular fluid collection and distorted cortical structure. This represents a subacute hematoma of the kidney.

distinguish fresh blood from urine extravasation; therefore, stable patients should undergo CT.

A fracture of the kidney may be suspected when a hematoma of the kidney parenchyma is present. An organ hematoma will usually be isoechoic in the acute phase, making the ultrasound diagnosis difficult. A fresh hematoma may occasionally appear as an echogenic, heterogeneous, subcapsular mass. Over time, a parenchymal hematoma will become more obvious on ultrasound and hypoechoic relative to the surrounding tissue (Figure 12-33). Using color or power

Doppler, absence of perfusion will be seen in the portion of the kidney containing the hematoma.

If the suspicion for renal injury is high, carefully inspect the pararenal compartments. Fluid in the anterior pararenal space is often difficult to visualize with ultrasound due to overlying bowel gas and lack of a distinct interface with solid organs. Hematomas involving the posterior pararenal compartment of the retroperitoneum (Figure 12-34) must be differentiated from intraperitoneal fluid in Morison's pouch, which in the setting of trauma suggests intra-abdominal organ injury. A high-grade renal injury such as fractured kidney with retroperitoneal hematoma may appear as disorganized renal architecture surrounded by mixed echogenic material.[83] Renal vascular injuries may show abnormal Doppler flow over the hilum. Segmental infarcts may appear as wedge-shaped areas of cortex without perfusion.

► COMMON VARIANTS AND OTHER ABNORMALITIES

SONOLUCENT PYRAMIDS

In some patients, the medullary pyramids appear so sonolucent that they may be mistaken for the anechoic collections of urine seen with hydronephrosis.[56] They can be differentiated from distended calyces by the presence of cortex between them, by their triangular shape, and sometimes by the appearance of arcuate arteries, which appear as bright hyperechoic dots at the base of the pyramids (Figure 12-35).

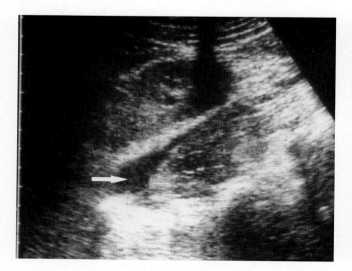

Figure 12-34. Coronal view of the kidney and psoas muscle demonstrates fluid in the posterior pararenal space (arrow). (Courtesy of James Mateer, MD)

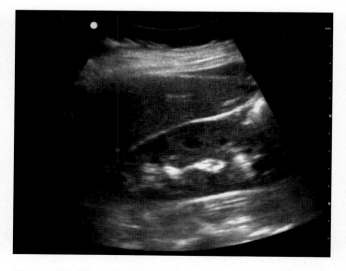

Figure 12-35. Left kidney in long axis with sonolucent renal pyramids. This corresponds with the medullary portions of the kidney.

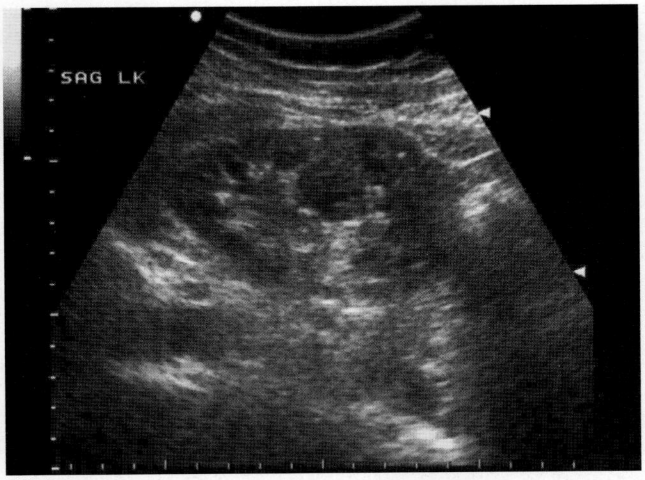

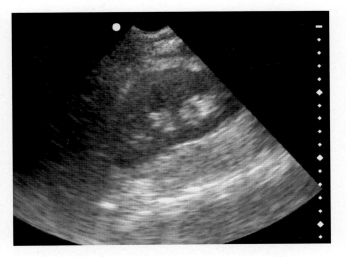

Figure 12-36. Long-axis view of the left kidney demonstrating a column of Bertin displacing the sinus structures. (Courtesy of Lori Sens, Gulfcoast Ultrasound)

Figure 12-37. Long-axis view of the left kidney demonstrating the typical morphology of a dromedary hump. (Courtesy of James Mateer, MD)

HYPERTROPHIED COLUMNS OF BERTIN

Although identification of renal masses is not a goal of focused point-of-care ultrasound of the kidney, there is one common anomaly that deserves special mention because of its potential to be mistaken for a renal mass. A "hypertrophied column of Bertin" refers to an invagination of renal cortical tissue into the renal sinus (Figure 12-36). This can mimic a mass because it may cause an indentation and splaying of the sinus structures. It does, however, have the same echogenicity as the renal cortex and can be seen to be continuous with the cortex in real time. In addition, these columns should not alter the outer contour of the kidney as commonly occurs with RCC.[51,56,57,82]

DROMEDARY HUMP

The dromedary (splenic) hump occurs most commonly on the lateral part of the left kidney as a normal variant and resembles the hump of a dromedary camel. This will appear as a focal, symmetrical, rounded enlargement of the central portion of the cortex with homogenous echotexture. Since the contour of the kidney is altered, it is more difficult to confidently exclude RCC and a follow-up study is recommended (Figure 12-37).

DUPLICATION OF THE COLLECTING SYSTEM

A duplex collecting system is one of the most common congenital renal anomalies and the degree of duplica-

tion can vary. A duplex collecting system may be sonographically detected as two central echogenic sinuses with normal bridging renal parenchyma between them (Figure 12-38). Hydronephrosis of the upper pole sinus and visualization of two distinct collecting systems and ureters is diagnostic of this condition.

ECTOPIC KIDNEY

If the kidney has an abnormal contour or is not found on the flank examinations as described above, then

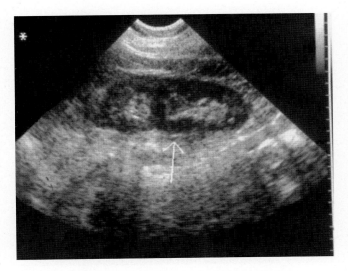

Figure 12-38. Partial duplex collecting system. Long-axis view of the kidney shows a distinct separation between the upper and lower portions of the collecting system within the kidney. (Courtesy of Lori Sens and Lori Green, Gulfcoast Ultrasound)

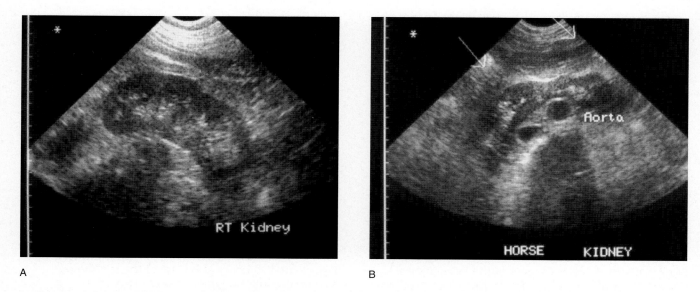

A

B

Figure 12-39. Horseshoe kidney. (A) Longitudinal view of the right kidney shows a slightly unusual shape and an indistinct lower pole. The horseshoe kidney could have been missed if transverse views had not been done (B). Transverse views clearly demonstrated a connection of the lower poles of both kidneys in the midline over the aorta (labeled). (Courtesy of Lori Sens and Lori Green, Gulfcoast Ultrasound)

congenital abnormalities such as horseshoe kidney (Figure 12-39), pelvic kidney (Figure 12-40), or congenital absence of a kidney must be entertained. In any of these circumstances, consideration of comprehensive imaging and specialty consultation is indicated. All of these abnormalities place the patient with obstructive uropathy and other renal pathologies at increased risk for complications.

KIDNEY TRANSPLANT

Transplanted kidneys are usually placed in an extraperitoneal location in the iliac fossa, making them easily accessible for evaluation by ultrasound. Because of the relatively superficial location of a transplanted kidney, anatomical structures are more pronounced and well defined (Figure 12-41). Identification of intrarenal

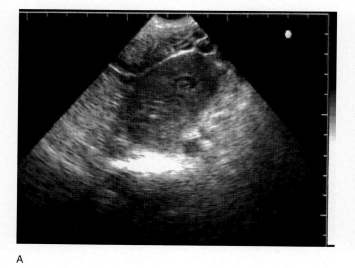

A

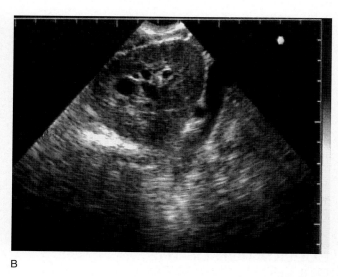

B

Figure 12-40. Pelvic kidney. Endovaginal image with a 7.5 MHz transducer. Left adnexal mass is noted to be kidney shaped (A). Detailed views demonstrated normal renal architecture and a position adjacent to the iliac vein (B). (Courtesy of James Mateer, MD)

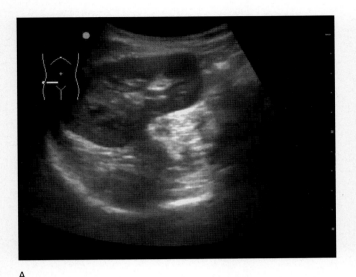

A

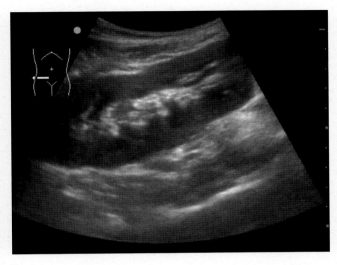

B

Figure 12-41. Transplanted kidney. Right pelvic transplanted kidney in iliac fossa (A). Longitudinal view (B) shows no fluid collection, mass, or hydronephrosis.

vasculature and prominent hypoechoic medullary pyramids is much more common. Additionally, the boundary between cortex and medulla is accentuated. Evaluate transplanted kidneys for hydronephrosis, which may be a sign of ureteric compression by hematoma or abscess. Hydronephrosis may also be a result of ureteric stenosis, which is a late complication of renal transplant. Hematomas may be identified after transplant or biopsy. Urinary leaks may appear as peri-ureteric anechoic fluid collections. Scan the parenchyma for abscesses in the setting of infection. Transplanted kidneys can also develop cysts and tumors that should be evaluated with complementary imaging. Acute rejection is a major concern and should be considered in patients with deteriorating renal function; the ultrasound findings are nonspecific in the acute phase. Vascular complications such as thrombosis and stenosis may be evaluated using Doppler imaging; comprehensive imaging is indicated in these cases.

PROSTATE ENLARGEMENT

An enlarged prostate gland may be seen while imaging the bladder on transabdominal ultrasonography. It may be recognized as a hyperechoic ovular mass at the bladder neck and should be considered enlarged when the transverse diameter is more than 4 cm (Figure 12-42). Volume measurements of the prostate are a more accurate way to evaluate prostate size. As the specific gravity of prostate tissue is 1.050, the prostate weight in grams can be estimated by calculating the volume in

cubic centimeters. The normal prostate volume is less than 25 mL.

POLYCYSTIC KIDNEYS

PCKD can be recognized as an abundance of cysts of varying sizes that both enlarge and distort the regular renal architecture (Figure 12-43). Patients with PCKD will often also have hepatic cysts. Follow-up is recommended for these patients.

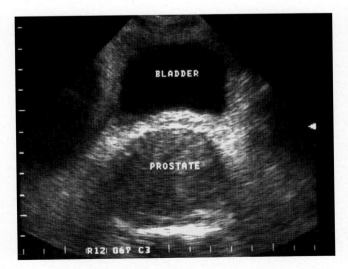

Figure 12-42. Enlarged prostate. Transverse view of the bladder shows an enlarged prostate posteriorly.

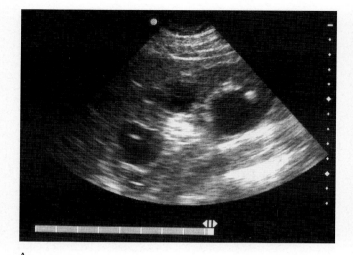

A

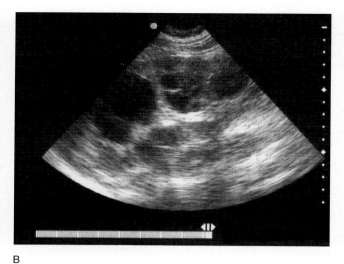

B

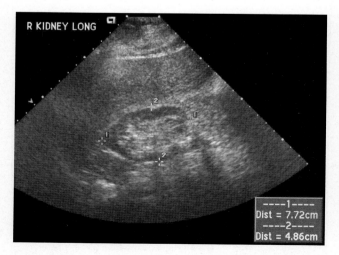

C

Figure 12-43. Adult polycystic kidney disease. Coronal views of the right (A) and left (B) kidneys demonstrate adult polycystic kidney disease. CT scan of the same patient (C) for comparison. (Courtesy of James Mateer MD).

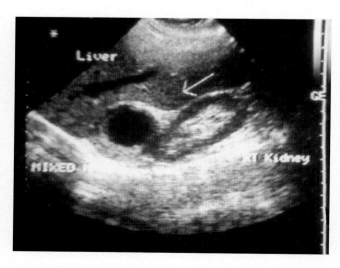

Figure 12-44. Chronic renal disease. This kidney demonstrates thinning of the cortex, and a contracted size, from chronic renal disease.

Figure 12-45. Adrenal mass. The right adrenal mass (arrow) has a thickened ring of tissue surrounding a cystic central portion. (Courtesy of Lori Sens and Lori Green, Gulfcoast Ultrasound)

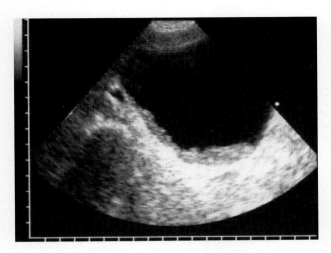

Figure 12-46. Bladder wall tumor. Transverse view of the bladder reveals a localized irregular thickening of the posterolateral bladder wall. (Courtesy of James Mateer, MD)

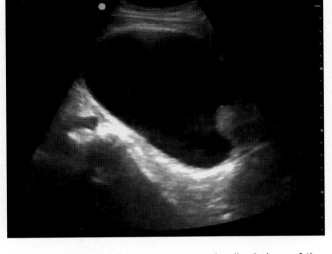

Figure 12-47. Bladder mass. Longitudinal view of the bladder shows a polypoid mass in a patient with acute urinary retention. The mass was subsequently diagnosed as benign prostatic hyperplasia.

CHRONIC RENAL DISEASE

The most common sonographic findings in chronic renal failure are that of bilateral small and hyperechoic kidneys. A variety of pathologic processes ranging from diseases of the glomerulus (e.g., glomerulonephritis), infection (e.g., chronic pyelonephritis), and renal vascular disease may result in these sonographic findings. They are not specific to any particular etiology (Figure 12-44).

ADRENAL MASS

Although the normal adrenal glands may not be visualized during focused ultrasound of the urinary tract in the acute care setting, moderate and large adrenal masses

may be seen anteromedially to the superior pole of the kidney. Because of the excellent acoustic window provided by the liver, right-sided masses are often better visualized. The appearance of adrenal masses is varied, as is the underlying pathology. Additional imaging with CT and biopsy may both be required to make a definitive pathologic diagnosis (Figure 12-45).

BLADDER MASS

Bladder masses, both benign and malignant, may present as focal bladder wall thickening (Figure 12-46) or as an irregular echogenic mass projecting into the lumen (Figure 12-47 and 12-48). If such a mass is

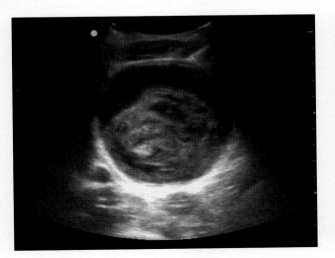

A

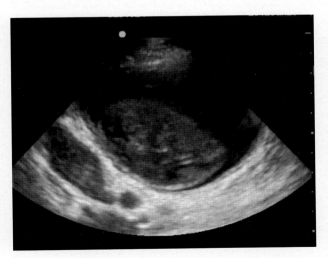

B

Figure 12-48. Bladder mass. Transverse (A) and longitudinal (B) views of the bladder demonstrate a large heterogenous bladder mass representing metastatic prostate cancer.

visualized, address the possibility of upper tract obstruction by visualizing the kidneys as well as examining for hydronephrosis. Further imaging and biopsy are required to make a definitive diagnosis.

▶ PITFALLS

1. Point-of-care ultrasound is limited in scope. Any abnormalities that are recognized require close follow-up.
2. Several fairly common processes may mimic the presence of hydronephrosis, including prominent medullary pyramids, renal cortical cysts, renal vessels, an overdistended bladder, and pregnancy. Color Doppler is useful to differentiate renal vessels. Renal parapelvic cysts are less common but are easily confused with hydronephrosis due to their central location within the renal sinus. They can be differentiated from hydronephrosis due to their round shape and

their lack of communication with the fluid-filled renal pelvis. Extrarenal pelvis is a congenital variant in which the renal pelvis lies outside of the kidney. It can also be confused with hydronephrosis. The visible anechoic area will be anatomically related to the sinus but will lie outside of the body of the kidney.[93] Always scan both kidneys for comparison and evaluate the bladder for degree of filling.
3. Presence of hydronephrosis may be masked by dehydration. If ureterolithiasis is suspected, obtain images after the patient receives either an IV or an oral fluid bolus.
4. The absence of hydronephrosis does not rule out a ureteral stone. Small stones and early presentations of acute obstruction may not cause significant enough obstruction to produce hydronephrosis.
5. Absence of ureteral jets must be confirmed with prolonged ultrasound imaging. The combination of hydronephrosis and absent ureteral jets

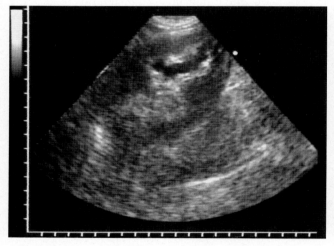

A

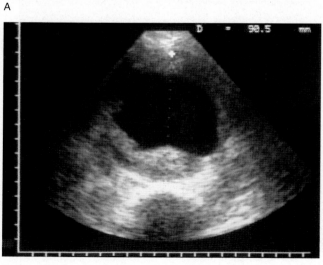

C

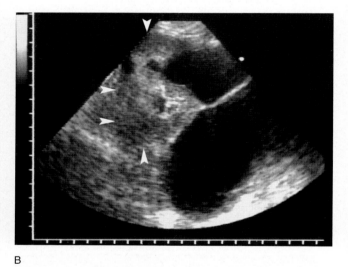

B

Figure 12-49. Hydronephrosis from AAA. A coronal view of the inferior pole of the left kidney reveals mild hydronephrosis (A). A coronal view of the lower flank (angled superiorly) in the same patient shows a septated fluid collection that communicates with the collecting system of the kidney (B). The renal borders are outlined (arrowheads). The contained fluid collection is a perinephric urinoma secondary to ureteral compression with calyceal rupture from a large (9.0 cm) AAA (C). (Courtesy of James Mateer MD)

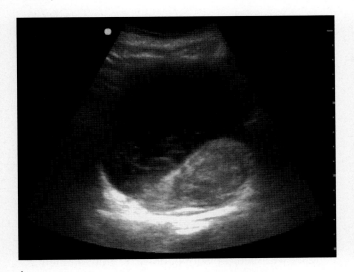

A

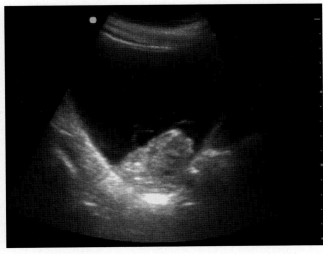

B

Figure 12-50. Bladder hematoma. Transverse (A) and longitudinal (B) views of the bladder in a patient with gross hematuria show a posterior mass that resolved following bladder irrigation. (Courtesy of Thomas Mailhot, MD)

suggests high-grade urinary tract obstruction. However, evaluation of ureteral jets may require up to 10 minutes of scanning in order to determine absence of flow.[94]

6. Patients with an acute AAA often present with flank pain. A ruptured AAA can present with a clinical picture suggesting acute renal colic. A large AAA can potentially compress the ureter and cause hydronephrosis. In patients older than 50 years with suspected renal colic, always scan the aorta in addition to the urinary tract (Figure 12-49).

7. A bladder mass may be a hematoma. In patients with gross hematuria, blood may accumulate in the bladder and appear as a mass on ultrasound. When suspected, this can be confirmed by resolution of the mass following bladder irrigation (Figure 12-50).

► CASE STUDIES

CASE 1

Patient Presentation

A 38-year-old man presented to the ED at 3 AM after 2 hours of excruciating left flank pain and vomiting. He had similar pain the day prior, but it was not as intense and subsided after a short period of time. He denied hematuria or dysuria. He had no previous history of renal colic.

On physical examination, he was noted to be in significant pain with difficulty getting comfortable. His blood pressure was 140/80 mm Hg, heart rate 110 beats per minute, respirations 16 per minute, and his temperature 37.5°C. Head, neck, chest, and CV examinations were within normal limits. Examination of the abdomen revealed no significant anterior abdominal tenderness, but he was noted to have tenderness at the left costovertebral angle. External GU examination was normal.

Management Course

The patient was administered an IV narcotic for acute pain control and an antiemetic. IV saline was initiated and basic laboratory tests were sent, including urinalysis. While awaiting laboratory tests, a bedside-focused ultrasound of the kidneys was performed by the treating physician. Ultrasound revealed moderate hydronephrosis of the left kidney confirming the clinical impression of acute renal colic (Figure 12-51). Two hours later, he was pain-free and urinalysis revealed 10–20 RBCs/hpf with no pyuria. He was given urology follow-up for the following day and oral analgesics on discharge.

Commentary

Case 1 is a classic presentation of acute renal colic in a young adult. Many authors would recommend no testing except urinalysis in this scenario, while others would argue for an imaging study for all cases. Even in classic presentations, a confirmatory test is desirable. Of the available modalities, ultrasound is the least expensive

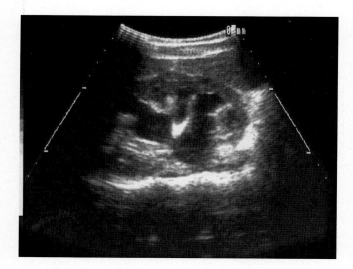

Figure 12-51. Case 1. Moderate hydronephrosis of the left kidney.

and fastest, and requires no ionizing radiation. This patient presented at 3 AM, which further complicates the case because of the limited imaging resources usually available at this hour in many practice settings. This patient may need further definitive imaging, but point-of-care ultrasound provides enough information for acute diagnosis and disposition for emergency purposes.

CASE 2

Patient Presentation

A 56-year-old woman presented to the ED with 1 week of dysuria, nausea, and fevers. She was treated with a 3-day outpatient course of an antibiotic she was unable to recall. She recently had worsening left flank pain and vomiting. Her past medical history was significant for poorly controlled diabetes and hypertension. She denied chest pain, shortness of breath, or any vaginal complaints.

Physical examination revealed an obese female in moderate distress. Vitals signs revealed a blood pressure of 90/60 mm Hg, heart rate 110 beats per minute, respirations 18 per minute, and temperature 39.8°C. Blood glucose was 450. She had dry mucous membranes. Abdominal examination revealed an obese abdomen with diffuse tenderness that was worse in the suprapubic region. Back examination revealed bilateral flank tenderness without signs of hematoma. Chest and GU examinations were within normal limits.

Management Course

IV access was established immediately and a fluid bolus was given. Blood and urine samples were obtained

and sent to the lab. A urine pregnancy test was negative. Labs and urinalysis confirmed the diagnosis of urosepsis and antibiotics were given in addition to a second fluid bolus. The patient continued to deteriorate despite resuscitation so a point-of-care ultrasound was performed to evaluate for an infectious complication of nephrolithiasis. The right kidney, gallbladder, and aorta all appeared normal. The left kidney showed hyperechoic areas within the sinus with "dirty" posterior shadows (Figure 12-27). The diagnosis of emphysematous pyelonephritis was made, and the patient was admitted to the intensive care unit where she underwent percutaneous drainage by urology.

Commentary

Patients with acute pyelonephritis do not routinely require renal ultrasound. However, if the presentation is atypical or extreme as in this case, a point-of-care ultrasound exam to screen for concomitant urinary obstruction or signs of gas formation is warranted. Infected ureterolithiasis with obstruction and emphysematous pyelonephritis are urologic emergencies that benefit from early consultation and surgical intervention. Mortality from emphysematous pyelonephritis is high if the diagnosis is not recognized and treated promptly. The patient in this case was too unstable for CT, but point-of-care ultrasound allowed early diagnosis and appropriate treatment.

CASE 3

Patient Presentation

A 35-year-old man presented to the ED with 1 week of low back pain radiating to both legs. History was significant for chronic low back pain secondary to a work-related injury and IV drug abuse, although he denied any recent use. He denied trauma, fever, weakness, or sensory changes. He said he urinated on himself this morning because he could not make it to the bathroom in time.

On physical examination, he was in mild pain. His vital signs revealed a blood pressure of 124/70 mm Hg, heart rate 90 beats per minute, respirations 16 per minute, and temperature 37.8°C. He had normal gait, strength, sensation, and reflexes. He had midline pain over the lower lumbar area. He refused rectal examination or catheterization to measure postvoid residual.

Management Course

Blood and urine samples were collected. IV analgesia was administered. Lumbar radiographs were unremarkable. MRI was unavailable overnight except for emergent cases. The patient agreed to point-of-care ultrasound, which revealed a postvoid residual urine volume of 139 mL (Figure 12-26). After discussion with the radiologist, a radiology technician was called in for an emergent MRI of the spine. This showed a lumbar spinal epidural abscess at L4–5 causing compression of the cauda equina. Antibiotics were started and the patient was taken to surgery emergently for decompression and evacuation. He was discharged 8 days later with a Foley catheter, but without any additional neurologic deficits.

Commentary

Clinical presentation of cauda equina syndrome is variable and diagnosis relies on immediate MRI, which may not be readily available. Early diagnosis is critical to prevent progression of nerve damage. Point-of-care ultrasound allows noninvasive and painless measurement of postvoid residual urine volume, which provides critical data when attempting to obtain emergent imaging and consultation.

REFERENCES

1. ACEP: *Emergency Ultrasound Imaging Criteria: Renal.* Statement Approved by ACEP Board, 2006.
2. Brown DF, Rosen CL, Wolfe RE: Renal ultrasonography. *Emerg Med Clin North Am* 15:877–893, 1997.
3. American College of Emergency Physicians. Use of ultrasound imaging by emergency physicians. *Ann Emerg Med* 38:469–470, 2001.
4. Noble VE, Brown D: Renal ultrasound. *Emerg Med Clin North Am* 22:641–659, 2004.
5. Kiely EA, Hartnell GG, Gibson RN, et al.: Measurement of bladder volume by real-time ultrasound. *Br J Urol* 60:33–35, 1987.
6. Krupnick AS, Teitelbaum DH, Geiger JD, et al.: Use of abdominal ultrasonography to assess pediatric splenic trauma. Potential pitfalls in the diagnosis [see comments]. *Ann Surg* 225:408–414, 1997.
7. Mainprize TC, Drutz HP: Accuracy of total bladder volume and residual urine measurements: Comparison between real-time ultrasonography and catheterization. *Am J Obstet Gynecol* 160:1013–1016, 1989.
8. Topper AK, Holliday PJ, Fernie GR: Bladder volume estimation in the elderly using a portable ultrasound-based measurement device. *J Med Eng Technol* 17:99–103, 1993.
9. Poston GJ, Joseph AE, Riddle PR: The accuracy of ultrasound in the measurement of changes in bladder volume. *Br J Urol* 55:361–363, 1983.
10. Hartnell GG, Kiely EA, Williams G, et al.: Real-time ultrasound measurement of bladder volume: A comparative study of three methods. *Br J Radiol* 60:1063–1065, 1987.
11. Chan H: Noninvasive bladder volume measurement. *J Neurosci Nurs* 25:309–312, 1993.
12. Ireton RC, Krieger JN, Cardenas DD, et al.: Bladder volume determination using a dedicated, portable ultrasound scanner. *J Urol* 143:909–911, 1990.
13. Chen L, Hsiao AL, Moore CL, et al.: Utility of bedside bladder ultrasound before urethral catheterization in young children. *Pediatrics* 115:108–111, 2005.
14. Milling TJ Jr, Van Amerongen R, Melville L, et al.: Use of ultrasonography to identify infants for whom urinary catheterization will be unsuccessful because of insufficient urine volume: Validation of the urinary bladder index. *Ann Emerg Med* 45:510–513, 2005.
15. Spouge AR, Wilson SR, Wooley B: Abdominal sonography in asymptomatic executives: Prevalence of pathologic findings, potential benefits, and problems. *J Ultrasound Med* 15:763–767; quiz 769–770, 1996.
16. Ozen H, Colowick A, Freiha FS: Incidentally discovered solid renal masses: What are they?. *Br J Urol* 72:274–276, 1993.
17. Zagoria RJ, Dyer RB: The small renal mass: Detection, characterization, and management. *Abdom Imaging* 23:256–265, 1998.
18. Mandavia DP, Pregerson B, Henderson SO: Ultrasonography of flank pain in the emergency department: Renal cell carcinoma as a diagnostic concern. *J Emerg Med* 18:83–86, 2000.
19. Henderson SO, Hoffner RJ, Aragona JL, et al.: Bedside emergency department ultra-sonography plus radiography of the kidneys, ureters, and bladder vs intravenous pyelography in the evaluation of suspected ureteral colic. *Acad Emerg Med* 5:666–671, 1998.
20. Dalla Palma L, Stacul F, Bazzocchi M, et al.: Ultrasonography and plain film versus intravenous urography in ureteric colic. *Clin Radiol* 47:333–336, 1993.
21. Rosen CL, Brown DF, Sagarin MJ, et al.: Ultrasonography by emergency physicians in patients with suspected ureteral colic. *J Emerg Med* 16:865–870, 1998.
22. Haddad MC, Sharif HS, Shahed MS, et al.: Renal colic: Diagnosis and outcome. *Radiology* 184:83–88, 1992.
23. Ghali AM, Elmalik EM, Ibrahim AI, et al.: Cost-effective emergency diagnosis plan for urinary stone patients presenting with ureteric colic. *Eur Urol* 33:529–537, 1998.
24. Fielding JR, Silverman SG, Rubin GD: Helical CT of the urinary tract. *AJR Am J Roentgenol* 172:1199–1206, 1999.
25. Spencer BA, Wood BJ, Dretler SP: Helical CT and ureteral colic. *Urol Clin North Am* 27:231–241, 2000.
26. Rao PN: Imaging for kidney stones. *World J Urol* 22:323–327, 2004.
27. Boulay I, Holtz P, Foley WD, et al.: Ureteral calculi: Diagnostic efficacy of helical CT and implications for treatment of patients. *AJR Am J Roentgenol* 172:1485–1490, 1999.
28. Chen MY, Zagoria RJ: Can noncontrast helical computed tomography replace intravenous urography for evaluation of patients with acute urinary tract colic? *J Emerg Med* 17:299–303, 1999.
29. Chen MY, Zagoria RJ, Saunders HS, et al.: Trends in the use of unenhanced helical CT for acute urinary colic. *AJR Am J Roentgenol* 173:1447–1450, 1999.
30. Dalrymple NC, Verga M, Anderson KR, et al.: The value of unenhanced helical computerized tomography in the management of acute flank pain. *J Urol* 159:735–740, 1998.
31. Fielding JR, Steele G, Fox LA, et al.: Spiral computerized tomography in the evaluation of acute flank pain: A

replacement for excretory urography. *J Urol* 157:2071–2073, 1997.

32. Sheley RC, Semonsen KG, Quinn SF: Helical CT in the evaluation of renal colic. *Am J Emerg Med* 17:279–282, 1999.

33. Sheafor DH, Hertzberg BS, Freed KS, et al.: Nonenhanced helical CT and US in the emergency evaluation of patients with renal colic: Prospective comparison. *Radiology* 217:792–797, 2000.

34. Smith RC, Verga M, McCarthy S, et al.: Diagnosis of acute flank pain: Value of unenhanced helical CT. *AJR Am J Roentgenol* 166:97–101, 1996.

35. Vieweg J, Teh C, Freed K, et al.: Unenhanced helical computerized tomography for the evaluation of patients with acute flank pain. *J Urol* 160:679–684, 1998.

36. Fowler KA, Locken JA, Duchesne JH, et al.: US for detecting renal calculi with nonenhanced CT as a reference standard. *Radiology* 222:109–113, 2002.

37. Westphalen AC, Hsia RY, Maselli JH, et al.: Radiological imaging of patients with suspected urinary tract stones: National trends, diagnoses, and predictors. *Acad Emerg Med* 18:700–707, 2011.

38. Lindqvist K, Hellstrom M, Holmberg G, et al.: Immediate versus deferred radiological investigation after acute renal colic: A prospective randomized study. *Scand J Urol Nephrol* 40:119–124, 2006.

39. Denton ER, Mackenzie A, Greenwell T, et al.: Unenhanced helical CT for renal colic—Is the radiation dose justifiable? *Clin Radiol* 54:444–447, 1999.

40. Katz SI, Saluja S, Brink JA, et al.: Radiation dose associated with unenhanced CT for suspected renal colic: Impact of repetitive studies. *AJR Am J Roentgenol* 186:1120–1124, 2006.

41. Gaspari R, Horst K: Emergency ultrasound and urinalysis in the evaluation of flank pain. *Acad Emerg Med* 12:1180–5, 2005.

42. Watkins S, Bowra J, Sharma P, et al.: Validation of emergency physician ultrasound in diagnosing hydronephrosis in ureteric colic. *Emerg Med Australas* 19:188–195, 2007.

43. Patlas M, Farkas A, Fisher D, et al.: Ultrasound vs CT for the detection of ureteric stones in patients with renal colic. *Br J Radiol* 74:901–904, 2001.

44. Sheafor DH, Hertzberg BS, Freed KS, et al.: Nonenhanced helical CT and US in the emergency evaluation of patients with renal colic: prospective comparison. *Radiology* 217:792–797, 2000.

45. Goertz JK, Lotterman S: Can the degree of hydronephrosis on ultrasound predict kidney stone size?. *Am J Emerg Med* 28:813–816, 2010.

46. Zagoria RJ: *Genitourinary Radiology: The Requisites.* St Louis, MO: Mosby-Yearbook, Inc, 1997:418.

47. Corradi F, Brusasco C, Vezzani A, et al.: Hemorrhagic shock in polytrauma patients: Early detection with renal Doppler resistive index measurements. *Radiology* 260:112–118, 2011.

48. Cramer JS, Forrest K: Renal lithiasis: Addressing the risks of austere desert deployments. *Aviat Space Environ Med* 77:649–653, 2006.

49. Surange RS, Jeygopal NS, Chowdhury SD, et al.: Bedside ultrasound: A useful tool for the on-call urologist?. *Int Urol Nephrol* 32:591–596, 2001.

50. Park SJ, Yi BH, Lee HK, et al.: Evaluation of patients with suspected renal calculi using sonography as an initial diagnostic tool: How can we improve diagnostic accuracy?. *J Ultrasound Med* 18;27:1441–1450, 2008.

51. Thurston W, Wilson S: The urinary tract. In: Rumack C, Wilson S, Charboneau J, et al. eds. *Diagnostic Ultrasound.* St. Louis, MO: Mosby, 1997.

52. Lanoix R, Leak LV, Gaeta T, et al.: A preliminary evaluation of emergency ultrasound in the setting of an emergency medicine training program. *Am J Emerg Med* 18:41–45, 2000.

53. Kartal M, Eray, O, Erdogru T, et al.: Prospective validation of a current algorithm including bedside US performed by emergency physicians for patients with acute flank pain suspected for renal colic. *Emerg Med J* 23:341–344, 2006.

54. Sinclair D, Wilson S, Toi A, et al.: The evaluation of suspected renal colic: Ultrasound scan vs excretory urography. *Ann Emerg Med* 18:556–559, 1989.

55. Ather MA, Jafri AH, Sulaiman MN: Diagnostic accuracy of ultrasound compared to unenhanced CT for stone and obstruction in patients with renal failure. *BMC Medical Imaging* 4:2, 2004.

56. Anderhub B: *General Sonography: A Clinical Guide.* St. Louis, MO: Mosby-Yearbook, Inc, 1995:414.

57. Williamson M: Renal ultrasound. In: Williamson M, ed. *Essentials of Ultrasound.* Philadelphia, PA: WB Saunders, 1996.

58. Burge HJ, Middleton WD, McClennan BL, et al.: Ureteral jets in healthy subjects and in patients with unilateral ureteral calculi: comparison with color Doppler US. *Radiology* 180:437–442, 1991.

59. Strehlau J, Winkler P, de la Roche J: The uretero-vesical jet as a functional diagnostic tool in childhood hydronephrosis. *Pediatr Nephrol* 11:460–467, 1997.

60. Alnaif B, Drutz HP: The accuracy of portable abdominal ultrasound equipment in measuring postvoid residual volume. *Int Urogynecol J Pelvic Floor Dysfunct* 10:215–218, 1999.

61. Riccabona M, Nelson TR, Pretorius DH, et al.: In vivo three-dimensional sonographic measurement of organ volume: Validation in the urinary bladder. *J Ultrasound Med* 15:627–632, 1996.

62. Marks LS, Dorey FJ, Macairan ML, et al.: Three-dimensional ultrasound device for rapid determination of bladder volume. *Urology* 50:341–348, 1997.

63. Ozawa H, Chancellor MB, Ding YY, et al.: Noninvasive urodynamic evaluation of bladder outlet obstruction using Doppler ultrasonography. *Urology.* 56:408–412, 2000.

64. Rosseland LA, Bentsen G, Hopp E, et al.: Monitoring urinary bladder volume and detecting postoperative urinary retention in children with an ultrasound scanner. *Acta Anaesthesiol Scand* 49:1456–1459, 2005.

65. Rosseland LA, Stubhaug A, Breivik H: Detecting postoperative urinary retention with an ultrasound scanner. *Acta Anaesthesiol Scand* 46:279–282, 2002.

66. Van Os AF, Van der Linden PJ: Reliability of an automatic ultrasound system in the post partum period in measuring urinary retention. *Acta Obstet Gynecol Scand* 85:604–607, 2006.

67. Bozsa S, Poto L, Bodia J, et al.: Assessment of postoperative postvoid residual bladder volume using three-dimensional

ultrasound volumetry. *Ultrasound Med Biol* 37:522–529, 2011.

68. Yen DH, Hu SC, Tsai J, et al.: Renal abscess: Early diagnosis and treatment. *Am J Emerg Med* 17:192–197, 1999.

69. Huang JJ, Tseng CC: Emphysematous pyelonephritis: Clinicoradiological classification, management, prognosis, and pathogenesis. *Arch Intern Med* 160:797–805, 2000.

70. Wan YL, Lo SK, Bullard MJ, et al.: Predictors of outcome in emphysematous pyelonephritis. *J Urol* 159:369–373, 1998.

71. Stone SC, Mallon WK, Childs JM, et al.: Emphysematous pyelonephritis: Clues to rapid diagnosis in the emergency department. *J Emerg Med* 28:315–319, 2005.

72. Siepel T, Clifford DS, James PA, et al.: The ultrasound-assisted physical examination in the periodic health evaluation of the elderly. *J Fam Pract* 49:628–632, 2000.

73. Ueda T, Mihara Y: Incidental detection of renal carcinoma during radiological imaging. *Br J Urol* 59:513–515, 1987.

74. Tosaka A, Ohya K, Yamada K, et al.: Incidence and properties of renal masses and asymptomatic renal cell carcinoma detected by abdominal ultrasonography. *J Urol* 144:1097–1099, 1990.

75. Lanctin HP, Futter NG: Renal cell carcinoma: Incidental detection. *Can J Surg* 33:488–490, 1990.

76. Sweeney JP, Thornhill JA, Graiger R, et al.: Incidentally detected renal cell carcinoma: Pathological features, survival trends and implications for treatment. *Br J Urol* 78:351–353, 1996.

77. Smith SJ, Bosniak MA, Megibow AJ, et al.: Renal cell carcinoma: Earlier discovery and increased detection. *Radiology* 170:699–703, 1989.

78. Charboneau JW, Hattery RR, Ernst EC, III, et al.: Spectrum of sonographic findings in 125 renal masses other than benign simple cyst. *AJR Am J Roentgenol* 140:87–94, 1983.

79. Helenon O, Correas JM, Balleyguier C, et al.: Ultrasound of renal tumors. *Eur Radiol* 11:1890–1901, 2001.

80. Belldegrun A, deKernion J: Renal tumors. In: Campbell M, Walsh P, eds. *Campbell's Urology*. Philadelphia, PA: WB Saunders Company, 1998.

81. Forman HP, Middleton WD, Melson GL, et al.: Hyperechoic renal cell carcinomas: Increase in detection at US. *Radiology* 188:431–434, 1993.

82. Drago J, Cunningham J: Ultrasonography of renal masses. In: Resnick M, Rifkin M, eds. *Ultrasonography of the Urinary Tract*. Baltimore, MD: Williams & Wilkins, 1991.

83. McGahan JP, Richards JR, Jones CD, et al.: Use of ultrasonography in the patient with acute renal trauma. *J Ultrasound Med* 18:207–213; quiz 215–216, 1999.

84. McGahan PJ, Richards JR, Bair AE, et al.: Ultrasound detection of blunt urological trauma: A 6-year study. *Injury* 36:762–770, 2005.

85. Jalli R, Kamalzadeh N, Lotfi M, et al.: Accuracy of sonography in detection of renal injuries caused by blunt abdominal trauma: A prospective study. *TJTES* 15:23–27, 2009.

86. Catalano O, Lobianco R, Sandomenico F, et al.: Real-time, contrast-enhanced sonographic imaging in emergency radiology. *Radiol Med (Torino)* 108:454–469, 2004.

87. Fang YC, Tiu CM, Chou YH, et al.: A case of acute renal artery thrombosis caused by blunt trauma: Computed tomographic and Doppler ultrasonic findings. *J Formos Med Assoc* 92:356–358, 1993.

88. Poletti PA, Platon A, Becker CD, et al.: Blunt abdominal trauma: Does the use of a second-generation sonographic contrast agent help to detect solid organ injuries?. *AJR Am J Roentgenol* 183:1293–1301, 2004.

89. Valentino M, Serra C, Zironi G, et al.: Blunt abdominal trauma: Emergency contrast-enhanced sonography for detection of solid organ injuries. *AJR Am J Roentgenol* 186:1361–1367, 2006.

90. Tempkin B: *Ultrasound Scanning: Principles & Protocols*. Philadelphia, PA: WB Saunders, 1993.

91. Cox IH, Erickson SJ, Foley WD, et al.: Ureteric jets: Evaluation of normal flow dynamics with color Doppler sonography. *AJR Am J Roentgenol* 158:1051–1055, 1992.

92. Curtis LA, Dolan TS, Cespedes RD: Acute urinary retention and urinary incontinence. *Emerg Med Clin North Am* 19:591–619, 2001.

93. Hagen-Ansert S: Urinary system. In: Hagen-Ansert S, ed.: *Textbook of Diagnostic Ultrasound*. St. Louis, MO: Mosby, 1995.

94. Delair SM, Kurzrock EA: Clinical utility of ureteral jets: disparate opinions. *J Endourol* 20:111–114, 2006.

CHAPTER 13

Testicular

Srikar Adhikari

Acute testicular pain represents about 0.5% of ED complaints.[1] Causes of acute testicular pain include trauma, epididymitis, orchitis, torsion of the testicular appendage, and hernia; however, testicular torsion is the diagnosis of the greatest concern in the emergency setting.

The traditional teaching was that most patients presenting to an ED or urgent care with a complaint of acute testicular pain had testicular torsion.[2] This misconception has been dispelled and it is now known that the most common etiology of acute testicular pain is epididymitis.[2] However, the evaluation of acute testicular pain presents a considerable challenge for emergency providers, since 50% of patients presenting with testicular torsion have delayed seeking care for >6 hours and are at high risk of losing the torsed testicle.[3]

The issue of acute testicular pain is further complicated by the high potential for litigation associated with infertility after testicular loss due to torsion or disruption of the testicle from severe trauma. When the diagnosis of testicular torsion is missed, the majority of patients have been incorrectly diagnosed with epididymitis.[4]

▶ CLINICAL CONSIDERATIONS

High-resolution color Doppler ultrasonography has become widely accepted as the test of choice for evaluating acute scrotal pain, replacing scintigraphy in most institutions.[5] While scintigraphy requires less technical skill on the part of the radiologist consulted to evaluate the patient, there are major drawbacks to the technique.

Scintigraphy is a time-consuming process that can add an hour or more to the evaluation of a patient who may already be several hours into the testicular torsion process.[5] Furthermore, the resultant hyperemia of the scrotal skin during testicular torsion can mask a lack of blood flow to the testicle itself and lead to a misdiagnosis in less experienced hands.[6] This nuclear medicine study also provides no information regarding testicular anatomy, which is a critical issue if pathology other than torsion is present. MRI is a promising imaging modality for detecting acute scrotal problems, including ischemia caused by torsion. However, MRI is expensive and time consuming.

Traditionally the history and physical examination were thought to be the keys to diagnosing or ruling out testicular torsion.[3] However, the historical features of several disease processes may be similar. For example, the duration of pain in testicular torsion, epididymitis, orchitis, and torsion of a testicular appendage frequently overlap.[7] Also, only 50% of patients with torsion have sudden onset of pain and about 20% of have pain associated with trauma or physical exertion, such as heavy lifting.[8,9] Adding to the difficulty using the history is the fact that many young men do not provide an accurate history of trauma. The physical exam can be similarly misleading, because it is frequently limited by pain, edema, and patient compliance. In addition, findings such as absent cremasteric reflex, abnormal testicular lie (present in <50% of testicular torsion cases), and epididymal tenderness are not reliable in differentiating torsion from other causes of acute scrotal pain.[10]

The classic clinical features of epididymitis, such as dysuria and urethral discharge, are not consistent. Up to

50% of patients with acute epididymitis do not have dysuria or urethral discharge.[4] Furthermore, many patients with epididymitis complain of acute onset of pain. This is probably due to poor recall or the need for a threshold of discomfort to be crossed prior to the patient's recognition of pain. Another complicating factor is that if the body or tail of the epididymis is inflamed without affecting the head, the pain and swelling will be in a different location from where most clinicians expect with epididymitis. Most clinicians learn to feel for the head of the epididymis on their physical examination and do not realize that it may not be involved. Patients with testicular torsion who are initially misdiagnosed with epididymitis are most commonly misdiagnosed because of the presence of dysuria, pyuria, or urethral discharge, or because of a vague history of pain onset, giving the impression of a less acute process.[1] Because of the time-sensitive nature of testicular torsion, ultrasound is an ideal diagnostic test for the evaluation of testicular pain.

► CLINICAL INDICATIONS

The clinical indications for point-of-care testicular ultrasound are as follows:

- Acute testicular pain
- Acute scrotal mass
- Trauma

ACUTE TESTICULAR PAIN

The most serious cause of acute testicular pain is testicular torsion. Testicular torsion can occur at any age; however, the majority of cases occur between 12 and 18 years of age. The most common underlying cause of testicular torsion is a congenital malformation known as bell clapper deformity, where the tunica vaginalis completely encircles the epididymis, spermatic cord, and testis instead of attaching to the posterolateral aspect of the testis. This allows the testicle to twist about its own axis compressing the vasculature and resulting in ischemia. The bell clapper deformity is most often found to be bilateral (50–80% of cases) upon surgical exploration.[11] Further increasing the likelihood of testicular torsion is a history of an undescended testicle.[12] Once blood flow is interrupted to the testicle, infarction and loss of the testicle can occur quickly. Testicular salvage rates are approximately 100% prior to 3 hours, 83–90% at 5 hours, 75% at 8 hours, and 50–70% at 10 hours. When a testicle has been torsed for longer than 10 hours, the rates of salvage decrease to 10–20%. After 24 hours, salvage of a testicle is rarely seen unless there has been intermittent detorsion.[13] In general, urologists are reluctant to take patients to the operating room and

explore a painful scrotum based solely on the clinical examination. Studies argue that such patients should not be routinely explored and that accurate diagnosis can be provided with Doppler ultrasound of the involved testicle.[14]

For the detection of acute testicular torsion, ultrasonography has a sensitivity of 80–98% and a specificity of 97–100%.[15] Data regarding testicular ultrasound use by clinicians at the bedside are relatively limited.[16–21] Testicular ultrasound carries a stigma of being a difficult and advanced level examination that will lead to dire consequences if misinterpreted, but the data do not support this notion. One study evaluated 36 patients with acute testicular pain who underwent point-of-care testicular ultrasound by an emergency physician, and demonstrated a sensitivity and specificity of 95% and 94%, respectively, for testicular torsion when surgical follow-up and radiology imaging were used as the criterion standard.[16] All patients with testicular torsion were correctly identified. Other diagnoses found included epididymitis, orchitis, hemorrhage, and herniation. Another study demonstrated good accuracy of point-of-care ultrasound for a variety of testicular pathology encountered in the emergency setting.[21]

Patients at institutions without 24/7 radiology ultrasound capabilities will benefit the most from clinician-performed point-of-care testicular ultrasound. Also, when clinicians can quickly confirm lack of blood flow to a painful testicle they are more likely to attempt manual detorsion, which may significantly improve testicular salvage rates.

A major limitation for clinicians attempting to gain experience with testicular ultrasound is the infrequency of patients presenting with acute scrotal pain. However, one study demonstrated that testicular torsion could be easily simulated for training purposes by digital compression of the spermatic cord. This technique holds great promise as an educational tool that could quickly increase clinician confidence and expand the use of point-of-care testicular ultrasound.[19]

ACUTE SCROTAL MASS

Painless scrotal masses are unlikely to represent an acute disease process. Patients often describe that the involved testicle has been slowly enlarging for some time, but they had simply ignored it or grew accustomed to the difference until some factor finally made them seek medical assistance. Firm, nontender testicular masses commonly represent neoplasms that should be directed for expeditious follow-up with a urologist. When the patient presents complaining of pain from the testicular mass, it may be from hemorrhage into the neoplasm itself. The vast majority of soft, nontender testicular masses are hydroceles that may develop because of a number of disease processes or idiopathically. Many are congenital and result from a direct communication with the abdominal cavity. Hydroceles may result from trauma, infection, neoplasm, radiation therapy, and undiagnosed torsion.[22] Hernias can present with complaints of acute scrotal mass, and are generally painful. The presentation can be similar to that of torsion if the scrotum is erythematous.

TRAUMA

Blunt trauma can lead to injury of the testicle or associated structures. Assault, athletic injury (about 50% of blunt trauma cases), bicycle crashes, and motor vehicle crashes are the most common causes of blunt testicular trauma.[23] Injuries can be in the form of laceration, hemorrhage, or contusion of the testicle. Clinical features of testicular injury are a tender swollen testicle, often accompanied by ecchymosis. Accurate diagnosis by physical examination alone is often difficult secondary to marked swelling and pain in the traumatized scrotum, thus making ultrasound imaging a requisite. The goal of point-of-care ultrasound in patients presenting with acute trauma to the scrotum is to determine whether the testicle is injured and requires operative intervention. Although a contusion or focal hemorrhage may simply require follow-up, fracture through the capsule of the testicle necessitates surgical intervention. Furthermore, since trauma can lead to testicular torsion, blood flow should be evaluated as well. Ultrasound is sensitive for detecting major trauma to the testicle and, therefore, can be useful for screening patients. While the accuracy of ultrasound is operator dependent, the diagnosis of a significant testicular injury is relatively straightforward.[24, 25]

▶ ANATOMICAL CONSIDERATIONS

The scrotum is divided into two separate compartments by a midline septum called the median raphe. Each compartment of the scrotum contains a testis, epididymis, vas deferens, and spermatic cord. The normal adult testes are located in the scrotum and are oval in shape. Average testicular measurements obtained by ultrasound are 4 cm × 3 cm × 2.5 cm. Each adult testicle weighs between 10 and 19 grams. The size of the testicle changes with age; it increases in size up to puberty and decreases later in life. The testis is surrounded by a fibrous capsule known as tunica albuginea, which is covered by tunica vaginalis. The tunica vaginalis has two layers: the outer parietal and inner visceral, which merge at the posterolateral aspect of the testis (Figure 13-1). These two layers are separated by small amount of fluid. The tunica albuginea projects posteriorly into the testis to form an incomplete septum called mediastinum testis.

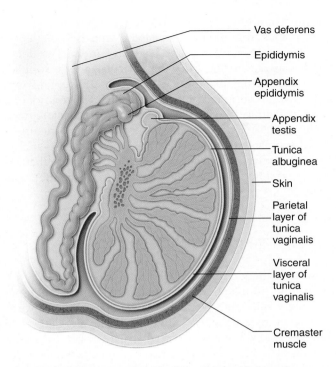

Figure 13-1. Normal testicular and scrotal anatomy.

Labels: Vas deferens; Epididymis; Appendix epididymis; Appendix testis; Tunica albuginea; Skin; Parietal layer of tunica vaginalis; Visceral layer of tunica vaginalis; Cremaster muscle

Multiple septations arise from the tunica albuginea and run through the testicle. These septations result in the separation of the testicle into multiple lobules. The testicular parenchyma is made up of numerous seminiferous tubules that converge toward mediastinum testis and open into rete testis, which drains into the epididymal head.[26, 27]

The epididymis is a tubular structure located along the posterolateral aspect of each testis. It measures approximately 6–7 cm in length and consists of a head, body, and tail. The head of the epididymis lies superolaterally to the testis, the body adjacent to the posterolateral margin of the testis, and the tail at the inferior pole of the testis. The tail of the epididymis turns into the vas deferens as it travels superiorly out of the scrotum. The vas deferens, in turn, travels in the spermatic cord. The spermatic cord contains a number of structures, including the testicular artery, cremasteric artery, deferential artery, pampiniform venous plexus, lymphatic structures, nerves, and vas deferens. The appendix testis and the appendix epididymis are found toward the superior pole of the testis. The appendix testis, an oval structure about 5 mm in length, usually lies in the groove between the testis and the epididymis. The appendix epididymis is attached to the head of the epididymis and is of the same approximate dimensions as the appendix testis. The appendix epididymis has been identified unilaterally in 34% and bilaterally in 12% of testes.[26, 27]

Most of the arterial blood supply received by a testicle comes from the abdominal aorta through the testicular artery. A small portion of the arterial supply comes from the deferential and cremasteric arteries, which anastomose with the testicular artery. The deferential artery, arising from the vesicular artery, supplies the epididymis and the vas deferens. The epididymis, however, is supplied predominantly by the superior epididymal artery, which is a branch of the testicular artery. The cremasteric artery arises from the epigastric artery and supplies the peritesticular tissues. There is variability in normal anatomy and, in general, anything that appears abnormal should be compared to the contralateral side.[26]

▶ GETTING STARTED

Ensure patient comfort when performing a testicular ultrasound examination. The main issue is having the patient lay still when performing power and pulsed-wave Doppler measurements. Both of these modalities are very sensitive to motion artifact. Thus, provide adequate analgesia and reassurance. Explain the examination details and its goals to the patient. Disrobe the patient from the waist down and scan in the supine position. A frog leg position allows good access to the scrotum and it may help to prop pillows or blankets under each bent knee to allow relaxation of the legs. Place the scrotum in a sling and support it on a rolled towel placed between the patient's thighs to isolate the scrotum for scanning (Figure 13-2). Position the penis over the suprapubic region and cover it with a towel.

Place the ultrasound machine on the patient's right. Use a generous amount of warmed ultrasound gel. Cold gel may make the patient more uncomfortable by elic-

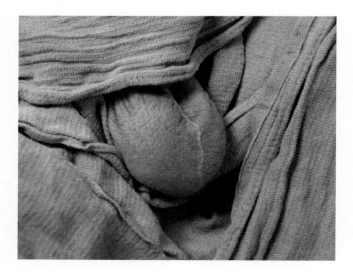

Figure 13-2. A properly exposed and draped patient with the scrotum supported in a sling of towels for improved patient comfort and visualization.

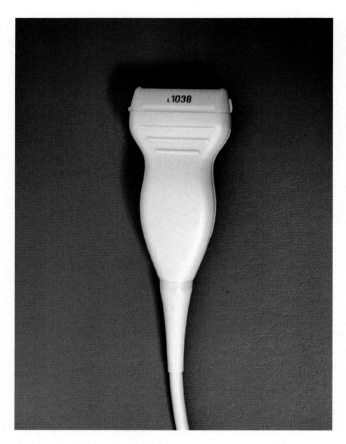

Figure 13-3. An example of a high-resolution linear array transducer that can be used for testicular sonography.

iting a cremasteric reflex. In cases of significant inflammation or torsion, activation of the cremasteric reflex may cause considerable pain. Cold gel can also result in contraction and thickening of the scrotal skin, making it difficult to see scrotal contents. When evaluating the testes, select a high-frequency (7.5–10 MHz) broadband linear transducer, or a 5.0 MHz transducer for large masses or very edematous scrotum (Figure 13-3). The resolution provided by high-frequency linear transducers is crucial for examining not only the parenchyma of the testicle but also the blood flow within it. Some clinicians will even utilize 12–15 MHz transducers to obtain the best Doppler resolution. This may not be possible if significant swelling exists and the testicle itself is several centimeters from the skin surface. Select a small part or testes preset on the machine. In addition to a high-resolution transducer, color, power and spectral Doppler modes are required when evaluating a patient for torsion. Power Doppler, a nondirectional version of color Doppler, is highly sensitive for detecting vessels with low blood flow, and its signal is independent of Doppler angle correction. The disadvantages of power Doppler are its susceptibility to motion and omission of directional information. Power Doppler is used for

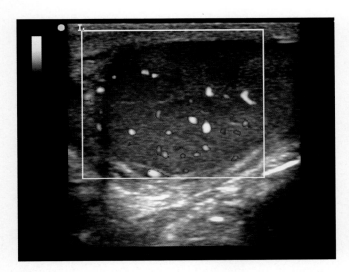

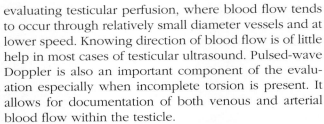

Figure 13-4. Power Doppler box superimposed on the B-mode image of testis.

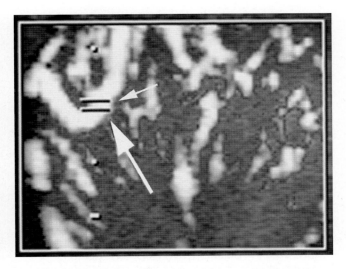

Figure 13-5. A close-up of the pulsed-wave Doppler gate is shown by arrows in this image.

evaluating testicular perfusion, where blood flow tends to occur through relatively small diameter vessels and at lower speed. Knowing direction of blood flow is of little help in most cases of testicular ultrasound. Pulsed-wave Doppler is also an important component of the evaluation especially when incomplete torsion is present. It allows for documentation of both venous and arterial blood flow within the testicle.

Power Doppler activation will bring up a box-like window the size of which may or may not be adjustable (Figure 13-4). This box can be moved around the screen to the portion of the testicle or scrotum of interest. If the size of the power Doppler box or window is adjustable, it may or may not be helpful to enlarge it, so that it covers the entire testicle. The drawback of enlarging the color box is that this decreases the frame rate, which may make it more difficult to detect higher velocity arterial blood flow. Typically, a balance has to be achieved between a power Doppler window that is too small, requires frequent movement and does not capture the overall blood flow of the testicle, and a window that is too large and does not allow the machine to refresh the image frequently enough. Simply turning on the power Doppler box may not be adequate if the presets on the machine are not set correctly. Adjusting the sensitivity setting as low as possible without having power Doppler signal everywhere will allow for more accurate detection of blood flow.

Once reliable power Doppler signals are visualized in the unaffected testicle, use the pulsed-wave Doppler. A small gate, often two parallel lines, will appear on the screen (Figure 13-5). It is guided with a trackball or touch pad to the power Doppler signals inside the power Doppler box. Typically, an update button will have to be pushed (or the pulsed-wave button may have

to be pushed a second time) when the parallel lines are placed over the power Doppler signal. Once activated, a tracing will appear showing the pulsed-wave Doppler signal. Adjust the size of the sampling gate, otherwise a poor waveform will be obtained. Turning up the pulsed-wave gain is acceptable to a point where the background around the graph baseline becomes brighter and shows some noise. This will allow the exam to be more sensitive for detecting pulsed-wave venous and arterial flow. Venous flow in the testis is typically continuous with minimal variation in velocity (Figure 13-6). Arterial flow to the testes has pulsatility, with a low-resistance, high-flow waveform pattern (Figure 13-7). Sampling should occur in multiple areas in the testicle. Once the settings have been properly adjusted on the unaffected

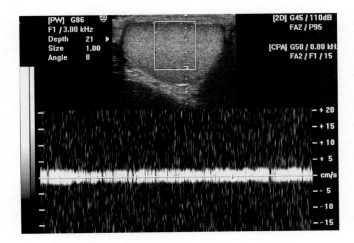

Figure 13-6. A pulsed-wave Doppler tracing is obtained from a testicle. A typical venous waveform is shown.

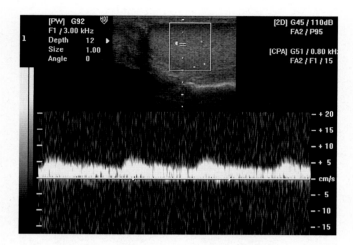

Figure 13-7. A pulsed-wave Doppler tracing is obtained from a testicle. A typical arterial waveform with a systolic and diastolic flow component is shown.

side, move the transducer to the painful testicle. If the machine's settings are identical to those used for the unaffected testicle, the clinician will quickly appreciate if blood flow in the affected testicle is similar, decreased, or absent. In addition, gray scale comparison can quickly be made between the two testicles (Figure13-8). A side-by-side comparison of the two testes can be helpful and illustrates any difference in power Doppler blood flow or echogenicity in a single image

▶ TECHNIQUE AND NORMAL ULTRASOUND FINDINGS

Scan the scrotum and its contents in two orthogonal planes, along the longitudinal and transverse axes. Scan

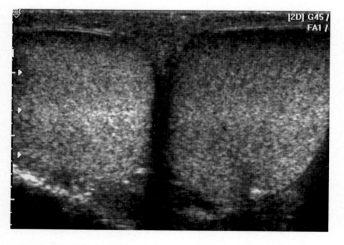

Figure 13-8. A side-by-side comparison image is shown. Both testicles are scanned at once with one linear transducer.

the asymptomatic side first to familiarize the patient with the process; it also provides a comparison of sonographic anatomy and blood flow. Anchoring the scanning hand to patient's thigh will keep it from moving unintentionally. Scan the unaffected testicle in the longitudinal plane from medial to lateral (Figure 13-9A). At this point the indicator on the transducer is typically pointed toward the patient's torso; however, if the testicle has an oblique lie, it is appropriate to orient the indicator toward the upper pole of the testicle. Pay attention to the gray scale abnormalities such as edema, focal masses, or disruptions, and measure the length and thickness of the testes. Evaluate the epididymis in this view. In the long-axis view with the indicator directed cephalad, the epididymis is seen on the left side of the screen. Any epididymal abnormalities will often become evident on the longitudinal views. Turning transverse, still on the unaffected side, scan the testicle from top to bottom, again looking for any gray scale abnormalities (Figure 13-9B and 13-9C). Measure the width in the central portion of the testicle. Scan the spermatic cord from the inguinal canal to the posterosuperior aspect of the testes. After evaluating the testes, assess the scrotal skin thickness and the remaining scrotal contents. Adjust the gain, depth, and resolution settings as appropriate for optimal gray scale image acquisition.

Perform the Doppler examination after the gray scale evaluation of the scrotum to assess blood flow. Scan the asymptomatic side first to adjust Doppler settings to display low-flow velocities. Orient the transducer in the longitudinal plane of the testicle with the power Doppler feature turned on. Unless the machine presets happen to already be optimized for the testicular examination, some adjustments in gain, wall filter, scale, and pulse repetition frequency (PRF) will have to be made. Low wall filter (100 KHz), low PRF (1–2 Hz), and 70–90% color gain output settings are ideal for testicular scanning. The goal of these adjustments is to demonstrate as much blood flow as possible without introducing more than minimal artifact. Power Doppler is highly sensitive to any movement of the testicle or the clinician's hand. Once areas of power Doppler signal are visualized, appreciate the amount of blood flow in the testicle. With experience it will be obvious when there is too much blood flow, as in cases of inflammation, or too little blood flow, as in possible ischemia. Even in experienced hands, however, it is prudent to reserve judgment until the two sides can be compared, as long as the other testicle is present for comparison. At this point, activate the pulsed-wave Doppler and place its sampling gate over areas of power Doppler signal until both venous and arterial waveforms are obtained in multiple areas within the body of the testicle. Blood flow seen on the edge of the testicle may be misleading and should not be reassuring. After evaluating testicular perfusion, a complete ultrasound examination of the

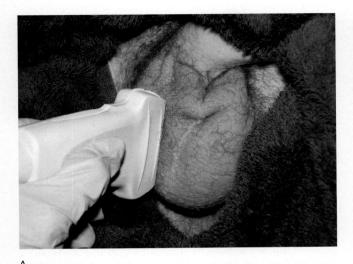

A

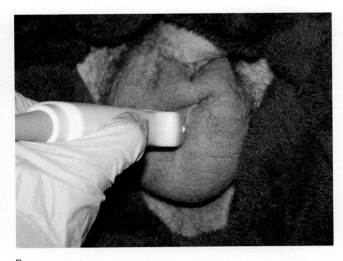

B

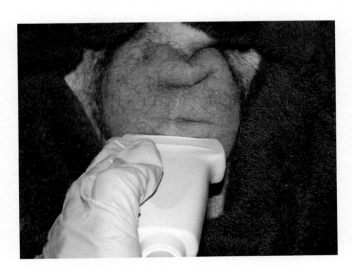

C

Figure 13-9. A longitudinal orientation to the transducer is shown on the right testicle (A). The transducer is held in transverse orientation of the right testicle and moved from upper pole (B) to lower pole (C).

scrotum includes confirmation of epididymal blood flow using power Doppler and spectral Doppler waveform analysis. Quantification of outflow resistance can be accomplished by determining the resistive index (RI). RI is defined as the peak systolic velocity minus the end-diastolic velocity, divided by the peak-systolic velocity, and is easily calculated by the ultrasound machine's software.

Repeat the entire process on the affected side; however, the examination is typically not finished at this point. In the majority of cases, it is helpful to perform a transverse scan of both testes simultaneously to identify differences in size, echogenicity, and blood flow (Figure 13-10). With the transducer turned horizontal through the midportion of both testes and indicator toward the patient's right hip, scan the testes from upper to lower pole for comparison in gray scale. Turn on power Doppler to evaluate the testes. This will often mean enlarging the power Doppler box, thus slowing the motion on the screen. This view is ideal for demonstrating any

Figure 13-10. The transducer is held in transverse orientation across both testicles. This generates a comparison view of both testicles on the screen for gray scale and Doppler evaluation.

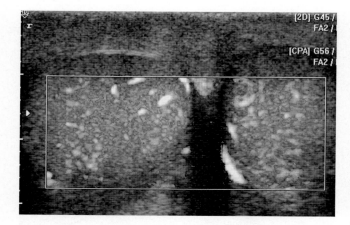

A

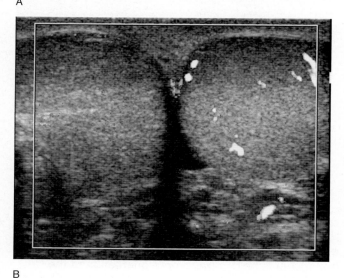

B

Figure 13-11. Power Doppler evaluation (gray scale copy). An equal amount of flow is shown in this comparison view of both testicles with power Doppler (A). In this side-by-side view, no flow is seen in the right testicle, which is displayed on the left side of the screen (B). Torsion was confirmed in the operating room.

similarities or differences between testes in both gray scale and power Doppler. This is especially illustrative in cases of torsion, with one side showing ample blood flow and the affected side showing no blood flow in the same power Doppler box (Figure 13-11A and 13-11B). Similarly, when one testicle has significantly increased blood flow due to inflammation and the other has normal blood flow, the diagnosis is difficult to dispute when such an image is obtained (Figure 13-12). Despite which order one chooses to perform the individual steps, perform the examination the same way each time for consistency.

Sonographically, a testicle has mid-gray or medium-level echoes and appears quite homogeneous in echo-

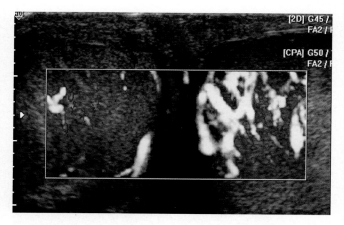

Figure 13-12. A side-by-side comparison view with power Doppler is shown. The left testicle, shown on the right side of the screen, has markedly increased flow in this example of orchitis.

texture (Figure 13-13). The echogenicity of the testes is somewhat similar to liver and thyroid tissue. The normal scrotal wall thickness varies between 2 and 8 mm, depending on the state of contraction of the cremasteric muscle.[26] The tunica albuginea is seen as one echogenic stripe encircling the testis. The epididymis can be readily differentiated from the rest of the testicle in normal as well as pathologic instances. It has similar echogenicity to the testicle but can appear slightly brighter. While the head of the epididymis is readily seen, the body (2–4 mm in diameter) and tail (2-5 mm in diameter) may be harder to differentiate when no inflammation is present. The mediastinum testis is seen as a linear echogenic band extending across the testes in a craniocaudal direction (Figure 13-14). The thickness and

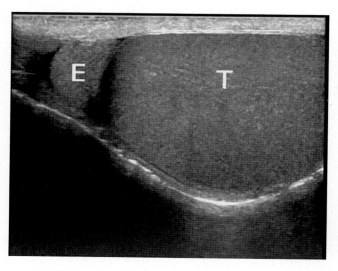

Figure 13-13. Longitudinal view of the normal testis. E = head of the epididymis, T = testicle.

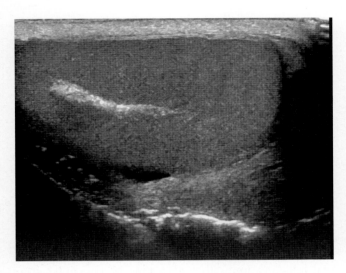

Figure 13-14. Longitudinal view of the normal testis with an echogenic mediastinum testis extending craniocaudally.

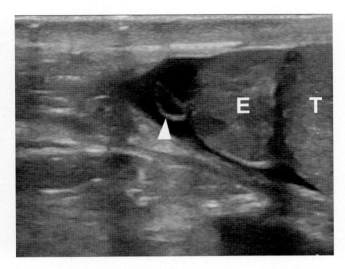

Figure 13-16. An appendix epididymis (arrowhead) outlined by hydrocele is seen adjacent to the head of the epididymis. E = head of the epididymis, T = testicle.

length of mediastinum testis are variable. Adjacent to the mediastinum testis, the normal rete testis is seen as a hypoechoic area with a striated configuration in approximately 18% of patients.[26] The appendix testis (5 mm in length) is a small oval structure and is normally hidden by the epididymal head, thus making it nearly impossible to differentiate in normal examinations. On B-mode, the appendix testis appears isoechoic to the testis. If a hydrocele is present, the appendix testis often becomes outlined by the fluid and is seen as a defined structure (Figure 13-15). When torsed, it may cause not only local inflammation but also an epididymitis-like appearance due to diffuse inflammation of the epididymal head. The appendix testes may be located in different areas on the testicle. Additionally, the epididymis can have appendages. The appendix epididymis is approxi-

mately the same size as the appendix testis but is usually pedunculated and located at the head of the epididymis (Figure 13-16) Sonographically, the spermatic cord is seen as multiple hypoechoic linear structures in the long axis and circular hypoechoic structures in the transverse axis (Figure 13-17). The normal thickness of the spermatic cord in the inguinal canal is approximately 4 mm. The normal spectral waveform of the intratesticular arteries and arteries supplying the epididymis (deferential and cremasteric arteries) have a low-resistance, high-flow pattern. However, the arteries supplying the scrotal

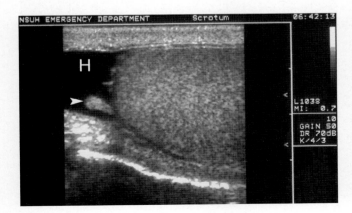

Figure 13-15. A small hydrocele outlines the appendix testis (arrowhead) in this patient presenting for chronic testicular pain. H: hydrocele.

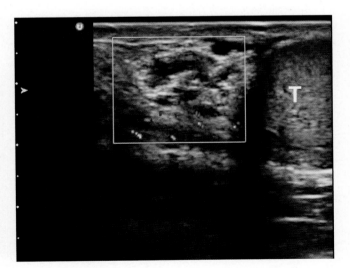

Figure 13-17. Spermatic cord is shown as multiple hypoechoic structures (within the power Doppler box) superior to the testis (T) in the long-axis view.

wall have a low-flow, high-resistance pattern. The RI of normal testicular artery ranges from 0.5 to 0.8.[15]

► COMMON AND EMERGENT ABNORMALITIES

EPIDIDYMITIS

Epididymitis is the most common cause of scrotal pain in adolescents and adults.[28] The disease is insidious in nature; however, a significant proportion of patients present with sudden onset of pain mimicking testicular torsion. Infection of the epididymis or testicle usually results from retrograde spread of bacteria from the bladder or prostate via the vas deferens.[28] Another disease process that can present with signs and symptoms of epididymitis in prepubertal males is torsion of the testicular appendage. In fact, it is believed that many cases of appendiceal torsion are misdiagnosed as epididymitis in prepubertal males.

The epididymal head is the most commonly affected region, but the entire epididymis may be involved in acute epididymitis. Infection usually starts in the head or tail of the epididymis, and then spreads to the entire epididymis and the testis. Comparison with the contralateral testis is crucial to make an accurate diagnosis. Sonographically, the affected epididymis appears enlarged, which is usually confirmed by comparing both the affected and unaffected sides (Figure 13-18). It will often have decreased echogenicity on standard B-mode examination due to associated edema. Although the epididymis is diffusely involved, focal inflammation of a region of the epididymis is seen in one-third of the patients leading to an area of well-defined swelling or enlarge-

ment. This is usually either the head or the body of the epididymis. Scrotal wall thickening is frequently seen, which is an indirect sign of inflammation. Epididymitis can cause accumulation of a reactive hydrocele similar to testicular torsion or torsion of the appendix testis. Thus, the presence of a small or moderate amount of fluid in the hemiscrotum is not a reliable sign for differentiating between the disease processes. In cases with isolated epididymitis, the testis looks normal on ultrasound.[26]

The sensitivity of color Doppler ultrasound in detecting scrotal inflammation is almost 100%.[26] In the majority of cases, the color Doppler confirms the gray scale findings typical of acute epididymitis. However, in 20% of patients with epididymitis, the gray scale appearance of the epididymis is completely normal and the inflammation is only detected using color Doppler.[29] Epididymal inflammation, either idiopathic or infectious, usually leads to increased blood flow that is easily noted on power Doppler when compared to the unaffected side (Figure 13-19). With Doppler technology, minimal blood flow is seen in the normal epididymis, and the detection of any significant vascularity in epididymis should be considered abnormal. It is important to realize that focusing on the head of the epididymis may cause novice operators to overlook the body and tail of the epididymis, which may be the site of isolated inflammation (Figure 13-20). The vas deferens may actually be inflamed first, before the epididymal tail, and would have markedly increased blood flow on power Doppler in its posterior location at the inferior pole of the testicle and epididymal tail. The tail of the epididymis can remain prominent after infection even with appropriate antibiotic therapy. Power Doppler should help differentiate between an acutely inflamed epididymal tail and a prominent leftover from previous infection. Spectral

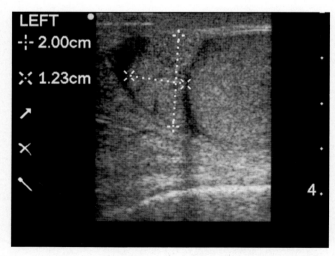

A

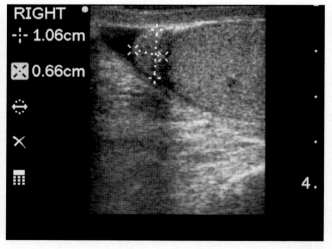

B

Figure 13-18. Epididymitis. The left epididymal head is enlarged (A). Measurements for normal comparison on the right are included (B). (Courtesy of James Mateer, MD)

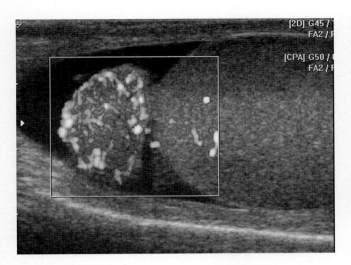

Figure 13-19. The enlarged epididymis is shown on the left side of the image with prominent blood flow shown by power Doppler (gray scale copy).

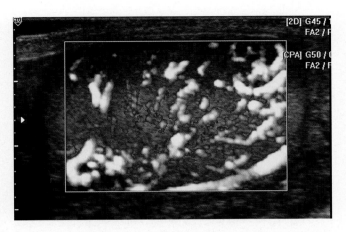

Figure 13-21. Marked increase in blood flow is seen with power Doppler throughout this testicle due to the presence of orchitis.

waveform analysis and RI can also provide additional information because epididymitis is associated with decreased vascular resistance compared with that seen in healthy men. The RI is rarely <0.5 in healthy individuals, but in >50% of patients with epididymo-orchitis, the RI is <0.5. Peak systolic velocity is increased in epididymal arteries, and use of a peak systolic velocity threshold of 15 cm/s results in a diagnostic accuracy of 93% for epididymitis.[26] What clearly separates epididymitis from testicular torsion is the presence of increased blood flow in the testicle when compared to the contralateral side.

ORCHITIS

Orchitis is an acute infection of the testicle; most cases follow an initial episode of epididymitis.[3] Isolated orchi-

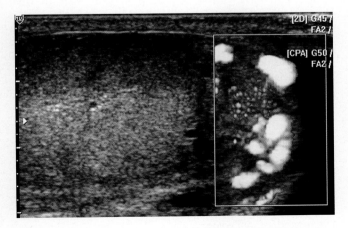

Figure 13-20. Prominent blood flow is shown in the power Doppler box located over the inflamed tail of the epididymis.

tis without epididymal involvement is rare and is usually viral in etiology. Testicular inflammation from mumps occurs in approximately 30% of cases and involvement is often bilateral. Orchitis develops in 20–40% of cases due to direct spread of infection from epididymis. It is usually diffuse. Patients present with a painful testicle must be differentiated from testicular torsion or other causes.

Sonographically, diffuse testicular involvement is usually seen as enlarged hypoechoic testicle due to edema, whereas a focal process usually manifests as multiple hypoechoic lesions. Other gray scale findings of orchitis include reactive hydrocele and scrotal skin thickening. In both orchitis and testicular torsion, inflammation and edema can lead to decreased echogenicity of the testis. B-mode ultrasound is not a reliable method to differentiate between orchitis and torsion unless torsion is advanced and prominent changes are noted. Power Doppler can assist in differentiating between the two diagnoses since testicular blood flow will increase as a result of inflammation (Figure 13-21). In approximately 40% of cases of orchitis, gray scale findings are normal and hyperemia on the color Doppler is the diagnostic finding.[29] The inflammation and associated increase in blood flow seen on power Doppler may be regionalized, especially early in the process. Significant inflammation may be seen in one portion of the testicle (e.g., the inferior pole), but not in the rest of the testicle. The clinician should take time to investigate the areas without markedly increased blood flow to make sure that flow is not absent in these regions. Necrosis in one part of the testicle could lead to inflammation and increased flow in an adjacent portion, which should prompt a urologic consultation. In addition, an area of absent blood flow may be due to an abscess, which should also prompt a urologic consultation (Figure 13-22).

Spectral Doppler can provide additional diagnostic clues such as increased intratesticular peak systolic

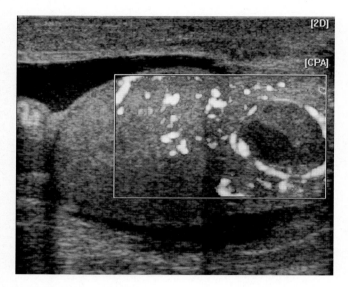

Figure 13-22. A complex hypoechoic area is shown in the testicle on the right side of the image. Power Doppler (gray scale copy) reveals flow in its periphery and elsewhere, but not inside this suspicious mass.

velocity, RI <0.5, and easily detectable and increased venous flow. The use of a peak systolic velocity threshold of 15 cm/s yields a diagnostic accuracy of 90% for orchitis.[26]

The increased blood flow of orchitis can mimic hyperemia seen after detorsion; if clinically suspicious, the clinician may simply rescan the patient in 15 minutes. The hyperemia from a recent detorsion should have resolved and the pain should also have resolved. Conversely, increased blood flow from orchitis will not resolve and pain will continue. Diffuse testicular hyperemia is also seen with infiltrative malignant diseases such as lymphoma and leukemia. In such cases, the clinical history can help differentiating infection from neoplasm. In cases with focal hypoechoic hypervascular lesion, involvement of the epididymis may distinguish the lesion from a testicular tumor. When focal lesions of heterogeneous echogenicity are diagnosed as epididymo-orchitis, a follow-up ultrasound examination after antibiotic treatment is recommended to confirm the resolution of the lesions so that other causes such as tumor, infarction, and metastasis can be ruled out. The complications of epididymo-orchitis include testicular infarction, scrotal abscess, pyocele, infertility, chronic pain, and atrophy.[28]

TESTICULAR TORSION

Torsion more often affects the left testes than right due to the greater length of the spermatic cord on the left side.[30] The sonographic findings of testicular torsion vary with the degree of rotation and duration of obstruction. The

▶ **TABLE 13-1. GRAY SCALE FEATURES OF TESTICULAR TORSION**

Normal appearance on gray scale (early torsion)
Enlarged and diffusely hypoechoic testis (Figure 13-23)
Hypoechoic pattern that may be partial
Hyperechoic and heterogeneous pattern (advanced finding)
Hypoechoic and small testis (chronic torsion)
Reactive hydrocele
Epididymal swelling
Thickening of the scrotal wall

gray scale features of testicular torsion are summarized in Table 13-1. The gray scale findings are nonspecific for testicular torsion and may be subtle or absolutely normal early in the course of testicular torsion. The edema and change in echogenicity of testes and epididymis may take 6 hours to develop.[15,30,31] Thus, always use Doppler to assess testicular perfusion. The Doppler features of testicular torsion are summarized in Table 13-2. When blood flow is absent or severely compromised in the affected testicle, the diagnosis of testicular torsion is clear. When the degree of flow is similar between the affected and comparison testicle, obtain pulsed-wave Doppler tracings to confirm both arterial and venous flow. Power Doppler alone should not assure the clinician that both venous and arterial flow are present. Additionally, the presence of arterial flow does not always exclude testicular torsion. The absence of a venous pattern by pulsed-wave Doppler on the affected side may be the only finding in early torsion. This is better understood by reviewing the mechanism of torsion and loss of blood supply to the testicle. During torsion, the testicle begins to twist around the axis of the spermatic cord. As the twisting progresses, venous flow is initially lost because of easily collapsible vessel walls in the low-pressure venous system. Venous obstruction is followed by a decrease in arterial inflow that eventually progresses to complete arterial obstruction. Thrombosis occurs in the arteries and veins and results in necrosis of testicular tissue. Experimental studies have shown that complete arterial occlusion occurs at about 450–540 degrees of torsion.[32] Once the spermatic cord

▶ **TABLE 13-2. DOPPLER PATTERNS OF TESTICULAR TORSION**

Absent or decreased venous flow
Absent or decreased arterial flow
Increased resistive index
Decreased arterial velocity
Decreased diastolic flow
Reversed diastolic flow

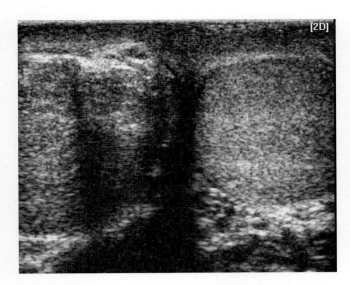

Figure 13-23. A side-by-side B-mode comparison view showing the right testicle (on the left side of the image) to be enlarged and less echogenic than the normal side (shown on the right side of the image).

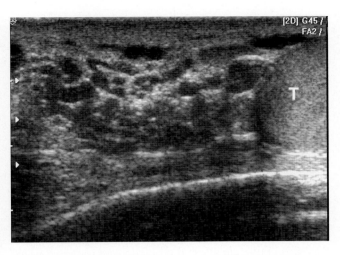

Figure 13-25. The transducer has been moved up proximal to the testicle (T) and cord vessels now fill the screen.

is fully torsed and no blood flow is present, the testicle takes on a diffusely edematous appearance (Figure 13-23), but this may take several hours to develop. The best way to diagnose complete torsion is to document the lack of power Doppler signal within the affected testicle (Figure 13-24).

Another abnormality that may be visualized in patients with testicular torsion is a spiral twisting of the spermatic cord above the level of the testicle. This may

appear as a round or oval extratesticular mass at the level of the torsion. This finding is known as the whirlpool sign and has been described as having the appearance of a doughnut, a target with concentric rings, a snail, a snail shell, or a storm on a weather map.[33] To detect this abnormality, advance the transducer proximally from the superior pole of the testicle and follow the incoming vessels up to the inguinal canal (Figure 13-25). When proceeding up the inguinal canal with the transducer oriented from the patient's feet to the head, the whirlpool mass may be seen (Figure 13-26). Adding power Doppler may show flow in blood vessels approaching the mass from the pelvis but no flow leaving

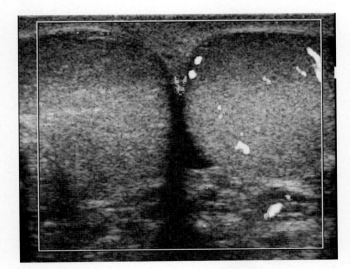

Figure 13-24. The same side-by-side comparison view as shown in Figure 13-23 but now with power Doppler (gray scale copy). The right testicle (shown on the left side of the image) is devoid of blood flow and was torsed at exploration.

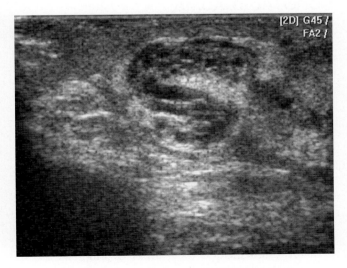

Figure 13-26. A longitudinal section above the testicle shows a complex area of knotting or twisting of the spermatic cord (whirlpool mass) in a patient with torsion.

the mass and heading toward the testicle. This confirms the diagnosis of torsion. Conversely, being able to trace cord vessels proximally into the inguinal canal and showing blood flow throughout their course help exclude the diagnosis of testicular torsion. The whirlpool sign is highly specific for testicular torsion; however, this finding can be misinterpreted as an enlarged epididymis and the patient can be misdiagnosed with epididymitis. Doppler can distinguish these entities by demonstrating decreased blood flow distal to a whirlpool mass and increased flow to the epididymis and testicle in cases of epididymitis.[33]

If the diagnosis is in doubt due to continued pain or if torsion–detorsion is suspected, performing serial point-of-care examinations is helpful. Closely following the blood flow can allow the practitioner to detect worsening torsion or the presence of torsion and detorsion in a patient who may otherwise have been sent home. Repeated color, power, and spectral Doppler examination could detect subtle progression of torsion in a patient with continued pain but with a normal initial exam. However, the presence of both venous and arterial blood flow in the testicle means it is not actively undergoing necrosis. Therefore, while continuing pain may be concerning, severe organ injury is not ongoing.

Torsion is not the only cause of testicular ischemia. Ischemia can result from spontaneous thrombosis of varicoceles or after corrective surgery. Severe edema following surgery or accidental vessel ligation during a vasectomy can also lead to vascular congestion and ischemia. The findings will be the same as in classic testicular torsion. A knot in the spermatic cord will not be identifiable in such cases.

SCROTAL TRAUMA

Scrotal trauma may result in damage to both the testes and the extratesticular structures. Visualization of a normal testicle on ultrasound examination virtually excludes any significant injury. Since surgical intervention is required for rupture of a testicle, the clinician should have a heightened awareness for any abnormalities seen within the testicle on ultrasound. In these cases, further investigation or urology consultation is warranted. The timely diagnosis of testicular rupture based on ultrasound findings is critical because prompt surgical intervention results in salvage of the testis in 80–90% of rupture cases.[23,34] Delayed diagnosis could result in ischemic necrosis of the testis, abscess, and loss of spermatogenesis. Ultrasound findings that suggest testicular rupture include focal areas of inhomogeneous echogenicity (Figure 13-27). These usually signal an area of hemorrhage or focal infarction. With larger hemorrhage, the testicle will lose its smooth contour (Figure 13-28). If the capsule of the testicle is intact, conserva-

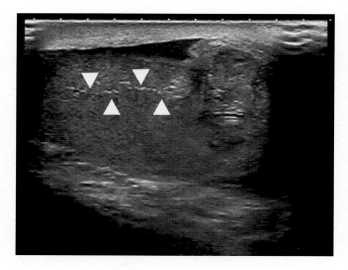

Figure 13-27. Arrow heads point to small focal hemorrhages in the testis after a baseball injury.

tive treatment will often suffice. However, if discontinuity of the echogenic tunica albuginea is seen, then surgical intervention is required. A testicular fracture is seen as a linear hypoechoic band crossing the testicular parenchyma, which represents a break in the normal testicular architecture. In fewer than 20% of cases, actual

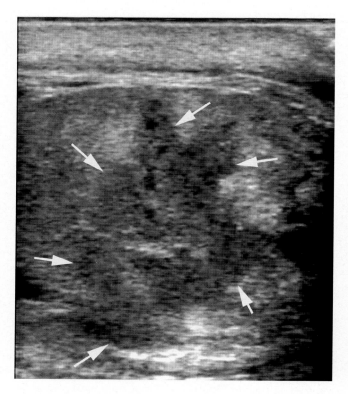

Figure 13-28. Testicular rupture has occurred after a sporting injury. Arrows outline an area of hemorrhage and testicular capsule appears violated.

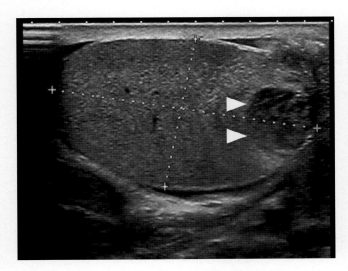

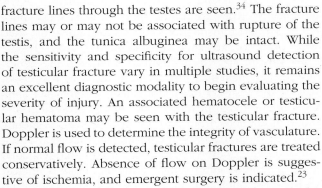

Figure 13-29. A focal intratesticular hematoma (arrow heads) is shown at the inferior pole of the testis after blunt testicular trauma.

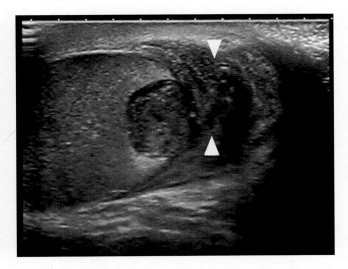

Figure 13-30. Adjacent to intratesticular hematoma and external to the testis, echogenic fluid collection representing hematocele (arrow heads) is seen.

fracture lines through the testes are seen.[34] The fracture lines may or may not be associated with rupture of the testis, and the tunica albuginea may be intact. While the sensitivity and specificity for ultrasound detection of testicular fracture vary in multiple studies, it remains an excellent diagnostic modality to begin evaluating the severity of injury. An associated hematocele or testicular hematoma may be seen with the testicular fracture. Doppler is used to determine the integrity of vasculature. If normal flow is detected, testicular fractures are treated conservatively. Absence of flow on Doppler is suggestive of ischemia, and emergent surgery is indicated.[23]

Hematomas can involve the testis or extratesticular soft tissues such as the epididymis or the scrotal wall. The intratesticular hematomas are generally focal but can be multiple (Figure 13-29). The appearance of the hematoma within the testicle can vary depending on the age and size of the bleed. Acute hematomas appear inhomogeneously echogenic, but will later develop large anechoic regions within it. If the hematoma is large and involves entire testis, the testicular parenchyma has heterogeneous appearance. Doppler ultrasound can help assess the potential viability of the testis in these cases. Although gray scale sonography can occasionally confuse hematomas and tumors, the use of color Doppler may differentiate the two processes. Tumors are often hypervascular while hematomas will not reveal blood flow internally. A mixture of findings can occur when a patient hemorrhages into a testicular mass.

Testicular hematomas may be associated with a hematocele and scrotal wall injuries. Scrotal wall hematoma is seen as echogenic focal thickening of the wall with absent or decreased vascularity. Hematoceles are complex fluid collections within the potential space

between the visceral and parietal layers of the tunica vaginalis. The appearance of hematocele varies depending on the length of time since the trauma occurred. Acute hematoceles are hyperechoic, and subacute and chronic hematoceles appear as complex fluid collections with loculations and septations (Figure 13-30). Hydroceles are also seen with scrotal trauma. Approximately 50% of acquired hydroceles are secondary to trauma.[23,34]

Testicular dislocation is a very rare condition after scrotal trauma. Dislocated testis can be found anywhere along a circle, the center of which is located in the external inguinal ring and the spermatic cord being the radius. The most common site reported is the superficial inguinal area, and other less common sites include the perineum, retrovesical, and acetabular regions. Ultrasound helps to exclude intratesticular injuries, and Doppler assessment confirms the viability of the testis. If the testis is viable, a manual reduction in the dislocated testis is recommended. If unsuccessful, emergent surgical reduction and fixation should be performed. Posttraumatic testicular torsion is a well-recognized entity, with an incidence of about 4–8%. The described mechanism of testicular torsion is a forceful contraction of cremasteric muscles. Perform color Doppler ultrasound assessment of testes to rule out torsion during scrotal injury evaluation.[23,34]

FOURNIER'S GANGRENE

Fournier's gangrene is another potential emergency that can present with acute scrotal pain and swelling. Fournier's gangrene is a rapidly progressing necrotizing fasciitis of the perineum and scrotum. It is a life-threatening polymicrobial infection that more commonly affects patients with impaired immune function.[35,36] Fournier's gangrene may be diagnosed solely on clinical grounds in advanced stages, where morbidity and mortality are highest. Since early detection and treatment are essential for decreasing morbidity and mortality, early imaging modalities may be required to differentiate Fournier's gangrene from scrotal cellulitis. Any delay in differentiating Fournier's gangrene from cellulitis or idiopathic scrotal edema may increase morbidity and mortality.

Ultrasound can aid in the early diagnosis of Fournier's gangrene before it is apparent clinically. It can provide valuable clues to differentiate between Fournier's gangrene and a benign cellulitis. Subcutaneous air on plain radiographs is not universally present, especially early in the disease process. CT does not visualize the scrotal structures as well as ultrasound, but more accurately detects small amounts of subcutaneous gas and may reveal the underlying cause of Fournier's gangrene, such as a perianal abscess, fistulous tract, intraabdominal infectious process, or incarcerated inguinal hernia.[37]

Sonographic findings seen with early Fournier's gangrene include thickening of the scrotal skin and multiple hyperechoic foci with dirty shadowing within the scrotal wall, which is pathognomonic for Fournier's gangrene (Figure 13-31).[20] The hyperechoic foci and associated dirty shadowing represent gas within the scrotal wall, not in the testicle. The presence of gas in the scrotal wall should not be confused with gas sometimes seen in herniated bowel in the scrotum. The characteristic gas pattern seen in Fournier's gangrene is parallel to the transducer face in the subcutaneous tissue of the scrotal wall. However, the gas visualized in the bowel lumen is located away from the scrotal wall and is not parallel to the transducer surface.[37] The testes are rarely involved in Fournier's gangrene because the blood supply to the scrotum is different from that to the testes. Since Fournier's gangrene may result from prostatitis or orchitis, signs of epididymo-orchitis may also be seen.

► COMMON VARIANTS AND SELECTED ABNORMALITIES

TESTICULAR CYSTS

Simple testicular cysts are usually asymptomatic, nonpalpable, and found in the testicular parenchyma. These benign cysts are filled with clear serous fluid. The cysts are usually solitary, but they can be multiple and bilateral. They are associated with extratesticular spermatoceles and epididymal cysts. The causes of simple testicular cysts are trauma, surgery, and prior inflammation. Sonographically, they are thin-walled, well-defined, have good through transmission, and contain anechoic fluid with posterior acoustic enhancement (Figure 13-32). They vary in size from 2 mm to 2 cm and are generally located near the mediastinum testis in the upper half of the testis. Tunica albuginea cysts have a similar sonographic appearance but tend to be smaller and range in diameter from 2 to 5 mm. They are frequently found in older patients and brought to medical attention when a patient presents with a palpable testicular lump. The etiology of tunica albuginea cysts is unclear and is most often a result of trauma, hemorrhage, and infection. They are well-defined cysts located within the

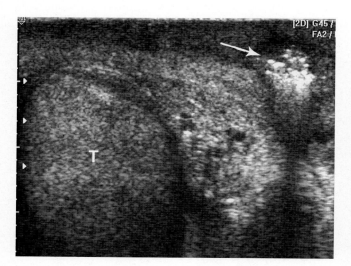

Figure 13-31. B-mode image showing testis (T) with thickened scrotal skin. A small area of subcutaneous gas is seen (arrow). This patient was found to have a scrotal abscess that was progressing to Fournier's gangrene.

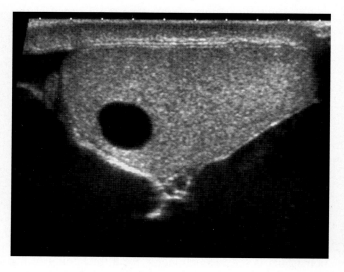

Figure 13-32. A well-defined intratesticular cyst shown in the long-axis view of the testis.

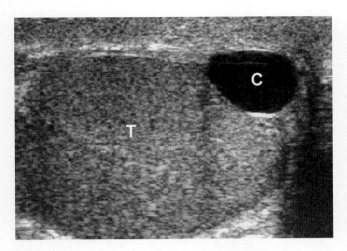

Figure 13-33. A cyst is shown in the tunica albuginea (C), in contact with the testicle (T).

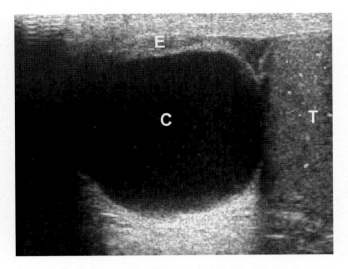

Figure 13-35. A large cyst (C) is shown in the epididymal head. A small wedge of compressed epididymal tissue (E) is shown just above the cyst. The testicle (T) is shown on the right side of the image.

tunica at the upper anterior or lateral aspects of the testicle (Figure 13-33). They are generally solitary and unilocular but can be multiple or multilocular. Rarely, they can have a complex appearance mimicking a testicular neoplasm.[27,38,39]

SPERMATOCELE/EPIDIDYMAL CYST

Spermatoceles are thought to result from cystic dilatations of the tubules of the efferent ductules and may be associated with a prior vasectomy. They are generally unilocular but can be multilocular. Sonographically, they are well-defined anechoic lesions measuring in size from subcentimeter to several centimeters, located within the

head of the epididymis (Figure 13-34). They have low-level echoes with posterior acoustic enhancement. They are difficult to differentiate from epididymal cysts on ultrasound. Epididymal cysts are less common than spermatoceles. They contain clear serous fluid and arise throughout the length of the epididymis. An increased incidence of epididymal cysts was reported in boys who are exposed to diethylstilbestrol in utero (Figures 13-35 and 13-36). Both lesions are thought to be the result of prior episodes of epididymitis and trauma.[11,27,39]

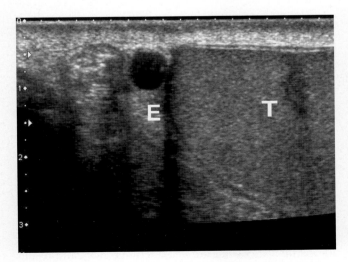

Figure 13-34. A small spermatocele is shown within the head of the epididymis. E = head of the epididymis, T = testicle.

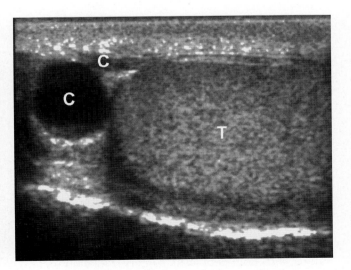

Figure 13-36. A medium-sized cyst is shown in the epididymal head (C) next to the testicle (T) as well as another smaller one just above and to the right of it.

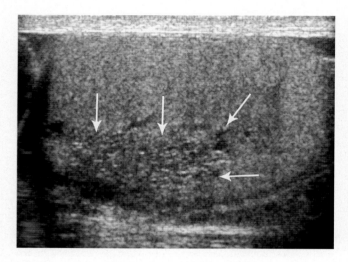

Figure 13-37. An area of dilated Rete testis is shown (arrows) in the long-axis view of the testicle.

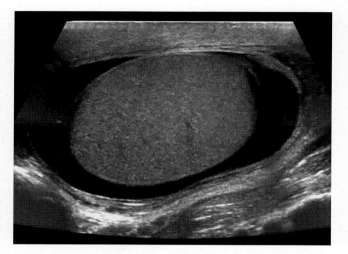

Figure 13-38. B-mode image showing testis outlined by serous fluid of moderate-sized hydrocele.

TUBULAR ECTASIA OF RETE TESTIS

Tubular ectasia of rete testis is an anatomical variant that may be more commonly found because of improved resolution on new ultrasound equipment. The majority of cases occur in men older than 55 years of age and are associated with spermatoceles or epididymal cysts. It is generally associated with obstruction in the epididymis from prior inflammation or trauma. Sonographically, dilated rete testis appears as a collection of multiple small cysts or channels in the region of mediastinum testis (Figure 13-37). Power Doppler will reveal them to be avascular. These lesions are often bilateral but are frequently asymmetric. Dilated rete testis can be mistaken for testicular tumor.[27]

HYDROCELE

There is a potential space between the visceral and parietal layers of the tunica vaginalis that can collect fluid, resulting in a hydrocele. A hydrocele is an abnormal collection of large amount of serous fluid in between the two layers of tunica vaginalis. It is the most commonly reported cause of painless scrotal swelling. Hydroceles are usually visualized in the anterolateral aspect of the scrotum and may be bilateral or unilateral. Their location is due to the attachment of the tunica to the testicle and scrotum posteriorly. Many hydroceles are congenital and result from a persistent communication between the scrotal sac and the abdominal cavity via a patent processus vaginalis. Acquired hydroceles can result from trauma, infection, neoplasm, surgery, radiation therapy, and undiagnosed torsion.[22]

Sonographically, a simple hydrocele appears as an anechoic or dark area surrounding the testicle

(Figure 13-38). Occasionally low-level echoes are visualized secondary to high protein content or deposition of cholesterol crystals. Complex hydroceles can contain septations and loculations, especially when an inflammatory process is present. Most acute hydroceles that form in reaction to infection are thin walled. The collections of fluid seen as a result of trauma or torsion also tend to be small. Chronic hydroceles (hematocele or pyocele) that have developed slowly from a secondary process are larger and may have irregular septations, which reflect previous hemorrhage or infection. As in most cases with ultrasonography, blood cannot always be differentiated from serous fluid. A history of trauma, previously diagnosed neoplasm, or surgery would suggest a hematocele. Pyoceles are the result of untreated epididymo-orchitis or rupture of an intratesticular abscess into the potential space between the two layers of the tunica vaginalis. A large number of echoes with septations and loculations in the hydrocele may suggest the presence of pus in the proper clinical setting (Figure 13-39).[8,26–28]

VARICOCELE

Varicocele represents abnormal dilation and tortuosity of the veins in the pampiniform plexus located in the spermatic cord. There are two types of varicoceles: primary (idiopathic) and secondary (acquired). Idiopathic varicocele is believed to be caused by incompetent valves in the internal spermatic vein, which results in retrograde flow of blood into pampiniform plexus. Nearly 99% of idiopathic varicoceles are left-sided but they can present bilaterally.[20] The spermatic vein on the right drains directly into the inferior vena cava. The left spermatic vein first drains into the left renal vein at nearly a 90° angle.

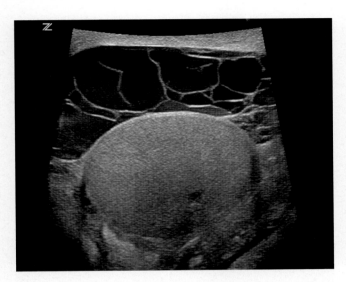

Figure 13-39. B-mode image demonstrating pyocele with multiple septations and echogenic fluid surrounding the testicle. On exploration, the scrotum was filled with pus that may have started with epididymitis. (Courtesy of Michelle Vaughn, RDMS)

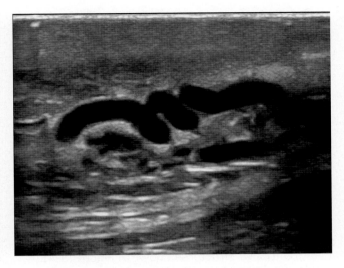

Figure 13-40. Serpiginous dilated vessels characteristic of varicocele are shown on this image running from left to right (toward the testicle).

The left-sided predominance of varicoceles is due to the greater length of the left internal spermatic vein in comparison with the right and increased venous pressure on the left side caused by the junction of the left internal spermatic vein with the left renal vein at a right angle. Secondary varicoceles are due to increased pressure on the spermatic vein caused by various disease processes such as hydronephrosis, cirrhosis, or a mass in the abdomen or retroperitoneal space. Secondary varicoceles may also occur with thrombosis of the inferior vena cava and in the nutcracker phenomenon, which is characterized by compression of the left renal vein in the fork between the abdominal aorta and proximal superior mesenteric artery that leads to retrograde blood flow from the left renal vein into the internal spermatic vein causing varicocele.[40] A right-sided varicocele, non-decompressible varicocele, and a newly discovered varicocele in a patient older than 40 years should prompt an investigation for a neoplasm. In men over 40 years of age, a non-decompressible varicocele is classically caused by a renal malignancy invading the renal vein.

Patients usually present with a palpable scrotal mass, dull scrotal pain, or discomfort or feeling of heaviness. Perform ultrasound assessment with the patient in both a supine and a standing position. Varicocele becomes more noticeable in the standing position and when the patient performs a Valsalva maneuver. Normally, the diameter of veins of the pampiniform plexus veins range from 0.5 to 1.5 mm. Gray scale findings include multiple, hypoechoic, serpiginous, tubular structures with diameters exceeding 2 mm that are usually best seen superior and lateral to the testis (Figures 13-40

and 13-41). Color Doppler ultrasound is almost 100% sensitive and specific in diagnosing varicocele.[26] The addition of power Doppler, especially with a concomitant Valsalva maneuver, will demonstrate blood flow in the characteristic pattern (Figure 13-42). Doppler will reveal a phasic venous blood flow pattern and retrograde filling with Valsalva maneuver. Varicoceles increase in size and show increased color Doppler flow with the patient in standing position.

Occasionally, varicoceles may be confused with inflammation of the epididymal tail or bowel content in the scrotum. Having the patient perform a Valsalva maneuver should cause distention of the varices, and an

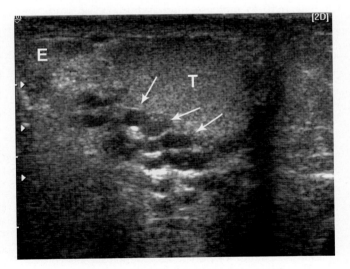

Figure 13-41. Extended varicocele. Tubular structures (arrows) are shown in the lower left corner of the testicle (T). The typical testicular architecture is disrupted. E = Epididymis.

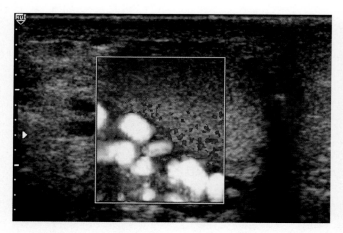

Figure 13-42. A power Doppler window now sits over the tubular structures shown in Figure 13-41. A significant amount of venous flow is shown with a Valsalva maneuver.

obvious increase in blood flow through the venous structures. On rare occasions, a varicocele may be seen extending into the testicle itself. It can be followed from its origin to differentiate it from other pathologic processes.

HERNIATION

Herniation of abdominal contents into the scrotum may cause acute scrotal pain. The clinical presentation may simulate testicular torsion, epididymitis, or orchitis. Ultrasound is especially helpful in patients with equivocal clinical findings. To identify a hernia, it may not be sufficient to just scan patients in the supine position. It may help to increase intra-abdominal pressure with a Valsalva maneuver. Ultrasound can help identify the testes and often allows the examiner to visualize abdominal contents (Figure 13-43). Occasionally, a fluid or air-filled loop of bowel can be clearly visualized. In other cases, artifacts from bowel gas may be the only sign of a hernia. It is critical not to confuse Fournier's gangrene with bowel gas in a hernia. The viability of a bowel segment within the hernia sac can be grossly assessed with ultrasound. Obvious peristalsis typically means that the bowel has not yet infarcted. An akinetic dilated loop of bowel has high sensitivity (90%) and specificity (93%) for bowel strangulation.[26] Clinicians should be aware of the possibility of contraction of the Dartos mimicking peristalsis. Also, power Doppler identification of blood flow in the bowel wall suggests viability. Absence of peristalsis, edematous bowel wall, and lack of blood flow on power Doppler suggest infarction. Increased power Doppler flow (hyperemia) may be seen in the early stages of strangulation. Omental fat can also be herniated into the scrotum and become

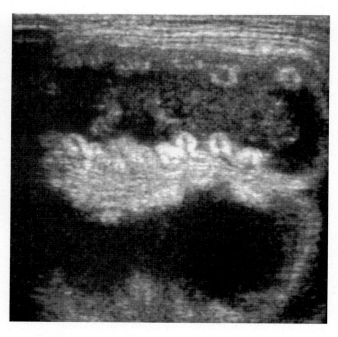

Figure 13-43. Scrotal hernia. Two loops of bowel are shown in the scrotum. Some fecal matter is shown in the near-field loop.

strangulated. Sonographically, omental fat is seen as a complex echogenic paratesticular mass in the hernia sac. In addition, testicular ischemia can occur due to vascular compression from a hernia. Manipulation of hernia contents may result in compression of vascular structures within the inguinal canal. Consider post-reduction testicular ultrasound when patients have ongoing pain after reduction in an inguinal hernia.[41]

TESTICULAR TUMORS

The incidence of testicular tumors in prepubertal boys is estimated at 0.5–2.0 cases per 100,000. Most patients present with a painless scrotal swelling. Testicular tumors are uncommon causes of acute painful scrotum. Approximately 10% of the patients present with acute scrotal pain due to hemorrhage into the tumor or necrosis of the tumor. This acute presentation may mimic testicular torsion or epididymo-orchitis. The majority (95%) of the testicular tumors are germ cell neoplasms.[42] Seminoma accounts for approximately 50% of these cases. In most cases, patients with testicular tumors need early urologic follow-up, not an emergent procedure. However, if a large intratumoral hemorrhage is detected, then immediate urologic consultation is prudent. Patients who present with large painless testicular masses that may have been developing for years require careful consideration prior to discharge (Figure 13-44).

The sensitivity of ultrasound for detecting testicular tumors approaches 100%. Sonographically, testicular

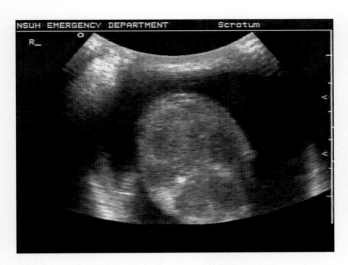

Figure 13-44. Testicular tumor. A long-axis view of the testicle reveals a surrounding hydrocele and multiple hypoechoic areas that replace the normal architecture. This tumor was discovered in a patient complaining of acute testicular enlargement. On further questioning, the patient admitted that his testicle was slowly enlarging for over 2 years.

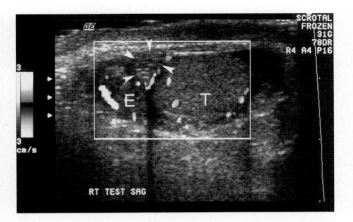

Figure 13-45. While increased flow was shown in the epididymis and testicle of this 8-year-old patient, no flow was noted within the suspected torsed appendix testis outlined by arrowheads. E = epididymis, T = testicle.

tumors appear as focal or diffuse areas of hypoechogenicity in enlarged testicles. An area of heterogeneous echogenicity is suggestive of intratumoral hemorrhage and necrosis. Calcifications and cysts may also be found. Color Doppler imaging of suspected tumors is unreliable since the hypervascularity detected in testicular tumors is not distinguishable from the hypervascularity seen in testicular inflammation. The absence of enlargement of epididymis and edema of scrotal skin should favor the diagnosis of a tumor rather than an inflammatory process.

TORSION OF THE APPENDIX TESTIS

The appendix testis is a remnant of the paramesonephric duct. Torsion of the appendix testis is the most common cause of acute scrotal pain in children before puberty. In the pediatric population, appendiceal torsion is nearly as common as testicular torsion, accounting for 20–40% of acute scrotal pain cases.[28,29] It is more frequently seen on the left side. Torsion of the appendix testis can present with similar symptoms to testicular torsion, but is often noted in a younger age group. It is important to distinguish appendicial torsion from testicular torsion because appendicial torsion is a self-limiting condition and does not require surgery. The sensitivity of ultrasound for the detection of appendiceal torsion is approximately 90%. Sonographically, the torsed appendix is visualized as a small hyper- or hypoechoic mass adjacent to the superior aspect of the testis or epi-

didymis, depending on the evolution time. The testicular appendage larger than 5.6 mm is suggestive of torsion. Color Doppler demonstrates no internal blood flow in a torsed testicular appendage, and marked hyperemia in the adjacent tissues and diffusely throughout the testis and epididymis (Figure 13-45). Other ultrasound findings include reactive hydrocele, enlarged epididymal head, and scrotal skin edema.[28,29]

CALCIFICATIONS

Calcifications in the scrotum are most often in the testicle or tunica albuginea, or within a hydrocele. "Scrotal pearls" are mobile hyperechoic calculi within a hydrocele resulting in a discrete acoustic shadow. These calcified bodies are the result of inflammation of the tunica vaginalis testis, hematoma, or torsion of the appendix testis or the epididymis. Scrotal pearls are usually of no clinical significance and no further workup is warranted. Small testicular calcifications are known as microlithiasis (Figure 13-46). Testicular microlithiasis refers to the presence of multiple nonshadowing echogenic foci that are 1–3 mm in size within the testicular parenchyma. The presence of five or more echogenic foci per transducer field in one testis is considered abnormal.[26,43] These echogenic foci represent calcified hydroxyapatite concretions within the lumen of the seminiferous tubules. Most are discovered incidentally by ultrasound examinations done for symptoms such as pain, swelling, trauma, varicocele, hydrocele, or infertility.[26,43] Testicular microlithiasis is usually benign, but it is found in 50% of patients with germ cell neoplasms, and the significance of this association is unclear.

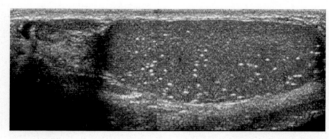

A

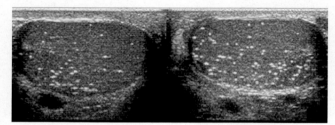

B

Figure 13-46. Longitudinal view of one testicle (A) and transverse views of both testicles (B) reveal multiple small symmetrical echogenic foci consistent with microlithiasis.

UNDESCENDED TESTICLE

Patients may occasionally present with scrotal pain and are found to have only one testicle. While there can be congenital or surgically related absence of a testicle, it may be worthwhile to check for an undescended testicle, even in young adults. An undescended testicle may increase the risk of both infertility and testicular cancer. It is associated with a 50-fold increased risk of testicular cancer. Additionally, there is a 10-fold increase in the incidence of torsion of an undescended testis.[30] Some patients may not be aware that one testicle has not descended. The majority (80%) of undescended testes lie within the inguinal canal and are often (25%) bilateral. Ultrasound has an accuracy of approximately 90% for localizing the undescended testicle. The undescended testis is frequently small and hypoechoic, and it might be difficult to differentiate from a lymph node. Assess blood flow since the risk of torsion is high in patients with painful undescended testicles (Figures 13-47 and 13-48).[27]

▶ PITFALLS

1. **Contraindication.** There are no absolute contraindications to evaluating the testicle with ultrasound. Examinations may be limited by pain, and analgesia will occasionally be required. Since minimal pressure is applied during the

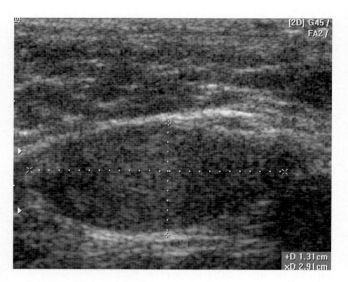

Figure 13-47. This small, prepubescent appearing testicle was located proximal to the scrotum in the patient's pelvis.

evaluation of the acute testicle, damage to a fractured testicle is not a concern.

2. **Neonates and prepubescent boys.** Testicular blood flow in prepubescent boys and neonates can be very difficult to detect, which may lead to inaccurate diagnoses. Doppler can demonstrate blood flow in only 32% of pediatric patients with a testicular volume <1 mL. In neonates, it is difficult to detect blood flow in about 10%

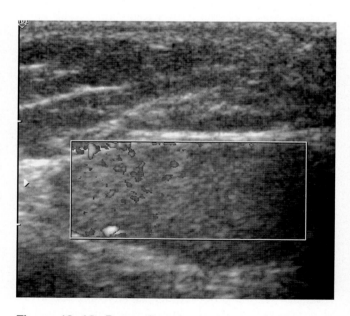

Figure 13-48. Power Doppler (gray scale copy) detected some flow in the undescended testicle with both venous and arterial flow patterns confirmed on pulsed-wave Doppler.

▶ **TABLE 13-3. SPECTRAL DOPPLER FEATURES OF PARTIAL TESTICULAR TORSION**

Decreased intratesticular flow compared to the unaffected testis

Asymmetry in the spectral Doppler arterial waveform

Absence of a dicrotic notch in the arterial waveform

Drop in diastolic flow velocities on the affected side

Reversal of diastolic flow

Asymmetry in resistive indices

of normal testes.[30] It may require very sensitive equipment and considerable expertise to evaluate prepubescent testes.

3. **Incomplete torsion.** Complete torsion occurs at approximately 450° of twisting of the spermatic cord. Venous flow initially disappears followed by arterial blood flow. The presence of blood flow on Doppler only excludes complete testicular torsion. The sonographic findings of incomplete torsion may be subtle and careful comparison between the two sides is important to exclude incomplete or partial torsion. Diagnosing torsion early, when it is incomplete, can be challenging with color Doppler alone, as this method relies on subtle differences between the testes. The use of spectral Doppler to document both venous and arterial waveforms is optimal. The spectral Doppler findings suggestive of partial torsion are summarized in Table 13-3. The whirlpool sign, ipsilateral hydrocele, and scrotal thickening may also be found. If the suspicion

for torsion is high and the initial ultrasound is normal, serial point-of-care ultrasound examinations should be considered.[15,30,31]

4. **Intermittent torsion.** A history of intermittent episodes of testicular pain that resolve spontaneously is highly suggestive of intermittent testicular torsion and detorsion. Approximately 50% of patients presenting with acute testicular torsion report previous episodes of recurrent scrotal pain. Ultrasound may not always be helpful since torsion may resolve before imaging is performed and ultrasound may show normal appearing testes. Unfortunately, intermittent testicular torsion can result in testicular damage seen histologically as peritubular fibrosis, atrophic seminiferous tubules, and decreased spermatogenesis. If this clinical entity is suspected, a urology consultation and orchiopexy is recommended in the near future before another acute event occurs. Approximately 10% of patients with history of intermittent torsion develop acute testicular torsion while waiting for orchiopexy.[15,30,31]

5. **Postischemic hyperemia/Torsion–detorsion.** Some patients may exhibit torsion and spontaneous detorsion. This entity can make for a challenging diagnosis if the ultrasound examination is performed during a period of detorsion. Shortly after detorsion, compensatory postischemic hyperemia may be detected as increased blood flow in the affected testicle (Figure 13-49). This can be confused with epididymo-orchitis. This paradoxical increase in blood flow will usually not last much longer

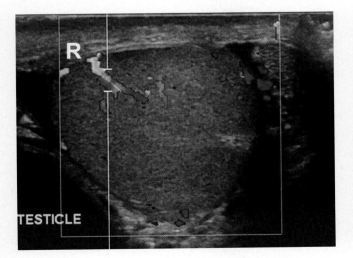
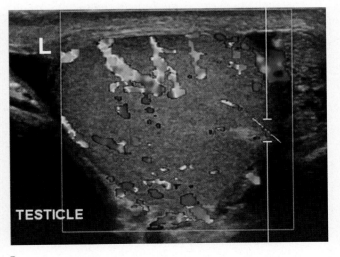

A   B

Figure 13-49. Color Doppler ultrasound performed shortly after detorsion shows normal flow in right testicle (A) compared to increased flow in the left (affected) testicle (B) from compensatory postischemic hyperemia.

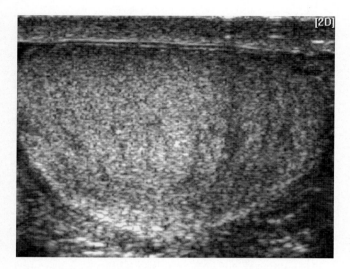

Figure 13-50. The testicle appears to have multiple vertical striations running through it. This was not a pathologic state, rather the normal appearance of a testicle of this 55-year-old diabetic patient.

than 15 minutes and returns to normal again at the site of detorsion. Point-of-care ultrasonography may be helpful in this setting because it allows for serial examinations. With the clinical acumen to observe the patient and perform serial ultrasound examinations, clinicians should be able to avoid this pitfall.[15,30,31]

6. **Striated testis.** With the aid of modern high-resolution equipment, providers are more likely than ever to see details of testicular structure not previously noted on ultrasound. In fact, the technological advances in imaging have created dilemmas, in which differentiation between normal anatomic variants and pathologic conditions can become challenging. One such example is striated testes, which presents as multiple hypoechoic linear bands radiating within the testis perpendicular to its long axis, similar in orientation to the testicular interlobar fibrous septae (Figure 13-50). Striated testes are most likely the result of interstitial fibrosis in asymptomatic older men and require no further evaluation. However, the differential diagnosis of striated testes also includes neoplasm, infection, infarction, and trauma. Narrowing the differential diagnoses depends on clinical presentation (age, history of malignancy, palpable testicular mass), and additional sonographic findings such as size of the testicle, focal mass, and Doppler abnormalities. In the absence of risk factors, relevant clinical findings, and Doppler abnormalities, a striated testicle is of no clinical significance. It is most likely due to fibrosis from

aging or prior infection and probably needs no further follow-up.[44]

► CASE STUDIES

CASE 1

Patient Presentation

A 21-year-old man presented to the ED with a complaint of right testicular pain. He stated that the pain started suddenly 5 hours prior to presentation. Since then, he also noted some swelling on the right side. The patient denied being sexually active but did note being struck in the genitals the day before during a basketball game. He had an unremarkable medical history and did not smoke. The patient denied any history of sexually transmitted diseases and stated he was not having any urinary symptoms or urethral discharge.

Physical examination revealed a healthy young male in mild distress with normal vital signs. The abdominal examination was unremarkable, with no obvious hernias or costovertebral angle tenderness. Testicular examination revealed an erythematous right hemiscrotum with moderate swelling. The right testicle was enlarged and painful to the touch. The epididymis was tender and slightly enlarged on examination. The right testicle had a horizontal lie and the cremasteric reflex could not be elicited. The left testicle was normal size and nontender to palpation.

Management Course

A urinalysis was normal. No urology service was available and a tertiary care hospital was approximately 90 minutes away by ambulance. Point-of-care emergency ultrasonography was available to the emergency physician. She performed an examination of the scrotum, noting enlargement and greatly increased blood flow to the right testicle and epididymis, with the epididymis twice the width compared to the contralateral side. A diagnosis of epididymitis with orchitis was made and the patient was discharged home with antibiotics, analgesics, and close follow-up and return instructions.

Commentary

Case 1 represents an example of the nonspecific signs, symptoms, and history that may be associated with the presentation of acute scrotal pain. The patient acutely became aware of testicular discomfort and swelling, although the disease process was probably slower in onset. The history of minor testicular trauma was coincidental, but could not be ignored. The physical examination is often less helpful than described in many textbooks, especially when orchitis is present and the entire testicle is tender and swollen. Without the availability of point-of-care ultrasound, the emergency physician would have had to transfer the patient. If a lack of blood flow was seen in the testicle, arrangements could have been made for immediate transfer to a urology consultant and manual detorsion could have been attempted. In this case, Doppler ultrasound showed increased blood flow to the testicle and epididymis, which is consistent with orchitis and epididymitis. An unnecessary transfer was avoided and the patient was discharged home with appropriate treatment and follow-up instructions.

CASE 2

Patient Presentation

An 18-year-old man presented to the ED 3 days after being kicked in the groin during a soccer match. The patient was seen at an outside facility shortly after the injury at which time an evaluation, including an ultrasound examination, revealed a small-to-moderate-sized area of hemorrhage and no rupture through the testicular capsule. The patient was evaluated by an urologist and discharged home. He presents today because of increased swelling of the testicle. The scrotal skin is firm and erythematous, according to the mother, who is a pediatrician. The hydrocodone the patient was prescribed no longer relieves his pain. He denies any hematuria or other urinary symptoms.

Physical examination revealed an uncomfortable appearing male with normal vital signs. The cardiac, lung, and abdominal examinations were normal. Testicular examination revealed an enlarged and erythematous left hemiscrotum that was markedly tender to palpation. The testicle was clearly enlarged but difficult to differentiate within the scrotum. The contralateral testicle was nontender and appeared to be of normal size. A urinalysis was normal. The mother insisted that something had changed since his injury; however, when she contacted the urologist, he suggested a follow-up appointment in 2 days and recommended increasing the patient's analgesic dose.

Management Course

An ultrasound examination in the medical imaging department was not available after hours. The emergency physician performed a point-of-care ultrasound examination, and this revealed a large heterogeneous testicle with areas of acute and old hemorrhage. Normal color Doppler flow was present in the portion of the testicle that appeared normal. A fracture line could be defined through the parenchyma of the testicle and appeared to go through the capsule of the testicle. The urologist on call was contacted. After a brief evaluation and re-

view of the point-of-care ultrasound examination clips, the patient was taken to the operating room for scrotal exploration. Exploration revealed several areas of hemorrhage and a testicular rupture that were repaired. The patient was admitted overnight. Follow-up showed slow resolution of the injury with 80% function of the testicle at 30 days. No further surgical intervention was required.

Commentary

Case 2 illustrates the utility of ultrasound in defining testicular anatomy. The patient had already been scanned 3 days ago and no severe pathology was noted. However, he bled more into the testicle and a fracture line going through the capsule was better defined on reexamination. The patient had findings that led directly to operative intervention. It would have been tempting to simply discharge him home for follow-up with his urologist as planned. Point-of-care ultrasound helped the patient avoid ongoing pain and further disability.

CASE 3

Patient Presentation

A 34-year-old man presented to the ED, complaining of left scrotal pain. The patient noted awaking with severe pain approximately 6 hours prior to the admission. His medical history was remarkable for recent surgery to "fix" some varicoceles that had been causing him pain for years. He complained of scrotal pain, which was different from the incisional pain.

Physical examination revealed an afebrile patient in moderate distress. Examination of the abdomen was unremarkable. The GU examination showed a slightly erythematous scrotum, more prominent on the left. There was moderate swelling of the left testicle and it was exquisitely tender. It had a normal lie and the epididymis could not be reliably palpated. The cremasteric reflex was elicited with difficulty bilaterally. There was no evidence of infection at the incision site.

Management Course

A urinalysis showed three RBCs per high-powered field and five WBCs per high-powered field. No bacteria were seen. An ultrasound examination performed by the emergency physician revealed the right testicle to have normal echotexture, size, and blood flow. The left testicle was found to be moderately enlarged and appeared less echogenic than the unaffected testicle. The right testicle had normal blood flow with color and power Doppler imaging. No blood flow was seen within the left testicle with either color or power Doppler. The on-call urologist was consulted and immediately took the patient for surgical exploration of the scrotum. He was found to have an ischemic left testicle as a result of diffuse thrombosis of veins in the spermatic cord with resultant vascular congestion.

Commentary

This case illustrates the difficulty in making a diagnosis of testicular ischemia without imaging in patients with scrotal pain. Clinicians who use point-of-care ultrasound are likely to make more accurate and confident diagnoses.

► ACKNOWLEDGMENT

The author gratefully acknowledges the contributions of Michael Blaivas, who authored this chapter in the previous edition.

REFERENCES

1. Lewis AG, Bukowski TP, Jarvis PD: Evaluation of acute scrotum in the emergency department. *J Pediatric Surg* 30:277–280, 1995.
2. Fernandez MS, Dominguez C, Sanguesa C: The use of color Doppler sonography of the acute scrotum in children. *Cir Pediatr* 10:25–27, 1997.
3. Zoller G: Genitourinary trauma. In: Rosen P, Barkin R, eds. *Emergency Medicine Concepts and Clinical Practice.* 4th ed. St. Louis, MO: Mosby, 1997:2243–2245.
4. Knight PJ, Vassy LE: The diagnosis and treatment of the acute scrotum in children and adolescents. *Ann Surg* 200:664–666, 1984.
5. Albrecht T, Lotzof K, Hussain HK, et al.: Bruyn: Power Doppler US of the normal prepubertal testis: Does it live up to its promises? *Radiology* 203:227–231, 1997.
6. Fenner MN, Roszhart DA, Texter JH: Testicular scanning: Evaluating the acute scrotum in the clinical setting. *Urology* 10:25, 1991.
7. Jefferson RH, Perez LM, Joseph DB: Critical analysis of the clinical presentation of acute scrotum: A 9-year experience at a single institution. *J Urol* 158:1198–1201, 1997.
8. Aso C, Enríquez G, Fité M, et al.: Gray-scale and color Doppler sonography of scrotal disorders in children: An update. *Radiographics* 25:1197–1214, 2005.
9. Cos LR, Rabinowitz R: Trauma-induced testicular torsion in children. *J Trauma* 22:223–225, 1982.
10. Schmitz D, Safranek S: Clinical inquiries. How useful is a physical exam in diagnosing testicular torsion?. *J Fam Pract* 58:433–434, 2009.
11. Gorman B: The scrotum. In: Rumack C, Wilson S, Charboneau W, Levine D, eds. *Diagnostic Ultrasound.* Philadelphia, PA: Elsevier, 2011:840–877.
12. Prater JM, Overdorf BS: Testicular torsion: A surgical emergency. *Am Fam Emerg Physician* 44:834–840, 1991.
13. Lee TF, Winter DB, Madsen FA, et al.: Conventional color Doppler velocity sonography versus color Doppler energy sonography for the diagnosis of acute experimental torsion of the spermatic cord. *AJR* 167:785–790, 1996.
14. Kass EJ, Stone KT, Cacciarelli AA, et al.: Do all children with an acute scrotum require exploration? *J Urol* 150:667–669, 1993.
15. Prando D: Torsion of the spermatic cord: The main gray-scale and Doppler sonographic signs. *Abdom Imaging* 34:648–661, 2009.
16. Blaivas M, Sierzenski P, Lambert M: Emergency evaluation of patients presenting with acute scrotum using bedside ultrasonography. *Acad Emerg Med* 8:90–93, 2001.
17. Blaivas M, Sierzenski P: Emergency ultrasonography in the evaluation of the acute scrotum. *Acad Emerg Med* 8:85–89, 2001.
18. Blaivas M, Batts M, Lambert M: Ultrasonographic diagnosis of testicular torsion by emergency physicians. *Am J Emerg Med* 18:198–200, 2000.
19. Sierzenski P, Blaivas M, Belden M, et al.: Manual compression of the spermatic cord to simulate testicular torsion on ultrasound. A teaching model for emergency physicians. *Acad Emerg Med* 7:493, 2000.
20. Morrison D, Blaivas M, Lyon M: Emergency diagnosis of Fournier's gangrene with bedside ultrasound. *Am J Emerg Med* 23:544–547, 2005.
21. Blaivas M, Lyon M, Theodoro D: A two-year experience with bedside emergency ultrasound for acute scrotal pain in the emergency department. *Ann Emerg Med* 44:S82, 2004.
22. Stewart R, Carroll B: The scrotum. In: Rumack CM, Wilson SR, Charboneau JW, eds. *Diagnostic Ultrasound*, vol 1. St. Louis, MO: Mosby, 1991:565–589.
23. Deurdulian C, Mittelstaedt CA, Chong WK, et al.: US of acute scrotal trauma: Optimal technique, imaging findings, and management. *Radiographics* 27:357–369, 2007.
24. Micallef M, Ahmad I, Ramesh N, et al.: Ultrasound features of blunt testicular injury. *Injury* 32:23–26, 2001.
25. Corrales JG, Corbel L, Cipolla B, et al.: Accuracy of ultrasound diagnosis after blunt testicular trauma. *J Urol* 150:1834–1836, 1993.
26. Dogra VS, Gottlieb RH, Oka M, et al.: Sonography of the scrotum. *Radiology* 227:18–36, 2003.
27. Akin EA, Khati NJ, Hill MC: Ultrasound of the scrotum. *Ultrasound Q* 20:181–200, 2004.
28. Turgut A, Bhatt S, Dogra V: Acute painful scrotum. *Ultrasound Clin* 3:93, 107, 2008.
29. Coley B: The acute pediatric scrotum. *Ultrasound Clin* 1:485–496, 2006.
30. Prando D: Torsion of the spermatic cord: sonographic diagnosis. *Ultrasound Q* 18:41–57, 2002.
31. Dogra V, Bhatt S, Rubens D: Sonographic evaluation of testicular torsion. *Ultrasound Clin* 1:55–66, 2006.
32. Netter F: *Scrotum: Reproductive System.* West Caldwell, NJ: CIBA; 1989:73.
33. Vijayaraghavan SB: Sonographic differential diagnosis of acute scrotum: Real-time whirlpool sign, a key sign of torsion. *J Ultrasound Med* 25:563–574, 2006.
34. Bhatt S, Ghazale H, Dogra V: Sonographic evaluation of scrotal and penile trauma. *Ultrasound Clin* 2:45–56, 2007.

35. Benziri E, Fabiani P, Migliori G, et al.: Gangrene of the perineum. *Urology* 47:935–939, 1996.

36. Carroll PR, Cattolica EV, Turzan CW, et al.: Necrotizing soft-tissue infections of the perineum and genitalia: Etiology and early reconstruction. *West J Med* 144:174–178, 1996.

37. Levenson RB, Singh AK, Novelline RA: Fournier gangrene: Role of imaging. *Radiographics* 28:519–528, 2008.

38. Dogra VS, Gottlieb RH, Rubens DJ, et al.: Benign intratesticular cystic lesions: US features. *Radiographics* 21:S273–S81, 2001.

39. Bhatt S, Rubens DJ, Dogra VS: Sonography of benign intrascrotal lesions. *Ultrasound Q* 22:121–136, 2006.

40. Mohammadi A, Ghasemi-Rad M, Mladkova N: Varicocele and nutcracker syndrome: Sonographic findings. *J Ultrasound Med* 29:1153–1160, 2010.

41. Turgut AT, Olcucuoglu E, Turan C, et al.: Preoperative ultrasonographic evaluation of testicular volume and blood flow in patients with inguinal hernias. *J Ultrasound Med* 26:1657–1666, 2007.

42. Hill MC, Sanders RC: Sonography of benign disease of the scrotum. In: Sanders RC, Hill M, eds. *Ultrasound Annual*. New York, NY: Raven Press, 1986:197–237.

43. Carkaci S, Ozkan E, Lane D, et al.: Scrotal sonography revisited. *J Clin Ultrasound* 38:21–37, 2010.

44. Loberant N, Bhatt S, McLennan GT, et al.: Striated appearance of the testes. *Ultrasound Q* 26:37–44, 2010.

CHAPTER 14

First Trimester Pregnancy

Robert F. Reardon, Jamie Hess-Keenan, Chad E. Roline, Liberty V. Caroon, and Scott A. Joing

Ultrasound is the primary imaging modality used in pregnancy.[1-4] In the first-trimester, pregnant patients who present with vaginal bleeding or abdominal pain, ultrasound can be used to distinguish ectopic pregnancy from threatened abortion or embryonic demise. The primary goal of emergency sonography of the pelvis in the first trimester is to identify an intrauterine pregnancy, which usually excludes the diagnosis of ectopic pregnancy.[5] Secondary objectives are to detect extrauterine signs of an ectopic pregnancy, estimate the viability of an intrauterine pregnancy, clarify gestational age, and characterize other causes of pelvic pain and vaginal bleeding. In addition, sonographic detection of free fluid outside of the pelvis can help emergency physicians expedite the care of a patient with a ruptured ectopic pregnancy.[6] Emergency point-of-care sonography is not intended to define the entire spectrum of pelvic pathology in early pregnancy. A follow-up comprehensive pelvic ultrasound examination may be indicated after the initial focused point-of-care examination, the timing of which is dictated by the clinical scenario.

▶ CLINICAL CONSIDERATIONS

Abdominal or pelvic pain and vaginal bleeding are common complaints during early pregnancy. Challenges to emergency or acute care physicians include making the diagnosis of pregnancy and then using available diagnostic tools to determine the etiology of the patient's complaint.

The development of sensitive pregnancy tests has made a missed diagnosis of early pregnancy unlikely. Modern qualitative urine tests for human chorionic gonadotropin (β-hCG) have a threshold of about 20 IU/L and allow detection of pregnancy as early as 1 week postconception (3 weeks' gestational age). False-negative urine tests may occur when the urine is highly dilute (specific gravity <1.010), and obtaining a quantitative serum β-hCG should be considered in such cases.[7]

Once pregnancy is recognized in a symptomatic or high-risk patient, complications of early pregnancy, particularly ectopic pregnancy, must be considered. Those patients with pelvic or abdominal pain, vaginal bleeding, dizziness, syncope, or any risk factors for ectopic pregnancy need to have the status of their pregnancy evaluated. The location, viability, and gestational age of the pregnancy are important factors in establishing a diagnosis. Other findings such as free intraperitoneal fluid in the pelvis or a pelvic mass may also impact the patient's management.

Many diagnostic tests can be used to detect complications of early pregnancy. Serum β-hCG and progesterone levels, suction curettage, culdocentesis, and laparoscopy yield some information, but none can identify the entire spectrum of pathology like pelvic sonography. Furthermore, other imaging modalities, like CT and MRI, are not commonly used for detecting complications of early pregnancy.

The hormone β-hCG is produced by the trophoblasts during early pregnancy. Serum β-hCG levels rise exponentially in early pregnancy and can be used as a marker to date normal pregnancies. However, abnormal pregnancies have widely varying β-hCG levels, so a single level cannot differentiate a normal intrauterine pregnancy from an ectopic pregnancy or other abnormality.[8]

Progesterone is produced by the corpus luteum in early pregnancy and serum levels remain relatively high during a normal pregnancy. Serum levels are generally lower in abnormal pregnancies, including ectopic pregnancy, and fall with pregnancy failure. Clinicians who do not have point-of-care ultrasound immediately available have utilized progesterone levels to help differentiate between a normal pregnancy and a possible ectopic with some success.[9,10] These methods, however, have not been proven to be as efficient or as accurate as protocols that incorporate initial transvaginal sonography. Reports suggest that progesterone may have a role in further categorizing patients who have an initial indeterminate transvaginal ultrasound. One study found that patients with a progesterone level ≥11 ng/mL are significantly more likely to have an early intrauterine pregnancy rather than an ectopic or an abortion (sensitivity 91%, specificity 84%).[11] Another study demonstrated a progesterone level <5 ng/mL to be 88% sensitive (although only 40% specific) in detecting ectopic pregnancy in the setting of an indeterminate (nonspecific free fluid or empty uterus) ultrasound.[12]

Suction curettage of the uterus can provide a definitive diagnosis of an intrauterine pregnancy if chorionic villi are identified. However, this test terminates an intrauterine pregnancy, making it applicable only when termination is desired or the pregnancy has obviously failed. Because it is invasive and other tests can provide similar information, suction curettage is rarely useful in the initial emergency evaluation during early pregnancy.

Culdocentesis is needle aspiration of the pelvic cul-de-sac through the posterior fornix of the vagina. Aspiration of blood is considered indicative of an ectopic pregnancy, although blood in the cul-de-sac can be seen with an intrauterine pregnancy. However, culdocentesis is invasive and lacks sensitivity for detecting nonruptured ectopic pregnancies.[5,13-15] It now has a very limited role and is recommended only when ultrasound is not available.[16]

Laparoscopy is an excellent test for visualizing extrauterine pelvic pathology, especially ectopic pregnancy.[17] However, it does not give any information about intrauterine contents or fetal viability. Laparoscopy has been utilized less frequently because sonography is noninvasive and can provide more information.[14] Laparoscopy can be used as a therapeutic tool and a diagnostic adjunct when sonography is nondiagnostic.

There are many advantages of using ultrasound in the first trimester of pregnancy. It is an ideal diagnostic tool in this setting, since it can visualize both intrauterine contents and potentially extrauterine pelvic pathology.

When used judiciously, ultrasound has no known adverse effects on the embryo and can be repeated as needed. Unlike curettage or culdocentesis, ultrasound is noninvasive and well tolerated by most patients.[18] In contrast to curettage or laparoscopy, ultrasound can directly visualize the intrauterine or extrauterine location of a pregnancy.[19] Unlike serum markers, ultrasound can immediately identify an abnormal pregnancy or evaluate fetal viability. Also, ultrasound can accurately measure the gestational age of a pregnancy, whereas serum markers can only give a gross estimation. Finally, patients with an ectopic pregnancy can be risk-stratified using ultrasound by estimating the size of an extrauterine mass or the amount of free intraperitoneal blood.

A disadvantage of using ultrasound in early pregnancy is that a pregnancy may not be visible between 3 and 5 weeks' gestational age. During this time, sensitive urine pregnancy tests are positive, but the gestation is usually too small to identify, even with transvaginal ultrasound. Another disadvantage of using ultrasound is that it is both equipment and operator dependent. Clinicians who make important patient management decisions based on ultrasound results must know the limitations of each study based on who is performing the examination and what type of equipment is being used.

▶ CLINICAL INDICATIONS

Any patient who is at risk of complications of early pregnancy is a candidate for pelvic sonography. Symptoms and physical examination findings include pelvic or abdominal pain or tenderness, vaginal bleeding, dizziness, syncope, a pelvic mass, or uterine size that does not correlate with the gestational age. Risk factors for ectopic pregnancy include pelvic inflammatory disease, tubal ligation, tubal surgery, increased maternal age, intrauterine contraceptive devices, prior ectopic pregnancy, and a history of infertility.[20] Classically, patients with an ectopic pregnancy present with abdominal or pelvic pain, vaginal bleeding, or dizziness, but some are relatively asymptomatic. Since no specific sign or symptom is absolute, physicians must have a high index of suspicion so that subtle presentations are not overlooked. Also, any woman of childbearing age who presents with shock of unknown etiology should have an immediate abdominal and pelvic ultrasound examination, even before a pregnancy test is completed.[6]

The main indication of emergency pelvic sonography in the first trimester is to differentiate an intrauterine pregnancy from an ectopic pregnancy. Point-of-care ultrasound can immediately establish one of these diagnoses in most patients with first trimester complaints.[19]

- Intrauterine pregnancy
- Ectopic pregnancy

Emergency pelvic sonography is also useful for the diagnosis of the following conditions in the first trimester of pregnancy:

- Pregnancy loss
- Multiple pregnancy
- Pelvic mass
- Ovarian torsion
- Gestational trophoblastic disease (GTD)

INTRAUTERINE PREGNANCY

A normal intrauterine pregnancy is the most common sonographic finding during the first trimester. Pelvic ultrasound can be used effectively by clinicians with varying degrees of experience because identifying an intrauterine pregnancy is straightforward (Figure 14-1).[21] In general, finding an intrauterine pregnancy virtually eliminates the possibility of an ectopic pregnancy. However, a patient undergoing fertility treatment has a significantly increased risk of heterotopic pregnancy, with both an intrauterine and ectopic pregnancy occurring simultaneously. While no further workup for ectopic is required in a low-risk patient with an obvious intrauterine pregnancy, a woman undergoing fertility treatment who has symptoms concerning for ectopic pregnancy should have more careful screening for heterotopic pregnancy.

About 70% of patients who present with abdominal pain or vaginal bleeding in the first trimester will have an intrauterine pregnancy visualized with point-of-care ultrasound and will not require further testing.[22] Care must be taken when using sonography between 3 and 5 weeks' gestational age because it is easy to confuse sonographic signs of an early intrauterine pregnancy with those of an ectopic pregnancy.

Identifying an intrauterine pregnancy with cardiac activity can give patients some reassurance about the outcome of their pregnancy. Those patients with a finding of embryonic cardiac activity have a lower incidence of pregnancy loss than other patients with similar symptoms.[23,24] However, clinicians should be careful

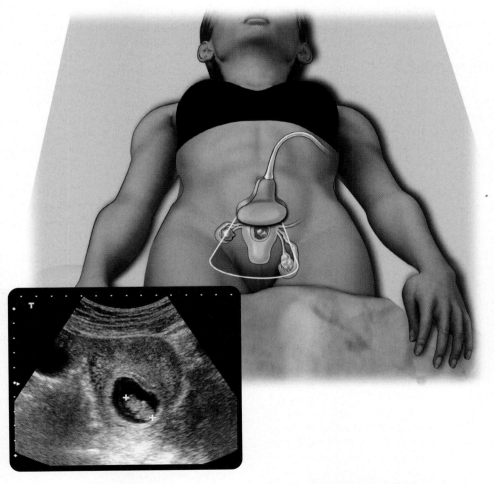

Figure 14-1. Intrauterine pregnancy. Ultrasound techniques and findings are outlined in the corresponding sections of this chapter.

not to give patients false hope about their pregnancy. Even when a normal intrauterine pregnancy is discovered, it is prudent to inform patients that point-of-care sonography is a focused examination only and will not detect fetal anomalies. Also, patients with abdominal pain or vaginal bleeding still have a significant chance of pregnancy loss.

Dating an intrauterine pregnancy is not as important as excluding an ectopic pregnancy. However, when the uterine size does not correlate with the gestational age or when the last menstrual period is unknown, sonography is indicated to date the pregnancy. This is very common because about half of all pregnant women cannot remember their last menstrual period. Pregnancy dating is simple and rapid with modern ultrasound equipment. Sonographic dating during the first trimester is more accurate than dating later in pregnancy. A few minutes spent measuring an embryo will be much appreciated by the patient's obstetrician, especially in patients who have unclear menstrual dates or are noncompliant with prenatal care. This early measurement becomes more important when determining fetal viability after 24 weeks and also near term when the obstetrician is considering induction of labor in a patient whose uterine size does not correlate with gestational age.

ECTOPIC PREGNANCY

Ectopic pregnancy occurs in about 2% of all pregnancies in the United States.[13,14,25] However, symptomatic patients who present to an emergency setting have a much higher incidence, as high as 4.5–13% in some reports.[9,26–28] The incidence of ectopic pregnancy has quadrupled in the last 20 years.[13] During the same period of time, the case-fatality rate for ruptured ectopic pregnancies has decreased significantly. This decrease is due to earlier diagnosis and treatment secondary to increased awareness and improved diagnostic capabilities, such as transvaginal sonography.[14] Despite these improvements, a significant percentage of ectopic pregnancies are still missed.[29] Also, ectopic pregnancy remains the leading cause of maternal death during the first trimester of pregnancy.[30]

Heterotopic pregnancy, which is a concomitant intrauterine and extrauterine pregnancy, has also become more common in the last few decades. In 1948, the incidence of heterotopic pregnancy was estimated to be 1 per 30,000 pregnancies, based on a theoretical calculation and assuming an ectopic pregnancy rate of 0.37%.[31] Now that the ectopic pregnancy rate is about 2%, it is reasonable to expect that the rate of heterotopic pregnancy is higher than previously estimated. There is some suggestion that the incidence of heterotopic pregnancy may be as high as 1 in 8000 pregnancies, but this may be practice specific.[31–36] The incidence is much higher in patients taking ovulation-inducing medications or undergoing in vitro fertilization (as high as 1 per 100 pregnancies).[37–39]

Emergency or acute care physicians have an important role in preventing morbidity and mortality from ectopic pregnancy.[40] Early diagnosis of ectopic pregnancy allows conservative treatment options, like methotrexate therapy.[14,41] Pelvic ultrasound is the main diagnostic modality that allows an early diagnosis to be made (Figure 14-2). Emergency physicians have been shown to be effective at performing and interpreting pelvic ultrasound examinations to rule out ectopic pregnancy. In an analysis of 10 studies with over 2000 patients, ultrasound examinations performed by emergency physicians were 99.3% sensitive for ectopic pregnancy, with a negative predictive value of 99.96%.[42]

In addition, transvaginal ultrasound is relatively straightforward to learn. A study assessed an emergency medicine residency program that conducted a single didactic lecture and 10 supervised ultrasound examinations. The residents were able to accurately identify the absence or presence of an intrauterine pregnancy in 93.3% of cases when compared to the emergency medicine ultrasound director.[43]

When emergency physicians perform point-of-care transvaginal sonography, pregnant patients have a shorter length of stay in the ED.[44–46] Also, point-of-care pelvic ultrasound screening by clinicians is more cost-effective than ordering comprehensive pelvic sonography on every patient with a possible ectopic pregnancy.[47] Most importantly, a protocol, which includes point-of-care transvaginal ultrasound by emergency physicians, has been shown to decrease the incidence of discharged patients returning with a subsequent ruptured ectopic pregnancy.[22,27,48]

Algorithm with Transvaginal Sonography and β-hCG Discriminatory Zone

Prior to the development of ectopic pregnancy algorithms and the widespread use of transvaginal sonography, the diagnosis of about half of all ectopic pregnancies was missed, and about half of those ruptured prior to their next presentation.[27,49,50] In the 1980s, ectopic pregnancy was one of the leading causes of emergency physician malpractice suits.[51,52] Algorithms that incorporate transvaginal sonography and a β-hCG discriminatory zone have improved diagnostic accuracy and reduced the incidence of patients who are discharged and subsequently present with a ruptured ectopic pregnancy.[19,27]

One algorithm utilizes emergency point-of-care transvaginal sonography as the initial diagnostic step for all patients at risk of ectopic pregnancy before a quantitative serum β-hCG is obtained (Figure 14-3).[1,27,48,50,53–62] Transvaginal sonography can establish a diagnosis of intrauterine pregnancy or ectopic

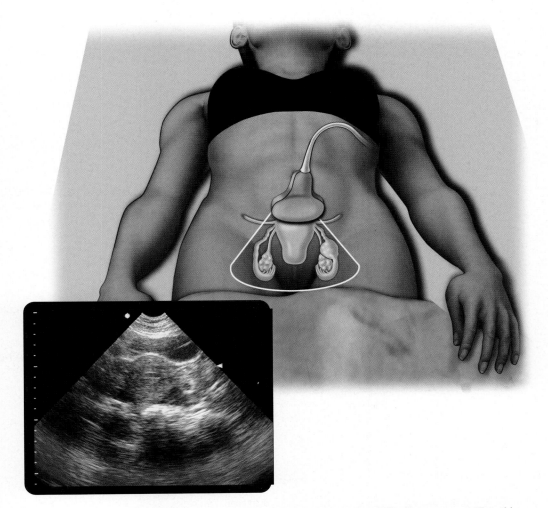

Figure 14-2. Ectopic pregnancy. Ultrasound techniques and findings are outlined in the corresponding sections of this chapter.

pregnancy in 75% of patients at the time of their initial presentation.[19] If emergency point-of-care sonography demonstrates an intrauterine pregnancy or an ectopic pregnancy, then the workup is complete. When no intrauterine pregnancy or ectopic pregnancy is identified, then the point-of-care ultrasound examination is indeterminate, and at this point a quantitative serum β-hCG level and a comprehensive pelvic ultrasound examination should be ordered. Again, if the comprehensive study shows an intrauterine pregnancy or an ectopic pregnancy, then the workup is complete. If either the point-of-care or comprehensive ultrasound examination demonstrates nonspecific signs of an ectopic pregnancy, then the risk is very high. Therefore, this situation should be managed in the same manner as a clear ectopic pregnancy, and an obstetrics consultation should be obtained. If both sonograms show no intrauterine pregnancy and no signs of an ectopic pregnancy, then the management is more complex. Traditionally, the next step is to obtain a serum β-hCG

level. Patients with an indeterminate ultrasound examination and a β-hCG level above the discriminatory zone (β-hCG >1000 mIU/mL) have a presumed ectopic pregnancy or embryonic demise and require an immediate obstetrics consultation.

Patients with an indeterminate ultrasound examination and a β-hCG level below the discriminatory zone (β-hCG <1000 mIU/mL) may have a small ectopic pregnancy, a very early intrauterine pregnancy, or embryonic demise. If hemodynamically stable and with an unremarkable physical examination, these patients can be discharged home without an obstetrics consult, but they should be given clear ectopic pregnancy discharge instructions and scheduled for close follow-up in 2–3 days for a repeat ultrasound examination and serum β-hCG level.[63]

Similar algorithms, incorporating point-of-care transvaginal sonography, have been shown to improve the quality of patient care and to be more cost-effective than other approaches.[19,27,47,48]

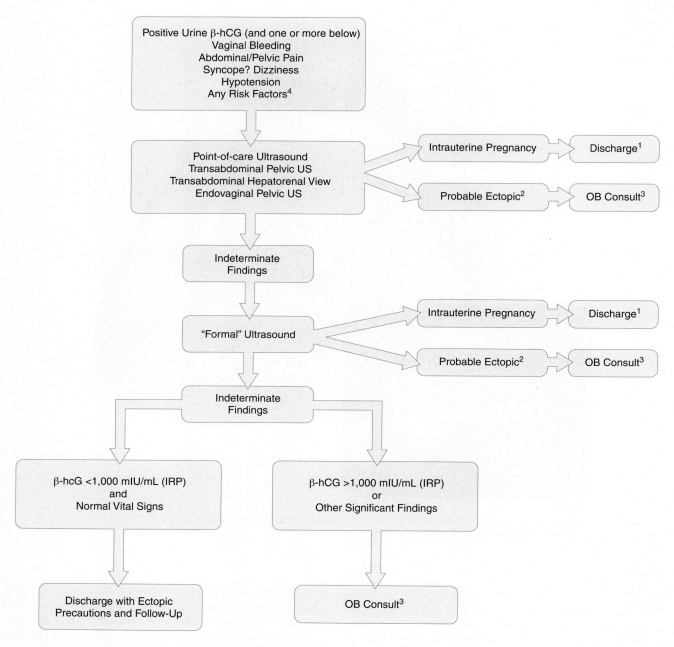

Figure 14-3. Ectopic pregnancy algorithm.

1. Unless patient is on fertility medications or undergoing IVF.
2. US criteria for probable ectopic pregnancy: extrauterine yolk sac or embryo, tubal ring, complex mass, or free fluid.
3. Surgery may be required if the patient has hypotension, a large ectopic sac (>4 cm), a large amount of pelvic free fluid, or hepatorenal fluid.
4. Risk factors include: PID, tubal surgery or ligation, IUD's, prior ectopic, infertility, advanced age.

Quantitative Serum β-hCG and Discriminatory Zone

Serum β-hCG rises exponentially and predictably during the first 6–8 weeks of pregnancy and peaks at about 100,000 mIU/mL in a normal pregnancy. Serial β-hCG levels are useful for differentiating normal pregnancies from abnormal pregnancies. The serum level should increase by at least 66%, multiplying by 1.6, every 48 hours, and may even double between 36 and 48 hours. An abnormally slow rise in β-hCG indicates an abnormal pregnancy, either an ectopic pregnancy or embryonic demise. A normal or expected rise in β-hCG, however, does not necessarily exclude an ectopic pregnancy.

Quantitative β-hCG measurements are currently standardized in relation to the International Reference Preparation (IRP). The reference standard for all β-hCG levels discussed in this chapter is the IRP. The standard method for reporting IRP β-hCG levels is in mIU/mL. Other reference standards are referred to in the literature, and it is important to distinguish between them since they are not equivalent. The Second International Standard is roughly equal to one half of the IRP and the Third International Standard is roughly equal to the IRP. In this chapter, β-hCG concentrations are reported in relation to the IRP, in mIU/mL.

A single serum β-hCG level is not as useful as serial levels because it does not differentiate a normal early intrauterine pregnancy from an ectopic pregnancy.[64] A common misconception is that a very low β-hCG level rules out ectopic pregnancy. Studies show that about 40% of ectopic pregnancies present with a β-hCG level <1000 mIU/mL and about 20% present with a β-hCG level <500 mIU/mL.[19,65] In fact, patients who present with a β-hCG level <1000 mIU/mL have a higher risk of ectopic pregnancy than other patients.[19,66,67] Furthermore, a low β-hCG level does not predict a benign course. Approximately 30–40% of ectopic pregnancies with a β-hCG level <1000 mIU/mL will be ruptured at the time of diagnosis.[19,65,66]

The "discriminatory zone" is a concept that was developed to allow the complementary use of pelvic ultrasound and a single serum β-hCG level to help determine the likelihood of ectopic pregnancy. The discriminatory zone is the β-hCG level above which an intrauterine pregnancy should be consistently visualized by pelvic sonography. Patients with a β-hCG level above the discriminatory zone who do not have an intrauterine pregnancy on ultrasound examination are presumed to have an ectopic pregnancy until proven otherwise. This is the concept that led to the use of the discriminatory zone in previous ectopic pregnancy algorithms. Older algorithms used the β-hCG discriminatory zone to limit the use of pelvic sonography since it was thought that only patients with levels >1000 mIU/mL would benefit from an ultrasound examination.[50,55] When outdated algorithms are applied, however, a significant percentage of ectopic pregnancies will be missed.[50]

Studies clearly show the benefit of performing pelvic sonography on all patients with a possible ectopic pregnancy, regardless of their β-hCG level.[19,27,61,65,66,68] Although a normal pregnancy will not be visualized when the β-hCG level is low, many ectopic pregnancies are easily identified when the β-hCG level is <1000 mIU/mL. In fact, transvaginal sonography can detect about half of ectopic pregnancies with β-hCG levels <1000 mIU/mL.[19,63,65,66,69–71]

Indeterminate Ultrasound Examinations

An "indeterminate" ultrasound examination in early pregnancy demonstrates no signs of intrauterine pregnancy or an ectopic pregnancy. One study attempted to subclassify patients with an indeterminate ultrasound examination based on their intrauterine findings.[72] Patients with a completely empty uterus and normal thin midline stripe had a 27% chance of an ectopic pregnancy and a 10% chance of an intrauterine pregnancy. Those with a nonspecific endometrial fluid collection had a 13% chance of an ectopic pregnancy and a 25% chance of an intrauterine pregnancy. Patients with intrauterine echogenic material had a 5% chance of ectopic pregnancy and none had an intrauterine pregnancy.

Approximately 15% of patients who are evaluated for a possible ectopic pregnancy have a β-hCG level >1000 mIU/mL and an indeterminate ultrasound.[19,72] Roughly 20% of these patients have an ectopic pregnancy.[56,58,72,73]

Management and Disposition

Patients diagnosed with an ectopic pregnancy have traditionally required surgery, which is usually a laparoscopic procedure. Although less successful compared to surgery,[74,75] medical therapy has become increasingly popular, with single-dose IM methotrexate therapy being the most common regimen.[76] This regimen has a success rate ranging from 64% to 94%.[14,77–79] Clinical and sonographic criteria can help obstetricians decide which patients are candidates for medical therapy instead of surgery. Higher serum β-hCG levels, especially above 10,000 mIU/mL, the presence of a yolk sac, and endometrial stripe thickness >12 mm are associated with failure of methotrexate therapy.[41,78,80–83] Also, an adnexal mass >4 cm in diameter, the presence of embryonic cardiac activity, a large amount of pelvic free fluid, and severe pain should be considered relative contraindications to medical management.[14,84] Clinical signs of shock along with free intraperitoneal fluid outside of the pelvis, such as in the hepatorenal space, are indications of surgery and contraindications to medical therapy.[6,14,30] Routinely scan Morison's pouch for free fluid when assessing for ectopic pregnancy. Free intraperitoneal fluid identified in Morison's pouch is predictive of the need for operative intervention. This can be rapidly performed and can significantly change management so it is recommended as a routine component of ultrasound for ectopic pregnancy.[85]

Patients with an unclear diagnosis of ectopic pregnancy need serial sonography and serial β-hCG levels. Obstetricians may be unwilling to initiate therapy in such patients for fear of interrupting an intrauterine pregnancy. Patients with concerning signs or symptoms and unclear or questionable sonographic findings should ideally be observed in the hospital. Repeat sonography and β-hCG level at 12–24 hours will make the diagnosis more clear. Those with minimal symptoms, no mass, free fluid, or other signs of ectopic pregnancy are safe to be discharged with early follow-up for repeat sonography and β-hCG level in 24–48 hours.[13,45,48,55]

The majority, up to 70% of all ectopic pregnancies, will spontaneously resolve without any treatment.[86,87] Therefore, expectant management may be reasonable in selected cases. Candidates for expectant management must have minimal symptoms, a small ectopic mass, and a low β-hCG level. Excellent clinical, sonographic, and laboratory follow-up must be ensured if expectant management is attempted.

PREGNANCY LOSS

Diagnosing pregnancy loss is not as urgent as excluding an ectopic pregnancy. It is important, however, for emergency or acute care physicians to be aware of the sonographic features of pregnancy loss. It is helpful to know the risks of pregnancy loss related to specific ultrasound findings. This information will allow physicians to do a better job of counseling patients and making reasonable management plans for those with a threatened abortion.

Vaginal bleeding is a very common presentation and occurs in about 25% of all clinically apparent early pregnancies.[88–90] About 40–50% of these patients will eventually be diagnosed with pregnancy loss.[19,30,91–93] A threatened abortion is a significant source of anxiety for pregnant patients. Concern for the viability of the pregnancy is usually the primary reason for presentation. Pelvic sonography is very useful in patients with a threatened abortion because it provides an immediate diagnosis in about half of all patients with subsequent pregnancy loss.[91] Those without a definitive diagnosis require serial pelvic sonography and β-hCG levels.

Spontaneous abortion refers to expulsion of a nonviable pregnancy from the uterus before 20 weeks' gestational age. Microscopic identification of chorionic villi or obvious products of conception are required to make a definitive diagnosis. A completed spontaneous abortion can be diagnosed when all products of conception have been expelled. This usually occurs shortly after embryonic demise but may be delayed for days to weeks. Sonographically, an empty uterus should be seen after a completed spontaneous abortion. This finding indicates that the patient can be managed expectantly without curettage.[94–96]

Incomplete abortion is a nonspecific term used when a pregnancy has failed but all of the products of conception have not been expelled from the uterus. The terms embryonic demise, blighted ovum, and retained products of conception are all synonymous with incomplete abortion. Patients with an incomplete abortion may experience continued bleeding, infection, and anxiety, so it is important to make the diagnosis as soon as possible after embryonic demise has occurred. Patients with an incomplete abortion may require suction and curettage to remove retained products of conception.[96,97] Sonography is the only diagnostic modality that can directly assess intrauterine contents before a curettage is performed.

The term inevitable abortion implies that expulsion of uterine contents is in progress. Patients with an inevitable abortion have an open cervical os on physical examination. Pelvic sonography may show a separated gestational sac lying low within the uterus.[89] It is reasonable for physicians to use point-of-care pelvic sonography to help make initial management decisions in patients with a threatened abortion. However, it is prudent to confirm the diagnosis of embryonic demise with a comprehensive pelvic ultrasound prior to evacuation of intrauterine products. Also, it is important not to give patients false reassurance. Even when a completely normal intrauterine pregnancy is seen, they should be aware that there is still a chance of subsequent pregnancy loss.

Sonographic signs of a normal intrauterine pregnancy are reassuring and decrease the likelihood that a pregnancy will be lost.[23,91,98–100] In asymptomatic patients, those without threatened abortion, the rate of first trimester pregnancy loss decreases as the gestational age increases and as more normal structures can be identified with sonography. The rate of loss after only a gestational sac is identified is 11.5%. The rate decreases to 8.5% after a yolk sac is identified and to 7.2% after an embryo (2–5 mm) is identified. When a larger embryo is seen, the loss rate is even lower: 3.3% with a 6- to 10-mm embryo and 0.5% with an embryo >10 mm. In addition, there is a 2% risk of pregnancy loss after the first trimester in pregnancies that previously appeared viable by ultrasound.[99]

As stated above, patients presenting with a first trimester threatened abortion have a 40–50% chance of pregnancy loss.[19,30,91–93] If embryonic cardiac activity can be seen, however, the rate of subsequent pregnancy loss is lower at 15–20%.[23,91] Also, as the gestational age and the size of the embryo increase, cardiac activity is more reassuring. Very early in the first trimester, when the embryo is <5 mm long, patients with a threatened abortion and cardiac activity have a loss rate of about 24%.[100] Those with a threatened abortion and cardiac activity near the end of the first trimester have a very low rate of pregnancy loss.[24]

MULTIPLE PREGNANCY

Characterizing a multiple pregnancy (twins, triplets, etc.) is typically not in the realm of emergency medicine. However, timely pelvic sonography is indicated when menstrual dates do not correlate with the size of the patient's uterus. In such cases, sonographic pregnancy dating and evaluation for multiple pregnancy or molar pregnancy should be performed. Also, multiple pregnancies are often an incidental finding when sonography is performed for other indications, such as ruling out an ectopic pregnancy. Regardless of the indication for the sonogram, finding a multiple pregnancy is significant since the pregnancy will then be categorized as high risk and the patient will need close follow-up with an obstetrician.

Twin pregnancies are more likely to have fetal anomalies, premature delivery, and low birth weight. Early sonographic evaluation of a multiple pregnancy is important because differentiating dichorionic from monochorionic twins is much easier during the first trimester. Fraternal (dizygotic) twins are always dichorionic and diamnionic but identical (monozygotic) twins may be dichorionic, monochorionic, diamnionic, or monoamnionic, depending on when the zygote splits. Determining chorionicity is important since monochorionic twins have a mortality rate two to three times higher than dichorionic twins. Monochorionic twins share a single placenta, so they are at risk of twin transfusion syndrome, twin embolization syndrome, and acardiac parabiotic twin syndrome. In addition, determining amnionicity is important since monoamniotic twins are at risk of cord knots, wrapping of the cord around a co-twin, or locking of twins during delivery.

When imaging a multiple pregnancy, physicians should try to record quality images that clearly show the chorionicity and amnionicity. If chorionicity and amnionicity cannot be determined, then the patient should have a comprehensive ultrasound examination within several days. Also, it is important to inform patients that about 25% of twin pregnancies diagnosed during the first trimester will become singleton pregnancies by the second trimester.[101,102]

PELVIC MASSES

A pelvic mass may be noted in the first trimester of pregnancy during the physical examination or routine pelvic ultrasound examination. Physicians who perform point-of-care sonography need to have some basic knowledge of pelvic masses so they can make reasonable management plans. Most pelvic masses found in the first trimester are benign and require no treatment. They all, however, require close follow-up with serial sonography because some masses are at risk of hemorrhage, torsion, rupture, dystocia, and malignancy. Surgery will be required in about 1 per 1,300 pregnancies to exclude malignancy or to deal with one of the above complications. About 3% of all masses discovered during pregnancy have malignant potential.[103]

In general, patients with masses <5 cm in diameter in early pregnancy are treated conservatively and followed with serial sonography. Those presenting with peritoneal signs or severe pain may need immediate surgery because of rupture or torsion of a mass. Masses that are large, cause pain, or grow rapidly may require surgery. Those containing large solid areas, solid irregular areas, papillary excrescences, and irregular septae are at higher risk of malignancy. Also, the presence of ascites, in addition to a cystic pelvic mass, increases the chance of malignancy.[104] If surgery is required, then the optimal period is during the second trimester, when maternal and fetal risks are smallest.

The most common mass seen in early pregnancy is a corpus luteum cyst. The corpus luteum secretes progesterone to support the early pregnancy. A corpus luteum cyst is usually <5 cm in diameter and appears as a thin-walled unilocular structure surrounded by normal ovarian parenchyma. The appearance may vary substantially and the size may be >10 cm. Hemorrhage into a corpus luteum cyst can cause the appearance of internal echogenic debris and septae.[30] Corpus luteum cysts usually regress spontaneously prior to 18 weeks of gestation.

A theca lutein cyst is an exaggerated corpus luteum and occurs in patients with very high β-hCG levels. Theca lutein cysts are commonly seen in patients with GTD and ovarian hyperstimulation from fertility medications. They appear as large multiseptated cystic masses. Theca lutein cysts usually resolve spontaneously once the abnormal stimulus is removed.

Uterine leiomyomas, or fibroids, are solid pelvic masses that are very common and may enlarge during pregnancy because of increased estrogen levels. They usually appear as relatively hypoechoic masses within the uterine wall and are sometimes confused with a simple muscular contraction of part of the uterine wall. Fibroids can have many different appearances, depending on the amount of smooth muscle and hyaline they contain and whether they have undergone hemorrhagic degeneration. They may contain calcifications or cystic areas of degeneration. Small fibroids tend to enlarge during the first and the second trimesters but larger fibroids tend to enlarge only during the first trimester.[105] All fibroids tend to decrease in size during late pregnancy. Patients with multiple fibroids have a higher risk of bleeding, premature contractions, malpresentation, and retained products.[104] Large fibroids located in the lower part of the uterus during late pregnancy can obstruct labor and necessitate a cesarean section.

The most common complex mass seen in early pregnancy is a teratoma, or dermoid cyst.[103,104] These tumors arise from germ cells within the ovary and contain heterologous tissue like fat, skin, hair, and teeth. Sebaceous material within a dermoid can appear as a fluid-fluid level and teeth are very echogenic with distal shadowing. Dermoids are prone to torsion and rupture. Leaking of dermoid fluid can cause granulomatous peritonitis and sudden rupture can cause an acute abdomen.[104]

Mucinous and serous cystadenomas are ovarian epithelial neoplasms; they are the most common cystic tumors that enlarge during pregnancy.[106] Both of these tumors can appear as multicystic masses. Mucinous cystadenomas usually contain multiple thick internal septations and serous cystadenomas usually appear as unilocular structures. Again, pelvic masses that have internal septations and papillary excrescences are more likely to be malignant.[104]

Emergency and acute care physicians typically do not attempt to characterize pelvic masses using sonography. However, these physicians will inevitably discover pelvic masses as incidental findings. When this occurs, most patients will need a comprehensive ultrasound examination and close follow-up with an obstetrician. Patients should be informed when a mass is found, and they should understand that point-of-care sonography is a screening tool and that further workup is needed.

ADNEXAL TORSION

Adnexal torsion is uncommon but about 20% of all cases occur during pregnancy.[107,108] Also, most cases occur during the first trimester.[105,109] Pregnant patients may be predisposed to torsion because of increased ovarian arterial flow and decreased ovarian venous flow, causing ovarian edema and enlargement. Torsion almost always occurs in the setting of an enlarged ovary or an ovarian mass; torsion rarely occurs in a normal size ovary. Ovarian hyperstimulation from fertility medications has been recognized as a risk factor for adnexal torsion because of ovarian enlargement.

Pain is the most common symptom of adnexal torsion. The diagnosis of torsion may be easily missed during pregnancy because pain may be attributed to the gravid uterus, the round ligament, or an adnexal mass. Further delay may occur because of the poor accuracy of Doppler ultrasound, which may miss up to 60% of cases of adnexal torsion.[110] Also, when a cystic ovarian mass is present, blood flow to the ovary may be difficult to visualize using pulse wave Doppler, even though torsion has not occurred.

Simple gray scale pelvic sonography may be of some help in diagnosing adnexal torsion.[111,112] Finding a unilaterally enlarged ovary with multifollicular enlargement or any adnexal mass makes torsion more likely. Most patients with torsion have free fluid in the pelvic cul-de-sac, probably as a result of obstruction of venous and lymphatic drainage.[111,113] Finding normal-size ovaries and no pelvic free fluid makes the diagnosis of adnexal torsion highly unlikely.

Most diagnoses of adnexal torsion are delayed because of atypical clinical presentations and poor sensitivity of diagnostic modalities.[114] This may be especially detrimental in pregnancy causing maternal morbidity and fetal mortality. Therefore, it is prudent to have a high index of suspicion when there is no clear etiology for abdominal, pelvic, flank, or groin pain. Also, when the diagnosis is strongly suspected, negative diagnostic studies should not deter consultation and further evaluation.[115] Laparoscopy has been used during pregnancy as both a diagnostic and therapeutic modality.

GESTATIONAL TROPHOBLASTIC DISEASE

GTD is a proliferative disease of the trophoblast. It occurs in about 1 per 1,700 pregnancies in the United States but is much more common in some other parts of the world.[116] GTD may occur with an intrauterine pregnancy or an ectopic pregnancy, or after a spontaneous abortion or full-term pregnancy. Most cases of GTD (80%) present as a benign hydatidiform mole. More malignant forms of GTD, invasive mole (12–15%), and choriocarcinoma (5–8%) may develop after a hydatidiform mole. Hydatidiform moles usually involve the entire placenta but a mole involving only part of the placenta can be associated with a live pregnancy.

Early in pregnancy, GTD may present with vaginal bleeding, uterine size that is too large for dates, persistent severe hyperemesis gravidarum, or early preeclampsia. Sometimes, the first clue to the diagnosis is a markedly elevated serum β-hCG level, usually >100,000 mIU/mL. It has been shown that qualitative β-hCG urine assays may be falsely negative in the setting of GTD with markedly elevated serum β-hCG.[117] GTD is often discovered during routine pelvic sonography for pregnancy dating or other indications.

Ultrasound is the preferred modality for diagnosing GTD and both transabdominal and transvaginal sonography are usually diagnostic.[118] The classic finding, described as having a grape-like appearance, is an intrauterine echogenic mass containing diffuse small hypoechoic vesicles. In the first trimester, GTD may not be as obvious and can be confused with an incomplete abortion. In about half of cases of GTD, a theca lutein cyst is seen in the adnexa.

Early diagnosis and prompt treatment are the key to a favorable outcome. A hydatidiform mole usually resolves completely with evacuation of the uterus. Choriocarcinoma can metastasize to the lung, liver, and brain. It is very sensitive to chemotherapy, but morbidity and mortality depend on the extent of metastases and early aggressive treatment.

► ANATOMICAL CONSIDERATIONS

The uterus is located in the center of the true pelvis between the bladder anteriorly and the rectosigmoid colon posteriorly. The uterus is a thick-walled muscular structure that is about 6–7 cm long and about 3–4 cm in transverse and anterior–posterior diameters. It is shaped like an inverted pear and the uterine body is the widest portion. The cervix is the narrowest portion and is anchored to the posterior bladder by the parametrium. The cervix meets the vagina at the level of the bladder angle and protrudes into the anterior wall of the vagina. When the uterus is in the normal anteflexed position, the longitudinal axes of the uterus and vagina create an angle of about 90°. The fallopian tubes enter the body of the uterus laterally, in an area called the cornua. The fundus is the most superior portion of the uterine body above the cornua.

The uterine body and fundus lie inside the peritoneal cavity; intraperitoneal potential spaces exist both anterior and posterior to the uterus. The anterior cul-de-sac, between the bladder and uterus, is usually empty but can contain loops of bowel or free fluid. The posterior cul-de-sac, between the uterus and the rectosigmoid colon, is also known as the "pouch of Douglas" and it usually contains bowel loops. The posterior cul-de-sac is the most dependent intraperitoneal region when the patient is supine; therefore, it is the most common site for pooling of free pelvic fluid.

Lateral to the uterus, the peritoneal reflection forms the two layers of the broad ligament. The broad ligament extends from the uterus to the lateral pelvic sidewalls. The fallopian tubes extend laterally from the body of the uterus in the upper free margin of the broad ligament. The ovaries are attached to the posterior surface of the broad ligament. They are also attached to the body of the uterus by the ovarian ligaments and to the lateral pelvic sidewalls by the suspensory ligaments of the ovary. Normal ovaries are about 2 cm wide and 3 cm long. The ovaries are usually located in a depression on the lateral pelvic walls called the ovarian fossa. However, since the ligaments are not rigid structures, the ovaries may be seen in a number of other locations, especially in women who have previously been pregnant.

▶ GETTING STARTED

While working with a stable patient in need of early first trimester pregnancy evaluation in the ED, ultrasonography of the pelvis is most efficiently accomplished immediately following the pelvic examination. This allows for uninterrupted presence of a chaperone that may have assisted with the pelvic examination. Sonographic findings of very early pregnancy and nonpregnant patients can be difficult to distinguish. Therefore, it is often advisable to wait to perform the pelvic examination and subsequent ultrasound evaluation after pregnancy status has been confirmed, usually by urine qualitative β-hCG. Occasionally patients will communicate that they are pregnant when in reality they are not. Waiting for

laboratory confirmation of pregnancy status helps avoid the misuse of time and resources looking for a pregnancy that does not exist. However, if the patient's last menstrual period suggests a sufficiently advanced gestational age, immediate transabdominal ultrasonography can confirm pregnancy and eliminate the need for urine or serum β-hCG. Immediately scan any patient who has signs and symptoms suggestive of possible ectopic pregnancy without waiting for the β-hCG level.

During the transabdominal pelvic ultrasound examination, the bladder should be full. Initially obtain a longitudinal image of the uterine midline to determine the location of the body of the uterus, the cervix, and the pouch of Douglas. Apply axial pressure to produce the best images if this can be tolerated by the patient. After imaging the long axis of the uterus, rotate the transducer transversely 90° in its long axis to find the ovaries and scan the adnexa. The ovaries are located lateral to the widest portion of the uterus in the transverse plane next to the internal iliac artery and vein. Follow the broad ligament laterally from the cornual region of the uterus to the ovary on each side.

During the transvaginal ultrasound examination, the bladder should be empty. The uterus and cervix should serve as anatomic landmarks and initially be visualized longitudinally. Because of anatomic variability, the midline of the uterus may not be in the same plane and consistent with the midline of the patient's body. Ovaries are most easily visualized in the transverse plane after following the broad ligament laterally from the cornual region of the uterus. Evaluation of specific structures such as the uterus, ovaries, or adnexal masses may be enhanced by placement of the transducer tip directly over the area of interest. Just as the examiner's hand is used to palpate structures during a routine physical examination, gentle application of axial force on the transducer may elicit tenderness and provide important diagnostic information.

▶ TECHNIQUE AND NORMAL ULTRASOUND FINDINGS

Transabdominal and transvaginal sonography are complementary imaging techniques and should be used together. In general, transvaginal imaging should not be performed without also performing a transabdominal scan, but this may not be practical in a busy clinical setting. Transvaginal imaging allows the transducer tip to be placed very close to the organ of interest so that high-frequency transducers can be used to generate high-resolution images. However, transvaginal transducers have a limited field of view, and objects more than a few centimeters away from the transducer tip may not be seen. Transabdominal sonography uses lower frequency transducers so the field of view is much larger, and a better overview of pelvic structures can be

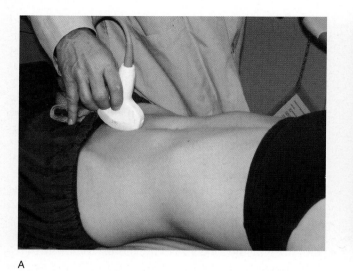

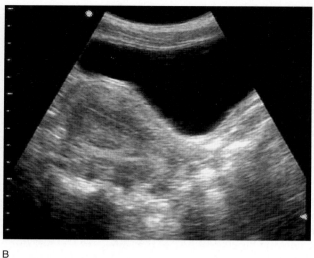

A   B

Figure 14-4. Transabdominal midline sagittal view of the normal pelvis. Transducer position (A) and corresponding ultrasound image (B). (A, Courtesy of James Mateer, MD)

obtained. The main drawback of transabdominal scanning is that the resolution is lower, so details of small pelvic structures are not as discernible, particularly ovaries and early pregnancies.

NORMAL NONPREGNANT PELVIS

Transabdominal Scanning

Transabdominal scanning is usually accomplished using a 3.5–5 MHz ultrasound transducer. The bladder is used as a window in transabdominal scanning, so it should be full to obtain optimal images. In the emergency setting, transabdominal scanning may be performed without a full bladder because it is not practical to have patients drink fluid and wait for an hour while their bladders fill. IV fluid administration will typically lead to rapid bladder filling. Quality images are usually obtained without bladder filling in thin women and those with an anteflexed uterus. Apply gentle pressure with the transducer to produce good-quality transabdominal images without filling the bladder (See Video 16-1).

The best transabdominal view for evaluating the uterus and its contents is the standard midline sagittal view (Figure 14-4). To obtain this view, place the transducer on the abdominal wall in the midline just above the pubic bone, with the transducer indicator pointing cephalad (Figure 14-5). By convention, the indicator on the transducer should correlate with the left side of the

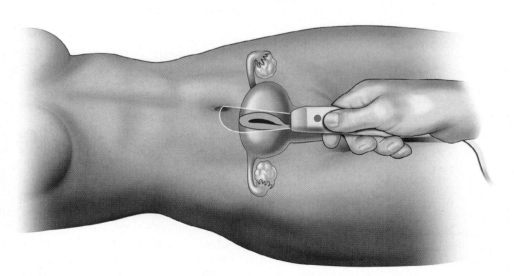

Figure 14-5. Scan plane for the transabdominal midline sagittal view. The marker dot is pointed cephalad.

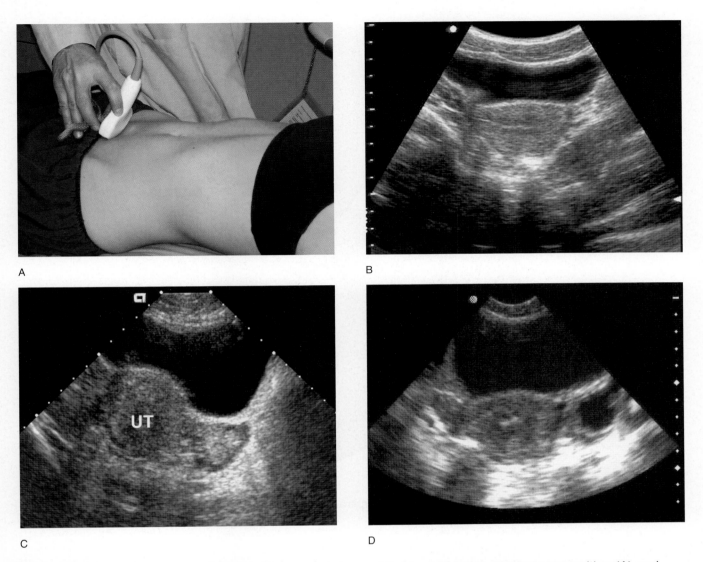

Figure 14-6. Transabdominal transverse ultrasound views of the normal pelvis. Transducer position (A) and corresponding transverse midline ultrasound view (B). Transverse view of left adnexa and left ovary (C). Transverse ultrasound view of the uterus and both ovaries (D). The right ovary is small and of similar echogenicity as the uterus, and the left ovary is more prominent because of a contained cyst. UT = uterus. (A, D, Courtesy of James Mateer, MD; C, Courtesy of Waukesha Memorial Hospital)

monitor so that in sagittal images cephalad structures are on the left side. This view provides a longitudinal image of the uterus, and the entire midline stripe should be visible. The cervix is seen just posterior to the bladder angle with the body of the uterus to the left of the angle and the vaginal stripe to the right. View the ovaries by sliding the transducer laterally, with the transducer indicator still pointing cephalad, and aiming the beam toward the contralateral adnexa, using the bladder as a window. Sometimes when the bladder is very full or a large pelvic mass is present, better images can be obtained by placing the transducer directly over the adnexa.

In some cases, it may be easier to visualize the ovaries and other adnexal structures with the standard transabdominal transverse view (Figure 14-6). This view is obtained by placing the transducer in the midline of the abdominal wall just above the pubic bone, with the transducer indicator pointing to the patient's right side. This view provides a transverse image of the uterus and allows the midline of the uterus and the adjacent adnexa to be seen in the same image if the anatomy cooperates. In transverse images, anatomic structures have the same orientation as on a CT scan: right-sided structures are on the left side of the monitor and left-sided structures are on the right. To examine the entire pelvis in

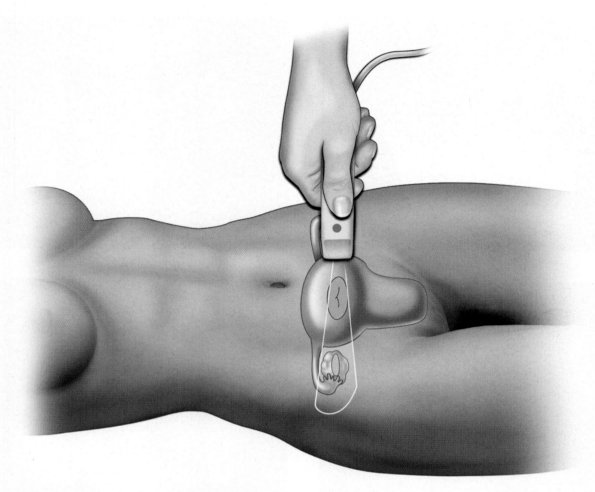

Figure 14-7. Scan plane for the transabdominal transverse view. The marker dot is pointed toward the patient's right side.

transverse planes, place the transducer in the midline suprapubic region with the transducer indicator pointed to the patient's right and aim the beam caudad and cephalad (Figure 14-7). This motion will allow the uterus to be viewed in transverse sections from the cervix to the fundus, respectively.

The ovaries are most commonly found between the body of the uterus and the pelvic sidewall. In their normal location, the ovaries are bound posteriorly by the internal iliac artery and superiorly by the external iliac vein. These structures can be identified and used to help locate the ovaries. Normal ovaries appear as small discrete hypoechoic structures. Individual ovarian follicles are usually not visible with transabdominal imaging. Normal ovaries are not always seen with transabdominal sonography because they are relatively small and may be camouflaged by bowel or other surrounding structures with similar echogenicity. However, adnexal masses are frequently larger and very easy to identify with transabdominal imaging (Figure 14-6D).

Transvaginal Sonography

Transvaginal scanning is different from other ultrasound techniques because the ultrasound transducer is placed inside the vagina and very close to the organs of interest. The transvaginal technique is referred to as "endovaginal" sonography by some authors. Transvaginal sonography is accomplished using a specialized 5–7.5 MHz transducer. The transducer has an indicator, similar to other ultrasound transducers, which should correlate to the left side of the monitor screen. The sound beams may emanate straight out from the tip of the transducer (end-fire) or at an angle from the tip of the transducer (offset). End-fire transducers are more versatile and make imaging planes easier to understand. This discussion of scanning planes will assume that an end-fire transducer is being used.

Before using the transvaginal transducer, thoroughly clean and disinfect it (per manufacturer and CDC recommendations) and cover it with a rubber or vinyl

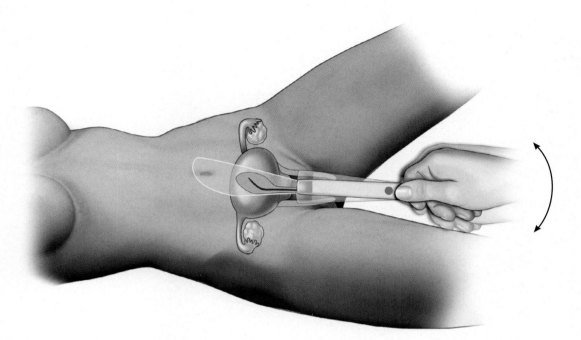

Figure 14-8. Scan plane for the transvaginal sagittal view (frontal perspective). The marker dot is pointed toward the ceiling.

sheath. Place conducting gel inside the sheath before the transducer is covered for appropriate sound transmission. Most clinicians use specially made latex condoms as transducer covers, although vinyl gloves can be used as well.[119] Use a water-based lubricant, not conducting gel, to lubricate the outside of the sheath before insertion into the vagina because ultrasound conducting gel may be irritating to the vaginal mucosa. Patients should empty their bladder before transvaginal scanning is performed. A full bladder will straighten the angle between the uterus and vagina and move the body of the uterus away from the transducer and produce artifacts. Patient positioning is important in obtaining good transvaginal scans. The operator must be able to aim the transducer anterior enough to see the fundus of an anteverted uterus. Scanning is best accomplished while the patient is in lithotomy stirrups or by elevating her pelvis on a pillow while she is in a frog-leg position. Many clinicians prefer to use lithotomy stirrups and perform transvaginal sonography as part of their pelvic examination, after the speculum and bimanual examinations.

Before inserting the transvaginal transducer, explain the procedure to the patient. It is usually best to explain that transvaginal sonography is similar to the bimanual pelvic examination but visual rather than tactile information is obtained. Transvaginal sonography should not be painful and is usually very well tolerated by patients. Anxious patients may be given the option of inserting the transducer into the vagina themselves.

Initially insert the transducer with the transducer indicator pointed toward the ceiling (Figures 14-8 and 14-9). The uterus is easily recognized upon insertion of the transducer. This is the standard transvaginal sagittal view; it produces a longitudinal image of the uterus similar to the transabdominal sagittal view but rotated 90° counterclockwise (Figure 14-10). Visualize the entire uterine midline stripe in this view. If the uterus is not seen immediately, then it may be extremely anteverted and the transducer should be aimed upward toward the anterior abdominal wall, keeping the indicator pointed toward the ceiling. Lateral movement of the transducer can be used to scan from side to side through the entire pelvis (Figure 14-8). The uterus appears as a relatively hypoechoic structure with thick walls and a well-defined border. The endometrial midline stripe is thin during the proliferative phase and thick during the secretory phase of the menstrual cycle (Figures 14-11 and 14-12). Visualize the cervix by pulling the transducer back a few centimeters and aiming the transducer tip downward toward the patient's back (Figure 14-13). In this view, inspect the posterior cul-de-sac for any evidence of free fluid.

After the uterus is identified, the ovaries can be found by their position relative to the uterus. They are usually found just lateral and posterior to the body of the uterus, between the uterus and the lateral pelvic wall. The sonographic appearance of the ovaries is distinct. They are relatively hypoechoic structures containing multiple anechoic follicles (Figures 14-14, 14-15, and 14-16).

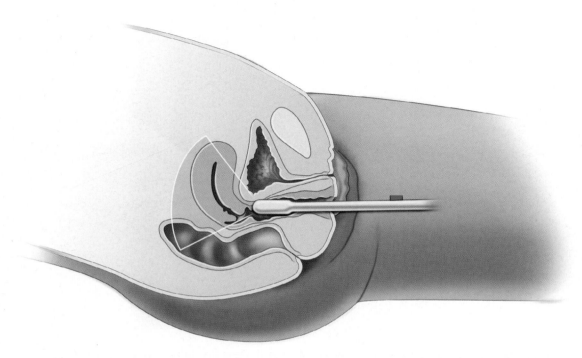

Figure 14-9. Scan plane for the transvaginal sagittal view (sagittal perspective). The marker dot is pointed toward the ceiling.

To find the ovaries in sagittal oblique planes, aim the transducer laterally, with the transducer indicator still toward the ceiling (Figure 14-8). The internal iliac artery and vein can often be identified and used as a guide because the normal position of the ovary is adjacent to these structures. Sometimes the ovaries cannot be identified with transvaginal sonography.[120]

The standard transvaginal coronal view may be better for surveying the entire pelvis. This view is obtained by turning the transducer indicator toward the patient's right side (Figures 14-17). The coronal view gives a transverse image of the uterus and allows the uterus and ovaries to be seen in the same plane. The entire pelvis can be explored with oblique coronal planes

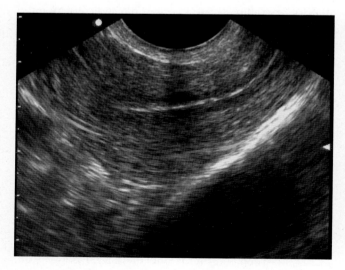

Figure 14-10. Transvaginal midline sagittal ultrasound view of the normal pelvis. The thin endometrial stripe represents the early proliferative phase.

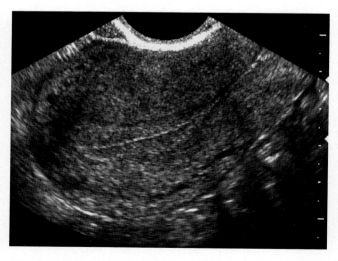

Figure 14-11. Transvaginal midline sagittal ultrasound of the uterus during the late proliferative menstrual phase. The endometrial stripe is slightly thickened, but not very echogenic.

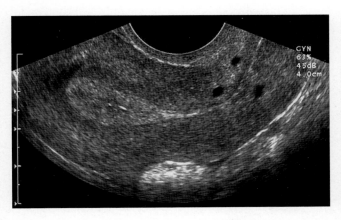

Figure 14-12. Transvaginal midline sagittal ultrasound of the uterus during the secretory menstrual phase. The endometrium is thickened and echogenic. Three nabothian cysts are shown in the cervix.

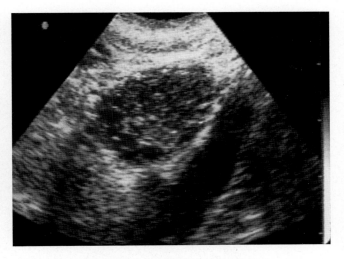

Figure 14-14. Transvaginal view of a normal left ovary. The ovary is recognized by the oval shape, peripheral follicles, and echogenicity similar to the myometrium of the uterus. This ovary is adjacent to the iliac vein. (Courtesy of James Mateer, MD)

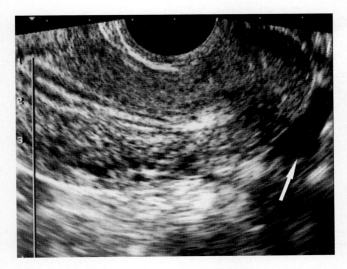

Figure 14-13. Transvaginal sagittal view of the uterine body and cervix. A small (physiologic) fluid collection is present in the posterior cul-de-sac (arrow).

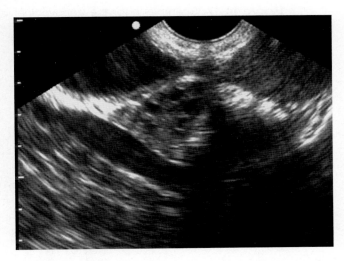

Figure 14-15. Transvaginal view of a normal ovary. This ovary (center of the image) is surrounded by the bladder (above-left), iliac vein (below), intestine with gas and shadows (below-right), and the uterus (above-right).

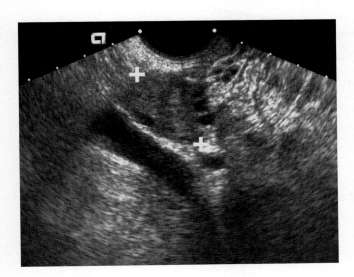

Figure 14-16. Transvaginal ultrasound of the normal right ovary (long axis marked by cursors). The external iliac vein is below and to the left of the ovary on the image, while a cross section of the internal iliac artery (or vein) is directly below and to the right. (Courtesy of James Mateer, MD, Waukesha Memorial Hospital)

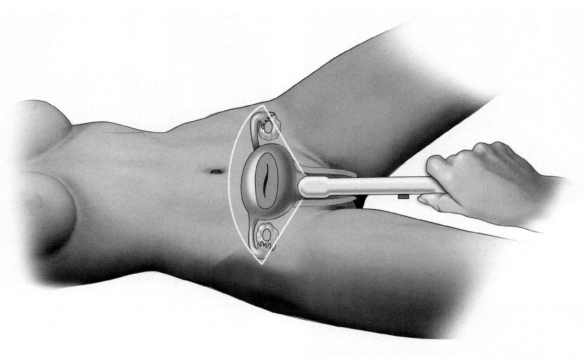

Figure 14-17. Scan plane for the transvaginal coronal view (frontal perspective). The marker dot is pointed toward the patient's right side.

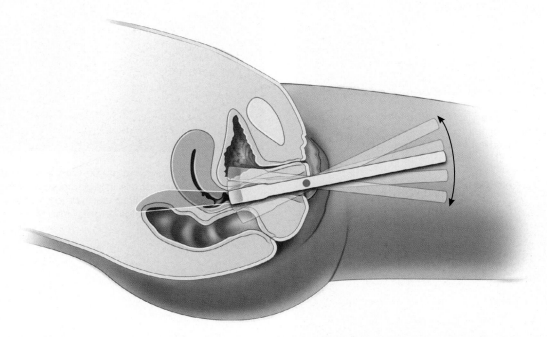

Figure 14-18. Scan plane for the transvaginal coronal view (sagittal perspective). The marker dot is pointed toward the patient's right side.

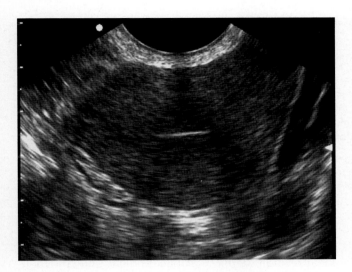

Figure 14-19. Transvaginal coronal ultrasound view of the normal pelvis.

by aiming the transducer up toward the anterior abdominal wall and down toward the patient's back, keeping the transducer indicator pointing toward the patient's right side (Figures 14-18 and 14-19).

Transvaginal sonography is a dynamic imaging technique. To visualize structures, they need to be very close to the tip of the transducer. When structures are not readily visualized, operators should use their free hand to palpate the patient's anterior abdominal wall, similar to performing a bimanual pelvic examination.[30,91,119] Pressure on the anterior abdominal wall will often bring an ovary or a mass into the field of view. Also, use the hand on the abdominal wall and the transvaginal transducer together to manipulate pelvic contents and observe how the organs move in relation to one another. An ovary may be easier to identify if it is seen as a discrete structure moving independently from adjacent loops of bowel. Also, structures that appear as complex masses may be comprised of multiple smaller structures that move independently of each other. Holding the transvaginal transducer very still and observing for bowel peristalsis is a good method for differentiating bowel from other pelvic structures. Finally, the tip of the transvaginal transducer can be used to try to localize pelvic pain. This may help the physician narrow the differential diagnosis when a mass or other abnormality is visualized.

Although several standard imaging planes have been described, the pelvis can often be scanned without concern for specific planes. Once an organ or a mass is identified, turn the transducer in any direction that helps obtain better images. Also, as long as the entire pelvis is imaged in a systematic organized manner, the use of specific planes is probably not crucial.[121]

NORMAL EARLY PREGNANCY

Both transvaginal and transabdominal sonography can be used to detect an early intrauterine pregnancy. Transvaginal ultrasound can identify an intrauterine pregnancy at about 5 weeks' gestational age (3 weeks' postconception) and about 7–10 days earlier than transabdominal ultrasound. The convention when referring to the age of a pregnancy is gestational age, which is the date from conception plus 2 weeks. An approximate correlation can be made between gestational age, β-hCG level, and pelvic ultrasound findings (Table 14-1).[1,30,62,89,122–128]

Transvaginal sonography is now the standard modality for evaluating early pregnancy. The following descriptions pertain to transvaginal sonography, except where specifically noted. The first sonographic sign of early pregnancy, the intradecidual sign, can be seen at 4–5 weeks (Figure 14-20). The intradecidual sign is a small sac, only a few millimeters in diameter, which is completely embedded within the endometrium on one side of the uterine midline, not deforming the midline stripe.[30,128,129] There is a focal echogenic thickening of endometrium surrounding the sac. The intradecidual sign can be seen only by using a high-resolution transducer (5 MHz or higher) and is not a universally accepted indicator of intrauterine pregnancy.[129]

A gestational sac can be clearly identified at about 5 weeks. With transvaginal sonography, a gestational sac can be seen in most patients with β-hCG levels of 1000–2000 mIU/mL and in all patients with levels above 2000 mIU/mL.[127] A gestational sac is characterized by a sonolucent center (chorionic sac) surrounded by a thick symmetric echogenic ring, known as the chorionic rim. This finding is seen in most intrauterine pregnancies but can also be seen surrounding a pseudogestational sac associated with an ectopic pregnancy.[89] Doppler ultrasound can be used to measure peritrophoblastic flow in order to distinguish a true gestational sac from a pseudogestational sac.[130] However, since this is outside the realm of point-of-care sonography, identification of a simple gestational sac should not be used as definitive evidence of an intrauterine pregnancy.

Many experts consider a clear double decidual sign as the first definitive evidence of an intrauterine pregnancy.[30,89,131] The double decidual sign is two concentric echogenic rings surrounding a gestational sac (Figure 14-21). The inner ring is the same structure as the chorionic ring and is called the decidua capsularis. The outer ring is called the decidua vera, derived from the stimulated endometrium of the uterus, while the thin hypoechoic layer between them is the endometrial canal.[30,131,132] A gestational sac with a vague or an absent double decidual sign is not diagnostic of an intrauterine pregnancy and may be a pseudogestational sac. If two clear rings are seen, an intrauterine pregnancy

▶ **TABLE 14-1. CORRELATION OF GESTATIONAL AGE, β-HCG LEVEL, AND PELVIC ULTRASOUND FINDINGS**

Gestational Age	β-hCG[*,†,‡] (mIU/mL)	Transvaginal U.S. Findings	Transabdominal U.S. Findings
4–5 weeks	<1,000	Intradecidual sac	N/A
5 weeks	1,000–2,000	Gestational sac (±DDS)	N/A
5–6 weeks	>2,000	Yolk sac (±embryo)	Gestational sac (±DDS)
6 weeks	10,000–20,000	Embryo with cardiac activity	Yolk sac (±embryo)
7 weeks	>20,000	Embryonic torso/head	Embryo with cardiac activity

*Significant individual variation in β-hCG levels at a given gestational age may occur.
†In multiple pregnancy (twins, triplets, etc.), β-hCG levels will be much higher at a given gestational age.
‡β-hCG reference standard is the International Reference Preparation (IRP).

is very likely. Unfortunately, the double decidual sign is present in only about half of all intrauterine pregnancies and is not 100% accurate.[133]

The yolk sac is the first structure that can be seen inside the gestational sac (Figure 14-22). Some experts consider the yolk sac the first definitive evidence of intrauterine pregnancy.[62,128] It is probably prudent for

most clinicians to visualize the yolk sac before making a diagnosis of an intrauterine pregnancy, avoiding misinterpretation of more subtle findings like the double decidual sign. The yolk sac is a symmetric circular echogenic structure at the edge of the gestational sac. The yolk sac has a role in the transfer of nutrients to the embryo during the first trimester and early

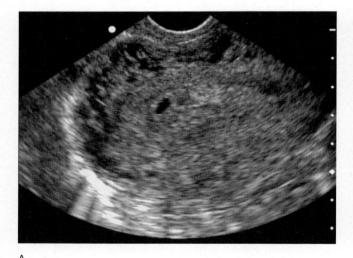

A

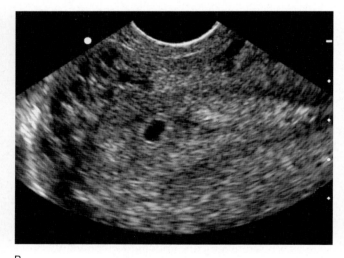

B

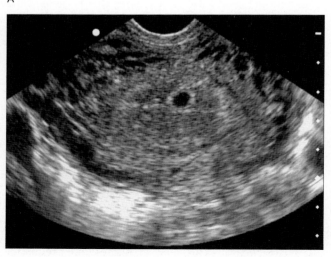

C

Figure 14-20. Intradecidual sign. Longitudinal transvaginal view of the uterus at 7.5 MHz (A). Magnified long-axis view of the endometrium shows a 5-mm gestational sac within a slightly thickened endometrium (B). Transverse view of the same patient demonstrates the location within the upper portion of the endometrium and the lack of deformation of the midline stripe (C). All views show a prominent arcuate venous plexus (a variant of normal) within the myometrium of the uterus for this patient. (Courtesy of James Mateer, MD)

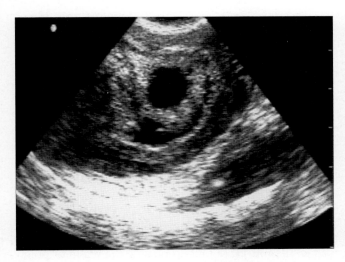

Figure 14-21. Transvaginal image of double decidual sign surrounding an intrauterine gestational sac in normal early pregnancy. This sign is often subtle and usually only noticeable along one side of the gestational sac but is very distinct in this example. (Courtesy of James Mateer, MD)

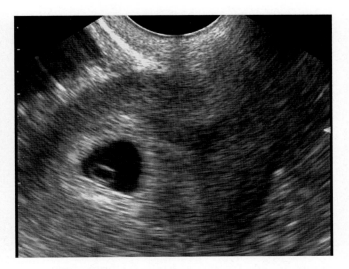

Figure 14-22. Transvaginal image of yolk sac within an intrauterine gestational sac in normal early pregnancy.

hematopoiesis takes place there. The yolk sac can first be seen by transvaginal sonography at about 5–6 weeks and then shrinks and disappears by about 12 weeks.[134]

The embryo appears as a thickening or small mass that is seen at the margin of the yolk sac between 5 and 6 weeks (Figure 14-23A). The normal embryo will grow rapidly, about 1 mm per day. The embryo can first be seen when it is only 2–3 mm and cardiac activity may not be detectable initially. By 6 weeks, the embryo is a distinct structure separate from the yolk sac

(Figure 14-23B). Also, the tiny vitelline duct, which connects the yolk sac to the base of the cord, can sometimes be seen between the yolk sac and the embryo.

Cardiac activity should be detected within the embryo at about 6 weeks. Any embryo measuring >5 mm should have cardiac activity when transvaginal sonography is used. At 7 weeks, the embryo will be about 12 mm and the head of the embryo will be clearly distinguished. At this age, the embryo's head contains a single large cerebral ventricle and has an appearance similar to the yolk sac.[89] At 8 weeks, the head of the embryo is about the same size as the yolk sac and limb buds begin

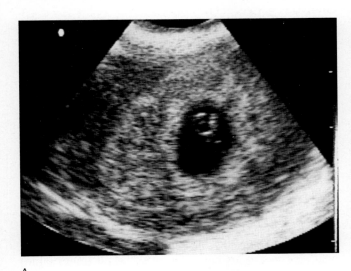

A

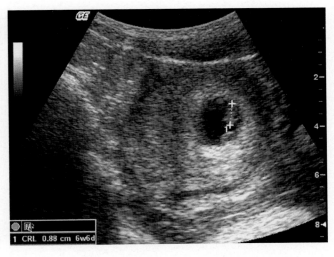

B

Figure 14-23. Small embryo and yolk sac within an intrauterine gestational sac (A). The 5-mm embryo is positioned along the right side of the yolk sac in this image and cardiac pulsations were visible during real-time sonography. Transvaginal image at 7.5 MHz (courtesy of James Mateer, MD). Embryonic pole is separated from the yolk sac and measures 6 weeks ± 6 days via crown-rump length (B). Transabdominal longitudinal view with empty bladder. (Courtesy of Hennepin County Medical Center)

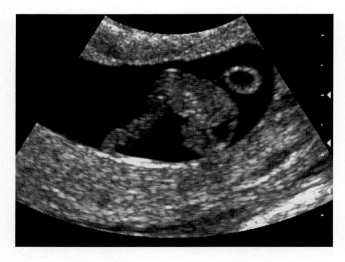

Figure 14-24. Transvaginal image of intrauterine embryo and yolk sac in normal pregnancy at 8 weeks.

to appear (Figure 14-24). Also, the physiologic midgut herniation can be visualized as an echogenic mass anterior to the trunk of the embryo. The bowel becomes intra-abdominal and the hernia disappears by 12 weeks. At 8 weeks and beyond, a thin echogenic line, the amnionic sac, may be seen surrounding the embryo.

At 10 weeks, organogenesis is complete and the embryo is now referred to as a fetus (Figure 14-25). Between 10 weeks and the end of the first trimester, the contours of the fetus become much more obvious. The fingers and toes can be identified and counted. Limb movements can be observed and bones and joints can be recognized. In the head, the falx cerebri becomes

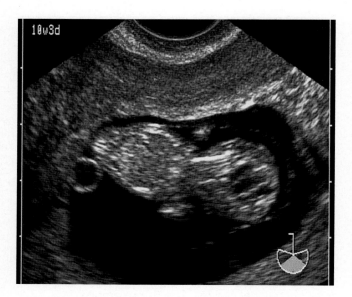

Figure 14-25. Transvaginal image of intrauterine fetus and yolk sac with surrounding amnion. Normal pregnancy at 10 weeks.

very distinct and the prominent choroid plexus can be seen in each of the lateral ventricles. The kidneys and bladder can be evaluated at 12 weeks. The heart and the stomach can also be identified inside the trunk and a four-chamber heart can be recognized by the end of the first trimester. Finally, the face and palate can be easily recognized late in the first trimester.

Routine screening for fetal abnormalities is not typically performed during the first trimester; the optimal time for this is at 18–20 weeks. However, some obvious abnormalities may be identified and it is important to know which structures are usually seen during the first trimester. There is some utility to evaluating nuchal thickness with transvaginal sonography, between 11 and 14 weeks, as a screening test for exomphalos and trisomies 18 and 13, but this is outside the realm of point-of-care sonography.

PREGNANCY DATING

Measurements of both the gestational sac and the embryo are accurate in the first trimester. Tables and formulas are available for calculating the gestational age using these measurements.[1,135] However, modern ultrasound software automatically calculates gestational age when calipers are placed on the structures of interest and appropriate presets are used.

The earliest measurement that can be used for pregnancy dating is mean sac diameter (MSD) of the gestational sac. MSD is the average of three orthogonal measurements of the gestational sac: (length + width + depth)/3. Pregnancy dating using MSD is only useful at 5–6 weeks, when the gestational sac is present but an embryo is not yet seen.

When an embryo is visible, at about 6 weeks, use measurement of the crown-rump length (CRL) of the embryo to date the pregnancy.[62] When measuring CRL, measure the maximal embryo length, excluding the yolk sac (Figure 14-26). Errors can occur when the calipers are not carefully placed at the margins of the embryo. Also, the embryo can flex and extend slightly, changing the measurement. Nevertheless, gestational age determination by CRL is accurate to within 5–7 days.[30]

Measurement of the biparietal diameter (BPD) of the fetal skull is used for pregnancy dating at the end of the first trimester and during the second trimester. The BPD is a transverse measurement of the diameter of the skull at the level of the thalamus. Position the calipers from the leading edge of the skull (outer table) on the near side to the leading edge of the skull (inner table) on the far side (Figure 14-27). Errors can be made by measuring the wrong part of the skull or if the image plane is not a true transaxial section through the fetal head. Pregnancy dating by BPD is also very accurate, especially prior to 20 weeks.[89]

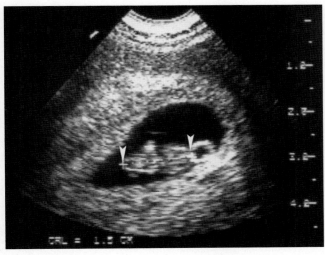

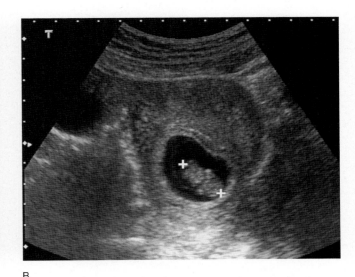

A

B

Figure 14-26. Crown-rump length. Transvaginal ultrasound that shows proper placement of cursors for CRL measurement (A). Measure the maximal embryo length, excluding the yolk sac. Transabdominal transverse ultrasound of a 9-week IUP (B). (A, Courtesy of James Mateer, MD; B, Courtesy of Hennepin County Medical Center)

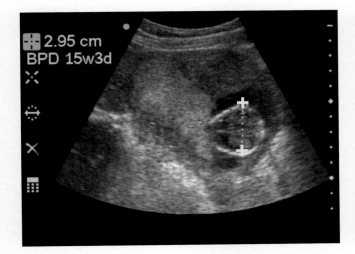

Figure 14-27. Biparietal diameter. Endovaginal ultrasound shows correct imaging plane of the head and cursor placement for accuracy. (Courtesy of James Mateer, MD)

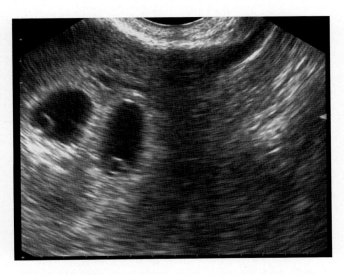

Figure 14-28. Dichorionic twins. Two chorionic sacs and two yolk sacs are clearly seen (transvaginal image).

MULTIPLE PREGNANCY

Documentation of the chorionicity and amnionicity of a multiple pregnancy is important early in the pregnancy because it may be hard to determine later in pregnancy. There are several sonographic criteria that can be used to determine chorionicity and amnionicity in the first trimester. Two clear gestational (chorionic) sacs may be seen as early as 6 weeks; this is good evidence of dichorionic twins (Figure 14-28). Later in the first trimester,

dichorionicity can be established by finding a thick septum separating the two chorionic sacs (Figure 14-29). If the septum separating the two pregnancies is thin, then it may be difficult to determine whether it is the wall of a chorionic sac or an amnionic membrane. When the septum is thin, identification of a chorionic peak can confirm a dichorionic twin pregnancy. A chorionic peak is a triangular projection of tissue, of the same echogenicity as the placenta, emanating from the placenta and tapering to a point in the intertwin membrane.[30]

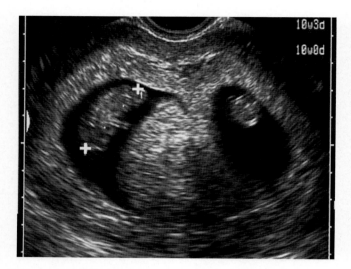

Figure 14-29. Dichorionic twins. Calipers mark the crown-rump length of one of the embryos. Gestational age is 10 weeks 0 days (transvaginal image).

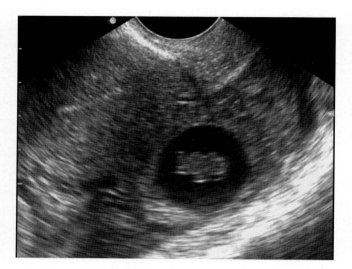

Figure 14-30. Ectopic pregnancy. Living embryo in the adnexa and empty uterus (endometrial echo is visible in the left upper portion of the image). Embryonic cardiac activity was present on real-time imaging (transvaginal image).

The amnionicity of a monochorionic pregnancy can also be determined by first trimester sonography. Counting the number of yolk sacs is the easiest way to determine amnionicity; if there are two yolk sacs, then there must be two amnions.[89] After about 8 weeks, amnionic membranes should be visible and diamnionic pregnancies should have a separate amnion surrounding each twin.

► COMMON AND EMERGENT ABNORMALITIES

ECTOPIC PREGNANCY

Definite Ectopic Pregnancy

A live extrauterine embryo with cardiac activity can be seen with transvaginal sonography in up to 15–20% of ectopic pregnancies (Figure 14-30).[56,57] An extrauterine gestational sac containing an embryo or yolk sac is also diagnostic and is seen in a significant percentage of ectopic pregnancies (Figure 14-31; Video 14-1: Evaluation for Ectopic Pregnancy).[56]

Nonspecific Signs of Ectopic Pregnancy: Free Fluid, Tubal Ring, and Complex Mass

There are several nonspecific sonographic findings that are not diagnostic but are highly suggestive of an ectopic pregnancy in pregnant patients with an empty uterus (Table 14-2).[27,56–58,60,61,136–138] Some of these findings are subtle and may be easily missed, especially if transvaginal sonography is not available. Therefore, emergency physicians should obtain a comprehensive

ultrasound examination if no intrauterine pregnancy or ectopic pregnancy is identified with point-of-care sonography.

Free Pelvic or Intraperitoneal Fluid

Free fluid in the posterior pelvic cul-de-sac or in other intraperitoneal sites is suggestive of ectopic pregnancy (Figure 14-32).[58,60,137,139] Transvaginal sonography is very sensitive for detecting free fluid in the posterior cul-de-sac.[30] Only about one-third of ectopic pregnancies have no free fluid in the cul-de-sac.[140] Also, free fluid is the only abnormal sonographic finding in about 15% of ectopic pregnancies.[137] The greater the volume of free intraperitoneal fluid, the greater the likelihood of ectopic pregnancy (Figures 14-33 and 14-34).[89,139] In fact, patients with a moderate-to-large amount of free pelvic fluid have about an 86% chance and those with hepatorenal free fluid have a nearly 100% chance of having an ectopic pregnancy.[58] Although a large amount of fluid predicts ectopic pregnancy, it is not a reliable indicator of tubal rupture. Only about 60% of those with

► **TABLE 14-2. NONSPECIFIC SONOGRAPHIC SIGNS OF ECTOPIC PREGNANCY**

Sonographic Findings	Likelihood of Ectopic Pregnancy (%)
Any free pelvic fluid	52
Complex pelvic mass	75
Moderate or large free pelvic fluid	86
Tubal ring	>95
Mass and free fluid	97
Hepatorenal free fluid	~100

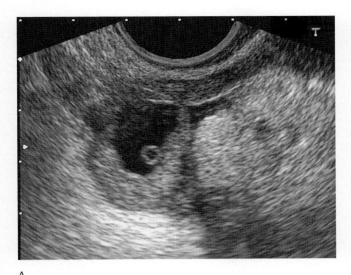

A

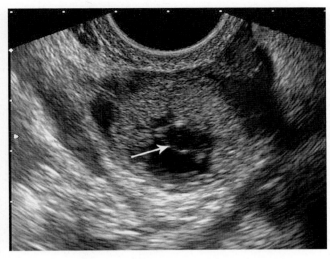

B

Figure 14-31. Ectopic pregnancy. Extrauterine gestational sac with a thick echogenic ring containing a yolk sac (A). A small stripe of free fluid is present as well as bowel gas artifact surrounding the structure (transvaginal image). A thick concentric echogenic ring in the adnexa is surrounded by free fluid (B). A subtle yolk sac is contained within the structure (arrow). (Courtesy of Hennepin County Medical Center)

a large amount of free fluid have a ruptured tube.[60,141] Free fluid may be due to leaking of blood from the end of the fallopian tube, which can occur slowly.

Echogenic fluid is more likely to represent blood, and this also increases the chances of an ectopic pregnancy (Figure 14-32). If bleeding is brisk, clots may be seen in the pelvic cul-de-sac instead of fluid. Although a small amount of hypoechoic free pelvic fluid may be normal, it must be considered suspicious in the setting of a pregnant patient with an empty uterus.[58,60,61,137]

The definition of "small amount" is fluid that is confined to the cul-de-sac and covering less than one-third of the inferior posterior uterus. As stated, anything more than a small amount is almost always associated with an ectopic pregnancy.[56,58,60]

Visualize the hepatorenal potential space (Morison's pouch) on every patient with a possible ectopic pregnancy.[30,89] Free fluid in the hepatorenal space

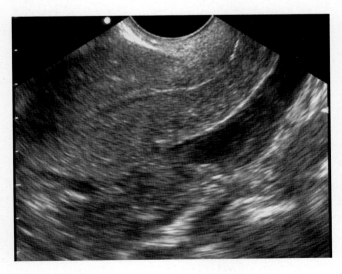

Figure 14-32. Ectopic pregnancy. Transvaginal sagittal image of empty uterus and echogenic free fluid in the posterior cul-de-sac.

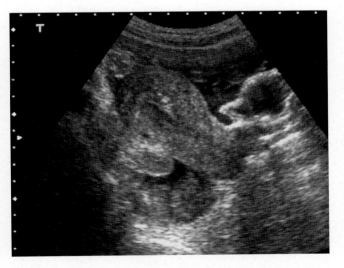

Figure 14-33. Ectopic pregnancy. Transabdominal longitudinal view shows an empty uterus. Complex fluid from liquid and clotted blood is present in both the anterior and posterior cul-de-sac areas. The bladder is collapsed around a Foley catheter balloon. (Courtesy of Hennepin County Medical Center)

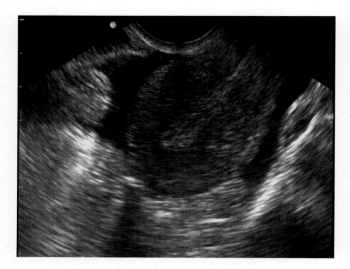

Figure 14-34. Ectopic pregnancy. Transvaginal image of free fluid surrounding an empty uterus.

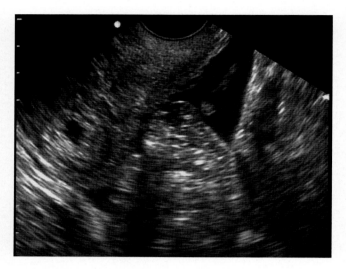

Figure 14-36. Ectopic pregnancy. Tubal ring (2 cm). Transvaginal image of free pelvic fluid with floating bowel.

(Figure 14-35), or elsewhere outside the pelvis, is evidence of a large amount of intraperitoneal fluid.[142] In a pregnant woman with an empty uterus, this must be considered bleeding secondary to an ectopic pregnancy. Finding free fluid in the hepatorenal space with point-of-care sonography reduces the time to diagnosis and treatment of ectopic pregnancy.[6] A finding of hepatorenal free fluid "should give the surgeon a greater sense of urgency."[30]

Tubal Ring

A tubal ring is nearly diagnostic of ectopic pregnancy.[56,57,136,137] A tubal ring is a concentric hyperechoic structure found in the adnexa (Figures 14-36, 14-37, and 14-38). It is created by the trophoblast of the

ectopic pregnancy surrounding the chorionic sac and is the equivalent of a gestational sac.[30] A tubal ring, in general, has a different sonographic appearance than a corpus luteum or other ovarian cysts because it has a relatively thick and brightly echogenic, round, symmetric wall. Ovarian cysts have walls of varying thickness and are surrounded by normal ovarian follicles. With transvaginal sonography, it may be possible to identify a tubal ring in >60% of ectopic pregnancies.[56,57] When a tubal ring is seen, the likelihood of ectopic pregnancy is >95%.[56]

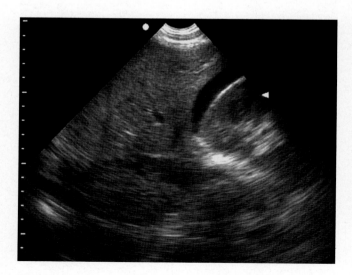

Figure 14-35. Ectopic pregnancy. Transabdominal image of free fluid in the hepatorenal space.

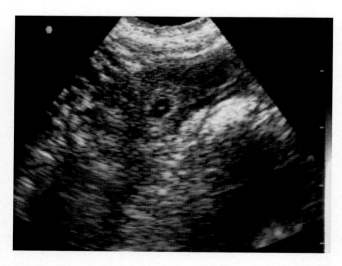

Figure 14-37. Tubal ring. Transvaginal view of the right adnexa shows a tiny (7 mm), brightly echogenic ring-like structure. This was determined to be a very early ectopic pregnancy. (Courtesy of James Mateer, MD)

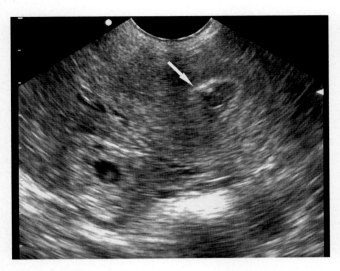

Figure 14-38. Ectopic pregnancy. Transvaginal image of pseudogestational sac in the uterus (arrow) and 2.5 cm brightly echogenic tubal ring in the adnexa.

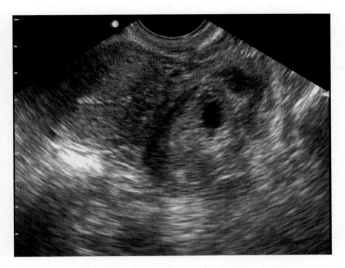

Figure 14-40. Ectopic pregnancy. An empty uterus is shown in transverse transvaginal view and is identified by the endometrial stripe. The complex mass is in the left adnexa and adjacent to the uterus.

Complex Mass

The most common sonographic finding in ectopic pregnancy is a complex adnexal mass (Figures 14-39 and 14-40).[55] A complex adnexal mass may represent a tubal hematoma, ectopic trophoblastic tissue, or distorted contents of an ectopic gestational sac.[56–58,89,137,138] A complex mass contains a mixture of cystic and solid components. This is a sensitive sonographic sign of ectopic pregnancy. It may be seen in up to 85% of cases on transvaginal scanning.[56] However, a complex mass may be subtle and easily missed.[89] The mass may blend into adjacent structures with similar echogenicity and may have an appearance similar to the bowel or ovaries.

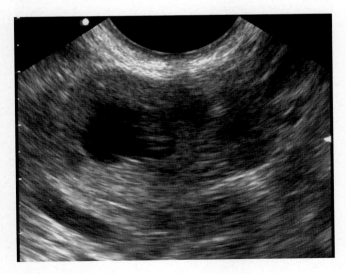

Figure 14-39. Ectopic pregnancy. Transvaginal image of complex right adnexal mass located above the iliac vein.

Several sonographic signs may help differentiate a complex mass from the surrounding pelvic structures. Identifying the ovaries and then searching between the ovaries and the uterus is the best technique for locating an adnexal mass. To differentiate a mass from other pelvic structures, gently press down on the patient's lower abdomen with the free hand during transvaginal scanning in a manner similar to performing a bimanual pelvic examination. This will cause pelvic structures to move in relation to one another and examiners can recognize a mass as a separate structure, moving independently from the ovary and bowel. Also, if the transvaginal transducer is held very still, peristalsis of the bowel can be seen, differentiating it from other pelvic structures.

Color Doppler has been used in an attempt to differentiate surrounding structures from an adnexal mass. High-velocity, low impedance trophoblastic flow can sometimes be seen surrounding an ectopic sac; this is referred to as the "ring of fire"[143] (Figure 14-41). Some authors suggest that color Doppler provides little additional information and is not more accurate than gray scale sonography for determining whether an adnexal mass is an ectopic pregnancy.[30,108,144] Some studies and case reports suggest asymmetric adnexal color Doppler flow is a useful clue.[145,146]

PREGNANCY LOSS

Embryonic Demise

There are several sonographic signs that can reliably predict embryonic demise. The earliest sign is a gestational

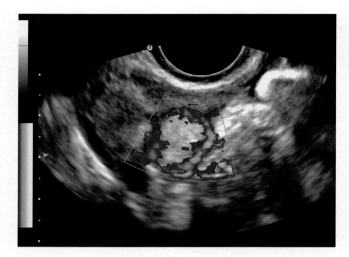

Figure 14-41. Ring of fire. Transvaginal ultrasound of the adnexa demonstrates ectopic mass with surrounding power Doppler signal. (Courtesy of J. Christian Fox, MD)

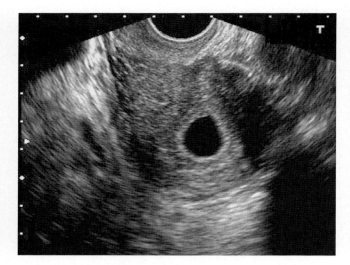

Figure 14-42. Early embryonic demise. Transvaginal image of empty intrauterine sac consistent with 6.5 weeks' gestational sac size contains no yolk sac or embryo. (Courtesy of Hennepin County Medical Center)

sac without a yolk sac or embryo (Figure 14-42). With high-resolution transvaginal sonography ($\geq$6.5 MHz), a yolk sac is usually seen within the gestational sac when MSD is $\geq$10 mm and an embryo is usually seen when MSD is $\geq$16 mm.[30,125,147,148] However, with transvaginal or transabdominal scanning, a yolk sac may not be seen until the MSD is $\geq$20 mm.[89,149,150] For the purposes of point-of-care transvaginal sonography, an empty gestational sac $\geq$20 mm is a good predictor of embryonic demise; this is referred to as a blighted ovum. The nonobstetrics clinician should refrain from proclaiming

this to the patient and simply note that normal structures are not seen and it may be too early to make a firm diagnosis.

Another good indicator of embryonic demise is lack of embryonic cardiac activity (Figure 14-43). With transvaginal sonography, cardiac activity should be seen in all embryos >5 mm long by CRL.[30,89,100,151] With transabdominal sonography, cardiac activity should be seen in all embryos >10 mm long.[89] When searching for embryonic cardiac activity, it is important to be sure that

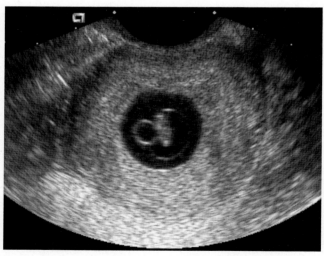

A

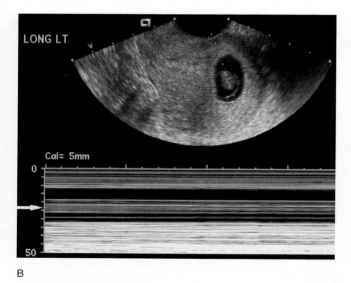

B

Figure 14-43. Embryonic demise. Transvaginal image of the fetal pole that measured 7 weeks via CRL (A). The yolk sac appears slightly enlarged and the amnion is clearly visible. There was no cardiac activity on real-time sonography and this was documented by the M-mode examination (B). Note the lack of any motion in the fetal band (arrow). (Courtesy of James Mateer, MD, Waukesha Memorial Hospital)

the embryo is clearly seen. This is easier at 7–8 weeks when the embryonic head and torso can be identified. Also, it is essential to use a high frame rate and turn off the frame-averaging mode when looking for cardiac activity.[30]

Several more subtle signs are also suggestive of embryonic demise or poor fetal outcome. Embryonic bradycardia predicts a poor prognosis.[152,153] The normal heart rate for an embryo longer than 5 mm by CRL (6.3 weeks' gestational age) is >120 beats per minute (bpm). The lower the heart rate is below 120 bpm, the lower the survival rate of the embryo. Embryos longer than 5 mm with heart rates below 100 bpm have a survival rate of only 6%.[153] Very early pregnancies, with embryos <5 mm in length, normally have slower heart rates, but a rate <90 bpm is nearly always associated with embryonic demise.[152,153]

An abnormal yolk sac is another subtle sign of demise or abnormal pregnancy. A very small yolk sac (<2 mm diameter) between 8 and 12 weeks is usually associated with an abnormal pregnancy.[154] A very large yolk sac (>6 mm diameter) between 5 and 12 weeks is predictive of embryonic demise or a significant chromosomal abnormality.[30,155] Also, prior to 12 weeks, inability to visualize the yolk sac when an embryo is clearly present is strong evidence of impending embryonic demise.[155] Yolk sac shape is not associated with adverse pregnancy outcome. Pregnancies with a normal size but irregularly shaped yolk sac have a normal outcome in nearly all cases.[30]

An odd-shaped or grossly distorted gestational sac is reportedly a good indicator of pregnancy failure, but this finding is subjective (Figure 14-44).[149] A gestational sac low in the uterus, with or without a yolk sac or embryo, is generally considered a sign of inevitable abor-

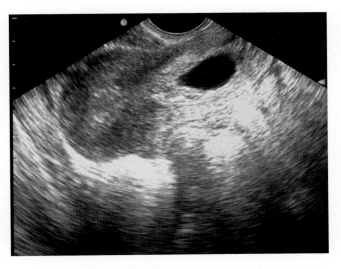

Figure 14-45. Inevitable abortion. The fundus is on the left of the image and the gestational sac is approaching the cervical portion of the uterus (transvaginal image).

tion (Figures 14-45 and 14-46). Also, a weakly echogenic or thin (<2 mm wide) trophoblastic reaction surrounding a gestational sac may indicate imminent demise. Finally, a gestational sac, with a MSD not >5 mm larger than the CRL of the embryo, is probably abnormal.[150,156]

Subchorionic hemorrhage is bleeding between the endometrium and chorionic membrane. This is a common finding late in the first trimester. Sonographically, part of the chorionic membrane and placenta are separated from the decidua vera (the endometrium) (Figure 14-47).[30] Acutely, the hemorrhage may appear

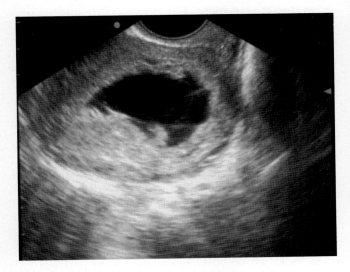

Figure 14-44. Embryonic demise. Transvaginal image of distorted gestational sac.

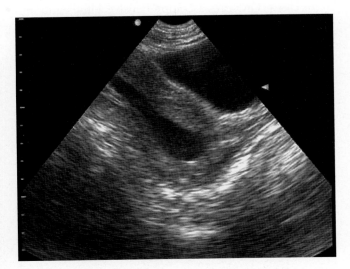

Figure 14-46. Embryonic demise with inevitable abortion. Large empty distorted intrauterine sac that is bulging toward the cervical canal. Transabdominal longitudinal view with the bladder and vaginal stripe along the right side of the image.

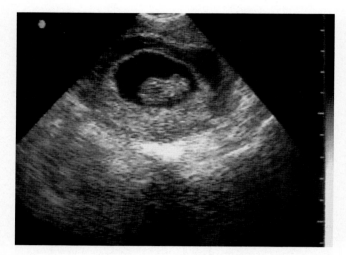

Figure 14-47. Subchorionic hemorrhage. An echolucent crescent-shaped stripe is located between the decidua capsularis and the decidua vera (endometrium) from implantation hemorrhage (transvaginal images). (Courtesy of James Mateer, MD)

hyperechoic or isoechoic relative to the placenta, with only slight elevation noted. Over the next week or two, the blood becomes hypoechoic. Patients who present with threatened abortion and have a subchorionic hemorrhage probably have a higher incidence of embryonic demise.[157,158] Those with large subchorionic hemorrhages may have a much higher rate of pregnancy loss.[157]

Interpret findings of embryonic demise conservatively and give the pregnancy the benefit of the doubt in all cases. Ordering a comprehensive ultrasound and

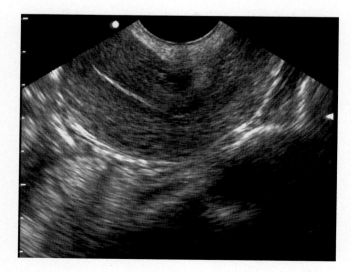

Figure 14-48. Transvaginal image of empty uterus after a completed spontaneous abortion.

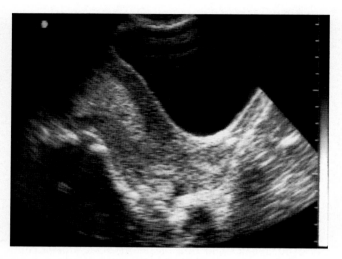

Figure 14-49. Transabdominal longitudinal image of intrauterine echogenic material (2–3 cm thick), consistent with retained products of conception. (Courtesy of James Mateer, MD)

obtaining an obstetrics consult is prudent when the diagnosis is unclear.

Completed Spontaneous Abortion
The uterus should be empty after a completed spontaneous abortion (Figure 14-48). A small amount of blood or clot may be present.

Retained Products of Conception
Patients with intrauterine echogenic material or a thickened midline stripe (≥10 mm wide) after a spontaneous abortion probably have retained products of conception (Figure 14-49).[94,96,159] When curettage is performed in such cases, chorionic villi are identified in about 70%.[96] Many patients with retained products will do well with expectant management, but they may require curettage and should be followed closely for bleeding and infection.[160]

► COMMON VARIANTS AND SELECTED ABNORMALITIES

Several normal anatomic variants may make transabdominal and transvaginal pelvic sonography more difficult. Retroversion of the uterus occurs in about 10% of women. It has little clinical significance, but it makes transabdominal imaging difficult. Retroversion means that the body of the uterus bends posterior toward the rectosigmoid colon instead of toward the anterior abdominal wall. The body of the uterus is then too far away from the transabdominal transducer and resolution is poor (Figure 14-50A). Transvaginal sonography is much better for imaging a retroverted uterus because

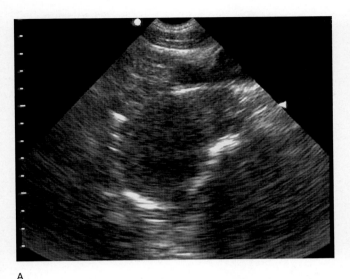

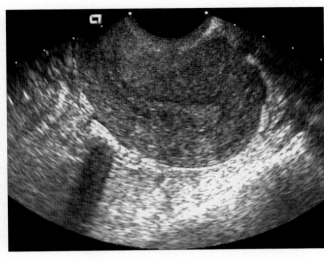

A   B

Figure 14-50. Transabdominal sagittal view of a retroverted uterus (A). The uterine body and fundus are not well visualized because of the uterine position and empty bladder. A transvaginal longitudinal view of the uterus (B) provides improved resolution. Note that with a retroverted uterus, the fundus is projected to the right side of the image and the cervix to the left. (B, Courtesy of James Mateer, MD, Waukesha Memorial Hospital)

the transducer can still be placed close to the body of the uterus (Figure 14-50B). When the uterus is retroverted, the ovaries usually lie anterior and lateral to the body of the uterus.

Lateral deviation of the uterus is another normal variant that makes pelvic ultrasound difficult. When transabdominal or transvaginal scanning is performed and the uterus is not seen in the midline, then aim the transducer laterally and obtain sagittal oblique images. It is not uncommon to find the body of the uterus bending toward the lateral pelvis. If this is the case, then the midline stripe may be difficult to see in just one plane. Lateral and coronal images may be helpful in this situation. When the uterus is deviated laterally, it may displace the ovary out of its usual location. The ovary may then be found superior to the uterus or in the posterior cul-de-sac.

Variation in the location of the ovaries can also make pelvic ultrasound difficult. Transvaginal sonography is required to visualize most normal ovaries. Even with transvaginal scanning, however, they may be difficult to find. In women who have previously been pregnant, the ovaries may be found lateral, posterior, or superior to the uterus. In patients with an enlarged uterus, those who are pregnant or have uterine fibroids, the ovaries are often displaced superior to the uterus. When the ovaries are superior to the uterus, they are difficult to see with transvaginal sonography.

The fallopian tubes are not normally seen on transabdominal ultrasound. If the tubes are filled with fluid secondary to scarring or pelvic inflammatory disease, then they may be easily recognized. They will be found

in the adnexa lateral to the uterine body. When imaged longitudinally, the fallopian tubes will appear as anechoic tubal structures; when imaged transversely, they will appear as cystic structures. If multiple redundant loops of the tube are adjacent to one another, then this may be misinterpreted as a large multicystic mass. Using the endovaginal approach, healthy fallopian tubes are frequently imaged at their uterine origin and may be traced near each ovary if there is no bowel gas interference.

A small amount of fluid in the posterior cul-de-sac can be normal. This fluid may not be seen with transabdominal sonography but is easily visualized with transvaginal imaging (Figure 14-51).

PELVIC MASSES

Corpus Luteum Cyst

Corpus luteum cysts are the most common pelvic masses found in early pregnancy. They are usually unilocular and have thin walls (Figure 14-52). Internal hemorrhage may result in internal septations and echogenic material (Figure 14-53). The corpus is solid in appearance in up to 50% of cases.

Leiomyomas

Uterine fibroids are very common and may grow during pregnancy. They are located in the uterine wall and have a variable sonographic appearance. They often cause

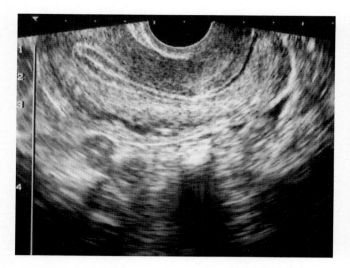

Figure 14-51. Transvaginal sagittal view of the normal anteflexed uterus. Note that the fundus is displayed on the left side of the monitor. Minimal (physiologic) free fluid can be seen in the posterior cul-de-sac below the cervix. The patient has a moderately prominent arcuate venous plexus that does not represent free fluid.

dispersion of ultrasound and distortion of pelvic images (Figure 14-54).

Malignant Pelvic Masses

The most common tumors that enlarge during pregnancy are ovarian cystadenomas. Internal septations and papillary excrescences are suggestive of malignancy (Figure 14-55).

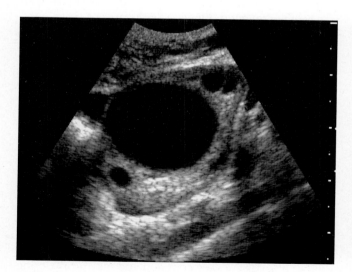

Figure 14-52. Transvaginal image of corpus luteum cyst.

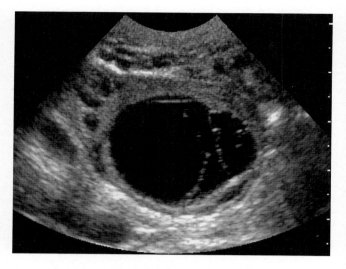

Figure 14-53. Transvaginal image of corpus luteum cyst with fine septations from internal hemorrhage..

ADNEXAL TORSION

Most cases of adnexal torsion occur in the presence of an enlarged ovary or an ovarian mass. Finding a normal ovary makes the diagnosis much less likely.

GESTATIONAL TROPHOBLASTIC DISEASE

Most cases of GTD present as a benign molar pregnancy. Those with an invasive mole or choriocarcinoma usually have a history of a molar pregnancy. The classic finding is the appearance of a cluster of "grapes," an intrauterine mass with diffuse hypoechoic vesicles (Figure 14-56).

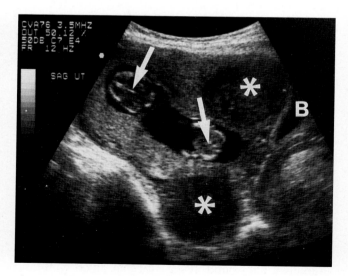

Figure 14-54. Transvaginal image of uterine fibroids (∗) with pregnancy (arrows).

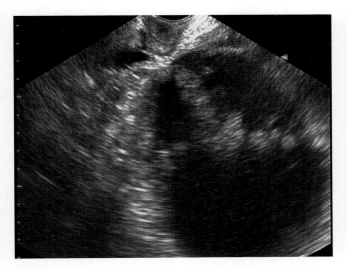

Figure 14-55. Transvaginal image of large complex pelvic mass with papillary excrescences and septations with possible malignancy.

The appearance is not always classic in the first trimester, and the diagnosis may be missed (Figure 14-57).

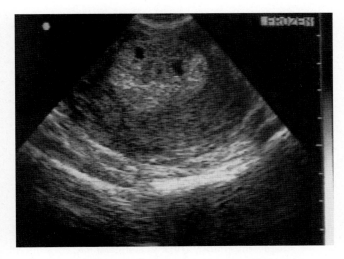

Figure 14-57. Early molar pregnancy. Transverse transvaginal image reveals a thick, echogenic endometrial echo with a few scattered irregular cystic areas in a patient with a high hCG level. (Courtesy of James Mateer, MD)

▶ PITFALLS

ECTOPIC PREGNANCY

1. **Not performing pelvic sonography because of a recent last menstrual period or a low β-hCG.** Patients with a positive pregnancy test who present with abdominal pain or vaginal bleeding should undergo a pelvic ultrasound examination regardless of their reported last menstrual period or β-hCG level. Patients may misinterpret vaginal spotting during pregnancy for a menstrual period; thus, obtaining a menstrual history is not an accurate method for excluding ectopic pregnancy. Also, it is not uncommon for patients to have a low β-hCG level and a ruptured ectopic pregnancy.

2. **Attributing an empty uterus to a very early intrauterine pregnancy or a completed spontaneous abortion.** More than 40% of ectopic pregnancies have a β-hCG level <1000 mIU/mL; therefore, an empty uterus with a low β-hCG level should not be considered normal

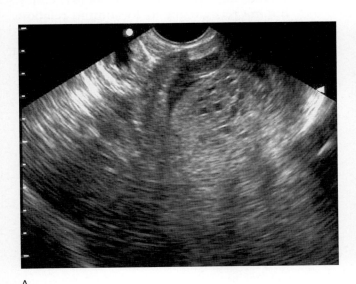

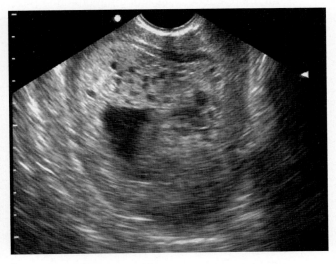

A

B

Figure 14-56. Transvaginal images (A and B) of molar pregnancy.

and the entire pelvis should be scanned for signs of an ectopic pregnancy.[65] Also, the only definitive evidence of a completed spontaneous abortion is passage of obvious products of conception or chorionic villi. Without definitive evidence of a completed abortion, the diagnosis of ectopic pregnancy must be ruled out.[49]

3. **Mistaking a pseudogestational sac for a gestational sac.** Visualizing an intrauterine pregnancy essentially excludes the diagnosis of ectopic pregnancy in most patients. The intradecidual sign and gestational sac are early signs of an intrauterine pregnancy, but neither is 100% reliable.[125,128,129] Be careful not to mistake a pseudogestational sac associated with an ectopic pregnancy for a gestational sac.[30,89,130] A pseudogestational sac, also known as a decidual cast, is an intrauterine fluid collection surrounded by a single decidual layer (Figures 14-38). A pseudogestational sac occurs in 5–10% of ectopic pregnancies and appears as an elongated and odd-shaped sac in the center of the endometrial cavity with inconsistent thickening of the endometrium.[89] A pseudogestational sac can usually be differentiated from a gestational sac using transvaginal sonography.[104] Also, Doppler ultrasound may help by finding high-velocity, low impedance peritrophoblastic flow surrounding a true gestational sac, but the reliability of this is not 100%.[130,143]

4. **Misidentifying an early intrauterine pregnancy.** Avoid making the diagnosis of an intrauterine pregnancy when only a small gestational sac is visible. A clear double decidual sign is the first reliable evidence of an intrauterine pregnancy.[30,131] A yolk sac and embryo are more tangible signs of an intrauterine pregnancy and should be seen when making the diagnosis of an intrauterine pregnancy.[125] Cardiac activity should be seen in all embryos >5 mm long, and this is regarded as the best evidence of an intrauterine pregnancy. It may be prudent for clinicians early in their ultrasound training to see cardiac activity before diagnosing an intrauterine pregnancy.

5. **Overestimating the ability to identify subtle signs of ectopic pregnancy.** Although an empty uterus, free intraperitoneal fluid in the hepatorenal space, and free fluid in the pelvis are easy to identify, complex adnexal masses and tubal rings may be subtle to identify. Repeat indeterminate point-of-care scans to look for these subtle signs or obtain a comprehensive ultrasound examination.

6. **Performing a transvaginal ultrasound without a transabdominal scan.** The transabdom-

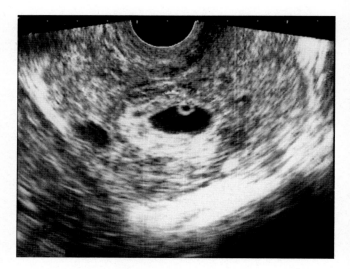

Figure 14-58. Ectopic pregnancy. Transvaginal image of extrauterine gestational sac with a bright, thick echogenic ring and a yolk sac within. A cursory examination could mistake the surrounding mid-level echoes as uterine tissue, but note the absence of any endometrial echo.

inal pelvic view allows a broader view of the pelvis and may detect masses that are outside the field of view of the transvaginal transducer and may be a helpful starting point in some patients. Also, always scan the hepatorenal space to evaluate for free intraperitoneal fluid.[89] Some patients may have minimal symptoms and normal vital signs despite a ruptured ectopic pregnancy with a large amount of intraperitoneal blood.

7. **Identifying a normal appearing pregnancy but not recognizing its location in relation to the uterus.** An ectopic pregnancy may appear to be an intrauterine pregnancy if its extrauterine location is not carefully noted (Figure 14-58). Also, an interstitial ectopic pregnancy may appear to be intrauterine but careful imaging will reveal that it lies on the margin of the uterine wall and not in the intrauterine cavity. Transabdominal sonography will help clarify the big picture in cases of possible ectopic pregnancy.

8. **Mistaking an interstitial pregnancy for an intrauterine pregnancy.** An interstitial pregnancy may be mistaken for an intrauterine pregnancy.[161] Interstitial pregnancies comprise about 2–5% of all ectopic pregnancies.[89] Most ectopic pregnancies occur in the ampullary segment of the fallopian tube, but interstitial ectopic pregnancies occur in the cornual region (Figure 14-59). They are partially enveloped by

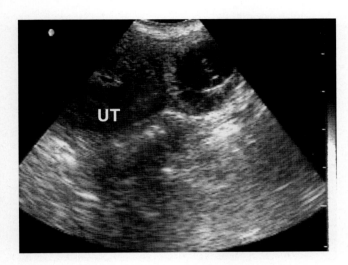

Figure 14-59. Interstitial ectopic. Transverse transvaginal ultrasound reveals a small fluid collection within the endometrium of the uterus (UT). The round echogenic ectopic ring was partially imbedded within the uterine myometrium. (Courtesy of James Mateer, MD)

the myometrium. Because of the rich myometrial blood supply, an interstitial pregnancy can grow larger and rupture later than most ectopic pregnancies. When rupture occurs, intraperitoneal bleeding (potentially arterial) and vaginal bleeding may be brisk and profuse. Many of these patients exsanguinate and die before reaching the hospital. It may be difficult to identify an interstitial pregnancy because the gestational sac may be completely surrounded by the uterus. However, an interstitial pregnancy usually appears to be at the margin of the uterine wall rather than inside the uterine cavity.[162] The eccentrically located gestational sac is surrounded by an asymmetric myometrial mantle with a free wall thickness usually <5–8 mm. The "interstitial line sign" is a fine echogenic line extending from the endometrial stripe to the interstitial gestational sac. This finding is diagnostic of an interstitial ectopic pregnancy. If the diagnosis is not made early, prior to rupture, up to 50% of patients may require a hysterectomy.[89]

9. **Failure to identify heterotopic pregnancy.** Failure to obtain a history of fertility medications or in vitro fertilization may lead to this pitfall. The risk of heterotopic pregnancy in such patients is as high as 1%, so finding an intrauterine pregnancy does not exclude the diagnosis of ectopic pregnancy. Also, patients without these risk factors may have a heterotopic pregnancy.[33,163] Therefore, it is prudent to scan the entire pelvis looking for free pelvic fluid

or an adnexal mass, even after an intrauterine pregnancy has been identified.

▶ OTHER PITFALLS

1. **Fetal anomalies.** Failure to diagnose fetal anomalies by ultrasound has become a significant source of malpractice litigation. To avoid this problem, patients should be informed that point-of-care sonography is a focused examination only and is not designed to detect embryonic abnormalities.

2. **Embryonic demise.** Many potential pitfalls are associated with the diagnosis of embryonic demise. When poor resolution or poor quality scans are obtained, normal structures may not be visualized, leading to the errant diagnosis of a blighted ovum. Also, inability to identify embryonic cardiac activity can occur secondary to mistaking another structure for the embryo or using a frame-averaging ultrasound mode. These pitfalls can be avoided by positively identifying the embryo and by using a high frame rate setting when searching for embryonic cardiac activity. Before the diagnosis of embryonic demise is made, the pregnancy should be given the benefit of the doubt. Sonography by an experienced operator and consultation with obstetrics is prudent before the patient is informed of the definitive diagnosis.

3. **Multiple pregnancy.** When twins are identified by point-of-care ultrasound, it is important to inform the patient that about 25% of twin pregnancies diagnosed in the first trimester will become singleton pregnancies by the second trimester.

4. **Pelvic masses.** The most common pitfall when identifying a pelvic mass is neglecting to arrange close follow-up and informing the patient of the finding. Pelvic masses may enlarge during pregnancy and are usually incidental findings on pelvic sonography. Ovarian malignancy may rarely present during pregnancy.

5. **Pelvic pain.** Pelvic pain is a common complaint in early pregnancy. A common pitfall of using pelvic ultrasound in these patients is that the finding of an intrauterine pregnancy often ends the workup for the etiology of the patient's symptoms. Once ectopic pregnancy is excluded, the patient's pelvic pain may be attributed to the pregnancy and diagnoses such as appendicitis or adnexal torsion may not be considered. Physicians should remember that appendicitis is relatively common in pregnancy

and 20% of adnexal torsion occurs during pregnancy.

6. **Gestational trophoblastic disease.** Molar pregnancy is usually obvious on pelvic ultrasound. However, early in pregnancy, the findings may be subtle. Serum β-hCG will always be very high in GTD. A potential pitfall is assuming that this diagnosis is excluded because it is not seen on point-of-care ultrasound. Such patients need close follow-up and repeat ultrasound examinations.

► CASE STUDIES

CASE 1

Patient Presentation

A 20-year-old woman, gravida 3, para 0, at about 3–6 weeks' gestation (unsure of the date of her last menstrual period) presented with several hours of heavy vaginal bleeding and low, central abdominal cramping. She denied any history of sexually transmitted disease, intrauterine device, ectopic pregnancy, or pelvic surgery. Previous pregnancies ended in early spontaneous abortions. She denied vomiting, fever, and urinary symptoms.

On physical examination, her blood pressure was 105/71 mm Hg, heart rate 87 bpm, respirations 14 per minute, and temperature 36.8°C. She was in no distress. Her head, neck, pulmonary, CV, and back examinations were unremarkable. Abdominal examination revealed a soft abdomen with mild suprapubic tenderness. Speculum examination revealed a closed cervical os with a small amount of blood in the vaginal vault. Bimanual pelvic examination revealed no tenderness or mass.

Management Course

Urinalysis was unremarkable, but the urine pregnancy test was positive. Point-of-care transvaginal ultrasound performed by the emergency physician immediately after the pelvic examination showed an empty uterus and a 3 × 3 × 4 cm right adnexal mass adjacent to the right ovary, containing a gestational sac, yolk sac, and embryo (Figure 14-60). Estimated gestational age by CRL was 6 weeks and 2 days. Trace free fluid was noted in the right adnexa, but the pouch of Douglas and the pouch of Morison were negative for free fluid. IV access was obtained, and the obstetrics service was consulted. The serum β-hCG level was 14,358 mIU/mL and the blood type was B positive. A repeat ultrasound examination in the radiology department confirmed the above bedside findings. The patient was taken to the operating room where a laparoscopic right salpingectomy was

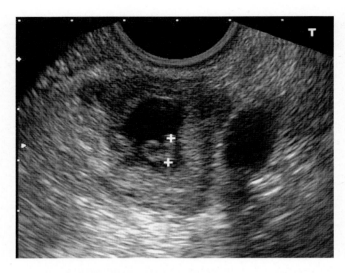

Figure 14-60. Case 1. Point-of-care transvaginal ultrasound showed an empty uterus and a 3 × 3 × 4 cm right adnexal mass adjacent to the right ovary, containing a gestational sac, yolk sac, and embryo. (Courtesy of Hennepin County Medical Center)

performed without complications. The patient recovered well and subsequently was discharged home.

Commentary

Case 1 is an example of a patient presenting with an unruptured ectopic pregnancy. This diagnosis was made rapidly by the emergency physician using point-of-care transvaginal ultrasound immediately after the routine pelvic examination. This case demonstrated that the bimanual pelvic examination is unreliable for detecting significant pelvic pathology. Given the patient's serum β-hCG level >10,000 mIU/mL and adnexal mass diameter of 4 cm, medical therapy with methotrexate would likely fail.

CASE 2

Patient Presentation

A 36-year-old woman, gravida 2, para 1 at 11 weeks stated gestational age, presented to the ED via ambulance 15 minutes after the acute onset of painless vaginal bleeding. She reported that she had been dealing with multiple episodes of vomiting over the previous 5 days, which was unlike her previous pregnancy. She denied any other significant symptoms or medical history.

On physical examination, her blood pressure was 110/68 mm Hg, heart rate 110 bpm, respirations 20 per minute, and temperature 36.7°C. She appeared older than her stated age. Her head, neck, pulmonary, CV, and back examinations were unremarkable. Abdominal

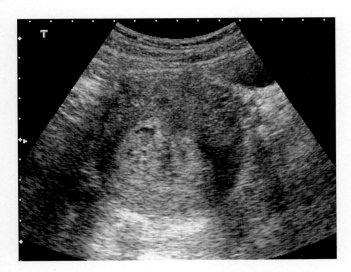

Figure 14-61. Case 2. Point-of-care transabdominal pelvic ultrasound showed a "snowstorm" appearance of the uterus and cystic structures within the endometrium consistent with gestational trophoblastic disease. (Courtesy of Hennepin County Medical Center)

examination revealed a prominently gravid abdomen, noted to appear larger than expected for the patient's stated gestational age. Mild epigastric tenderness was present. ED pelvic examination was deferred in consideration of vaginal bleeding and advanced gestational age.

Management Course

A urine pregnancy test was positive. The patient received IV fluids and an antiemetic. Point-of-care transabdominal pelvic ultrasound in the ED showed a "snowstorm" appearance with cystic structures within the uterus, concerning for GTD (Figure 14-61). Serum β-hCG measured 2,354,000 mIU/mL. The patient's blood type was A positive. The obstetrics service was consulted and a comprehensive ultrasound examination detailed an enlarged uterus filled with tissue and cysts consistent with complete molar pregnancy. The patient underwent a suction dilation and curettage. Her nausea and vomiting improved and she was discharged home on postoperative day 1 with plans for serial β-hCG measurements and clinic follow-up.

Commentary

Case 2 exemplifies the utility of point-of-care ultrasound in the rapid diagnosis of pathologic conditions not routinely encountered in the ED. Recognition of normal and abnormal findings on point-of-care ultrasound helped focus on the differential diagnosis. Although hyperemesis, a prominently gravid abdomen, and a markedly elevated serum β-hCG level were clues to this patient's final diagnosis, definitive diagnosis and management would not have taken place without ultrasound imaging.

CASE 3

Patient Presentation

A 28-year-old woman arrived in the ED late in the evening, complaining of nausea, weakness, and episodic loss of consciousness over the past few hours. She did not know when her last menstrual period was. She felt confused, but denied any significant pain. She was unwilling to provide any further history, citing nausea and weakness.

Upon physical examination, her blood pressure was 82/40 mm Hg, heart rate 86 bpm, respirations 22 per minute, and temperature 36.9°C. The patient was diaphoretic and appeared uncomfortable. Her head, neck, pulmonary, and back examinations were unremarkable. Cardiac examination revealed a grade I/VI systolic murmur. Abdominal examination was significant for mild bilateral lower quadrant tenderness with no rebound or guarding. GU examination revealed a closed cervical os and no bleeding. She had mild cervical motion and bilateral adnexal tenderness.

Management Course

A urine pregnancy test was ordered as the emergency physician performed a transabdominal ultrasound examination. This revealed a hypoechoic sac in the uterus, a tubal ring in the left adnexa, and a small amount of free pelvic fluid (Figure 14-62). A scan of the upper abdomen revealed free fluid in the hepatorenal space. A urine pregnancy test was positive. After 2 L of IV normal saline, the patient's blood pressure was 94/52 mm Hg with a heart rate of 84 bpm; infusion of O negative packed red blood cells was initiated. The on-call obstetrician was immediately contacted and the operating room was prepared. While the obstetrician was en route, a point-of-care transvaginal ultrasound examination by the emergency physician confirmed a definite ectopic pregnancy with a yolk sac in the left adnexa. The patient was taken directly to the operating room when the obstetrician arrived. A ruptured ectopic pregnancy and 2–3 L of free intraperitoneal blood were found at surgery. The patient required a left salpingectomy. Her serum β-hCG level was 917 mIU/mL.

Commentary

Case 3 illustrates a patient with a ruptured ectopic pregnancy. She was in hemorrhagic shock and required immediate resuscitation. She could not provide a reliable

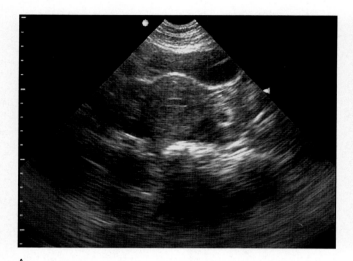

A

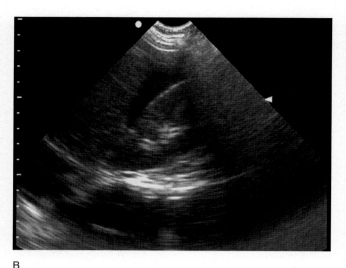

B

Figure 14-62. Case 3. Pseudogestational sac within the uterus and tubal ring in the left adnexa. Transabdominal transverse image (A). Free fluid in the hepatorenal space. Transabdominal right upper quadrant image (B).

history and was not aware that she was pregnant. She had relatively mild abdominal symptoms and was not tachycardic, which is not uncommon with acute intraperitoneal blood loss. Transabdominal sonography revealed hepatorenal free fluid and a tubal ring. Hepatorenal free fluid alone, in a young pregnant woman with nontraumatic hypotension, is nearly diagnostic of a ruptured ectopic pregnancy and was enough evidence to proceed to surgery. In addition, this patient had a tubal ring, which is also nearly diagnostic of an ectopic pregnancy. Immediate point-of-care transvaginal scanning by the emergency physician allowed a more detailed view of the mass and revealed a definite ectopic pregnancy. This case also illustrates the potential limitation of quantitative β-hCG for guiding immediate management decisions in patients with complications of early pregnancy.

REFERENCES

1. Jehle D: Ectopic pregnancy. In: *Emergency Medicine: A Comprehensive Study Guide.* New York, NY: McGraw-Hill, 2000:737–748.
2. Physicians: ACoE. Clinical policy for the initial approach to patients presenting with a chief complaint of vaginal bleeding. American College of Emergency Physicians. *Ann Emerg Med* 29:435–458, 1997.
3. Physicians: ACoE. American College of Emergency Physicians. ACEP emergency ultrasound guidelines-2001. *Ann Emerg Med* 38:470–481, 2001.
4. Physicians: ACoE. American College of Emergency Physicians. Use of ultrasound imaging by emergency physicians. *Ann Emerg Med* 38:469–470, 2001.
5. Brennan DF: Ectopic pregnancy–Part II: Diagnostic procedures and imaging. *Acad Emerg Med: Official Journal of the Society for Academic Emergency Medicine* 2:1090–1097, 1995.
6. Rodgerson JD, Heegaard WG, Plummer D, et al.: Emergency department right upper quadrant ultrasound is associated with a reduced time to diagnosis and treatment of ruptured ectopic pregnancies. *Acad Emerg Med: Official Journal of the Society for Academic Emergency Medicine* 8:331–336, 2001.
7. Cartwright PS, Victory DF, Moore RA, et al.: Performance of a new enzyme-linked immunoassay urine pregnancy test for the detection of ectopic gestation. *Ann Emerg Med* 15:1198–1199, 1986.
8. Marill KA, Ingmire TE, Nelson BK: Utility of a single beta HCG measurement to evaluate for absence of ectopic pregnancy. *J Emerg Med* 17:419–426, 1999.
9. Stovall TG, Kellerman AL, Ling FW, et al.: Emergency department diagnosis of ectopic pregnancy. *Ann Emerg Med* 19:1098–1103, 1990.
10. Stovall TG, Ling FW, Andersen RN, et al.: Improved sensitivity and specificity of a single measurement of serum progesterone over serial quantitative beta-human chorionic gonadotrophin in screening for ectopic pregnancy. *Hum Reprod* 7:723–725, 1992.
11. Valley VT, Mateer JR, Aiman EJ, et al.: Serum progesterone and endovaginal sonography by emergency physicians in the evaluation of ectopic pregnancy. *Acad Emerg Med: Official Journal of the Society for Academic Emergency Medicine* 5:309–313, 1998.
12. Dart R, Ramanujam P, Dart L: Progesterone as a predictor of ectopic pregnancy when the ultrasound is indeterminate. *Am J Emerg Med* 20:575–579, 2002.
13. Janicke K: *Emergency Medicine: A Comprehensive Study Guide.* New York, NY: McGraw-Hill, 2000:686.
14. Lipscomb GH, Stovall TG, Ling FW: Nonsurgical treatment of ectopic pregnancy. *N Engl J Med* 343:1325–1329, 2000.
15. Vermesh M, Graczykowski JW, Sauer MV: Reevaluation of the role of culdocentesis in the management of ectopic pregnancy. *Am J Obstet Gynecol* 162:411–413, 1990.

16. Vande Krol L, Abbott JT: The current role of culdocentesis. *Am J Emerg Med* 10:354–358, 1992.

17. Brennan DF: Diagnosis of ectopic pregnancy. *J Flor Med Assoc* 84:549–556, 1997.

18. Pelsang RE: Diagnostic imaging modalities during pregnancy. *Obstet Gynecol Clin North Am* 25:287–300, 1998.

19. Kaplan BC, Dart RG, Moskos M, et al.: Ectopic pregnancy: Prospective study with improved diagnostic accuracy. *Ann Emerg Med* 28:10–17, 1996.

20. Peterson HB, Xia Z, Hughes JM, et al.: The risk of ectopic pregnancy after tubal sterilization. U.S. Collaborative Review of Sterilization Working Group. *N Eng J Med* 336:762–767, 1997.

21. Loffredo AJ, Dyne PL: Emergency medicine residents can perform bedside ultrasound with a high degree of sensitivity and specificity to detect intrauterine pregnancy with cardiac activity. *Acad Emer Med: Official Journal of the Society for Academic Emergency Medicine* 8:547, 2001.

22. Durham B, Lane B, Burbridge L, Balasubramaniam S: Pelvic ultrasound performed by emergency physicians for the detection of ectopic pregnancy in complicated first-trimester pregnancies. *Ann Emerg Med* 29:338–347, 1997.

23. Cashner KA, Christopher CR, Dysert GA: Spontaneous fetal loss after demonstration of a live fetus in the first trimester. *Obstet Gynecol* 70:827–830, 1987.

24. Wilson RD, Kendrick V, Wittmann BK, et al.: Spontaneous abortion and pregnancy outcome after normal first-trimester ultrasound examination. *Obstet Gynecol* 67:352–355, 1986.

25. Van Den Eeden SK, Shan J, Bruce C, et al.: Ectopic pregnancy rate and treatment utilization in a large managed care organization. *Obstet Gynecol* 105:1052–1057, 2005.

26. Condous G, Okaro E, Khalid A, et al.: A prospective evaluation of a single-visit strategy to manage pregnancies of unknown location. *Hum Reprod* 20:1398–1403, 2005.

27. Mateer JR, Valley VT, Aiman EJ, et al.: Outcome analysis of a protocol including bedside endovaginal sonography in patients at risk for ectopic pregnancy. *Ann Emerg Med* 27:283–289, 1996.

28. Tayal VS, Cohen H, Norton HJ: Outcome of patients with an indeterminate emergency department first-trimester pelvic ultrasound to rule out ectopic pregnancy. *Acad Emerg Med: Official Journal of the Society for Academic Emergency Medicine* 11:912–917, 2004.

29. Braen Krause WA: Harwood-Nuss' clinical practice of emergency medicine. In: Harwood-Nuss, ed. *Harwood-Nuss' Clinical Practice of Emergency Medicine*. Philadelphia, PA: Lippincott Williams & Wilkins, 2005:500.

30. Lyons LD: Diagnostic ultrasound. In: Rumack C, Wilson SR, Charboneau JW, eds. *Diagnostic Ultrasound*. St. Louis: Mosby; 1999:975–1011.

31. De VR, Pratt JH: Simultaneous intrauterine and extrauterine pregnancy. *Am J Obstet Gynecol* 56:1119–26, 1948.

32. Bright DA, Gaupp FB: Heterotopic pregnancy: A reevaluation. *J Am Board Fam Pract* 3:125–128, 1990.

33. Jerrard D, Tso E, Salik R, Barish RA: Unsuspected heterotopic pregnancy in a woman without risk factors. *Am J Emerg Med* 10:58–60, 1992.

34. Reece EA, Petrie RH, Sirmans MF, et al.: Combined intrauterine and extrauterine gestations: A review. *Am J Obstet Gynecol* 146:323–30, 1983.

35. Richards SR, Stempel LE, Carlton BD: Heterotopic pregnancy: Reappraisal of incidence. *Am J Obstet Gynecol* 142:928–930, 1982.

36. Richards SR, Stempel LE, Carlton BD: Heterotopic pregnancy. *Am J Obstet Gynecol* 148:227–228, 1984.

37. Berger MJ, Taymor ML: Simultaneous intrauterine and tubal pregnancies following ovulation induction. *Am J Obstet Gynecol* 113:812–813, 1972.

38. Gamberdella FR, Marrs RP: Heterotopic pregnancy associated with assisted reproductive technology. *Am J Obstet Gynecol* 160:1520–1522; discussion 2–4, 1989.

39. Tal J, Haddad S, Gordon N, Timor-Tritsch I: Heterotopic pregnancy after ovulation induction and assisted reproductive technologies: A literature review from 1971 to 1993. *Fertil Steril* 66:1–12, 1996.

40. Nederlof KP, Lawson HW, Saftlas AF, et al.: Ectopic pregnancy surveillance, United States, 1970–1987. MMWR CDC Surveill Summ: Morbidity and mortality weekly report CDC surveillance summaries/Centers for Disease Control 39:9–17, 1990.

41. Lipscomb GH, McCord ML, Stovall TG, et al.: Predictors of success of methotrexate treatment in women with tubal ectopic pregnancies. *N Engl J Med* 341:1974–1978, 1999.

42. Stein JC, Wang R, Adler N, et al.: Emergency physician ultrasonography for evaluating patients at risk for ectopic pregnancy: A meta-analysis. *Ann Emerg Med* 56:674–683, 2010.

43. Macvane CZ, Irish CB, Strout TD, et al.: Implementation of transvaginal ultrasound in an emergency department residency program: An analysis of resident interpretation. *J Emerg Med* 43:124–128, 2012.

44. Burgher SW, Tandy TK, Dawdy MR: Transvaginal ultrasonography by emergency physicians decreases patient time in the emergency department. *Acad Emerg Med: Official Journal of the Society for Academic Emergency Medicine* 5:802–807, 1998.

45. Schlager D, Whitten D, Tolan K: Emergency department ultrasound: Impact on ED stay times. *Am J Emerg Med* 15:216–217, 1997.

46. Shih CH: Effect of emergency physician-performed pelvic sonography on length of stay in the emergency department. *Ann Emerg Med* 29:348–351; discussion 52, 1997.

47. Durston WE, Carl ML, Guerra W, et al.: Ultrasound availability in the evaluation of ectopic pregnancy in the ED: Comparison of quality and cost-effectiveness with different approaches. *Am J Emerg Med* 18:408–417, 2000.

48. Mateer JR, Aiman EJ, Brown MH, et al.: Ultrasonographic examination by emergency physicians of patients at risk for ectopic pregnancy. *Acad Emerg Med: Official Journal of the Society for Academic Emergency Medicine* 2:867–873, 1995.

49. Abbott J, Emmans LS, Lowenstein SR: Ectopic pregnancy: Ten common pitfalls in diagnosis. *Am J Emerg Med* 8:515–522, 1990.

50. Barnhart K, Mennuti MT, Benjamin I, et al.: Prompt diagnosis of ectopic pregnancy in an emergency department setting. *Obstet Gynecol* 84:1010–1015, 1994.

51. Holbrook J: A computerized audit of 15,009 emergency department records. *Ann Emerg Med* 19:139–144, 1990.

52. Trautlein JJ, Lambert RL, Miller J: Malpractice in the emergency department—Review of 200 cases. *Ann Emerg Med* 13:709–711, 1984.

53. Barnhart K, Coutifaris C: Diagnosis of ectopic pregnancy. *Ann Emerg Med* 29:295–296, 1997.

54. Barnhart KT, Simhan H, Kamelle SA: Diagnostic accuracy of ultrasound above and below the beta-hCG discriminatory zone. *Obstet Gynecol* 94:583–587, 1999.

55. Braffman BH, Coleman BG, Ramchandani P, et al. Emergency department screening for ectopic pregnancy: A prospective US study. *Radiology* 190:797–802, 1994.

56. Brown DL, Doubilet PM: Transvaginal sonography for diagnosing ectopic pregnancy: Positivity criteria and performance characteristics. *J Ultrasound Med: Official Journal of the American Institute of Ultrasound in Medicine* 13:259–266, 1994.

57. Cacciatore B: Can the status of tubal pregnancy be predicted with transvaginal sonography? A prospective comparison of sonographic, surgical, and serum hCG findings. *Radiology* 177:481–484, 1990.

58. Mahony BS, Filly RA, Nyberg DA, et al.: Sonographic evaluation of ectopic pregnancy. *J Ultrasound Med: Official Journal of the American Institute of Ultrasound in Medicine* 4:221–228, 1985.

59. Nyberg DA, Filly RA, Laing FC, et al.: Ectopic pregnancy. Diagnosis by sonography correlated with quantitative HCG levels. *J Ultrasound Med: Official Journal of the American Institute of Ultrasound in Medicine* 6:145–150, 1987.

60. Sadek AL, Schiotz HA: Transvaginal sonography in the management of ectopic pregnancy. *Acta Obstetricia et Gynecologica Scandinavica* 74:293–6, 1995.

61. Shalev E, Yarom I, Bustan M, et al.: Transvaginal sonography as the ultimate diagnostic tool for the management of ectopic pregnancy: Experience with 840 cases. *Fertil Steril* 69:62–65, 1998.

62. Timor-Tritsch. Transvaginal sonography of the normal and abnormal fetus. In: Zimmer B, ed. *Transvaginal Sonography of the Normal and Abnormal Fetus.* New York, NY: Parthenon Publishing, 2001:7–34.

63. Clinical policy: critical issues in the initial evaluation and management of patients presenting to the emergency department in early pregnancy. *Ann Emerg Med* 41:123–133, 2003.

64. Stovall TG, Ling FW: Ectopic pregnancy. Diagnostic and therapeutic algorithms minimizing surgical intervention. *J Reprod Med* 38:807–812, 1993.

65. Dart RG, Kaplan B, Cox C: Transvaginal ultrasound in patients with low beta-human chorionic gonadotropin values: How often is the study diagnostic? *Ann Emerg Med* 30:135–140, 1997.

66. Counselman FL, Shaar GS, Heller RA, et al.: Quantitative B-hCG levels less than 1000 mIU/mL in patients with ectopic pregnancy: Pelvic ultrasound still useful. *J Emerg Med* 16:699–703, 1998.

67. Kohn MA, Kerr K, Malkevich D, et al.: Beta-human chorionic gonadotropin levels and the likelihood of ectopic pregnancy in emergency department patients with abdominal pain or vaginal bleeding. *Acad Emerg Med: Official Journal of the Society for Academic Emergency Medicine* 10:119–126, 2003.

68. Condous G, Kirk E, Lu C, et al.: Diagnostic accuracy of varying discriminatory zones for the prediction of ectopic pregnancy in women with a pregnancy of unknown location. *Ultrasound Obstet Gynecol: Official Journal of the International Society of Ultrasound in Obstetrics and Gynecology* 26:770–775, 2005.

69. Bernaschek G, Rudelstorfer R, Csaicsich P: Vaginal sonography versus serum human chorionic gonadotropin in early detection of pregnancy. *Am J Obstet Gynecol* 158:608–612, 1988.

70. Kadar N, Bohrer M, Kemmann E, et al.: The discriminatory human chorionic gonadotropin zone for endovaginal sonography: A prospective, randomized study. *Fertil Steril* 61:1016–20, 1994.

71. Nyberg DA, Mack LA, Laing FC, et al.: Early pregnancy complications: Endovaginal sonographic findings correlated with human chorionic gonadotropin levels. *Radiology* 167:619–622, 1988.

72. Dart R, Howard K: Subclassification of indeterminate pelvic ultrasonograms: Stratifying the risk of ectopic pregnancy. *Acad Emerg Med: Official Journal of the Society for Academic Emergency Medicine* 5:313–319, 1998.

73. Parvey HR, Maklad N: Pitfalls in the transvaginal sonographic diagnosis of ectopic pregnancy. *J Ultrasound Med: Official Journal of the American Institute of Ultrasound in Medicine* 12:139–144, 1993.

74. Lewis-Bliehall C, Rogers RG, Kammerer-Doak DN, et al.: Medical vs. surgical treatment of ectopic pregnancy. The University of New Mexico's six-year experience. *J Reprod Med* 46:983–988, 2001.

75. Sowter MC, Farquhar CM: Ectopic pregnancy: An update. *Curr Opin Obstet Gynecol* 16:289–293, 2004.

76. ACOG Practice Bulletin. Medical management of tubal pregnancy. Number 3, December 1998. Clinical management guidelines for obstetrician-gynecologists. American College of Obstetricians and Gynecologists. *Inter J Gynecol Obstet: Official organ of the International Federation of Gynaecology and Obstetrics* 65:97–103, 1999.

77. Potter MB, Lepine LA, Jamieson DJ: Predictors of success with methotrexate treatment of tubal ectopic pregnancy at Grady Memorial Hospital. *Am J Obstet Gynecol* 188:1192–1194, 2003.

78. Stika CS, Anderson L, Frederiksen MC: Single-dose methotrexate for the treatment of ectopic pregnancy: Northwestern Memorial Hospital three-year experience. *Am J Obstet Gynecol* 174:1840–1846; discussion 6–8, 1996.

79. Stovall TG, Ling FW: Single-dose methotrexate: An expanded clinical trial. *Am J Obstet Gynecol* 168:1759–1762; discussion 62–65, 1993.

80. Bixby S, Tello R, Kuligowska E: Presence of a yolk sac on transvaginal sonography is the most reliable predictor of single-dose methotrexate treatment failure in ectopic pregnancy. *J Ultrasound Med: Official Journal of the American Institute of Ultrasound in Medicine* 24:591–598, 2005.

81. Hung TH, Shau WY, Hsieh TT, et al.: Prognostic factors for an unsatisfactory primary methotrexate treatment of cervical pregnancy: A quantitative review. *Hum Reprod* 13:2636–2642, 1998.

82. Nazac A, Gervaise A, Bouyer J, et al.: Predictors of success in methotrexate treatment of women with unruptured

tubal pregnancies. *Ultrasound Obstet Gynecol: Official Journal of the International Society of Ultrasound in Obstetrics and Gynecology* 21:181–185, 2003.

83. Takacs P, Chakhtoura N, De Santis T, et al.: Evaluation of the relationship between endometrial thickness and failure of single-dose methotrexate in ectopic pregnancy. *Arch Gynecol Obstet* 272:269–272, 2005.

84. Milad H: Gynecology and obstetrics. In: Sciarra ed. *Gynecology and Obstetrics*. Philadelphia, PA: Lippincott Williams & Wilkins, 2000:1–14.

85. Moore C, Todd WM, O'Brien E, et al.: Free fluid in Morison's pouch on bedside ultrasound predicts need for operative intervention in suspected ectopic pregnancy. *Acad Emerg Med: Official Journal of the Society for Academic Emergency Medicine* 14:755–758, 2007.

86. Shalev E, Peleg D, Tsabari A, et al.: Spontaneous resolution of ectopic tubal pregnancy: Natural history. *Fertil Steril* 63:15–19, 1995.

87. Elson J, Tailor A, Banerjee S, et al.: Expectant management of tubal ectopic pregnancy: Prediction of successful outcome using decision tree analysis. *Ultrasound Obstet Gynecol: Official Journal of the International Society of Ultrasound in Obstetrics and Gynecology* 23:552–556, 2004.

88. Everett C: Incidence and outcome of bleeding before the 20th week of pregnancy: Prospective study from general practice. *BMJ* 315:32–34, 1997.

89. Weston M: The first trimester. In: Dewbury K, Meire H, Cosgrove D, eds. *Clinical Ultrasound: A Comprehensive Text*. 3rd ed. London: Churchill Livingstone, 2001:151–187.

90. Wilcox AJ, Weinberg CR, O'Connor JF, et al.: Incidence of early loss of pregnancy. *N Engl J Med* 319:189–194, 1988.

91. Falco P, Milano V, Pilu G, et al.: Sonography of pregnancies with first-trimester bleeding and a viable embryo: A study of prognostic indicators by logistic regression analysis. *Ultrasound Obstet Gynecol: Official Journal of the International Society of Ultrasound in Obstetrics and Gynecology* 7:165–169, 1996.

92. Filly. Ultrasonography in obstetrics and gynecology. In: Callen, ed. *Ultrasonography in Obstetrics and Gynecology*. Philadelphia, PA: WB Saunders, 1994:63–85.

93. Scott DH: Spontaneous abortion. In: Scott DH, ed. *Danforth's Obstetrics and Gynecology*. Philadelphia, PA: Lippincott; 1994:175.

94. Cetin A, Cetin M: Diagnostic and therapeutic decision-making with transvaginal sonography for first trimester spontaneous abortion, clinically thought to be incomplete or complete. *Contraception* 57:393–397, 1998.

95. Mansur MM: Ultrasound diagnosis of complete abortion can reduce need for curettage. *Eu J Obstet, Gyneco Reprod Biol* 44:65–69, 1992.

96. Rulin MC, Bornstein SG, Campbell JD: The reliability of ultrasonography in the management of spontaneous abortion, clinically thought to be complete: A prospective study. *Am J Obstet Gynecol* 168:12–15, 1993.

97. Jurkovic D, Ross JA, Nicolaides KH: Expectant management of missed miscarriage. *Br J Obstet Gynaecol* 105:670–671, 1998.

98. Goldstein SR: Early detection of pathologic pregnancy by transvaginal sonography. *J Clin Ultrasound* 18:262–273, 1990.

99. Goldstein SR: Embryonic death in early pregnancy: A new look at the first trimester. *Obstet Gynecol* 84:294–297, 1994.

100. Levi CS, Lyons EA, Zheng XH, et al.: Endovaginal US: Demonstration of cardiac activity in embryos of less than 5.0 mm in crown-rump length. *Radiology* 176:71–74, 1990.

101. Landy HJ, Weiner S, Corson SL, et al.: The "vanishing twin": ultrasonographic assessment of fetal disappearance in the first trimester. *Am J Obstet Gynecol* 155:14–19, 1986.

102. Sampson A, de Crespigny LC: Vanishing twins: The frequency of spontaneous fetal reduction of a twin pregnancy. *Ultrasound Obstet Gynecol: Official Journal of the International Society of Ultrasound in Obstetrics and Gynecology* 2:107–109, 1992.

103. Whitecar MP, Turner S, Higby MK: Adnexal masses in pregnancy: A review of 130 cases undergoing surgical management. *Am J Obstet Gynecol* 181:19–24, 1999.

104. Fleischer AC, Shah DM, Entman SS: Sonographic evaluation of maternal disorders during pregnancy. *Radiol Clin North Am* 28:51–58, 1990.

105. Lev-Toaff AS, Coleman BG, Arger PH, et al.: Leiomyomas in pregnancy: Sonographic study. *Radiology* 164:375–380, 1987.

106. Beischer NA, Buttery BW, Fortune DW, et al.: Growth and malignancy of ovarian tumours in pregnancy. *Aust N Z J Obstet Gynaecol* 11:208–220, 1971.

107. Bider D, Mashiach S, Dulitzky M, et al.: Clinical, surgical and pathologic findings of adnexal torsion in pregnant and nonpregnant women. *Surg Gynecol Obstet* 173:363–366, 1991.

108. Fleischer. Ultrasound: A practical approach to clinical problems. In: Bluth A, Benson, Ralls, Siegel, eds. *Ultrasound: A Practical Approach to Clinical Problems*. New York: Thieme, 2000:273–280.

109. Grendys EC Jr, Barnes WA: Ovarian cancer in pregnancy. *Surg Clin North Am* 75:1–14, 1995.

110. Pena JE, Ufberg D, Cooney N, et al.: Usefulness of Doppler sonography in the diagnosis of ovarian torsion. *Fertil Steril* 73:1047–1050, 2000.

111. Albayram F, Hamper UM: Ovarian and adnexal torsion: Spectrum of sonographic findings with pathologic correlation. *J Ultrasound Med: Official Journal of the American Institute of Ultrasound in Medicine* 20:1083–1089, 2001.

112. Lambert MJ, Villa M: Gynecologic ultrasound in emergency medicine. *Emerg Med Clin North Am* 22:683–696, 2004.

113. Warner MA, Fleischer AC, Edell SL, et al.: Uterine adnexal torsion: Sonographic findings. *Radiology* 154:773–775, 1985.

114. Houry D, Abbott JT: Ovarian torsion: A fifteen-year review. *Ann Emerg Med* 38:156–159, 2001.

115. Thickman A: Diagnostic radiology in emergency medicine. In: Rosen, ed. *Diagnostic Radiology in Emergency Medicine*. St. Louis, Missouri: Mosby-Yearbook, 1992:581–589.

116. Freedman RS, Tortolero-Luna G, Pandey DK, et al.: Gestational trophoblastic disease. *Obstet Gynecol Clin North Am* 23:545–571, 1996.

117. Davison CM, Kaplan RM, Wenig LN, et al.: Qualitative beta-hCG urine assays may be misleading in the presence

of molar pregnancy: A case report. *J Emerg Med* 27:43–47, 2004.

118. Teng FY, Magarelli PC, Montz FJ: Transvaginal probe ultrasonography. Diagnostic or outcome advantages in women with molar pregnancies. *J Reprod Med* 40:427–430, 1995.

119. Bronshtein Z: Transvaginal sonography of the normal and abnormal fetus. In: Zimmer B, ed. *Transvaginal Sonography of the Normal and Abnormal Fetus*. New York, NY: Parthenon Publishing; 2001:48–50.

120. DiSantis DJ, Scatarige JC, Kemp G, et al.: A prospective evaluation of transvaginal sonography for detection of ovarian disease. *AJR Am J Roentgenol* 161:91–94, 1993.

121. Rottem S, Thaler I, Goldstein SR, et al.: Transvaginal sonographic technique: Targeted organ scanning without resorting to "planes". *J Clin Ultrasound: JCU* 18:243–247, 1990.

122. Filly. Ultrasonography in obstetrics and gynecology. In: Callen, ed. *Ultrasonography in Obstetrics and Gynecology*. Philadelphia, PA: WB Saunders; 1988:19–46.

123. Fossum GT, Davajan V, Kletzky OA: Early detection of pregnancy with transvaginal ultrasound. *Fertil Steril* 49:788–791, 1988.

124. Keith SC, London SN, Weitzman GA, et al.: Serial transvaginal ultrasound scans and beta-human chorionic gonadotropin levels in early singleton and multiple pregnancies. *Fertil Steril* 59:1007–1010, 1993.

125. Nyberg DA, Mack LA, Harvey D, et al.: Value of the yolk sac in evaluating early pregnancies. *J Ultrasound Med: Official Journal of the American Institute of Ultrasound in Medicine* 7:129–135, 1988.

126. Pellicer A, Calatayud C, Miro F, et al.: Comparison of implantation and early development of human embryos fertilized in vitro versus in vivo using transvaginal ultrasound. *J Ultrasound Med: Official Journal of the American Institute of Ultrasound in Medicine* 10:31–35, 1991.

127. Sengoku K, Tamate K, Ishikawa M, et al.: Transvaginal ultrasonographic findings and hCG levels in early intrauterine pregnancies. *Nihon Sanka Fujinka Gakkai Zasshi* 43:535–540, 1991.

128. Yeh HC, Goodman JD, Carr L, et al.: Intradecidual sign: A US criterion of early intrauterine pregnancy. *Radiology* 161:463–467, 1986.

129. Laing FC, Brown DL, Price JF, et al.: Intradecidual sign: Is it effective in diagnosis of an early intrauterine pregnancy? *Radiology* 204:655–660, 1997.

130. Dillon EH, Feyock AL, Taylor KJ: Pseudogestational sacs: Doppler US differentiation from normal or abnormal intrauterine pregnancies. *Radiology* 176:359–364, 1990.

131. Nyberg DA, Laing FC, Filly RA, et al.: Ultrasonographic differentiation of the gestational sac of early intrauterine pregnancy from the pseudogestational sac of ectopic pregnancy. *Radiology* 146:755–759, 1983.

132. Bradley WG, Fiske CE, Filly RA: The double sac sign of early intrauterine pregnancy: Use in exclusion of ectopic pregnancy. *Radiology* 143:223–226, 1982.

133. Parvey HR, Dubinsky TJ, Johnston DA, et al.: The chorionic rim and low-impedance intrauterine arterial flow in the diagnosis of early intrauterine pregnancy: Evaluation of efficacy. *AJR Am J Roentgenol* 167:1479–1485, 1996.

134. Stampone C, Nicotra M, Muttinelli C, et al.: Transvaginal sonography of the yolk sac in normal and abnormal pregnancy. *J Clin Ultrasound: JCU* 24:3–9, 1996.

135. Kurtz. Ultrasonography in obstetrics and gynecology: A practical approach. In: Benson AB, ed. *Ultrasonography in Obstetrics and Gynecology: A Practical Approach*. New York, NY: Thieme, 2000:112–121.

136. Fleischer AC, Pennell RG, McKee MS, et al.: Ectopic pregnancy: Features at transvaginal sonography. *Radiology* 174:375–378, 1990.

137. Nyberg DA, Hughes MP, Mack LA, et al.: Extrauterine findings of ectopic pregnancy of transvaginal US: Importance of echogenic fluid. *Radiology* 178:823–826, 1991.

138. Nyberg DA, Mack LA, Jeffrey RB Jr, et al.: Endovaginal sonographic evaluation of ectopic pregnancy: A prospective study. *AJR Am J Roentgenol* 149:1181–1186, 1987.

139. Dart R, McLean SA, Dart L: Isolated fluid in the cul-de-sac: How well does it predict ectopic pregnancy? *Am J Emerg Med* 20:1–4, 2002.

140. Russell SA, Filly RA, Damato N: Sonographic diagnosis of ectopic pregnancy with endovaginal probes: What really has changed? *J Ultrasound Med: Official Journal of the American Institute of Ultrasound in Medicine* 12:145–151, 1993.

141. Frates MC, Brown DL, Doubilet PM, et al.: Tubal rupture in patients with ectopic pregnancy: Diagnosis with transvaginal US. *Radiology* 191:769–772, 1994.

142. Abrams BJ, Sukumvanich P, Seibel R, et al.: Ultrasound for the detection of intraperitoneal fluid: The role of Trendelenburg positioning. *Am J Emerg Med* 17:117–120, 1999.

143. Taylor KJ, Ramos IM, Feyock AL, et al.: Ectopic pregnancy: Duplex Doppler evaluation. *Radiology* 173:93–97, 1989.

144. Achiron R, Goldenberg M, Lipitz S, et al.: Transvaginal Doppler sonography for detecting ectopic pregnancy: Is it really necessary. *Isr J Med Sci* 30:820–825, 1994.

145. Blaivas M: Color Doppler in the diagnosis of ectopic pregnancy in the emergency department: Is there anything beyond a mass and fluid? *J Emerg Med* 22:379–384, 2002.

146. Ramanan RV, Gajaraj J: Ectopic pregnancy—The leash sign. A new sign on transvaginal Doppler ultrasound. *Acta Radiol* 47:529–535, 2006.

147. Kobayashi F, Sagawa N, Konishi I, et al.: Spontaneous conception and intrauterine pregnancy in a symptomatic missed abortion of ectopic pregnancy conceived in the previous cycle. *Hum Reprod* 11:1347–1349, 1996.

148. Levi CS, Lyons EA, Lindsay DJ: Early diagnosis of nonviable pregnancy with endovaginal US. *Radiology* 167:383–385, 1988.

149. Nyberg DA, Laing FC, Filly RA: Threatened abortion: Sonographic distinction of normal and abnormal gestation sacs. *Radiology* 158:397–400, 1986.

150. Rowling SE, Coleman BG, Langer JE, et al.: First-trimester US parameters of failed pregnancy. *Radiology* 203:211–217, 1997.

151. Pennell RG, Needleman L, Pajak T, et al.: Prospective comparison of vaginal and abdominal sonography in normal early pregnancy. *J Ultrasound Med: Official Journal of the American Institute of Ultrasound in Medicine* 10:63–67, 1991.

152. Doubilet PM, Benson CB: Embryonic heart rate in the early first trimester: What rate is normal? *J Ultrasound Med: Official Journal of the American Institute of Ultrasound in Medicine* 14:431–434, 1995.

153. Doubilet PM, Benson CB, Chow JS: Long-term prognosis of pregnancies complicated by slow embryonic heart rates in the early first trimester. *J Ultrasound Med: Official Journal of the American Institute of Ultrasound in Medicine* 18:537–541, 1999.

154. Green JJ, Hobbins JC: Abdominal ultrasound examination of the first-trimester fetus. *Am J Obstet Gynecol* 159:165–175, 1988.

155. Lindsay DJ, Lovett IS, Lyons EA, et al.: Yolk sac diameter and shape at endovaginal US: Predictors of pregnancy outcome in the first trimester. *Radiology* 183:115–118, 1992.

156. Bromley B, Harlow BL, Laboda LA, et al.: Small sac size in the first trimester: A predictor of poor fetal outcome. *Radiology* 178:375–377, 1991.

157. Bennett GL, Bromley B, Lieberman E, et al.: Subchorionic hemorrhage in first-trimester pregnancies: Prediction of pregnancy outcome with sonography. *Radiology* 200:803–806, 1996.

158. Nyberg DA, Cyr DR, Mack LA, et al.: Sonographic spectrum of placental abruption. *AJR Am J Roentgenol* 148:161–164, 1987.

159. Kurtz AB, Shlansky-Goldberg RD, Choi HY, et al.: Detection of retained products of conception following spontaneous abortion in the first trimester. *J Ultrasound Med: Official Journal of the American Institute of Ultrasound in Medicine* 10:387–395, 1991.

160. Nielsen S, Hahlin M, Platz-Christensen J: Randomised trial comparing expectant with medical management for first trimester miscarriages. *Br J Obstet Gynaecol* 106:804–807, 1999.

161. DeWitt C, Abbott J: Interstitial pregnancy: A potential for misdiagnosis of ectopic pregnancy with emergency department ultrasonography. *Ann Emerg Med* 40:106–109, 2002.

162. Jafri SZ, Loginsky SJ, Bouffard JA, et al.: Sonographic detection of interstitial pregnancy. *J Clin Ultrasound: JCU* 15:253–257, 1987.

163. Somers MP, Spears M, Maynard AS, et al.: Ruptured heterotopic pregnancy presenting with relative bradycardia in a woman not receiving reproductive assistance. *Ann Emerg Med* 43:382–385, 2004.

CHAPTER 15

Second and Third Trimester Pregnancy

Donald V. Byars and Barry J. Knapp

Over the last 30 years, ultrasound has played an essential role in the care of the obstetric patient. The body of knowledge and expertise in obstetric sonography is robust. Ultrasound is the primary imaging modality for evaluation of uterine, cervical, and amniotic fluid abnormalities; placental and umbilical cord problems; and determination of gestational age, fetal congenital abnormalities, multiple gestation, and fetal presentation.[1] While many parts of the examination are not relevant in the emergency setting, there are some findings that may be critical to the acute care of an obstetric patient. This chapter discusses the use of point-of-care ultrasound to evaluate pregnant patients in their second and third trimesters. During this time period, the major indications for its use are in the initial assessment of vaginal bleeding, labor, trauma, and abdominal pain. Emphasis will be placed on a focused or goal-directed ultrasound examination to rapidly measure fetal cardiac activity, estimate gestational age, and exclude placenta previa. Additional applications include assessment of cervical length and fetal position, and for the evaluation of traumatic and nonobstetrical causes of abdominal pain.

► CLINICAL CONSIDERATIONS

In early pregnancy, point-of-care ultrasound is commonly used to help rule out ectopic pregnancy by confirming an intrauterine pregnancy. The clinical indications for point-of-care ultrasound in early pregnancy, the limited information sought, and the recommended technique are widely agreed upon and well described (see

Chapter 14, "First Trimester Pregnancy"). In contrast, the role of point-of-care ultrasound in the second and third trimesters of pregnancy is not as well established. Yet, emergency care providers are frequently faced with evaluating patients who are in the latter part of pregnancy and present to the ED with trauma, vaginal bleeding, or abdominal pain. Depending on the practice setting, obstetrical consultation may not be readily available and patients may not have had prenatal care. Increasingly, point-of-care ultrasound is readily available in the emergency setting and clinicians are adept at its use. There are clearly a number of clinical situations during the second and third trimesters of pregnancy where a rapid, goal-directed ultrasound examination can expedite the diagnosis and improve the care of mother and fetus.

A discussion of the use of point-of-care ultrasound in the second and third trimesters of pregnancy must begin by addressing the following questions:

1. What are clinical indications for point-of-care ultrasound in the second and third trimesters of pregnancy?
2. Which focused ultrasound applications are reasonable for acute care providers to perform during late pregnancy?
3. What are the goals of the point-of-care ultrasound exam in the second and third trimesters of pregnancy?
4. Is ultrasound safe, and what are the alternative diagnostic modalities in pregnancy?

What are the clinical indications for point-of-care ultrasound in the second and third trimesters

of pregnancy? The concept that point-of-care ultrasound should remain goal-directed helps define its appropriate use in the latter part of pregnancy. In this setting, the focused concept takes on particular importance for the following reasons. First, since the scope and quantity of information potentially available using ultrasound in late pregnancy are enormous, the clinician performing ultrasound in the emergency setting must have a distinct, clinically relevant goal in mind before performing the exam. It would be inappropriate, for example, to assess fetal cardiac morphology in the emergency setting. Second, the medicolegal ramifications of basing clinical decisions on point-of-care ultrasound in the obstetric patient mandate caution. In one analysis of malpractice claims involving diagnostic ultrasound, obstetric ultrasound constituted 75% of the cases.[2] Not only should the information sought with each application be carefully limited, but ultrasound should be used only for emergency indications where the immediate benefit of the information outweighs the possibility of a missed diagnosis.

Major clinical indications for the use of point-of-care ultrasound that seem to satisfy these constraints include the initial evaluation of a pregnant trauma patient, mid- and late-trimester vaginal bleeding, labor, and abdominal pain during pregnancy.

Which focused ultrasound applications are reasonable for acute care providers to perform during late pregnancy? Several standard point-of-care ultrasound applications are indicated in late pregnancy and are considered safe and accurate in this setting. These include the focused assessment with sonography for trauma (FAST) examination to assess for significant hemoperitoneum, a right upper quadrant ultrasound examination to assess for gallstones and signs of cholecystitis, and a renal ultrasound examination to evaluate for severe hydronephrosis. Ultrasound may also be used to rapidly visualize fetal cardiac activity. It is also reasonable to estimate gestational age by measuring biparietal diameter (BPD) or femur length. In addition, transabdominal ultrasound can be used to evaluate for possible placental abruption, to exclude placenta previa, and to ascertain the position of the fetus. Transvaginal ultrasound may be used to clarify the relationship of the placenta to the internal os and to measure cervical length.

What are the goals of the point-of-care ultrasound exam in the second and third trimesters of pregnancy? In other words, given the patient's clinical problem, what clinically important question(s) can be answered rapidly with a focused ultrasound examination? For example, in a trauma patient who is comatose and appears to be pregnant, the following questions may be answered with point-of-care ultrasound: Is the patient pregnant? Is there evidence of free intraperitoneal fluid (from hemoperitoneum or uterine rupture)? Is the fetus alive? What is the gestational age of the fetus (and might

it survive in the extrauterine environment)? (Figure 15-1) Is there obvious retroplacental hematoma? Figure 15-2 presents a goal-directed approach to point-of-care ultrasound in the second or third trimester of pregnancy based on the patient's clinical problem.

Is ultrasound safe, and what are the alternative diagnostic modalities in pregnancy? The emergence of ultrasound as the main imaging modality in pregnancy is based, in part, on it being considered extremely safe for the fetus. Human organogenesis largely takes place before the 10th week of gestation, the time period when diagnostic ultrasound is often used. The absence of an association between ultrasound and fetal structural anomalies supports its safety in early pregnancy.[3] The critical period of brain development occurs during the 14th–22nd week of gestation. The theoretical adverse affect of ultrasound on the fetal brain, due to production of thermal energy and cavitation, has been the topic of several important epidemiologic studies, all of which have found no deleterious effects on cognitive development.[4,5] By contrast, the risk to the fetus associated with exposure to ionizing radiation, particularly from abdominal CT, is considered significant.[1]

For assessment of fetal well-being, alternatives to sonography include the handheld Doppler stethoscope for measurement of fetal heart tones and continuous cardiotocography. Cardiotocography is a form of fetal assessment that simultaneously records fetal heart rate, fetal movements, and uterine contractions to investigate fetal well-being.

In the absence of a reliable menstrual history, a very rough estimate of gestational age can be obtained by measuring fundal height. This crude test represents the only alternative to sonography for estimating gestational age when the history is unclear.

For the evaluation of vaginal bleeding in late pregnancy, sonography has supplanted the traditional double setup and potentially harmful physical examination for excluding the diagnosis of placenta previa. Placental abruption is usually diagnosed using clinical information, by excluding the diagnosis of placenta previa with ultrasound, and with the assistance of cardiotocography. The use of magnetic resonance imaging has been described in the workup of relatively stable patients with unexplained vaginal bleeding, but it is not widely used.[6]

Ultrasound provides information that is complimentary to the physical examination and cardiotocography in the evaluation and management of preterm or precipitous labor. Ultrasound is the only imaging modality used in this setting to assess cervical length, amniotic fluid volume, and fetal position.

Abdominal pain of unclear etiology is an important clinical indication for use of point-of-care ultrasound in late pregnancy where alternative imaging modalities—such as plain radiography and CT—are commonly employed in nonpregnant patients with similar complaints.

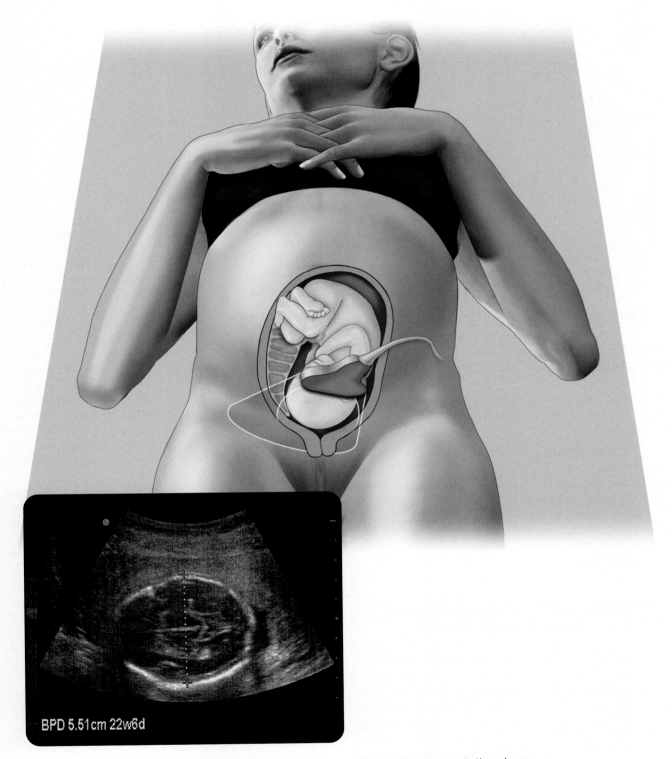

BPD 5.51cm 22w6d

Figure 15-1. Biparietal diameter used to estimate gestational age.

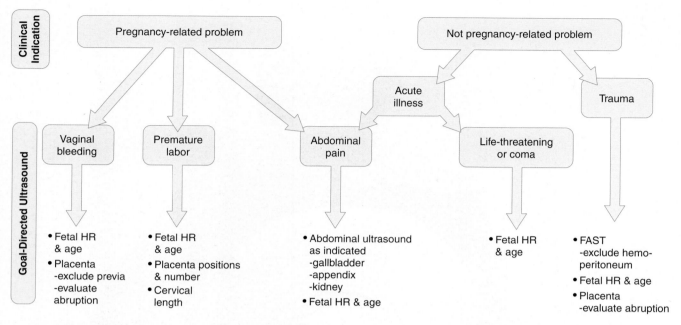

Figure 15-2. Goal-directed ultrasound in the second and third trimesters based on the clinical indication.

► CLINICAL INDICATIONS

The clinical indications for performing point-of-care ultrasound in the second and third trimesters of pregnancy are as follows:

1. Determination of gestational age and fetal heart rate
2. Assessment of obstetrical causes of abdominal pain and vaginal bleeding
3. Evaluation of labor
4. Evaluation of traumatic injuries
5. Assessment of nonobstetrical causes of abdominal pain

DETERMINATION OF GESTATIONAL AGE AND FETAL HEART RATE

Fetal assessment begins with measurement of fetal cardiac activity to establish fetal viability. This step is recommended early, not only in evaluation of the pregnant trauma patient[7] but also in patients with vaginal bleeding[8] and preterm labor.[9] The normal fetal heart rate following the first trimester is 120–160 beats per minute (bpm). Sustained bradycardia is often associated with fetal hypoxia and acidemia. Historically, in emergency medicine, fetal cardiac activity was established by measuring fetal heart tones with a handheld Doppler stethoscope.

Point-of-care ultrasound is an attractive alternative to the handheld Doppler stethoscope for initial detec-

tion of fetal cardiac activity. Using B-mode scanning of the gravid uterus, locating the fetal heart, and assessing the presence of cardiac motion is relatively straightforward. Using M-mode scanning, the waveform produced by cardiac motion can be recorded. Fetal heart rate is then determined rapidly and accurately with the aid of obstetrics software contained in most ultrasound machines.

Knowledge of gestational age is critical in many clinical settings. This information may be used to guide the decision to perform an emergency cesarean section, such as in the setting of maternal cardiac arrest.[10] In addition, gestational age and fetal maturity often influence the management of placenta previa, preterm labor, rupture of membranes, eclampsia, and other severe medical illnesses in late pregnancy. In the setting of trauma, sonographic assessment of gestational age, along with fetal heart rate, can be performed as an adjunct to the initial E-FAST examination. In a stable trauma patient, gestational age may influence the decision to proceed to exploratory laparotomy.[11]

When assessing gestational age, consider the following general points. By current convention, obstetric dating begins with the first day of the last normal menstrual period, referred to as gestational age or menstrual age, and is equal to the fetal or conceptual age plus 14 days. Assume fetal viability when the gestational age is >24 weeks. The pregnancy is considered "term" at 38 weeks. Sonographic estimates of gestational age are progressively less accurate in later pregnancy due to natural variations in the size of the fetus (Table 15-1). A simple rule that reinforces this principle is that the

▶ **TABLE 15-1. VARIABILITY OF GESTATIONAL AGE ESTIMATES**[*]

Parameter Measured	Gestational Age Interval (weeks)			
	14–20	20–26	26–38	32–42
BPD	1.4	2.1	3.8	4.1
HC	1.2	1.9	3.4	3.8
FL	1.4	2.5	3.1	3.5

[*]Two standard deviations, in weeks.
BPD = biparietal diameter; FL = femur length; HC = head circumference.
Adapted with permission from Benson CB, Doubilet PM: Sonographic prediction of gestational age: accuracy of 2nd and 3rd trimester measurements. *Am J Radiol* 157:1275–1277, 1991.

variability (2 SD from the mean) of a gestational age estimate is equal to approximately 8% of the predicted age.[12] An ultrasound measurement of BPD that yields a gestational age of 32 weeks has a variability of ±19 days. Nevertheless, estimates based on BPD, obtained as late as 20 weeks, still outperform menstrual history for predicting onset of labor.[13] If possible, base gestational age on results of an ultrasound examination performed prior to 20 weeks or on a reliable menstrual history. Beyond 20 weeks, point-of-care ultrasound may be used to estimate gestational age if menstrual dates are unreliable or when the patient cannot provide a history.

In the first trimester, crown-rump length is the preferred biometric measurement for establishing gestational age. In the second and third trimesters, measurements commonly used to estimate gestational age include BPD, head circumference (HC), and femur length. Modern ultrasound machines contain software that will automatically calculate gestational age based on any one of these parameters. In choosing which biometric parameter to measure, the established predictive validity of the parameter (Table 15-1) should be considered, and the ease and speed with which it can be obtained. A parameter that has excellent predictive validity according to the obstetric literature, but is difficult to measure and therefore prone to error, may not be well suited to the emergency setting.

In the second trimester, BPD and HC are the most widely used measurements to determine gestational age.[12,14] Although in expert hands, HC has a somewhat better predictive validity than BPD, measurement of BPD is preferable in the emergency setting because of the relative ease with which it is obtained. While HC must be calculated in a particular plane, BPD can be measured in any plane, provided the line of measurement intersects the thalamus and third ventricle.[12,15] Of particular relevance to emergency medicine providers is a study that directly correlated neonatal survival in premature infants with various biometric measurements obtained

by ultrasound shortly before birth. Based on analysis of receiver operator curves, a BPD of >54 mm was the single best predictor of survival.[16]

In the third trimester, femur length is a frequently used alternative to BPD for estimating gestational age.[12,17] In late pregnancy, measurement of BPD may be difficult because the fetal skull is frequently located within the maternal pelvis and can be obscured by acoustic shadowing. The predictive validity of femur length is slightly better than BPD at this stage.[14] Femur length is relatively easy to measure because the transducer need only be parallel to the long axis of the femur.[12,18]

In the late third trimester, identification of an ossified distal femoral epiphysis represents a potentially rapid means of estimating gestational age, and may be useful in the emergency setting. The appearance of this ossification center indicates a gestational age of 29 weeks or greater, whereas its absence means that the gestational age is <34 weeks.[19] Similarly, the appearance of an ossified proximal tibial epiphysis suggests a gestational age of at least 35 weeks indicating the fetus is at or very near term.[12]

ASSESSMENT OF OBSTETRICAL CAUSES OF ABDOMINAL PAIN AND VAGINAL BLEEDING

The primary pregnancy-related causes of abdominal pain in the second and third trimesters are preterm labor, placental abruption, and chorioamnionitis.[20–24] Chorioamnionitis refers to an infection of the amniotic fluid, typically following a rupture of membranes, or rarely as a complication of diagnostic amniocentesis. In rare cases, infection may occur without membrane rupture, causing pain, preterm labor, and systemic signs of infection. The diagnosis can be made by ultrasound-guided amniocentesis.[25]

There are several disorders unique to pregnancy that may cause abdominal pain. Severe pregnancy-induced hypertension can be complicated by HELLP syndrome in 5–10% of cases, which is characterized by hemolysis, elevations in liver function tests, and low platelets. Midepigastric or right upper quadrant pain is present in 25% of cases.[25] Spontaneous liver or spleen subcapsular hematomas can also develop, usually, but not always, in association with pregnancy-induced hypertension. Patients may experience right or left upper quadrant pain and mild coagulopathy, but have normal liver function tests. Hematoma rupture results in peritonitis and hemorrhagic shock.[24] The diagnosis is often difficult, since this condition may resemble uterine rupture or abruption, and ultrasound may be helpful in differentiating these conditions.

Patients with vaginal bleeding in the second and third trimesters are at high risk, with fetal mortality or adverse outcomes in up to one-third of all cases.[25,26,27] Vaginal bleeding beyond 20 weeks' gestational age complicates 5% of all pregnancies. In 13% of those with bleeding, placental abruption is the cause, and in 7% placenta previa is the cause.[28,29] Placenta previa and abruption account for the vast majority of cases requiring transfusion or cesarean section, as opposed to cases of vaginal bleeding caused by early labor, lower genital lesions, or other diagnoses.

Placenta Previa

The term placenta previa refers to a placenta that completely covers the internal cervical os. Placenta previa has traditionally been subdivided into complete, meaning that the entire os is covered by placenta, and partial, meaning the os is partially covered. When the placental edge is located within 3 cm of the internal os, it is termed marginal placenta previa. The term low-lying placenta is useful for describing the case of a placenta located in the lower portion of the uterus in which the exact os–placenta relationship cannot be defined, or for describing an apparent placenta previa when seen in the second trimester (Figure 15-3).

Placenta previa is present at term in only approximately 0.5% of pregnancies. Yet, routine ultrasound in early second trimester has found low-lying placenta in up to 45% of patients and an apparent placenta previa in 5%.[30–32] The explanation for this paradox is widely referred to as placental migration, the relatively rapid elongation of the lower uterine segment during the third trimester, which effectively moves the placenta away from the os.[33]

Maternal risk factors for placenta previa include advanced age, multiparity, non-Caucasian race, previous cesarean section, and prior history of placenta previa.[33,34] Placenta previa usually presents as painless vaginal bleeding. However, pain from contractions sometimes accompanies the hemorrhage. The first episode of bleeding typically occurs in the third trimester, but may not occur until after the 36th week in up to one-third of cases.[33]

The evaluation of possible placenta previa begins with transabdominal scanning as it is rapid, noninvasive, and reliable for locating the placenta (Figure 15-4) A digital vaginal examination can precipitate severe hemorrhage in the presence of placenta previa. Ultrasound can be used to locate the placenta and exclude placenta previa prior to vaginal examination. The sensitivity for ultrasound diagnosing placenta previa is 92–98%.[35,36] When the placenta is visualized at or near the fundus by transabdominal ultrasound, placenta previa is effectively excluded. After excluding the diagnosis of placenta previa, the clinician can then proceed to evaluate the patient for placental abruption. However, if the placenta is clearly seen covering the entire cervical os, particularly in the third trimester, the diagnosis of placenta previa is confirmed. When the placenta appears to be low lying or partially covering the os, or when an adequate view cannot be obtained with transabdominal ultrasound, further evaluation with transvaginal or translabial ultrasound is generally indicated. The diagnosis of placenta previa by transabdominal ultrasound has a high false-positive rate, up to 17% in one large study.[37] Placenta previa is often overdiagnosed in the second trimester because it is mimicked by two conditions: (1) an overdistended bladder that compresses the lower uterine segments and (2) focal contractions.[38] With the transabdominal approach, the relationship of the inferior edge of the cervix to the internal os is frequently obscured by patient obesity, an overdistended bladder, myometrial contractions, a posterior placenta, or the ossified fetal skull.[39,40] In one study of patients with suspected previa, assessment of the placenta–os relationship was impossible in 31%

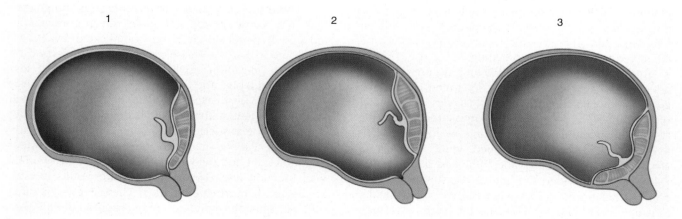

1   2   3

Figure 15-3. Classification of placenta previa: 1 = marginal, 2 = low lying, 3 = complete.

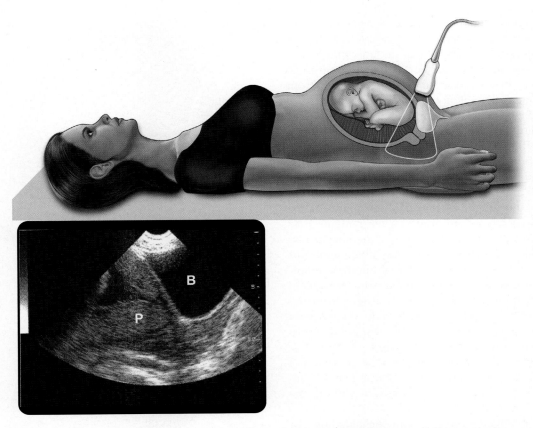

Figure 15-4. Placenta previa. Transabdominal longitudinal ultrasound demonstrates partial previa. B = bladder; P = placenta. (Sonogram courtesy of Lori Sens and Lori Green, Gulfcoast Ultrasound)

of transabdominal studies.[41] Nevertheless, in the case of severe hemorrhage, if findings on transabdominal ultrasound appear to be consistent with placenta previa, the patient should proceed directly to the operating room. A double setup examination may then be performed in the operating room at the obstetrician's discretion.

The approach to management of placenta previa depends largely on the sonographic assessment of fetal well-being and gestational age. Although cesarean section is the definitive treatment, vaginal bleeding due to confirmed placenta previa is frequently managed in an expectant fashion. The rationales for expectant management are as follows: (1) bleeding prior to the third trimester is often self-limited and can be treated by transfusion, if necessary; (2) vaginal bleeding represents little direct risk to the fetus in the absence of significant abruption or maternal shock; and (3) delaying delivery, to maximize fetal maturity, improves perinatal outcome.[33] Confirmation of fetal well-being is a prerequisite to expectant management. A rapid initial measurement of fetal cardiac activity can be performed in the emergency setting with transabdominal ultrasound, although cardiotocography is then required for ongoing fetal monitoring. Other measures of fetal well-being,

such as amniotic fluid volume and biophysical profile, may have an impact on management.

A determination of gestational age also is required to guide treatment decisions.[8] The following general guidelines have been proposed with regard to management of previa based on gestational age. When gestational age is <24 weeks, delivery is indicated only for hemorrhage that is life threatening to the mother. Between 24 and 34 weeks, fetal distress and life-threatening hemorrhage are indications for delivery. Beyond 34–37 weeks, delivery is indicated for fetal distress, significant bleeding, or labor.[33]

Placental Abruption

Any abnormal separation of the placenta occurring after 20 weeks' gestation is defined as a placental abruption. Prior to this date, placental separation is considered part of the process of a spontaneous abortion. While it affects <1% of all pregnancies, abruption accounts for more than a quarter of all perinatal mortality.[8,33] The epidemiology of placental abruption suggests that a variety of risk factors contribute to its development, many of which relate to more general microvascular disease. One of the strongest associations is with maternal hypertension, both chronic and pregnancy induced.[42] Cigarette smoking and cocaine abuse have also been linked to higher rates of abruption.[43,44] Trauma is an uncommon but important cause of abruption. Particular attention must be given to victims of motor vehicle crashes, falls from height, and domestic violence.[28,33,45]

Hemorrhage from abruption begins at the point of separation between the placenta and the uterus, or the placenta and the amnion. The timing and degree of subsequent bleeding from the cervix are dependent on the size of the hemorrhage and its location relative to the placenta. The amount of vaginal bleeding is not a reliable guide to the degree of placental abruption or the severity of hemorrhage. In some cases, patients may experience no vaginal bleeding despite significant placental separation. The amount of vaginal bleeding must never be taken as a guide to degree of internal hemorrhage. Also, the presence of abdominal pain, considered a hallmark symptom for abruption, is absent in nearly half of all cases.[8,33] Therefore, when evaluating patients with painless vaginal bleeding in pregnancy, the possibility of abruption must be considered.[7,33] The most consistent finding in abruption will be the presence of uterine irritability and contractions.[7] These may be unappreciated by both patient and physician without the aid of cardiotocography.

Because neither the character of the bleeding nor the presence of pain can be relied upon to differentiate placental abruption from placenta previa, it is recommended that the evaluation of vaginal bleeding in the second and third trimesters begins with an ultrasound examination to exclude placenta previa. Once the diagnosis of placenta previa is excluded, abruption becomes the major diagnostic consideration.

During placental abruption, hemorrhage occurs within a layer of the placenta causing separation from the adjacent uterine wall.[33] This hemorrhage and separation may remain partial and self-limited or progress on to complete abruption. The clinical manifestations of abruption and its prognosis are directly determined by the extent to which placental circulation is compromised, which in turn depends on both its size and location. Hemorrhage confined to the edge of the placenta is referred to as a marginal abruption. The degree or size of placental-uterine separation is graded as mild (grade 1), partial (grade 2), or complete (grade 3) (Figure 15-5).[27,46] These categories correlate reasonably well with the clinical presentation and prognosis. Grade 1 separations are usually marginal, involve less than a few centimeters of the placental border, and are usually not clinically significant. In contrast, grade 3 abruption can be fatal to both the fetus and the mother. Abruption is further categorized by the anatomic location of the hematoma relative to the placenta: retroplacental (in the decidua basalis, between placenta and uterine wall), subchorionic (between decidua and the membranes),

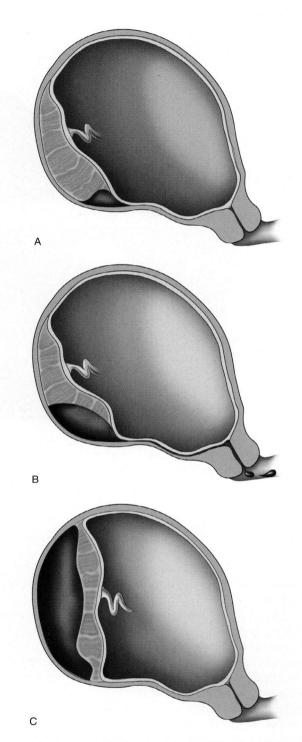

Figure 15-5. Classification of placental abruption.
(A) Grade 1, mild abruption—as in this diagram, usually marginal in location. Presentation may be subtle or subclinical, affords best prognosis.
(B) Grade 2, partial abruption—presentation and prognosis determined by location of separation and degree of compromise of maternal–fetal circulation.
(C) Grade 3, complete abruption—worst prognosis. In this diagram, the hemorrhage is concealed by the tamponading effect of the placental margins.

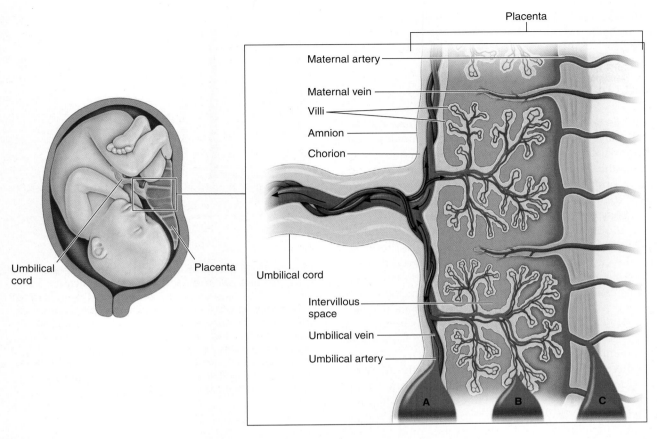

Figure 15-6. Diagram of the anatomy of the third trimester placenta. The location of three types of placental abruption is also shown: (A) preplacental, (B) subchorionic, and (C) retroplacental.

and preplacental (between placenta and amniotic fluid, immediately beneath the amnionic membrane) (Figure 15-6).[47] These distinctions also have significant prognostic implications, but primarily for fetal outcome. A retroplacental hemorrhage of 60 mL or more results in a 50% fetal mortality rate, but a similar-sized subchorionic hemorrhage results in a 10% fetal mortality rate. Preplacental hemorrhage is often self-limited and clinically silent, with 30% detected only after delivery.[27,47] They appear sonographically as an irregular bulge along the inner border of the placenta. Rupture of these hematomas results in the classic "port-wine" staining of the amniotic fluid.

Ultrasound is not a sensitive test for placental abruption and the diagnosis remains largely clinical, beginning with a meticulous search for evidence of vaginal bleeding, uterine tenderness, labor, or fetal distress. Signs of labor and fetal distress are the keys to making the diagnosis. Uterine contractions are present in nearly all cases of abruption, although they may be difficult to appreciate by either the physician or the patient. Contractions are characteristically of high frequency but low amplitude. It has been demonstrated that 6 hours

of cardiotocographic monitoring after trauma is 100% sensitive for predicting all subsequent complications.[7] Even rare cases of late-onset abruption or fetal distress after trauma are heralded by early abnormalities on cardiotocography.[48] Hence, the absence of uterine irritability or fetal distress remains an excellent indicator of maternal–placental well-being, suggesting that abruption is either absent or clinically insignificant. Cardiotocography should be a routine part of the initial evaluation where there is a concern for abruption, even in those who are asymptomatic. The stable patient without evidence of uterine irritability for 6 hours may be discharged home with appropriate instructions and follow-up.

Once placental abruption is diagnosed, an immediate cesarean section remains the definitive treatment. Decisions regarding the manner and timing of any intervention depend on an overall assessment of maternal–fetal well-being. If the fetus is immature and the abruption is judged to be mild, an expectant approach may be attempted. Signs of preterm labor may be difficult to distinguish from mild abruption.[33] A term fetus or evidence of uterine irritability refractory to medical management should prompt expedited delivery. Similarly, fetal distress or maternal signs of abruption indicate a need for immediate cesarean section.[25,33]

EVALUATION OF LABOR

Approximately 7% of newborns are premature at birth, which may result in mental or physical impairment.[49] Preterm labor is defined as regular uterine contractions accompanied by characteristic changes in the cervix, occurring prior to 37 weeks' gestation. Assessing the potential for premature delivery is the main goal of the emergency evaluation for preterm labor.

Ultrasound is a safe, rapid, and accurate method of evaluating the cervix for signs of labor. As labor begins, the cervix undergoes effacement followed by dilation. While the digital examination has traditionally been used to evaluate such cervical changes, ultrasound has emerged as a safer and more accurate means to evaluate cervical changes.[50] Sonographic measurement of cervical length represents an objective way to quantify effacement.

There are several justifications for using an ultrasound examination rather than the digital examination in this setting. First, a direct contraindication to digital examination may exist, such as placenta previa or ruptured membranes, and digital examination in these settings can produce life-threatening bleeding or chorioamnionitis. A transabdominal or translabial ultrasound examination may negate the need for a digital examination. Second, an ultrasound examination has been shown in numerous studies to be more accurate than digital examination in estimating cervical length and predicting preterm labor.[50]

An advantage of using ultrasound is that it can visualize the internal cervical os and detect funneling. Funneling is dilatation of the internal cervical os without dilation of the external cervical os, and it is one of the earliest signs of labor. A digital examination cannot palpate the internal os, so it cannot detect funneling. An ultrasound examination is the only practical way to detect this important finding.[50–55]

There are three methods for imaging the cervix with ultrasound: transabdominal, transvaginal, and translabial. The transabdominal approach is the least reliable method, with successful imaging of the cervix in only 46% of patients without a full bladder and 86% with a full bladder.[56] Presenting fetal parts and a large maternal habitus may obscure visualization of the cervix. The transvaginal technique produces the most consistent findings, with visualization of the cervix in up to 100% of patients.[51] The translabial ultrasound is considered the most technically difficult method. In the hands of a skilled operator, however, this approach provides an adequate view of the cervix in up to 95% of

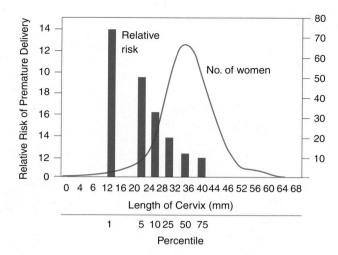

Figure 15-7. Relative risk of premature delivery (solid bars) versus cervical length, measured by transvaginal ultrasound at 24 weeks. Cervical length is expressed both in millimeters and percentiles of the normal distribution. The number of subjects versus cervical length is also shown (solid curve). (Reprinted, with permission, from Lams JE, Goldenberg RL, Meis PJ, et al.: The length of the cervix and the risk of spontaneous premature delivery. *N Engl J Med* 334:567, 1996.)

patients.[51,57] In the emergency setting, it is reasonable to begin with transabdominal ultrasound and then proceed to transvaginal or translabial imaging if the cervix cannot be well visualized.

From studies of all three ultrasound methods, it is clear that cervical measurements can predict the risk of preterm delivery. In one study of nearly 3000 patients at 24–28 weeks' gestation, it was demonstrated that a positive correlation exists between short cervical length (<30 mm) and risk for preterm birth before 35 weeks (Figure 15-7).[53] Another study of patients between 16 and 28 weeks' gestation found a 79% rate of preterm delivery in those with cervical funneling of >50%.[58] Subsequent studies have confirmed the predictive value of both short cervical length and the presence of funneling, and have extended the findings to twin pregnancies.[55,59] For the most part, patients in these studies were asymptomatic so applicability in the emergency setting is unclear. Also, the impact of such findings on clinical management, such as the need for cervical cerclage, remains uncertain.

The use of ultrasound in determining the presence or absence of cervical changes can help the emergency physician risk stratify patients with symptoms suggestive of labor. The goal of such an evaluation is to identify patients who would benefit from admission and tocolysis versus candidates for outpatient follow-up. The utility of cervical sonography in the management of preterm labor was retrospectively evaluated at one facility.

Women were hospitalized only if they had a cervical length <30 mm. This protocol produced a decrease in hospital days of 48% without affecting the rate of preterm births.[60] The critical cervical length appears to be 30 mm, with preterm delivery much more likely in patients with a shorter cervical measurement by ultrasound.[60] Apply cervical sonography in conjunction with clinical variables—such as the results of a biophysical profile (discussed below), the gestational age, and a history of preterm births—to influence management decisions.

Lie refers to the relationship of the fetus to the long axis of the uterus, while presentation describes what fetal part is nearest the cervix. In normal deliveries, the fetal lie is longitudinal and the presentation is cephalic. Transverse lie and breech presentation—where the fetal sacrum and feet, respectively, are engaged in the pelvis—are referred to as malpresentations. The classification of breech presentations is demonstrated in Figure 15-8.

In the emergency setting, it is absolutely essential to know the presenting fetal part. Even with good prenatal care, fetal presentation is often unknown because prior to 25 weeks the fetus frequently changes position. Breech presentations, which account for 3–4% of all deliveries, are fraught with complications such as asphyxia, cord prolapse, and spinal cord injuries to the fetus.[61] Knowledge of the presentation allows the emergency physician to mobilize the appropriate equipment and support staff needed for delivery. In an emergency vaginal delivery, the presenting part is discovered easily by physical examination of the vagina or perineum. Prior to this point, determining fetal position by palpation may be difficult, particularly for a nonobstetrician. Moreover, vaginal examination is contraindicated when preterm labor is accompanied by vaginal bleeding. In such cases, an ultrasound examination can be used to establish fetal position.

Just as important as fetal position is the determination of the number of fetuses prior to delivery. Ultrasound is invaluable for identifying the "surprise twin." Perinatal death occurs seven times more frequently in twin deliveries compared to singletons.[62] Like breech presentations, delivery of twins requires additional expertise, support, and equipment.

There are multiple noninvasive measures to evaluate the health of the unborn child. Traditionally, nonstress testing and amniotic fluid volume measurement have been used. The biophysical profile is a more sophisticated instrument that combines nonstress testing and amniotic fluid volume with three additional sonographic parameters—fetal tone, movement, and breathing—to derive an objective score that reflects overall fetal well-being (Table 15-2).[63-65] The idea behind the biophysical profile is that the CNS, which is very sensitive to hypoxia, controls all of the measured parameters. Thus, a low biophysical profile score may indicate either acute or chronic fetal hypoxia.[66,67] Results of the

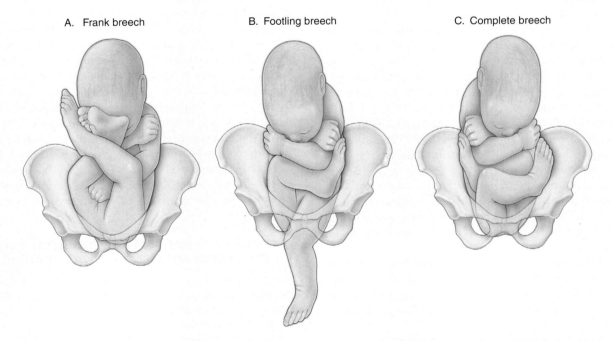

A. Frank breech   B. Footling breech   C. Complete breech

Figure 15-8. Types of breech presentation. In a frank breech presentation (the most common), the thighs are flexed at the hips with the legs and knees extended. In complete breech (the least common), the thighs are flexed at the hips, and there is flexion of the knees as well. One or both hips and knees are extended in the footling breech. The risk of cord prolapse is greatest with footling breech and least with a frank breech.

▶ TABLE 15-2. **CRITERIA FOR FIVE COMPONENTS OF THE FETAL BIOPHYSICAL PROFILE***

Biophysical Variable	Normal (Score = 2)	Abnormal (Score = 0)
Fetal breathing movements	One or more episode of ≥20 s duration in 30 min	Absent or no episode of ≥20 s in 30 min
Gross body movements	Two or more discrete body/limb movements in 30 min (episodes of active continuous movement considered as single movement)	Less than two episodes of body/limb movements in 30 min
Fetal tone	One or more episode of active extension with return to flexion of fetal limb(s) or trunk (opening and closing of hand considered normal tone)	Slow extension with return to partial flexion, movement of limb in full extension, absent fetal movement, or partially open fetal hand
Reactive fetal heart rate	Two or more episodes of acceleration of ≥15 bpm and of >15 s associated with fetal movement in 20 min	One or no episode of acceleration of fetal heart rate or acceleration of <15 bpm in 20 min
Qualitative amniotic fluid volume	One or more pockets of fluid measuring ≥2 cm in vertical axis	Either no pockets or largest pocket <2 cm in vertical axis

*A score of 8 or more is considered normal.
Reprinted with permission from Manning FA: Fetal biophysical profile. *Obstet Gynecol Clin North Am* 26(4):557, 1999.

biophysical profile are always considered together with gestational age and maternal and fetal comorbidities, but in general, lower scores have increased risk of fetal hypoxia, and scores >8 are considered normal.[65−72]

EVALUATION OF TRAUMATIC INJURIES

Trauma occurs in 6% of pregnant patients[73] and is the leading cause of nonobstetrical maternal mortality.[74] Furthermore, fetal loss as a result of trauma far exceeds maternal mortality.[75] Point-of-care ultrasound has the potential to play a critical role in the initial evaluation of pregnant trauma patients. Use of the E-FAST examination to evaluate maternal intra-abdominal hemorrhage has been shown to be beneficial.[11] The sensitivity and specificity of the E-FAST examination in pregnant trauma patients are similar to the sensitivity and specificity in nonpregnant trauma patients.[76] Because fetal well-being is dependent on adequate maternal circulation, a tenant of trauma care is that resuscitation of the mother and assessment of maternal injuries is the initial priority.

Besides maternal shock, processes that contribute to fetal loss include direct fetal injury, uterine rupture, placental abruption, ruptured membranes, and premature labor. Factors associated with fetal loss after maternal trauma are listed in Table 15-3.[77−82]

Placental abruption is the most common cause of fetal loss in pregnant trauma patients, and may occur after relatively minor trauma and in the absence of other injuries.[7] While cardiotocography and observation for the occurrence of frequent contractions remain the cornerstone of the evaluation,[73] ultrasound may sometimes be able to confirm the presence of significant abruption.[7] In addition, point-of-care ultrasound may be used to rapidly demonstrate fetal cardiac activity and determine gestational age.[11]

Perform the E-FAST examination either immediately following or, preferably, contemporaneously with the primary survey of the pregnant trauma victim. The sonographic evaluation of pregnant trauma victim is a combination of the E-FAST exam as well as three other rapid and goal-directed scanning protocols. In order to perform this combination of ultrasound studies, the preferred transducer is the curvilinear, due to its lower frequency range and obstetric preset calculations. First and foremost is the sonographic assessment of potential maternal life threats with the E-FAST examination. This will allow the emergency provider to rapidly determine the presence of intraperitoneal fluid, pericardial fluid, pleural fluid, or pneumothorax (see Chapter 5, "Trauma"). Following the E-FAST exam, change the machine settings to OB and answer four questions: (1) Does the

▶ TABLE 15-3. **FACTORS ASSOCIATED WITH FETAL LOSS AFTER MATERNAL TRAUMA**

Ejection from vehicle
Pedestrian struck by vehicle
Maternal Injury Severity Score >9
Maternal tachycardia
Maternal hypotension
Maternal hypoxia
Maternal contractions
Abnormal fetal heart rate
Penetrating uterine injuries

patient have a sonographically visible intrauterine pregnancy?; (2) What is the gestational age?; (3) Is there fetal cardiac activity?; and (4) What is the fetal heart rate?

ASSESSMENT OF NONOBSTETRICAL CAUSES OF ABDOMINAL PAIN

Abdominal pain in the second and third trimesters of pregnancy represents a significant challenge for clinicians. The differential diagnosis must include obstetrical and nonobstetrical causes of abdominal pain, and the impact of diagnostic and management decisions on both the mother and the fetus must be considered. The anatomic and physiologic changes of pregnancy may alter the traditional presentation of many disorders, and the symptomatology of pregnancy itself may overlap with that of nonobstetrical abdominal pathology. Concerns over ionizing radiation or medication-induced teratogenicity may limit choices of diagnostic imaging or therapy. All of these elements may confuse the clinical picture and delay definitive diagnosis, increasing the risk of morbidity to the mother and the fetus. Ultrasound offers a safe and effective first step for the evaluation of abdominal pain in pregnancy.

Nonobstetrical causes of abdominal pain in pregnancy occur at rates similar to that of the nonpregnant population. Similarly, the need for urgent abdominal surgery during pregnancy parallels that of the general population when ectopic pregnancies and cesarean sections are excluded.[20,21] However, the morbidity associated with virtually every abdominal emergency is higher in pregnancy, mostly due to the difficulty in making an early diagnosis.[22]

The evaluation of abdominal pain in the second and third trimesters demands that clinicians maintain a broad differential and an awareness of the altered presentation of common abdominal disorders in pregnancy. Table 15-4 lists the common obstetrical and nonobstetrical causes of abdominal pain. Every workup begins with a careful history and physical examination that should significantly narrow the differential. Laboratory tests must be interpreted in the context of pregnancy-induced changes (e.g., leukocytosis and relative anemia) and are frequently of limited diagnostic value.

Sonography is a reasonable first diagnostic step in most cases and helps to substantially narrow the differential diagnosis, if not confirm the diagnosis. As an example, right upper quadrant pain in the third trimester engenders a broad differential that should include biliary disease, liver disease, nephrolithiasis, pyelonephritis, and appendicitis. Normal laboratory tests and urinalysis may help to reduce the list of likely possibilities to biliary colic and appendicitis. Ultrasound could then be used to confirm or exclude both of these disorders while providing additional information on the pregnancy itself.

▶ **TABLE 15-4. DIFFERENTIAL DIAGNOSIS OF ABDOMINAL PAIN IN THE SECOND AND THIRD TRIMESTER**

Obstetric causes
  Labor
  Placental abruption
  Placenta previa
  Chorioamnionitis
  Pre-eclampsia/HELLP
Nonobstetric causes
  Appendicitis
  Cholecystitis
  Pyelonephritis
  Nephrolithiasis
  Hepatitis
  Peptic ulcer disease and reflux

Ultrasound is the traditional first-line imaging modality for abdominal pain in pregnancy because it provides anatomic and functional information about the mother and fetus without exposing either to the effects of ionizing radiation. Intrauterine exposure to radiation may have both oncologic and teratogenic effects. Case-controlled studies of childhood cancer show a slight but significant increase in relative risk among the children of female radiologists exposed to 1000 mrems of radiation.[21] The potential for teratogenicity and carcinogenesis appears to be greatest in the period of 2–15 weeks and decreases proportionally as the fetus nears term. In the first trimester, *in utero* radiation exposure is graded as low, moderate, or high depending on the total dose, with the clearest evidence of harm above a threshold level of 150 mGy (Table 15-5).[23] Significant variability exists, however, depending on gestational age, body habitus, and the type of radiographic study. Exposure in the second and third trimesters is less critical with

▶ **TABLE 15-5. QUALITATIVE RADIATION RISK CATEGORIES AND ESTIMATED FETAL DOSE BY TYPE OF RADIOGRAPH**

Qualitative radiation risk categories	
Risk category	Dose range (mGy)*
Low	<10
Intermediate	10–250
High	>250
Fetal dose estimation by type of radiograph	
Diagnostic procedure	Estimated dose (mGy)*
Conventional radiograph	2 mGy/exposure
CT (abdomen or pelvis)	5 mGy/slice
Fluoroscopy (pelvis or abdomen)	10 mGy/min

*10 mGy = 1 rad.
Reprinted with permission from Mann F, Nathens A, Langer S, et al.: Communicating with the family the risks of medical radiation to conceptuses in victims of major blunt-force trauma. *J Trauma* 48(2):354, 2000.

an estimated relative increase in cancer risk of 64% per rad (10 mGy), which corresponds to a 0.05% relative increase in the rate of childhood malignancies. Fortunately, the majority of radiographic tests fall well below the threshold level (150 mGy or 15 rads) and plain radiography and CT remain potential diagnostic tools in pregnant patients with abdominal pain.[23] That said, the decision to use radiography in a pregnant patient must take into account a number of competing elements: the risk of radiation to the developing fetus, the risk of delayed diagnosis if available imaging techniques are not used, and the relative suitability of alternative imaging or management strategies. There are also the intangible concerns about radiation exposure that may not be supported by data, but nevertheless push providers toward using alternative imaging modalities. The use of diagnostic radiography in the pregnant patient is appropriate provided the risks and benefits are weighed in a manner that ensures the best outcome for the mother and fetus. Regardless of the relative risks and benefits of radiography, ultrasound is a valuable initial tool in the evaluation of the pregnant patient with abdominal pain, given its safety and unique ability to assess fetal well-being.

As pregnancy advances into the second and third trimesters, a number of anatomic and physiologic changes occur. These changes alter the way a variety of common disease processes present. The primary sonographic approach to these disorders must change accordingly. As the uterus enlarges, the intestinal tract is displaced upward, backward, and to the sides. The appendix moves to the right upper quadrant and away from the omentum (Figure 15-9). Increased intra-abdominal pressure leads to increased gastroesophageal reflux, and the gravid uterus compresses the ureters, inferior vena cava, and bladder.[20,21] Pregnant women commonly experience varying degrees of anorexia, nausea, vomiting, and back and flank pain, which are all related to the compressive and postural effects of the gravid uterus. Serious intra-abdominal processes can cause similar symptoms.

Appendicitis

Appendicitis is the most common surgical emergency in pregnancy, accounting for two-thirds of all laparotomies.[25,83] In the first half of pregnancy, the clinical presentation of appendicitis is similar to that in nonpregnant patients. Thereafter, the clinical picture becomes more atypical.[25] As mentioned above, early constitutional symptoms of appendicitis are often subtle and dismissed as normal symptoms of pregnancy. The abdominal pain is predominantly right-sided and corresponds to the location of the appendix in different stages of pregnancy (Figure 15-9). Leukocytosis is a common but unreliable finding, and 20% of pregnant patients with

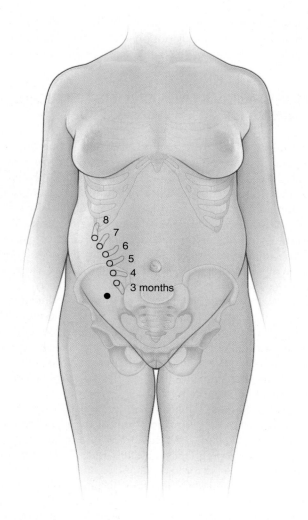

Figure 15-9. Location of the appendix during succeeding months of pregnancy.

appendicitis have sterile pyuria.[84] The differential diagnosis includes ovarian mass, ovarian torsion, and other sources of right upper quadrant pain, specifically cholecystitis, pyelonephritis, or hepatitis.[20,21,85]

If appendicitis is suspected on clinical grounds, the diagnosis may be confirmed by graded compression ultrasound, which is highly accurate for the diagnosis of appendicitis during pregnancy. In one study of 45 pregnant women with abdominal pain, graded compression ultrasound demonstrated a sensitivity of 100% and specificity of 96% for the diagnosis of appendicitis.[86] However, earlier studies found a considerably lower sensitivity of 75–89%, although with similar specificities.[87,88] These results, along with its well-established diagnostic performance in nonpregnant patients, would suggest that ultrasound for appendicitis in pregnancy should be regarded as a diagnostic test that is specific, but may have limited sensitivity. A positive finding would allow surgical management without the need for other diagnostic testing, but a negative ultrasound exam, in the setting of an intermediate or high pretest probability, would require further testing.

The sonographic evaluation for appendicitis is challenging and highly operator dependent. During pregnancy, this assessment is further complicated by the upward and outward displacement of the appendix by the growing uterus. A graded compression test is performed with special attention paid to the overall diameter of the appendix, wall thickening, or the presence of surrounding fluid and debris. The specific sonographic findings of appendicitis are discussed in Chapter 11, "General Surgery Applications." In the third trimester, the size of the uterus may preclude adequate visualization of the appendix, despite a proper high-lateral approach.[86] Placing the patient in the left lateral decubitus position may make visualization of the appendix more likely.

Laparoscopy or laparotomy, without any diagnostic testing, may be indicated. It has been recommended that surgeons maintain a lower threshold for surgical exploration in pregnant patients with possible appendicitis, given the variability of clinical signs and the increased morbidity associated with diagnostic delay. Negative exploration rates as high as 40% in the third trimester are commonplace and may be acceptable.[88]

The functional absence of the omentum in pregnancy means that a ruptured appendix is less likely to be walled off, resulting in early peritonitis. Perinatal mortality rises from 4.8% in nonperforated appendicitis to 27.8% when the appendix ruptures. The perforation rate prior to diagnosis is as high as 30% during the third trimester.[83] Since the risk of fetal loss and maternal morbidity from a delayed diagnosis of appendicitis is considerable, clinical vigilance is required even in the absence of classic signs and symptoms.[21]

Cholelithiasis and Cholecystitis

Acute gallbladder disease is more common in pregnancy than in the nongravid population, which reflects a higher prevalence of gallstones in fertile women (3.5–11%).[89,90] Signs and symptoms are essentially the same as in the general population: abrupt onset of stabbing or colicky right upper quadrant abdominal pain accompanied by nausea and vomiting. While the presence of fever and Murphy's sign suggests acute cholecystitis, mild elevations in the WBC, amylase, and alkaline phosphatase can be normal during pregnancy. The differential diagnosis includes appendicitis, pyelonephritis, nephrolithiasis, and rare entities such as the HELLP syndrome or subcapsular hematoma.

Pregnant patients suspected of having biliary disease should invariably have a right upper quadrant ultrasound exam (see Chapter 10, "Hepatobiliary"; Videos 10-1 and 10-2). As in the nonpregnant population, sonography is the imaging modality of choice for biliary disease, and its technique and diagnostic performance are essentially unaltered by pregnancy. Oral cholecystograms and HIDA scans are effective but less attractive options in the pregnant patient due to the risks of radiation exposure. Ultrasound will identify nearly all gallstones when the exam is performed carefully.[90] The presence of gallbladder wall thickening or pericholecystic fluid are strong indicators of gallbladder inflammation. Many patients with acute cholecystitis during pregnancy can be managed conservatively with IV hydration, analgesia, and antibiotics. The risk of fetal loss with cholecystectomy approaches 5%, but appears to be lowest when performed in the second trimester. Surgical intervention should not be delayed if the patient becomes toxic or develops pancreatitis, since the fetal loss rate may reach 50% in these patients.[90]

▶ ANATOMICAL CONSIDERATIONS

By the 13th week of gestation, or the beginning of the second trimester, the fundus of the gravid uterus is easily palpable above the pelvic brim and, by 20 weeks, it normally reaches the level of the umbilicus. The distance in centimeters from the pubic symphysis to the fundus approximates gestational age in weeks (Figure 15-10). As the uterus and developing fetus grow, the intestines are displaced posteriorly, superiorly, and toward the flanks. As a result, by the third trimester, the appendix is normally found in the right upper quadrant (Figure 15-9). The growing uterus also compresses the ureters, frequently resulting in asymptomatic hydronephrosis, which occurs more often on the right side.

Familiarity with the anatomy of the lower uterine segment, the cervix, and surrounding pelvic structures is essential for sonographic evaluation of cervical length and placenta previa (Figure 15-11). The normal cervix is 3–5 cm long and cylindrical in shape. The long axis of the cervix normally lies at a right angle to the long axis of the vagina. In late pregnancy, the inner one-third of the cervix, or isthmus, elongates to form the lower uterine segment. The passageway between the uterine cavity and the external os is referred to as the endocervical canal. An area of glandular tissue, which may be hypoechoic or hyperechoic, surrounds the endocervical canal. This glandular zone disappears after 31 weeks' gestation, indicating cervical ripening, and making the canal difficult to locate sonographically.[51,91] The bladder lies anterior to the vagina and cervix. As the bladder distends, it impinges on the anterior wall of the lower uterine segment. The rectum and sacral promontory lie posterior to the cervix and lower uterus.

Understanding the sonographic appearance of placental pathology requires familiarity with the underlying

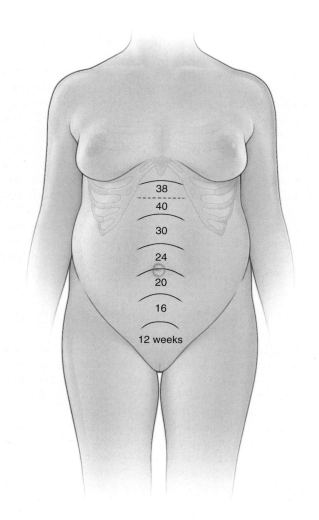

Figure 15-10. Estimation of gestational age of a singleton pregnancy by height of the fundus (cm).

uterine and placental anatomy. The placenta is primarily a fetal organ, and its size, thickness, and texture reflect the health and gestational age of the developing fetus. In the early part of the second trimester, the placenta is easily visible sonographically as a homogeneous, hyperechoic rim of tissue adjacent to the gestational sac (Figure 15-12).[35] The thickness of the placenta in millimeters approximates the gestational age in weeks and rarely exceeds 4 cm.[92]

By the latter part of the second trimester, the relevant anatomic segments of the placenta become more established. These include (from outside in) the myometrium, decidua basalis (endometrial–placental interface), intervillous space (area of maternal–fetal exchange), chorion (membrane that envelopes the fetal vessels), and amnion (membrane that overlies the placenta, separating it from amniotic fluid) (Figure 15-6). Fetal (umbilical) vessels course within the chorion, whereas maternal (endometrial) vessels are located within the decidua.

The sonographic appearance of these layers is variable. Prominent endometrial arteries and veins within the decidua may appear as hypoechoic bands of tissue separating the myometrium from the fetal placenta, which is termed the retroplacental hypoechoic complex.[35] In the intervillous space, sonolucent pools of maternal blood, called villous lakes, can lend a heterogeneous appearance to this middle layer. The addition of Doppler in both of these regions may help determine the vascular nature of a sonolucent area. Lastly, the subchorionic segment may undergo cystic changes associated with fibrin deposition in up to 20% of patients. These echogenic, cyst-like lesions can grow to 1 cm in size but are of no clinical significance.[35,92] The normal occurrence of these lesions limits the specificity of the ultrasound in the evaluation of possible abruption.

A discussion of fetal anatomy and development is beyond the scope of this chapter and has limited relevance to point-of-care ultrasound. Fetal anatomic landmarks that must be recognized for the BPD and femur length measurements are described in the "Technique and Normal Ultrasound Findings" section.

► GETTING STARTED

Most modern ultrasound machines are capable of imaging for the entire range of pregnancy-related complaints. It is recommended that both abdominal (3.5–5 MHz) and transvaginal (5.0–8.0 MHz) transducers be available. Ultrasound gel (preferably warmed) is a requirement for both scanning techniques. For abdominal scanning, position patients in either the supine or in the left lateral decubitus position. For transvaginal scanning, a dedicated pelvic exam bed (with foot holders and breakaway bottom) will allow for optimal scanning conditions. Sterile setup and transducer covers are required. For transvaginal scanning, place ultrasound gel on the transducer's scanning surface and then cover with a sterile cover. Place sterile surgical lubricant on the transducer cover over the scanning area of the transducer.

► TECHNIQUE AND NORMAL ULTRASOUND FINDINGS

FETAL HEART RATE DETERMINATION

Determine fetal heart rate by transabdominal scanning using a 3.5–5 MHz transducer. Set the ultrasound machine for simultaneous B-mode and M-mode recording and obstetrical measurements. The specific scanning plane is unimportant, although fanning the transducer in a plane transverse to the fetal spine is a good method of rapidly locating the heart. Position the M-mode sampling line through the heart. Freeze the image when a

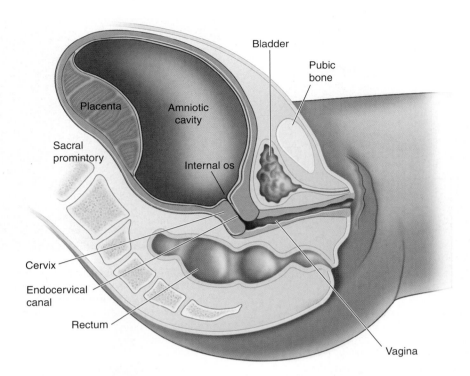

Figure 15-11. Diagram of cervix and surrounding structures (sagittal view).

continuous waveform is evident on the M-mode tracing at a depth corresponding to cardiac movement. Measure the distance between one- or two-cycle lengths (depending on the ultrasound machine's software); the computer will calculate and display the fetal heart rate (Figure 15-13). Avoid using pulsed-wave, continuous-wave, or color Doppler, particularly in the first trimester, because these modalities transmit higher energy.

ESTIMATION OF GESTATIONAL AGE

Biparietal Diameter

Because of its predictive validity and relative ease of measurement, BPD is the biometric measurement of

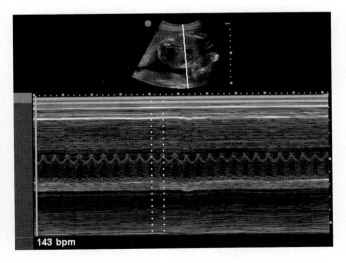

Figure 15-13. Fetal heart rate determination. B-mode image and M-mode tracing are simultaneously displayed. M-mode sampling line passes through fetal heart. Cardiac oscillations are evident on M-mode tracing. With image frozen, a cardiac cycle length is automatically calculated and displayed with obstetrics measurement software.

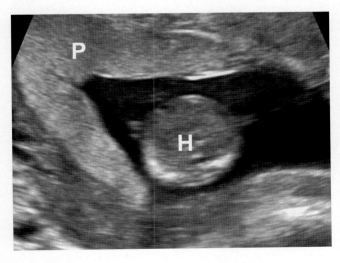

Figure 15-12. Ultrasound appearance of the placenta (P) and fetal head (H) in the early second trimester.

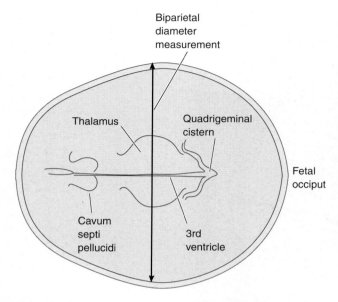

Biparietal diameter measurement

Thalamus

Quadrigeminal cistern

Fetal occiput

Cavum septi pellucidi

3rd ventricle

Figure 15-14. Schematic diagram of fetal anatomic landmarks used to locate the correct plane for biparietal diameter measurement. The "arrow sign" arises from the junction of third ventricle (shaft of the "arrow") and quadrigeminal cistern (forms the "arrowhead"), which points toward the fetal occiput.

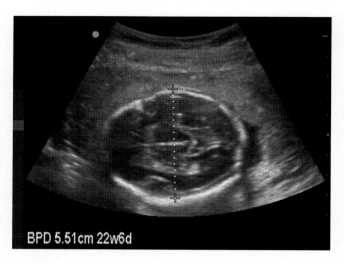

BPD 5.51cm 22w6d

Figure 15-15. Biparietal diameter to estimate gestational age. Measurement is taken from outer wall of calvarium to inner wall (see marker cursors), in a line that crosses the paired thalami and third ventricle.

choice for estimating gestational age after 14 weeks. Perform determinations of gestational age during the second and third trimesters by transabdominal scanning using a 3.5–5 MHz transducer. Measure the BPD at the level of the third ventricle, paired thalami, quadrigeminal cistern, and cavum septi pellucidi.[14,17] Although it is counterintuitive, the fetal ventricles and subarachnoid space are echogenic compared to brain due to the relative prominence of the choroid plexus and pia-arachnoid matter. The junction of the hyperechoic third ventricle and quadrigeminal cistern forms an easily recognizable sonographic landmark, referred to as the arrow sign (Figure 15-14). It has been proposed that the BPD can be measured in any plane as long as the line of measurement crosses the thalami and the third ventricle.[15] Points of measurement should be from the outer edge of the near calvarial wall to the inner edge of the far wall. The near and far calvarial walls should appear symmetric. Be careful not to include overlying soft tissue and scalp in the measurement (Figure 15-15).[15]

Femur Length

Beyond 26–32 weeks' gestation femur length is an alternative to BPD, and may be easier to measure. Femur length is actually a measurement of the ossified portion of the diaphysis and metaphysis only, and does not include the cartilaginous portions of the bone. Points of measurement are the junction of the ossified metaph-

ysis and the cartilaginous diaphysis at either end of the femur. The distal femoral epiphysis, a secondary ossification center, is not included. Femur length can be measured in any plane as long as it is parallel to the long axis of the bone and includes the accepted end points. To avoid an oblique, falsely short measurement, the plane of section should include the femoral head or greater trochanter and the distal femoral condyle, all of which are cartilaginous (Figure 15-16).[18] Further information about gestational age can be obtained by noting

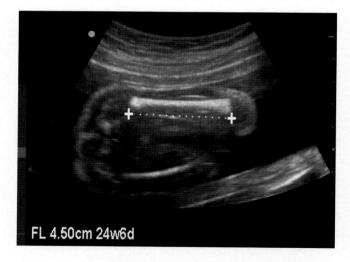

FL 4.50cm 24w6d

Figure 15-16. Femur length to estimate gestational age. Inclusion of cartilaginous greater trochanter and lateral condyle in the image assures proper long-axis plane. However, measurement includes only the ossified (brightly hyperechoic) portion of bone (cursors).

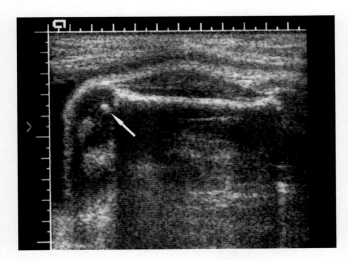

Figure 15-17. Distal femoral epiphysis. Longitudinal view of the femoral shaft with bent knee on the left. Appearance of a distal femoral epiphysis (arrow) indicates that the gestational age is at least 29 weeks.

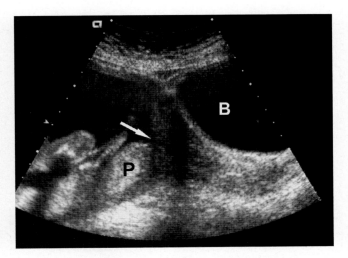

Figure 15-18. Posterior marginal placenta previa (P). Transabdominal approach, sagittal plane. The endocervical canal (arrow) is obscured by edge artifact emanating from the bladder (B).

whether the distal femoral and proximal tibial epiphyses are ossified (Figure 15-17).

LOCATION OF THE PLACENTA

Transabdominal Approach

Begin the sonographic evaluation of vaginal bleeding in the second and third trimester by determining the location of the placenta. Begin with transabdominal scanning using a 3.5–5.0 MHz transducer. Locate the placenta and scan in the sagittal plane to determine whether it extends into the lower uterine segment (Figure 15-18). If so, perform transverse and oblique scanning to determine whether it is centrally or laterally located. When the placenta is low lying, measurement of the os–placenta distance by transabdominal ultrasound is often difficult because the endocervical canal and inferior placental edge may not be visible in the same sagittal plane.[33]

The bladder should be full for optimal visualization of the lower uterine segment and internal os. However, if the placenta appears to be close to the internal os when the bladder is full, repeat scanning after the patient has voided. A full bladder may create a false impression of placenta previa by pushing the anterior wall of the lower uterus against the posterior wall, artificially elongating the cervix and shortening the distance between the placenta and the internal os (Figure 15-19). Myometrial contractions, which in the second trimester may not be felt by the mother, may also result in a false-positive diagnosis of placenta previa. A myometrial thickness >2 cm is suggestive of a contraction.[35] Repeat scanning in 20–30 minutes has been suggested

to avoid a false-positive diagnosis of placenta previa due to contractions; however, this option may be unrealistic in the emergency setting.

Transvaginal Approach

Use transvaginal or translabial sonography to clarify the internal os–placenta relationship when transabdominal scanning is nondiagnostic. The main contraindication to these techniques is ruptured or bulging membranes.[35] Transvaginal ultrasound is considered safe in the setting of second and third trimester bleeding because optimal images are usually obtained with the transducer

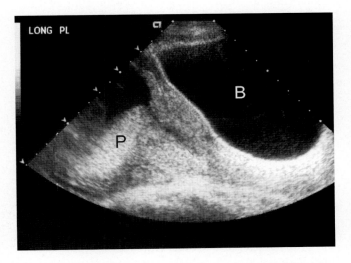

Figure 15-19. Posterior marginal placenta previa (P). Transabdominal approach, sagittal plane. In this case, an overdistended bladder (B) may be compressing the lower uterine segment, causing a false-positive impression of previa.

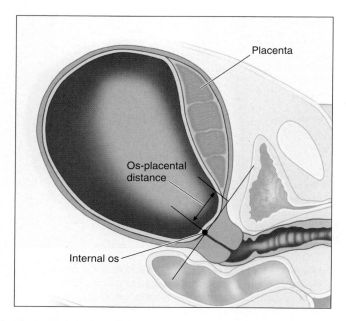

Figure 15-20. Diagram of measurement of os–placental distance. (Redrawn with permission from Cunningham FG, Leveno K, and Bloom SL, et al.: *Williams Obstetrics*. 21st ed. New York, NY: McGraw-Hill, 2001.)

inserted only about 2.5 cm beyond the introitus and no closer than 3 cm to the cervix.[93,94] Also, the angle between the transducer and the cervix is usually sufficient to prevent the transducer from inadvertently entering the cervix. Perform the technique using a 5.0–8.0 MHz endovaginal transducer covered by scanning medium and a sterile transducer cover. Begin the examination with sagittal scanning; the transducer may subsequently be rotated and its angle changed to obtain a longitudinal view of the placenta. Visualize the walls of the lower uterine segment in two orthogonal planes. Measure the os–placental distance if the inferior edge of the placenta is near the internal os. To do so, the endocervical canal, which appears sonographically as a faint, hyperechoic or hypoechoic line, must first be located. The junction between the amniotic fluid and the endocervical canal is designated as the internal os. Angle and rotate the transducer until the imaging plane contains both the internal os and the lowest part of the placenta, at which point freeze the image and make the measurement (Figure 15-20).

Translabial Approach

Perform a translabial (or transperineal) ultrasound examination by using a 3.5–5.0 MHz transducer to which scanning medium is applied, then a sterile cover, and finally a thin layer of sterile surgical lubricant over the cover. If available, a phased array transducer with a small footprint is preferable. The bladder should be empty. Place

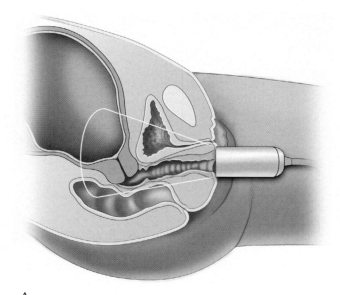

A

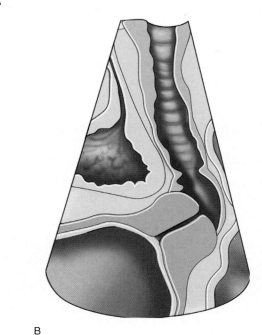

B

Figure 15-21. (A) Diagram of translabial transducer position and (B) correlation with the standard image projection on the monitor.

the transducer over or between the labia majora, posterior to the urethra, and anterior to the vaginal introitus. Perform scanning in a sagittal plane, with the bladder to the left on the monitor (Figure 15-21). Once the cervical os and placenta are visualized, laterally angle the transducer to image the entire surface of the cervix and lateral walls of the lower uterine segment.

Measure the os–placenta distance when a low-lying placenta is visualized. It has been proposed that placenta previa can be excluded by translabial scanning when a fetal part is visualized directly adjacent to the cervix or when the cervix is separated from a fetal part only by amniotic fluid without intervening placental tissue.[37]

The advantage of translabial scanning over transvaginal scanning is that it does not require an endovaginal transducer. Translabial scanning can be performed immediately after an apparently positive or nondiagnostic transabdominal scan without changing transducers, which may be an advantage in the emergency setting. However, there is no evidence that the translabial approach is safer than transvaginal ultrasound for patients with placenta previa, and transvaginal scanning is more familiar, provides better resolution, and is technically easier to perform.

CERVICAL LENGTH ASSESSMENT

Cervical length assessment using ultrasound is a valuable tool in predicting preterm birth.[51] The three scanning approaches available for measuring cervical length—transabdominal, transvaginal, and translabial—are identical to those described for assessing placenta previa. The transabdominal approach tends to suffer from various impediments to visualizing the entire cervix, such as large maternal habitus, intervening presenting part, or a shadow from the pubic bone. A distended bladder provides a good acoustic window, but may create an artificially lengthened cervix by pushing the anterior wall of the lower uterine segment against the posterior wall. The cervical canal is visualized posterior to the angle of the bladder (Figure 15-22). If transabdominal scanning fails to provide an adequate view of the cervix, transvaginal or translabial scanning is required.

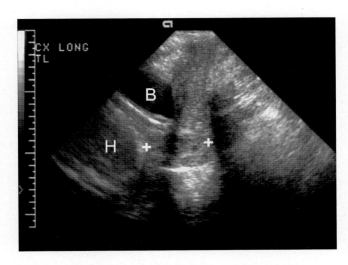

Figure 15-23. Translabial ultrasound showing the fetal head and bladder. The vaginal canal is visualized in the near field and the cervix lies at a right angle to the vaginal canal. Normal cervical length measurement (5 cm by cursors) is also indicated. B = bladder, H = fetal head.

The translabial approach to measuring cervical length generally requires more experience because proper image acquisition and interpretation are somewhat difficult (Figure 15-23). With the presenting part on the left side of the image, adjust the imaging plane so that the vagina courses directly away from the transducer between the bladder and the rectum. With the translabial approach, rectal gas can obscure the distal cervix and the pubic symphysis can obscure the proximal cervix. A left-side-down decubitus position and partially full bladder may facilitate translabial scanning. Translabial scanning of the cervix is particularly difficult prior to 20 weeks or with a posteriorly directed cervix.[51]

Regardless of the approach employed, cervical measurements are made in a sagittal plane, from internal os to external os. Begin by locating the endocervical canal, which may appear hypo- or hyperechoic. The internal os is located at the junction between the amniotic fluid and the endocervical canal. To locate the external os, visualize both the endocervical canal and the vaginal stripe. The cervix may be dynamic, especially in patients at risk for preterm labor, so observe it for 3–5 minutes before any measurements are made. In general, record the shortest cervical length (Figure 15-22). The normal cervix measures between 2.9 and 5 cm in length.[51]

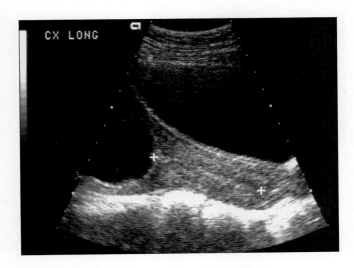

Figure 15-22. Normal cervical length measurement—transabdominal approach, sagittal plane. Correct measurements are indicated from the external os to the internal os (see cursors).

FETAL POSITION AND NUMBER

Perform assessment of the fetal number and position by point-of-care ultrasound carefully and systematically. Missing the diagnosis of a breech presentation or twins

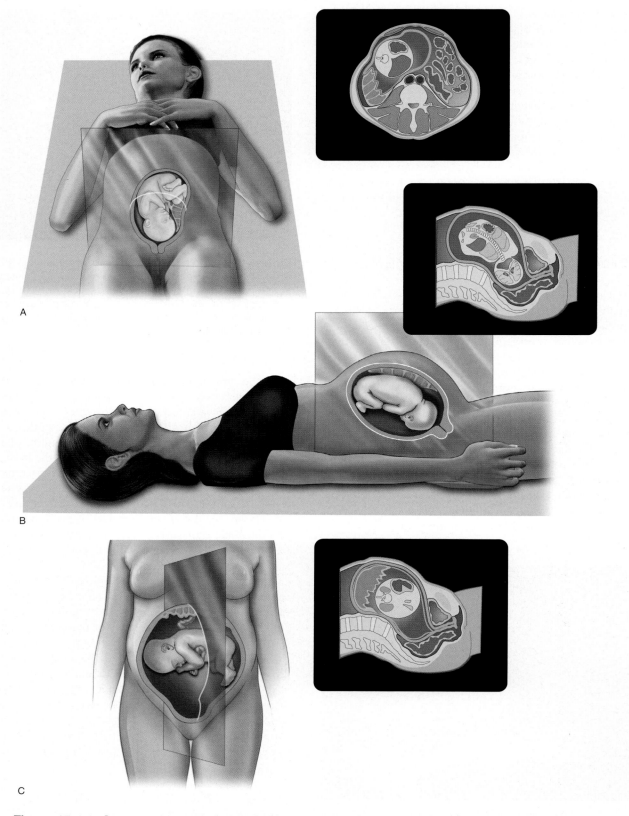

Figure 15-24. Sonographic technique for determining fetal position as described by Callen.[1] (A) Transverse scan of longitudinal lie, vertex presentation. (B) Sagittal scan of longitudinal lie, vertex presentation. (C) Sagittal scan of transverse lie.

may result in significant morbidity or mortality. Also, correctly interpreting sonographic images of a moving, near term fetus can be difficult. Document fetal position using the maternal bladder as a reference point. Scrutinize the presenting part in multiple imaging planes to confirm a cephalic or breech presentation versus a transverse lie. Deliberately scan the fetal spine in both a long axis and transverse plane (Figure 15-24). In the case of a known breech presentation, attempt to characterize it as a frank, complete, or footling breech (Figure 15-8). To avoid missing multiple gestations, systematically interrogate the entire uterine cavity and scan the full length of the fetus in two orthogonal planes.[45]

► COMMON ABNORMALITIES

PLACENTA PREVIA

Optimal imaging is usually obtained by transvaginal sonography with the endovaginal transducer no closer than 3 cm to the cervix,[41] and there have been no reported cases of transvaginal ultrasound precipitating or worsening hemorrhage. The sensitivity of transvaginal ultrasound for the diagnosis of placenta previa is nearly 100% (Figures 15-25 and 15-26).[36,37,93–95] In a study that is particularly relevant in the emergency setting, it was demonstrated that when the distance from the placenta edge to the internal os was >2 cm, a vaginal delivery was possible in every case, and a cesarean section for vaginal bleeding was required in 7 of 8 cases in which the distance was less than or equal to 2 cm.[93]

Translabial or transperineal sonography is an increasingly accepted alternative to transvaginal scanning.[33,96] As with transvaginal scanning, the os–

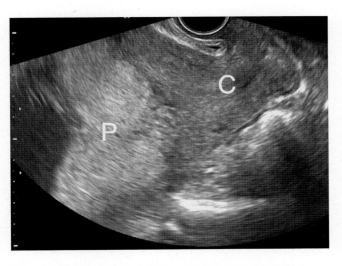

Figure 15-26. Transvaginal ultrasound showing a placenta (P) *completely* overlying the cervix (C).

placenta relationship is almost always well visualized, so it provides better diagnostic accuracy than transabdominal scanning[39,97] and a full bladder is not required (Figure 15-27). In the case of complete placenta previa, however, a transabdominal ultrasound may be diagnostic (Figure 15-28).

PLACENTAL ABRUPTION

The most consistent sonographic finding in placental abruption is hemorrhage and hematoma, the appearance of which will depend not only on its quantity and location but also on the timing of the ultrasound

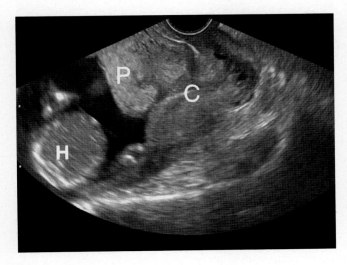

Figure 15-25. Transvaginal ultrasound showing a placenta (P) partially overlying the cervix (C). H = head.

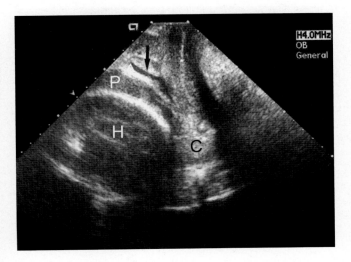

Figure 15-27. Translabial ultrasound showing the fetal head (H) overlying the internal os, and a low-lying placenta (P). The bladder is collapsed (black arrow) and the vaginal stripe is seen between the transducer and cervix (black C).

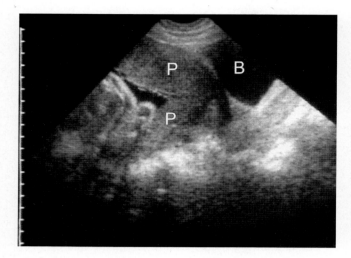

Figure 15-28. Placenta previa. Transabdominal longitudinal ultrasound demonstrates complete previa. B = bladder; P = placenta. (Courtesy of Gulfcoast Ultrasound)

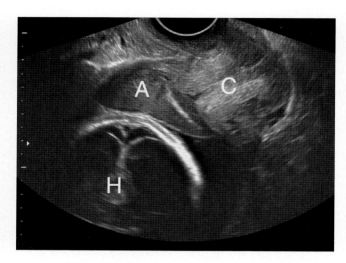

Figure 15-29. Hematoma from placental abruption (A) overlying cervix (C) — transvaginal ultrasound. H= fetal head.

in relation to the onset of hemorrhage (Figure 15-29). Acute hemorrhage appears isoechoic to slightly hyperechoic relative to the highly vascular normal placenta (Figure 15-30).[98,99] Gradually over 1–2 weeks, the hematoma becomes sonolucent and more easily distinguished from the adjacent placenta. Therefore, sonograms obtained 1–2 weeks after the onset of abruption may identify sonolucent hematomas that are not apparent on earlier studies. Isoechoic hematomas may be suspected if a portion of the placenta appears unusually thick or heterogeneous in texture. Because of their variable appearance, hematomas of abruption are occasionally mistaken for uterine leiomyomas. Another obstacle to sonographic diagnosis is that acute hemorrhage may spontaneously decompress to an adjacent area or into the vagina, such that the amount of retroplacental blood remaining is inadequate for visualization by ultrasound examination.[27,28] It cannot be overemphasized that ultrasound is not considered the primary diagnostic modality for placental abruption.

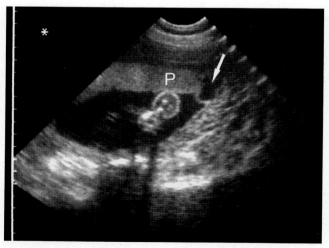

A

B

Figure 15-30. (A) Placental abruption. Transabdominal long-axis scan shows an anterior placenta with a contained marginal abruption (arrow). (B) Placental abruption. Transabdominal scan, sagittal plane, demonstrating retroplacental hematoma (H) in an 18-week pregnancy. The placenta (P) is located on the posterior wall. A myometrial contraction (M) of the anterior wall is evident. (A: Courtesy of Gulfcoast Ultrasound.)

▶ OTHER SELECTED ABNORMALITIES

UTERINE RUPTURE

Uterine rupture is most often diagnosed by ultrasound when it occurs in the setting of trauma.[11,100] Sonographic findings associated with uterine rupture include free intraperitoneal fluid, which may represent amniotic fluid or blood, and lack of fetal cardiac activity. In addition, the uterus may be empty, with the fetus found in the peritoneal cavity. There are numerous case reports describing the use of sonography to diagnose uterine rupture during labor.[101,102] Sonographic findings include a visible defect in the uterine wall, fetal membranes intact, and ballooning through the uterine wall, subchorionic hematoma adjacent to a scar in the lower uterine segment, and evidence of blood layering within amniotic fluid. When uterine rupture during labor is strongly suspected on clinical grounds, an ultrasound examination should not delay cesarean section.[10]

▶ PITFALLS

PLACENTA PREVIA

1. **Full bladder.** Although it provides an acoustic window, a full bladder may create a false impression of placenta previa by pushing the anterior wall of the lower uterine segment against the posterior wall, which makes the cervix appear longer and the internal os appear closer to the placenta (Figure 15-19).
2. **Myometrial contractions.** These contractions may lead to a false-positive diagnosis of placenta previa by thickening and shortening the lower uterine wall.
3. **Incomplete examination.** A false-negative diagnosis may result from failure to examine the entire lower uterine segment, thereby overlooking placental tissue that encroaches on the lateral aspect of the internal os.

PLACENTAL ABRUPTION

The diagnosis of placental abruption cannot be excluded by an ultrasound examination. The specificity of ultrasound is hampered by the common occurrence of prominent endometrial vessels, subchorionic cysts, and villous lakes. These sonolucent or hyperechoic structures may mimic the appearance of abruption but are of no clinical significance. Cardiotocographic monitoring is required for all patients when placental abruption is considered.

CERVICAL LENGTH ASSESSMENT

1. **Full bladder.** A full bladder may create an artificially lengthened cervix by pushing the anterior wall of the lower uterine segment against the posterior wall (Figure 15-19).
2. **Pseudodilatation of the cervix.** A contracting lower uterine segment can produce pseudodilatation of the cervix. This can be distinguished from true dilatation by the following findings: length of the cervix is >5 cm; the distal cervix is normal; there is thickened myometrium adjacent to the cervix; and the dilatation passes after the contraction ceases.[50]

GESTATIONAL AGE ESTIMATE

The main pitfalls for gestational age estimation are failure to carefully follow the guidelines for measurement; failure to recognize the inherent variability of estimates; and measurement of femur length in an oblique plane relative to the long axis of the bone, which may result in a falsely short measurement.

▶ CASE STUDIES

CASE 1

Patient Presentation

A 23-year-old obese woman presented to the ED with complaints of severe abdominal pain after a motor vehicle crash. The patient was the restrained driver in a rear impact collision. On arrival, her vital signs were blood pressure 80/50 mm Hg, heart rate 125 bpm, and respirations 22 per minute. Her physical examination revealed significant right-sided abdominal tenderness to palpation. The patient was unsure of her last menstrual period and indicated that she "might be pregnant."

Management Course

Upon arrival, a 1-L bolus of normal saline was initiated and blood was sent for type and crossmatch. The E-FAST exam revealed normal lung sliding bilaterally and no evidence of either pleural or pericardial fluid. However, the abdominal portion of the exam revealed a significant amount of free fluid in Morison's pouch. A rapid transabdominal pelvic ultrasound exam revealed an intrauterine pregnancy with a fetal heart rate of 186 bpm. The BPD of the fetal skull indicated a gestational age of 18 weeks.

Packed red blood cells and fresh frozen plasma were ordered and the patient was expeditiously transported to the operating room for exploratory laparotomy without further diagnostic testing.

Commentary

This case typified the axiom of "save the mother in order to save the baby." The initial maternal vital signs were indicative of shock. The patient's presentation demanded immediate investigation with the E-FAST exam. A significant amount of intraperitoneal free fluid raised the concern for solid organ injury. Exploratory laparotomy was indicated because the patient was hemodynamically unstable. Measurement of gestational age at 18 weeks indicated a previable fetus; therefore, all efforts were appropriately focused on resuscitation of the mother. The fetal heart rate was indicative of fetal distress; however, optimal therapy was treatment of maternal hypovolemic shock.

CASE 2

Patient Presentation

An 18-year-old pregnant woman, G1P0 with unknown gestational age, presented to the ED with complaints of painless vaginal bleeding and having not felt the baby move over the last several hours. The bleeding started 2 hours prior to presentation. She described changing four feminine pads during the last hour. The patient had not received any prenatal care. The hospital she presented to did not have an on-call obstetrician or labor and delivery capacity.

The patient's blood pressure was 100/78 mm Hg, heart rate 114 bpm, and respirations 14 per minute. She did not appear to be in distress. Physical examination revealed a gravid uterus with a fundal height 15 cm above the umbilicus. The abdomen was nontender to palpation.

Management Course

The emergency physician recognized the initial concern for placenta previa or abruption and deferred an initial pelvic exam. A large bore IV line was established and blood work was sent for CBC and type and screen. A transabdominal ultrasound was used initially to confirm fetal viability and gestational age. Fetal movement was noted and fetal heart rate confirmed at 140 bpm. Gestational age was estimated to be 36 weeks by femur length measurement. The transabdominal ultrasound exam failed to visualize the placental location. A transvaginal ultrasound was performed, and the placenta was visualized overlying the internal cervical os,

confirming the diagnosis of placenta previa (Figure 15-26).

The patient remained stable and was emergently transferred to the nearest hospital with an obstetrics staff. The patient had continued bleeding and underwent cesarean section the next morning.

Commentary

The physician in this case determined fetal viability by estimating gestational age using femur length, and by observing fetal cardiac activity and measuring the heart rate. Understanding that transvaginal ultrasound was safe and accurate in the setting of placenta previa, and that digital examination of the cervix was contraindicated, the physician was able to make the diagnosis of placenta previa. By determining fetal viability and gestational age and by making the diagnosis of placenta previa, the emergency physician was able to safely, efficiently, and accurately evaluate this patient. This allowed the patient to be appropriately transferred for specialized obstetrical care. It is critical for emergency providers to consider placenta previa as an etiology for vaginal bleeding in the second and third trimesters of pregnancy.

CASE 3

Patient Presentation

A 23-year-old woman, G2P1 at 32 weeks gestation, presented to the ED after having fallen down two steps. She fell on her side and did not strike her abdomen. She complained initially of abdominal cramping that resolved prior to arrival. Her blood pressure was 114/80 mm Hg, hear rate 98 bpm, respirations 14 per minute. Her abdominal examination revealed a gravid uterus with minimal tenderness to palpation and no other signs of trauma.

Management Course

The emergency physician performed a point-of-care E-FAST exam and did not note any abnormalities. Fetal viability and movement were noted on point-of-care transabdominal pelvic ultrasound, with a fetal heart rate of 158 bpm. No placental abruption was visualized. The patient was transferred to labor and delivery for cardiotocographic monitoring. After 6 hours without signs of contractions or fetal distress, the patient was discharged with routine obstetric follow-up.

Commentary

It is important to emphasize that placental abruption can occur in the setting of minor trauma. Abdominal pain may or may not be present. Emergency care providers must be keenly aware that ultrasound is not an accurate tool for making the diagnosis of abruption. Cardiotocographic monitoring can identify signs of fetal distress or subclinical uterine contractions that are not noticed by the patient or detectible on physical examination. Six hours of cardiotocographic monitoring without abnormal findings essentially rules out placental abruption.

▶ ACKNOWLEDGMENTS

The authors acknowledge Drs. Bradley Frazee, Chandra Auban, Katie Bakes, and Eric Snoey for their contributions to prior editions of this chapter, and Dr. Alfred Abuhamad and Stephanie Greenside for their contributions to this edition.

REFERENCES

1. Callen PW: The obstetric ultrasound examination. In: Callen PW, ed. *Ultrasonography in Obstetrics and Gynecology*. 5th ed. Philadelphia, PA: WB Saunders, 2008:3, 808–810.

2. Sanders RC: Legal problems related to obstetrical ultrasound. *Ann NY Acad Sci* 847:220–227, 1998.

3. Bioeffects Report Subcommittee: Bioeffects considerations for the safety of diagnostic ultrasound. *J Ultrasound Med* 7:s1–s38, 1998.

4. Stark CR, Orleans M, Haverkamp AD, et al.: Short and long-term risks after exposure to diagnostic ultrasound in utero. *Obstet Gyncecol* 63:194–200, 1984.

5. Salvensen KA, Bakketeig IS, Elk-Nes SH, et al.: Routine ultrasonography in utero and school performance at age 8–9 years. *Lancet* 62:339–342, 1992.

6. Kay HH, Spritzer CE: Preliminary experience with magnetic resonance imaging in patients with third trimester bleeding. *Obset Gynecol* 78:424, 1991.

7. Pearlman MD, Tintinalli JE, Lorenz RP: A prospective controlled study of outcome after trauma during pregnancy. *Am J Obstet Gynecol* 162:1502–1510, 1990.

8. Van De Kerkhove K, Johnson TRB: Bleeding in the second half of pregnancy: Maternal and fetal assessment. In: Pearlman MD, Tintinalli JE, eds. *Emergency Care of the Woman*. New York, NY: McGraw-Hill, 1998:77–98.

9. Anderson HF: Emergency management of preterm labor. In: Pearlman MD, Tintinalli JE, eds. *Emergency Care of the Woman*. New York, NY: McGraw-Hill, 1998:704.

10. Katz VL, Dotters DJ, Droegemueller W: Perimortem cesarean delivery. *Obstet Gynecol* 68:571–576, 1986.

11. Ma OJ, Mateer JR, DeBehnke DJ: Use of ultrasonography for the evaluation of pregnant trauma patients. *J Trauma* 40:665–668, 1996.

12. Galan HL, Pandipati S, Filly RA, et al.: Ultrasound evaluation of fetal biometry and normal and abnormal fetal growth. In: Callen PW, ed. *Ultrasonography in Obstetrics and Gynecology*. 5th ed. Philadelphia, PA: WB Saunders, 2008:225–247.

13. Waldenstrom U, Axelsson O, Nilsson S: A comparison of the ability of a sonographically measured biparietal diameter and the last menstrual period to predict the spontaneous onset of labor. *Obstet Gynecol* 76:336–338, 1990.

14. Benson CB, Doubilet PM: Sonographic prediction of gestational age: Accuracy of second and third trimester fetal measurements. *AJR* 157:1275–1277, 1991.

15. Shepard M, Filly RA: A standardized plane for biparietal diameter measurement. *J Ultrasound Med* 1:145–150, 1982.

16. Smith RS, Bottoms SF: Ultrasound prediction of neonatal survival in extremely low birth weight infants. *Am J Obstet Gynecol* 169:490–493, 1993.

17. Wolfson RN, Peisner DB, Chik LL, et al.: Comparison of biparietal diameter and femur length in the third trimester: Effects of gestational age and variation in fetal growth. *J Ultrasound Med* 5:145–149, 1986.

18. Goldstein RB, Filly RA, Simpson G: Pitfalls in femur length measurements. *J Ultrasound Med* 6:203–207, 1987.

19. Mahony BS, Callen PW, Filly RA: The distal femoral epiphyseal ossification center in the assessment of third-trimester menstrual age: Sonographic identification and measurement. *Radiology* 155:201–204, 1985.

20. Nathan L, Huddleston J: Acute abdominal pain in pregnancy. *Obstet Gynecol Clin North Am* 22:55, 1995.

21. Morrison LJ: General approach to the pregnant patient. In: Marx JA, Hockberger RS, Walls RM, et al., eds. *Rosen's Emergency Medicine: Concepts and Clinical Practice*. Philadelphia, PA: Mosby/Elsevier, 2010:2771–2774.

22. Cunningham F, McCubbin J: Appendicitis complicating pregnancy. *Obstet Gynecol* 45:415, 1975.

23. Mann F, Nathens A, Langer S, et al.: Communicating with the family the risks of medical radiation to conceptuses in victims of major blunt-force trauma. *J Trauma* 48(2):354, 2000.

24. Manas KJ: Hepatic hemorrhage without rupture in preeclampsia. *NEJM* 312:424, 1985.

25. Houry DE, Salhi BA: Acute complications of Pregnancy. In: Marx JA, Hockberger RS, Walls RM, et al., eds. *Rosen's Emergency Medicine: Concepts and Clinical Practice*. Philadelphia, PA: Mosby/Elsevier; 2010:2286–2296.

26. Nyberg DA, Cyr DR, Mack L: Sonographic spectrum of placental abruption. *AJR* 148:161, 1987.

27. Ananth CV, Savitz DA, Luther ER: Maternal cigarette smoking as a risk factor for placental abruption, placenta previa and uterine bleeding in pregnancy. *Am J Epidemiol* 144:881–889, 1996.

28. Scott J: Placenta previa and abruption. In: Dansforth J, ed. *Obstetrics and Gynecology*. 8th ed. Philadelphia, PA: Lippincott Williams & Wilkins, 1999:407.

29. Baron F, Hill WH: Placenta previa, placenta abruption. *Clin Obstet Gynecol* 41:527–532, 1998.

30. Wexler P, Gottesfeld K: Early diagnosis of placenta previa. *Obstet Gynecol* 54:231–234, 1979.

31. Rizos N, Doran TA, Miskin M, et al.: Natural history of placenta previa ascertained by diagnostic ultrasound. *Am J Obstet Gynecol* 133:287–291, 1979.

32. Iyasu S, Saftlas AK, Rowley DL, et al.: The epidemiology of placenta previa in the United States, 1979 through 1987. *Am J Obstet Gynecol* 168:1424–1429, 1993.

33. Hull AD, Resnik R: Placenta previa and abruptio placentae. In: Creasy F, Resnick R, eds. *Maternal–Fetal Medicine.* 6th ed. Philadelphia, PA: WB Saunders, 2009:725–733.

34. Faiz AS, Ananth CV: Etiology and risk factors for placenta previa: An overview and meta-analysis of observational studies. *J Matern Fetal Neonatal Med* 13(3):175–190, 2003.

35. Feldstein VA, Harris RD, Machin, GA: Ultrasound of the placenta and umbilical cord. In: Callen PW ed. *Ultrasonography in Obstetrics and Gynecology.* 4th ed. Philadelphia, PA: WB Saunders, 2008:725–726.

36. Leerentveld RA, Gilberts EC, Marinua JCW, et al.: Accuracy and safety of transvaginal sonographic placental localization. *Obstet Gynecol* 76:759–762, 1990.

37. Tan NH, Abu M, Woo JL, et al.: The role of transvaginal sonography in the diagnosis of placenta previa. *Aust NZ J Obstet Gynaecol* 35:42–45, 1995.

38. Artis AA, Bowie JD, Rosenberg ER, et al.: The fallacy of placental migration: Effect of sonographic techniques. *AJR* 144:799, 1985.

39. Hertzberg BS, Bowie JD, Carroll BA, et al.: Diagnosis of placenta previa during the third trimester: Role of transperineal sonography. *AJR* 159:83–87, 1992.

40. Brown JE, Thieme GA, Shah DM, et al.: Transabdominal and transvaginal endosonography: Evaluation of the cervix and lower uterine segment in pregnancy. *Am J Obstet Gynecol* 155:721–726, 1986.

41. Farine D, Fox HE, Jakobson S, et al.: Vaginal ultrasound for diagnosis of placenta previa. *Am J Obstet Gynecol* 159:566–569, 1988.

42. Pritchard J, Mason R, Coley M, et al.: Genesis of severe placental abruption. *Am J Obstet Gynecol* 108:22, 1970.

43. Landy HJ, Hinson K: Placenta abruption associated with cocaine use. *Repro Toxicol* 1:203, 1987.

44. Ananth CV, Smulian JC, Vintileos AM: Incidence of placental abruption in relation to cigarette smoking and hypertensive disorders during pregnancy: A meta analysis of observational studies. *Obstet Gynecol* 93:622, 1999.

45. Callen PW: The obstetric ultrasound examination. In: Callen PW, ed. *Ultrasonography in Obstetrics and Gynecology.* 5th ed. Philadelphia, PA: WB Saunders, 2008:14.

46. Kuhlman RS, Warsof S: Ultrasound of the placenta. *Clin Obstet and Gynecol* 39:519, 1996.

47. Ananth CV, Berkowitz G, Savitz D, et al.: Placental abruption and adverse outcomes. *JAMA* 282:1646, 1999.

48. Curet MJ, Schermer CR, et al.: Predictors of outcome in trauma during pregnancy: Identification of patients who can be monitored for less than 6 hours. *J Trauma* 49:18, 2000.

49. Cunningham FG, MacDonald PC, Leveno KJ, et al., eds: Parturition: Biomolecular and physiologic processes. In: Williams *Obstetrics.* 19th ed. Norwalk, CT: Appleton & Lange, 1993:297–361.

50. Berghella V, Tolosa JE, Kuhlman K, et al.: Cervical ultrasonography compared with manual examinations a predictor of preterm delivery. *Am J Obstet Gynecol* 177(4):723, 1997.

51. Bega G, Berghella V: Ultrasound evaluation of the cervix. In: Callen PW, ed. *Ultrasonography in Obstetrics and Gynecology.* 5th ed. Philadelphia, PA: WB Saunders, 2008:699–708.

52. Sonek JD, Iams JD, Blumenfeld M, et al.: Measurement of cervical length in pregnancy: Comparison between vaginal ultrasound and digital examination. *Obstet Gymecol* 76(2):172–175, 1990.

53. Iams JE, Goldenberg RL, Meis PJ, et al.: The length of the cervix and the risk of spontaneous premature delivery. *N Engl J Med* 334:567, 1996.

54. Timor-Tritsch LE, Boozarjomehri F, Masakowski Y, et al.: Can a "snapshot" sagittal view of the cervix by transvaginal ultrasonography predict active preterm labor? *Am J Obstet Gynecol* 174:990, 1996.

55. Crane JM, Van Den Hof M, Armson BA, et al.: Transvaginal ultrasound in the prediction of preterm delivery: Singleton and twin gestations. *Obstet Gynecol* 90:357, 1997.

56. Anderson HF: Transvaginal and transabdominal ultrasonography of the uterine cervix during pregnancy. *J Clin Ultrasound* 19:77, 1991.

57. Mahony BS, Nyberg DA, Luthy DA, et al.: Translabial ultrasound of the third-trimester uterine cervix. *J Ultrasound Med* 9:717, 1990.

58. Berghella V, Kuhlman K, Weiner S, et al.: Cervical funneling: Sonographic criteria predictive of preterm delivery. *Ultrsound Obstet Gynecol* 10:161, 1997.

59. Mercer BM, Goldenberg RL, Meis PJ, et al.: The preterm prediction study: Prediction of preterm premature rupture of membranes through clinical findings and ancillary testing. The National Institute of Child Health and Human Development maternal–fetal medicine units network. *Am J Obstet Gynecol* 183(3):738, 2000.

60. Rageth JC, Kernen B, Saurenmann E, et al.: Premature contractions: Possible influence of sonographic measurement of cervical length on clinical management. *Ultrasound Obstet Gynecol* 9:183, 1997.

61. Fontenot T, Compbell B, Mitchell-Tutt E, et al.: Radiographic evaluation of breech presentation: Is it necessary? *Ultrasound Obstet Gynecol* 10:338, 1997.

62. Benson CB, Doubilet PM: Sonography of multiple gestations. *Radiol Clin North Am* 28:149, 1990.

63. McGrath-Ling M: Fetal well-being and fetal death. In: Sanders RC, Miner NS, eds. *Clinical Sonography: A Practical Guide.* 3rd ed. Philadelphia, PA: Lippincott, 1998:173.

64. Manning FA: Dynamic ultrasound-based fetal assessment: The fetal biophysical profile score. *Clin Obstet Gynecol* 38:26, 1995.

65. Walkinshaw SA: Fetal biophysical profile scoring. *Br J Hosp Med* 47:444, 1992.

66. Manning FA: Fetal biophysical profile. *Obstet Gynecol Clin North Am* 26(4):557, 1999.

67. Babbitt NE: Antepartum fetal surveillance. *SDJ Med* 49:403, 1996.

68. Garmel SH, D'Alton ME: Diagnostic ultrasound in pregnancy: An overview. *Semin Perinatol* 18(3):117, 1994.

69. Manning FA, Morrison I, Harman CR, et al.: Fetal assessment by fetal BPS: Experience in 19,221 referred high-risk pregnancies: The false negative rate by frequency and etiology. *Am J Obstet Gynecol* 157:880, 1987.

70. Alfirevic Z, Neilson JP: Biophysical profile for fetal assessment in high-risk pregnancies. *Cochrane Database Syst Rev* (2):CD000038, 2000.

71. Ghidine A, Salafia CM, Kirn V, et al.: Biophysical profile in predicting acute ascending infection in preterm rupture

of membranes before 32 weeks. *Obstet Gynecol* 96:201, 2000.

72. Lewis DF, Adair CD, Weeks JW, et al.: A randomized clinical trial of daily nonstress testing versus biophysical profile in the management of preterm premature rupture of membranes. *Am J Obstet Gynecol* 181:1495, 1999.

73. Pearlman MD, Tintinalli JE, Lorenz RP: Blunt trauma in pregnancy. *N Eng J Med* 323:1609–1613, 1990.

74. Varner MW: Maternal mortality in Iowa from 1952–1986. *Surg Gynecol Obstet* 168:555–562, 1989.

75. Agran PF, Dunkle DE, Winn DG, et al.: Fetal death in motor vehicle accidents. *Ann Emerg Med* 16:1355–1358, 1987.

76. Sugrue ME, O'Connor MC, D'Amours SK: Trauma during pregnancy. *ADF Health* 5:24–28, 2004.

77. Shah KH, Simons RK, Holbrook T, et al.: Trauma in pregnancy: Maternal and fetal outcomes. *J Trauma* 45:83–86, 1998.

78. Curet MJ, Schermer CR, Demarest GB, et al.: Predictors of outcome in trauma during pregnancy: Identification of patients who can be monitored for less than 6 hours. *J Trauma* 49:18–24; discussion 24–26, 2000.

79. Theodorou DA, Velmahos GC, Souter I, et al.: Fetal death after trauma in pregnancy. *Am Surg* 66:809–812, 2000.

80. Baerga-Varela Y, Zietlow S, Bannon M, et al.: Trauma in pregnancy. *Mayo Clin Proc* 75:1243–1248, 2000.

81. Hoff WS, D'Amelio LF, Tinkoff GH, et al.: Maternal predictors of fetal demise in trauma during pregnancy. *Gynecol Obstet Surg* 172:175–180, 1991.

82. Rogers FB, Rozycki GS, Osler TM, et al.: A multi-institutional study of factors associated with fetal death in injured pregnant patients. *Arch Surg* 134:1274–1277, 1999.

83. Weingold AB: Appendicitis in pregnancy. *Clin Obstet Gynecol* 26:801, 1983.

84. Mourad J, et al: Appendicitis in pregnancy: New information that contradicts long-held clinical beliefs. *Am J Obstet Gynecol* 185:259, 2000.

85. Lim HK, Bae SH, Seo GS: Diagnosis of acute appendicitis in pregnant women: Value of sonography. *AJR* 159:539, 1992.

86. Abu-Yousef MM, Bleichen JJ, Maher JW, et al.: High-resolution sonography of acute appendicitis. *AJR* 149:53, 1987.

87. Gomez A, Wood M: Acute appendicitis during pregnancy. *Am J Surg* 137:180, 1979.

88. Mahmoodian S: Appendicitis complicating pregnancy. *South Med J* 85:19, 1992.

89. Williamson S, Williamson M: Cholecystosonography in pregnancy. *J Ultrasound* 3:329, 1984.

90. Simon JA: Biliary tract disease and related surgical disorders during pregnancy. *Clin Obstet Gynecol* 26:810, 1983.

91. Hassan SS, Chaiworapongsa T, Vaisbuch E, et al.: In: Fleischer AC, Toy E, Lee W, eds. *Sonography in Obstetrics & Gynecology: Principles and Practice.* 7th ed. New York, NY: McGraw-Hill, 2011:816–819.

92. Hoddick W, Mahoney B, Collen P, et al.: Placental thickness. *J Ultrasound Med* 4:479, 1985.

93. Oppenheimer LW, Farine D, Ritchie K, et al.: What is a low-lying placenta? *Am J Obstet Gynecol* 165:1036–1038, 1991.

94. Taipale P, Hiilesmaa V, Ylostalo P, et al.: Diagnosis of placenta previa by transvaginal sonographic screening at 12–16 weeks in a nonselected population. *Obstet Gynecol* 89:364–367, 1997.

95. Laurie MR, Smith RS, Treadwell CH, et al.: The use of second-trimester transvaginal sonography to predict placenta previa. *Ultrasound Obstet Gynecol* 8(5):337–340, 1996.

96. Doubilet PM, Benson CB: Emergency obstetrical ultrasonography. *Semin Roentgenol* 33:339–350, 1998.

97. Dawson WB, Dumas MD, Romano WM, et al.: Translabial ultrasonography and placenta previa: Does measurement of the os–placenta distance predict outcome? *J Ultrasound Med* 15:441–446, 1996.

98. Nyberg DA, Mack LA, Benedetti TJ: Placental abruption and placental hemorrhage: Correlation of sonographic findings with fetal outcome. *Radiology* 358:357, 1987.

99. Nyberg DA, Cyr DR, Mack L: Sonographic spectrum of placental abruption. *AJR* 148:161, 1987.

100. Ripley D: Uterine emergencies: Atony, inversion and rupture. *Obstet Gynecol Clin* 26:419–434, 1999.

101. Shrout AB, Kopelman JN: Ultrasonographic diagnosis of uterine dehiscence during pregnancy. *J Ultrasound Med* 14:399–402, 1995.

102. Gale JT, Mahony BS, Bowie JD: Sonographic features of rupture of the pregnant uterus. *J Ultrasound Med* 5:713–714, 1996.

CHAPTER 16

Gynecologic Concepts

J. Christian Fox and Michael J. Lambert

Female patients with acute lower abdominal or pelvic pain often represent a diagnostic challenge. The differential diagnosis is broad (Table 16-1), and the workup often requires multiple diagnostic tests. Ultrasound is the initial diagnostic imaging modality of choice in the majority of cases. Point-of-care ultrasound, performed and interpreted by the clinician, and completed at the time of the initial physical examination, helps narrow the differential diagnosis and may eliminate the need for further diagnostic testing.

▶ CLINICAL CONSIDERATIONS

Imaging the pelvis is a crucial step in the evaluation of women with lower abdominal pain or pelvic pain. Accurate management is predicated on choosing the most effective diagnostic tool. Four diagnostic modalities are available for evaluating the pelvis: ultrasound, CT, MRI, and laparoscopy.

Ultrasound has proven to be a rapid, noninvasive, portable, repeatable, inexpensive, and accurate method for visualizing and diagnosing pathology within the pelvis. Several advantages over CT, MRI, and even the bimanual pelvic examination have made ultrasound the first-line diagnostic imaging modality in patients with acute pelvic pain or masses.[1-3] Both transabdominal and endovaginal ultrasound can be used by the clinician at the bedside during the initial physical examination. The use of point-of-care ultrasound has far-reaching benefits to patient care. It may identify specific diseases in the differential diagnosis and often elimi-

nates the need for expensive and time-consuming diagnostic tests (Figure 16-1). In addition, ultrasound does not expose patients to ionizing radiation. Since the clinician performs the point-of-care ultrasound examination,

▶ TABLE 16-1. DIFFERENTIAL DIAGNOSIS OF LOWER ABDOMINAL PAIN IN FEMALE PATIENTS

GI
Appendicitis
Inflammatory bowel disease
Irritable bowel syndrome
Constipation
Gastroenteritis
Diverticulitis

URINARY TRACT
Cystitis
Pyelonephritis
Nephrolithiasis

REPRODUCTIVE
Ectopic pregnancy
Intrauterine pregnancy
Pelvic inflammatory disease
Tubo-ovarian abscess
Ovarian cyst
Hemorrhagic functional cysts
Ovarian torsion
Mittelschmerz
Dysmenorrhea
Endometriosis

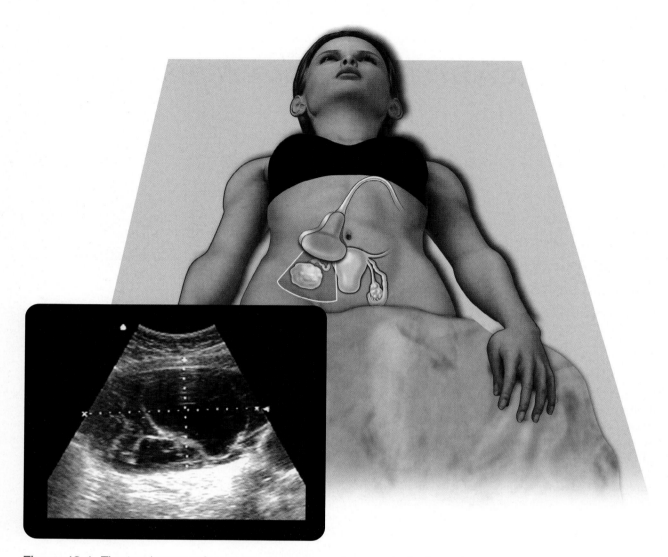

Figure 16-1. The top image refers to the transverse placement of a large footprint curved array transducer. The bottom image depicts a complex ovarian mass, one of the many entities that lies within the differential diagnosis for women presenting with acute pelvic pain.

patients perceive this as more time spent with their physician. This serves to improve patient satisfaction, provides them with more time to ask questions, and ultimately increases their confidence in the physician and their understanding of the diagnosis. Another advantage unique to ultrasound is the ability of color flow Doppler to evaluate pelvic organs for adequacy of blood flow.

The main disadvantage of ultrasound with respect to the other imaging modalities is its limited scope. Other imaging modalities, such as CT and MRI, may yield valuable information about other organ system pathology and the extent to which a disease process may have progressed. Also, sonograms are sometimes technically inadequate due to interference from bowel gas.

While CT is used routinely for the preoperative evaluation of masses that are suspicious for malignancy, it is generally considered a second-line imaging modality to

ultrasound for the evaluation of pelvic pain. The advantage of CT is its ability to image the full extent of a large adnexal lesion that cannot be visualized in its entirety with sonography alone. Another advantage of CT is its usefulness in diagnosing GI sources of pain, such as appendicitis and diverticulitis. The major disadvantages to CT are radiation exposure and cost. CT emits ionizing radiation.[4]

Although MRI is also considered a second-line imaging modality, it has several advantages over CT and ultrasound. MRI does not expose the patient to radiation and provides more detailed information for the detection of subtle tissue differentiation of pelvic organs. MRI has better tissue resolution than ultrasound, and is therefore more accurate in diagnosing pelvic inflammatory disease (PID) and pelvic masses. A 1999 study compared MRI with endovaginal ultrasound for the diagnosis of laparoscopy-proven PID. Of the 21 patients proven to have PID, MRI diagnosed 20 (95%) patients while endovaginal ultrasound correctly diagnosed 17 (81%) patients.[5] Many of the same disadvantages of CT—cost, availability, lack of portability—apply to MRI as well.

While laparoscopy remains the gold standard for the diagnosis of PID and pelvic masses, its use may not be readily available or justified in screening patients with vague symptoms. It is invasive, costly, time-consuming, results in scarring, and requires the small but real risk of general anesthesia. The advantage of laparoscopy, however, is the ability to reveal other pathologic conditions that have been misdiagnosed as PID. In one study, 12% of patients diagnosed with PID revealed other pathologic findings during laparoscopy, such as appendicitis or endometriosis.[6] Another advantage of laparoscopy is the ability to intraoperatively intervene in a pathologic process, such as the untwisting or resection of a torsed ovary, drainage of an abscess, or appendectomy.

▶ CLINICAL INDICATIONS

Clinical indications for performing pelvic ultrasound include:

- Acute pelvic pain
- Acute pelvic inflammatory disease
- Evaluation of pelvic or adnexal masses

ACUTE PELVIC PAIN

Acute pelvic pain in women is a common complaint in the emergency or ambulatory care setting. The differential diagnosis is vast. Although life-threatening conditions such as ectopic pregnancy are in the differential, the majority of patients can be treated and discharged home. While the definitive evaluation of these patients ultimately may involve CT, pelvic sonography is the diagnostic imaging modality indicated in their initial evaluation.

Ovarian Torsion

This entity should be considered in the differential diagnosis of any woman with lower abdominal pain (Table 16-2). Ovarian torsion is a GYN emergency that can result in both reproductive and hormonal compromise if not promptly diagnosed and treated. Because the diagnosis is often elusive and sufficiently delayed, detorsion of the ovary is rarely an option. A twisting of the ovarian attachments through the utero-ovarian ligament to the uterus and through the infundibulopelvic ligament to the pelvic sidewall results in congestion of the ovarian parenchyma and eventual hemorrhagic infarction from decreased ovarian blood supply.[7] The "classic" symptoms of acute, severe, unilateral lower abdominal or

▶ **TABLE 16-2. DIFFERENTIAL DIAGNOSIS OF OVARIAN TORSION**

Appendicitis
Adnexal mass
Pelvic mass
Myoma
Ectopic pregnancy
Tubo-ovarian abscess
Ruptured viscus

pelvic pain are present only in approximately one-third of the patients with confirmed ovarian torsion. Ovarian torsion is frequently missed on the preoperative diagnosis; the two most common incorrect preoperative diagnoses are tubo-ovarian abscess (TOA) and ruptured corpus luteum cyst.[8]

Torsion can occur in normal ovaries, but this would be an unusual occurrence. In general, for torsion to take place, the ovary or tube must be enlarged such as in the case of a mass or cyst as part of or immediately adjacent to the ovary or fallopian tube. These masses are thought to act as a fulcrum by which torsion can propagate. One study demonstrated that ovarian torsion was associated with palpable adnexal masses in over 90% of adults compared with only 50% of children.[9] Others reported that a unilaterally enlarged ovary with small peripherally located cysts (1–6 mm) was the most common finding (56%) in young and adolescent girls.[10] In 1985, it was reported that ovarian masses were associated with cases of torsion in only 50% of patients. Pregnancy appears to be a risk factor as well; 20% of all cases can be found to occur during pregnancy.[8]

Abnormal blood flow detected by Doppler sonography is highly predictive of ovarian torsion and is therefore useful in the diagnosis of ovarian torsion. Failure to identify arterial waveforms is highly suggestive of ovarian torsion. When normal flow is detected by Doppler sonography, it does not necessarily *exclude* ovarian torsion. In fact, ovarian torsion is missed in 60% of these cases, and time to diagnosis is therefore delayed. In patients undergoing hormonal therapy for ovarian stimulation, the sensitivity of Doppler for ovarian torsion increases to 75%.[11] Despite being intuitively similar to other organs, such as the testicle, lack of blood supply to the ovary cannot be adequately excluded using Doppler. The reason for this is twofold. First, Doppler flow may be present in one part of the ovary (peripheral or central) but not in the other because the ovary has a dual blood supply. Second, thrombosis of venous structures produces the symptoms of ovarian torsion prior to the arterial system becoming occluded. While some authors have suggested that absent blood flow on spectral Doppler and color Doppler is specific for torsion,[12,13] others suggest that observing blood flow to the ovary should not be relied upon to definitively exclude this diagnosis.[14] One study reported that the presence of a Doppler signal was present in 9 of 14 patients ultimately proven to have ovarian torsion.[10]

Gray scale findings may be useful in diagnosing ovarian torsion by identifying a large ovary with enlarged follicles or an enlarged complex cystic adnexal mass. Conversely, it has been suggested that normal ovarian size and texture may be helpful in excluding this diagnosis. One study evaluated 41 patients suspected of having ovarian torsion who had undergone transabdominal ultrasound. Of the 11 patients who had ovarian torsion proven at surgery, 7 were correctly diagnosed by ultrasound. Ovarian enlargement was detected in all 11 patients. This study (albeit a very small sample size) yielded a positive predictive value of 87.5%. In the other 28 patients, sonography correctly excluded the diagnosis, yielding a specificity of 93%. All patients were followed for 63 months on an outpatient basis.[7]

Vaginal Conditions

Some GYN procedures involve instrumentation that result in postoperative complications. These patients may present with vaginal bleeding, acute pelvic pain, and unstable vital signs. Ultrasound can play a crucial role in the timely diagnosis and management of these patients. For example, ultrasound can localize and diagnose a vaginal hematoma in a hypotensive patient who recently underwent a dilatation and curettage procedure. Typically, the ultrasound examination is performed transabdominally in an attempt to localize the hematoma within the vaginal tissue planes.

ACUTE PELVIC INFLAMMATORY DISEASE

Acute PID, defined as an infection in the upper genital tract, represents a spectrum of disease entities, including any combination of endometritis, salpingitis, oophoritis, pelvic peritonitis, and TOA.[15] More than 1 million women are diagnosed with PID annually and 25% of them proceed to suffer at least one sequela of PID, which include infertility, ectopic pregnancy, or chronic abdominal pain.[16] The severity of clinical presentation corresponds poorly with the damage to the fallopian tubes. Many young women with PID have mild and vague symptoms.[17] Therefore, the diagnosis of PID on clinical grounds has been notoriously difficult and was shown to be only 66% accurate in one study.[18] It is not surprising that endovaginal ultrasound was demonstrated to be superior to bimanual examination alone in the diagnosis of findings consistent with PID.[19]

Early sonographic signs of PID are increased adnexal volume and periovarian inflammation with fluid collections. On ultrasound, this appears as structures that lack the distinct margins that are normally identified. Another sonographic sign of PID is the decreased ability of the ovary to slide smoothly in the adnexa (sliding organ sign) when the ultrasound transducer is inserted and withdrawn from the vagina. This sign suggests that the ovary has been tethered to the fallopian tube by inflammatory adhesions. These sonographic findings were correlated with laparoscopic evidence of periovarian exudates and adhesions.[20] In 1992, it was demonstrated that sonographic evidence of free fluid had a sensitivity of 77% and specificity of 79% in culture-proven PID. Finally, the presence of "polycystic-like" ovaries containing increased stroma with several follicles scattered throughout the stroma has been found to be indicative of PID; one study demonstrated a sensitivity of 100% and a specificity of 71% for this finding.[21]

Another study evaluated four ultrasound markers to suggest evidence of PID: free fluid in the cul-de-sac, multicystic ovaries, visualization of fallopian tube or tubal fluid, and presence of an adnexal mass or TOA. This study found that in patient populations that have a high prevalence of PID, an endovaginal ultrasound examination positive for these markers is useful for suggesting the diagnosis of PID, and thus helping avoid laparoscopy. A negative ultrasound examination, however, should not be viewed by the clinician as being reliable for excluding the diagnosis of PID in a patient who appears clinically ill. In this subset of patients, laparoscopy may be required to make the diagnosis.[22]

EVALUATION OF PELVIC OR ADNEXAL MASSES

Hydrosalpinx

Since hydrosalpinx is present only in abnormal conditions such as PID, TOA, or ectopic pregnancy, its finding should immediately raise a red flag. Fluid in the fallopian tube can be encountered after tubal ligation.

Tubo-Ovarian Abscess

Women who present with a pelvic mass may have a TOA, tubo-ovarian complex, uterine fibroid, hydrosalpinx, ovarian cyst, or a variety of other complex adnexal masses. Clinicians cannot rely solely on their bimanual examination to accurately detect pelvic masses; 70% of pelvic masses found on ultrasound examination were initially missed during the bimanual examination.[23] A pelvic mass detected on physical examination is an indication for a pelvic ultrasound examination. If a cystic structure is found within the ovary, this may provide a finding for the clinician to explain the patient's symptoms and a clear disposition that often negates further workup during that visit. The presence of a cystic structure on the ovary, however, is very common and does not exclude the presence of other concomitant pathology. Furthermore, if the cyst is large enough, typically over 3.5 cm, ovarian torsion may need to be considered.

Pelvic ultrasonography is indicated in cases of severe, recurrent PID with or without the presence of a mass on physical examination. It is critically important that a distinction be made between PID and TOA to direct specific treatment regimens. Since the same clinical diagnostic difficulties of PID apply to TOA, ultrasound plays a crucial role in the diagnosis. Understanding that the development of a TOA occurs through a stepwise fashion will aid the clinician with the ultrasound examination. The first stage involves inflammation of the tubal mucosa. The wall eventually thickens and purulent material fills the lumen and spills into the cul-de-sac. If either end of the fallopian tube becomes blocked, a pyosalpinx can occur. As the pressure within the lumen increases, the walls are stretched thin and the tube becomes distended. In some patients, the process stops at this stage, resulting in chronic hydrosalpinx. When the remnants of the endosalpingeal folds become fibrotic, they appear as spokes outlined by anechoic fluid ("cogwheel sign"). When interrogated using power Doppler, marked hyperemia is seen throughout this complex structure. As the acute inflammatory process continues to proceed, it erodes through the distended wall. If the ovary has a recent defect from the ruptured corpus luteum, it becomes exposed to this inflammation and purulent material enters this space. The final stage of abscess formation occurs when the pus walls itself off, fusing the tube and ovary together.

The incidence of PID developing into TOA has been reported to be between 4%[24] and 30%.[25] TOA requires a different treatment regimen than PID since it forms an abscess, tends to be polymicrobial, and consists of anaerobes.[26] Since the mid-1970s, ultrasonography has been shown to be an accurate, sensitive, and noninvasive imaging technique for diagnosing TOA.[27,28] Furthermore, serial ultrasound examinations have proven to be useful in following a TOA that is managed nonoperatively. Pelvic ultrasound also assists in the selection of the most effective treatment regimen.[26,29] In a study of 106 patients with clinically suspected PID, ultrasound findings demonstrated 19 patients with pyosalpinx and 4 patients with hydrosalpinx. These 23 patients had their medical therapy directly altered as a result of the endovaginal ultrasound.[30]

Uterine Fibroids

Uterine fibroids represent the most common GYN tumor. Leiomyomas start as a mass of smooth muscle proliferation in a whorled spherical configuration. Atrophy and vascular compromise eventually ensue, which result in necrosis and calcification. These patients can present with pelvic pain, dysuria, dysmenorrhea, constipation, or low back pain (from compression of lumbar plexus).

▶ ANATOMICAL CONSIDERATIONS

To understand the pelvic anatomy, it may be helpful to think of the pelvis as two distinct regions: the true pelvis and false pelvis. The true pelvis has a basin-shaped contour and is bounded anteriorly by the pubic symphysis and pubic rami. It is bounded posteriorly by the sacrum and coccyx and inferiorly by the perineal musculature. The false pelvis is located superior to the true pelvis. The abdominal wall represents its anterior border, the iliac bones define its lateral border, and the sacral promontory outlines its posterior border. The empty bladder lies within the true pelvis and, when distended, enters the false pelvis (Figure 16-2A and B).

The uterus is a thick-walled, muscular structure whose shape can vary with cyclical menstrual changes and distention of the bladder. Typically, the uterus is found in the anteverted position in its relationship with the bladder; in 25% of women, it is retroflexed. During the reproductive years, the uterus measures up to 7 cm × 4 cm × 5 cm. The postmenopausal uterus measures 7 cm in length and 1–2 cm in transverse. The endometrial thickness varies with the menstrual cycle from 6 mm to less than 1 mm following menstruation.

The ovaries are elliptical-shaped structures and are found in a range of positions in the parous woman. In the nulliparous woman, the ovaries are typically located on the posterolateral wall of the true pelvis, adjacent to the internal iliac vessels. The menstrual cycle is categorized into two phases: the proliferative phase, which culminates in ovulation, followed by the secretory phase, which ends in menstruation. Cystic follicles regularly occur during the proliferative phase and are not technically termed a "cyst" until they reach a diameter of 2.5 cm. A corpus luteum then forms at the site of ovulation during the secretory phase, but rarely lasts for more than 6 weeks in the nonpregnant patient. Therefore, in the absence of ovulation, these cysts cannot occur. Once ruptured, the only evidence of their existence may be the presence of free fluid in the posterior cul-de-sac or near the ovary.[31]

The pouch of Douglas is a term that refers to the potential space in the posterior cul-de-sac of the pelvis. It consists of the peritoneal reflection posterior to the uterus and anterior to the rectosigmoid colon. Because this is the most dependent portion of the supine woman, a trace of free fluid is normally seen here, especially in the 5 days prior to menstruation.[32] The anterior cul-de-sac lies between the bladder (anterior) and the uterus (posterior). Since this potential space is not dependent, it only contains free fluid when a significant amount is present in the pelvis.

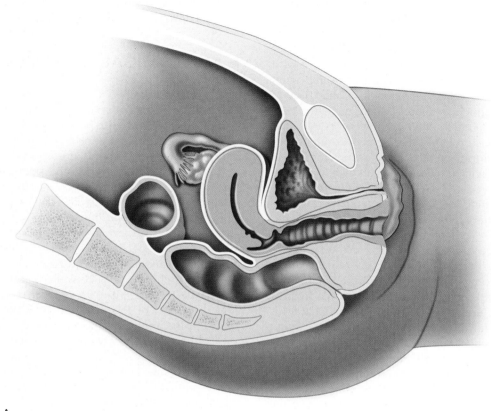

A

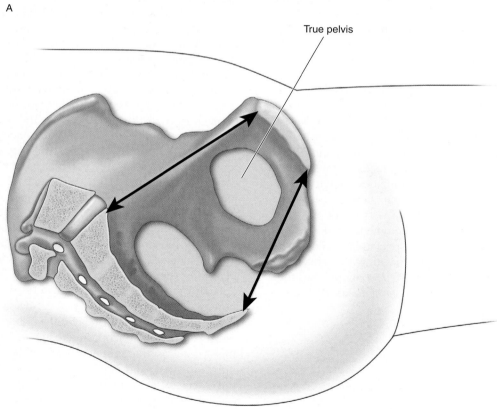

True pelvis

B

Figure 16-2. (A) Normal pelvic anatomy and (B) borders of the true pelvis.

► GETTING STARTED

Foremost in importance is patient positioning. Failure to allow for a full range of motion of the transducer handle will often result in inadequate imaging. Allowing the buttocks to come to the edge of a lithotomy table while the feet are securely placed in stirrups is the ideal position for endovaginal scanning. In lieu of an available GYN gurney, one can elevate the patient's hips by placing several towels under the buttocks. This will allow for full transducer handle movement when attempting to visualize anterior structures. The second most important factor in endovaginal ultrasound is instructing the patient to empty her bladder. Even small amounts of urinary volume can move the uterus and ovaries away from the tip of the endovaginal transducer and signifi-

cantly alter image quality. Conversely, scanning via the transabdominal route is facilitated by urinary bladder volume.

Endovaginal pelvic ultrasound may initially be confusing, but it is actually more straightforward than transabdominal pelvic ultrasound. It is important to learn the standard transducer orientations and understand the very different views used for transabdominal versus endovaginal imaging. Transabdominal views are usually obtained with a full bladder (Figure 16-3A,B), and endovaginal views are usually obtained with an empty bladder (Figure 16-3C,D). It is crucial to understand that an anteverted uterus changes position significantly depending on the volume of urine in the bladder. This explains how the tip of the transducer can touch the lateral wall of the uterus during endovaginal scanning

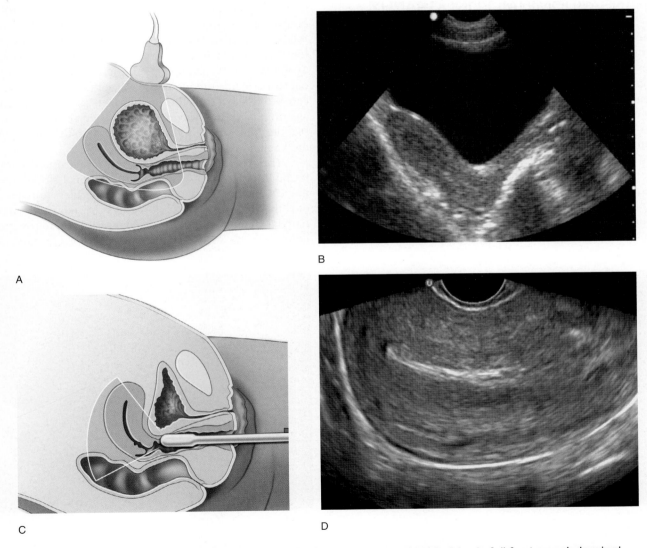

A

B

C

D

Figure 16-3. (A) Position of the uterus and imaging sector when the bladder is full for transabdominal ultrasound and (C) empty for endovaginal ultrasound. Comparison of ultrasound resolution of the uterus in the same patient using transabdominal (B) and endovaginal (D) longitudinal views.

despite the fact that the vaginal stripe and the body of the uterus are not adjacent structures in transabdominal images.

The ability to touch the pelvic organs with the tip of the transducer allows the use of higher frequency transducers, which produce significantly better images than the transabdominal approach. The key to endovaginal ultrasound is to consider the body of the uterus the main landmark and then find other structures based on their positions relative to the body of the uterus. Using this simple approach can make endovaginal ultrasound easier to learn.

▶ TECHNIQUE AND NORMAL ULTRASOUND FINDINGS

TRANSABDOMINAL SONOGRAPHY

The advantage of transabdominal sonography is that it is rapid and noninvasive, and provides a good overall view of the pelvis. The disadvantage is that the pelvic organs are several centimeters away from the ultrasound transducer head and a lower frequency transducer must be utilized.

Employing transabdominal sonography, place the transducer on the lower aspect of the midline abdominal wall just superior to the pubic symphysis (Video 16-1: Female Pelvic Transabdominal Normal). A low-frequency transducer (3.5–5.0 MHz range) is advantageous to penetrate to the desired depth in the pelvis. Filling the bladder will likewise enhance the quality of sonographic images by displacing the air-filled bowel

out of the true pelvis thereby aligning the solid organs perpendicular to the transducer. Avoid overfilling the bladder as the bladder can actually push the uterus and ovaries out of the way enough to make visualization difficult.

Scan the pelvic structures in two planes: longitudinal and transverse. In the longitudinal plane, place the transducer vertically with the indicator toward the patient's head (Figure 16-4A). In this plane, the bladder has a triangular appearance. The uterus is pear-shaped and typically measures 5–7 cm in length in the menstruating female (Figure 16-4B). The initial goal is to visualize the midline of the uterus, which is not necessarily in the midline of the pelvis, so the transducer may need to be adjusted when the uterus is tilted off the midline. The endometrial stripe is a thin hyperechoic line running down the center of the uterus along its length, and it fluctuates with the menstrual cycle. It appears thin and less echogenic just following menses in the proliferative phase, and becomes thick and more echogenic following ovulation during the secretory phase. In this longitudinal plane, the endometrial stripe is visualized as the transducer is fanned from left to right. The vaginal stripe that is unique to the transabdominal approach can be visualized in the longitudinal plane. It appears as a thin echo bright curved stripe seen posterior to the bladder. The cervix is visualized between the uterus and the vagina.

The majority of women have an anteverted uterus found angulated 90° to the midline vaginal stripe when the bladder is empty. Filling the bladder straightens out the uterus so that it comes to lie in a more parallel alignment to the vaginal stripe. A retroverted uterus can be seen extending in an opposite direction

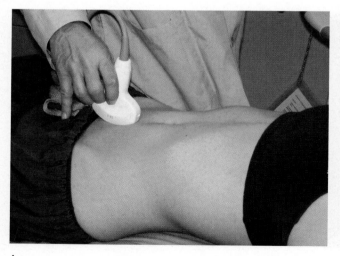

A

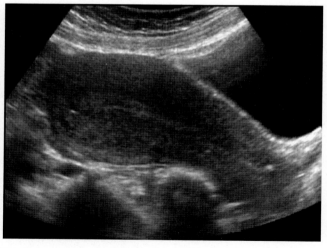

B

Figure 16-4. Transabdominal longitudinal view of the pelvis. Transducer position (A) and ultrasound image in a thin model with a partially filled bladder (B).

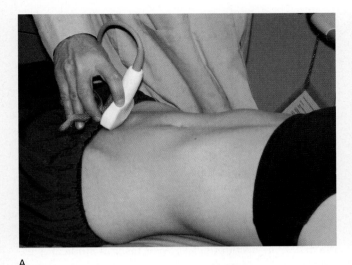

A

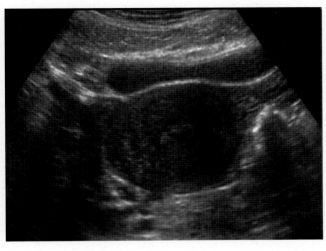

B

Figure 16-5. Transabdominal transverse view of the pelvis. Transducer position (A) and ultrasound image in a thin model with a partially filled bladder (B).

to the bladder and appears linear when the bladder is full.

In the transverse view, orient the transducer horizontally with slight caudal angulation and with the indicator pointed toward the patient's right side (Figure 16-5A). The uterus appears as an oval structure in the transverse plane (Figure 16-5B). Scan the uterus from the fundus to the cervix by fanning the ultrasound beam in superior to inferior movement. In this plane, the ovaries can be identified on either side of the uterus. Normal fallopian tubes generally cannot be visualized by transabdominal sonography unless surrounded by fluid.

The ovaries are best viewed in this plane and are typically found posterior and lateral to the uterus. In the multiparous patient, ovaries may be found in a variety of positions, from as posterior as the pouch of Douglas to as anterior as the uterine fundus. Typical ovaries measure 2 cm × 2 cm × 3 cm in adults and are characterized by anechoic follicular structures in the periphery (cortex).

ENDOVAGINAL SONOGRAPHY

Endovaginal ultrasound allows the provider to touch the pelvic organs with the tip of the transducer. The advantage of this approach is that high-frequency transducers (5–9 MHz) can be used, resulting in much better resolution compared to transabdominal imaging. Also, endovaginal ultrasound is well tolerated and preferable to transabdominal ultrasound by most patients. Even among adolescent patients undergoing evaluation for PID, 28% preferred endovaginal over transabdominal

ultrasound.[30] The advantage of not requiring patients to have a full bladder and the small diameter of endovaginal transducers (compared to a speculum) helps to explain why endovaginal ultrasound is preferred by most patients.

Disinfect the endovaginal transducer with standard bactericidal agents between each usage. Apply a proper acoustic medium on both sides of a protective cover. Displace any air bubbles within the condom to avoid beam scattering artifacts. In patients undergoing infertility therapy, the ultrasound gel should not contain any spermicidal agent; in these cases, tepid sterile water is suitable for lubrication.

There are two main types of endovaginal transducers (Figure 16-6A,B). One type is referred to as an "end-fire" transducer in which the handle and the shaft are in a straight line and the ultrasound waves exit the transducer surface along this line. The other type has an angulated handle and an ultrasound beam that fires askew. The authors will refer to these transducer types as "end-fire" and "angulated" in the following discussion.

Place the patient in the lithotomy position. A gynecology table is preferable to elevation of hips on a stack of towels. In a systematic fashion, scan the entire pelvis in both sagittal and coronal planes. With the handle of the endovaginal transducer being held in a "pistol-grip" fashion, gently insert the endovaginal transducer with the indicator pointed toward the ceiling. While inserting the transducer, confirm the bladder as a landmark anterior to the uterus. It should be clearly discerned from any fluid collection in the anterior cul-de-sac. Clearly identify the endometrial stripe in a midline sagittal view of the uterus (Figure 16-7A). Maintaining this sagittal plane,

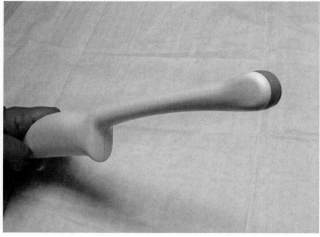

A

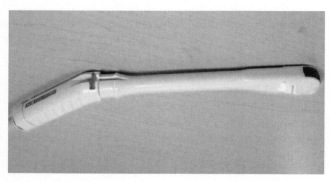

B

Figure 16-6. Endovaginal transducer. End-fire type (A) and angulated type (B).

evaluate the entire uterus. Lifting the handle toward the ceiling will direct the sound inferiorly enabling visualization of the cervix. Define the boundaries of the uterus by extending into both lateral projections. To scan patients with a retroverted uterus, it may be necessary to slightly remove the transducer and then severely angle the transducer face posteriorly (handle toward the ceiling). This allows the beam to be directed in a posterior fashion, which permits sound waves to access the fundus. If the fundus still lies beyond the angle of the beam, and if the angulated transducer type is used, rotate the handle 180°, reversing the on-screen direction of fundal image while allowing for adequate (and more comfortable) uterus evaluation.

From the midline sagittal plane, rotate the transducer 90° in a counterclockwise fashion (indicator toward the patient's right) to view structures in the coronal plane. The coronal plane can also be thought of as axial, or transverse, and simply refers to the short-axis view of the uterus. Obtain views by fanning through the entire uterus from cervix to fundus. The uterus and endometrial stripe assume a round appearance in this projection (Figure 16-7B).

Ovaries are typically identified by their size, oval shape, and the presence of circular hypoechoic follicles. These follicles can be confused with cross-sectional uterine vessels (arcuate arteries) that become tubular when the transducer is rotated. Normal ovaries are mobile and may be found in different positions during the same examination (Figure 16-8). To view the left ovary, start in the sagittal plane with the top of the transducer pointed toward the ceiling. Starting at the fundus, scan until the iliac vessels are seen to stretch across the screen in their long axis. Then, follow this structure into the patient's left adnexa until the characteristic follicles of the left ovary are identified. Similarly identify the right ovary

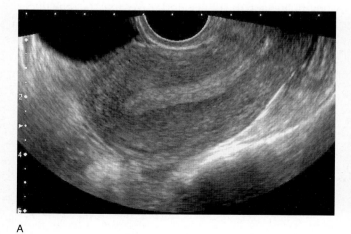

A

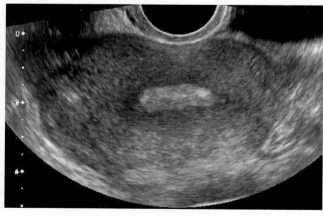

B

Figure 16-7. (A) Midline sagittal endovaginal view of the uterus with thickened (secretory) endometrium. (B) Transverse view of the uterus in the same patient.

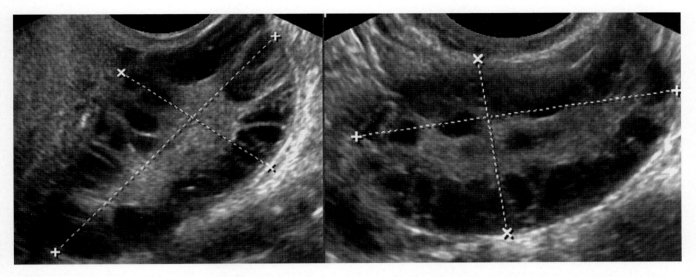

Figure 16-8. Endovaginal ultrasound of bilateral ovaries with normal follicles. Note that these are good-quality images because the transducer is very close to the ovaries.

except turning the transducer toward the patient's right. Another technique for finding the ovaries is to scan in the transverse plane and search for the ovaries adjacent to the cornual region of the uterus. Identify the cornual region by directing the transducer to the widest part of the body of the uterus and visualizing where the myometrium tapers as it connects to the fallopian tube. The ovary will usually be just lateral or posterior to the cornual region of the uterus.

The normal fallopian tube is a poor sonic reflector, which makes it virtually impossible to scan in a transabdominal approach. Utilizing an endovaginal approach, the healthy fallopian tubes may be appreciated by tracing them from their origin at the cornual areas of the uterus. A clearly seen lumen of the fallopian tube should increase the suspicion of a pathologic process. The tubal lumen is not normally visualized unless it is filled with fluid. Once the entire tubal lumen is filled, only then can the fimbriae be identified. In the longitudinal axis, the tortuous fallopian tube varies in length. Similarly the transverse axis may vary in width depending on the plane in which it is cut with the ultrasound beam. The width typically approximates 1 cm in normal individuals. The proximal (myometrial) portion of the fallopian tube may occasionally be visualized as a hyperechoic line as it enters the uterus.

► COMMON AND EMERGENT ABNORMALITIES

FUNCTIONAL SIMPLE CYSTS

These cysts are the most common ovarian masses in nonpregnant young women. Sonographically, they ap-

pear as thin-walled, unilocular anechoic spheres. Using specific criteria, a thin-walled, anechoic structure within the ovary is a physiologic cyst until it reaches a diameter greater than 2.5 cm. Follicular cysts can range from 2.5 cm to over 15 cm. As opposed to the anechoic interior of simple cysts, those containing internal echoes may be hemorrhagic cysts (Figure 16-9). Typical follicular cysts are unilateral, but they may be found in both ovaries, especially in patients with polycystic ovarian disease (Figure 16-10).[31] Ovarian cysts contain heterogeneous tissue, with peripheral follicles frequently identified along its border. It is not uncommon for these simple ovarian cysts to rupture. This event, however, is a clinical diagnosis and not a sonographic one. Regardless, maintain a high clinical suspicion for a ruptured

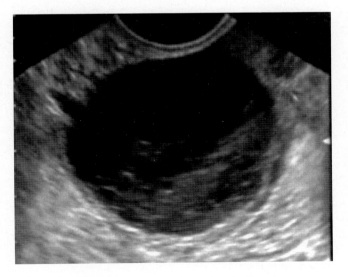

Figure 16-9. Endovaginal ultrasound of a hemorrhagic ovarian cyst.

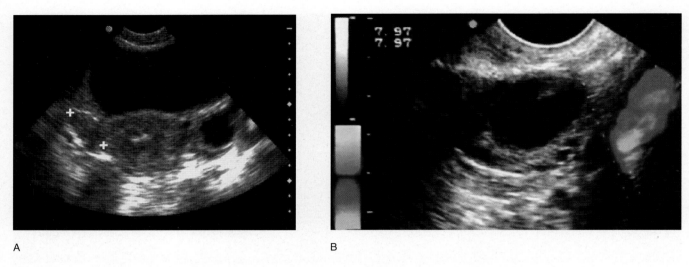

Figure 16-10. (A) Transverse transabdominal ultrasound of a simple ovarian cyst. Right ovary length is indicated (cursors). Left ovary contains 2-cm cyst outlined by ovarian tissue. (B) Endovaginal ultrasound of a simple ovarian cyst (follicular cyst). A 2.7-cm simple cyst is identified within the left ovary (bordered by a rim of ovarian follicular tissue). The external iliac vein is identified with color Doppler.

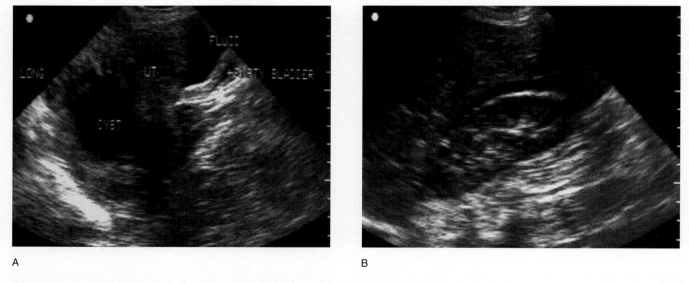

Figure 16-11. Ruptured corpus luteum cyst. (A) Long-axis transabdominal image shows a collapsed bladder with fluid in the anterior cul-de-sac and a large cyst in the posterior cul-de-sac. (B) A small stripe of free fluid was noted in Morison's pouch. (Courtesy of James Mateer, MD)

cyst in any patient who presents with severe lower abdominal pain and free fluid in the pelvis with or without an ovarian cyst (Figure 16-11).

CORPUS LUTEUM CYST

When a patient becomes pregnant, a corpus luteum cyst can persist up to 16 weeks' gestation and enlarge significantly because of failure to rupture or internal hemorrhage.[31] The corpus luteum cyst should not separate from the ovary on probing with the ultrasound transducer and abdominal palpation with the free hand. However, the vast majority of tubal rings will separate. The corpus luteum cyst can have a variety of appearances (Figure 16-12). Similar to a functional simple cyst of the ovary, corpus luteum cysts may also rupture resulting in severe abdominal pain.[33]

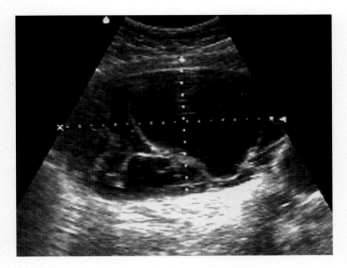

A

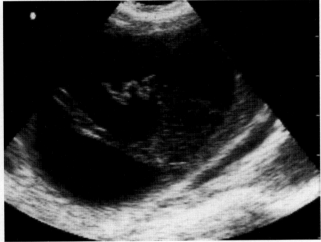

B

Figure 16-12. (A) Transabdominal ultrasound of a corpus luteal cyst. (B) Endovaginal ultrasound of a corpus luteal cyst. Endovaginal view provided improved detail of the ovary compared to the transabdominal view Figure 16-11A in the same patient. (Courtesy of James Mateer, MD)

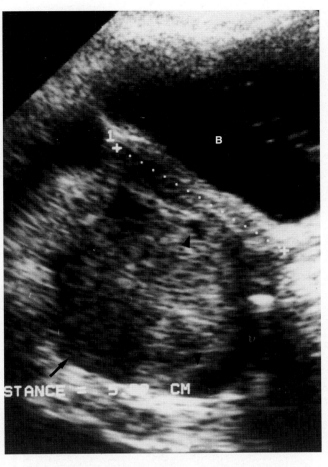

Figure 16-13. Ovarian torsion. Pelvis. Longitudinal plane. The uterus is marked off by measurement points. It is 5 cm in length. Posterior to it is a large solid mass (arrows) with a few peripheral cysts (arrowheads). This is a relatively classic image for ovarian torsion, although the echogenicity of the ultrasound image is related to the variable internal contents of the torsed ovary. This mass, which is the patient's torsed left adnexa, was much larger than the patient's normal right adnexa. B = bladder. (Reproduced from Cohen HL, Sivit CJ: *Fetal and pediatric ultrasound.* New York: McGraw-Hill, 516, 2001).

OVARIAN TORSION

The only specific gray scale sonographic sign of ovarian torsion is demonstration of multiple follicles in the cortical part of a unilaterally enlarged ovary. Transudative fluid flows into the multiple follicles as the ovary becomes congested from circulatory impairment. Ovarian enlargement, when present, is relatively obvious. It has been reported that a torsed ovary is at least 3 to 4 times larger than the average *prepubescent* ovary and 8 times larger than the average *adult* ovary[7] (Figure 16-13).

Doppler can be helpful in making the diagnosis of ovarian torsion when there is complete absence or asymmetric blood flow to one ovary (Figure 16-14). To reduce operator error, it is important to scan in several different planes when examining the ovary for presence of blood flow. Optimizing power Doppler settings to detect slow flow is critical. While it is difficult to exclude ovarian torsion with power and pulse wave Doppler, torsion can be diagnosed when no flow is detected. By changing the scanning angle, the clinician decreases the

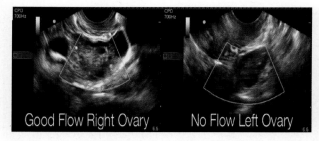

A

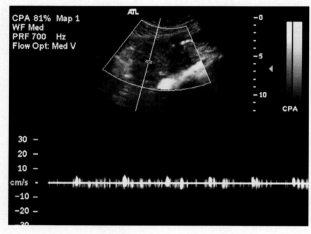

B

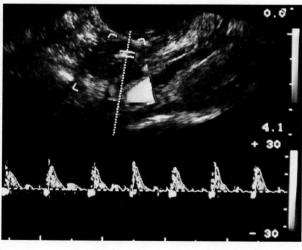

C

Figure 16-14. (A) Absent blood flow to the left ovary and positive flow in the right ovary by power Doppler imaging. (B) Inadequate ovarian arterial flow seen on spectral Doppler. (C) Normal ovarian arterial flow seen on spectral Doppler.

likelihood that the finding of absent blood flow is due to the angle at which the blood was moving in relation to the ultrasound beam.[34] Absence of ovarian enlargement due to a mass or cyst or effect from a nearby mass makes torsion very unlikely.

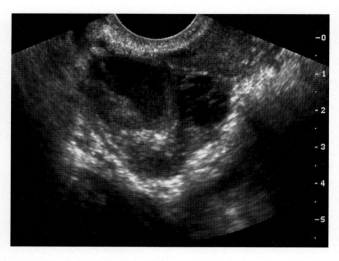

Figure 16-15. Endovaginal ultrasound demonstrating lack of distinct adnexal margins consistent with PID.

ACUTE PELVIC INFLAMMATORY DISEASE

Early sonographic signs of PID are increased adnexal volume and periovarian inflammation. On ultrasound, this appears as structures that lack the distinct margins that are normally identified (Figure 16-15) and an abnormal organ sliding sign (ovary becomes adhered to surrounding structures and is immobile when gentle transducer pressure is applied. Four ultrasound markers that suggest evidence of PID include (Figure 16-16) free fluid in the cul-de-sac, multicystic ovaries, visualization of fallopian tube or tubal fluid, and presence of an adnexal mass or TOA. An endovaginal ultrasound examination positive for these markers is useful for suggesting the diagnosis of PID.

TUBO-OVARIAN ABSCESS

Imaging the TOA has several caveats. First, the process of TOA formation usually occurs bilaterally, but not necessarily in step; therefore, bilateral TOA may appear "out of phase" with one another. Second, there often is absence of the sliding organ sign. Third, organisms producing gas result in highly echogenic reflectors within the abscess. Finally, the fallopian tube surrounds the ovary causing it to lose the typical appearance of anechoic follicles in the periphery. This appears sonographically as an ovary connected to, or embraced by, the fluid-filled fallopian tube (tubo-ovarian complex).[21,33] (Figure 16-17). When interrogated using power Doppler, marked hyperemia is seen throughout this complex structure. As the acute inflammatory process continues to proceed, it

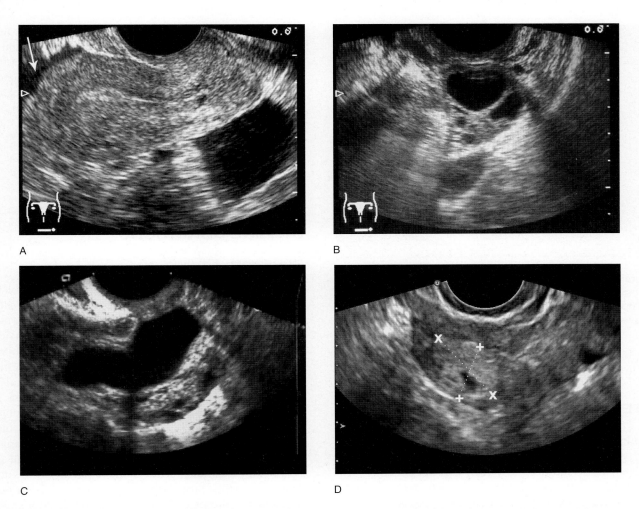

Figure 16-16. Four markers of PID. Endovaginal views. (1) Longitudinal ultrasound showing significant free fluid (A) in the posterior cul-de-sac (pouch of Douglas) and a small amount of fluid in the anterior cul-de-sac (arrow); (2) endovaginal ultrasound demonstrating multicystic ovary (B); (3) hydrosalpinx (C) endovaginal ultrasound shows fluid-filled fallopian tube; (4) adnexal mass (D) is outlined by the measurement cursors.

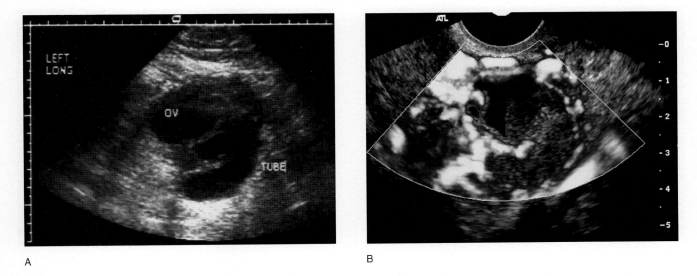

Figure 16-17. Tubo-ovarian complex. Endovaginal image of the left adnexa (A) shows a distorted ovary (OV) partially encircled by a fluid-filled hydrosalpinx (TUBE). Power Doppler (B) shows marked hyperemia throughout this similar complex structure.

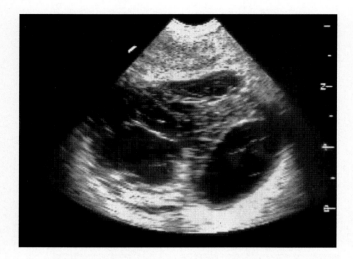

Figure 16-18. Tubo-ovarian abscess. Endovaginal transverse view of the cul-de-sac area shows a complex septated cystic mass 4 × 6 cm in size that proved to be a TOA. (Courtesy of James Mateer, MD)

erodes through the distended wall creating a localized or an expanding TOA (Figure 16-18).

UTERINE FIBROIDS

A uterus with multiple fibroids appears heterogeneous and globular, with discrete masses embedded in the uterine wall (Figure 16-19). They can be isoechoic, hyperechoic, or hypoechoic. Fibrotic changes and calcifications cause sonographic attenuation and loss of definite margins, which make size estimations problematic. Color Doppler can identify those fibroids containing a vascular supply, which may be responsive to hormonal therapy.[33] Because fibroids tend to reflect the sound waves, there is usually significant shadowing distal to the mass. In fact, the shadowing is often dense enough that it interferes with high-frequency imaging of the endovaginal approach. For this reason, patients with large or multiple fibroids may require a transabdominal, full bladder technique to obtain adequate images of the pelvic structures.

► COMMON VARIANTS AND SELECTED ABNORMALITIES

UTERINE CONDITIONS

Bicornate Uterus

One relatively common anatomic variant is the bicornate uterus. This can be very subtle ranging from a slight widening of the endometrial stripe to two separate entire uteruses each containing their own endometrial cavities (uterine didelphys). In the coronal plane, a partial bicornate uterus can be easily identified as having a widening of the fundus with separate endometrial stripes tracing away from each other in a Y-type of pattern (Figure 16-20). For a complete bicornate uterus, as the operator fans the ultrasound beam from left to right, the uterine fundus will appear to "re-grow." It is important to note that in this longitudinal plane both fundi will not be visualized simultaneously, but rather in succession. Switching to the coronal plane makes it possible for both horns of the uterus to be examined simultaneously. As the sonologist fans anterior to posterior coronally, each horn is seen to grow and recede together including their respective endometrial stripes seen in short axis.

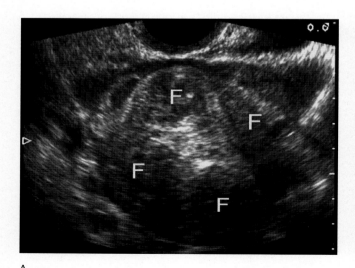

A

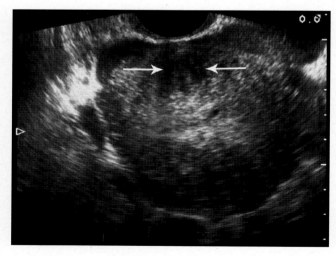

B

Figure 16-19. Fibroid uterus. Endovaginal ultrasound reveals multiple isoechoic discrete masses embedded in the uterine wall (A). A single hypoechoic fibroid with posterior linear shadowing (B) is outlined (arrows). F = Fibroids.

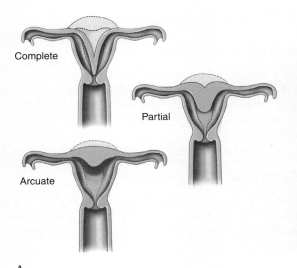

Complete

Partial

Arcuate

A

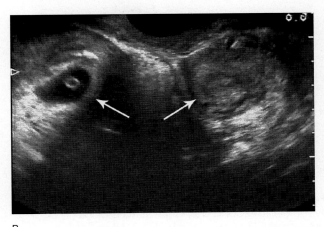

B

Figure 16-20. Bicornate uterus. (A) Illustration of a complete and partial bicornate uterus. (B) An extreme form of complete bicornate uterus is termed uterine didelphys. This is a transverse endovaginal view of uterine didelphys with each horn (arrows) separated by a loop of bowel. The patient's right horn contains an early IUP and yolk sac. (Part A redraw with permission from Cunningham FG, Leveno, KL, and Bloom, S et al., *William's Obstetrics,* 21st ed. New York, NY: McGraw-Hill, 2001; Part B courtesy of J. Christian Fox, MD).

Intrauterine Device

Occasionally, patients present to the ED or acute care clinic because of concerns that an intrauterine device (IUD) has been dislodged. This becomes further complicated when the string normally attached to the IUD has broken off or is missing. Sonographically, the IUD is strongly reflective and easily identified on endovaginal views unless located outside the uterus (Figure 16-21).[35] It is important to note that even though they represent a highly echoic structure, an IUD may not be distinguishable from the endometrial stripe using the transabdominal approach.

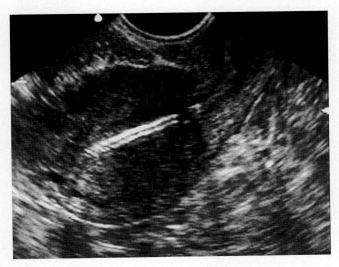

Figure 16-21. Intrauterine device (IUD). The IUD is strongly reflective and easily identified on this longitudinal endovaginal view.

Endometritis

This condition is most often seen with PID, during postpartum or after instrumentation. The endometrial stripe appears prominent or irregularly shaped. Fluid, gas, or debris can often be visualized.

Endometriosis

This ectopic endometrial tissue is usually found in the cul-de-sac, ovaries, and fallopian tubes. During menses, this tissue hemorrhages, resulting in multiple small fluid collections (endometriomas) that generally are not easily visualized by ultrasound. An enlarged endometrioma (termed "chocolate cyst") appears on ultrasound as a cystic structure with thickened walls and containing mid-level echogenic centers.[33] The viscous-fluid center can be mistaken for a solid ultrasound mass, but is identified as a cyst by posterior acoustical enhancement distal to the structure.

Uterine Polyps

Uterine polyps, found in 10% of women, are pedunculated sections of endometrial tissue that can occur as a single lesion or as multiple lesions. They may become so large that they protrude through the cervical os. The endometrium is thickened with areas of focal echogenicity or endocavitary masses surrounded by fluid.

Endometrial Hyperplasia

This condition results from the unopposed estrogen stimulation of endometrial proliferation without the

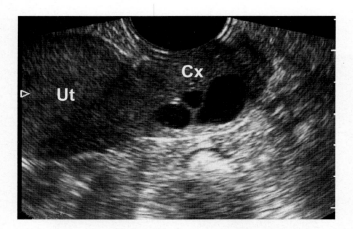

Figure 16-22. Nabothian cysts. Longitudinal endovaginal ultrasound demonstrating multiple benign nabothian cervical cysts. UT = Uterus, Cx = Cervix.

shedding effects of progesterone. The sonographic findings are nonspecific but do suggest a thickened endometrial stripe often greater than 5 mm. Postmenopausal patients with greater than 1 cm of endometrial thickness usually indicate hyperplasia or carcinoma.[36]

Endometrial Neoplasm

These tumors range in echogenicity from hyper- to hypoechoic. Some tumors may simply stretch the endometrium without directly invading it, making them difficult to visualize on ultrasound. Tumors larger than 1 cm in anterior–posterior dimension or ones larger than 10 mL in volume may warrant endometrial biopsy. Hyperplasia, in general, is a known precursor to carcinoma.[35]

CERVICAL CONDITIONS

Nabothian Cysts

Nabothian cysts occur when the endocervical glands become obstructed and dilated. This is a benign condition that frequently occurs without symptoms and has no clinical or pathologic significance. They appear sonographically within the cervix as a thin-walled, anechoic cystic structure up to 1 cm in diameter (Figure 16-22).

Cervical Malignancy

The majority (90%) of cervical malignancies are squamous cell and appear as bulky heterogeneous material within the cervix. This entity is seen best in the sagittal view.

ADNEXAL CONDITIONS

Ovarian cysts are common in all age groups, but especially in women of menstrual age. There exists a great deal of overlap in the sonographic appearance of the various masses found in the ovary and the adnexa. Their sonographic characteristics become even more similar when one considers the subset of masses with a complex morphology. It is the task of the clinician to sort through which findings require immediate diagnostic evaluation and which can be monitored on an outpatient basis.

Mucinous Cystadenomas

Mucinous cystadenomas are benign masses that represent the largest part of the ovarian neoplasms. They are capable of growing to occupy the entire abdominal cavity such that patients appear gravid (Figure 16-23A).

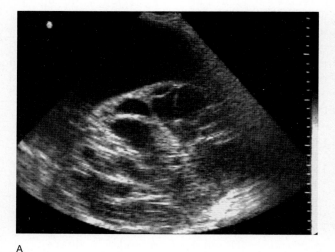

A

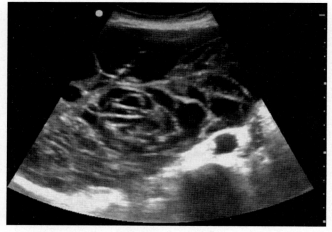

B

Figure 16-23. Cystadenoma. (A) Mucinous cystadenoma. The transabdominal ultrasound is at maximum viewing depth for a 3.5-MHz probe. A 38-pound seromucinous cystadenoma was confirmed at laparotomy. (B) Ovarian neoplasm. Transabdominal ultrasound of a large (12 × 20 cm) complex adnexal mass. (Part A courtesy of James Mateer, MD)

They contain mucinous material, which may appear sonographically as multiple fine, low-level echoes.[33]

Serous Cystadenomas

Serous cystadenomas, constituting approximately 20% of all benign neoplasms of the ovary, appear sonographically as a multilocular cystic mass containing few or no internal echoes. Septations are sufficiently thin so as to undulate with gentle transducer palpation. In the benign form, nodularity is typically absent; therefore, any solid tissue noted should raise concern for malignancy.

Cystadenocarcinoma

Ultrasound distinction between benign cystadenomas and malignant cystadenocarcinoma is difficult. Unfortunately when a biopsy of the ovary is performed, the histology is not conclusive up to 15% of the time.[37] Sonographic characteristics that suggest malignant histology include thick septa, increased mural nodularity, presence of solid tissue, and ascites (Figure 16-23B). The presence of ascites was noted in over 50% of malignant epithelial neoplasms of the ovary and is completely absent with benign disease.[38]

Dermoid Cysts

Dermoids (also known as teratomas) are the second most common cause for ovarian mass. They have a wide range of appearance and size and may contain hair, teeth, and fat. Calcified structures, such as teeth, produce strong shadows and are easily identified on plain films.[35] It is ideal to recognize these early as they tend to enlarge and replace the normal ovarian tissue over time. A solid teratoma often contains fatty tissue that is echogenic on ultrasound. A cystic teratoma (dermoid cyst) can be mostly cystic or complex—containing both solid and cystic components. Malignant transformation can occur (Figure 16-24).

Polycystic Ovaries

Polycystic ovaries are represented as multiple immature follicles smaller than 1 cm packed along the periphery. They are sometimes described as "beads on a string" in morphology.[33] When stimulated with hormones, they

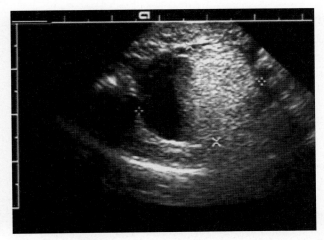

B

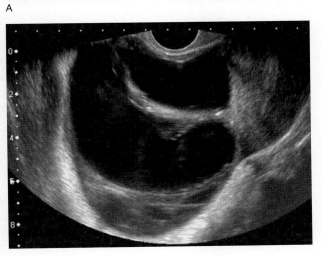

C

Figure 16-24. (A) Early dermoid. Endovaginal view of the right ovary reveals a small (2-cm) echogenic mass within the borders of the ovary. (B) Dermoid. Endovaginal image of the right adnexa shows the typical appearance of a dermoid demonstrating the echogenic solid component and a cystic portion. (C) Ovarian teratoma. Transvaginal ultrasound of a large (8 × 10 cm) complex adnexal mass with small areas of calcification. (Part A courtesy of James Mateer, MD)

A

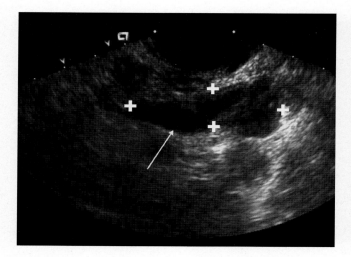

Figure 16-25. Hydrosalpinx. Endovaginal ultrasound of a fallopian tube (cursors) filled with anechoic fluid (arrow).

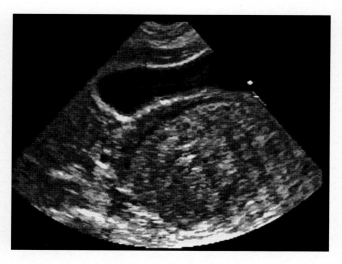

Figure 16-27. Vaginal hematoma. Transabdominal ultrasound view of a vaginal hematoma in patient who recently underwent a dilatation and curettage procedure.

have an exaggerated appearance resembling a stained glass window.

Hydrosalpinx and Pyosalpinx

Normal fallopian tubes are not visualized; however, when filled with fluid they become dilated and are prominently visualized on ultrasound due to their fluid-filled nature (Figure 16-25). They may be mistaken for ovarian pathology, such as an ovarian cyst or TOA (Figure 16-26). The way to distinguish fallopian tube pathology from ovarian pathology is to locate the ovary as a separate entity, and the fallopian tube will be seen *between* the ovary and the uterus.

VAGINAL CONDITIONS

Ultrasound can be helpful for identifying a vaginal hematoma. This finding is often incidentally recognized on transabdominal sonography, and the etiology of the pelvic mass can be initially confusing (Figure 16-27).

▶ PITFALLS

1. **Presence of blood flow in the involved ovary does not necessarily exclude the diagnosis of ovarian torsion.** Absence of ovarian blood flow is helpful in diagnosing ovarian torsion. The converse has not been shown to be reliable for excluding ovarian torsion. In other words, in the correct clinical setting, the index of suspicion for ovarian torsion should be maintained even if blood flow is present in the involved ovary.

2. **The uterine vasculature may appear cystic on cross-sectional image planes and are frequently mistaken for follicles within an ovary.** The ovary can be confirmed by these cystic structures lacking blood flow. These structures should remain circular in different scanning planes when the transducer is rotated. Vascular structures contain blood flow and lengthen out when viewed in alternate scanning planes.

3. **Large ovarian follicles may be mistaken for fallopian tubes.** These ovarian follicles will change during the cycle and be localized within the ovary.

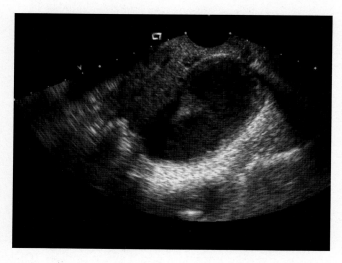

Figure 16-26. Pyosalpinx. Endovaginal ultrasound of a fallopian tube filled with echogenic material (pus).

4. **Small ovarian cysts can falsely appear as a thin-walled hydrosalpinx.** The finding of ovarian tissue in the periphery helps exclude this diagnosis.
5. **Retained mucous secretions can imitate tumors by appearing to have endometrial thickening.**
6. **Other disease processes, such as tuberculosis and various GYN malignancies, can cause peritoneal implantation to the uterine serosa.** These disease entities are easily identified sonographically when surrounded by fluid.
7. **Imaging the shrunken postmenopausal ovary is difficult because of its lack of follicles, decreased pelvic fluid, and decreased vaginal elasticity inhibiting transducer movement.**

▶ CASE STUDIES

CASE 1

Patient Presentation

A 22-year-old nulliparous woman presented to the ED with a 1-day history of severe right lower quadrant abdominal pain and scant vaginal discharge. The patient was seen by her primary care physician 4 days previously and was treated for a urinary tract infection. She reported having unprotected sex with one sexual partner for the past several months. Her medical history and surgical history were unremarkable. Review of systems was significant for tactile fever and decreased oral intake.

On physical examination, the patient had a blood pressure 110/70 mm Hg, heart rate 123 beats per minute, respiratory rate 18 per minute, and temperature 39.8°C. She appeared toxic. The abdominal examination revealed severe right lower quadrant tenderness slightly inferior to McBurney's point, no rebound or guarding, normoactive bowel sounds, and no costovertebral angle tenderness. The rectal examination lateralized tenderness to the right, and the stool was guaiac negative. Sterile speculum examination revealed a friable cervix with scant purulent discharge. Bimanual examination revealed right adnexal tenderness, cervical motion tenderness, but no evidence of fullness or masses. A urinalysis specimen was unremarkable, and the urine pregnancy test was negative. The WBC was 15,000 cells/mL with a left shift.

Management Course

At this stage in the workup, acute appendicitis was suspected. A general surgeon ordered a CT scan of the abdomen and pelvis with triple contrast. This test was read as negative for appendicitis but did reveal a complex structure associated with the right ovary. A point-of-care endovaginal ultrasound revealed a cogwheel formation of the right ovary, absence of the sliding ovary sign, and heterogenic material within the right fallopian tube. A diagnosis of TOA was made, triple antibiotic therapy was initiated, and the gynecologist was consulted. The patient was taken to the operating room for laparoscopy with abscess drainage.

Commentary

Case 1 illustrates the diagnostic role that ultrasonography can have in the workup of a young woman with lower abdominal pain. Ectopic pregnancy and urinary tract disease had been excluded by the urine sample. Appendicitis initially was at the top of the differential diagnosis. A negative CT scan, however, is not 100% accurate for excluding appendicitis, and the general surgeon continued to entertain thoughts of taking the patient to the operating room to perform an appendectomy. The pelvic ultrasound examination confirmed the diagnosis of TOA and the patient's care was expedited by having the gynecologist perform the laparoscopic procedure for abscess drainage.

CASE 2

Patient Presentation

A 16-year-old nulliparous woman presented to the ED with the sudden onset of severe left lower quadrant abdominal pain. The symptoms started 30 minutes before the arrival and were associated with nausea, three episodes of vomiting, and chills. The patient denied vaginal bleeding or discharge and any prior history of sexual intercourse. Medical history and surgical history were unremarkable.

On physical examination, the patient had a blood pressure 120/70 mm Hg, heart rate 118 beats per minute, respiratory rate 20 per minute, and temperature 37.8°C. She appeared in severe distress secondary to the pain and nausea. Abdominal examination revealed moderate tenderness in left lower quadrant without rebound or guarding. Bowel sounds were normal. There were no masses or costovertebral tenderness. Rectal examination was nontender, and stool was guaiac negative. Sterile speculum examination was unremarkable and bimanual examination revealed left adnexal tenderness, cervical motion tenderness, normal right adnexa, and no masses or fullness. The WBC was normal, and the urinalysis and urine pregnancy test were negative.

Management Course

The emergency physician's differential diagnosis included ovarian torsion, ruptured ovarian cyst with chemical peritonitis, and TOA. The physician's point-of-care endovaginal ultrasound examination showed no evidence of free fluid, ovarian mass, or TOA. There was, however, an enlarged left ovary with complete absence of any discernible blood flow despite evaluation in multiple planes. The right ovary had normal appearing blood flow. A gynecologist was immediately called to the bedside for suspected ovarian torsion, and she took the patient to the operating room for laparoscopy. Her ovary was immediately detorsed with intraoperative visual evidence of good perfusion.

Commentary

Case 2 illustrates a young woman who presented with acute ovarian torsion. This case demonstrates that the pelvic ultrasound examination could be performed rapidly at the patient's bedside, which are two of the main advantages of ultrasonography. The emergency physician was able to expedite the patient's disposition to the operating room. This helped the gynecologist salvage the young woman's left ovary.

CASE 3

Patient Presentation

A 32-year-old, gravida 4, para 4 woman presented to the ED with worsening right lower quadrant abdominal pain over the past several days. She admitted that this pain felt like the same pain she has had in the past with her ovarian cysts. She denied vaginal discharge, vaginal bleeding, fever, chills, nausea, or vomiting. She had no medical history or surgical history.

On physical examination, the patient had a blood pressure 110/70 mm Hg, heart rate 92 beats per minute, respiratory rate 16 per minute, and temperature 37.2°C. She appeared in mild distress secondary to abdominal pain. Abdominal examination revealed moderate tenderness to deep palpation in her right lower quadrant. No rebound or guarding was appreciated, and there were no masses or costovertebral tenderness. Rectal examination was nontender, and the stool was guaiac negative. Sterile speculum examination was unremarkable; however, bimanual examination revealed adnexal fullness on the right side with moderate tenderness. No cervical motion tenderness was elicited and the left adnexa was normal. The WBC was normal, and the urinalysis and urine pregnancy test were negative.

Management Course

The differential diagnosis included appendicitis, ovarian torsion, PID, and TOA. The emergency physician performed a screening point-of-care endovaginal ultrasound examination that revealed a 4-cm right ovarian cyst and evidence of normal appearing blood flow to the surrounding ovarian tissue and trace free fluid in the posterior cul-de-sac. The patient's symptoms were alleviated with oral ibuprofen and she was discharged home. Arrangements were made with her gynecologist to schedule a repeat ultrasound examination later that week in her office. This follow-up ultrasound examination revealed resolution of the cyst with a moderate amount of free fluid in the posterior cul-de-sac.

Commentary

Case 3 demonstrates how utilization of point-of-care emergency ultrasound allowed the physician to avoid ordering expensive, time-consuming diagnostic tests for the evaluation of the patient's complaint. While the patient's differential diagnosis included several worrisome disease entities, the physician was able to match the patient's clinical picture to a finding on the ultrasound examination, and then initiated the appropriate therapy.

REFERENCES

1. Close RJ, Sachs CJ, Dyne PL: Reliability of bimanual pelvic examinations performed in emergency departments. *West J Med* 175:240–244; discussion 244–245, 2001.
2. Padilla LA, Radosevich DM, Milad MP: Accuracy of the pelvic examination in detecting adnexal masses. *Obstet Gynecol* 96:593–598, 2000.
3. Padilla LA, Radosevich DM, Milad MP: Limitations of the pelvic examination for evaluation of the female pelvic organs. *Int J Gynaecol Obstet: The Official Organ of the International Federation of Gynaecology and Obstetrics* 88:84–88, 2005.
4. Brenner DJ, Hall EJ: Computed tomography—An increasing source of radiation exposure. *N Engl J Med* 357:2277–2284, 2007.
5. Tukeva TA: MR imaging in pelvic inflammatory disease: Comparison with laparoscopy and US. *Radiology* 210:209–216, 1999.
6. Jacobson L, Westrom L: Objectivized diagnosis of acute pelvic inflammatory disease. Diagnostic and prognostic value of routine laparoscopy. *Am J Obstet Gynecol* 105:1088–1098, 1969.
7. Graif M, Itzchak Y: Sonographic evaluation of ovarian torsion in childhood and adolescence. *AJR* 150:647–649, 1988.
8. Hibbard L: Adnexal torsion. *Am J Obstet Gyn* 152:456–460, 1985.
9. Schultz LR, Newton WA, Clatoworthy HW: Torsion of previously normal tube and ovary in children. *N Engl J Med* 268:343–346, 1963.
10. Stark J, Siegel M: Ovarian torsion in prepubertal and pubertal girls: Sonographic findings. *AJR* 163:1479–1482, 1994.
11. Pena JE: Usefulness of Doppler sonography in the diagnosis of ovarian torsion. *Fertil Steril* 73(5):1047–1050, 2000.

12. Surratt J, Siegel J: Imaging of pediatric ovarian masses. *Radiographics* 11:533–548, 1991.

13. Van Hoorhis B, Schwaiger J, Syrop C, et al.: Early diagnosis of ovarian torsion by color Doppler sonography. *Fertil Steril* 58:215–217, 1992.

14. Rosado W, Trambert M, Gosink B, et al.: Adnexal torsion: Diagnosis by using Doppler sonography. *AJR* 159:1251–1253, 1992.

15. Centers for Disease Control and Prevention: 1998 guidelines for treatment of sexually transmitted diseases. *MMWR* 47:79, 1998.

16. Washington AE, Katz P: Cost of and payment source for pelvic inflammatory disease: Trends and projections, 1983 through 2000. *JAMA* 226:2565, 1991.

17. Lawson MA, Blythe MJ: Pelvic inflammatory disease in adolescents. *Pediatr Clin North Am* 46:4, 1999.

18. Jacobson L: Objectivized diagnosis of acute PID. *Am J Obstet Gynecol* 105:1088–1098, 1969.

19. Arbel-DeRowe Y, Tepper R, Rosn DJ, et al.: The contribution of pelvic ultrasonography to the diagnostic process in pediatric and adolescent gynecology. *J Pediatr Adolesc Gynecol* 10:3, 1997.

20. Patten RM: PID: Endovaginal sonography and laparoscopic correlation. *J Ultrasound Med* 9:681–689, 1990.

21. Cacciatore B, Leminen A: Transvaginal sonographic findings in ambulatory patients with suspected pelvic inflammatory disease. *Obstetr Gynecol* 80(6):912–916, 1992.

22. Boardman L, Peipert J, Brody J, et al.: Endovaginal sonography for the diagnosis of upper genital tract infection. *Endovagin Sonogr* 90:54–57, 1997.

23. Teisala K, Heinonen PK, Punnonen R, et al.: Transvaginal ultrasound in the diagnosis and treatment of tubo-ovarian abscess. *Br J Obstet Gynecol* 77:178–180, 1990.

24. Roberts W, Dockery JL: Management of tubo-ovarian abscess due to pelvic inflammatory disease. *S Med J* 77:7, 1984.

25. Reed S, Landers D, Sweet RL: Antibiotic treatment of tuboovarian abscess: Comparison of broad-spectrum beta-lactam agents versus clindamycin-containing regimens. *Am J Obstet Gynecol* 164:1556–1562, 1991.

26. Landers DV: Tubo-ovarian abscess complicating pelvic inflammatory disease. In: Landers DV, Sweet RL, eds. *Pelvic Inflammatory Disease*. New York, NY: Springer Verlag, 1996:94.

27. Taylor KJW: Accuracy of grey-scale ultrasound diagnosis of abdominal and pelvic abscesses in 220 patients. *Lancet* 1:83–84, 1978.

28. Uhrich PC, Sanders RC: Ultrasound characteristics of pelvic inflammatory masses. *Clin Ultrasound* 4:199–204, 1976.

29. McNeeley SG: Medically sound, cost-effective treatment for pelvic inflammatory disease and tuboovarian abscess. *Am J Ob Gyn* 1786:1272–1278, 1998.

30. Bulas DI, Ahlstrom PA, Sivit CJ, et al.: Pelvic inflammatory disease in the adolescent: Comparison of transabdominal and transvaginal sonographic evaluation. *Radiology* 183:435–439, 1992.

31. Holt SC, Levi CS, Lyons EA, et al.: Normal anatomy of the female pelvis. In: Callen P, ed. *Ultrasonography in Obstetrics and Gynecology*. St. Louis, MO: WB Saunders, 1993:550–551, 555, 561–562.

32. Davis JA, Gosnick BB: Fluid in the female pelvis: Cyclic patterns. *J Ultrasound Med* 5:75–79, 1986.

33. Rottem S, Timor-Tritsch I: Ovarian pathology. In: Timor-Trisch I, Rottem S, eds. *Transvaginal Sonography*. New York, NY: Elsevier, 1991:155–157.

34. Zagebski J: Doppler instrumentation. In: *Essentials of Ultrasound Physics*. St. Louis, MO: Mosby, 1996:90.

35. Comstock C: Ultrasonography of gynecologic disorders. In: Pearlman M, Tintinalli J, eds. *Emergency Care of the Woman*. New York, NY: McGraw Hill, 1998:669, 671.

36. Fleischer A, Kepple D, Entman A: Transvaginal sonography of uterine disorders. In: Timor-Trisch I, Rottem S, eds. *Transvaginal Sonography*. New York, NY: Elsevier, 1991:119.

37. Mendelson EB, Bohm-Velez M, Joseph N, Neiman HL: Gynecologic imaging: Comparison of transabdominal and transvaginal sonography. *Radiology* 166:321–324, 1988.

38. Cramer DW, Welch WR: Determinants of ovarian cancer risk. Inferences regarding pathogenesis. *J Natl Cancer Inst* 71:717, 1983.

CHAPTER 17

Deep Venous Thrombosis

Thomas G. Costantino, Harry J. Goett, and Michael A. Peterson

Ultrasound evaluation for deep venous thrombosis (DVT) is one of the 11 core ultrasound applications for emergency physicians as listed in the 2008 American College of Emergency Physicians guidelines.[1] This evaluation typically consists of a limited compression ultrasound of the proximal lower extremities. Although different from a typical "duplex" examination performed in many vascular laboratories in the United States, which consists of a combination of whole leg compression ultrasound and Doppler ultrasound, limited compression ultrasound has been widely studied as the initial investigative tool for the diagnosis of DVT.[2,3]

► CLINICAL CONSIDERATIONS

If left untreated, DVT can lead to significant morbidity and mortality, including pulmonary embolism (PE) and post-phlebotic syndrome. The annual incidence of venous thromboembolism is approximately 1 in 1,000 and increases with age. Since two-thirds of patients with venous thromboembolism are initially diagnosed as proximal lower extremity DVT, this leads to an annual incidence in the United States of DVT of approximately 200,000 cases.[4] Without treatment, 50% of these will progress to PE with a resultant 30 days mortality of approximately 15%.[4] With treatment, the complications of DVT are reduced to less than 5%. However, anticoagulation causes major bleeding in almost 2% of patients and mortality in 0.2%, so treatment should be limited to only those diagnosed with the disease.[5] Therefore, diagnostic strategies need to have a high sensitivity and specificity.

The vast majority of DVTs (>90%) are diagnosed in the proximal veins of the lower extremity (common femoral vein, superficial femoral vein, and popliteal vein). The iliac veins account for about 2% of DVTs.[6] Upper extremity veins account for a small share of DVTs, unless a venous catheter is present.

The approach to isolated calf vein DVTs is still a source of great controversy. The tendency of these to propagate proximally is at the center of the debate concerning the best approach, including (1) repeat ultrasound in 1 week, (2) D-dimer testing for patients with a negative limited compression ultrasound, and (3) a single whole leg ultrasound.[3] Superficial thrombophlebitis had been thought to never progress to DVT, though some studies are challenging that and even suggesting treatment for superficial thrombophlebitis involving the proximal greater saphenous vein.[7]

Clinical signs and symptoms of DVT consist of leg swelling and tenderness; however, only about 20% of patients who are clinically suspected of having a DVT actually have one. High-sensitivity D-dimer assays, when negative, have been shown to help rule out DVT in patients with a low clinical suspicion.[8] Ultrasound of the proximal lower extremities has become the gold standard imaging test for diagnosing DVT. Most current algorithms for assessing patients with suspected lower extremity DVT involve using a combination of clinical suspicion, high-sensitivity D-dimer assays, and compression ultrasound of the lower extremity.[8,9]

Emergency medicine providers are uniquely qualified to use a combination of clinical suspicion, lab testing, and limited compression ultrasound to rapidly diagnose patients with DVT and safely discharge low-risk patients who do not have evidence of DVT.

▶ CLINICAL INDICATIONS

The clinical indications for performing a venous ultrasound examination are as follows:

- Suspicion of a lower extremity DVT
- Suspicion of an upper extremity DVT

SUSPICION OF A LOWER EXTREMITY DVT

Virchow's triad—hypercoagulability, venous stasis, and vessel injury—is the main risk factor for developing a DVT. The pathophysiology behind the development of venous thrombosis is not as well understood as arterial thrombosis, although both involve similar elements of the coagulation cascade. Once thrombus has occurred, reorganization of the clot begins. This process allows clefts to form between the clot and the vein wall, beginning about 1 week after initial clot formation; this is thought to be when the risk of PE is greatest. Over the next several weeks, the clot may be lysed and recanalized, leaving a thickened intima.

Only about half of all patients with DVT have any noticeable signs or symptoms. Risk factors for DVT are listed in Table 17-1. The combination of risk factors, physical examination findings, and clinician judg-

▶ **TABLE 17-1. RISK FACTORS FOR DEEP VENOUS THROMBOSIS**

Age >60 years
Cancer
Central venous catheter insertion
Genetic causes of hypercoagulability
History of DVT
Immobilization
Obesity
Pregnancy
Smoking
Trauma or recent surgery
Use of birth control pills or hormone replacement therapy

▶ **TABLE 17-2. WELLS CRITERIA: SIMPLIFIED CLINICAL MODEL FOR ASSESSMENT OF DEEP VEIN THROMBOSIS***

Clinical Variable	Score
Active cancer (treatment ongoing or within previous 6 months or palliative)	1
Paralysis, paresis, or recent plaster immobilization of the lower extremities	1
Recently bedridden for 3 days or more, or major surgery within the previous 12 weeks requiring general or regional anesthesia	1
Localized tenderness along the distribution of the deep venous system	1
Entire leg swelling	1
Calf swelling at least 3 cm larger than that on the asymptomatic leg (measured 10 cm below the tibial tuberosity)	1
Pitting edema confined to the symptomatic leg	1
Collateral superficial veins (nonvaricose)	1
Previously documented DVT	1
Alternative diagnosis at least as likely as DVT	−2

*Scoring method indicates high probability if score is 3 or more; moderate if score is 1 or 2; and low if score is 0 or less.

ment has been developed into a clinical prediction model (Table 17-2).[8,9] This clinical prediction model is often combined with a high-sensitivity D-dimer assay to decide who should undergo ultrasound evaluation for DVT.

There are different views about how ultrasound should be used to assess for DVT. Historically, whole leg ultrasound has been performed in vascular laboratories. This is often referred to as duplex ultrasound, which combines compression ultrasound with multiple measurements using color and pulse wave Doppler. The entire leg is usually scanned, with measurements taken every few centimeters from the inguinal ligament down to and including the calf veins. This technique is time consuming, taking an average of 37 minutes to perform in one study.[10]

Another school of thought is to perform limited compression ultrasound concentrating on the common femoral vein and the popliteal vein. This technique seems best suited for emergency care providers because it can be performed rapidly at the patient's bedside and has been shown to be safe and effective. One study compared limited compression ultrasound to contrast venography in 220 patients clinically suspected of having DVT. Limited compression ultrasound was found to be 100% sensitive and 99% specific for clinically relevant DVT (popliteal and above).[11] Numerous studies since then have confirmed the high sensitivity and specificity of a limited compression ultrasound technique.[12–17] Others have raised a theoretical concern that there may be isolated DVT present in the superficial femoral vein that could be missed by this technique, but the preponderance of data do not support this belief.[18]

Several large studies have followed outcomes of patients at 3 and 6 months looking for venous thromboembolic events. They have all pointed to the safety of limited compression ultrasound for the diagnosis of DVT. A 2002 study performed a limited compression ultrasound on 1756 patients with suspected DVT.[19] They combined this with a high-sensitivity D-dimer assay and limited repeat ultrasound in 1 week for patients with a positive D-dimer. Twenty-two percent of patients were diagnosed with a proximal DVT initially. Of patients with a negative initial ultrasound and D-dimer assay, only 6/828 (0.7%) had a venous thromboembolism at 3 months. Patients with a low pretest probability and a negative D-dimer assay had a 1.8% incidence of venous thromboembolism at 3 months, similar to previous validations of Wells criteria. Patients with a negative initial ultrasound and positive D-dimer had a 3% incidence of DVT in 1 week and an additional 2.1% at 3 months. At no point during this study were calf veins evaluated.

A 2008 study sought to directly compare a limited compression ultrasound evaluation plus D-dimer testing versus a whole leg duplex evaluation.[3] It randomized 2098 patients to either approach, with death and DVT/PE at 3 months as the end point. In the limited compression pathway, 0.9% of patients had an untoward event at 3 months versus 1.2% in the whole leg group, which was considered equivalent. The whole leg approach diagnosed 20.4% proximal DVT initially, with 6% calf vein thrombosis; all were treated with anticoagulation. The limited compression ultrasound approach diagnosed 20.8% DVT initially. Of those with a normal initial ultrasound, 30.9% had a positive D-dimer and underwent repeat ultrasound after 1 week. No patients developed PE during this week and none were anticoagulated. After 1 week, an additional 5.5% of patients were found to have a proximal DVT. This study demonstrated that a limited compression ultrasound combined with 1-week repeat ultrasound in patients with a positive D-dimer was equivalent to a whole leg duplex study. This was presumably because the undiagnosed calf vein thrombi that will lead to proximal DVT tend to do so within 1 week. The limited compression ultrasound technique used in these studies included a single compression of the common femoral vein at the inguinal ligament, and two compressions of the popliteal vein, one at the midpoint of the popliteal fossa and the other at the distal popliteal fossa just proximal to its trifurcation.

Several studies have demonstrated that emergency medicine physicians can perform limited compression ultrasound in a few minutes with excellent results.[12–17] A 2008 meta-analysis showed that emergency physicians can perform limited compression ultrasound for DVT with accuracy similar to radiology-performed ultrasound.[20] In addition, a 2010 study demonstrated that emergency physicians who learned to perform simple compression ultrasound in just 10 minutes had 100% accuracy for diagnosing DVT compared to a whole leg duplex ultrasound performed by radiology.[17]

Most algorithms for the evaluation of DVT assume ultrasound is an expensive and time-consuming procedure, and so more emphasis is placed on clinical prediction models and D-dimer assays to exclude patients from requiring ultrasound[21] (Figure 17-1). However, as emergency physicians become more adept at the technique, a limited compression ultrasound examination can be performed much more swiftly than a D-dimer assay. Using an ultrasound-first algorithm, all patients with clinically suspected DVT (whether low, moderate, or high) can have a limited compression ultrasound examination performed with the plan to have a repeat ultrasound performed in 1 week (Figure 17-2).

Limited compression ultrasound is often of greatest value to emergency providers on evenings, nights, weekends, and holidays when diagnostic imaging services are delayed or unavailable. Although calf vein thrombosis is not assessed with a limited compression ultrasound exam, managing patients based on the results of the limited compression exam has been shown to be safe and effective. A DVT will be diagnosed in about 10–20% of patients who are assessed with limited compression ultrasound, depending on how it is used. Patients who do not have a DVT may have incidental findings that lead to another diagnosis. About 15% of patients suspected of having DVT are eventually diagnosed with a Baker's cyst, knee effusion, or cellulitis, all of which can be visualized with ultrasound.

SUSPICION OF AN UPPER EXTREMITY DVT

Upper extremity DVT is thought to account for about 5% of all DVT cases.[22] The most common causes of this disease process are malignancy, central venous catheters, and pacemaker wires. The vast majority of upper extremity DVTs is due to indwelling catheters and many occur in the subclavian vein. Other sources of DVT are the axillary and internal jugular veins. External jugular vein thrombosis is extremely rare.

While simple compression ultrasound works well in the lower extremities, the subclavian vein does not lend itself to compression. Therefore, excluding an upper

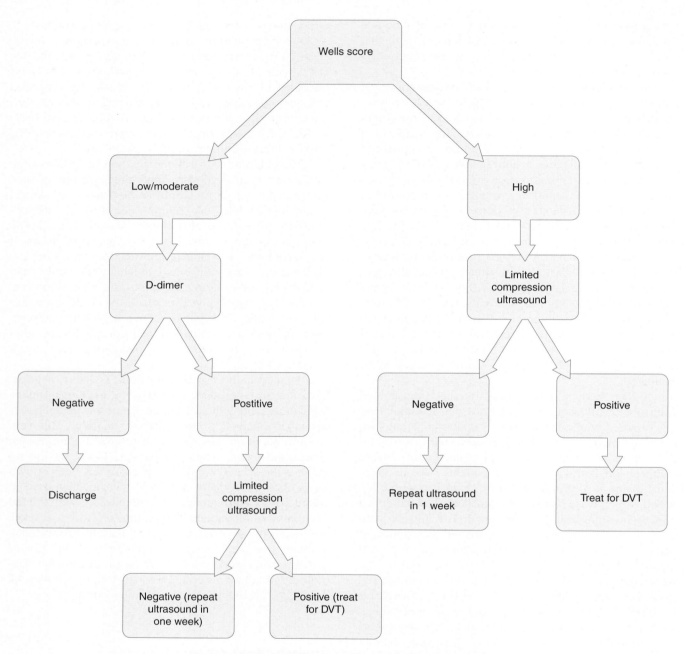

Figure 17-1. Typical algorithm for evaluating DVT.

extremity DVT depends on Doppler ultrasound and in-direct confirmation of vein patency in a major venous segment. Although it has not been well studied, this suggests that ruling out an upper extremity DVT may be more difficult for less experienced providers. It may be prudent for less experienced providers to use upper extremity ultrasound to rule in the diagnosis of DVT, but

not to try to rule it out. It is often straightforward to rec-ognize a positive finding, so it is reasonable to do a brief point-of-care exam. However, patients with a negative point-of-care exam may need further evaluation with a comprehensive ultrasound exam or a CT scan, depend-ing on the experience of the provider and the quality of the initial exam.

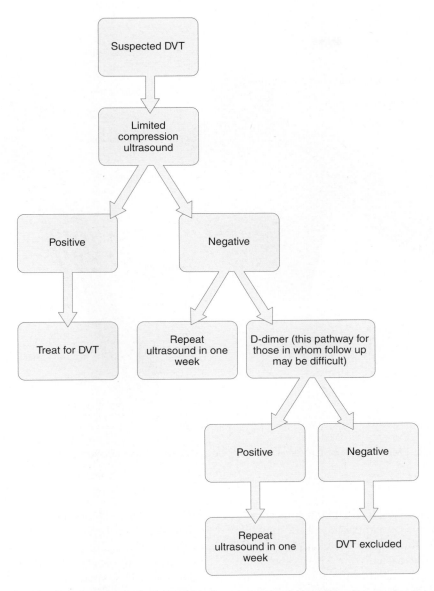

Figure 17-2. A clinician-performed ultrasound-based algorithm for evaluating DVT.

SUPERFICIAL THROMBOPHLEBITIS

Although data are lacking, upper extremity DVT is generally considered thrombosis involving the axillary and subclavian veins. Clot in the brachial and basilic veins is generally considered superficial thrombophlebitis, but some believe that this should be treated with anticoagulation. In the leg, the greater saphenous vein is considered a superficial vein, but some believe that thrombosis at this location also requires anticoagulation.[7] Superficial venous thrombosis at other locations is considered to be of no significant risk for PE and is treated conservatively

and without anticoagulation. On ultrasound, the appearance of superficial venous thrombosis is similar to that of a DVT with failure to compress the vein as the diagnostic criteria.

▶ ANATOMICAL CONSIDERATIONS

The upper extremity veins include the radial and ulnar veins, which arise from the palmar venous plexus (Figure 17-3). The radial and ulnar veins run next to the radial and ulnar arteries and join in the antecubital area

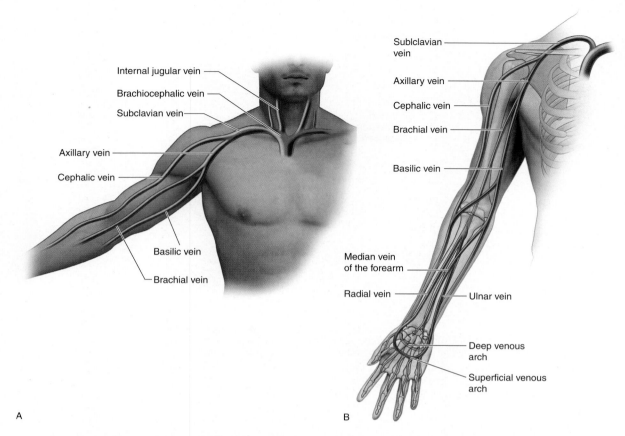

Figure 17-3. Deep veins of the arm (A) and deep veins of the proximal arm and thorax (B).

to form the brachial vein. The brachial vein runs superiorly, usually as two veins on either side of the brachial artery, and flows into the axillary vein approximately where it is joined by the basilic vein. The axillary vein flows into the thorax and becomes the subclavian vein. The subclavian vein is then joined by the internal jugular vein to form the brachiocephalic vein.

The venous system of the lower extremity is quite simple in a proximal to distal examination from the inguinal ligament to the level of the upper calf. Although many clinicians may feel they know the location and anatomy of the femoral vessels, few truly understand the details of the anatomy and variations that may be present. Historically, clinicians are taught that the femoral vein is located just medial to the femoral artery; however, ultrasound examination often reveals that vein and artery overlap rather than lie side by side. When this occurs, the typical arrangement is for the femoral artery to lie on top of the femoral vein.

Proceeding proximal to distal, the first segment after the external iliac vein is the common femoral vein. The first branch of the femoral vein after the inguinal ligament is the greater saphenous vein, which diverges medially and courses superficially down the medial as-

pect of the leg. The common femoral artery usually bifurcates several centimeters proximal to the bifurcation of the common femoral vein. Often a small innominate vein will be the second branch of the common femoral vein and will course laterally between the superficial and deep femoral arteries. The common femoral vein then bifurcates into the deep femoral and superficial femoral veins. This nearly always occurs within 10 cm of the inguinal crease (Figure 17-4). The name "superficial femoral vein" is deceptive because it is considered part of the deep vein system. There have been efforts to change the name of the superficial femoral vein because inexperienced clinicians have sometimes mistaken reports of thrombus in this location to be outside of the deep venous system.

The deep femoral vein travels deep into the thigh and is difficult to visualize by ultrasound. The superficial femoral vein proceeds distally until it dives into the obturator canal above the knee. In this region, the vein is difficult to access until it emerges behind the knee as the popliteal vein. The popliteal vein travels for about 5 cm in the popliteal fossa before trifurcating into the anterior and posterior tibial veins and the peroneal vein.

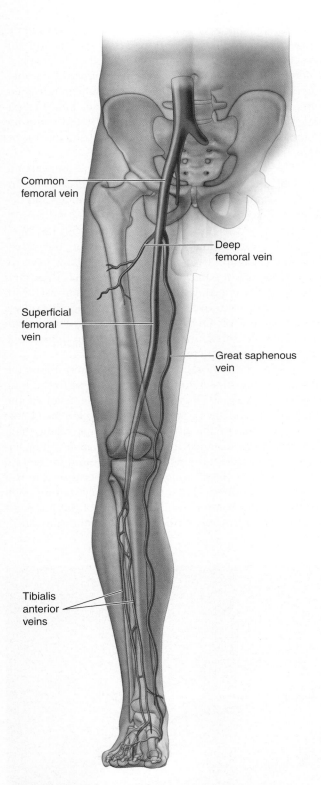

Common femoral vein

Deep femoral vein

Superficial femoral vein

Great saphenous vein

Tibialis anterior veins

Figure 17-4. The deep femoral and superficial femoral veins are seen to come together, forming the common femoral vein. DFV = deep femoral vein, CFV = common femoral vein, SFV = superficial femoral vein.

▶ GETTING STARTED

Place the ultrasound machine to the right side of the patient, although convenience, clinician comfort, and patient positioning can dictate on which side of the patient it is placed (See Video 17-1). Many ultrasound machines have multiple attached transducers. Select a high-frequency linear array, 5–10 MHz transducer since it provides optimal venous compression and image resolution. Other transducers, such as a large curved array transducer, may be used if a linear array transducer is not available or deeper imaging is required. A curved array transducer, however, may compromise venous compression and superficial image resolution. A linear array transducer is ideal because the linear footprint provides more even compression over the vessel of interest than curved transducers. Controls that select various transducer frequencies and focus for a given transducer are available on most machines, and these settings may be adjusted once the examination has begun to further improve image quality (depending on the depth of the veins being examined).

Raise the head of the bed 15–30° or place the patient in a reverse Trendelenburg position in order to assure that the veins of the lower extremity are filled. Adjust bed height to a level comfortable for the clinician. Use an adequate amount of ultrasound gel during the examination. Finally, dim the lights in the examination room to improve image visualization (contrast resolution).

▶ TECHNIQUE AND NORMAL ULTRASOUND FINDINGS

LOWER EXTREMITY

Select a 5–10 MHz linear array transducer for lower extremity scanning (Figure 17-5). Many ultrasound machines have settings that allow the clinician to adjust the frequency of the transducer. Higher frequency settings allow for better spatial resolution and improved viewing of more superficial structures, which maximizes image quality in thin patients. Alternatively, the lower frequency settings can optimize imaging in larger patients or deeper structures. Color Doppler and pulse wave Doppler may also aid in differentiation of arterial versus venous blood flow if the anatomy is difficult to identify. However, unlike the duplex ultrasound performed in most vascular laboratories, Doppler functions are used as an adjunct for identifying anatomy or assessing structures that cannot be compressed, and not as a primary modality in the limited compression ultrasound exam.

While venous compression is the most important method to evaluate the patency of veins in the lower

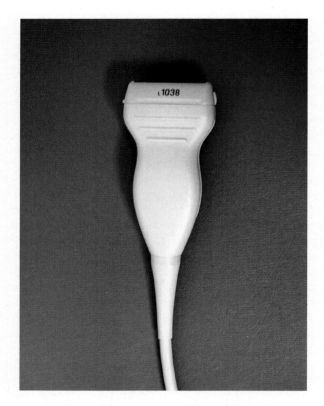

Figure 17-5. A linear array transducer.

extremity, some clinicians may choose to utilize color flow Doppler or spectral Doppler. Doppler techniques can be used to evaluate spontaneity, phasicity, direction, and augmentation of flow. In normal patent veins, flow is spontaneous and the velocity of flow varies (phasic-ity) with the changing intrathoracic pressures during the respiratory cycle. Typically, flow is anterograde and uni-directional unless there is venous valvular insufficiency. Additionally, venous flow can be augmented by applying pressure to the calf. Increase flow in the anterograde direction when performing this maneuver indicates patency of the vein. If an abnormality is noted using the Doppler adjuncts, have a heightened suspicion of venous thrombosis.

Place the patient in the supine position with the head of the bed raised 30–45° (Figure 17-6). This increases venous pooling in the lower extremities and distends the veins of the lower extremity. Extend the leg of interest and slightly externally rotate with the knee bent for the examination of the vessels in the proximal thigh (Figure 17-7). Obese patients may have an abdominal pannus that covers the proximal thigh and this should be raised. Usually, the patient can assist with this, but if unable, an assistant may be needed. Apply a liberal amount of ultrasound gel to the proximal thigh and place the ultrasound transducer on the thigh at the level of the inguinal crease.

Locate the femoral artery and vein and adjust the ultrasound transducer so that it is transverse to the long axis of the vessels (Figure 17-8). At the level of the inguinal crease, the common femoral vein is almost always medial to the artery, though this relationship can change as distance from the inguinal ligament increases. Visualize the junction of the common femoral vein and the greater saphenous vein because this is a common location for clot and the proximal starting point for the limited compression ultrasound of the leg veins (Figure 17-9A). Apply firm pressure to the transducer

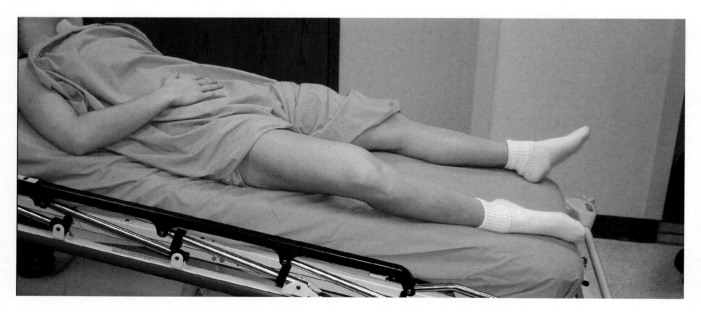

Figure 17-6. A bed angle of 30–45° allows lower extremity veins to fill and makes them easier to locate. (Courtesy of James Mateer, MD)

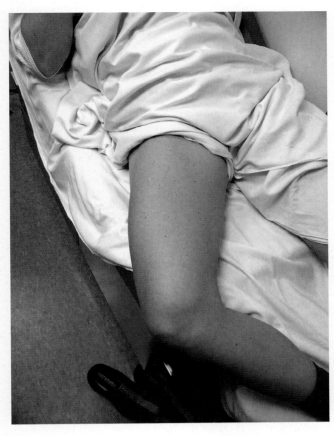

Figure 17-7. The leg is bent at the knee and rotated outward to allow best exposure of popliteal fossa as well as the junction of the common, deep, and superficial femoral veins.

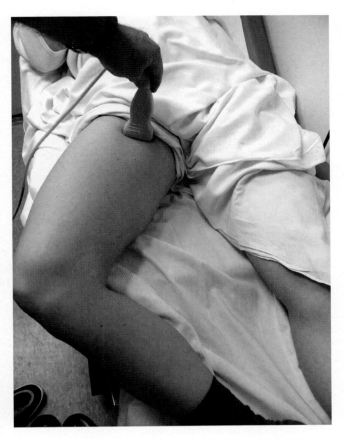

Figure 17-8. The approximate position of the linear transducer is shown transversely over the common femoral vein. The transducer handle is being held near the cord for demonstration.

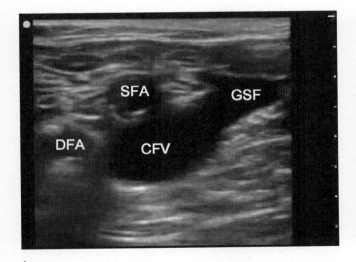

A   B

Figure 17-9. Right femoral vessels—Transverse view, linear array transducer: Baseline view (A) shows that the common femoral artery has already bifurcated into the deep femoral artery (DFA) and superficial femoral artery (SFA). Compression view (B) demonstrates complete collapse of the common femoral vein (CFV). The greater saphenous vein (GSV) can be seen branching anteromedially and is mostly collapsed in this view (slight probe repositioning and pressure should be applied to ensure complete collapse if subtle thrombus is to be excluded in this vessel).

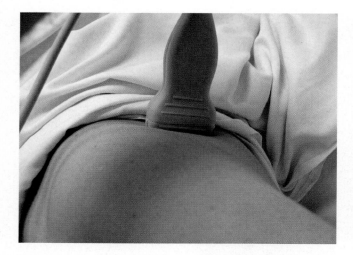 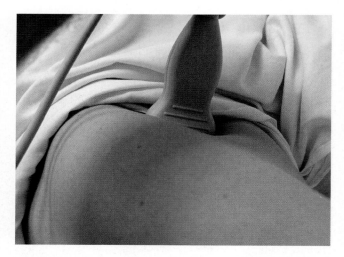

Figure 17-10. A moderate amount of pressure is applied to the leg as shown on the right in this figure. Inadequate pressure can lead to incomplete collapse of the vein.

(Figure 17-10). Both the common femoral vein and the proximal portion the greater saphenous vein should be compressible (Figure 7-9B). Complete apposition of the walls of the vein excludes DVT. Adequate force must be applied to the ultrasound transducer to achieve complete compression. In the setting of DVT, the femoral artery can often be seen to compress and is an indication that adequate force has been applied. Novice clinicians may have difficulty fully compressing a normal femoral vein. This is most often due to either inadequate force of compression or compression at an angle oblique, rather than truly transverse, to the vessel.

Some experts think it is best to follow the common femoral vein distally and compress it every 2 cm until the bifurcation of the superficial and deep femoral veins (Figure 17-11) or 10 cm distal to the inguinal ligament if it is difficult to visualize the bifurcation. However, it may not be necessary to follow the vein distally because most studies are based on just one compression at the level of the inguinal ligament

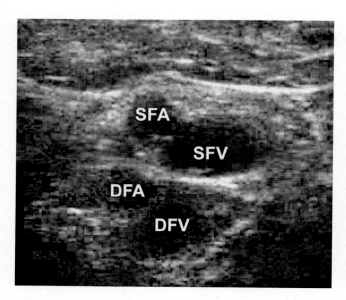 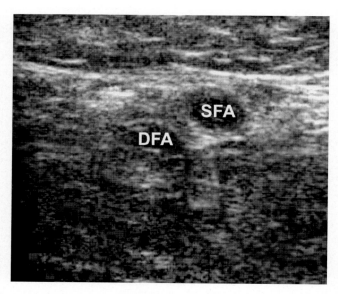

Figure 17-11. On the left side of the image, the transducer is positioned over the superficial and deep femoral arteries (SFA and DFA, respectively) and the superficial and deep femoral veins (SFV and DFV, respectively). On the right side, pressure has been applied and both veins have collapsed completely leaving only the two arteries visible.

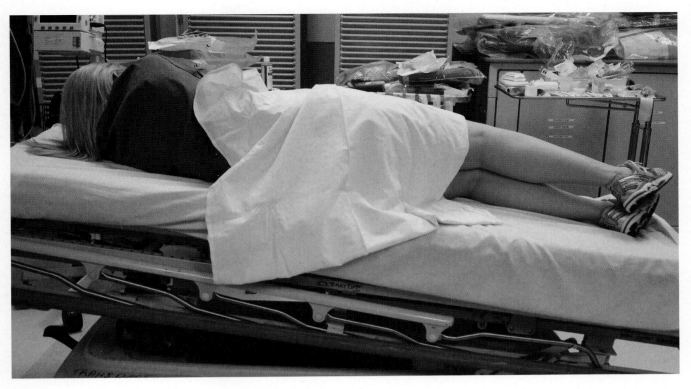

A

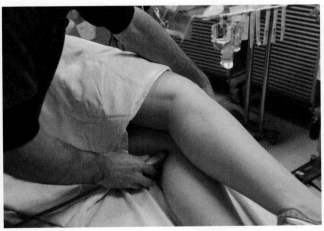

B

Figure 17-12. Ideally, the patient should be placed with their affected side down in reverse Trendelenburg to maximize distension of the popliteal vein (A). The other hand can be used to aid in compression by holding the knee in place (B).

(Figure 17-9).[2,3,11,23] Once examination of the common femoral vein is complete, proceed to evaluation of the popliteal vessels.

For evaluation of the popliteal vein, patient positioning is often more challenging (Figure 17-12). Gaining adequate access to the popliteal fossa is more difficult than the inguinal region in many patients, especially the obese. One common approach is to have the patient move to a lateral recumbent position with the examined leg in a dependent position and the knee slightly flexed. This position allows access to the popliteal fossa and optimal venous distention in the extremity.

The popliteal vein is located adjacent and superficial to the popliteal artery in the mid popliteal fossa (Figure 17-13A). Complete collapse of the vein lumen demonstrates patency of the vein and an absence of clot (Figure 17-13B). The popliteal fossa is a small area, and compression of the vein in more than one location can be quickly performed. We recommend compression of the proximal, mid, and distal popliteal fossa with the

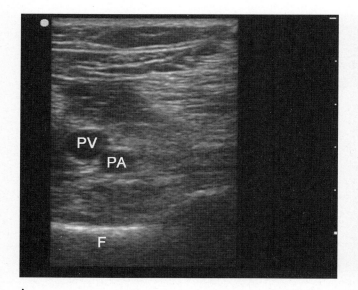
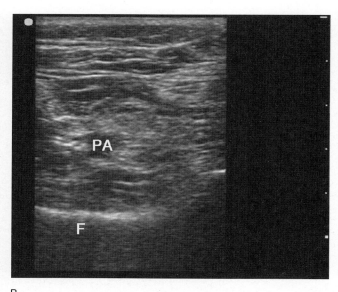

A

B

Figure 17-13. Left popliteal vessels—Transverse view, linear array transducer: Baseline view (A). Pressure applied to the transducer (B) results in complete collapse of the popliteal vein (PV), which is located superficial to the popliteal artery (PA). Showing the femur (F) at the bottom of the screen ensures that the vessels being imaged are the popliteal and not superficial or duplicated vessels.

latter being identified as the popliteal vein reaches its trifurcation.

It is common to see smaller veins adjacent or superficial to the popliteal vessels and 5% of patients have a truly duplicated popliteal vein. Identification of the popliteal vein may be difficult in morbidly obese patients due to vessel depth and poor patient positioning. It is important to recognize that the popliteal vein, whether normal or duplicated, superficial or deep, is always accompanied by the popliteal artery. Additionally, the popliteal vein is the deepest vein in the popliteal fossa when viewed from a posterior approach, so visualization of the femur deep to the vessel is further confirmation that the vein in question is in fact the popliteal and not a more superficial vessel. If this is not appreciated, superficial veins may be mistaken for the popliteal vein and a DVT may be missed.

Controversy exists regarding the need to routinely scan the contralateral leg in patients undergoing limited compression ultrasound for unilateral lower extremity complaints. The incidence of contralateral, asymptomatic leg thrombi is as high as 34% in some patient populations, especially hospitalized patients and those with active malignancy or other significant risk factors for DVT.[24] While some authors have argued that bilateral scanning should be the standard, others argue that scanning an asymptomatic extremity is not cost-effective and wastes resources.[25-27] It may be reasonable to scan both extremities in very high-risk patients and only the symptomatic extremity in most outpatients.[24] One study

recommends a unilateral lower extremity scan in outpatients and a scan of the contralateral leg if the patient is found to have a DVT in the symptomatic extremity.[28] Limited compression ultrasound is much faster compared to traditional vascular laboratory duplex scans, so the threshold for scanning both legs may be lower. However, in the setting of a busy ED, if only one lower extremity is symptomatic, scanning of the contralateral leg is generally not indicated.

UPPER EXTREMITY

Use a 5–10 MHz linear transducer for upper extremity vascular imaging. Place patients supine or in the Trendelenburg position, which increases neck and upper extremity venous engorgement, aiding in identification of anatomy and image acquisition. Begin the study by locating the distal portion of the internal jugular vein in the transverse plane (Figure 17-14). If there is difficulty locating the internal jugular vein, color Doppler may aid with identification. Apply gentle pressure with the transducer to completely collapse the vein in 1 cm increments while moving proximally. Minimize compression of the internal jugular vein only to that necessary to completely collapse the vein. Examine the internal jugular vein proximally to the point where it enters the brachiocephalic or subclavian vein. The proximal portion of the internal jugular vein becomes difficult to compress due to overlying bony structures; direct visualization of

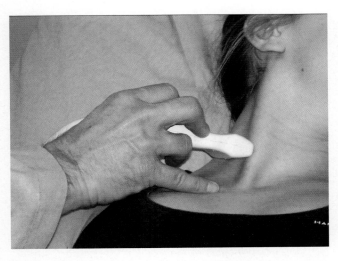

Figure 17-14. A linear transducer is held at the level of the internal jugular in transverse. The entire length of the jugular can be traced and evaluated for thrombus. Aggressive compression is avoided in this region, especially in elderly patients. Interrogation is started higher on the neck than shown here. (Courtesy of James Mateer, MD)

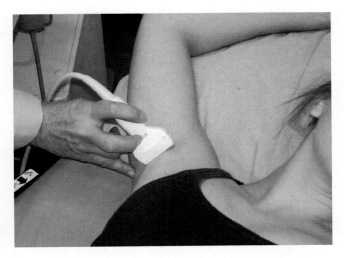

Figure 17-16. A linear transducer is held in the axilla. This allows transverse visualization of the vessels and compression. (Courtesy of James Mateer, MD)

thrombus or color Doppler may be helpful in identifying any abnormality. The proximal subclavian vein can usually be visualized using a supraclavicular window with transducer orientation longitudinal to the vessel. It is not possible to compress the proximal subclavian vein so the exam relies on direct visualization of thrombus or visualization of color Doppler flow (Figure 17-15). It may be difficult to visualize the distal subclavian and proximal axillary veins but they should be compressed where

possible. Resume a more direct examination when the distal axillary vein emerges in the axilla (Figure 17-16). Compress the brachial and basilic veins after they bifurcate from the axillary vein, moving distally to the level of the antecubital fossa. Compress these veins individually to ensure complete collapse. If there is a high suspicion of DVT in the axillary or subclavian veins and it cannot be visualized with ultrasound, then consider using CT to assist with the diagnosis.[29]

DOCUMENTATION AND BILLING

Document diagnostic ultrasound examinations for the medical record and billing purposes. Documentation of the study should generally include:[30]

- Indication for the examination
- Views obtained
- Relevant findings
- Physician interpretation

Obtain and store images of the relevant anatomy. When billing for the study, at least one image of the study must be recorded and stored permanently to satisfy CPT coding criteria. Two-point limited compression ultrasound of the lower extremity for DVT is coded as a limited duplex scan of the lower extremity veins (CPT code 93971).[31] Storing video clips of venous compression is the best way to document the study. If video is not available, split screen still images can be used to document vein compression (Figures 17-9 and 17-13).

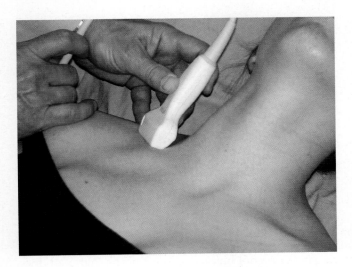

Figure 17-15. A linear transducer is held just above the clavicle, allowing a longitudinal view of the subclavian vein. (Courtesy of James Mateer, MD)

► COMMON AND EMERGENT ABNORMALITIES

The inability to fully compress the vein of interest with the ultrasound transducer indicates a thrombus within the vein. Normally, veins will compress easily while arteries can be difficult to compress. If pressure is inadequate or applied at an oblique angle, then the vein may not be fully compressed and a false positive interpretation may result.

ACUTE DVT

An acute DVT is best appreciated by the inability to completely compress the vein lumen (Figure 17-17). In general, an acute DVT is found centrally within the vein and may appear to be floating within the vein lumen (Figure 17-18). An acute DVT will also have smoother edges and be less echogenic than a chronic DVT, but the degree of echogenicity can be variable. Some acute DVTs may be echo lucent and can only be recognized by incomplete collapse of the vessel with compression (Figure 17-19). Occasionally, an obvious echogenic DVT will be noted within the vein prior to compression (Figure 17-20). Upper extremity clots may have a similar appearance (Figure 17-21). There have not been any reported iatrogenic complications, such as PE,

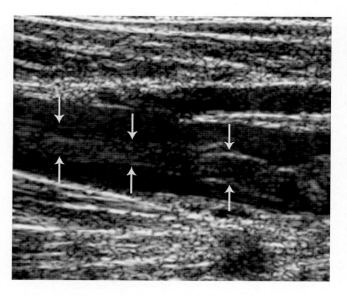

Figure 17-18. Arrows show a freely floating thrombus in the femoral vein. In this portion of the image, the clot does not come in contact with the anterior or posterior wall of the vein.

from compression of a DVT during a limited compression ultrasound exam. False positive studies can result if echogenic appearance alone is used to make the diagnosis.

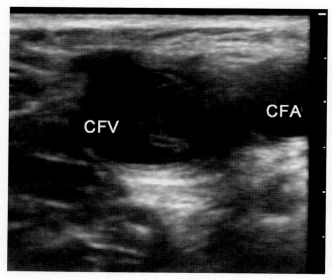

A

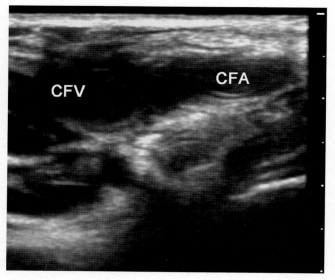

B

Figure 17-17. Acute DVT in the left common femoral vein (CFV). Thrombus can be seen as an echogenic mass in the baseline image (A). Relying on echogenic structures in the lumen as the only criteria for the diagnosis of DVT can lead to false positives due to artifacts. In the compression image (B), enough force has been applied to begin to compress the common femoral artery (CFA), yet the vein does not completely compress. Although the thrombus is not as readily visible on the compression view, the inability to completely collapse a vein with adequate force is most important for making the diagnosis of DVT. (Note: Overall gain of the image is high in order to enhance visualization of the thrombus.)

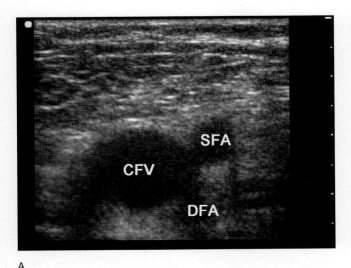

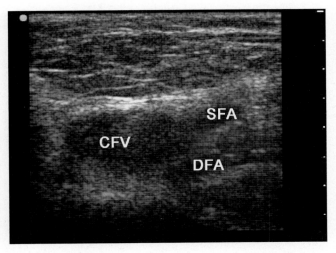

A   B

Figure 17-19. DVT in the left CFV. Clot is echolucent in the baseline view (A). Pressure is then applied to the transducer (B) with enough force to cause some compression of the SFA. The CFV walls are collapsing only partially in this view (B) diagnosing DVT. [Note also that in this example, compression reveals subtle echogenicity within the vein (thrombus).] DFA = deep femoral artery, CFV = common femoral vein, SFA = superficial femoral artery.

CHRONIC DVT

Chronic DVT refers to a condition where an acute DVT becomes recanalized over time, thus allowing venous blood to flow either through or around the thrombus. Prolonged presence of thrombus in the vein can cause damage to the venous valves resulting in venous hypertension, extremity swelling, erythema, and pain, which may mimic an acute DVT. A vein with a chronic DVT will not fully collapse, mimicking an acute DVT. In general, the thrombus of a chronic DVT is more echogenic and has a more ragged appearing edge than an acute DVT. Additionally, acute DVTs tend to recanalize centrally, leaving the thrombus of chronic DVT appearing to adhere to the walls of the vein (Figures 17-22 and 17-23). It is sometimes helpful to examine the vein in a sagittal view to differentiate acute versus chronic DVTs. Despite the differences between acute and chronic DVTs, both

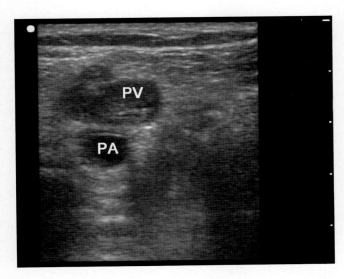

Figure 17-20. Acute DVT in popliteal vein (PV). There is increased echogenicity within the vein and failure to compress at all when compression is applied.

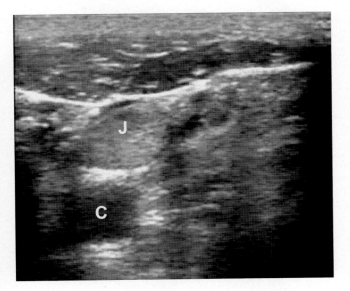

Figure 17-21. A transverse image shows a noticeable thrombus in this internal jugular vein (J), just superficial to the carotid artery (C). Compression was not necessary to verify that a DVT was present in this obvious case.

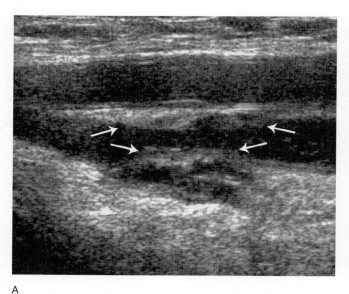

A

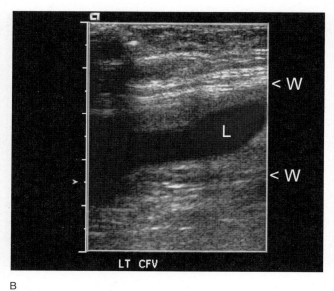

B

Figure 17-22. Chronic DVT. A DVT is seen in this deep femoral vein (A). Arrows point to areas of scarring that are echogenic and lie along the walls of the vein. A channel is open for blood flow in between the two areas of scar or chronic DVT. Longitudinal view of the common femoral vein (B) shows chronic echogenic clot along the walls (W) with central recannulation of the lumen (L). (B, Courtesy of James Mateer, MD, Waukesha Memorial Hospital)

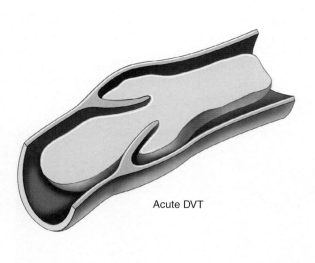

Acute DVT

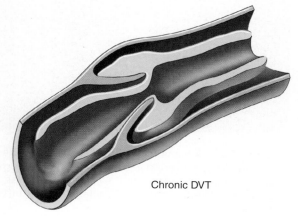

Chronic DVT

Figure 17-23. The illustration on the right shows a recanalized, old thrombus. The left image demonstrates an early acute thrombus that can enlarge and obstruct flow completely.

historically and in ultrasound appearance, it is important to remember that patients who have known chronic DVTs are more likely to develop acute DVTs within the same vessel. If there is uncertainty concerning chronicity, treat patients with positive ultrasound findings for acute DVT.

SUPERFICIAL VENOUS THROMBOSIS

Providers will occasionally note thrombosis of a superficial vein when performing a limited compression ultrasound of an extremity. This most commonly occurs in the saphenous vein, but may occur in any superficial vein of the upper or lower extremity. Depending on the vein involved, a follow-up study in 5–7 days may be warranted to evaluate for extension of the thrombus into the deep venous system. Most treatment protocols do not recommend anticoagulation in the instance of superficial thrombosis. One notable exception is when a thrombosis of the proximal saphenous vein is either near to or "hanging" into the common femoral vein (Figure 17-24). In this situation anticoagulation is recommended. In other situations, such as thrombus in the antecubital or brachial veins, there are no clear treatment recommendations other than to obtain close follow-up and repeat the examination within 1 week (Figure 17-25).

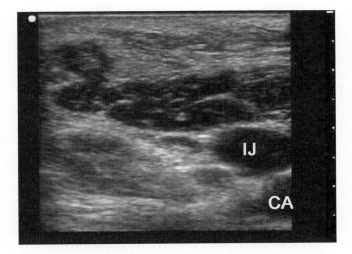

Figure 17-25. External jugular vein clots are extremely rare. Although this clot does not involve the internal jugular vein (IJ), this patient was anticoagulated. External jugular vein clots are considered by some as an exception to the usual conservative treatment of superficial venous thrombosis. CA = carotid artery.

► COMMON VARIANTS AND SELECTED ABNORMALITIES

When evaluating the lower extremity venous system, other rounded structures may be mistaken for normal and pathological findings. Lymph nodes may be encountered in the region of the common femoral vein, especially in ill patients (Figure 17-26). An inflamed lymph node can be initially mistaken for a noncollapsing vein due to similar echogenicity and cross-sectional structure.

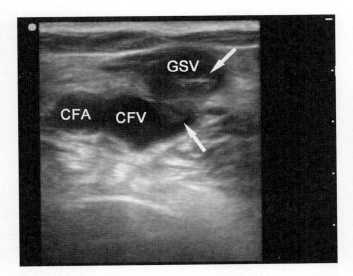

Figure 17-24. The greater saphenous vein (GSV) is seen branching from the common femoral vein (CFV). A clot is seen in the GSV "dangling" into the CFV (arrows). Even though the CFV completely compressed on transducer pressure (the GSV did not), the presence of a "dangling" clot should lead to anticoagulation. (Note: Overall gain of the image is high in order to enhance visualization of the thrombus.)

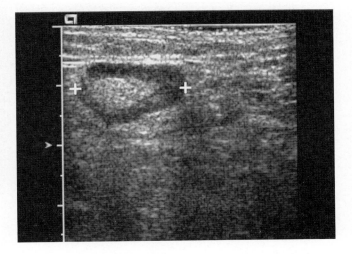

Figure 17-26. Typical appearance of an enlarged inguinal lymph node (2 cm). The thickened capsule is hypoechoic while the central hilum is echogenic. (Courtesy of James Mateer, MD, Waukesha Memorial Hospital)

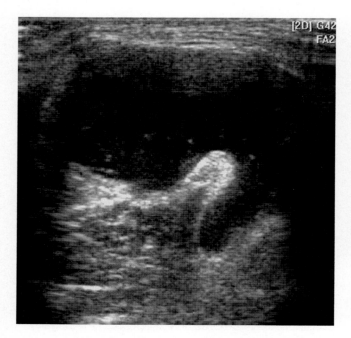

Figure 17-27. Longitudinal view of the posterior knee area demonstrates a large Baker's cyst.

Careful sonographic evaluation in transverse and sagittal planes will show its true shape to be spherical rather than a tubular vessel. Duplication of the femoral or popliteal vessels can occur, and it is important to identify any extra vessels and ensure their patency as well. Deep veins are always accompanied by an artery, while superficial or "tributary" veins are not.

Findings in the popliteal fossa include Baker's cysts (Figure 17-27), which can be confusing when small in

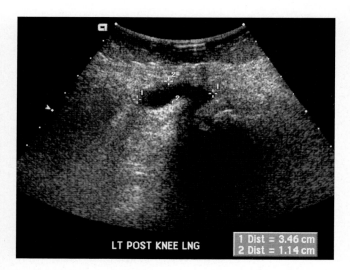

Figure 17-28. Longitudinal view of the posterior knee reveals a small Baker's cyst. (Courtesy of James Mateer, MD, Waukesha Memorial Hospital)

size (Figure 17-28). A Baker's cyst appears as a pocket of fluid with irregular borders that protrudes into the popliteal space and sometimes into the calf, and rarely, into the thigh. Careful examination of the structure should lead to its discrimination from the popliteal vessels. Consider rupture of a Baker's cyst in any patient with calf swelling who has a history of chronic arthritis or knee effusion. These can present with impressive swelling and pain and may present with fluid dissecting through soft tissue planes posterior to and below the knee on ultrasound (Figure 17-29). Popliteal artery aneurysms are occasionally encountered and may make

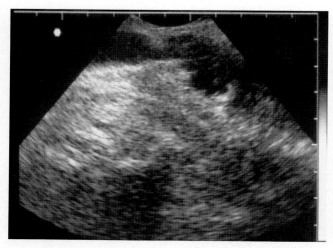

A

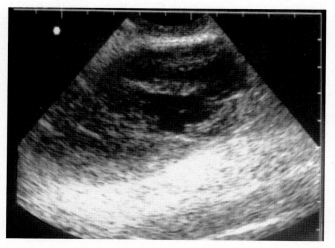

B

Figure 17-29. Ruptured Bakers's cyst. (A) Longitudinal view of the posterior knee shows a Baker's cyst (left upper image) communicating with subcutaneous fluid in the upper calf. (B) Longitudinal view over the mid calf of the same patient shows a significant amount of subcutaneous fluid dissecting inferiorly. (Courtesy of James Mateer, MD)

it harder to compress the popliteal vein. Aneurysms larger than 2 cm can cause complications and should be followed closely.

▶ PITFALLS

1. **Contraindication.** There are no absolute contraindications for evaluating the deep venous system of the lower extremities. Patient comfort or level of cooperation may limit the examination. Consider administering analgesia prior to the exam to facilitate compression. There have not been any documented cases of embolization of a DVT due to a compression ultrasound examination.

2. **Technically difficult exams.** Patients who are morbidly obese or have severe lower extremity edema may be very difficult to image. The ultrasound beam greatly deteriorates with increased fat as well as distance. A variety of adjustments or changes can be made on some equipment to optimize image quality. Options include tissue harmonics, spatial compounding, and other image processing features. Using a lower frequency transducer is also an option. In a large thigh, make sure the vessel of interest is positioned directly between the transducer and femur, otherwise it will be difficult to achieve complete compression.

3. **Segmental DVT.** One concern about the limited compression ultrasound examination is the possibility of segmental DVT; for instance, a DVT potentially may span several centimeters of the superficial femoral vein mid-thigh but cannot be found elsewhere. The true incidence of such an occurrence is not known, but evidence suggests that it is very rare. However, a repeat study in 5–7 days is often recommended after a negative limited compression ultrasound exam. This will detect propagation of an undetected calf thrombosis and a segmental clot. If a patient is able to identify a specific area of localized pain or swelling on his or her thigh, evaluating that area for possible DVT is reasonable and may be reassuring.

4. **Misunderstanding the limitations of ultrasonography.** Although ultrasound is now the method of choice for detecting the presence of lower extremity thrombosis, it is not 100% accurate. Practitioners should understand the limitation of ultrasound, especially when considering that the method described in this chapter does not attempt to evaluate veins in the calf. Furthermore, the use of ultrasound examination of bilateral lower extremities to exclude PE is

fraught with potential danger if the physician does not keep in mind that only a positive finding is helpful. Many patients with PE will not have a proximal DVT found on lower extremity ultrasound. This may be due to a nonlower extremity source or due to the thrombus completely embolizing to the lungs.[32]

5. **Mistaking artery for vein.** While this is not a common pitfall, novice operators should be aware that in some cases an artery may be pliable enough to collapse under moderate transducer pressure, while the vein lumen is held open by the presence of clot. If available, color and pulse wave Doppler may help simplify the identification of blood vessels.

6. **Femoral lymph nodes mistaken for a DVT.** Occasionally, lymph nodes encountered in the groin can be mistaken for a noncompressible deep vein. This is especially true for inflamed lymph nodes. Figure 17-30 shows an example of a large lymph node that was mistaken for a femoral DVT. The lymph node is an oval-shaped structure, and moving the transducer proximally or distally will allow the clinician to identify the edges of the lymph node. Rotating the transducer will also frequently show the boundaries of the lymph node as well as its atypical appearance for a blood vessel. Lymph nodes tend to be more superficial or closer to the skin surface than deep vessels.

7. **Pelvic vein thrombosis.** Thrombosis of the pelvic veins, such as the external iliac, frequently occurs in combination with DVT of the common femoral and more distal venous segments. Thus, identification of clot in the external

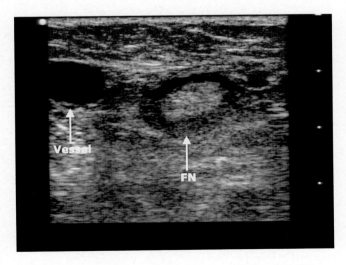

Figure 17-30. The femoral lymph node next to the actual vein has an uncanny resemblance to a lumen filled with thrombus. FN = Femoral lymph node.

iliac vein is not as crucial when a common femoral DVT is located and the patient is anticoagulated. However, in a small percentage of cases, thrombosis of the pelvic veins is an isolated event.[33] Isolated pelvic vein thrombosis may be quite challenging to diagnose and poses a high risk of embolization. Ultrasound interrogation of the external iliac, common iliac, and the proximal portion of the internal iliac vein is possible in few thin patients without interfering bowel gas. In a minority of patients, the external and common iliac can be seen and compressed. If suspicion for pelvic vein thrombosis exists and ultrasound will not provide adequate imaging, then other diagnostic measures such as CT with venous angiography will have to be employed. Even if the iliac veins cannot be visualized, a DVT may be suspected if there is a lack of respiratory variation in the venous flow in the common iliac vein. Normally, variation is seen in the baseline venous flow with respiration (Figure 17-31). If this variation is absent, it is suggestive of a proximal obstruction, such as a thrombus in the external or common iliac ipsilaterally. Conversely, if respiratory variation is observed, then there is unlikely to be a complete obstruction of proximal vein.

8. **Slow venous blood flow.** Occasionally, blood flow in a vein segment may be slow enough that swirling of the blood is actually seen within the lumen. This can have the appearance of echogenic material in the vein and be mistaken for a thrombus. It is important not to make this mistake by moving too quickly through the examination. Compression of the vein segment will reveal complete collapse of the vein and disappearance of the vein lumen.

9. **Mistaking the saphenous vein for the superficial femoral (deep) vein.** The saphenous vein runs superficially down the anterior and medial thigh after its takeoff from the common femoral vein. Its most prominent feature is the absence of a paired artery. If an examiner mistakes this vessel for the superficial femoral vein, a DVT in the femoral vein may be missed.

10. **Limited compression sonography for DVT.** There is a risk for abbreviating this exam too much. A limited exam is not exclusive of a thorough exam. Preparation of the patient and equipment is likely to take more time than the actual ultrasound examination. The ultrasound imaging is limited to two main areas in the lower extremity, but several compression segments of each area are recommended (see section 'Technique and Normal Ultrasound Findings'). Early thrombus formation is often associated with branching areas of the vein, so the clinician should also attempt to visualize and compress the confluence of these main branching areas (Figure 17-32).

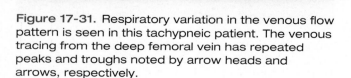

Figure 17-31. Respiratory variation in the venous flow pattern is seen in this tachypneic patient. The venous tracing from the deep femoral vein has repeated peaks and troughs noted by arrow heads and arrows, respectively.

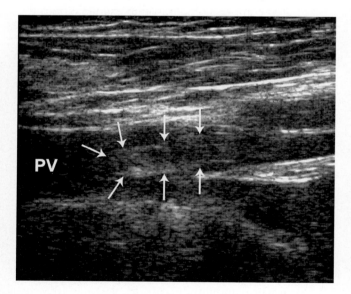

Figure 17-32. A longitudinal image of the popliteal vein (PV) on the left side of the image. On the right side the PV is splitting. Arrows outline a free-floating thrombus coming out of a calf vein into the very distal portion of the popliteal. This clot would not have been caught if compression had not included the proximal portion of popliteal trifurcation.

▶ CASE STUDIES

CASE 1

Patient Presentation

A 25-year-old woman presented to the ED with a complaint of right calf swelling and pain. The patient was a law school student who was studying for final examinations. She denied any strenuous activity and noted spending most of the last week sitting in the library. The patient was normally athletic and rides a stationary bicycle daily. She had an unremarkable medical history and did not smoke. She thought her older sister had a "blood clot" several years ago.

Physical examination revealed a healthy young woman with normal vital signs, including an oxygen saturation of 98% on room air. She had a moderately tender right calf without any visible erythema or palpable cord. The patient had moderate discomfort on manipulation of her foot at the ankle. Her right calf measured approximately 2.5 cm larger than the left, a fact the patient attributed to a left knee injury while playing soccer in college.

Management Course

The vascular laboratory was not open on Saturday. Previous department policy suggested anticoagulation until ultrasound was available on Monday, but the emergency physicians had recently become credentialed in limited compression ultrasonography. The emergency physician performed an ultrasound examination of the patient's right leg. The common femoral and saphenous vein junction and the deep femoral and superficial femoral veins were located. All were noncompressible. The popliteal vein was visualized behind the knee and also did not compress. Because of the extensive nature of her DVT, a vascular surgeon was consulted for consideration of thrombolytics and/or mechanical clot retrieval. The patient was eventually discharged on low molecular weight heparin injections. A follow-up appointment with a vascular surgeon was made for the following week.

Commentary

Case 1 represents an example of a fairly low-risk patient who can still inspire considerable angst for the treating physician. With her suggestive symptoms and family history, the patient might present a medicolegal risk if she was discharged home without definitive diagnostic imaging and had a complication from anticoagulation that was later determined to be unnecessary. Treating the patient presumptively with low molecular weight heparin as an outpatient may seem attractive, but it has some limitations. The patient must be

taught how to administer the injections. Also, there was a risk of bleeding even if it was relatively low. Discovering the extent of her clot changed the management from simple anticoagulation to consideration of more aggressive therapy. With increasing concerns about post-thrombotic syndrome in patients treated with anticoagulation alone, and with recognition that thrombolysis and/or mechanical clot retrieval may both reduce the risk of post-thrombotic syndrome and return patients to full function sooner, it is prudent to consider these treatment modalities in facilities where such expertise is available.[34]

This scenario is quite realistic in many facilities. Staffing a vascular laboratory 24 hours a day, 7 days a week, can be very expensive, especially when coupled with a shortage of sonographers. In this case, the emergency physician was able to confidently demonstrate an extensive DVT, justify the risk of anticoagulant treatment, and seek an appropriate consultation.

CASE 2

Patient Presentation

A 32-year-old woman with no previous medical history presented to the ED with dizziness and dyspnea. She reported her last normal menstrual period to be 7 weeks ago. On physical examination, her blood pressure was 70/50 mm Hg, heart rate of 135 beats per minute, and respirations 26 per minute. She was a diaphoretic young woman, pale, and in moderate distress. Her examination was otherwise unremarkable, including nontender, nonedematous legs.

Management Course

Her point-of-care pregnancy test was negative. The emergency physician performed bilateral lower extremity ultrasound exams, which showed a DVT in the left popliteal vein. Despite anticoagulation and fluid resuscitation, the patient's vital signs continued to rapidly deteriorate, so a systemic thrombolytic agent was administered for her presumed PE. The patient's clinical status gradually improved in the ICU.

Commentary

Emergent management of critically ill patients with known or suspected PE goes beyond anticoagulation and includes systemic thrombolysis, local catheter directed thrombolysis, or mechanical thrombectomy.[35] Case 2 illustrates the benefit of critical information in time-sensitive situations, especially when therapies have risk (anticoagulation, thrombolysis) or require significant and rapid coordination of care (emergent interventional radiology consult). Delaying these interventions for an ultrasound examination by the vascular lab or diagnostic imaging service presents significant increased risk to the patient.

CASE 3

Patient Presentation

A 22-year-old woman with a history of sickle cell disease presented with a complaint of left lower leg swelling and pain. The patient stated that she first began to notice discomfort in the leg 4 days ago and today noticed swelling, redness, and increased pain. She denied any history of trauma and stated that her typical sickle cell pain is higher in the leg and that this pain has a different quality.

Physical examination revealed normal vital signs with a temperature of 100.0°F. The examination was within normal limits except for the patient's lower left leg. She had erythema and increased temperature of the anterior shin as well as nonpitting edema. The area was sensitive to the touch. The calf was mildly tender and slightly swollen. The patient's ankle was also swollen but no deformity was noted. She had diffuse pain in the ankle and anterior shin with flexion and extension of the foot. Distal pulses were present and equal to the contralateral side.

Management Course

A point-of-care ultrasound examination of the left leg was performed using the diagnostic algorithm in Figure 17-2 for clinician-performed ultrasound. The femoral and popliteal veins were completely compressible. The patient had planned on traveling next week and wished to avoid a repeat study. A D-dimer assay was positive, and the patient was counseled about the importance of returning in 5–7 days for a repeat study. A diagnosis of cellulitis was made with the patient being discharged home on oral antibiotics. She did follow up 1 week later and the repeat ultrasound exam was also negative.

Commentary

The primary goal of point-of-care ultrasound is to rapidly provide quality clinical information to assist in clinical decision making. Because of concerns about patient follow-up, the physician sent a D-dimer assay instead of just scheduling a repeat ultrasound in 1 week. Because the D-dimer assay was positive, the patient was instructed about the importance of the follow-up study. Alternatively, if the physician used the algorithm in Figure 17-1, the patient would be at low risk per the Wells criteria (Table 17-2), but the positive D-dimer assay would have led to the limited compression ultrasound in the

ED, and subsequently the follow-up ultrasound exam in 5–7 days with the identical outcome.

REFERENCES

1. American College of Emergency Physicians. Emergency ultrasound guidelines 2008. www.acep.org/WorkArea/DownloadAsset.aspx?ID=32878. February 2012.
2. Cogo A, Lensing AW, Koopman MM, et al.: Compression ultrasonography for diagnostic management of patients with clinically suspected deep vein thrombosis: Prospective cohort study. *BMJ* 316(7214):17–20, 1998.
3. Bernardi E, Camprese G, Buller HR, et al.: Serial 2-point ultrasonography plus D-dimer vs whole-leg color-coded Doppler ultrasonography for diagnosing suspected deep vein thrombosis. *JAMA* 300(14):1653–1659, 2008.
4. White RH: The epidemiology of venous thromboembolism. *Circ* 107:I4–I8, 2003.
5. Carrier M, Le Gal G, Wells PS, et al.: Systematic review: Case-fatality rates of recurrent venous thromboembolism and major bleeding events among patients treated for venous thromboembolism. *Ann Intern Med* 152(9):578, 2010.
6. Carpenter JP, Holland GA, Baum RA, et al.: Magnetic resonance venography for the detection of deep venous thrombosis: Comparison with contrast venography and duplex Doppler ultrasonography. *J Vasc Surg* 18:734–741, 1993.
7. Blumenberg RM, Barton E, Gelfand ML, et al.: Occult deep venous thrombosis complicating superficial thrombophlebitis. *J Vasc Surg* 27:338–343, 1998.
8. Wells PS, Owen C, Doucette S, et al.: Does this patient have deep venous thrombosis? *JAMA* 295(2):199–207, 2006.
9. Wells PS, Anderson DR, Bormanis J, et al.: Value assessment of pretest probability of deep-vein thrombosis in clinical management. *The Lancet.* 351:1795–1798, 1997.
10. Poppiti R, Papanicolaou G, Perese S, et al.: Limited B-mode venous imaging versus complete color-flow duplex venous scanning for detection of proximal deep venous thrombosis. *J Vasc Surg* 22:553–557, 1995.
11. Lensing AWA, Prandoni P, Brandjes D, et al.: Detection of deep-vein thrombosis by real-time B-mode ultrasonography. *N Engl J Med* 320:342–345, 1989.
12. Blaivas M, Lambert MJ, Harwood RA, et al.: Lower-extremity Doppler for deep venous thrombosis—Can emergency physicians be accurate and fast? *Acad Emerg Med* 7:120–126, 2000.
13. Frazee BW, Snoey ER, Levitt A: Emergency department compression ultrasound to diagnose proximal deep vein thrombosis. *J Emerg Med* 20:107–112, 2001.
14. Jang T, Docherty M, Aubin C, et al.: Resident-performed compression ultrasonography for the detection of proximal deep vein thrombosis: Fast and accurate. *Acad Emerg Med* 11:319–322, 2004.
15. Theodoro D, Blaivas M, Duggal S, et al.: Real-time B-mode ultrasound in the ED saves time in the diagnosis of deep vein thrombosis (DVT). *Am J Emerg Med* 22:197–200, 2004.
16. Jacoby J, Cesta M, Axelband J, et al.: Can emergency medicine residents detect acute deep venous thrombosis

with a limited, two-site ultrasound examination? *J Emerg Med* 32:197–200, 2007.

17. Crisp JG, Lovato LM, Jang TB: Compression ultrasonography of the lower extremity with portable vascular ultrasonography can accurately detect deep vein thrombosis in the emergency department. *Ann Emerg Med* 56:601–610, 2010.

18. Cogo A, Lensing AWA, Prandoni P, et al.: Distribution of thrombosis in patients with symptomatic deep vein thrombosis: implications for simplifying the diagnostic process with compression ultrasound. *Arch Intern Med* 153(24):2777–2780, 1993.

19. Kraaijenhagen RA, Piovella F, Bernardi E, et al.: Simplification of the diagnostic management of suspected deep vein thrombosis. *Arch Intern Med* 162(8):907–911, 2002.

20. Burnside PR, Brown MD, Kline JA: Systematic review of emergency physician performed ultrasonography for lower extremity deep vein thrombosis. *Acad Emerg Med* 15(6):493–498, 2008.

21. Goodacre S, Stevenson M, Wailoo A, et al.: How should we diagnose suspected deep-vein thrombosis? *QJM* 99(6):377–388, 2006.

22. Lechner D, Wiener C, Weltermann A, et al.: Comparison between idiopathic deep vein thrombosis of the upper and lower extremity regarding risk factors and recurrence. *J Thromb Haemost* 6:1269–1274.

23. Lensing AWA, Doris CI, McGrath FP, et al.: A comparison of compression ultrasound with color Doppler ultrasound for the diagnosis of symptomless postoperative deep vein thrombosis. *Arch Intern Med* 157:765–768, 1997.

24. Pennell RC, Mantese VA, Westfall SG: Duplex scan for deep vein thrombosis—Defining who needs an examination of the contralateral asymptomatic leg. *J Vasc Surg* 48:413–416, 2008.

25. Naidich JB, Torre JR, Pellerito JS, et al.: Suspected deep venous thrombosis: Is US of both legs necessary? *Radiology* 200:429–431, 1996.

26. Sheiman RC, McArdle CR: Bilateral lower extremity US in the patient with unilateral symptoms of deep venous thrombosis: Assessment of need. *Radiology* 194:171–173, 1995.

27. Strothman G, Blebea J, Fowl RJ, et al.: Contralateral duplex scanning for deep vein thrombosis is unnecessary in patients with symptoms. *J Vasc Surg* 22:543–547, 1995.

28. Garcia ND, Morasch MD, Ebaugh JL, et al.: Is bilateral ultrasound scanning of the legs necessary for patients with unilateral symptoms of deep vein thrombosis? *J Vasc Surg* 34:792–797, 2001.

29. ACR Appropriateness Criteria Suspected Upper Extremity Deep Vein Thrombosis 2011. http://www.acr.org/acet/Suspected-Upper-Extremity-Deep-Vein-Thrombosis-ET.pdf. February 2012.

30. Emergency Ultrasound Standard Reporting Guidelines 2011. www.acep.org/WorkArea/DownloadAsset.aspx?ID=82705. February 2012.

31. Emergency Ultrasound Coding and Reimbursement 2010. www.acep.org/WorkArea/DownloadAsset.aspx?ID=33016. February 2012.

32. Kluetz PG, White CS: Acute pulmonary embolism: imaging in the emergency department. *Radiol Clin North Am* 44:259–271, 2006.

33. Carpenter JP, Holland GA, Baum RA, et al.: Magnetic resonance venography for the detection of deep venous thrombosis: Comparison with contrast venography and duplex Doppler ultrasonography. *J Vasc Surg* 18(5):734–741, 1993.

34. Pollack CV: Advanced management of acute iliofemoral deep venous thrombosis: Emergency department and beyond. *Ann Emerg Med* 57:590–599, 2011.

35. Kearon C, Kahn SR, Agnelli G, et al.: Antithrombotic therapy for venous thromboembolic disease: American College of Chest Physicians evidence-based clinical practice guidelines (8th edition). *Chest* 133:454S–545S, 2008.

CHAPTER 18

Musculoskeletal, Soft Tissue, and Miscellaneous Applications

Andreas Dewitz

Beyond the well-known primary applications of emergency ultrasound lies a veritable smorgasbord of clinically useful ultrasound applications. Some of these applications allow emergency care providers to rapidly evaluate and better manage common clinical problems. This chapter will focus on eight applications of point-of-care ultrasound that are useful in the acute care setting. These include (1) evaluation of abdominal wall pain and masses; (2) airway assessment; (3) evaluation of bony cortices for rapid fracture diagnosis and postreduction alignment; (4) subcutaneous foreign body diagnosis and localization; (5) imaging of selected tendons, joints, and muscles for common musculoskeletal complaints; (6) diagnosis of salivary gland disease; (7) point-of-care detection of maxillary sinusitis; and (8) evaluation of soft tissue infections, particularly for detection and accurate localization of subcutaneous abscesses prior to drainage.

► ABDOMINAL WALL

CLINICAL CONSIDERATIONS AND INDICATIONS

A surprisingly wide range of pathologic processes can occur in the abdominal wall, and a patient's abdominal pain may, on occasion, be discovered due to a lesion or defect within this anatomic region. Since the area of anatomic interest is quite superficial and free of shadowing artifacts, it is well suited to sonographic evaluation with a linear array transducer. When a palpable or indistinct abdominal wall mass is found on physical examination, or when a focal area of abdominal wall tenderness is encountered, a point-of-care ultrasound examination of the affected area may help provide immediate answers to a number of clinical questions. Is the region of tenderness due to a lesion within the abdominal wall itself or does it appear that an underlying structure (e.g., a metastatic lesion in the liver) is causing the discomfort? If a lesion is present, where is it and what are its sonographic characteristics? Is it solid, cystic, hypo, or hyperechoic, and is it a vascular structure? Is a fluid collection present, and if so, is the fluid simple or complex? Is a fascial defect noted in the abdominal wall, and if present, is a loop of bowel seen passing through the defect? Armed with the additional anatomic knowledge of the site and character of the sonographic findings, as well as the clinical history, the provider can then pursue a more targeted workup.

Ultrasound examination of the abdominal wall can provide valuable information when the diagnosis of an *abdominal wall hernia* is unclear. In one clinical series, 39% of 144 patients with an abdominal wall mass of unclear etiology (with or without pain) were found to have a hernia.[1] Incisional hernias occur as a delayed complication in up to 4% of abdominal surgeries[2], and ultrasound can sometimes detect the fascial defect early in its development. While many abdominal wall hernias are apparent on clinical examination alone and do not require sonographic evaluation for diagnosis, others can be difficult to diagnose because the fascial defect is small and difficult to appreciate clinically. The fascial defect in a Spigelian hernia (also known as an interstitial hernia) will be found along the lateral border of the rectus muscle and a focal defect will be present in the aponeuroses of the transversus abdominis and internal oblique muscles, but not in the aponeurosis of the external oblique muscle. Since the fascial defect lies beneath the external oblique aponeurosis, the defect may not be apparent on clinical examination. A Spigelian hernia will typically be found where the lateral rectus sheath intersects with the inferior margin of the rectus sheath at a region termed the arcuate line, located about halfway between the umbilicus and the pubis. Signs and symptoms of a Spigelian hernia can be nonspecific and the pain may be poorly localized. Peak incidence is at age 50, with men and women affected equally.[3] Additionally, ultrasound can play an important role in the evaluation of patients with inordinate pain or excessive swelling of the abdominal wall in the postoperative period after a herniorrhaphy.[1]

The femoral region may be host to a wide range of pathologic and postoperative entities ranging from inguinal and femoral hernias, reactive and metastatic lymph nodes, lipomas, abscesses, hematomas, seromas, lymphomas, soft tissue sarcomas, vascular bypass grafts, and pseudoaneurysms.[4] Ultrasound examination of the groin can narrow the differential diagnosis and help differentiate among the many pathologic processes that occur in this anatomic region. Ultrasound is more accurate than the physical exam for distinguishing inguinal adenopathy from other inguinal pathology.[2]

A patient's abdominal pain is sometimes discovered to be due to a spontaneous or posttraumatic *rectus sheath hematoma*, most frequently caused by sudden vigorous abdominal contractions in the setting of a seizure, a coughing or sneezing paroxysm, direct trauma, or recent surgery. Older patients on anticoagulant therapy are most prone to this malady. In one series of 16 cases, 73% were on anticoagulant therapy and the mean age was 64.5 years old.[5] Bleeding may occur because of rupture of an epigastric artery or vein or because of a tear of the rectus muscle fibers.[2] The resulting hematoma remains confined to the rectus sheath.

Abdominal wall endometriosis can occur at the site of a previous C-section or laparotomy and should be considered in the differential diagnosis of women presenting with recurrent focal abdominal wall pain near a surgical scar during menses; the frequency of this disorder is estimated at 0.8% of all C-sections.[6] In one series of 28 patients scar endometrioma sizes ranged from 0.7 to 6 cm and the average time since the last C-section ranged from 40 to 66 months. In the 12 patients with large scar endometriomas (3–6 cm), the hypoechoic lesions exhibited increased vascularity, solid and cystic portions, occasional fistulous tracts, and irregular shapes when compared with smaller scar endometriomas.[7] Although the sonographic finding of a hypoechoic mass within the region of the operative scar is nonspecific, this finding coupled with a characteristic history can help make the diagnosis.[8]

Other abdominal wall masses such as lipomas, sebaceous cysts, subcutaneous abscesses, cutaneous metastases, a primary malignant melanoma, hemangiomas, and pseudoaneurysms of the epigastric artery may all occur in the abdominal wall and should also be included in the differential diagnosis of a palpable or tender abdominal wall mass. Ultrasound has been used to help localize the injection port of intrathecal drug delivery pumps whose location in the abdominal wall cannot be found by physical examination.[9]

Ultrasound also improves the performance characteristics of selected nerve blocks of the abdominal wall (the transversus abdominis plane or TAP block, as well as ilioinguinal nerve blocks), and has been used to guide injection therapy of entrapped abdominal wall cutaneous nerves at the lateral border of the rectus abdominis.[10–12]

ANATOMICAL CONSIDERATIONS

The abdominal wall is composed of skin, subcutaneous tissue of varying thickness depending on patient habitus, muscular layers that also vary in thickness with patient habitus and conditioning, and finally a layer of extraperitoneal fat. The muscular layers are enclosed in fibrous fascial sheaths. The fascial sheaths or aponeuroses of the three lateral abdominal wall muscles (the external oblique, the internal oblique, and the transverses abdominis muscles) combine to form a thickened fascial layer known as the *Spigelian fascia* in the paramedian region just lateral to the paired midline rectus muscles. The region along the lateral border of the rectus muscles extending from the costal margin to the pubic bone is referred to as the linea semilunaris or Spigelius line. Moving medially, the Spigelian fascia divides into two layers to form the anterior and posterior rectus sheaths that surround the rectus muscles. In the midline, the anterior and posterior rectus sheaths from each rectus muscle combine and fuse into a single central fascial layer known as the linea alba. In long axis, the rectus muscles appear as paired bundles of muscle tissue with the muscle fibers aligned in a sagittal orientation, interrupted by three transversely oriented tendinous intersections. In cross section, the rectus muscles are ovoid in profile. Of note, the posterior layer of the each rectus sheath ends approximately midway between the umbilicus and the pubic symphysis. The thickened inferior edge of the rectus sheath at this level forms an anatomic region termed the arcuate line. Below the arcuate line, the posterior layer of the rectus sheath is composed only of a thin layer of tissue known at the transversalis fascia.

The anatomy of the inguinal region is more complex and the region immediately adjacent to the inguinal ligament is the area of anatomic interest. The inguinal ligament represents the thickened inferior border of the aponeurosis of the external oblique muscle and is located between the anterior superior iliac spine and the pubic tubercle of the pelvis. Beneath the inguinal ligament lie three important bony prominences. Moving medially from the laterally situated anterior superior iliac spine, the next bony ridge encountered will be the anterior inferior iliac spine. Continuing further medially, the large curved bony ridge of the iliopubic eminence will be noted. This ridge corresponds to the anterior rim of the acetabulum. Medial to the iliopubic eminence lies the bony prominence of the pubic crest, about 1 cm medial to the pubic tubercle. The iliopsoas muscle runs beneath the inguinal ligament in the space between the anterior superior and inferior iliac spines and the iliopubic eminence. Medial to lateral, the common femoral vein, the common femoral artery, and the femoral nerve are found just anterior to the iliopubic eminence. Lymph nodes can be found on either side of this neurovascular bundle. The deep inguinal ring lies superficial to the inguinal ligament in the region above the femoral vessels. From there, the inguinal canal courses medially and inferiorly toward the superficial inguinal ring that is found in close proximity to the pubic crest, still superficial to the inguinal ligament.

TECHNIQUE AND NORMAL ULTRASOUND FINDINGS

The abdominal wall is divided into three sonographically distinct regions.[4] Since the anatomic structures of interest are all superficially located, a high-frequency linear array transducer is best suited to this type of examination. If extended-field-of-view or panoramic imaging software is available, this feature can be used to demonstrate the lesion's anatomic relationship with adjacent structures in the abdominal wall (Figure 18-1).

The midline region is best scanned in short axis. The linea alba (representing the midline confluence

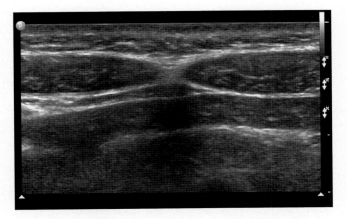

Figure 18-2. Transverse sonogram of the linea alba and adjacent rectus muscles. Skin and subcutaneous tissue are seen in the near field. The linea alba appears as a thickened, somewhat echogenic horizontal region in the midline. The hypoechoic conical or triangular regions on either side of the linea alba represent the medial portions of the adjacent rectus muscles.

of the anterior and posterior fascial sheaths from each rectus muscle) appears beneath the skin and subcutaneous tissue of the midline abdomen as a horizontally oriented and somewhat hyperechoic and thickened line. The linea alba is surrounded on either side by the hypoechoic triangular medial portions of each rectus muscle (Figure 18-2). The rectus muscles appear hypoechoic and speckled in short axis (Figure 18-3) and hypoechoic

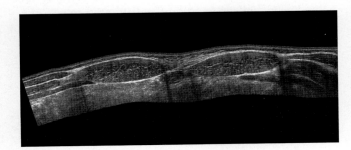

Figure 18-1. Extended-field-of-view or panoramic view of the upper anterior abdominal wall musculature. The external oblique, internal oblique, and transversus abdominis muscles can be seen just lateral to the rectus muscles in the upper abdomen.

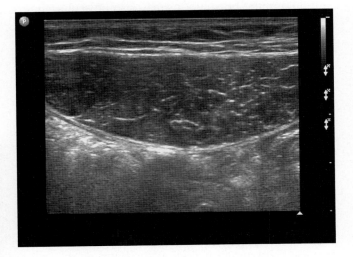

Figure 18-3. Transverse sonogram of a normal left rectus muscle above the umbilicus. The rectus muscle is seen as an ovoid, hypoechoic, and somewhat speckled structure in short axis, outlined by the echogenic anterior and posterior layers of the rectus sheath. In long axis, the muscle tissue appears striated.

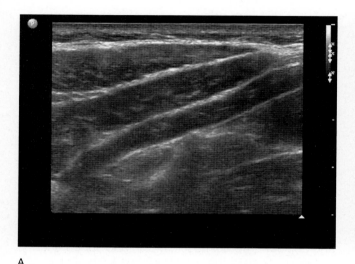
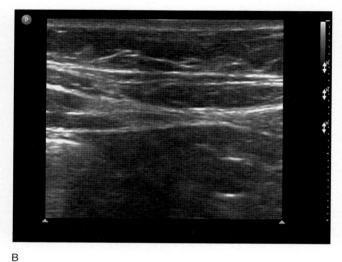

A

B

Figure 18-4. Oblique sonogram of the right paramedian upper abdominal wall just lateral to the rectus muscle (A). The external oblique, internal oblique, and transversus abdominis muscles appear as a succession of three hypoechoic layers surrounded by their respective hyperechoic fascial sheaths or aponeuroses. As they approach the rectus muscle, they taper to form the Spigelian fascia. More inferiorly (B) the Spigelian fascia is seen as a thickened hyperechoic line representing the combined aponeuroses of the three lateral abdominal wall muscles as they approach and then split to form the anterior and posterior rectus sheaths. The lateral portion of the right rectus muscle can be seen on the right side of the image.

and striated in long axis. The anterior and posterior rectus sheaths appear as thin hyperechoic lines surrounding the muscle bundles. The underlying peritoneal interface will usually be apparent on real-time scanning. The adjacent anterior bowel wall surface appears hyperechoic, and gliding of the bowel is usually noted with respiration or with bowel peristalsis. Comet-tail artifacts, or dirty shadowing, arising from pockets of admixed air and fluid in the bowel loops may also be seen (Figures 18-1 and 18-3).

In the paramedian region, the sonographic area of interest is at the lateral border of the rectus muscle at the confluence of the aponeuroses of the lateral abdominal wall muscles. In the paramedian region, the fascial layers surrounding the three lateral wall muscles (external oblique, internal oblique, and transverse abdominal) are conjoined into one fascial layer called the Spigelian fascia. Therefore, the landmarks for ultrasound of the paramedian region are the lateral border of the rectus muscle, the Spigelian facia, and the medial border of the three lateral wall muscles (Figure 18-4A and B). Spigelian hernias occur in the Spigelian fascia between the umbilicus and the pubis.

In the inguinal region, the area of sonographic focus will be along an oblique plane between the palpable bony landmarks of the anterior superior iliac spine and the pubic crest. The region should be scanned in a series of successive parallel planes several centimeters above and below the inguinal ligament. In the normal patient, the hypoechoic iliopsoas muscles will be seen occupying the region bounded by the anterior supe-

rior iliac spine laterally, the anterior inferior iliac spine below, and the edge of the iliopubic eminence medially. The hyperechoic curve of the iliopubic eminence will be noted just beneath the anechoic femoral vessels (Figure 18-5).

COMMON AND EMERGENT ABNORMALITIES

Postoperative Abdominal Wound Evaluation

As noted earlier, a wide range of postoperative pathology may occur in the abdominal wall. A wound abscess will typically appear as a hypoechoic, sometimes isoechoic, fluid collection at or near the surgical site with clinical signs suggesting that a wound infection is present. Swirling of the abscess fluid may be noted with gentle transducer pressure on the site. Deeper abscesses may be connected by a thin column of fluid rising up to the skin surface. A postoperative seroma will manifest as an anechoic collection of easily compressible fluid with no associated clinical signs to suggest infection (Figure 18-6). Liquefying hematomas will often exhibit both simple and complex features with layering.

Lymph Node

Focal tenderness in the inguinal region may be due to a reactive inguinal lymph node. A lymph node will appear as a lobulated elliptical structure in long axis,

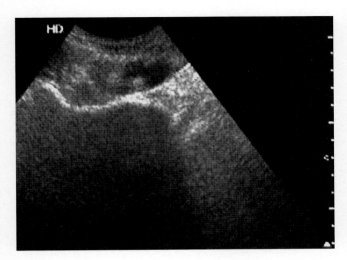

Figure 18-5. Oblique sonogram of the inguinal region with a curved array transducer. The scan plane is along the inguinal ligament. The curved hyperechoic line represents the shape of the bony pelvis beneath the inguinal ligament. The anterior superior iliac spine is not seen in this image and lies just beneath the skin off to the left of the sonogram. The first bony convexity seen on the left side of the image represents the anterior inferior iliac spine. The next convexity is somewhat shallower and more elongated, is seen on the right side of the sonogram, and represents the iliopubic eminence (corresponding to the anterior rim of the acetabulum). Posterior acoustic shadowing is seen beneath these bony ridges. The hypoechoic femoral vessels are seen in short axis just above the curve of the iliopubic eminence. The iliopsoas muscle occupies the region to the left of the femoral vessels. The upsloping bony ridge that leads to the pubic tubercle is seen beneath the femoral vessels.

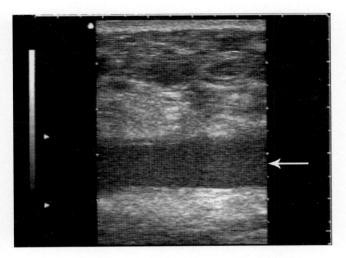

Figure 18-6. Transverse sonogram of an abdominal wall seroma in a patient several months after a hernia repair. A hypoechoic fluid collection (arrow) is seen beneath the subcutaneous tissues and is easily compressible. No clinical signs of infection were present.

hypoechoic at the periphery with a variably hyperechoic fatty central hilum (Figure 18-7).

Rectus Sheath Hematoma

On occasion, a patient may present with a focal region of abdominal tenderness and swelling due to a rectus sheath hematoma. Sonographically, the normally homogeneously hypoechoic rectus muscle will appear diffusely hyperechoic from hemorrhage into the muscle, and a focal homogeneous fluid collection consistent with a hematoma may also be present (Figure 18-8).

Hernia

A Spigelian hernia will appear as a hypoechoic fascial defect at or near the junction of the linea semilunaris and the arcuate line. A bowel loop may be seen extending laterally under the external oblique muscle. A small epigastric hernia will appear as a hypoechoic fascial defect in the linea alba; visualization of peristaltic movements

in the herniated bowel loop during real-time scanning will help confirm that a hernia is indeed present (Figure 18-9). Seen in cross section, a herniated loop of small bowel will have a rounded target-like appearance with a hypoechoic outer muscular layer, followed by a hyperechoic mucosal layer and, on occasion, strongly reflective central echoes that arise from admixtures of air and fluid in the bowel lumen (Figure 18-10). In long axis, a linear region of "dirty shadowing" and reverberation artifacts may be seen (Figure 18-10B). When obstructed, small

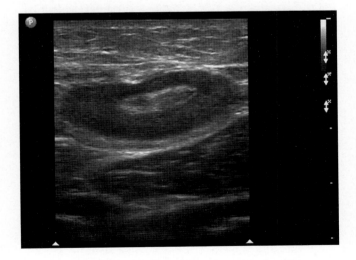

Figure 18-7. Long-axis sonogram of an inguinal lymph node. The oval-shaped lymph node appears hypoechoic at its periphery and echogenic at its fatty hilum. This patient's groin tenderness was attributable to a reactive adenopathy and not a hernia.

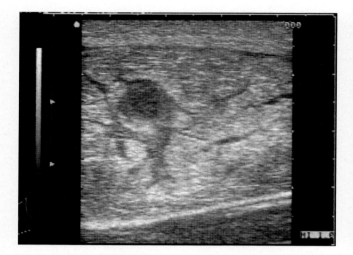

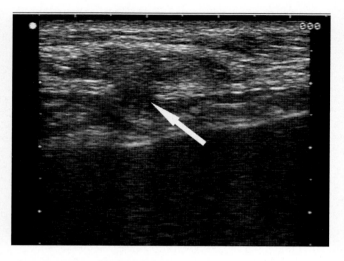

Figure 18-8. Transverse sonogram of a rectus sheath hematoma. The normally hypoechoic rectus muscle appears hyperechoic and quite thick in this patient. In the center, there is a hypoechoic region consistent with an inferior epigastric artery aneurysm. The hemorrhage dissects through the muscle tissue but is contained within the rectus sheath.

Figure 18-9. Transverse sonogram of an epigastric hernia. The patient had localized tenderness of the midline abdominal wall in the epigastric region but no fascial defect was appreciated clinically. A hypoechoic fascial defect (arrow) is seen on the sonogram in the otherwise echogenic linea alba. The hypoechoic mushroom-shaped region around and above the lesion represents a loop of small bowel that has herniated through the defect. On real-time imaging, peristalsis of the bowel loop was appreciated.

bowel loops will appear as dilated hypoechoic tubular fluid-filled structures with prominent hyperechoic valvulae conniventes.

Lipomas and Sebaceous Cysts

These masses typically appear as rounded or ovoid structures in the subcutaneous tissues. Palpation of the

lesion will guide the clinician to the region of sonographic interest. Lipomas appear similar in echotexture to the surrounding subcutaneous tissue. A subtle curved region of echogenicity will outline the border of the lipoma in what otherwise appears to be a homogenous

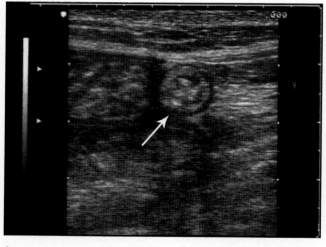

A

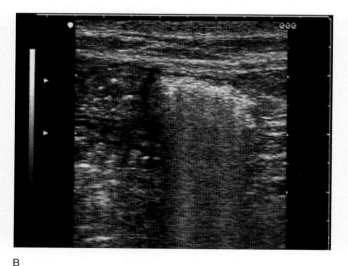

B

Figure 18-10. Transverse (A) and sagittal (B) sonograms of a small ventral hernia. A herniated loop of small bowel is seen within the abdominal wall between a fascial defect in the linea alba (to the right of the image) and the medial border of the rectus muscle (to the left). In short axis, the bowel segment has a characteristic circular and target-like appearance (arrow). In long axis, the sonographic pattern is one of "dirty shadowing" and reverberation artifacts.

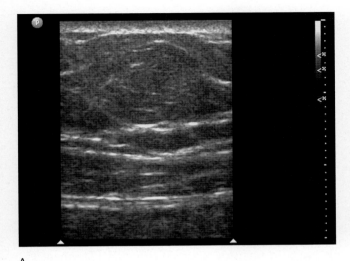

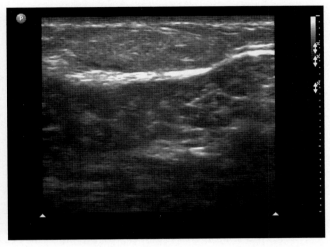

A

B

Figure 18-11. Transverse sonogram of abdominal wall lipomas. A firm and somewhat tender mass was appreciated clinically in both cases, but its etiology was unclear. The subtle curved outline of an ovoid structure is seen in the near field in both images. (A) The echogenicity of the lesions is similar to that of the fatty tissue in which it resides, consistent with the sonographic appearance of a lipoma. (B) The hyperechoic fascial layer below is distorted by the presence of the lipoma above.

layer of subcutaneous tissue (Figure 18-11) Angiolipomas exhibit somewhat increased echogenicity. A sebaceous (or epidermoid) cyst appears as a heterogeneous hypoechoic cystic mass, filled with a fatty cheese-like material (Figure 18-12). If the contents extravasate into the adjacent soft tissues, an abscess will frequently form.

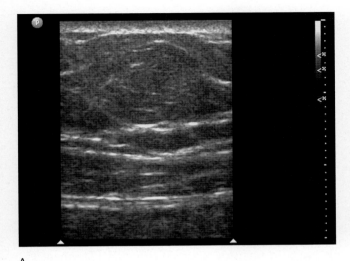

Figure 18-12. This abdominal wall mass was noted to be somewhat rubbery, somewhat deformable with pressure, with minimal tenderness to palpation. As opposed to the homogeneous appearance of a lipoma, this lesion appears as a discrete but sonographically heterogeneous ovoid mass. The sonographic characteristics are typical of a sebaceous cyst.

COMMON VARIANTS AND SELECTED ABNORMALITIES

Endometrioma

An abdominal wall endometrioma will be found at the site of a prior caesarean section or laparotomy and will appear as a solid hypoechoic mass and scattered internal echoes similar to the endometriomas that occur in the abdominal cavity.[8] An undescended testicle will appear as a homogenous mass smaller in size but similar in echotexture to a normal testicle, with its long axis parallel to the inguinal canal.

Pseudoaneurysm

A pseudoaneurysm represents an area of fibrous encapsulation around a pulsatile and expanding hematoma that occurs from arterial bleeding into adjacent soft tissue. Because there is a persistent communication between the vessel and the fluid space, to-and-fro flow will be noted between the mass and the adjacent artery and characteristic echogenic swirls will be seen on color Doppler examination. In contradistinction to a true aneurysm, the neck of a pseudoaneurysm is narrow.

PITFALLS

The major sonographic pitfalls of abdominal wall imaging are failure to consider a malignant etiology for any homogeneously hypoechoic solid lesion, especially in the groin, and failure to consider a vascular etiology for an anechoic lesion, particularly if aspiration is considered.

► AIRWAY

CLINICAL CONSIDERATIONS

The anatomic structures of the larynx and upper airway are superficially located and well suited for point-of-care sonographic assessment. Although airway ultrasound techniques are not widely used, there is growing evidence that ultrasound can provide valuable information about the anatomy of the upper airway and can be used to confirm proper placement of an endotracheal tube.

CLINICAL INDICATIONS

The indications for using point-of-care ultrasound for airway management are

1. Preintubation assessment of the upper airway
2. Assessment of anatomic structures for surgical airway management
3. Postintubation confirmation of endotracheal tube placement
4. Assessment of vocal cord function
5. Evaluation for epiglottitis

Preintubation Assessment of the Upper Airway

Airway ultrasound has been shown to be a useful tool for preintubation assessment in both adult and pediatric patients. Sonographic measurements of anterior soft tissue thickness at the level of the hyoid bone and thyrohyoid membrane can help predict difficult direct laryngoscopy better than clinical screening tests. Sonographic measurements of infrahyoid airway structures have been found to correlate well with CT or MRI.[13] Ultrasound imaging of the width of the air column at the level of the cricoid cartilage was found to have a correlation coefficient of 0.99 with MRI measurements taken in the same group of 19 patients. This parameter could help clinicians estimate proper endotracheal tube size and avoid the complications that occur when an excessively large endotracheal tube is employed. In a study of 192 pediatric patients 1 month to 6 years of age, sonographically measured subglottic airway diameter was better predictor of proper endotracheal tube size than standard age and height based formulas.[14]

Assessment of Anatomic Structures for Surgical Airway Management

Ultrasound of the upper airway can also play an important role when placement of a percutaneous cricothyrotomy or tracheostomy is contemplated. Surface landmarks are notoriously unreliable, especially in obese patients. In one review, percutaneous identification of the cricothyroid membrane by 18 anesthesiologists was found to be poor. Only 30% of 108 landmark assessments were located over the cricothyroid membrane and only 10% were over the desired target site.[15] In a study of percutaneous tracheotomies performed by 50 anesthesiologists on an inanimate model with unidentifiable anterior neck anatomy, ultrasound led to a significant increase in procedural success as well as a significant decrease in time to successful cannula placement (57 seconds vs. 110 seconds).[16] Also, a large human study showed that the mean time for emergency physicians to accurately visualize the cricothyroid membrane with ultrasound was 24 +/− 20 seconds.[17]

Postintubation Confirmation of Endotracheal Tube Placement

Numerous studies discuss the role of ultrasound for endotracheal tube placement confirmation. Recognition of the characteristic sonographic patterns of endotracheal or esophageal intubation on a transverse or longitudinal view of the trachea can be of significant clinical value for rapid identification of tracheal versus esophageal intubation.[18] Real-time imaging of the trachea on a transverse view at the level of the cricothyroid membrane was reported to be 99.7% sensitive and 97% specific for detection of endotracheal intubation. Real-time imaging during the intubation was found to be superior to a static imaging technique performed after the intubation. Evaluation of the static imaging technique alone revealed notably improved test characteristics when images were obtained at a suprasternal location (97% sensitivity and specificity) rather than at the cricothyroid membrane (73% sensitivity and 56% specificity).[19] In another study, transverse imaging just superior to the suprasternal notch confirmed tracheal versus esophageal tube placement in 150 patients with 100% sensitivity and specificity within 3 seconds of tube insertion.[20] In a cadaver model, a longitudinal scan plane was employed at the level of the cricothyroid membrane. Dynamic imaging was found to be 97% sensitive and 100% specific for endotracheal tube position confirmation. In contrast, static imaging at that site after the endotracheal tube had been placed was noted to be only 51% sensitive for confirming endotracheal tube location, which is consistent with other studies. In a randomized controlled trial, a transverse scan plane just above the suprasternal notch was employed dynamically during intubation, and correctly identified tracheal or esophageal intubations in all cases.[21] In pediatric patients, visualization of widening of the glottis with endotracheal tube passage and identification of lung sliding with initial ventilation were found to be reliable indicators of tracheal tube placement.[22] In one study, the combination of transverse dynamic ultrasound imaging at the cricothyroid membrane and lung sliding with initial ventilation was found to be 100% sensitive and 100% specific for endotracheal tube placement.[23]

Because of the large acoustic impedance mismatch between soft tissue and the air-filled trachea, visualization of an endotracheal tube within the airway may be difficult unless it is in direct contact with the tracheal wall. When a saline or foam-filled endotracheal tube cuff is utilized, the cuff will be in contact with the trachea and will exhibit a distinct sonographic pattern that assists in its identification. This technique was investigated in a series of 24 intubated patients and reached the following conclusions: (1) the saline or foam-filled cuff was best visualized in a long-axis view, (2) a slight longitudinal to-and-fro motion of the endotracheal tube further enhanced visualization of the cuff, and (3), when the cuff was visualized at the level of the suprasternal notch, the endotracheal tube was ideally situated midway between the vocal cords and the carina. The study concluded that this sonographic technique could be clinically useful for rapid assessment of endotracheal tube position in any situation where endotracheal tube movement, near extubation, or endobronchial intubation might have occurred.[24]

Ultrasound may also be used for secondary confirmation of endotracheal tube position either by direct observation of diaphragm motion or by identification of lung sliding during ventilation. One study of 59 emergently intubated patients ranging from newborn to 17 years of age utilized real-time B- and M-mode ultrasound and a subxiphoid window to evaluate diaphragm motion during ventilation. Of the 59 patients, 49 tracheal intubations, 2 esophageal intubations, and 8 right mainstem intubations were correctly identified with ultrasound. The authors concluded that ultrasound imaging of diaphragm motion was a "useful, quick, noninvasive, portable, and direct anatomic method for assessment of endotracheal tube position."[25] Diaphragmatic ultrasound has not been found to be a reliable indicator to distinguish mainstem endotracheal intubation, with only 50% specificity in one review.[26]

Using a cadaver model and a 4–2 MHz microconvex transducer, the identification of the lung sliding sign as a predictor of endotracheal tube placement was evaluated with 68 intubations in 9 cadavers.[27] For differentiating esophageal versus tracheal intubation, the sensitivity was 95–100% and the specificity was 100%. Visualization of lung sliding to rule out or identify mainstem intubation has not been well studied, but is used extensively in clinical practice. However, the unilateral absence of lung sliding in patients with mainstem intubation should not be confused with a pneumothorax.[28]

Assessment of Vocal Cord Function

A real-time image of the vestibular folds (the false vocal cords), the vocal folds (the true vocal cords), and the arytenoids can be obtained by scanning transversely though the thyroid cartilage. Ultrasound has been found to be a useful tool for evaluation of vocal cord function by a number of investigators.[29–31]

Evaluation for Epiglottitis

Ultrasound has also been used to assess the anteroposterior (AP) thickness of the epiglottis. One study examined 100 normal subjects using a subhyoid window and a transverse scan plane, and the epiglottis was visualized in all cases. There was little variation in the AP diameter of the normal adult epiglottis, with an average AP dimension of 2.39 ±0.15 mm in this report.[32] A long-axis view of the epiglottis may be obtained from either the midline or a paratracheal location at the level of the thyrohyoid membrane, but successful visualization of the epiglottis with this technique was noted to be only 71% compared with 100% when a transverse transducer orientation was employed. Another study touted the use of a long-axis sonographic technique as being a safe and practical way to noninvasively assess a patient for epiglottitis at the bedside. The study described a sonographic finding that they called the "alphabet P sign," the ultrasound equivalent to the "thumb print sign" seen on the lateral neck radiograph.[33] The use of ultrasound for rapid point-of-care assessment of a patient with suspected epiglottitis appears to be a promising technique.

ANATOMICAL CONSIDERATIONS

The thyroid and cricoid cartilages, the cricothyroid membrane, and the upper trachea are located within the superficial subcutaneous tissues of the anterior midline of the neck. The thyroid cartilage is composed of two broad rectangular laminae that meet in the anterior midline at about a 90° angle. Superiorly, the thyroid cartilage attaches to the hyoid bone via the thyrohyoid membrane. Posteriorly, the superior and inferior horns of the thyroid cartilage connect the thyroid cartilage with the hyoid bone and cricoid cartilages, respectively. Inferiorly and anteriorly, the thyroid cartilage connects to the cricoid ring via the cricothyroid ligament or membrane; in an adult, it averages about 2 × 1 cm in size. A V-shaped gap separates the upper aspects of the thyroid laminae in the midline and the base of this gap forms the superior thyroid notch or the laryngeal prominence. The strap muscles (the sternohyoid, omo-hyoid, and thyrohyoid muscles) lie just anterior to the thyroid cartilage. The cricothyroid muscles extend from the lower border of the thyroid cartilage to the lower aspect of the cricoid ring and surround the anterolateral portions of the cricothyroid membrane and cricoid cartilage. The thyroid gland surrounds the lateral portions of the cricoid ring, and extends superiorly to the lower border of the thyroid cartilage and anteriorly over the upper tracheal cartilages. The narrow rectangular midline segment of the thyroid gland is known as the thyroid isthmus.

The vestibular folds (also known as the false vocal cords or ventricular folds) are composed of a thick fold of mucous membrane and connective tissue. They lie just above and protect the more delicate vocal cords below. The vocal folds (or true vocal cords) are composed of the vocal ligaments medially and the laterally adjacent vocalis and thyroarytenoid muscles. They are covered by a mucous membrane and extend from the level of the mid-thyroid cartilage anteriorly to the paired arytenoid cartilages posteriorly. The arytenoids rest on the broad posterior cricoid ring and are attached to the thyroarytenoid muscles that adduct the vocal folds. The midline gap between the vocal ligaments is referred to as the rima glottidis.

The base of the epiglottis attaches to the upper border of the thyroid cartilage via the thyroepiglottic ligament; more superiorly the hyoepiglottic ligament provides the anterior support for the epiglottis. A preepiglottic fat pad separates the epiglottis from the thyrohyoid membrane. The epiglottis approaches its widest dimension just below the level of the hyoid bone.

The cricoid cartilage is the only complete ring of cartilage around the trachea and attaches distally to the first tracheal ring via the cricotracheal ligament. The upper five or six tracheal rings of the trachea lie just beneath the skin in the region between the cricoid cartilage and the lower aspect of the suprasternal notch. The diameter of the airway at the level of the cricoid ring governs the choice of endotracheal tube size, as this is the narrowest point in the upper airway.

TECHNIQUE AND NORMAL ULTRASOUND FINDINGS

Transducers

The superficial structures in the upper airway are best imaged with a high-frequency linear array, or hockey stick transducer. Use the short-axis midline, long-axis midline, or long-axis paratracheal views, depending on the airway application being performed. The length of the transducer face may limit its utilization in long axis if the neck is short or the transducer face is long. Gen-erous application of ultrasound gel may help with obtaining adequate images at the suprasternal notch. For submandibular views, a curved array transducer may be more appropriate and will provide a wider field of view of the many structures being imaged at that level.

Thyroid Cartilage

The thyroid cartilage is best imaged in a transverse scan plane in the upper neck with the neck slightly extended. Beneath the skin and subcutaneous tissues the thyroid cartilage appears as an inverted V-shaped structure that exhibits a variety of echogenic appearances, ranging from nearly isoechoic in younger patients to hyperechoic if the cartilage has become calcified. The hypoechoic strap muscles are seen overlying the laminae on each side of the thyroid cartilage. When the thyroid cartilage is hyperechoic, the region beneath will appear nearly anechoic (Figure 18-13) and when the thyroid cartilage is isoechoic with the surrounding muscles, the laryngeal structures beneath (arytenoids, vocal folds, and vocal cords) can frequently be identified (Figure 18-14). When scanning in cross section just above the superior thyroid notch, the anterior portion of the inverted V appears hypoechoic; a thin echogenic line corresponding to the anterior portion of the thyrohyoid ligament

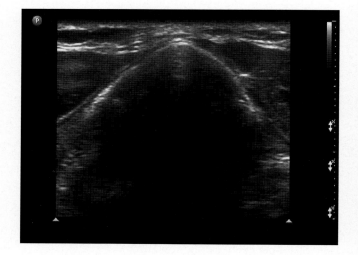

Figure 18-13. Short-axis sonogram of the thyroid cartilage below the level of the thyroid notch. Beneath a thin layer of skin and subcutaneous tissue, the two laminae of the thyroid cartilage meet in the anterior midline at about a 90° angle and appear as an inverted V-shape. In some subjects, as in this example, the cartilage will appear hyperechoic and the region beneath anechoic. The hypoechoic structures on either side of the cartilage are the strap muscles.

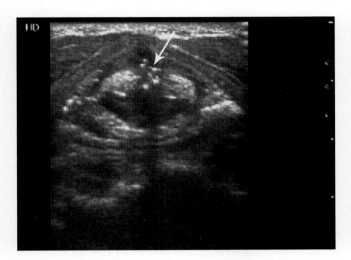

Figure 18-14. Short-axis sonogram of the thyroid cartilage. Here the thyroid cartilage is nearly isoechoic with the strap muscles on either side. The inverted V-shape is again apparent and visualization of the inner structures of the larynx is excellent. Seen here are the arytenoids (hyperechoic and rounded structures near the midline), the glottic opening (arrow) (echogenic anteriorly with posterior shadowing), and the posterior portion of the cricoid cartilage (moderately echoic curved structure deep to the arytenoids).

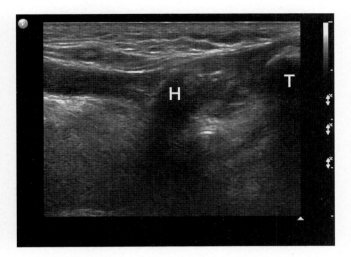

Figure 18-16. Long-axis sonogram of the upper midline neck. The echogenic anterior surface of the uppermost portion of the thyroid cartilage is seen to the right of the image. The hyoid bone with its prominent posterior acoustic shadow is seen in cross section in the middle of the image. The mylohyoid muscle (with an adjacent small lymph node) appears as a rectangular region of hypoechogenicity at the upper left side of the image. T = thyroid cartilage, H = shadow from hyoid bone.

may be noted (Figure 18-15). If the transducer is placed in long axis in the midline at the upper portion of the thyroid cartilage, the hyoid bone will be seen in cross section and its prominent posterior acoustic shadow will be noted (Figure 18-16)

Cricoid Cartilage and Cricothyroid Membrane

As the transversely oriented transducer face slides down the length of the thyroid cartilage, the inverted V-shape of the thyroid cartilage suddenly disappears, and the airway takes on a more rounded appearance. A prominent area of echogenicity will be noted in the anterior midline at the level of the cricothyroid membrane. When the insonating beam suddenly encounters the air-filled lumen of the airway, the large acoustic impedance mismatch gives rise to an echogenic periodic resonance artifact that makes identification of the cricothyroid membrane straightforward (Figure 18-17). The cricothyroid muscles surround the cricoid cartilage at this level and appear as anechoic crescents on either side of the slightly more echogenic outline of the cricoid ring. The cricoid ring is the only complete ring in the airway, is round in its transverse profile, wedge-shaped in a lateral profile, and becomes progressively taller as one moves laterally and posteriorly. The ring of the cricoid cartilage appears as a smaller circular structure in the center of the sonogram. The thyroid isthmus may be seen overlying the cricothyroid membrane and exhibits a homogenous mid-gray echotexture unless some thyroid gland pathology is present. The right and left lobes of the thyroid gland will be seen on either side of the trachea at this level and will typically exhibit a homogenous granular mid-gray echotexture (Figure 18-18). When scanning the

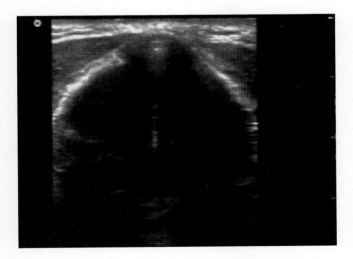

Figure 18-15. Short-axis sonogram of the thyroid cartilage *above* the level of the superior thyroid notch. A hypoechoic gap is seen in the space between the two laminae of the thyroid cartilage. The thin echogenic line in the center of the image corresponds to the vocal ligaments.

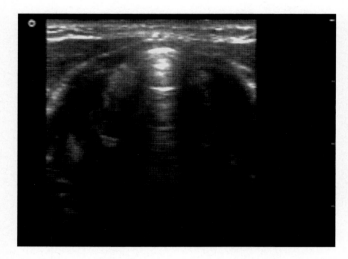

Figure 18-17. Short-axis sonogram at the level of the cricothyroid ligament or membrane. The airway has transitioned from an inverted V-shape to a more ovoid shape. In the center of the image, a prominent echo is seen with an associated periodic resonance artifact corresponding to the cricothyroid membrane and the air-filled tracheal lumen. The anechoic crescents on either side of the oval correspond with the cricothyroid muscles. A slightly echogenic circular structure is seen in the central half of the image and represents the cartilaginous cricoid ring.

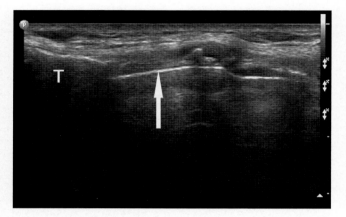

Figure 18-19. Long-axis sonogram of the anterior larynx centered over the cricothyroid ligament. To the upper left is a somewhat echogenic line that slants down toward the center of the image; this line corresponds to the anterior inferior surface of the thyroid cartilage. The cricothyroid membrane is seen as an echogenic horizontal line in the center of the image (arrow). The hypoechoic ovoid structure to its upper right corresponds to the anterior cricoid ring in cross section. Some internal calcifications are seen within the cricoid with some associated posterior acoustic shadowing. It is common to see a mirror image artifact of the cricoid ring on the other side of the cricothyroid membrane, giving the appearance of two adjacent hypoechoic ovals. The hypoechoic rectangular region to the right and slightly inferior to the cricoid cartilage represents the first tracheal cartilage. T = thyroid cartilage.

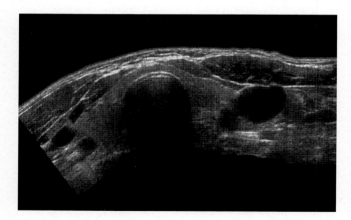

Figure 18-18. Panoramic view of the neck at the level of the thyroid gland. The normal thyroid gland and isthmus appear as a homogeneous, finely granular mid-gray echotexture structure on either side of the trachea. The sternocleidomastoid muscles can be seen just below the skin on either side of the neck. Strap muscles are noted just anterior to the thyroid isthmus. The common carotid arteries (more medial) and the internal jugular veins (more lateral) are noted lateral to the thyroid gland bilaterally. Note the marked asymmetry of the diameter of the internal jugular veins; this is a fairly common occurrence.

airway in a longitudinal midline or paramedian axis, the cricoid cartilage typically appears hypoechoic and ovoid in shape. It may, on occasion, contain areas of calcification that will appear echogenic. The cricothyroid membrane appears as a hyperechoic horizontal line located between the downward slanting thyroid cartilage on the left of the image, and the ovoid hypoechoic cross section of the cricoid cartilage on the right (Figure 18-19). Typically, two hypoechoic ovals will be noted on the caudal side of the image; the one immediately below the brightly echogenic cricothyroid membrane represents a mirror image artifact. A combination of first short- then long-axis views can be used for rapid and precise localization of the cricothyroid membrane.

Vocal Cords

Place the patient in a seated or supine position with the neck in a relaxed neutral position. Assuming that the thyroid cartilage is hypoechoic, scan the arytenoids and vocal cords with a linear array transducer held in a transverse orientation over the lower portion of the thyroid cartilage. The arytenoids appear as rounded echogenic structures that are easily identified by their posterior

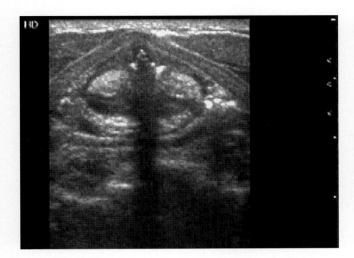

Figure 18-20. Short-axis sonogram through the lower larynx demonstrating the rima glottidis in normal respiration. The appearance is triangular anteriorly with posterior acoustic shadowing from the vocal ligaments. The rounded arytenoids appear on either side of the glottic opening, and the posterior cricoid ring is seen as a curved somewhat echogenic structure below.

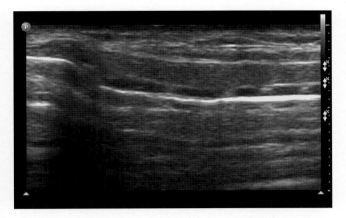

Figure 18-21. Long-axis midline sonogram of the upper tracheal cartilages in the neck. The cricoid cartilage is seen to the upper left of the image; the tracheal cartilages appear as hypoechoic rectangles in cross section and resemble a string of beads. The brightly echogenic surface below the rings represents the tracheal mucosal–air interface. A mirror image artifact of the hypoechoic tracheal rings is often seen below this bright line. If the tracheal cartilages are calcified, they will appear more echogenic and posterior acoustic shadowing will be noted.

paramedian location within the larynx and their characteristic movements on abduction and adduction (Figure 18-20).

The true vocal cords can be found by locating the hyperechoic anterior commissure; the inverted "V" of the vocal ligaments will appear as two centrally located narrow hyperechoic lines that abduct and adduct with respiration, and appear to flutter during phonation. The thicker hyperechoic false cords will be found somewhat more superiorly and will not move with phonation.

Trachea

In a midline or paratracheal long-axis orientation, identify the tracheal rings as small hypoechoic rectangular structures that appear like a string of beads in the near field. They may be either completely hypoechoic (in which case no shadowing will be seen) or somewhat calcified and have an echogenic surface with associated posterior acoustic shadowing. The tracheal lumen appears as a brightly echogenic line immediately beneath the cartilages (Figure 18-21). Identify the cricoid cartilage superiorly by its larger size and more ovoid profile allowing for accurate identification and numbering of the tracheal rings if needed.

Esophagus

Identify the esophagus just behind the left lobe of the thyroid gland. The normal gland has a uniformly fine-grained gray echotexture and the esophagus will be seen

as a somewhat flaccid to flattened circular or ovoid structure with alternating rings of hypo- and hyperechogenicity. It will usually be seen just anterior to the echogenic surface of the adjacent vertebral body and just medial to the carotid artery (Figure 18-22).

Confirmation of Endotracheal Intubation

Use both transverse and long-axis views for evaluation of endotracheal tube location and cuff position. Some investigators believe the real-time long-axis view to be best for visualizing the passage of the endotracheal tube into the trachea at the time of intubation. Slight to-and-fro movement of the endotracheal tube will further enhance its visualization (Figure 18-23). Filling the endotracheal tube cuff with 8–10 mL of saline can also enhance cuff visualization and assist with its accurate placement in the suprasternal notch (typically located midway between the vocal cords and the carina). The portion of the endotracheal tube that is in contact with the anterior tracheal wall will appear as two closely spaced parallel echogenic lines (curved in short axis, linear in long axis) representing the outer and inner anterior surfaces of the endotracheal tube. The tube will typically demonstrate a distinct comet-tail or reverberation artifact in contradistinction to the periodic resonance artifact of the unintubated airway. Although less distinct than a fluid-filled cuff, an air-filled cuff may be apparent by its curved profile and associated comet-tail

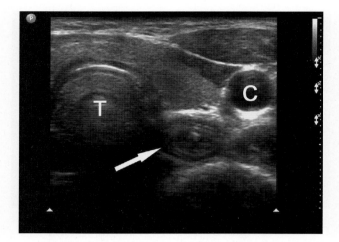

Figure 18-22. Transverse sonogram of the left upper trachea. The hypoechoic finely granular thyroid isthmus and gland are seen in the near field with the trachea immediately below. The left carotid artery is noted just beneath the hypoechoic sternocleido-mastoid muscle. The esophagus (arrow) is seen as an ovoid to flattened ring of alternating hypo and hyperechogenicity just beneath the left lobe of the thyroid gland and immediately anterior to the curved echogenic vertebral body below. The esophagus will most typically be found at this location. T = trachea, C = left carotid artery.

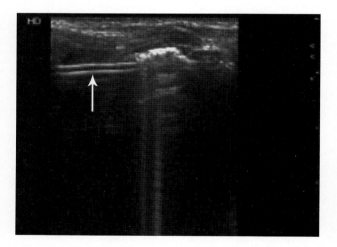

Figure 18-23. Long-axis sonogram of an endotracheal tube within the airway. The anterior endotracheal tube walls appear as two closely spaced echogenic parallel lines with an associated reverberation artifact below (arrow). The air-filled cuff appears as a distinctly different, somewhat curved, and brightly echogenic structure with associated comet-tail artifacts. The hypoechoic thyroid cartilage is seen slanting down on the left near field and the cricoid cartilage is seen in cross section to the right of the image just above the endotracheal tube cuff. The cuff needs to be moved further toward the supra-sternal notch; cuff placement at this location will typically result in the tube being in an ideal mid-tracheal position.

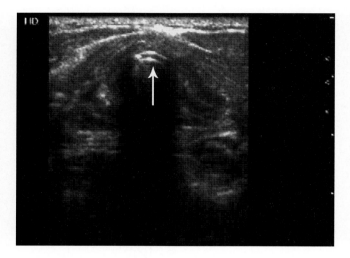

Figure 18-24. Short-axis sonogram of an intubated trachea at the level of the thyroid cartilage. The endotracheal tube is seen in the anterior airway as two parallel curved echogenic lines (arrow). Prominent posterior acoustic shadowing is present in this image.

artifacts (Figures 18-24 to 18-26). One recommended technique is to start in transverse orientation at the level of the cricothyroid membrane to quickly confirm that the endotracheal tube is not in the esophagus, then rotate to a long-axis orientation to confirm mid-tracheal cuff placement with a gentle to-and-fro movement of the tube. This technique has been touted as useful when supervising learner-performed intubations and might also be useful as a rapid confirmatory test in a postarrest situation when capnography is indeterminate.

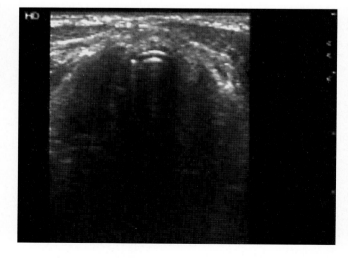

Figure 18-25. Short-axis sonogram of an intubated trachea about 1 cm below the cricoid cartilage. Two parallel curved echogenic lines are again seen in the anterior airway.

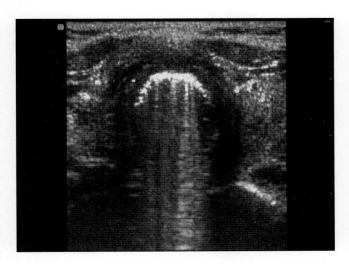

Figure 18-26. Short-axis sonogram of an intubated trachea at the level of the air-filled cuff. The hyperechoic signature of the air-filled endotracheal tube cuff appears different from that of the endotracheal tube: the cuff surface appears echogenic but irregular in contour and multiple comet-tail artifacts are prominent.

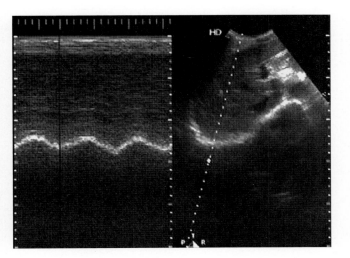

Figure 18-27. Combined B- and M-mode subxiphoid view of the right diaphragm with a curved array transducer during quiet respiration. The M-mode image traces the excursion of the echogenic diaphragm during the respiratory cycle; the diaphragmatic echo will be seen moving *toward* the transducer during inspiration and *away* during expiration. With an esophageal intubation, the diaphragm will move *away* from the transducer during ventilation. Asymmetric movement of the left and right diaphragms can indicate a mainstem intubation.

Secondary Confirmation of Endotracheal Tube Placement

Diaphragmatic movement may be observed in real time from a subxiphoid window using a standard curved array abdominal transducer. Use a wide sector angle so that both diaphragms may be easily visualized from a single scanning plane. When this is not feasible, use an oblique sagittal right or left chest view from the anterior to midaxillary line. Obtain a combined B- and M-mode image and observe the direction and depth of diaphragm motion in real time. With normal respirations or mechanical ventilation, the echogenic line corresponding to the diaphragm on the M-mode tracing will be seen to move toward the transducer with inspiration and away with expiration (Figure 18-27). With correct endotracheal tube placement, observe symmetrical movement toward the transducer with a delivered breath at both diaphragms. With an esophageal intubation, the air-filled stomach will push the diaphragm away from the transducer during inspiration. Asymmetry of movement of the two diaphragms may be seen with inadvertent right mainstem intubation. In an analogous fashion, evaluation of lung sliding may similarly be used to assess for correct tube placement (See Video 7-1). Absence of lung sliding implies that the hemithorax being assessed is either not being ventilated or that a pneumothorax is present.

Epiglottis

Scan the epiglottis from a subhyoid window in transverse orientation. Its sonographic appearance is that of a bird-like face or mask; the two ovoid hypoechoic "eyes" represent three of the four strap muscles (sternohyoid, omohyoid, thyrohyoid) in cross section; the hyperechoic triangular "nose" correlates with the preepiglottic fat pad located just deep to the thyrohyoid ligament, and the downturned hypoechoic "beak" or "mouth" represents the lower epiglottis in cross section (Figure 18-28). The posterior surface of the epiglottis is seen as a hyperechoic line due to the impedence mismatch at the mucosa–air interface.

COMMON AND EMERGENT ABNORMALITIES

Esophageal Intubation

With an esophageal intubation, the otherwise flaccid esophagus will be stented open by the endotracheal tube. On a short-axis view, the anterior surface of the endotracheal tube will appear as two closely spaced parallel curved echogenic lines with posterior acoustic shadowing. It may be detected either behind the left posterolateral inferior edge of the thyroid cartilage or just lateral to the trachea at the level of the cricothyroid membrane, directly behind the left lobe of the thyroid gland. As additional confirmation of an esophageal intubation, the lumen of the airway will not show any

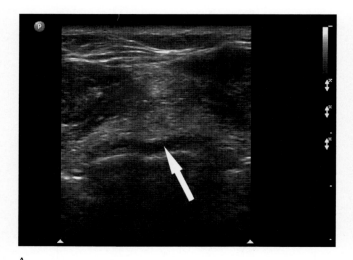

A

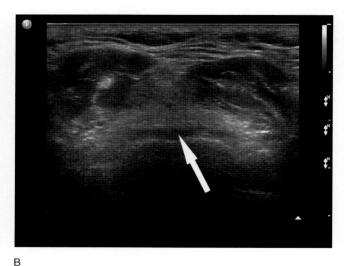

B

Figure 18-28. Short-axis sonograms of the normal upper neck taken through the thyrohyoid membrane. The sonograms in these two patients (A, B) have the appearance of a face or mask. The ovoid "eyes" represent the strap muscles in cross section. The hyperechoic "nose" represents the preepiglottic fat pad beneath the thyrohyoid membrane. The hypoechoic downturned "mouth" is the sonographic representation of the epiglottis (arrows) in cross section. The hyperechoic line beneath the epiglottis represents the air–mucosa interface.

evidence of endotracheal tube presence. Best visualization is reported to occur about 1 cm below the cricoid ring (Figure 18-29). Location of the esophagus can be somewhat variable, however. In two studies that commented on esophageal location at this level in the neck, the esophagus was noted to the left of the trachea in 85–88% of cases, and to the right or posterior to the trachea in 12–15% of cases.[20,21] A nasogastric tube will similarly stent open the normally flaccid and flattened esophagus but will appear as a smaller diameter structure with similar parallel anterior echoes and posterior acoustic shadowing (Figure 18-30).

Epiglottitis

In a patient presenting with epiglottitis, the transverse sonogram through the thyrohyoid membrane may reveal a dramatically altered picture from the usual bird-like image obtained at this location. The cross-sectional view of the normally thin and hypoechoic lower epiglottis (the "beak") will now be noted to be very thickened compared to normal, and the preepiglottic fat pad (representing the "nose") may appear enlarged due to localized edema. Instead of appearing like a bird, the image will have the appearance of a dog's snout (Figure 18-31).

Vocal Cord Palsy

Prolonged vocalization of a single vowel (such as "e") will enhance visualization of asymmetric vocal cord motion and abnormal arytenoid movement. Assuming the thyroid cartilage is not calcified, these findings should be readily apparent on a real-time examination. The affected vocal cord will appear shorter and in a lower position on the sonogram with anterior bowing of the flaccid vocal cord.[29]

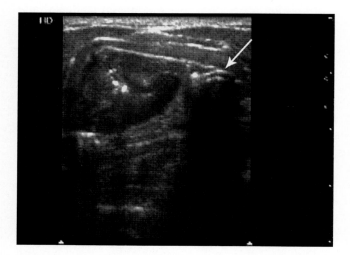

Figure 18-29. A somewhat-tilted transverse sonogram of an esophageal intubation seen at the level of the thyroid cartilage. The inverted V-shape of the thyroid cartilage is apparent in the near field and the vocal cords are adducted. The endotracheal tube (arrow) is seen lateral and posterior to the glottis and is recognizable by the paired parallel curved echoes anteriorly with posterior acoustic shadowing.

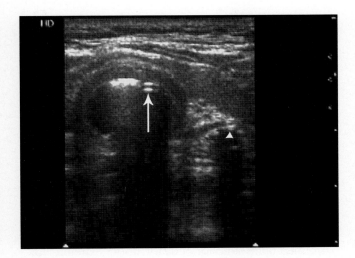

Figure 18-30. Short-axis sonogram of an intubated trachea at the level of the tracheal cartilages. A portion of the thyroid gland appears as a region of homogeneous mid-gray echogenicity anterior and lateral to the tracheal cartilage. The tracheal cartilage appears as a hypoechoic C that is open posteriorly. The signature double echo of the plastic wall of the endotracheal tube (arrow) is apparently adjacent to the tracheal ring; comet-tail artifacts are noted at the air–mucosa interface in the midline. A simultaneously placed nasogastric tube (arrowhead) demonstrates the lateral and somewhat posterior location of the esophagus relative to the airway. Both endotracheal and nasogastric tubes exhibit strong posterior acoustic shadowing.

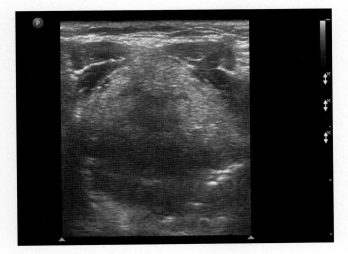

Figure 18-31. Transverse sonogram through the thyrohyoid membrane in a patient presenting with epiglottitis. Compared to the bird-like appearance of the normal image at this site, the image now has the appearance of a dog's snout. The hypoechoic "eyes" of the strap muscles appear similar to normal. The hyperechoic "nose" appears enlarged and more echogenic, and the hypoechoic "beak" of the epiglottis now appears considerably more thickened giving the overall image of the appearance of a dog's snout.

PITFALLS

1. Subcutaneous emphysema, significant neck edema, hemorrhage, or an open wound over the anterior neck can make sonography of the upper airway difficult or impossible.
2. Significant neck flexion may impair adequate scanning by making it difficult to place the transducer (especially in a long-axis orientation) on the anterior surface of the neck.
3. It may be difficult to obtain good images in the suprasternal notch because of poor transducer skin contact. Using a copious amount of gel may significantly improve image quality. A saline-filled endotracheal tube cuff may be difficult to visualize if air bubbles have entered the balloon along with the saline.
4. Real-time scanning during intubation may be difficult in a patient with a short neck and may interfere with the laryngoscope handle or with external laryngeal manipulation.

▶ BONY FRACTURE EVALUATION

CLINICAL CONSIDERATIONS AND INDICATIONS

Ultrasound excels at identifying the interface between soft tissue and bone due to the large difference in acoustic impedance between the two tissues. When perpendicular to a given bony surface, most of the incident ultrasound beam will be reflected back to the transducer and the interface will be represented by a brightly echogenic line that follows the contour of bony cortex being imaged. These cortical outlines on the sonogram can be used to identify precise locations for arthrocentesis as well as for finding landmarks for ultrasound-guided lumbar puncture. With the bony cortex so readily visible, sometimes to less than a millimeter resolution, ultrasound can also provide a rapid and portable means to assess for bony fractures. This section will focus on the identification of selected fractures, specifically ribs, sternum, zygomatic arch, nasal bones, and long bones.

Ultrasound has long been known to be considerably more sensitive for diagnosing *rib fractures* than standard chest radiography.[34–36] In one review of 103 patients with suspected rib injury, rib fractures were diagnosed about twice as often with ultrasound compared to standard chest radiography.[35] Ultrasound was also found to be useful for detecting coexisting small pleural effusions that were not demonstrated on the chest radiograph. The authors of this latter report opined that the ability to provide a definitive diagnosis of rib fracture (and thus better estimate the duration of work disability) was an important advantage that supported the use of ultrasound in this clinical setting. Ultrasound has particular utility in the ED workup of a patient with an isolated area of chest wall tenderness after trauma. The time-consuming nature of the examination in patients with larger areas of chest wall tenderness (from 10 to 15 minutes/patient reported in one study) and the inability to visualize retroscapular and infraclavicular rib injuries are some of the disadvantages for this particular ultrasound application.[34]

Although the diagnostic sensitivity of chest radiography and ultrasound for suspected *sternal fracture* is reported to be similar, the time required to make this diagnosis may be considerably less with the use of point-of-care ultrasound. In one report on 16 patients with radiographically documented sternal fractures, an examiner unfamiliar with the chest radiograph results was able to locate and diagnose the sternal fracture with ultrasound in each patient within 1 minute.[37] In a study of 31 patients with sternal fractures, ultrasound was found to be much more sensitive than radiography or bone scan. Twelve sternal fractures were noted on radiography, 18 with a bone scan, and 31 with ultrasound. Fracture distribution was noted as follows: 8 in the manubrium, 11 in the upper sternal body, 5 in the midsternal body, and 7 in the lower sternal body.[38]

Ultrasound may be most useful for diagnosis of *bony fractures in "austere" environments* where power, weight, and space requirements make conventional radiography impractical (e.g., battlefield or military settings, on a spacecraft or submarine, or in rural or wilderness medicine settings).[39–41] In an effort to evaluate the test characteristics of ultrasound for fracture diagnosis, one group of investigators trained cast technicians to assess ED patients for fractures after a 2-hour training program. One hundred fifty-eight ultrasound examinations were performed on 95 patients; the diagnostic accuracy was found to be greater in midshaft locations and least in the metacarpals, metatarsals, proximal femur, and hip. Leg and forearm fractures were found to be straightforward to diagnose with no missed injuries in patients with midshaft fractures of the radius, ulna, humerus, femur, tibia, or fibula. Of note, no false positives were reported in any location. The authors suggested that the FAST examination could be expanded to include both *extremity* assessment for fractures and *respiratory* assessment for pneumothorax, coining an alternate acronym: the "FASTER" examination.[39.] Requiring little added time to perform, such an extension of the FAST examination may provide useful and timely diagnostic information in the initial management of trauma patients.

Several studies have investigated the performance characteristics of ultrasound for fracture diagnosis in a turkey bone model with ED nurses, EMTs, and medics performing the exam. Sensitivities in these reports ranged from 98% to 100% and specificities from 90% to 93%.[42–44] Another group of investigators evaluated the accuracy of physician-performed ultrasound for the detection of *long bone fractures*. With only 1 hour of training, physicians with minimal prior ultrasound experience evaluated 58 ED patients using point-of-care ultrasound. Results were compared to plain films or CT as the gold standard. Ultrasound provided improved sensitivity with less specificity compared with physical examination. Ultrasound was found to be 100% sensitive for detecting humerus and midshaft femur fractures.[40.]

In pediatric patients, overall sensitivity of ultrasound was only 73%, with the highest accuracy noted at the diaphysis of long bones. The majority of diagnostic errors in this study (>85%) occurred at the ends of bones or near joints.[45] In a related review of physician-performed ultrasound for pediatric upper extremity fractures, there was 95% agreement between ultrasound and radiography for fracture identification.[46] In a series of 31 patients with hand fractures, ultrasound was noted to be 90% sensitive and 98% specific when compared with radiography.[47]

Ultrasound has also been employed as a diagnostic tool in the assessment of patients with *nasal trauma*. In a study of 63 patients seen in an ENT clinic with clinical signs of a nasal bone fracture, standard radiography employing lateral and occipitomental views was compared with ultrasound. Using a 10 MHz linear array transducer, images were obtained in three locations: on the left and right lateral nasal walls (for evaluation of the frontal processes of the maxillary bone) and on the nasal dorsum (for evaluation of the nasal bones proper). Of the 63 patients evaluated, 42 (67%) were diagnosed with nasal fractures. Ultrasound was found to be superior to radiography for assessment of the lateral nasal walls and radiography was superior for evaluation of the nasal dorsum.[48] Other authors have found ultrasound to be *more* sensitive than standard radiography for diagnosing fractures of the nasal dorsum (98% vs. 88%).[49]

High-resolution ultrasound is considered a reliable tool for the evaluation of nasal bone fractures, and several reports have advocated that this modality should be the first-line imaging modality in the setting of nasal trauma. Studies of high-resolution ultrasound have shown that it has better diagnostic accuracy than both CT[50] and standard radiography.[49] Higher frequency linear array transducers (20 MHz) normally used for the evaluation of skin tumors and skin thickness assessment have also been utilized for evaluation of nasal bone fractures.[51] Also, in a series of 32 patients, ultrasound was found to be useful for evaluation of intraoperative repositioning of the nasal bones when a closed reduction was being performed.[52]

Several additional applications of bony ultrasound have been reported in the medical literature. These include intraoperative postreduction confirmation of the position of zygomatic arch fracture fragments,[53] diagnosis of infant hip dislocation, diagnosis of pediatric skull fractures in children with scalp hematomas,[54] diagnosis of infant posterior shoulder dislocation,[55] diagnosis of posterior sternoclavicular dislocation,[56,57] diagnosis of subtle fractures of the clavicle and femur in infants,[58] and use of ultrasound as a procedural aid for closed reduction in displaced extra-articular distal radius fractures or pediatric forearm fractures.[59] In a series of 62 adults with distal radius fractures, the rate of repeat manipulation and reduction was significantly reduced (1.6% vs. 8.8%) when ultrasound was used compared with a standard "blind" technique. The ultrasound group was also noted to have an improved volar tilt and a reduced operative rate.[60] For each of these applications, identification of the bright bony cortical echo allows the provider to assess whether the bone and its relationship with surrounding structures is normal or abnormal.

ANATOMICAL CONSIDERATIONS

The location for ultrasound of the ribs is usually guided by the patient's complaint of pain; the rib segment in question will be found beneath skin, subcutaneous tissue, and the relevant chest wall musculature at the site being investigated. It is important to remember the curved course of the ribs when scanning. The sternum is superficially located beneath skin, subcutaneous tissue, and the medial portions of the pectoralis major muscles, and is composed of two flat bones, the manubrium superiorly and the sternal body inferiorly. The first seven ribs articulate with the manubrium and sternal body laterally, and the manubrium articulates with the sternal body at the sternal angle. The shafts of the long bones (humerus, radius, femur, and tibia) are fairly rounded in cross-sectional profile and become wider and flatter on their distal aspects. The bony support of the external nose is provided by the two nasal bones along the upper dorsum of the nose and the frontal processes of the maxillae laterally. The nasal bones are contiguous with the frontal bone above via the nasofrontal suture and the maxillae laterally via the nasomaxillary sutures (Figures 18-32 and 18-33). The frontal processes of the maxillae are contiguous with the frontal bone via the frontomaxillary sutures. The bony zygomatic arch sits beneath skin and subcutaneous tissue and is formed anteriorly by the temporal process of the zygoma and posteriorly by the zygomatic process of the temporal bone. The masseter muscle originates from the edge of the zygomatic arch and inserts on the ramus of the mandible below.

TECHNIQUE AND NORMAL ULTRASOUND FINDINGS

Use a linear array transducer (in the 7.5–12 MHz range) to assess for fractures of the ribs and costochondral carti-

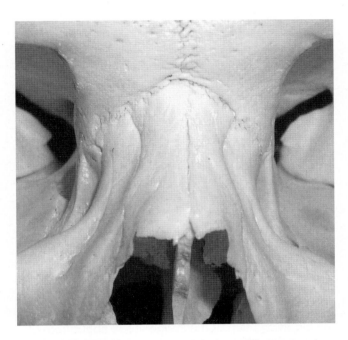

Figure 18-32. Frontal view of the nasal bones and nasal pyramid on a skull. The paired nasal bones are in the midline. The frontal processes of the maxillae make up the lateral walls of the nasal pyramid on either side. The frontomaxillary and nasofrontal sutures are seen at the top of the nasal pyramid.

lage. In short-axis orientation, a rib will be seen casting a dense posterior acoustic shadow beneath its echogenic superficial cortical surface (Figure 18-34). Slightly below the rib, the pleura will be seen as a brightly echogenic horizontal line. Pleural sliding and comet-tail artifacts will usually be noted at this interface on real-time

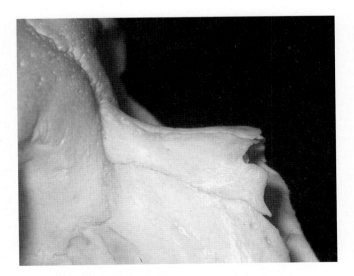

Figure 18-33. Lateral view of the right nasal bone, the nasomaxillary suture, and the right frontal process of the maxilla.

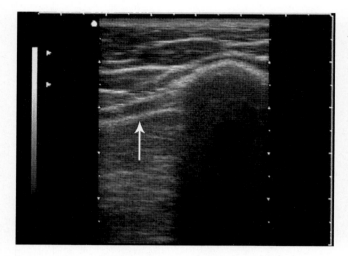

Figure 18-34. Short-axis sonogram of a rib. The curved echogenic surface of the rib appears on the right with dense posterior acoustic shadowing. The pleural line is seen as a horizontal echogenic line in the left midportion of the image; it lies about 1 cm deep to the most superficial aspect of the rib (arrow).

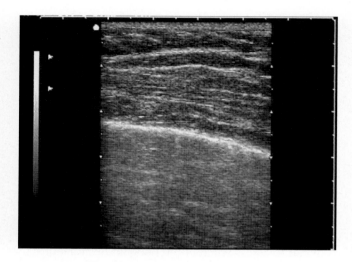

Figure 18-36. Long-axis sonogram of a rib interspace. The pleural line appears as a somewhat deeper, thicker, and more echogenic horizontal line beneath the skin, subcutaneous tissue, and intercostal muscle. Comet-tail artifacts and a positive sliding sign are typically seen when scanning this interface in real time.

scanning. At the site of maximal tenderness, align the transducer to evaluate the rib in the short-axis orientation in the center of the image. Then, turn the transducer parallel to the long axis of the rib. The superficial cortex of the normal rib and costal cartilage will appear as a thin echogenic line on the sonogram (Figure 18-35). Remain directly over the long axis of the rib since the pleural line will also appear as a horizontal echogenic line on the sonogram, albeit somewhat deeper and with pleural sliding and comet-tail artifacts usually apparent (Figure 18-36).

Use a 7.5–12 MHz linear array transducer for evaluation of a suspected sternal fracture. Scan the sternum in both long- and short-axis views, although the long-axis view is reported to be the most fruitful for fracture detection. The sternal surface will appear as a horizontal echogenic line with a slight elevation in the cortical surface noted at the level of the sternomanubrial junction. As with evaluation for suspected rib fractures, scanning at the area of maximal tenderness can help locate the fracture site quickly.

Ultrasound of long bones in the trauma setting can be undertaken with the same curved array transducer that is used for the FAST examination. A transverse orientation on the limb being scanned is best for quickly establishing the location and depth of the bone being examined (Figure 18-37). Once the lower end of the relevant bone has been located, rotate the transducer longitudinally and move the transducer up the extremity to evaluate for any cortical irregularities along the shaft (Figure 18-38). The cortical surface of the bone closest to the transducer will be seen as a smooth brightly echogenic line on the sonogram.

Use a 10 MHz or higher frequency linear array transducer for sonography of the nasal pyramid. Place the transducer along each side of the nose aiming medially along the lateral nasal pyramid to assess both the frontal process of the maxilla and ipsilateral proximal nasal bone, and along the left and right paramedian midline to assess the full length of the nasal bones proper (Figures 18-39 and 18-40). Set imaging depth to 3 cm and, as with all bone imaging, adjust the electronic focus to maximize

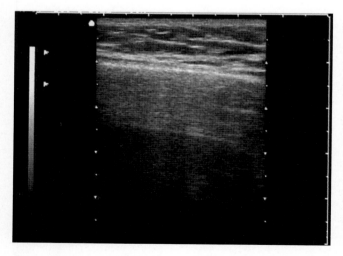

Figure 18-35. Long-axis sonogram of a rib. The cortical surface of the rib is seen as a thin, echogenic, superficially located horizontal line just beneath the skin and subcutaneous tissue in this image.

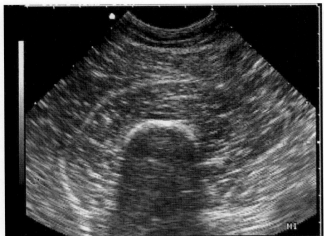

Figure 18-37. Short-axis sonogram of the proximal thigh. The hypoechoic and speckled appearing vastus muscles (vastus lateralis, intermedius, and medialis) are seen in cross section lateral, anterior, and medial to the femur. The anterior surface of the femur is seen in the center of the image as a brightly echogenic curved line with a prominent posterior acoustic shadow.

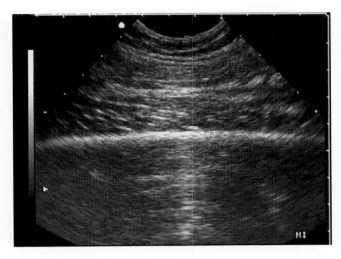

Figure 18-38. Long-axis sonogram of a normal femur. The anterior cortical surface of the femur appears as a smooth and regular echogenic line beneath the hypoechoic thigh muscles; a slight curvature of the image occurs when a curved array transducer is used.

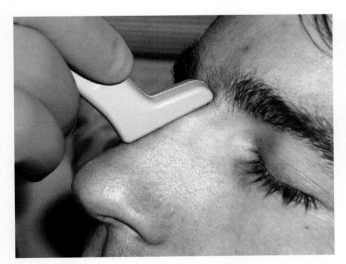

A

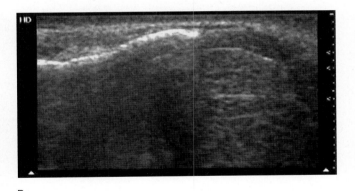

B

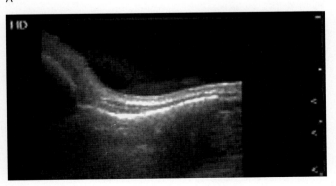

C

Figure 18-39. This image shows the anterior location where the ultrasound transducer should be placed when assessing the nasal pyramid for a fracture (A). Although a linear array transducer may also be used for this application, these images will be more easily obtained if a small parts (and hence, small footprint) transducer is used. Sonogram of a normal nasal bone (B). The nasofrontal border is not visualized in this image because the edge of a standard linear array transducer does not easily fit on the superior nasal bridge. Sonogram of the normal nasal bone and a portion of the frontal bone (C). A copious amount of gel was placed on the nasal bridge and the image now includes a portion of the frontal bone on the left, the nasofrontal suture, and the nasal bone proper.

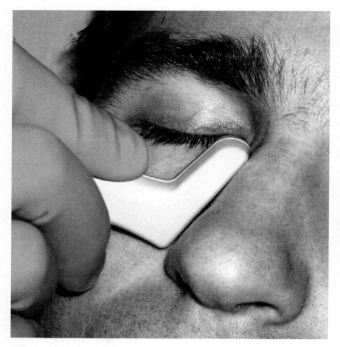

A

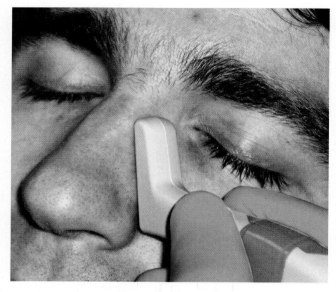

B

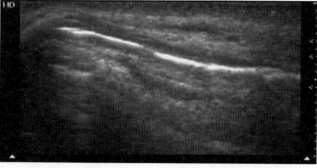

C

Figure 18-40. This sequence of images shows the two additional locations where the ultrasound transducer should be placed when assessing the nasal pyramid for a fracture (A, B). Sonogram of the normal lateral nasal pyramid (C). The echogenic surface of the nasal bone, the slightly hypoechoic nasomaxillary suture, and the frontal process of the maxilla are all seen on this sonogram of the lateral nasal wall.

resolution at the level of the cortex. Using transducers and settings similar to those used for nasal bone imaging, visualize the zygomatic arch by scanning the upper lateral cheek in a horizontal scan plane (Figure 18-41).

The same imaging techniques apply when ultrasound is used for reducing fractures (typically in the distal radius and forearm).

COMMON AND EMERGENT ABNORMALITIES

Rib Fractures

Fractures of the rib or costochondral junction will be recognized by a clear discontinuity of the anterior cortical echo of the rib, costochondral junction, or costal cartilage (Figure 18-42), or by real-time visualization of

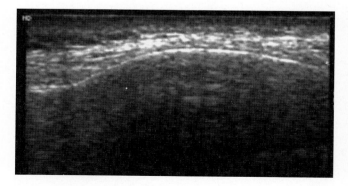

Figure 18-41. Sonogram of the bony contour of the normal zygomatic arch; the arch is seen as a thin echogenic line several millimeters below the skin surface.

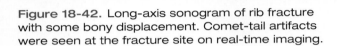

Figure 18-42. Long-axis sonogram of rib fracture with some bony displacement. Comet-tail artifacts were seen at the fracture site on real-time imaging.

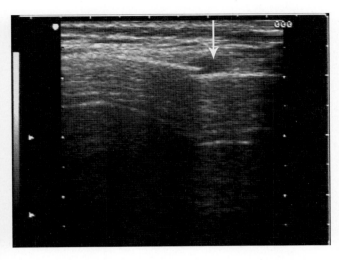

Figure 18-44. Long-axis sonogram of a sternal body fracture. There is an area of cortical discontinuity in the near field to the right of the image and there is a small associated hypoechoic fracture hematoma (arrow).

widening of the fracture line with local transducer pressure. Comet-tail artifacts may be noted to emanate posteriorly from the mobile fracture site (Figure 18-43), and a hypoechoic fracture hematoma will commonly be seen adjacent to the fracture.

Sternal Fractures

A sternal fracture will appear as a disruption in the cortical echo of the anterior sternum; movement of the sternum fracture fragments with respiration may be noted during real-time scanning. A hypoechoic fracture

hematoma may be seen adjacent to the fracture site (Figure 18-44).

Long Bones

Fractures of the femur, tibia, and humerus are best appreciated with a long-axis scanning technique and will be apparent as an obvious disruption in the echogenic line that corresponds to the cortical surface of the bone. Examples of common long bone fractures are demonstrated in Figures 18-44 to 18-47.

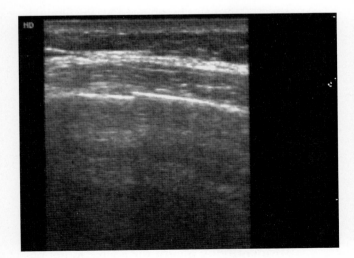

Figure 18-43. Long-axis sonogram of a rib fracture. Skin, subcutaneous tissue, fascia, and chest wall musculature are seen as distinct layers just above the thin echogenic rib surface. Even though the step-off at the fracture line is less than a millimeter, it is readily apparent on the sonogram.

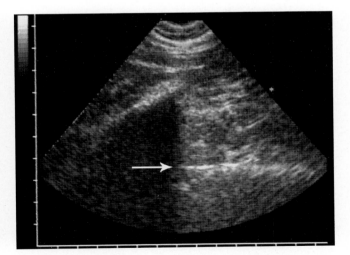

Figure 18-45. Long-axis sonogram of the proximal femoral shaft in a patient with femur fracture. The proximal fragment is seen to angulate anteriorly, and there is a prominent posterior acoustic shadow. The distal femur is seen as a horizontal echogenic line (arrow) about 4 cm deep to the anterior fragment.

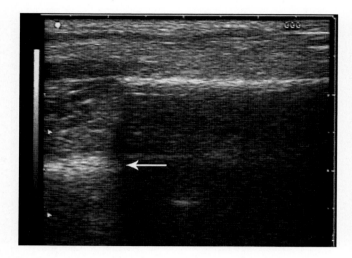

Figure 18-46. Long-axis sonogram of a tibial shaft fracture. About a centimeter of bony displacement is seen between the proximal (arrow) and distal fracture fragments in this image.

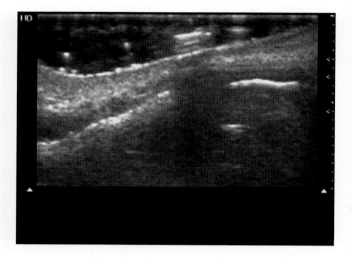

Figure 18-48. Sonogram of a nasal bone fracture. There is a region of obvious cortical discontinuity and a large gap is seen between the proximal nasal bone and the displaced distal fragment.

Nasal Bones

A nasal bone fracture is clearly demonstrated by the large hypoechoic gap in the normally echogenic cortical surface in Figure 18-48.

Zygomatic Arch

The normal contour of the zygomatic arch is clearly disrupted in Figure 18-49, and a prominent hypoechoic fracture hematoma is present.

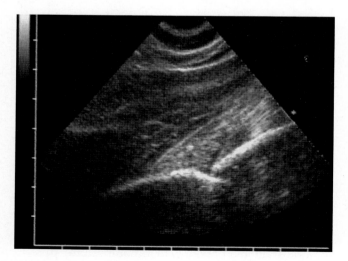

Figure 18-47. Long-axis sonogram of a humerus fracture. There is obvious disruption of the cortical surface in this image.

PITFALLS

1. **General pitfalls.** An important pitfall of fracture sonography was highlighted in an experimental study examining the sonographic profile of fractured cadaver bones. It was observed that fractures and bony defects were *not* well visualized when the transducer was oriented parallel to the fracture line or zone of bony impaction. Optimal imaging of a fracture and any associated bony displacement requires that the ultrasound transducer be oriented axially along the bone and, ideally, perpendicular to the fracture line.[61] Characteristically, an interruption of the normal cortical echo reflection and its associated posterior acoustic shadow will be noted; additionally, a dorsal band of comet-tail echoes may be seen at the fracture site.[62]

2. **Rib imaging pitfalls.** If the transducer is located partly over the rib and partly over an intercostal space (or over a portion of the scapula), the image obtained on the sonogram may be interpreted as representing a fracture when, in fact, none is present. Costal cartilage calcifications may also give rise to this "pseudofracture" phenomenon.

   Misidentifying pleura for a rib. Do not mistake the brightly echogenic pleural surface (seen when scanning along the long axis of an intercostal space) for the cortex of the rib. Initially scan the rib in question in short-axis orientation; it will be easily identified by its

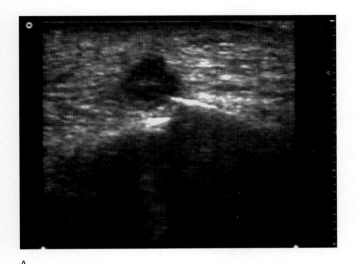

A

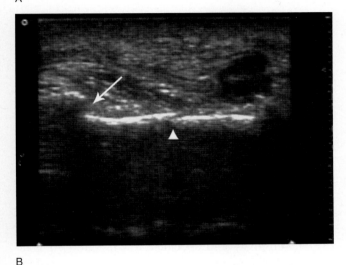

B

Figure 18-49. Sonogram of a right zygomatic arch fracture. This first image was taken near the zygomaticotemporal suture (A). The normally smooth contour of the cortical surface of the zygomatic arch has been disrupted and a hypoechoic fracture hematoma is seen at the fracture site. The overlying soft tissues are notably thicker than normal. The next image was taken over the zygomatic process of the temporal bone or the zygomatic arch proper (B). A depressed zygomatic arch fracture is apparent (arrow) and a fracture line is seen in the mid-arch (arrowhead). The hypoechoic fracture hematoma in the area of the zygomaticotemporal suture is now seen to the right of the image.

characteristic posterior acoustic shadowing. Note the location of the superficial surface of the rib and its depth within the soft tissues of the chest wall. Next, rotate the transducer into a long-axis orientation directly over the rib surface to assess for the presence of a fracture.

The brightly echogenic pleural line will usually be seen about a centimeter deep to the superficial surface of the rib. Careful observation during real-time scanning will typically reveal to-and-fro gliding movements ("lung sliding") at the brightly echogenic pleural interface. The lung sliding sign will be absent if a coexistent pneumothorax is present, however, and it may be the depth of this echogenic line alone that clarifies its identity as rib or pleural surface.

3. **Sternum fracture pitfalls.** The hypoechoic sternomanubrial junction may be confused with a fracture on the long-axis view. In general, a fracture of the sternum will appear as a sharply defined area of cortical discontinuity, whereas the sternomanubrial junction will appear as a gentle and smoothly edged ridge with a small hypoechoic joint space in between. Another reported pitfall, when imaging the sternum with ultrasound, is mistaking the hypoechoic pectoralis muscles for a hematoma on a short-axis view.[37]

4. **Long bone fracture pitfalls.** While generally excellent for diagnosing midshaft fractures of the long bones, diagnostic accuracy for fracture detection with ultrasound is limited by a number of factors. Diagnostic accuracy is notably poorer in the metacarpals, metatarsals, with small avulsion injuries, and injuries involving the joint space. Notably, imaging "at or above the intertrochanteric line of the femur" is felt to be fraught with difficulty, with a propensity for false positive studies to occur in this area.[40] These areas of poorer diagnostic accuracy are generally more challenging to image and interpret, likely due to the many irregular bony acoustic interfaces present. Subcutaneous air around an open fracture may also adversely affect image quality and therefore diagnostic accuracy.

5. **Nasal bone fractures pitfalls.** A large transducer head may be difficult to place on a small nose. In such cases, copious use of gel or an acoustic standoff such as a gel-filled portion of a rubber glove or a piece of a commercially available gel pad may prove helpful for obtaining an adequate image.

6. **Zygomatic arch fracture pitfalls.** The zygomatic arch is long and narrow and the transducer needs to be accurately aligned to image the arch fully. The length of the full contour of the arch may exceed the length of the transducer, and several images may be required to fully assess the arch for a fracture.

► FOREIGN BODY LOCALIZATION

CLINICAL CONSIDERATIONS

Correctly diagnosing and managing a wound that harbors a soft tissue foreign body can be challenging, especially when the foreign body is radiolucent. To further complicate matters, wounds that harbor foreign bodies often occur in the hand or foot where the likelihood of iatrogenic injury from blind wound exploration and the potential for subsequent infectious complications is high. Although usually located in superficial soft tissues, foreign bodies may cause no symptoms initially and can easily be overlooked. In a retrospective review of 200 patients referred for retained foreign bodies, 38% were misdiagnosed on the index visit.[63] Even with a high index of suspicion, liberal use of radiography, and exploration, a soft tissue foreign body can be missed. The possible infectious and medicolegal consequences of this missed diagnosis can be unfortunate for the patient and the provider alike. Missed foreign bodies have been reported to be one of the most common causes of malpractice claims against emergency physicians.[64]

While metal and glass are radio-opaque and usually apparent on standard two-view radiographs, other commonly encountered foreign bodies, particularly organic material such as wood or thorns, are nearly always radiolucent. Plastic is also typically radiolucent. CT or MRI may be useful in the assessment of suspected foreign bodies, but these modalities are expensive, time-consuming, and not always readily obtainable. Furthermore, the sensitivity of CT for the detection of wooden foreign bodies is low, reported to range from 0% to 60%.[65,66] Ultrasound offers some decided advantages in this setting. For detecting wooden foreign bodies—nearly always missed with plain radiography—ultrasound is 79–95% sensitive and 86–97% specific.[65,67,68] In a case where a radiolucent foreign body is suspected, an ultrasound evaluation of the wound should be considered in the ED workup. Whether radio-opaque or radiolucent, once a soft tissue foreign body has been identified, the next issue faced by the clinician is how best to remove it. As most experienced clinicians will confirm, removal of a subcutaneous foreign body can be enormously frustrating. Ultrasound can additionally be used to provide precise preoperative localization of the foreign body, or, if desired, the foreign body may be retrieved under direct sonographic guidance.

CLINICAL INDICATIONS

The clinical indications for the use of ultrasound in the management of a suspected soft tissue foreign body include:

- Detection and localization of a foreign body
- Foreign body removal

The literature on sonographic detection of soft tissue foreign bodies encompasses a wide range of specialties and methodologies.[65,67–80] The types of foreign bodies that have been described include metal, wood, graphite, plastic, gravel, sand, thorns, cactus spines, and bamboo twigs. Clinicians with varying levels of skill perform the ultrasound examinations in these studies, ranging from emergency physicians with no prior formal training, credentialed clinicians, and radiologists specially trained in musculoskeletal ultrasound. The ultrasound machines and transducers are different in nearly every study. While this literature is therefore somewhat difficult to synthesize, a number of useful conclusions can be drawn.

Success in detecting foreign bodies varies widely in the experimental literature, depending in part on the tissue model employed and foreign body type. Using a homogenous beef cube as a tissue model, ultrasound was 98% sensitive and specific in identifying a variety of embedded foreign bodies in one report,[70] whereas another study using a chicken thigh model (a model that more closely mimics the human hand) reported an overall sensitivity of only 79% for detecting a wooden foreign body.[67] In studies involving freshly thawed cadaver feet and hands, diagnostic sensitivities and specificities ranged from 90% to 94% and from 90% to 97%, respectively.[73,78] In contrast to such excellent results, another investigation that used ultrasound for detecting foreign bodies in chicken thighs reported an overall sensitivity and specificity of 43% and 70%, respectively, with a sensitivity of only 50% for detecting a 1-cm-long piece of wood.[72] Review of the methods employed in this study revealed that the chicken thighs were incised and systematically opened with a hemostat prior to foreign body placement. Such tissue disruption with the likely introduction of subcutaneous air probably exceeds that which occurs in natural wounding and may have made subsequent sonography more difficult. In a cadaveric study where 6 emergency physicians performed a total of 900 assessments looking for a <5 mm foreign body, the diagnostic sensitivity and specificity were found to be 53% and 47% respectively.[81] The model employed skin incision technique, depth of foreign body placement, and foreign body type and size as variables that can all dramatically affect outcome in such experimental studies. Of note, vigorous wound irrigation itself can introduce subcutaneous gas bubbles that can interfere with attempts to locate small glass fragments with ultrasound. However, in a study in which air was purposely injected into turkey breasts containing glass, metal, and bone, the soft tissue gas did not appear to diminish the ability to locate the foreign bodies.[82]

Success in soft tissue foreign body detection also depends on foreign body size. The test characteristics of ultrasound reported among various studies must therefore be interpreted with an awareness of the size of the experimental foreign body being imaged. Small glass fragments and cactus thorns were difficult to detect in one report, and may have exceeded the limits of the ultrasound transducer's resolution.[70] Variations in detection rates with two differing lengths of wooden toothpicks inserted into freshly thawed cadaver feet were reported. Sensitivity decreased from 93% for detecting a 5.0-mm-long fragment to 87% for detecting one that was 2.5 mm long.[73] Specificities were uniformly high across studies, indicating that it is uncommon to falsely identify a foreign body when none is present.

While it might appear intuitive that provider's experience and expertise would be a crucial determinant of success for foreign body localization, there is little experimental evidence to support this assumption. Only one study directly compared the ability of various types of clinicians to locate foreign bodies in a chicken thigh model with ultrasound.[67] It found no statistically significant difference in accuracy between a board-certified radiologist whose practice was limited to ultrasonography, two sonographers, and three emergency medicine residents. Sensitivity was 74% in the hands of the emergency physicians compared to 83% and 85%, respectively, for the radiologist and sonographers.

In clinical case series, wood is the most common radiolucent material reported. Hand, foot, calf, and forearm injuries predominate, and most foreign bodies are found to be superficial in location.[65,68,83] One series of 50 patients evaluated for radiolucent foreign bodies noted that 45 of the 50 injuries involved the hand or foot.[68] All of the 21 foreign bodies retrieved at surgery were found less than 2 cm from the skin surface in this report. In another case series of patients evaluated for suspected wooden foreign bodies in the feet, all 10 of the wooden foreign bodies discovered with ultrasound were located between 0.4 and 1.4 cm from the skin surface.[65] Ultrasound can also be utilized to detect and retrieve an errant piece of tongue or cheek piercing jewelry that has become accidently embedded beneath the skin surface or to detect a suspected radiolucent foreign body in a patient who has engaged in self-embedding behavior.

ANATOMICAL CONSIDERATIONS

Since hand and foot wounds are the most common injuries that may harbor a subcutaneous foreign body, a thorough familiarity with the anatomy of the hands and feet is essential for the clinician scanning these regions. Given the relatively shallow depth of the soft tissues in these anatomically intricate regions and the multi-ple acoustic interfaces present, clinicians should practice scanning on normal hands and feet to gain familiarity with the normal sonographic appearance of these commonly injured areas. The utility of examining the contralateral uninjured extremity for comparison when a confusing sonographic finding is encountered cannot be overemphasized.

TECHNIQUE AND NORMAL ULTRASOUND FINDINGS

Use the highest frequency linear array transducer available when searching for subcutaneous foreign bodies since most will be found located within 2 cm of the skin surface. A linear array transducer in the 7.5–12.0 MHz range is generally recommended. A 7.5 MHz curvilinear transducer, such as an endocavitary transducer, may also function adequately for this application and has the added advantage of having a smaller, rounded skin contact footprint for scanning in web spaces.[69,84] A 5.0 MHz transducer may be useful when searching for a deep foreign body. Higher frequency small parts transducers (typically in the 10–15.0 MHz range) offer the ability to discern very small foreign bodies; a 12.0 MHz transducer can reportedly detect a 1–2 mm foreign body. Small parts—"hockey stick"—transducers have become a more common addition to ultrasound equipment. The combination of high-resolution imaging with a small skin contact footprint makes these transducers particularly useful for imaging digits and web spaces for foreign bodies.

Use of an acoustic standoff pad may be necessary with some transducers to adequately image the superficial soft tissues. Standoff pads provide a sonolucent acoustic window, raise the transducer 1–2 cm above the skin surface, and move the subcutaneous region of interest beyond the extreme near field (and beyond the transducer's "dead zone") into a more suitable focal zone. Although incorporating the use of a standoff pad into the ultrasound examination requires additional technical agility and some practice, the effort can be amply rewarded with improved near-field image quality. Inexpensive and commercially available gel pads are available just for this purpose, and smaller chunks can be cut off for single patient use and then discarded. Other options include the use of a water- or gel-filled glove or glove finger. When using a water-filled glove, it is essential to exclude any air bubbles that may impede subsequent imaging. In the case of a large or gaping wound, copious sterile surgical gel can be applied onto the wound; after the ultrasound examination is completed, the wound should be thoroughly irrigated. A water bath technique, in which the affected extremity is submerged in a basin of water during scanning, represents an alternative to the use of a standoff pad or the copious use of sterile surgical gel. Compared to direct contact with gel, the water bath technique is easier to perform and provides superior images of tendons and foreign bodies.[85,86] The water bath technique also causes less patient discomfort since images may be obtained without direct contact between the patient and the transducer.[87] The provider should ensure that only the sealed portions of the transducer are immersed in the water bath or that a waterproof transducer cover is employed.

Optimizing depth and focus are particularly important when using ultrasound to search for a small, subcutaneous foreign body. Hold the transducer perpendicular to the skin surface and systematically scan the area of interest in two orthogonal imaging planes. Best visualization of a foreign body will occur when the transducer is aligned such that the long axis of the ultrasound beam is parallel to the long axis of the foreign body. Small objects can easily be missed when scanned in short-axis orientation alone. With a small wooden foreign body, however, it is sometimes the prominent posterior acoustic shadow on the *short-axis view* that alerts the provider to its presence. Because wounds containing foreign bodies can occur on any part of the body, a wide array of normal sonographic findings is therefore possible depending on the anatomic region being scanned. Most wounds suspected of harboring a foreign body occur in the hands and feet, however, where numerous anatomic structures and interfaces, each with a distinct sonographic appearance, will be encountered. The skin surface is the most superficial echogenic structure encountered, and is seen adjacent to the transducer surface (or, if an acoustic standoff is used, adjacent to the distant side of the anechoic standoff pad). In the hands and especially the feet, this layer is notably thicker than elsewhere on the body. Subcutaneous fat appears hypoechoic with a reticular pattern of echogenic connective tissue seen between the fat lobules. The thickness of this layer varies considerably with body location and habitus. Fascial planes appear as thin, echogenic, usually horizontal lines immediately adjacent to the muscle. Muscle tissue appears relatively hypoechoic with regular internal striations (linear or pennate in long axis and speckled in short axis due to the relative orientation of the muscle fibers). Tendons are moderately echogenic, appear ovoid and finely speckled in short axis, and rectangular with a characteristic fibrillar sonographic echotexture in long-axis orientation. Interestingly, tendons will appear considerably more hypoechoic when imaged obliquely; this characteristic of tendon imaging is known as *anisotropy* and is discussed in greater detail in the musculotendinous applications portion of this chapter. Tendon movement can be observed in real time when the corresponding joints are moved. Bone appears brightly echogenic

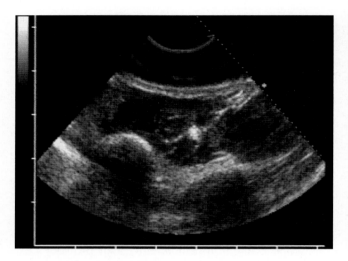

Figure 18-50. Sonogram of the thenar eminence of a normal hand using a 7.5 MHz annular array transducer and an acoustic standoff pad. The anechoic standoff appears first, then the hyperechoic skin surface, followed by the hypoechoic thenar eminence muscles below. The flexor pollicis longus tendon is seen in cross section as a hyperechoic circle in the middle of the image. The hyperechoic surfaces of the first and second metacarpals are seen in the far field with associated posterior acoustic shadowing.

on the cortical surface closest to the transducer, with prominent posterior acoustic shadowing. Joint spaces can be readily identified by a V-shaped discontinuity in the bright cortical echo of adjacent bones. Blood vessels are anechoic and have a circular or tubular profile when scanned in short or long axis, respectively. They can be further characterized with color flow Doppler, if necessary. In general, veins will compress easily with transducer pressure whereas arteries will remain pulsatile. Sonograms of the thenar eminence of a normal hand and a chicken thigh (commonly used as a tissue model for foreign body imaging) are shown in Figures 18-50 and 18-51.

COMMON AND EMERGENT ABNORMALITIES

Soft tissue foreign bodies exhibit a variety of sonographic patterns depending on the material involved, the size of the foreign body, and the length of time the foreign body has been present in the tissue. Common materials such as wood, glass, metal, plastic, and gravel will generally appear hyperechoic with variable amounts of posterior acoustic shadowing and associated artifacts that are material and shape dependent. A wooden

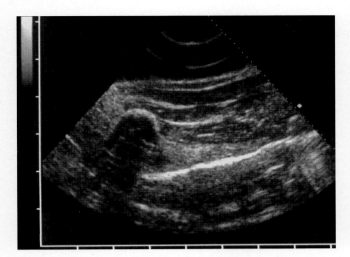

Figure 18-51. Sonogram of a chicken thigh using a 7.5 MHz annular array transducer and an acoustic standoff pad (a similar technique is used for all the experimental foreign body images that follow). Note the tissue thickness and appearance is similar to that of the hand. The skin has been removed, thigh muscle tissue appears hypoechoic, the thigh bone on the left of the image appears hyperechoic with posterior acoustic shadowing, and an echogenic horizontally oriented fascial plane is seen in the far field.

foreign body typically casts a hypoechoic posterior acoustic shadow that often facilitates its discovery (Figures 18-52 to 18-55). Linear metallic foreign bodies will typically display a reverberation artifact with bright, regularly spaced parallel lines seen distal to the actual object

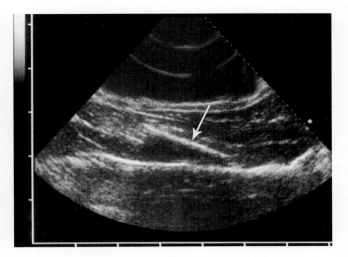

Figure 18-53. Long-axis sonogram of a wooden toothpick in a chicken thigh. The hyperechoic surface of the 2-cm wood fragment is seen in the near field in the center of the image (arrow points to center of toothpick); a posterior acoustic shadow is seen below.

(Figures 18-56 to 18-58). Metal objects that are small, or rounded, may display a comet-tail artifact (Figure 18-59). The acoustic profile of glass is less consistent, however, and acoustic shadowing, reverberation artifact, or diffuse beam scattering may all be encountered during scanning

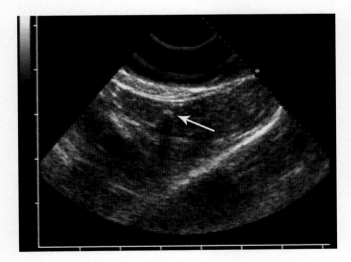

Figure 18-52. Short-axis sonogram of a wooden toothpick embedded in a chicken thigh. The hyperechoic wood fragment is seen in the near field. The posterior acoustic shadow draws the eye up to the location of the foreign body (arrow).

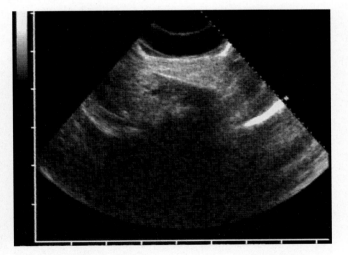

Figure 18-54. Long-axis sonogram of a wooden foreign body in a patient's foot. A 7.5 MHz annular array transducer and an acoustic standoff pad were used to obtain the image; the skin surface and immediate subcutaneous tissue appear hyperechoic. The wood fragment appears in the near field as a hyperechoic linear structure that slants to the right; a prominent posterior acoustic shadow is seen beneath the wood fragment.

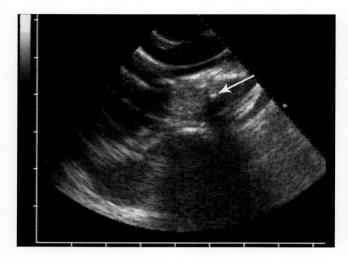

Figure 18-55. Short-axis sonogram of the wooden foreign body in Figure 18-54. The hyperechoic wood fragment appears in the near field on the right side of the image (arrow). The transducer is no longer entirely in contact with the foot because of the location being scanned. A prominent posterior acoustic shadow is again seen beneath the foreign body. More distally and in the center of the sonogram, the first metatarsal bone and its posterior acoustic shadow are seen in cross section.

(Figures 18-60 and 18-61). Foreign bodies retained for longer than 24 hours are frequently surrounded by a hypoechoic "halo," resulting from edema, pus, or granulation tissue. This hypoechoic region around the foreign body often facilitates identification and localization of the foreign body. In a similar fashion, a local anesthetic

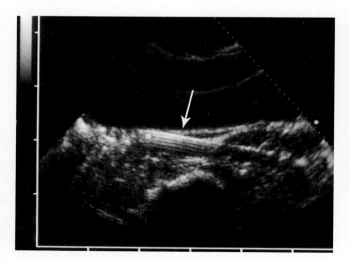

Figure 18-56. Long-axis sonogram of a needle in a chicken thigh. The needle appears hyperechoic (arrow) with a characteristic reverberation artifact seen below.

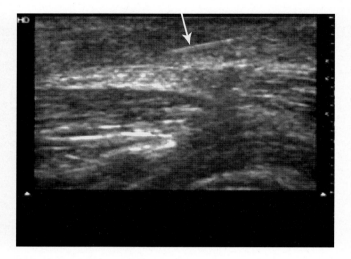

Figure 18-57. Long-axis sonogram of a broken needle fragment in the arm of an injection drug user. The needle appears hyperechoic (arrow). Although not appreciated on the sonogram, a fine reverberation artifact was seen on real-time imaging.

injected adjacent to a foreign body may improve the ability to visualize it. Sonograms of less commonly encountered foreign bodies such as plastic (with a prominent reverberation artifact) and gravel (with a prominent posterior acoustic shadow similar to a gallstone) are demonstrated in Figures 18-62 and 18-63.

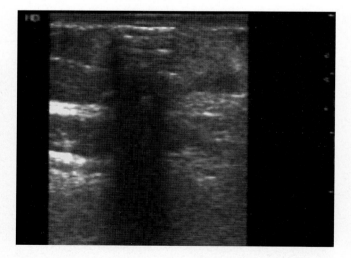

Figure 18-58. Clinically stable appearing victim of a gunshot wound to the right chest with a bullet seen on the *left* side in the chest radiograph. A mass was palpable beneath the skin on the left chest wall. A sonogram of the mass (the bullet) is notable for a reverberation artifact and posterior acoustic shadowing. The bullet was superficial in location and outside of the chest cavity (confirmed by CT).

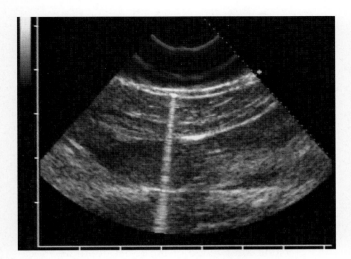

Figure 18-59. Sonogram of a BB in a chicken thigh. A prominent comet-tail artifact is seen.

COMMON VARIANTS AND SELECTED ABNORMALITIES

Various wound characteristics can complicate sonographic evaluation for a soft tissue foreign body. Air introduced into the wound by the injury itself, from the process of wound exploration or wound irrigation, or from bubbles inadvertently administered with the anesthetic agent can cause imaging difficulties. Air bubbles and associated artifacts may obscure the foreign body or may be mistaken for a foreign body when none is actually present. Air bubbles introduced during wound irrigation can complicate subsequent attempts to locate small glass fragments. Air pockets can sometimes be

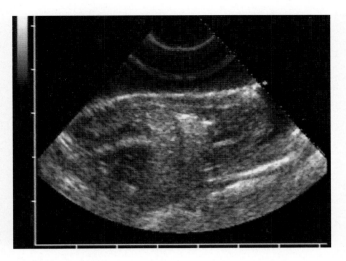

Figure 18-61. Sonogram of a piece of a broken glass bottle embedded in a chicken thigh. Although hyperechoic, the glass fragment in this image is indistinct with some dirty shadowing possibly due to air pockets surrounding the fragment.

obliterated by compression with the transducer, thereby improving image quality. Ultrasound examination of large open wounds may be difficult because of bleeding, associated tissue distortion, or patient discomfort.

PITFALLS

1. **Inadequate knowledge of the regional sonographic anatomy.** Lack of familiarity with normal sonographic anatomy, particularly of the hand and foot, can make correct interpretation

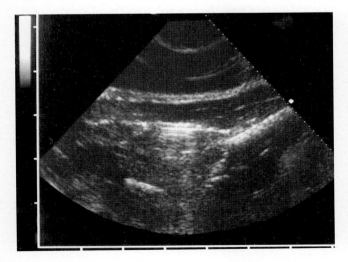

Figure 18-60. Sonogram of a linear glass shard embedded in a chicken thigh. The glass fragment in the center or the image appears hyperechoic with an associated reverberation artifact.

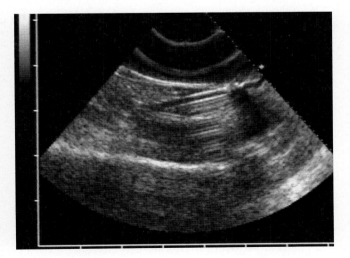

Figure 18-62. Long-axis sonogram of a plastic toothpick in a chicken thigh. The plastic surface of the toothpick appears hyperechoic with a prominent reverberation artifact seen below.

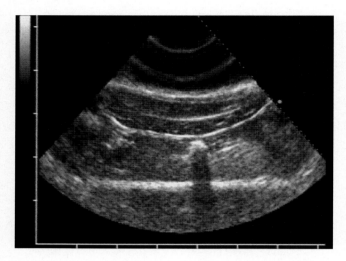

Figure 18-63. Sonogram of a piece of gravel in a chicken thigh. A prominent posterior acoustic shadow is seen beneath the hyperechoic surface of the gravel fragment.

of the ultrasound image difficult. Normal acoustic shadows from bone, brightly echogenic tissue interfaces and fascia, and artifacts arising from vascular calcifications, can all lead to misinterpretation of the image. Sesamoid bones may be falsely interpreted as a foreign body. Bony shadowing of the multiple carpal and metacarpal bones (or tarsal and metatarsal bones) and phalanges should not be confused with a foreign body.

2. **Failure to take necessary steps to optimize scanning of small superficial objects.** Scanning for subcutaneous foreign bodies, particularly in hands and feet, requires a significant investment in time, patience, and attention to certain scanning principles. A standoff pad or water bath may be required. Attention to transducer frequency, depth, and focus adjustment is crucial. In addition, the location of the wound and the transducer's skin contact footprint may make adequate imaging technically difficult. Scanning small curvilinear regions, such as a web space, may require a small parts (hockey stick) or endocavitary transducer, as well as standoff pad and the help of an assistant.

3. **Other pitfalls.** Small foreign bodies may exceed the limits of the transducer's resolution. Tissue interfaces in close proximity to one another may distort the image. A small foreign body adjacent to a bone may be hidden by the bone's posterior acoustic shadow. Scar tissue, air, ossified cartilage, and keratin plugs may all appear as small hyperechoic structures and be mistaken for foreign bodies.

4. **Foreign body removal.** Once a soft tissue foreign body has been located, an important clinical decision must be made as to whether retrieval is appropriate or even technically feasible. It is wise to set a time limit for exploration and foreign body removal and to have a plan for further evaluation or referral.[88] Various factors to consider include the skill of the operator, the body part injured, the time available, and the size and type of foreign body involved. With a deep wound, a poorly accessible foreign body, or closely adjacent neurovascular structures, consultation or referral to an appropriate surgical specialist is recommended. Advantages of real-time ultrasound use in this setting include knowledge of the exact depth and location of the foreign body as well as its proximity to other structures. Ultrasound-guided removal should be considered as "a first choice procedure for the extraction of foreign bodies" and can usually be successfully performed in 15–30 minutes.[89]

CASE STUDY

Patient Presentation

A 42-year-old man presented with a 10-day-old puncture wound of the finger with associated soft tissue swelling. The patient reported getting a splinter in his hand while sitting on a park bench. He thought he had removed the entire splinter at the time of the injury.

On physical examination, there was swelling over the volar proximal third phalanx but no definite fluctuance (Figure 18-64A). Distal neurocirculatory examination was intact, and there were no signs of lymphangitis or tenosynovitis.

Management

A radiograph of the affected digit was obtained and notable only for some soft tissue swelling (Figure 18-64B). An ultrasound was performed using a 7.5 MHz annular array transducer and an acoustic standoff to obtain the images in both longitudinal (Figure 18-64C) and transverse (Figure 18-64D) planes. A hyperechoic foreign body with an associated hypoechoic surrounding inflammatory response was seen above the PIP joint. The wood fragment was easily removed with a superficial skin incision along the PIP crease (Figure 18-64E).

Commentary

This case emphasizes the advantage of sonography over plain radiography for identification of wooden (and other radiolucent) foreign bodies. Foreign bodies

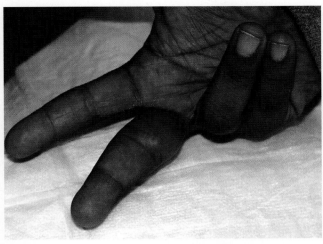

A

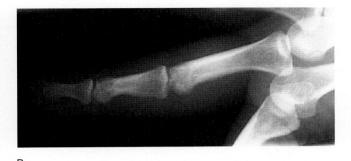

B

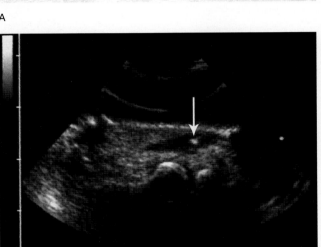

C

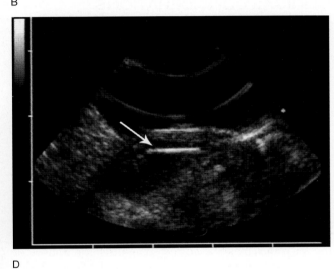

D

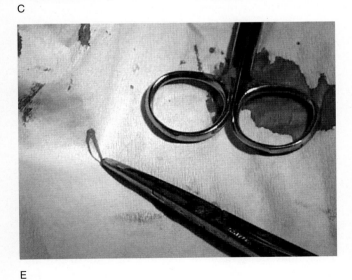

E

Figure 18-64. Case study. Image of swollen digit (A). Radiograph of the affected digit is notable only for some soft tissue swelling (B). Longitudinal sonogram on the volar surface of the third digit over the PIP joint shows a hyperechoic foreign body (arrow) in cross section (C). Note associated hypoechoic surrounding inflammatory response. Long-axis view of 1-cm splinter (arrow) (D). Wood fragment removed (E).

retained for longer than 24 hours will typically be surrounded by a hypoechoic "halo" resulting from edema, or early infection around the foreign body. This hypoechoic "halo" can facilitate identification and successful removal of a foreign body.

► MUSCULOTENDINOUS APPLICATIONS

CLINICAL CONSIDERATIONS

Technological advancements over the past decade have led to the increased use of diagnostic ultrasound for evaluation of a wide range of musculotendinous and rheumatologic conditions. Smaller, more portable ultrasound units, high-frequency small parts transducers with resolutions to a fraction of a millimeter, tissue harmonics, compound imaging technology, and extended-field-of-view features have helped promote ultrasound as a diagnostic tool for evaluating musculotendinous complaints by radiologists, orthopedists, rheumatologists, and emergency physicians. Ultrasound has emerged as "a powerful extension of the physical examination,"[90] especially in the setting of a musculotendinous complaint. Imaging of tendons, joints, and muscles can help the provider make a correct diagnosis for a host of painful musculoskeletal conditions and allow for optimal patient management. Self-teaching programs in musculoskeletal ultrasound have been promulgated for rheumatologists with excellent results reported after 24 hours of active scanning and 8–9 hours reviewing images with tutors.[91] A similar self-teaching program has been incorporated into the educational curriculum at a residency program in Physical Medicine and Rehabilitation.[92]

A myriad of musculoskeletal applications for diagnostic ultrasound has been described in the ultrasound literature. These include (1) evaluation of suspected partial or complete tendon tears (rotator cuff, triceps tendon, distal biceps tendon, Achilles tendon, quadriceps tendon, patellar ligament, and flexor tendons of the hand), (2) evaluation for suspected muscle tears (typically in the rectus femoris and gastrocnemius muscles), (3) diagnosis of occult ganglion cysts in the wrists or fingers[93] and diagnosis of soft tissue tumors of the hand,[94] (4) dynamic evaluation of flexor tendons of the hand (for evaluation of annular pulley ligament disruption or assessment of tendon location after flexor tendon avulsion), and (5) assessment of selected nerves for suspected entrapment or compression (e.g., the ulnar and median nerves in cubital and carpal tunnel syndromes). Some of these applications require expertise in ultrasound beyond that of most clinicians or they may require specialized transducers that are not generally available in the acute care setting. Since linear array and specialized small parts (hockey stick) transducers are available

on most point-of-care ultrasound units, a host of musculotendinous applications can be added to the diagnostic armamentarium of emergency care providers.

CLINICAL INDICATIONS

Clinical indications for performing a musculotendinous ultrasound examination may include

- Assessment of suspected partial/complete tendon or muscle tears
- Evaluation of suspected tenosynovitis and selected tendinopathies
- Precise needle guidance for aspiration and soft tissue injection procedures involving tendons and bursae

Assessment of Suspected Partial/ Complete Tendon or Muscle Tears

The use of ultrasound to image rotator cuff tears has encountered variable success.[95–97] A number of contributing factors have been identified to explain the wide range of reported accuracy for diagnosing rotator cuff tears with ultrasound (60–95%). The technical difficulty of the exam, the considerable experience required, the complex anatomy of the shoulder, and the occurrence of prominent beam propagation artifacts in the shoulder all combine to make sonographic evaluation of rotator cuff injuries a challenge.[98] Because of these difficulties, routine use of ultrasound to evaluate the shoulder for a suspected rotator cuff injury is uncommon. MRI provides excellent image quality without operator dependence and has become the diagnostic imaging technique most commonly used for these injuries. In general, sonography of the rotator cuff has little utility for the emergency evaluation of a shoulder injury since the clinical examination and radiography will usually adequately guide the direction of clinical care. Similarly, ultrasound is generally considered unsuitable for evaluation of meniscal or other ligamentous injuries of the knee, and MRI has become the imaging technique of choice for these injuries as well.

Complete disruptions of the biceps, triceps, quadriceps, or Achilles tendons are usually reliably diagnosed clinically and imaging is usually not required. However, ultrasound can be used to rapidly demonstrate the specific site of a tendon disruption at the bedside. Partial tendon tears present more of a diagnostic challenge. These may be difficult to diagnose on clinical grounds alone, and may therefore be misdiagnosed altogether. It is in this clinical scenario that ultrasound can help clarify the nature and extent of the suspected tendon injury. The Achilles, quadriceps, patellar, and triceps tendons all lend themselves to a point-of-care sonographic evaluation when a partial tendon tear is being considered. Each of these tendons is located in the superficial soft tissues and can therefore be examined in detail with a high-frequency transducer. The ability to both visualize the substance of the tendon and perform dynamic assessment of its function and integrity in real time can offer important diagnostic information that may not be appreciated on physical examination.

Evaluation of Suspected Tenosynovitis and Selected Tendinopathies

Ultrasound is felt to be at least as good as MRI for imaging selected tendon abnormalities.[99] In addition, ultrasound is very accurate for the diagnosis of tenosynovitis because its characteristic sonographic signature (hypoechoic fluid surrounding the tendon or tendons) is easy to recognize. In a patient with a swollen and painful hand or foot, the ability to rapidly and confidently make a diagnosis of tenosynovitis improves patient care and assists with the implementation of appropriate therapy. Similarly, selected tendinopathies can be diagnosed with a sonographic evaluation that reveals a characteristic focal area of hypoechogenicity of the tendon. Thickening of the plantar fascia insertion (more than 5 mm) on ultrasound is suggestive of plantar fasciopathy.[100]

Ultrasound is a useful diagnostic tool for screening soft tissue masses of the hand or forearm, allowing for characterization of a cystic versus solid mass, an accurate estimate of the lesion's volume, and precise 3D localization.[94] A ganglion cyst can be quickly diagnosed with the visualization of an anechoic saclike structure with a thin pedicle connecting it to a joint space or a tendon sheath. Use of ultrasound for the assessment of a host of painful arthritic joint conditions is discussed in more detail in the section on ultrasound-guided arthrocentesis (Chapter 22, "Additional Ultrasound-Guided Procedures").

Precise Needle Guidance for Aspiration and Soft Tissue Injection Procedures Involving Tendons and Bursae

Ultrasound guidance may be used for precise percutaneous injections of painful conditions of the musculotendinous system, specifically for injections of tendon sheaths, joints and bursae, and for fascial injections for the treatment of tendinitis, bursitis, arthritis, and fasciitis.[101] Inadvertent administration of corticosteroids within the substance of a tendon has long been known to put the patient at risk of tendon rupture. Real-time ultrasound imaging allows for continuous observation of both needle placement and medication delivery and is therefore ideally suited for precise deposition of the corticosteroids and local anesthesia that are used for treating these conditions. A specific example is the improved management of patients with subacromial bursitis. In a study investigating the treatment effectiveness of ultrasound-guided injections, a group of 40 pa-

tients with sonographically confirmed subacromial bursitis were given either standard blind injection or an ultrasound-guided injection.[102] The outcome measure was shoulder abduction range of motion preinjection compared with 1-week postinjection. No statistical differences were noted in shoulder range of motion at 1 week in the blind injection group, whereas a statistically significant difference was reported in the group that received the ultrasound-guided injections. The study concluded that ultrasound could be used to guide the injection needle accurately into the inflamed synovial bursa with significant therapeutic benefits. Ultrasound-guided injections may not be as useful for rotator cuff disease. In a randomized double blind study of 106 patients comparing ultrasound guided versus systemic steroid injection for rotator cuff disease, no significant difference in short-term outcome was detected.[103]

The sonoanatomy of trigger fingers has been described in detail by several investigators.[104, 105] Thickening and hypervascularization of the A1 pulley as well as distal flexor tendinosis ("dark tendon sign")[104] and tenosynovitis were found to be the sonographic hallmarks of this condition.[105] An ultrasound-guided A1 pulley steroid injection technique has been reported in a series of 24 patients and 50 trigger fingers. The technique described was found to be highly effective with a 90% success rate at 1 year for complete resolution of symptoms compared to the 57% success rate at 1 year reported for a blind injection technique.[106] In a cadaver model, the performance characteristics of peroneal tendon sheath injection were significantly improved when ultrasound was used for the procedure instead of a blind palpation technique (100% ultrasound vs. 60% with palpation).[107] Ultrasound-guided steroid injection has also been effectively used for the treatment of tenosynovitis of the first dorsal compartment of the wrist (DeQuervain's disease). In this report on a series of 17 patients with DeQuervain's disease, ultrasound guidance facilitated correct needle placement, thereby avoiding intratendinous injection as well as local complications such as fat atrophy and skin depigmentation.[108]

ANATOMICAL CONSIDERATIONS

Nearly all of the tendinous structures that are likely to be evaluated in an ED setting are superficial in location. Tendons consist of parallel fascicles of collagen fibers and may form a single homogenous bundle or they may be composed of multiple bundles or laminae in which case they are referred to as complex tendons. A thin layer of connective tissue, the peritenon, surrounds all tendons. A peritendinous synovial sheath usually surrounds tendons that take a more curvilinear course. This sheath contains a thin film of synovial fluid that helps reduce tendon friction and abrasions. Peritendinous bursae may additionally reduce friction between a tendon and adjacent bones during movements. Tendons are sparsely vascularized and receive their nourishment primarily from segmental vessels arising from the surrounding peritenon or through vincula.[109]

TECHNIQUE AND NORMAL ULTRASOUND FINDINGS

In general, perform musculotendinous ultrasound with high-frequency linear array or small parts transducers in the 7.5–15.0 MHz range. Sector transducers are generally not recommended for this application because the diverging beam of sector transducers can create undesirable beam scattering artifacts that leave only a small central portion of the image unaffected.[98] This draw-

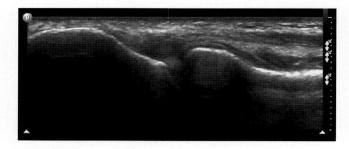

Figure 18-66. Sonogram of the lateral epicondyle of the elbow. The bony outline of the lateral epicondyle is seen on the left side of the image, then the joint line, followed by the bony contour of the radial head. The common extensor tendon, located just beneath the skin and scant subcutaneous tissue in this patient, appears variably echoic due to anisotropy; it is hyperechoic at the joint line, and hypoechoic at the right side of the image. The radial collateral ligament lies deep to the common extensor tendon, connects the lateral epicondyle to the radial head, and appears hyperechoic on the right side of this image.

back can be somewhat compensated for by narrowing the sector angle and using a standoff pad. When imaging very superficial structures, such as the Achilles tendon, patellar ligament, or structures within the finger, the use of an acoustic standoff pad may be helpful. Pay attention to proper frequency, focus, and depth settings to obtain optimal images. A split screen setup may be useful for comparing corresponding images from each side of the body.

The *epidermis and dermis* typically appear as a thin, slightly hyperechoic layer adjacent to the transducer or standoff pad. Subcutaneous tissue appears hypoechoic, is of variable thickness depending on body location and habitus, and has a fine reticular pattern of hyperechoic connective tissue between the fat lobules. Skeletal muscle is readily identified by its characteristic hypoechoic echotexture with echogenic internal striations that appear linear or pennate (feather-like) in long axis and speckled in short axis. Fascial planes are brightly echogenic and follow the surface contour of the muscle. Muscle fiber movement is often visible with muscle contraction in real time. In long axis, tendons appear as hyperechoic rectangular or linear structures that generally track on a parallel course with the long axis of the underlying bone. The tightly packed parallel echoes emanating from the collagen fibrils within the substance of the tendon give rise to a tendon's characteristic fibrillar echotexture. In short axis, tendons can appear round, ovoid, rectangular, or flat, depending on location, and will usually appear as a cluster of multiple small echogenic dots. A subtle anechoic rim will be seen in tendons that have an associated tendon sheath. Normal tendons are seen in Figures 18-65 to 18-69. A normal A1 flexor tendon pulley is demonstrated in Figure 18-70.

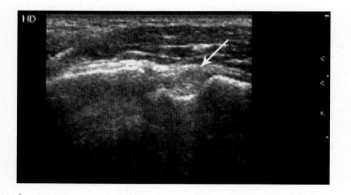

A

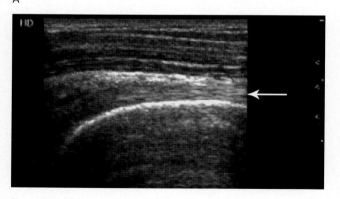

B

Figure 18-65. Short-axis sonogram of the biceps tendon (A). Skin and deltoid muscle appear in the near field. The anterior humeral head is seen in cross section as an echogenic line with a U-shaped depression known as the bicipital groove. The moderately echogenic biceps tendon (arrow) is located within the bicipital groove. Long-axis sonogram of the biceps tendon (B). Successive layers seen in this image are skin, hypoechoic deltoid muscle scanned along the long axis of its muscle fibers, the hyperechoic and fibrillar appearing biceps tendon (arrow), and the brightly echogenic surface of the anterior humerus.

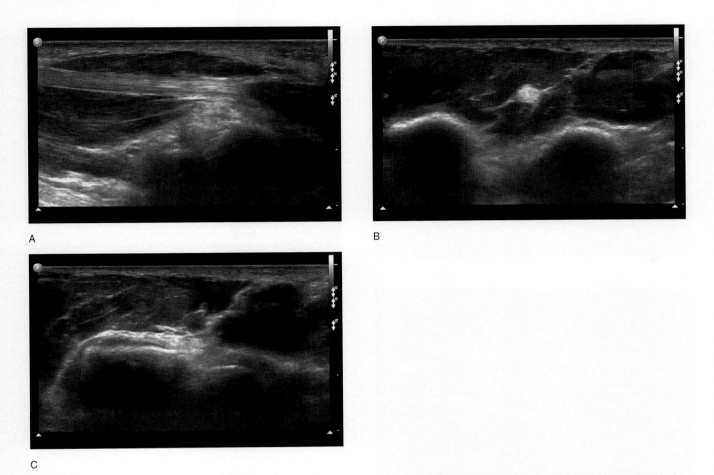

Figure 18-67. Sonograms of the flexor pollicis longus (FPL) tendon in the thenar eminence of the hand. In long axis (A), the somewhat hyperechoic skin and hypoechoic thenar muscles appear in the near field. Immediately beneath lies the FPL tendon, notable for its moderately echogenic and fibrillar appearance. The hyper and hypoechogenic portions of the tendon are due to anisotropy. Tendon motion within the tendon sheath can be observed with real-time imaging. In the first short-axis image (B), the tendon appears as a hyperechogenic circle when the insonating beam is perfectly perpendicular to the tendon fibers. The hypoechoic thenar muscles surround the tendon and the curved echogenic surface of the first and second metacarpal bones and their acoustic shadows are seen in the far field of the image. With a very small shift of the transducer away from a perpendicular plane, the FPL tendon becomes dark and is nearly isoechoic with the surrounding thenar muscles (C). Use of a fanning or heel toe technique is essential when performing tendon imaging.

Tendons exhibit an optical phenomenon known as *anisotropy* (i.e., the image obtained from the tendon is extremely dependent on the angle of the ultrasound beam) and a thorough understanding of this concept is essential for anyone engaged in musculotendinous imaging. A tendon will appear hyperechoic only when the insonating beam is precisely perpendicular to the tendon fibers. At all other angles, there is a significant reduction in the percentage of the ultrasound beam that is reflected back to the transducer and the tendon will therefore appear hypoechoic. Anisotropy is important because if a tendon is not properly imaged its internal structure cannot be adequately assessed.[109] It should be noted that most significant tendon pathology manifests itself sonographically as a hypoechogenic defect. If in-

adequate attention is paid to the imaging technique, a focal area of false hypoechogenicity may be interpreted as representing evidence of tendinosis or tendon rupture when in fact the hypoechogenicity is simply due to the insonating beam not being perfectly parallel with the tendon fibers at that region. A heel–toe imaging technique in long axis helps avoid this pitfall; the transducer is gently rocked in its long-axis plane from one end to the other while scanning the long axis over a tendon. In short axis, a dynamic fanning technique will achieve the same result. A focal area of hypoechogenicity that disappears with this technique is due to anisotropy; a defect that persists throughout changes in the angle of insonation likely represents true tendon pathology. Anisotropy is present in both long- and short-axis

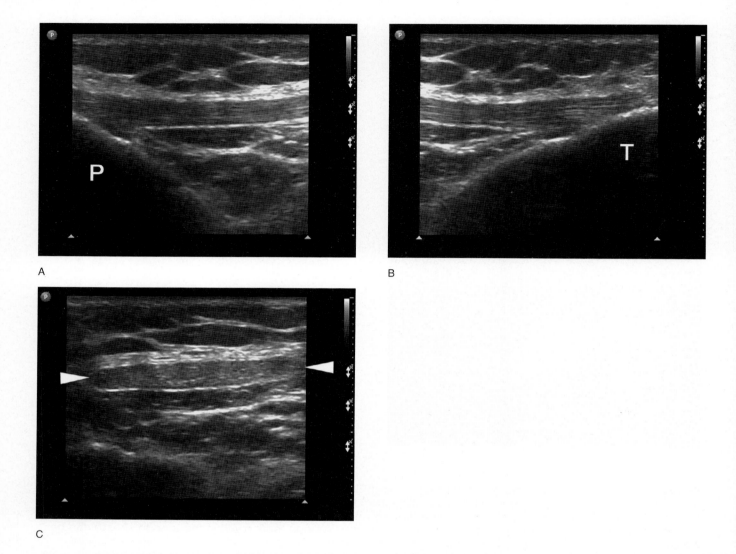

Figure 18-68. Sonogram of the patellar ligament. Long-axis view of the proximal aspect (A). The echogenic curved surface of the patella is seen on the left of the image with a sharply demarcated posterior acoustic shadow. The proximal portion of the patellar ligament is seen as a 3–4 mm thick, horizontal, fibrillar appearing band coming off the inferior pole of the patella. Hoffa's fat pad lies beneath the ligament. Long-axis view of the distal portion of the patellar ligament (B). The fibrillar ligament is now seen inserting on the tibial tuberosity to the right near field of the image. A small portion of Hoffa's fat pad is seen beneath the ligament on the left. An extended-field-of-view feature or a longer linear array transducer would allow the entire ligament to be demonstrated on one image. Short-axis view of the proximal patellar ligament (C). The ligament (arrowheads) is seen to be thick and generally rectangular in configuration with slightly curved edges. It sits immediately beneath the skin and subcutaneous tissue, extends almost the entire width of the image, and appears hyperechoic and speckled relative to the hypoechoic subcutaneous tissue above and fat pad below. P = patella, T = tibia.

planes, although it is more apparent when scanning the tendon in the long axis.

SPECIFIC IMAGING SCENARIOS

The biceps tendon is most easily found by scanning the upper arm in short axis just above the level of the axillary crease with the arm slightly externally rotated. The normal biceps tendon will be seen as a hyperechoic circular structure resting within the echogenic bicipital

groove of the proximal humerus. Once located in short axis, a long-axis view can easily be obtained by simply rotating the transducer.

The triceps tendon is best imaged from behind the patient with the transducer oriented in a midline long-axis orientation just above the olecranon process. This view is similar to that used when evaluating the elbow joint for an effusion. The triceps tendon will be seen in the near field as a moderately echogenic fibrillar structure that inserts on the echogenic olecranon process. The hypoechoic posterior fat pad and the echogenic

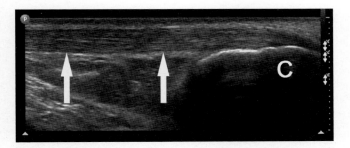

Figure 18-69. Long-axis sonogram of the Achilles tendon. The tendon is seen immediately beneath the skin, appears about 4 mm in thickness, and has a fibrillar appearance in this long-axis view (above arrows). A fat pad and posterior compartment muscles lie beneath the tendon. The tendon insertion on the echogenic posterior surface of the calcaneus is seen on the right side of this image. C = calcaneus.

outline of the posterior humerus, olecranon fossa, and olecranon will be seen in the far field of the image.

The lateral and medial epicondyles of the elbow are best imaged in long axis across the joint line with the arm and elbow in full extension, and the hand in either a "thumbs up" position for lateral epicondyle imaging or in a hypersupinated position for medial epicondyle imaging. The bony outlines of the respective epicondyles and either the radial head (lateral) or coronoid process (medial) will be noted on the sonogram. The radial and ulnar collateral ligaments are thin structures found adjacent to and crossing the joint line. The common extensor or flexor tendons will be seen lying superior to the collateral ligaments and their point of origin lies several centimeters above the joint line on their respective epicondyles.

Hand and foot tendons are quickly assessed for tenosynovitis by placing the transducer in the region

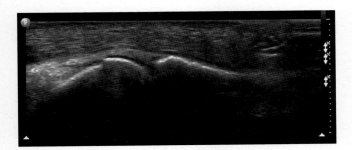

Figure 18-70. Volar MCP joint of a ring finger. The bony contour to the left represents the distal metacarpal. A thin layer of hypoechoic hyaline cartilage is seen at the joint surface and the volar surface of the proximal phalanx is seen to the right. The hyperechoic volar plate connects the proximal phalanx to the metacarpal. Immediately above lie the combined flexor tendons within a tendon sheath. The hypoechoic flattened A1 pulley is seen in the near field just above the flexor tendons at the level of the metacarpal head.

of clinical interest in a short-axis orientation relative to the direction of the tendon. Individual tendons are best examined in long axis when evaluating for tendon disruption.

Scan the patellar ligament in longitudinal and transverse planes with the knee held in 30° of flexion to avoid the "false hypoechogenicity" artifact that can occur in this location. This phenomenon is due to tendon anisotropy in the region adjacent to the patella. The contralateral knee should always be scanned for comparison.[98]

The Achilles tendon is best evaluated with the patient prone with the foot hanging over the edge of the examining table. Use of a standoff pad can be helpful, and the foot should be plantarflexed and dorsiflexed to observe dynamic tendon movement.

Soft Tissue Injection Techniques

Ultrasound imaging can provide real-time guidance for therapeutic injection of corticosteroids. A freehand technique is most commonly used for injection of tendon sheaths, joints, and bursae. The guiding principle is that the medication delivery needle should be oriented as perpendicular to the insonating beam as possible so that the needle will appear maximally reflective. The needle's position will be apparent by its strong reverberation or ring-down artifact. Needle tip localization can be further enhanced by (1) placing the needle bevel face up or face down and (2) injecting a small amount of anesthetic solution (the "hydrolocation" technique). The echogenic needle tip will be more clearly visualized within the hypoechoic anesthetic fluid pocket where it can then be redirected as needed. When a soft tissue injection procedure is undertaken, orient the tendons so that they display maximal anisotropy for best visualization. A short-axis orientation over the tendon and a long-axis orientation over the injection needle are recommended for avoiding intratendinous injections.[101]

COMMON AND EMERGENT ABNORMALITIES

General Ultrasound Findings

Partial tendon tears will appear as hypoechoic to anechoic regions within the substance of the tendon. Complete tendon tears will demonstrate obvious tendon discontinuity during real-time scanning; the tendon sheath may additionally contain a hypoechoic hematoma at the site of disruption. Synovial fluid will typically appear anechoic in an acute inflammatory process. The hallmark of tenosynovitis is an anechoic collection of inflammatory fluid seen surrounding the affected tendon. Additional sonographic features of tenosynovitis include tendon thickening, tendon sheath widening, and loss of the tendon's normal fibrillar echotexture. Tendonitis or tendinosis usually manifests as areas of patchy hypoechogenicity with loss of fibrillar echotexture within the affected portion of the tendon. Tendons without a sheath will appear thickened with altered echogenicity that varies according to the duration of the process.

Tenosynovitis

DeQuervain's disease is an overuse injury involving the two tendons in the first dorsal compartment of the hand (specifically, the abductor pollicis longus and extensor pollicis brevis tendons). Although a positive Finkelstein's test usually confirms the diagnosis, the tendon can be rapidly imaged in short axis to confirm the diagnosis in ambiguous cases. Fluid around the tendons, tendon thickening, and pain on "sonographic palpation" over the first dorsal compartment are typical (Figure 18-71). Bicipital tendonitis typically occurs as the result of overuse and repetitive stress on the tendon of the long head of the biceps. Sonographically, a hypoechoic fluid collection will be seen surrounding the biceps tendon and tenderness will be noted along the course of the tendon (Figure 18-72). Septic or reactive tenosynovitis may be encountered in the hands or feet, most commonly in injection drug users. The affected tendons in both entities typically appear thickened and hyperechoic with variable amounts of surrounding inflammatory synovial fluid (Figure 18-73).

Tendinopathies

Ultrasound can play a useful role in the evaluation of the athlete with chronic localized knee pain suggestive of tendinopathy of the proximal patellar ligament

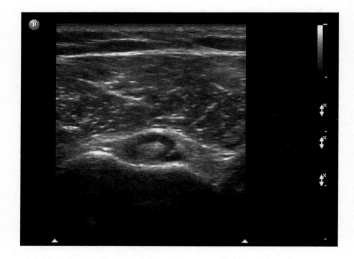

Figure 18-72. Short-axis sonogram of the biceps tendon at the bicipital groove. Beneath skin, hypoechoic subcutaneous tissue, and the speckled appearing deltoid muscle, the hyperechoic tendon of the long head of the biceps is seen surrounded by a hypoechoic fluid collection. The patient had palpable tenderness along the course of the tendon confirming the diagnosis of bicipital tendonitis.

("jumper's knee" or patellar tendinopathy). In a review of 25 surgically proven cases of "jumper's knee," ultrasound correctly identified the lesion in all patients. The authors advocated the use of ultrasound as "the method of choice for the evaluation of jumper's knee, as it is inexpensive, noninvasive, repeatable, and accurate."[110,111] Sonographically, the lesion appears as a localized area of hypoechogenicity in the central portion of the patellar ligament near its insertion on the patella. Patients with this condition will usually have exquisite tenderness to palpation at this site (Figure 18-74).

Partial and Complete Tendon Tears

The final common pathway for each of these lesions is excessive stress placed on the actively contracting muscle in question. Partial rupture of the proximal patellar ligament is apparent sonographically as a characteristic cone-shaped hypoechoic lesion, exceeding 0.5 cm in length, and found close to the origin of the patellar tendon at the inferior border of the patella. This hypoechoic lesion represents a focal discontinuity of the ligament in that anatomic area and an associated hematoma. An underlying tendonitis is often associated with this injury and is identified by thickening of the tendon and overall hypoechogenicity in the area of inflammation. A complete tear of the patellar ligament is usually clinically obvious. The disruption usually occurs at the point of attachment at the inferior edge of the patella. The discontinuity between the patellar ligament and the patella

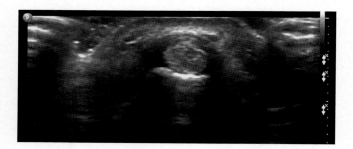

Figure 18-71. Short-axis sonogram of a patient with tenosynovitis of the first dorsal compartment of the hand (DeQuervain's tenosynovitis). The combined abductor pollicis longus and extensor pollicis brevis tendons appear hyperechoic and thickened, and fluid is seen surrounding the tendon. There is no skin contact with the transducer on either side of the image because the footprint of the transducer exceeds the relatively narrow curved surface of the radial wrist. Tenderness was present on "sonographic palpation."

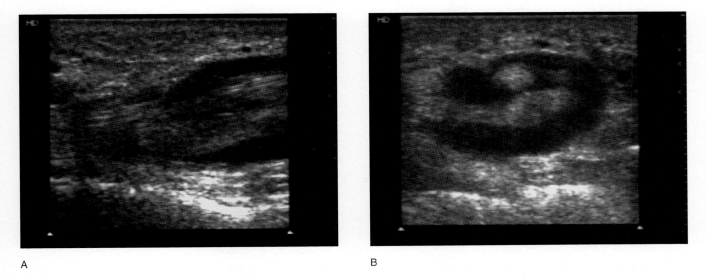

Figure 18-73. Long-axis sonogram of the thenar region in an injection drug user with a palmar tenosynovitis (A). The fibrillar flexor tendons of the hand are seen surrounded by a large amount of hypoechoic fluid. Short-axis sonogram of the same case in (B). Multiple flexor tendons are seen in cross section and a large amount of surrounding hypoechoic inflammatory fluid is noted.

will be apparent on ultrasound. An associated avulsion fracture fragment originating from the inferior pole of the patella may be seen attached to the proximal end of the ligament (Figure 18-75).

A partial tear of the triceps tendon will appear as a focal area of hypoechogenicity seen along the anterior insertion of the triceps tendon on the olecranon pro-

cess. The hypoechoic defect represents both torn tendon and an associated hematoma (Figure 18-76). Similarly, a partial tear of the Achilles tendon will appear as an obvious hypoechoic region of tendon discontinuity and hematoma. Dynamic imaging can help further clarify the extent and location of the tendon disruption (Figure 18-77).

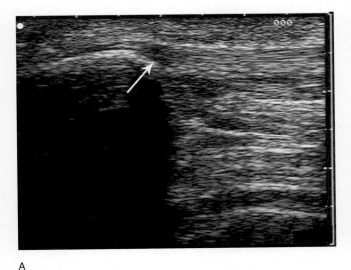

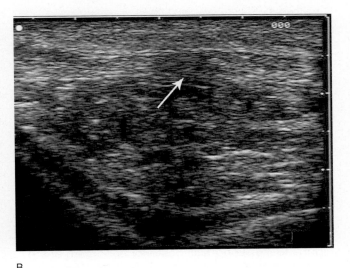

Figure 18-74. Long-axis sonogram of the proximal patellar ligament showing a hypoechoic tendon defect near the origin of the patellar tendon (A). The remainder of the tendon appears fibrillar and echogenic. A heel–toe insonating technique confirmed that a hypoechoic defect was present and that a tendinopathy ("jumper's knee") was present. Short-axis sonogram of the same patellar ligament (B). The ligament is seen as a somewhat echogenic horizontal structure about 5 mm beneath the skin surface and about 4 mm in width. In the central portion of the tendon, there is a focal area of hypoechogenicity that persists with careful imaging. This is the classic location and appearance of a "jumper's knee" or tendinopathy of the proximal patellar tendon.

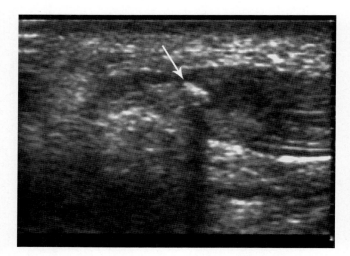

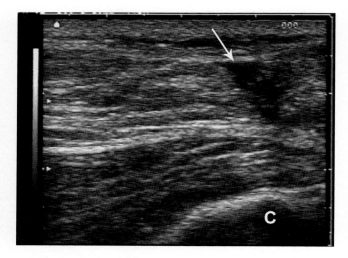

Figure 18-75. Long-axis sonogram of a patellar ligament rupture. The ligament is retracted and thickened with a hyperechoic avulsion fracture fragment attached to its proximal end (arrow). A high riding patella sits out of the field to the left of the image. The ligament has completely torn from its attachment at the lower pole of the patella.

Bursopathies

The Achilles tendon is surrounded anteriorly and posteriorly by two bursae near its point of insertion on the calcaneus. The superficial calcaneal bursa lies in the subcutaneous tissue posterior to the Achilles tendon,

Figure 18-77. Long-axis posterior sonogram of an "ankle sprain." The lower end of the Achilles tendon is seen in the near field about 5 mm beneath the skin. A large hypoechoic defect in the substance of the tendon is apparent (arrow), and on dynamic scanning the hypoechoic gap could be seen to widen. On short-axis views, some of the tendon was noted to still be intact. The hyperechoic curve of the posterior surface of the calcaneus (C) is seen in the right far field of the image.

and the retrocalcaneal bursa is found between the distal Achilles tendon and the calcaneus. These bursae are not typically seen on ultrasound in normal subjects, but can be visualized sonographically when they are inflamed (Figure 18-78).[112] Injection of the retrocalcaneal bursa is sometimes performed to relieve the pain of a chronic Achilles tendon bursitis. Scan the prone patient with the tendon and bursa in a transverse plane using a 7.5 or higher MHz transducer. Needle placement and steroid injection into the bursa are best accomplished with a lateral approach using an in-plane technique.

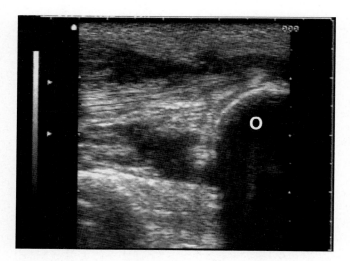

Figure 18-76. Long-axis posterior sonogram of the elbow in a patient with painful ROM after a fall on an outstretched arm. Plain radiographs were normal. The insertion of the triceps tendon onto the olecranon (O) reveals a large hypoechoic defect in the substance of the triceps tendon. Hypoechoic hematoma is seen extending around the tendon posteriorly. The hyperechoic posterior fat pad is seen in its normal position below the partial tendon tear; no joint effusion was detectable in the posterior recess.

COMMON VARIANTS AND SELECTED ABNORMALITIES

Ganglion Cysts

Assess a patient with a palpable mass in the hand, wrist, or digit with ultrasound to determine if a ganglion cyst is present. Ganglion cysts reportedly represent 50–75% of all soft tissue masses of the hand. They commonly appear as a sonolucent cystic or ovoid structure adjacent to a tendon sheath or the wrist joint. Typically, an anechoic linear duct will be seen extending from the ganglion cyst to the tendon sheath or joint giving the structure a "tadpole" appearance (Figure 18-79).[113]

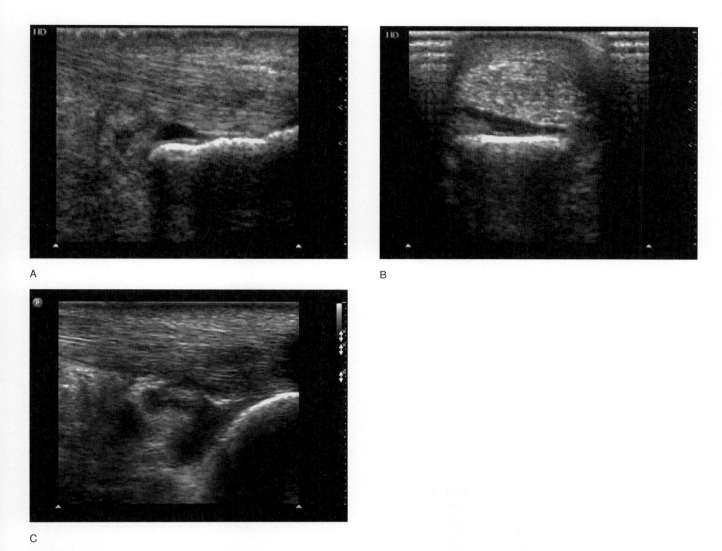

A

B

C

Figure 18-78. Long- and short-axis sonograms of the posterior heel in a patient with chronic heel pain (A and B). The Achilles tendon is seen in the near field as a thick fibrillar structure in long axis (A) or speckled in short axis (B) just beneath the skin surface. The echogenic line beneath the tendon represents the posterior surface of the calcaneus and the site of the Achilles tendon insertion. Between the Achilles tendon and the upper border of the calcaneus lies a hypoechoic saclike structure that represents the retrocalcaneal bursa. The bursal sac extends somewhat above and around the superior edge of the calcaneus and contains some echogenic debris within it, likely thickened synovium. In a second patient, the long-axis sonogram (C) shows a very thickened, enlarged, hypoechoic retrocalcaneal bursa with synovial thickening extending around the superior edge of the calcaneus. Light transducer pressure is advised to avoid collapsing the bursa while scanning. The short-axis view should be used when an intrabursal steroid injection is planned. The injection needle should be inserted from the lateral aspect of the ankle and the needle directed into the bursal sac under real-time guidance. The injection needle will appear maximally reflective in this orientation since it will be nearly perpendicular to the insonating beam.

Ultrasound-Guided Steroid Injections

The techniques employed for ultrasound-guided soft tissue injection therapy have been reviewed earlier. Injection of a common tendinopathy, lateral epicondylitis, is demonstrated in Figure 18-80. Medial or lateral epicondylitis is thought to occur as a result of chronic repetitive stress and microtrauma of the common flexor or common extensor tendons, respectively.[114,115] Sonographically, there may be some swelling of the extensor or flexor tendon near its origin on the epicondyle. With lateral epicondylitis, there is a reported predilection for deep tendon fiber injury. Intratendinous hyperemia may additionally be noted with color flow assessment.

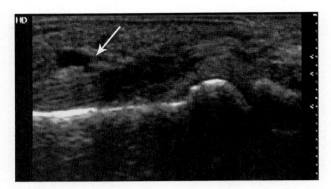

Figure 18-79. Long-axis sonogram of a volar index finger in a patient with atraumatic finger pain. The bony outline of the proximal phalanx and the PIP joint are apparent. The flexor tendons exhibit a finely fibrillar echotexture with a focal region of hypoechogenicity that persisted even when a heel–toe imaging technique was used to exclude anisotropy as the cause. A small hypoechoic ganglion cyst (arrow) is seen adjacent to this focal area of tendonitis and appears as a hypoechoic sac with a thin neck connecting it to the synovial sheath.

Ultrasound may also play a useful role in the management of patients with subacromial bursitis. On a subacromial scanning window (patient seated, arm behind the back with the elbow flexed), subacromial bursitis will appear as a hypoechoic fluid collection between the deltoid muscle and the supraspinatus tendon.

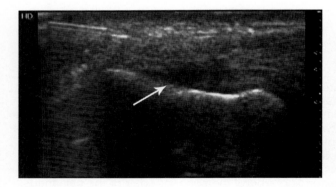

Figure 18-80. Long-axis sonogram over the lateral epicondyle in a patient with a clinical diagnosis of lateral epicondylitis. An ultrasound-guided steroid injection was performed at the site of maximal tenderness, several centimeters above the joint line (the joint line appears on the far right of the image, adjacent to the curve of the distal lateral epicondyle). The injection needle (located on upper left corner of image) is passed as perpendicular to the insonating beam as possible for maximal reflectivity and is readily identified by its reverberation artifact. The optimal injection site is immediately *above* the common extensor tendon; this avoids intratendinous administration of steroids that could lead to tendon rupture. The deeper fibers adjacent to the bony epicondyle (arrow) revealed a focal area of hypoechogenicity that is typical for lateral epicondylitis.

Other Musculotendinous Sonographic Findings

With biceps femoris, rectus femoris, or gastrocnemius muscle tears, a "clapper in the bell" sign may be seen on the sonogram where the retracted, ruptured upper portion of the muscle (the clapper) is surrounded by a hypoechoic hematoma (the bell). Obvious disruption of muscle fiber insertion on the adjacent aponeurosis may also be apparent in some of these injuries (Figure 18-81). A muscle tear due to penetrating trauma will appear as a focal region of discontinuity in the muscle. Dynamic imaging will widen the gap between the two ends of the now discontinuous muscle bundle, and a hypoechoic defect representing fresh blood or a hematoma will typically be noted at the site of the injury (Figure 18-82). Gouty tophi will demonstrate posterior acoustic shadowing, much like gallstones. Inflamed bursae will appear as superficial hypoechoic fluid collections. Limit transducer pressure on smaller bursae to avoid causing them to collapse. The diagnosis may be missed if the bursal fluid is displaced out of the field of view.

PITFALLS

The most important potentially misleading artifact in tendon sonography is the false hypoechogenicity that results from the slightest obliquity of the ultrasound beam in relation to the tendon fibers.[98] Since areas of

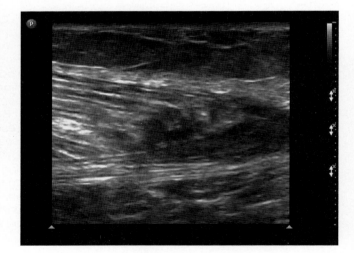

Figure 18-81. Long-axis sonogram of the distal medial gastrocnemius muscle in a patient presenting with acute calf pain after a misstep off a curb. Beneath the skin and hypoechoic subcutaneous tissue one can easily visualize the hyperechoic curved aponeurosis of the distal medial gastrocnemius muscle. The pennate distal muscle fibers have torn off their usual attachment site onto the aponeurosis; a hypoechoic hematoma is seen at the site of injury. This is the typical location for a gastrocnemius muscle tear.

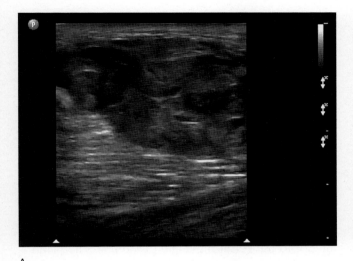

A

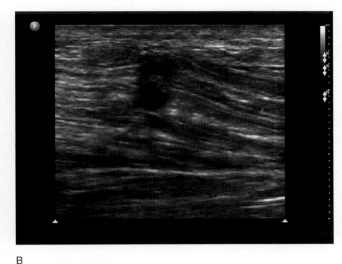

B

Figure 18-82. Penetrating trauma to the lateral calf with a large area of swelling. A large wound hematoma and disrupted muscle fibers were apparent on the sonogram (A). After local anesthesia, the area was squeezed, and a large clot was expressed. A repeat sonogram (B) demonstrates that the clot has been nearly entirely expressed; the region of superficial muscle fiber disruption is now clearly apparent.

hypoechogenicity provide the sonographic clues to tendon pathology (specifically, tendon disruption and tendonitis), optimal tendon imaging is paramount. The angle of insonation should ideally be as parallel to the course of the tendon fibers as possible to avoid this significant pitfall. Where areas of tendon hypoechogenicity are encountered, use a heel–toe scanning technique (or fanning of the transducer if imaging in short axis) to further clarify the true sonographic character of the area in question.

▶ SALIVARY GLANDS

CLINICAL CONSIDERATIONS AND INDICATIONS

When evaluating a patient with preauricular or submandibular swelling or tenderness, a point-of-care ultrasound examination of the area can rapidly determine if the source of the problem lies within the parotid or submandibular glands or if the swelling is unrelated to these structures. Although CT is the traditional imaging modality of choice for parotid and submandibular inflammatory conditions and MRI is considered the modality of choice for evaluation of parotid and submandibular tumors, ultrasound is now considered by many to be the initial imaging modality of choice for assessment of any palpable abnormalities in the region of the salivary glands.[116–118] Ultrasound can clarify if the lesion is intra- or extraglandular, provide information as to whether a focal process or diffuse glandular involvement is present, and help guide aspiration if an abscess is found in a case of acute bacterial sialadenitis.

It can also demonstrate if there is involvement of the surrounding lymph nodes.

Salivary gland disease can be broadly classified into four categories: acute sialadenitis (with viral and bacterial etiologies), chronic sialadenitis (with infective and noninfective etiologies), sialolithiasis, and tumors (benign and malignant).

Sialolithiasis is the most common salivary gland pathology encountered in the ED. Ultrasound is particularly useful in the evaluation of suspected sialolithiasis, where it has 96% diagnostic accuracy.[119] Salivary gland stones as small as 0.4 mm can be detected on ultrasound with 90% sensitivity.[117] Salivary gland calculi may occur in the parotid gland, but they will most commonly be found (80% of the time) in the submandibular gland, presumably because of the more mucinous content of submandibular gland secretions. Most of these calculi will be found in the submandibular duct; the remainder will be located within the gland or in the ductal hilum. Multiple stones are found in 25% of patients.[119] Most salivary gland tumors occur in the parotid gland. The vast majority (85–90%) of parotid tumors are benign pleomorphic adenomas. They are slow growing, painless masses, most commonly seen in middle-aged patients, and they are usually found in the superficial lobe of the parotid gland. By contrast, 50% of tumors discovered in the submandibular gland are malignant. Of note, neither CT nor MRI has been found to be superior to ultrasound in distinguishing benign from malignant tumors of the salivary glands.[117] In addition, ultrasound may be used to guide fine-needle aspiration of salivary gland tumors, and to guide intraglandular abscess drainage in advanced cases of bacterial sialadenitis. Finally, ultrasound-guided botulinum toxin injection into the salivary glands has recently been used as a therapy for patients with excessive salivation or drooling disorders.[117] Given the somewhat questionable reliability of the clinical examination[120] and the ready availability of point-of-care ultrasound equipment and high-frequency linear array transducers in most EDs, sonographic examination of the region of facial swelling or tenderness should be considered a routine part of the bedside workup of any patient with suspected salivary gland disease in the ED.

ANATOMICAL CONSIDERATIONS

The body of the parotid gland lies in a preauricular location, with its upper portion roughly in line with the external acoustic meatus and extending inferiorly and posteriorly to the angle of the jaw. The parotid duct (Stenson's duct) arises from the anterior border of the gland, lies superficial to the masseter muscle and about 1–2 cm below the zygomatic arch, courses horizontally at earlobe level through the buccal fat pad, and pierces the buccinator muscle to enter the mouth at the parotid papilla opposite the upper second molar. The normal duct is approximately 2–3 mm in diameter and 4–6 cm in length. On occasion, an accessory parotid gland may be seen lying anterior to and following the course of the parotid duct. The gland is broad and flattened superficially and wedge-shaped on its posterior and deep aspects. The bulk of the gland overlies the masseter and mandible. The facial nerve, the retromandibular vein, and the external carotid artery lie in a vertical orientation immediately deep to the gland. Small lymph nodes are commonly found within the substance of the parotid gland.

The submandibular glands are found beneath the superficial subcutaneous tissues of the submandibular triangle, lateral to the anterior belly of the digastric muscle. The much larger superficial lobe and the much smaller and more posterior deep lobe are C-shaped in long-axis profile and connect where they wrap around the posterolateral border of the mylohyoid muscle. Intraglandular ducts drain into the submandibular (or Wharton's) duct that emerges from the hilum of the submandibular gland. The submandibular duct passes medially, then up and over the posterolateral border of the mylohyoid muscle where it then courses medial to the sublingual glands to a papilla adjacent to the lingual frenulum in the anterior floor of the mouth. The submandibular duct is about 5 cm in length. Unlike the parotids, no intraglandular lymph nodes are found within the submandibular gland. The "Küttner" lymph node is reliably found in the space between the posterior border of the submandibular gland and the anterior border of the inferior aspect of the parotid gland.[119]

The sublingual glands are located below the mucous membranes of the floor of the mouth adjacent to the mandible and the genioglossus muscle. They drain via numerous small caliber ducts either directly into the floor of the mouth or into the submandibular duct.

TECHNIQUE AND NORMAL ULTRASOUND FINDINGS

Scan the parotid and submandibular glands with a 7.5–15 MHz linear array transducer. Scan the parotid gland in long axis in a vertical plane in front of the lower ear. Angle the superior portion of the transducer somewhat anteriorly to evaluate the portion of the gland that lies inferior to the ear at the angle of the jaw. The gland is predominantly superficial in location with some deeper portions of the gland hidden by the mandible. When evaluating the parotid duct in its long axis, use a transverse plane where transducer orientation is nearly horizontal from mid-earlobe level to the mid-cheek. The parotid duct appears as two closely spaced parallel echogenic lines with a thin region of lucency between them, and is found superficial to the masseter muscle. Because of the fatty glandular tissue composition of the gland, the normal parotid appears fairly homogeneous with a fine granular echotexture that appears similar to a fatty liver. Intraparotid ducts appear as echogenic linear structures within the substance of the gland. Intraparotid lymph nodes are common, especially in the preauricular region. Lymph nodes are typically elliptical in shape with a hypoechoic periphery and a hyperechoic fatty central hilum (Figures 18-83 to 18-85). When scanning the parotid in a long-axis orientation, the retromandibular vein and the external carotid artery will appear as two parallel hypoechoic channels beneath the gland; they are best appreciated with the use of color Doppler imaging. The facial nerve may be seen as a thin fibrillar structure overlying the more superficially located vein.

When scanning the submandibular gland, place the transducer in the submental region just medial to the mandible aiming toward the middle of the chin. Aim the orientation marker toward the operator's left. By doing so, the chin will appear on the right side of the image when scanning the right submandibular gland and on the left side of the image when scanning the left submandibular gland. The bulk of the gland is located inferior to the mylohyoid muscle and appears as a rounded and somewhat lobular structure with a homogeneous finely granular echotexture similar to but more distinct than the appearance of the more fatty parotid gland. The Küttner lymph node may be seen posterior and immediately adjacent to the submandibular gland in the space between the submandibular and the parotid glands (Figure 18-86). The mylohyoid muscle appears as a horizontally oriented and somewhat striated

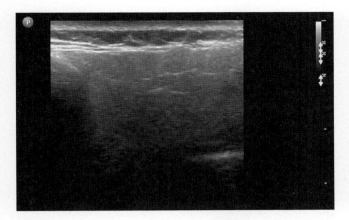

Figure 18-83. Long-axis sonogram of a normal parotid gland. The gland demonstrates a fine homogeneous mid-gray echotexture that appears similar to a fatty liver. Immediately beneath the gland lies the retromandibular vein, and beneath it the external carotid artery. Their locations are best appreciated with the use of color Doppler imaging and are not seen on this image.

appearing rectangular region of hypoechogenicity in the near field of the image, tapering as it approaches its insertion on the symphysis menti. The inferior aspect of the bony symphysis menti appears as a slightly curved region of hyperechogenicity in the near field with dense posterior acoustic shadowing below. The submandibular duct is somewhat narrower in caliber than the parotid duct, has a similar hyperechoic tubular appearance, and is best visualized when it is pathologically dilated. When scanning the submental region, remember that the patient's anatomy on the sonogram appears upside down;

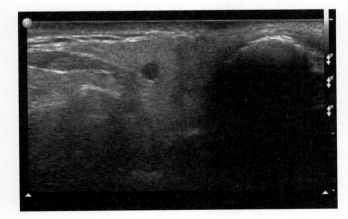

Figure 18-84. Short-axis sonogram of the left parotid. A small hypoechoic intraparotid lymph node is seen within the homogeneous, finely granular parotid tissue; this is a very common finding. The curved echo to the right of the image represents the mastoid process.

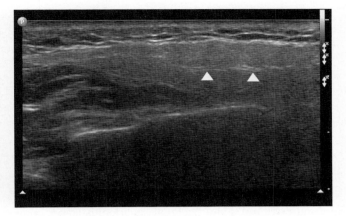

Figure 18-85. Transverse sonogram of a portion of the left parotid duct. The transducer is placed just in front of the ear in a horizontal orientation at the level of the mid-earlobe. The normal parotid duct (arrowheads) appears as two narrowly spaced echogenic lines; it courses anteriorly over the masseter before draining intraorally next to the maxillary second molar. A portion of the hypoechoic masseter muscle is seen in cross section beneath the gland. Deep to the masseter, the echogenic surface of a portion of the mandible is seen along with a dense posterior acoustic shadow.

the image obtained represents a somewhat oblique sagittal section of a patient standing on his or her head.

The sublingual glands are best visualized by scanning the anterior underside of the chin in a short-axis orientation. They appear as paired homogeneous

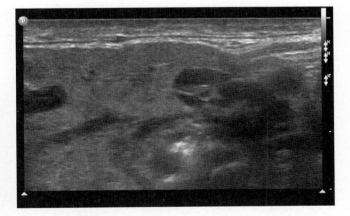

Figure 18-86. Long-axis sonogram of the left submandibular gland. Transducer marker points toward the symphysis menti. The gland is seen just beneath the skin and subcutaneous tissue and has a homogeneous mid-gray echotexture that appears somewhat more distinct than parotid tissue. The named Küttner lymph node is seen just to the right of the gland; a portion of the hypoechoic mylohyoid muscle is seen on the left. The submandibular gland is somewhat "C" shaped with a portion of the glandular tissue extending over and around the mylohyoid muscle.

triangular structures, just deep to the hypoechoic mylo-hyoid muscle, similar in echotexture to the submandibu-lar gland.

COMMON AND EMERGENT ABNORMALITIES

Sialadenitis

A variety of sonographic patterns may be encountered with parotid and submandibular gland disease. With acute viral sialadenitis (most commonly caused by mumps) and acute bacterial sialadenitis (most commonly caused by *Staphylococcus aureus* and *Streptococcus viridans*), the gland appears enlarged, hyperechoic compared to normal salivary glandular tissue, and has heterogeneous echotexture (Figures 18-87 and 18-88). With bacterial sialadenitis, air may be present within the intraglandular ducts and small hyperechoic foci with associated comet-tail artifacts may be seen. If an abscess has formed, it will usually appear hypoechoic or anechoic and demonstrate posterior acoustic enhancement similar to a subcutaneous abscess. Increased blood flow may be noted on color Doppler imaging with any acute inflammatory condition. Chronic sclerosing sialadenitis (also known as Küttner's tumor) occurs as a result of chronic infection and appears as a well-defined hypoechoic mass. The gland may appear normal to small in size and inhomogeneous in echotexture. In Sjögren's syndrome, a systemic autoimmune disorder that affects

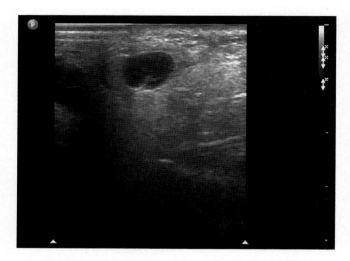

Figure 18-88. Transverse sonogram of a patient with viral sialadenitis. The right parotid gland appears enlarged and predominantly hyperechoic; an enlarged intraparotid lymph node is present.

exocrine glands, the salivary glands will exhibit varying degrees of parenchymal inhomogeneity, there will be reduced salivary gland volume, and hypoechoic foci of sialectasia will be present. Sonographic textural inhomogeneity scores are used as a tool to establish the diagnosis of Sjögren's syndrome.[117]

Masses

Most salivary gland tumors will be found in the parotid gland and most of these will be benign. Solid lesions will typically appear hypoechoic and demonstrate posterior acoustic enhancement. Cystic lesions will typically appear anechoic. A pleiomorphic adenoma is the most common benign solid parotid tumor, comprising 85–90% of parotid tumors. Sonographically, it appears rounded or lobular in shape, well circumscribed, and homogeneously hypoechoic with posterior acoustic enhancement. Fewer tumors are found in the submandibular glands, but the rate of malignancy there is much higher. While the tumor shape, boundary, and the posterior echoes are different when comparing benign and malignant salivary gland tumors, their internal echogenicity is similar.[121] Malignant neoplasms of the salivary gland are more likely to have irregular shapes, irregular borders, blurred margins, and a hypoechoic inhomogeneous structure, but they may be lacking these features and look similar to benign tumors.[122] The most common malignant solid tumor (mucoepidermoid carcinoma)[116] may initially appear sonographically similar to a pleiomorphic adenoma. Therefore, consider all solitary salivary gland masses to be neoplastic until proven otherwise and refer for definitive diagnosis. Prior trauma to the area and an occult salivary duct

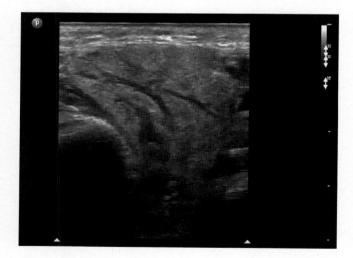

Figure 18-87. Transverse sonogram of a patient with bacterial sialadenitis. The left parotid gland appears enlarged, lobulated, and of heterogeneous echotexture. The parenchyma appears hyperechoic compared to the normal gland; hypoechoic areas correspond to regions of hypervascularity noted on Doppler imaging. Cloudy saliva was expressed from Stenson's duct.

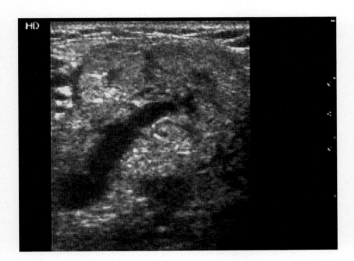

Figure 18-89. Left submandibular gland in a patient with calculus sialadenitis. The gland is enlarged and there are hypoechoic regions within the gland and hilum caused by ductal dilatation from the distal outflow obstruction caused by the stone. The salivary duct exits from the gland and courses up and over the posterolateral border of the mylohyoid muscle.

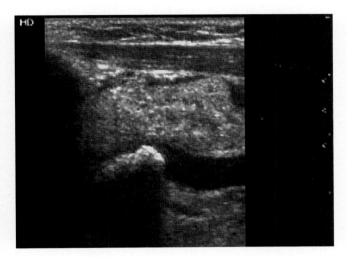

Figure 18-90. Long-axis sonogram of the distal left submandibular duct. The dilated submandibular duct is seen in long axis as an anechoic channel in the far field. A large echogenic salivary duct calculus is lodged in the distal duct; posterior acoustic shadowing is noted in the far field beneath the stone. The hypoechoic and striated mylohyoid muscle is seen just beneath the skin and subcutaneous tissue at the top of the image, and its insertion onto the mandible can be seen on the left side of the image. The inferior edge of the mandible appears as a curved echo with posterior acoustic shadowing on the far left of the image. For orientation purposes, it is important to remember that the top of the head is at the bottom of the image.

injury may give rise to a siaolocele, which will appear as a hypoechoic cystic mass.

Sialolithiasis

Salivary duct stones (or calculi) appear as hyperechoic foci with prominent posterior acoustic shadowing. Stones are usually found within the salivary duct of the submandibular gland and less frequently within the ductal hilum. Less commonly, calculi may be found within the parotid duct or gland. When complete obstruction occurs, the salivary duct becomes dilated and appears in long axis as a prominent anechoic tubular structure leading to the echogenic stone. The gland itself may appear enlarged with dilatation of the hilum giving the gland a somewhat "hydronephrotic" appearance (Figures 18-89 and 18-90).

Lymph Nodes

A preauricular mass or area of focal tenderness will sometimes be due to a reactive and enlarged lymph node. The lymph node has a characteristic elliptical shape with a hypoechoic periphery and an echogenic fatty central hilum (Figure 18-91).

PITFALLS

The major pitfall with ultrasound imaging of the salivary glands is failure to consider malignancy as the etiology for a solid lesion. The role of the point-of-care

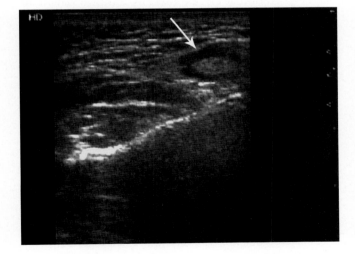

Figure 18-91. Longitudinal sonogram of an enlarged preauricular lymph node. A tender mass was clinically palpable in front of the ear; the sonogram demonstrates an enlarged intraparotid preauricular lymph node (elliptical in long axis with a hypoechoic periphery and a hyperechoic central hilum). The node is surrounded by a thin rim of granular mid-gray echogenicity that corresponds to normal parotid tissue.

ultrasound for potential salivary gland pathology is to determine if a focal lesion is present, establish whether it is intraglandular or not, and to determine if a salivary duct stone is the cause of the swelling or pain. With the exception of diffuse polyglandular enlargement (as seen with mumps), diffuse uniglandular enlargement and tenderness (as seen in acute sialadenitis), and a locally reactive lymph node, nearly all other salivary pathologies should be referred for further evaluation.

► MAXILLARY SINUSITIS

CLINICAL CONSIDERATIONS

Rhinosinusitis is one of the 10 most common diagnoses in ambulatory practice and the fifth most common diagnosis for which antibiotics are prescribed.[123] Accurately diagnosing bacterial sinusitis, for which antibiotics are recommended, is difficult with just the history and physical examination. At most, only 50% of patients presenting to acute care settings with sinus complaints have bacterial sinusitis.[124] Signs and symptoms of bacterial sinusitis are nonspecific and indistinguishable from the clinically similar presentation that occurs with viral rhinosinusitis. Although radiography improves diagnostic accuracy somewhat, neither plain radiography nor CT is recommended for evaluating uncomplicated sinusitis in ambulatory patients because of the additional time, cost, and radiation exposure associated with these tests.[125] Conversely, point-of-care ultrasound is a rapid and safe diagnostic tool that can be used by the provider to accurately identify a fluid-filled maxillary sinus.

Sinusitis is an important occult cause of fever and nosocomial pneumonia in patients undergoing prolonged mechanical ventilation.[126] In this setting, point-of-care sinus ultrasound is a well-established screening test for detecting maxillary sinusitis.

CLINICAL INDICATIONS

The primary indications for sinus ultrasound are

- Confirm or exclude clinically suspected maxillary sinusitis in patients with upper respiratory symptoms
- Detect maxillary sinus fluid in intubated ICU patients to screen for suspected nosocomial sinusitis

Maxillary Sinusitis

Although CT and MRI are sensitive imaging modalities for diagnosing sinusitis, the presence of sinus fluid or mucosal thickening alone does not necessarily indicate bacterial infection (low specificity and low positive predictive value). The true "gold standard" for diagnosing

bacterial sinusitis is a positive culture from fluid obtained on sinus puncture. Ultrasound, while less sensitive for mucosal changes and small amounts of fluid, is more specific for clinically important disease because a positive study requires the presence of a significant amount of fluid in the sinus. Studies evaluating the diagnostic characteristics of ultrasound for bacterial sinusitis vary substantially in terms of the population studied (general practice, subspecialty, or ICU), the criterion standard employed (sinus puncture, radiography, MRI), and methodological quality. A summary of studies conducted in the 1980s and 1990s in which sinus ultrasound was compared to sinus puncture found a weighted mean sensitivity and specificity for ultrasound of 85% and 82%, respectively. This compares favorably to the 87% sensitivity and 89% specificity found for plain radiography.[127] A systematic review of these early studies concluded that operator skill and experience had a large effect on how well ultrasound performed.[128]

Four studies have been conducted in ambulatory and emergency care settings comparing point-of-care ultrasound to radiography or MRI for diagnosing acute maxillary sinusitis. In one study, which used MRI as the gold standard, ultrasound was found to be 64% sensitive and 95% specific, compared to 73% sensitivity and 100% specificity for plain radiography.[129] The authors concluded that a positive ultrasound examination confirmed the diagnosis of maxillary sinusitis. If the ultrasound examination was negative and clinical suspicion was high, however, they recommended that plain radiographs be obtained. Another study found that ultrasound was 92% sensitive and 95% specific compared to plain radiography, and also noted that the addition of point-of-care sinus ultrasound to the history and physical examination would reduce antibiotic prescriptions for sinusitis by one half.[130] One study compared emergency physician-performed ultrasound to CT in 48 ED patients with suspected maxillary sinusitis.[131] It reported 86% agreement between the two techniques and noted that ultrasound was 81% sensitive and 89% specific compared to CT. Finally, in a prospective study of 67 pediatric patients (mean age 9 years 2 months +/− 3 years 9 months), 134 sinuses were imaged with both ultrasound and plain films.[132] There was 84% agreement between the two techniques, and compared to the plain films, ultrasound was found to be 95% sensitive and 98% specific.

Maxillary Sinus Fluid in Intubated Patients

In the ICU setting, point-of-care ultrasound has emerged as a convenient screening test for nosocomial sinusitis because plain radiographs are not accurate for visualizing sinus fluid in recumbent patients and CT is particularly time and labor intensive in intubated patients. Ultrasound can be used at the bedside to quickly and accurately assess for fluid in the maxillary sinuses. If fluid is present, rhinoscopy or sinus puncture is subsequently performed to obtain fluid for culture. The reported prevalence of true bacterial sinusitis varies widely among different studies, ranging from 5% to 60% of cases.[126,133,134] Among the three most robust studies of maxillary sinus ultrasound in the ICU setting, reported sensitivity ranged from 67–100% and specificity from 86–97%.[133,135,136] Specificity was 100% when all sinus walls were seen, which generally correlates with complete sinus opacification on radiography.

It is considered normal when the maxillary sinus ultrasound shows only an echo emanating from the front wall of the maxillary sinus; in such cases, the diagnosis of sinusitis can usually be eliminated. A complete sinusogram is defined as the sonographic visualization of all maxillary sinus walls (posterior, medial, and lateral), and this finding has a high specificity for the presence of sinusitis.

A diagnostic dilemma occurs in the case of a partial sinusogram when only the anterior and a portion of the posterior walls of the sinus are visualized. In such cases, a postural change test can be performed to help determine if an air-fluid level is present or if mucosal thickening is the cause of the partial sinusogram. An ICU study evaluated the test characteristics of a postural change test in patients in whom a partial sinusogram was found.[137] Maxillary sinus imaging was first performed with the patient in a "half-sitting" position. In patients with a partial sinusogram, a repeat sinusogram was subsequently performed with the patient supine. The test was considered positive for sinusitis if the partial sinusogram disappeared when the patient was supine (indicating the presence of fluid in the sinus). The test was considered negative if the partial sinusogram was visualized in both positions (indicating mucosal thickening). In the 300 sinuses scanned in this report, and using CT imaging as the criterion standard, results were reported as follows: (1) a complete sinusogram was found in 98 cases and all were radiologically confirmed to be sinusitis, (2) normal sinus ultrasound exams were found in 112 cases and CT confirmed the presence of a normal sinus in 95% of these patients, (3) a partial sinusogram was seen on ultrasound in 90 cases and CT confirmed the presence of sinusitis in 61%, and (4) the postural change test was performed in all patients who had a partial sinusogram, which increased the positive predictive value of sinus ultrasound from 61% to 91% in these patients. The same study also reported that proficiency in maxillary sinus imaging required performance of about 20 sinusograms.[137]

A-mode ultrasound has also been found to be useful for diagnosing maxillary sinusitis. In a series of 140 sinuses imaged in intubated ICU patients, A-mode sinus imaging was found to be 95% specific with a 92% negative predictive value.[138] In addition, all empty sinuses were correctly identified as being empty using this technique.

ANATOMICAL CONSIDERATIONS

The maxillary sinuses are paired and somewhat pyramid-shaped airspaces within the maxillary bone on either side of the nose. They are bordered by the orbital floor superiorly, the lateral nasal wall medially, the alveolar process and hard palate inferiorly, and the zygoma laterally. Mean maxillary sinus volume was noted to be $15.7 +/- 5.3$ cm^3 in an analysis of 120 maxillary sinuses measured on head CTs in one report.[139] The maxillary sinus is typically 2–4 cm in AP depth, and fluid within the sinus renders the posterior wall of the sinus visible by ultrasound. The ethmoid sinuses lie superomedially, and the sphenoid sinus lies in the midline deeper within the skull. The frontal sinuses, which would seem to be sonographically accessible, are usually not well visualized by ultrasound, likely because the anterior surface of the frontal bone is quite thick.

TECHNIQUE AND NORMAL ULTRASOUND FINDINGS

Maxillary sinus ultrasound may be performed with a wide array of transducers, ranging from a phased array or microconvex 3.5 MHz transducer (e.g., a typical cardiac transducer) to a 3–12 MHz linear array transducer. A small skin contact footprint is preferred, however, for scanning on the curved, relatively solid surface over the anterior maxilla. Although one might think that lower frequencies would be required to adequately penetrate the anterior bony wall of the sinus, this does not appear to be the case in practice, and a fluid-filled sinus can be visualized with either transducer type. The patient should sit upright or lean slightly forward to ensure that sinus fluid, if present, layers out against the anterior wall. Scan the sinus in both sagittal and transverse planes, midway between the nose and the zygoma, just below the orbital rim. When using a linear array transducer, the sagittal image is easier to obtain by angling the transducer slightly superomedially, parallel to the nasolabial fold. Pay attention to proper depth settings (typically 5–7 cm) so that the image of the sinus fills about 75% of the image. Adjust the transducer angle so that the anterior surface of the maxilla is represented as a horizontal line on the sonogram. Compare with the uninvolved sinus, especially in equivocal cases.

In the normal air-filled sinus, a prominent periodic resonance artifact will be apparent, consisting of an evenly spaced series of echogenic lines that parallel

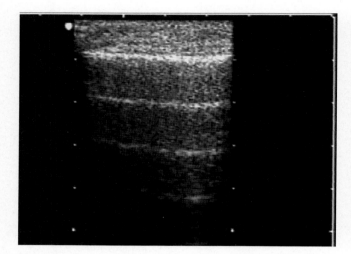

Figure 18-92. Sagittal sonogram of a normal sinus taken with a linear array transducer. Skin and subcutaneous tissue appear diffusely hyperechoic in the near field. A bright echo is seen at the level of the anterior surface of the maxillary sinus. The series of evenly spaced horizontal echoes that diminish in intensity at increasing depth represent a periodic resonance artifact emanating from the anterior wall of the sinus. A "snowstorm" pattern of echogenicity is normally seen within the nonopacified sinus.

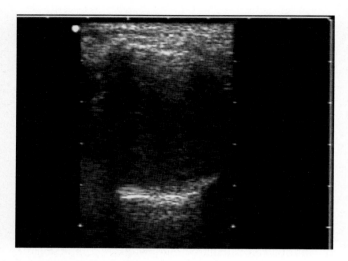

Figure 18-93. Sagittal sonogram of a patient with acute maxillary sinusitis. The brightly echogenic curve in the far field of the image represents the posterior wall of the sinus. The sinus cavity is hypoechoic and no periodic resonance artifacts are seen.

the shape of the anterior surface of the maxilla and diminish in intensity at increased depth. Beneath the distinct echo of the anterior wall of the sinus, an indistinct "snowstorm" appearance will be noted on the sonogram and the posterior wall of the sinus will *not* be apparent. It is essential not to confuse one of the deeper periodic resonance artifacts as representing the posterior wall of the sinus (Figure 18-92). These artifacts will always parallel the anterior surface of the maxilla, whereas the posterior wall of the sinus, when apparent, will always appear curved.

COMMON AND EMERGENT ABNORMALITIES

Acute viral rhinosinusitis produces abnormalities within the maxillary sinuses in up to 87% of cases, typically a thickening of the sinus mucosa along with some secretions. Occasionally, a significant amount of fluid will accumulate within the sinus and produce an air-fluid level on CT.[140] An ultrasound examination of the sinus at this point would appear positive for fluid and would represent a false-positive result for the diagnosis of bacterial maxillary sinusitis. Bacterial sinusitis is said to supervene in 1–2% of cases of viral rhinosinusitis[124] and typically occurs after 5–7 days of symptoms. It may be accompanied by mucopurulent nasal discharge and signs of maxillary inflammation (such as focal, often unilateral

sinus pain, and tenderness). As the inflammatory process evolves, pus accumulates in the sinus, giving rise to air–fluid levels or complete opacification on radiography, decreased transillumination, and a positive sinus ultrasound examination.

In the patient with a completely fluid-filled sinus, a curved, continuous, and brightly echogenic posterior sinus wall will be apparent in the far field of the sagittal sonogram, and typically no periodic resonance artifacts will be noted (Figure 18-93). In the transverse orientation, the medial and lateral walls of the sinus will also be clearly visualized. This constellation of sonographic findings is referred to as a complete sinusogram.[135] If the sinus is only partially filled with fluid, a mixed picture will be seen. The posterior wall of the sinus will be apparent only in the inferior fluid-filled portion of the sinus (right lower side of the image on the sagittal sonogram) and a periodic resonance artifact may be seen in the upper air-containing region of the sinus (left side of the image). A transverse view of the sinus will not show the presence of the medial or lateral walls of the sinus. This constellation of sonographic findings is referred to as a partial sinusogram.[133,135] As discussed, dynamic testing in both sitting and supine positions would then be indicated to clarify if the partial sinusogram represented fluid or mucosal thickening. An example of partial sinus opacification on CT and its corresponding sonographic representation are illustrated in Figure 18-94.

PITFALLS

The most important potential pitfall when evaluating suspected maxillary sinusitis with ultrasound is failure

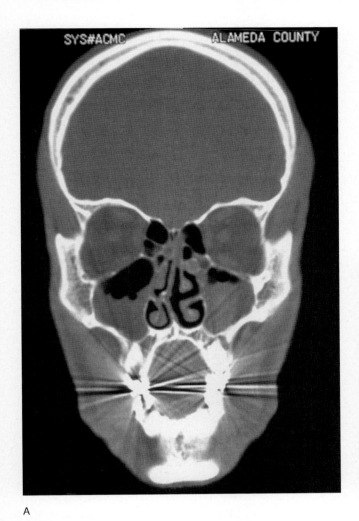

A

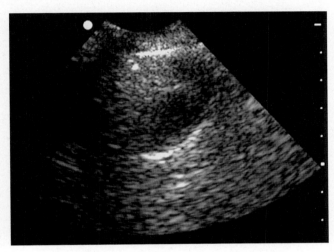

B

Figure 18-94. A *coronal* CT image of a patient with bilateral maxillary and ethmoid sinusitis (A). The left maxillary sinus is nearly completely fluid filled; the maxillary sinus on the right is only partially opacified. Although this is the preferred orientation for CT imaging of the sinuses, it should be noted that the sonogram obtained when scanning the maxillary sinus will be orthogonal to this scan plane. Sagittal sonogram of the partially opacified right maxillary sinus (B). Image taken with a microconvex 3.5 MHz transducer. On the right side of the image (corresponding with the inferior fluid-filled portion of the sinus), the posterior wall of the sinus is apparent as a brightly echogenic line. On the left side of the image (corresponding with the air-filled portion of the sinus), the image is indistinct and the posterior wall of the sinus is not apparent. A large amount of near-field artifact is present because gain settings are too high.

to consider the results of imaging in the context of the pretest likelihood of disease and other clinical indicators of severity. The weighted mean sensitivity of ultrasound for maxillary sinusitis is not more than 85% and involvement of other sinuses cannot be assessed. Therefore, in cases where there is a high clinical suspicion for sinusitis and when there are severe symptoms, especially in elderly or diabetic patients, obtain a more sensitive imaging study (CT) to provide a definitive diagnosis.

Note that a number of conditions other than sinusitis will allow transmission of the insonating beam

through the sinus and will result in visualization of the posterior wall of the sinus. Significant mucosal thickening, polyps, fluid filled cysts, solid masses, and blood from facial trauma and sinus fractures can all create a positive sinusogram (Figures 18-95 and 18-96).

Technical pitfalls include failure to accurately set the image depth to a level that includes the posterior wall of the sinus (usually 5–7 cm), misinterpreting a periodic resonance artifact for the posterior wall of the sinus (resonance artifacts are horizontal, the posterior sinus wall is curved), and only scanning the patient in

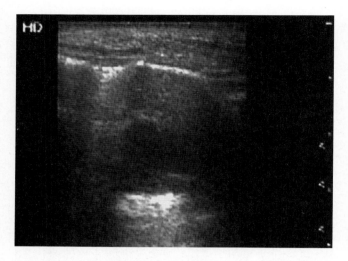

Figure 18-95. Sagittal sonogram of a patient with a polyp filling the lower half of the right maxillary sinus. The posterior wall of the sinus is visible in the inferior portion of the sinus (right side of the image), and posterior acoustic enhancement is evident. The upper portion of the sinus (left side of the image) has more of a "snowstorm" appearance with subtle reverberation (air) and periodic resonance (bone surface) artifacts and no visualization of the posterior wall of the sinus. The "partial sinusogram" image remained the same with both sitting and supine imaging.

a supine position (unless the sinusogram is clearly positive). A patient with a negative supine study may still have sinusitis, and further dynamic testing should be performed in such cases to see if a partial sinusogram is present in a "half-sitting" position as well.

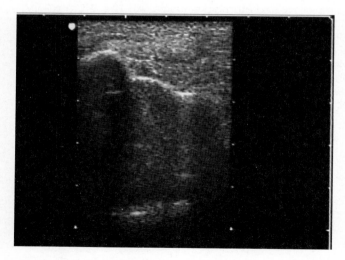

Figure 18-96. Sagittal sonogram of a patient with fractures of the anterior wall of the maxilla and a blood-filled maxillary sinus. Note the marked soft tissue swelling and the cortical irregularity of the anterior wall of the maxilla in the near field. The posterior wall of the sinus is apparent in the far field.

► SKIN AND SOFT TISSUE INFECTIONS

CLINICAL CONSIDERATIONS

Emergency and ambulatory care physicians evaluate patients with skin and soft tissue infections on a daily basis. These infections include cellulitis, abscesses, and necrotizing fasciitis. The diagnosis of cellulitis by physical examination alone is usually straightforward when erythema, warmth, and tenderness are present. Similarly, determining that a subcutaneous abscess exists is simple when fluctuance or focal skin necrosis is present. Clinical findings can be misleading, however, when a cutaneous abscess is small, deep to the skin surface, early in its formation, or where there is preexisting scar tissue from a prior abscess drainage procedure. An occult abscess may occasionally be present when the clinical presentation is consistent with simple cellulitis. Ambiguous clinical findings may direct the clinician away from performing a much needed drainage procedure. Ultrasound has emerged as a valuable tool for assessing soft tissue infections at the bedside. It is increasingly used in emergency and ambulatory care settings to detect occult abscesses, facilitate abscess drainage, and help providers avoid an unnecessary procedure in patients without true abscesses.

CLINICAL INDICATIONS

The clinical indications for the use of ultrasound in the management of soft tissue infections include

- Detection of an occult subcutaneous abscess when clinical findings are ambiguous
- Localization of an optimal site for incision and drainage or aspiration of an abscess
- Assessment of soft tissue inflammatory processes to determine if they are the result of an adjacent arthritis or tendonitis rather than cellulitis

Detection of Occult Subcutaneous Abscess

The ability of ultrasound to detect soft tissue abscesses and guide subsequent incision and drainage has been appreciated since the 1980s.[141–145] In reports focusing on injection drug users, particularly those with inflammatory lesions of the groin, ultrasound has been shown to successfully differentiate cellulitis from abscess, in addition to being useful for detecting adenitis, septic thrombophlebitis, and pseudoaneurysm.[141,144] Ultrasound has also been found to be of value in the diagnosis and treatment of odontogenic facial abscesses,[146] and in the assessment of patients with buccal space swelling.[147]

Four studies conducted in the ED setting have examined the utility of point-of-care ultrasound for evaluation of skin and soft tissue infections.[148–151] All four studies examined the impact of ultrasound assessment on the accuracy of abscess diagnosis, with cases stratified by the pretest likelihood of an abscess. Overall, ultrasound assessment led to a change in management of 17–56% of cases. A consistent finding was that among patients clinically categorized as unlikely to have an abscess, ultrasound frequently revealed an unsuspected abscess that was confirmed by a drainage procedure. This occurred in 14–58% of "low" likelihood cases.

Ultrasound is also useful when an abscess is thought to be present based on clinical factors. In such cases, a negative ultrasound evaluation often correctly excludes abscess, thereby preventing an unnecessary drainage procedure.

With the addition of ultrasound to physical examination alone, the positive predictive value in one study increased from 81% to 93%, and the negative predictive value increased from 77% to 97%.[149] Because of methodological limitations, the actual false-negative rate for detecting abscess cannot be determined with confidence from these studies. The conclusions that can be made from these four studies are as follows: (1) point-of-care ultrasound improves accuracy for detection of superficial abscesses in both adult and pediatric patients, (2) it helps prevent the performance of unnecessary invasive procedures, and (3) it provides guidance as to whether patients require further imaging or consultation.

Point-of-care ultrasound can also be used to guide other aspects of clinical care in patients with known or suspected cellulitis or soft tissue abscesses. In a study of 101 patients with superficial skin abscesses, incision and drainage were compared with ultrasound-guided needle aspiration. The success rate (sonographic and clinical resolution of the abscess by day 7) was reported to be 80% in the incision and drainage group and only 26% in the needle aspiration group leading to the clear conclusion that ultrasound-guided needle aspiration was insufficient therapy for skin abscesses.[152] Another study analyzed the utility of venous ultrasound in 240 patients with lower extremity cellulitis and found a DVT prevalence of only 6.25%. The study concluded that concurrent DVT and cellulitis are rare and that investigation for DVT in such patients has a low yield unless other risk factors are present.[153] In another report on patients with cellulitis, ultrasound examination of the affected area 4 days after initiation of antibiotic therapy revealed that patients with only subcutaneous thickening required a shorter duration of therapy and had a higher rate of early treatment response compared with patients who had subcutaneous cobblestoning.[154]

Assessment of Soft Tissue Inflammatory Processes

Localized pain and erythema over a joint may be due to an inflammatory condition in the joint rather than cellulitis. In a study of 54 patients with erythema, swelling, and joint pain, ultrasound was found to be a useful tool for differentiating soft tissue abnormalities from joint effusions and directing subsequent management. The study reported a statistically significant difference in treatment plans, with a 35% decrease in arthrocentesis procedures when ultrasound was used.[155] Ultrasound is useful in the evaluation and diagnosis of other soft tissue infections, including 1) Ludwig's angina,[156] (2) subcutaneous myiasis (maggot infiltration of human tissue),[157] and (3) muscular or subcutaneous cysticercosis. In cysticercosis, the characteristic sonographic finding is a cystic lesion with a mean diameter of 6 mm with pericystic inflammatory changes and an echogenic, eccentrically located pedunculated nodule attached to the inner wall of the cyst.[158]

ANATOMICAL CONSIDERATIONS

A thorough understanding of the regional anatomy of the area of interest is essential when evaluating for an abscess. Subcutaneous abscesses may be encountered nearly anywhere and are commonly seen on the hand, face, neck, forearm, groin, lower extremity, buttocks, and perianal region. They may be found in close proximity to veins, arteries, nerves, tendons, bones, and muscles. Awareness of the proximity of adjacent structures, familiarity with their normal sonographic appearance, and an understanding of the preferred lines for elective incision are essential.

TECHNIQUE AND NORMAL ULTRASOUND FINDINGS

Perform sonographic evaluation of the skin and subcutaneous tissue for a suspected abscess with a 7–12 MHz linear array transducer, although an annular array or sector transducer may also be utilized. An acoustic standoff pad may improve image resolution if a lower frequency transducer is being used or if the abscess is very superficial and a linear array transducer is not available. Adjust depth and focus settings to place the area of interest within the transducer's optimal focal zone. Keep transducer pressure to a minimum to avoid collapse and subsequent nonvisualization of superficial veins. Systematically scan the area of interest in two perpendicular planes.

One study demonstrated that *S. aureus* (including MRSA) frequently contaminates uncovered ultrasound transducers used in the ED for skin and soft tissue infection scanning. MRSA was reliably removed when a three-step cleaning and disinfection protocol was employed (wiping first with a dry gauze towel, then wiping with a sterile saline moistened gauze towel, and finally wiping with a quaternary ammonia germicidal wipe.)[159] If cleaning and disinfection is not consistent, it may be prudent to cover the ultrasound transducer with a sterile adhesive dressing when scanning patients with skin and soft tissue infections.

A study showed that pediatric emergency physicians without prior ultrasound training could learn to perform and interpret point-of-care ultrasound for assessment of skin and soft tissue infections with just a brief training program.[160] After 6 hours of training, these physicians were able to perform technically adequate studies with excellent agreement with an ultrasound expert (the interrater reliability of the clinician with the expert resulted in a kappa statistic of 0.8). Another study found that a training simulator using a chicken breast injected with "mock purulent material" is valuable for teaching sonographic diagnosis and management of superficial abscesses.[161]

Normal soft tissue ultrasound findings are reviewed as follows. Normal skin (epidermis and dermis) typically appears as a thin, homogeneous, and somewhat hyperechoic layer immediately beneath the transducer. Subcutaneous tissue, composed primarily of subcutaneous fat, lies immediately below and appears hypoechoic with a reticular pattern of thin echogenic connective tissue between the fat lobules. Fascia and connective tissue planes are usually seen as echogenic horizontal or gently curved lines that follow the contour of the underlying muscle. Arteries and veins appear as anechoic circular or tubular structures, depending on the orientation of the transducer relative to the vessel. The use of color flow or Doppler allows for further vessel characterization. Veins typically compress with light or moderate transducer pressure. Arteries will compress with significant pressure and a rhythmic arterial wall pulsation will be noted. Muscle appears relatively hypoechoic with a regular pattern of internal striations in long axis and a speckled appearance in short axis. The anterior cortex of bone is brightly echoic with far-field acoustic shadowing. The normal sonographic appearance of the various layers of soft tissue within the forearm is seen in Figure 18-97.

COMMON AND EMERGENT ABNORMALITIES

Cellulitis

Although nonspecific, familiarity with the sonographic appearance of cellulitis is important for two reasons. First, a rim of cellulitic tissue nearly always surrounds an abscess cavity, and second, cellulitis is the usual diagnosis of exclusion when performing ultrasound on an undifferentiated skin and soft tissue infection. Cellulitis is a diffuse infection of the skin and subcutaneous tissue, and the typical sonographic findings in cellulitis arise from the accumulation of edema fluid. Findings include thickened and abnormally hyperechoic skin and increased echogenicity of the subcutaneous tissue with poor detail resolution. "Cobblestoning" is also a common finding, characterized as areas of hypoechoic edema that traverse the subcutaneous fat in a reticular pattern (Figures 18-98 and 18-99).[162–164] Comparison to the unaffected limb or adjacent normal soft tissue may aid in the recognition of subtle findings. Sonographic findings in cellulitis are simply indicative of edema and are therefore nonspecific, and both necrotizing fasciitis and the inflamed tissue surrounding an abscess may take on the sonographic appearance of cellulitis. In patients with chronic lymphedema, the subcutaneous tissue appears hyperechoic relative to normal tissue but the skin is not thickened or as indistinct as in cellulitis. Additionally, prominent horizontal bands of hypoechoic

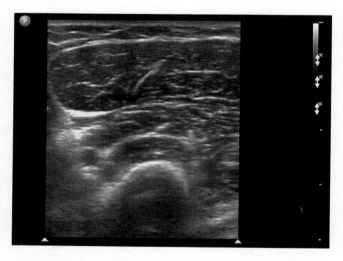

Figure 18-97. Short-axis sonogram of a normal arm. A thin layer of hyperechoic skin (epidermis and dermis) is seen adjacent to the transducer. Just below, a layer of hypoechoic subcutaneous tissue is noted with hyperechoic bands of connective tissue within the fat. A thin echogenic layer of muscle fascia is seen overlying the hypoechoic biceps and brachialis muscles below. The sonographic appearance of muscle tissue varies with the direction of the muscle fibers and will appear either striated (in long axis) or speckled (in short axis). A hypoechoic blood vessel is seen in short axis in the left far field of the image. The curved echogenic anterior surface of the humerus and an associated posterior acoustic shadow are seen in the midline far field.

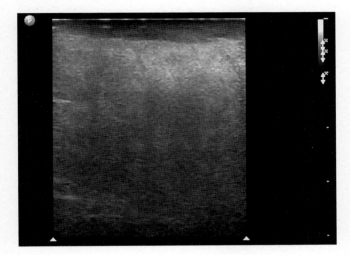

Figure 18-98. Sonogram of a region of cellulitis on a buttock. The skin and subcutaneous tissues appear diffusely hyperechoic and no soft tissue details can be appreciated.

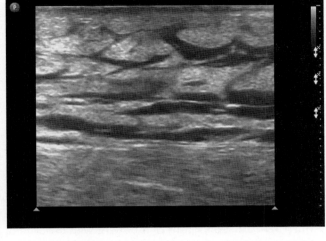

Figure 18-100. Long-axis sonogram of a patient with chronic lower extremity lymphedema. The skin is not thickened, the subcutaneous fat lobules are more hyperechoic than normal, but soft tissue detail is still apparent. Hypoechoic edema fluid surrounds the fat lobules, and horizontal bands of edema fluid are seen below the subcutaneous tissue. Muscle tissue is seen in long axis in the far field.

edema fluid will be seen traversing the subcutaneous tissue (Figure 18-100). Finally, regional lymph nodes in areas with soft tissue cellulitis will often become enlarged and very tender, and it is important to recognize their sonographic appearance and not confuse them with an abscess or other soft tissue mass (Figure 18-101).

Abscess

A subcutaneous abscess may have a variety of sonographic appearances,[144,162,164,165] but will almost uni-

versally be surrounded by a rim of edematous soft tissue or cellulitis that appears hyperechoic relative to normal subcutaneous tissue. Abscess cavities are most frequently spherical or elliptical shaped and the liquefied contents of the abscess cavity will typically demonstrate posterior acoustic enhancement. An abscess cavity may exhibit a wide range of sonographic patterns from

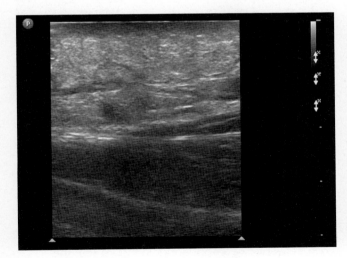

Figure 18-99. Long-axis sonogram of a region of lower extremity cellulitis. The skin is thickened and the subcutaneous tissues appear diffusely hyperechoic; fine reticular areas of hypoechoic stranding are noted giving the tissues a cobblestone appearance. Striated appearing muscle is noted in the far field.

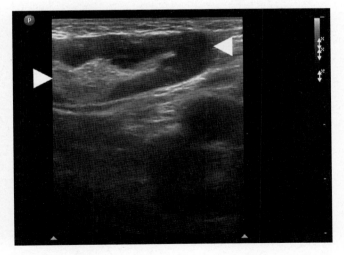

Figure 18-101. Long-axis sonogram of an enlarged, tender reactive lymph node (arrowheads) in a patient with a well-established thigh cellulitis. The hypoechoic periphery and the echogenic fatty central hilum are characteristic. Lymph nodes will often have a long-axis sonographic appearance similar to a kidney.

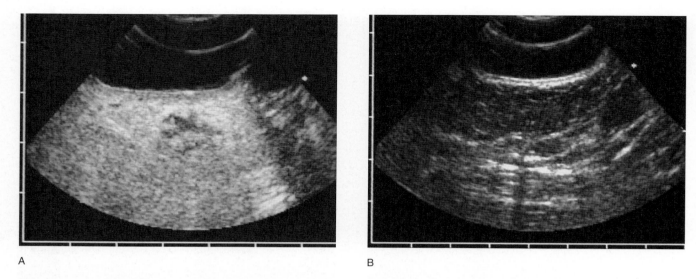

A

B

Figure 18-102. Sonogram of a patient with cellulitis of the lateral chest wall (A). The image was taken with an annular array transducer and an acoustic standoff. The tissues are diffusely hyperechoic with little detail resolution. A small region of hypoechogenicity is seen in the center of the image and represents early abscess formation. Sonogram of the contralateral normal chest wall of the same patient (B). The skin layer is hyperechoic and the subcutaneous tissue relatively hypoechoic with much greater detail resolution than the abnormal side.

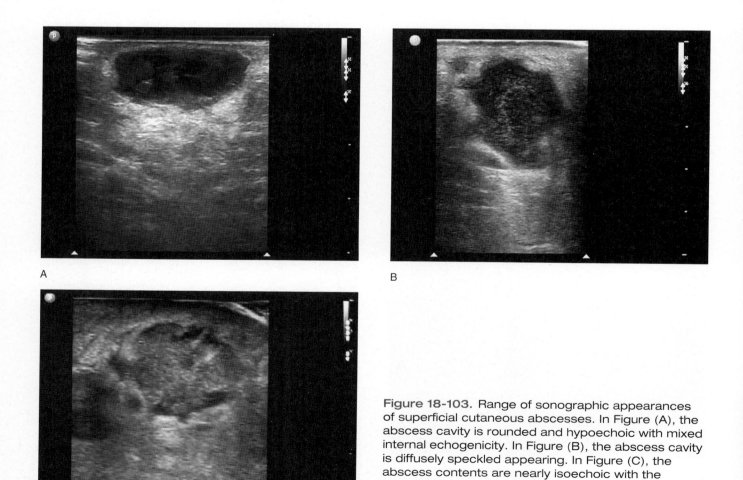

A

B

C

Figure 18-103. Range of sonographic appearances of superficial cutaneous abscesses. In Figure (A), the abscess cavity is rounded and hypoechoic with mixed internal echogenicity. In Figure (B), the abscess cavity is diffusely speckled appearing. In Figure (C), the abscess contents are nearly isoechoic with the surrounding soft tissues. In each of these cases, posterior acoustic enhancement is present (reflecting the liquid nature of the contents), and surrounding subcutaneous tissues appear hyperechoic with poor detail resolution due to cellulitis and tissue edema.

hypoechoic to isoechoic, but it will most commonly appear hypoechoic relative to surrounding soft tissues. On occasion the purulent abscess cavity may be isoechoic or even hyperechoic, making it more difficult to identify (Figures 18-102 to 18-105). Sometimes an abscess may appear irregular or lobulated, and the abscess cavity may interdigitate between tissue planes or take an irregular path within the surrounding hyperechoic cellulitic soft tissues (Figures 18-106 and 18-107). Occasionally, a subcutaneous abscess will be so large that the image will not fit within the field of view of the transducer. In such cases, an extended-field-of-view feature may be used to delineate the abscess's exact location and extent (Figure 18-108). Abscesses may contain hyperechoic debris, septae, or gas bubbles. Gas appears as brightly hyperechoic foci within the abscess cavity with an associated ring-down or reverberation artifact (Figure 18-109). Gentle transducer pressure over the abscess site may induce a swirling motion of the purulent material within the abscess cavity (referred to as "ultrasonic fluctuance") and helps confirm the liquid nature of the material (Figure 18-110). An abnormal fluid collection can be difficult to detect in cases where the abscess contents are isoechoic, and ultrasonic fluctuance can be of particular diagnostic value in such cases.[162] Color flow Doppler may demonstrate hyperemia adjacent to the abscess cavity and can help confirm absence of flow within it.[164] If a hypoechoic fluid collection is seen adjacent to a long bone, the diagnosis of osteomyelitis should be entertained. Finally, abscesses may be found situated

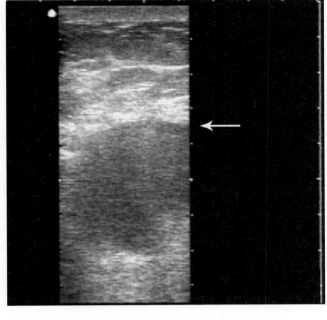

Figure 18-105. Long-axis sonogram of a deep midline buttock abscess in the region of the gluteal fold. The skin and immediate subcutaneous tissue exhibit relatively normal echogenicity. The deeper tissues surrounding the rounded abscess cavity appear more hyperechoic and edematous. Note that the superior edge of this large abscess cavity is 3.5 cm from the skin surface (arrow). Knowledge of the depth of this abscess cavity was crucial to the individual performing the drainage procedure.

adjacent to anatomic structures such as blood vessels, muscles, tendons, and bones. Recognition of adjacent structures is essential prior to embarking on a drainage procedure (Figure 18-111).

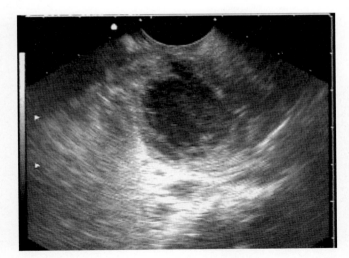

Figure 18-104. Sonogram of a peritonsillar abscess using a 7.5 MHz fingertip transducer. The abscess cavity appears rounded with hypoechoic contents of mixed echogenicity. There is posterior acoustic enhancement and two hypoechoic vessels are seen in short axis beneath the thick posterior wall of the abscess cavity. Peritonsillar abscesses are discussed in further detail in Chapter 22.

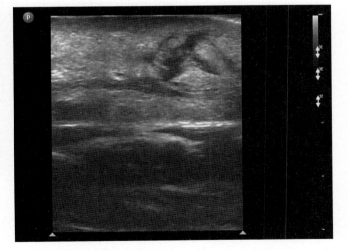

Figure 18-106. Sonogram of an irregularly shaped early hypoechoic abscess cavity surrounded by hyperechoic subcutaneous tissues.

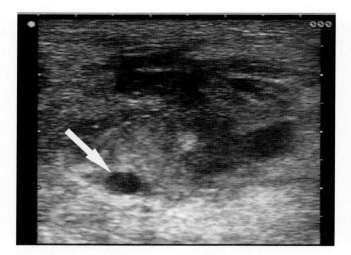

Figure 18-107. Short-axis sonogram of the antecubital fossa of an injection drug user with an abscess. The abscess cavity is large, irregular in shape, interdigitates between tissue planes, and has both hypoechoic and isoechoic components. Swirling of abscess contents was apparent on real-time scanning. The deep brachial artery is seen in short axis in the far field (arrow).

COMMON VARIANTS AND SELECTED ABNORMALITIES

Necrotizing Fasciitis

Necrotizing fasciitis is a rare soft tissue infection defined by tissue necrosis (particularly involving fascia) and a fulminant course. While rapid recognition and treatment can favorably affect outcome,[166] making the diagnosis of necrotizing fasciitis on clinical grounds alone is often

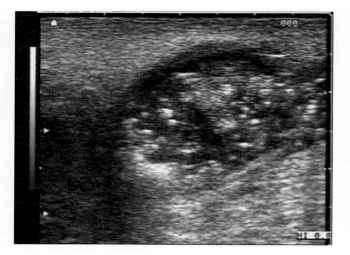

Figure 18-109. Hyperechoic foci with associated ring-down artifact are noted within the mixed echogenicity contents of this abscess cavity. These hyperechoic regions correspond to small gas bubbles within the abscess cavity.

challenging. The role of ultrasound as a diagnostic test for necrotizing fasciitis has never been studied systematically, and it should never be used to exclude the diagnosis. However, sonographic findings characteristic of the disease have been described by two groups of investigators in Taiwan, reporting on a total of 21 cases of necrotizing fasciitis in adults and children.[167,168] Invariably, the subcutaneous fascia, normally seen as a thin, brightly hyperechoic line, is greatly thickened and edematous

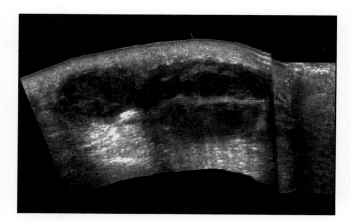

Figure 18-108. Long-axis extended-field-of-view sonogram of a very large buttock abscess in a diabetic patient. The size of the abscess cavity was significantly underestimated by clinical examination alone. The sonogram delineated the extent of the abscess and guided subsequent surgical intervention.

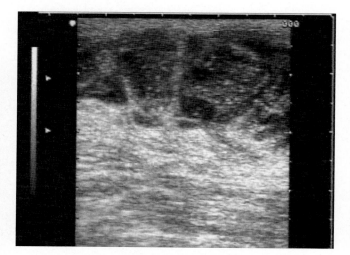

Figure 18-110. Sonogram of a postoperative abdominal wall wound infection. Multiple septae are seen within the hypoechoic collection immediately beneath the skin. Motion of the abscess contents was apparent with gentle transducer pressure on real-time scanning. Far-field hyperechogenicity is due to posterior acoustic enhancement.

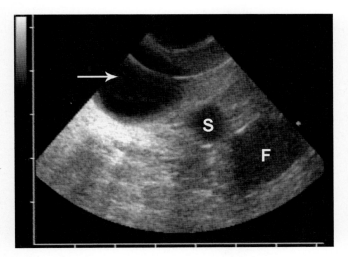

Figure 18-111. Short-axis sonogram of an abscess cavity in the left groin of an injection drug user. The thick-walled hypoechoic abscess cavity (arrow) is seen on the left near field of the image; adjacent are the hypoechoic saphenous (S) and common femoral veins (F). Although incision and drainage were ultimately simple, careful preprocedure ultrasound mapping provided essential anatomic information for safely performing a drainage procedure in this high-risk location.

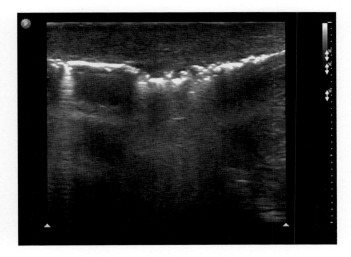

Figure 18-112. Sonogram of a patient with necrotizing fasciitis of the perineum and scrotum (Fournier's gangrene). The scrotal skin is noted to be markedly thickened compared to normal. Immediately below the skin an irregular layer of high amplitude echoes is evident. "Dirty" posterior acoustic shadowing and multiple areas of reverberation artifact are readily apparent. This is the sonographic signature of a subcutaneous gas collection. On CT scan, the entire hemiscrotum was noted to be filled with gas.

appearing, as is the overlying subcutaneous tissue. An anechoic fluid layer measuring greater than 4 mm adjacent to the deep fascia is considered by some authors to be diagnostic of necrotizing fasciitis.[167] In some cases, discreet masses are seen in and around the fascial plane, from which pus may be aspirated. Sonographic findings that may be present in cases of necrotizing fasciitis include (1) marked skin thickening, (2) swelling and increased echogenicity of the overlying fatty tissues with interlacing fluid collections, and (3) subcutaneous emphysema spreading along deep fascia.[169,170] The presence of a subcutaneous gas collection may be rapidly confirmed with a point-of-care ultrasound examination and will typically appear as a focal region of high amplitude echoes with "dirty" posterior acoustic shadowing as well as a reverberation artifact (Figure 18-112). Although small gas bubbles may occasionally be noted within an abscess cavity, the presence of subcutaneous gas that is not within a discreet abscess or gas following fascial planes should raise the index of suspicion for necrotizing fasciitis.

PITFALLS

1. **Abscesses are not always hypoechoic.** They can on occasion be sonographically subtle. An isoechoic collection of pus, especially one that is in or around muscle tissue, or an abscess that is deep and obscured by overlying hyperechoic soft tissues, may give rise to a false-negative ultrasound examination. Operator experience may also play a role. Optimization of the image with appropriate frequency, focus, and depth settings, and gentle transducer pressure to assess for ultrasonic fluctuance may help avoid this pitfall. In the face of strong clinical suspicion for an abscess and an apparently negative ultrasound result, performing a needle aspiration may be reasonable.

2. **Necrotizing soft tissue infections.** An uncommon but potentially disastrous pitfall is failure to consider a necrotizing soft tissue infection once an abscess has been excluded by ultrasound. Although studies examining the use of point-of-care ultrasound in the diagnosis of necrotizing fasciitis are limited, and although ultrasound should never be used to exclude the presence of necrotizing fasciitis, subcutaneous gas spreading along a fascial plane is an ominous finding and indicates the need for definitive imaging with CT as well as emergent surgical consultation.

3. **Failure to recognize adjacent structures.** Abscesses may occur in close proximity to tendons, nerves, arteries, and veins. Although

ultrasound is extremely helpful in diagnosing and mapping the location of an abscess, the decision to drain an abscess that is in close proximity to important structures should be guided by the experience and comfort level of the provider.

► ACKNOWLEDGMENTS

The author thanks Dr. Bradley W. Frazee for his contributions to this chapter in the previous edition.

► REFERENCES

1. Young J, Gilbert AI, Graham MF: The use of ultrasound in the diagnosis of abdominal wall hernias. *Hernia* 11(4):347–351, 2007.
2. Nguyen K, Sauerbrei E, Nolan R, et al.: The abdominal wall, In: Rumack C, Wilson S, Charboneau J, et al., eds. *Diagnostic Ultrasound*. 3rd ed. St. Louis, MO: Mosby, Inc., 2005:chap. 13.
3. Hodgson T, Collins M: Anterior abdominal wall hernias: Diagnosis by ultrasound and tangential radiographs. *Clin Radiol* 44:185–188, 1991.
4. Engel J, Deitch E: Sonography of the anterior abdominal wall. *AJR* 137:73–77, 1981.
5. Carkman S, Ozben V, Zengin K, et al:. Spontaneous rectus sheath hematoma: An analysis of 15 cases. *Ulus Travma Acil Cerrahi Derg* 16(6): 532–536, 2010.
6. Hensen JH, Van Breda Vriesman AC, Puylaert JB: Abdominal wall endometriosis: Clinical presentation and imaging features with emphasis on sonography. *AJR Am J Roentgenol* 186(3):616–620, 2006.
7. Francica G, Scarano F, Scotti L, et al.: Endometriomas in the region of a scar from cesarean section: Sonographic appearance and clinical presentation may vary with the size of the lesion. *J Clin Ultrasound* 37(4):215–220, 2009.
8. Alexiades G, Lambropoulou M, Deftereos S, et al.: Abdominal wall endometriosis-ultrasound research: A diagnostic problem. *Clin Exp Obst Gyn* 28:121–122, 2001.
9. Greher M, Eichenberger U, Gustorff B: Sonographic localization of an implanted infusion pump injection port: Another useful application of ultrasound in pain medicine. *Anesthesiology* 102:243, 2005.
10. Borglum J, Maschmann C, Belhage B, et al.: Ultrasound-guided bilateral dual transversus abdominis plane block: A new 4 point approach. *Acta Anaesthesiol Scand* 55(6): 658–663, 2011.
11. Kanakarajan S, High K, Nagaraja R: Chronic abdominal wall pain and ultrasound-guided abdominal cutaneous nerve infiltration: A case series. *Pain Med* 12(3):382–386, 2011.
12. Gofeld M, Christakis M: Sonographically guided ilioinguinal nerve block. *J Ultrasound Med* 25(12):1571–1575, 2006.
13. Lakhal K, Delplace X, Cottier JP, et al.: The feasibility of ultrasound to assess subglottic diameter. *Anesth Analg* 104(3):611–614, 2007.
14. Shibaski M, Nakajima Y, Ishii S, et al.: Prediction of pediatric endotracheal tube size by ultrasonography. *Anesthesiology* 113(4):819–824, 2010.
15. Elliott DS, Baker PA, Scott MR, et al.: Accuracy of surface landmark identification for cannula cricothyroidotomy. *Anesthesia* 65(9):889–894, 2010.
16. Dinsmore J, Heard M, Green RJ: The use of ultrasound to guide time-critical cannula tracheotomy when anterior neck airway anatomy is unidentifiable. *Eur J Anaesthesiol* 28(7):506–510, 2011.
17. Nicholls SE, Sweeney TW, Ferre RM, et al.: Bedside sonography by emergency physicians for the rapid identification of landmarks relevant to cricothyrotomy. *Am J Emerg Med* 26(8):852–856, 2008.
18. Drescher M, Conrad F, Schamban N: Identification and description of esophageal intubation using ultrasound. *Acad Emerg Med* 7:722–725, 2000.
19. Ma G, Chan TC, Vilke GM, et al.: Confirming endotracheal intubation using ultrasound. *Ann Emerg Med* 36:S20–S21, 2000.
20. Muslu B, Sert H, Kaya A, et al.: Use of sonography for rapid identification of esophageal and tracheal intubations in adult patients. *J Ultrasound Med* 30:671–676, 2011.
21. Werner, SL, Smith CE, Goldstein JR, et al.: Pilot study to evaluate the accuracy of ultrasonography in confirming endotracheal tube placement. *Ann Emerg Med* 49(1): 75–80, 2007.
22. Marciniak B, Fayoux P, Hebrard A, et al.: Airway management in children: Ultrasonography assessment of tracheal intubation in real time? *Anesth Analg* 108(2): 461–465, 2009.
23. Park SC, Ryu JH, Yeom SR, et al.: Confirmation of endotracheal intubation by combined ultrasonographic methods in the Emergency Department. *Emerg Med Australas* 21(4);293–297, 2009.
24. Raphael D, Conrad R: Ultrasound confirmation of endotracheal tube placement. *J Clin Ultrasound* 15:459–462, 1987.
25. Hsieh KS, Lee CL, Lin CC, et al.: Secondary confirmation of endotracheal tube position by ultrasound image. *Crit Care Med* 32:S374–S377, 2004.
26. Kerrey BT, Geis GL, Quinn AM, et al.: A prospective comparison of diaphragmatic ultrasound and chest radiography to determine endotracheal tube position in a pediatric emergency department. *Pediatrics* 123(6): e1039–e1044, 2009.
27. Weaver R, Lyon M, Blaivas M: Confirmation of endotracheal tube placement after intubation using the ultrasound sliding lung sign. *Acad Emerg Med* 13:239–244, 2006.
28. Blaivas M, Tsung JW: Point-of-care sonographic detection of left endobronchial main stem intubation and obstruction versus endotracheal intubation. *J Ultrasound Med* 27(5):785–789, 2008.
29. Friedman E: Role of ultrasound in the assessment of vocal cord function in infants and children. *Ann Otol Rhinol Laryngol* 106:199–209, 1997.
30. Sidhu S, Stanton R, Shahidi S, et al.: Initial experience of vocal cord evaluation using grey-scale, real-time, B-mode ultrasound. *ANZ J Surg* 71:737–739, 2001.

31. Ooi LL, Chan HS, Soo KC: Color Doppler imaging for vocal cord palsy. *Head Neck* 17:20–23, 1995.

32. Werner S, Jones R, Emerman C: Sonographic assessment of the epiglottis. *Acad Emerg Med* 11:1358–1360, 2004.

33. Hung TY, Li S, Chen PS, et al.: Bedside ultrasonography as a safe and effective tool to diagnose acute epiglottitis. *Am J Emerg Med* 29(3);359.e1–3, 2011.

34. Griffith JF, Rainer TH, Ching ASC, et al.: Sonography compared with radiography in revealing acute rib fracture. *AJR* 173:1603–1609, 1999.

35. Bitschnau R, Gehmacher O, Kopf A, et al.: Ultraschall-diagnostik von Rippen-und Sternumfrakturen. *Ultraschall Med* 18:158–161, 1997.

36. Wischhofer E, Fenkl R, Blum R: Sonographischer Nachweis von Rippenfrakturen zur Sicherung der Frakturdiagnostik. *Unfallchirurg* 98:296–300, 1995.

37. Fenkl R, Garrel T, Knaepler H: Notfalldiagnostik der Sternumfraktur mit Ultraschall. *Unfallchirurg* 95:375–379, 1992.

38. Jin W, Yang DM, Kim HC, et al.: Diagnostic values of sonography for assessment of sternal fractures compared with conventional radiography and bone scans. *J Ultrasound Med* 25(10):1263–1268, 2006.

39. Dulchavsky S, Henry S, Moed B, et al.: Advanced ultrasonic diagnosis of extremity trauma: The FASTER examination. *J Trauma* 53:28–32, 2002.

40. Marshburn T, Legome E, Sargsyan A, et al.: Goal-directed ultrasound in the detection of long-bone fractures. *J Trauma* 57:329–332, 2004.

41. Brooks A, Price V, Simms M, et al.: Handheld ultrasound diagnosis of extremity fractures. *J R Army Med Corps* 150:78–80, 2004.

42. Heiner JD, Proffitt AM, McArthur TJ: The ability of emergency nurses to detect simulated long bone fractures with portable ultrasound. *Int Emerg Nurs* 19(3):120–124, 2011.

43. Heiner JD, Baker BL, McArthur TJ: The ultrasound detection of simulated long bone fractures by U.S. Army Special Forces Medics. *J Spec Oper Med* 10(2);7–10, 2010.

44. Heiner JD, McArthur TJ: The ultrasound identification of simulated long bone fractures by prehospital providers. *Wilderness Environ Med* 21(2):137–140, 2010.

45. Weinberg ER, Tunik MG, Tsung JW: Accuracy of clinician-performed point-of-care ultrasound for the diagnosis of fractures in children and young adults. *Injury* 41(8):862–868, 2010.

46. Patel DD, Blumberg SM, Crain EF: The utility of bedside ultrasonography in identifying fractures and guiding fracture reduction in children. *Pediatr Emerg Care* 25(4):221–225, 2009.

47. Tayal VS, Antoniazzi J, Pariyadath M, et al.: Prospective use of ultrasound imaging to detect bony hand injuries in adults. *J Ultrasound Med* 26(9):1143–1148, 2007.

48. Thiede O, Kromer JH, Rudack C, et al.: Comparison of ultrasonography and conventional radiography in the diagnosis of nasal fractures. *Arch Otolaryngol Head Neck Surg* 131:434–439, 2005.

49. Gürkov R, Clevert D, Krause E: Sonography versus plain x rays in diagnosis of nasal fractures. *Am J Rhinol* 22(6):613–616, 2008.

50. Lee MH, Cha JG, Hong HS, et al.: Comparison of high-resolution ultrasonography and computed tomography in the diagnosis of nasal fractures. *J Ultrasound Med* 28(6);717–723, 2009.

51. Danter J, Klinger M, Siegert R, et al.: Ultrasonographische Darstellung von Nasenbeinfrakturen mit einem 20-MHz Ultraschallgerat. *HNO* 44:324–328, 1996.

52. Park CH, Houng HH, Lee JH, et al.: Usefulness of ultrasonography in the treatment of nasal bone fractures. *J Trauma* 67(6);1323–1326, 2009.

53. Akizuki H, Yoshida H, Michi K: Ultrasonographic evaluation during reduction of zygomatic arch fractures. *J Cranio-Maxillo-Facial Surg* 18:263–266, 1990.

54. Ramirez-Schrempp D, Vinci RJ, Liteplo AS: Bedside ultrasound in the diagnosis of skull fractures in the pediatric emergency department. *Pediatr Emerg Care* 27(4):312–314, 2011.

55. Hunter JD, Franklin K, Hughes PM: The ultrasound diagnosis of posterior shoulder dislocation associated with Erb's palsy. *Pediatr Radiol* 28:510–511, 1998.

56. Benson LS, Donaldson JS, Carrol NC: Use of ultrasound in management of posterior sternoclavicular dislocation. *J Ultrasound Med* 10:115–118, 1991.

57. Pollock RC, Bankes MJK, Emery RJH: Diagnosis of retrosternal dislocation of the clavicle with ultrasound. *Injury* 27:670–671, 1996.

58. Graif M, Stahl-Kent V, Ben-Ami T, et al.: Sonographic detection of occult bone fractures. *Pediatr Radiol* 18:383–385, 1988.

59. Chern TC, Jou IM, Lai KA, et al.: Sonography for monitoring closed reduction of displaced extra-articular distal radial fractures. *J Bone Joint Surg* 84-A:194–203, 2002.

60. Ang SH, Lee SW, Lam KY: Ultrasound-guided reduction of distal radius fractures. *Am J Emerg Med* 28, 1002–1008, 2010.

61. Durston W, Swartzentruber R: Ultrasound guided reduction of pediatric forearm fractures in the ED. *Am J Emerg Med* 18:72–77, 2000.

62. Grechenig W, Clement HG, Fellinger M, et al.: Scope and limitations of ultrasonography in the documentation of fractures—An experimental study. *Arch Orthop Trauma Surg* 117:368–371, 1998.

63. Anderson MA, Newmeyer WL, Kilgore ES, Jr: Diagnosis and treatment of retained foreign bodies in the hand. *Am J Surg* 144(1):63–67, 1982.

64. Trautlein JJ, Lambert RL, Miller J: Malpractice in the emergency department—Review of 200 cases. *Ann Emerg Med* 13(9, Pt 1):709–711, 1984.

65. Rockett MS, Gentile SC, Gudas CJ, et al.: The use of ultrasonography for the detection of retained wooden foreign bodies in the foot. *J Foot Ankle Surg* 34:478–484, 1995.

66. Graham DD, Jr: Ultrasound in the emergency department: Detection of wooden foreign bodies in the soft tissues. *J Emerg Med* 22(1):75–79, 2002.

67. Orlinsky M, Knittel P, Feit T, et al.: The comparative accuracy of radiolucent foreign body detection using ultrasonography. *Am J Emerg Med* 18:401–403, 2000.

68. Gilbert FJ, Campbell RSD, Bayliss AP: The role of ultrasound in the detection of non-radiopaque foreign bodies. *Clin Radiol* 41:109–112, 1990.

69. Turner J, Wilde CH, Hughes KC, et al.: Ultrasound-guided retrieval of small foreign objects in subcutaneous tissue. *Ann Emerg Med* 29:731–734, 1997.

70. Schlager D, Sanders AB, Wiggins D, Boren W: Ultrasound for the detection of foreign bodies. *Ann Emerg Med* 20(2):189–191, 1991.

71. Schlager D: The use of ultrasound in the emergency department. *Emerg Med Clin North Am* 15:895–912, 1997.

72. Manthey D, Storrow AB, Milbourn JM, et al.: Ultrasound versus radiography in the detection of soft-tissue foreign bodies. *Ann Emerg Med* 28:7–9, 1996.

73. Jacobson JA, Powell A, Craig JG, et al.: Wooden foreign bodies in soft tissue: Detection at US. *Radiology* 201:45–48, 1998.

74. Hill R, Conron R, Greissinger P, et al.: Ultrasound for the detection of foreign bodies in human tissue. *Ann Emerg Med* 29:353–356, 1997.

75. Ginsburg MJ, Ellis GL, Flom LL, et al.: Detection of soft-tissue foreign bodies by plain radiography, xerography, computed tomography, and ultrasonography. *Ann Emerg Med* 19(6):701–703, 1990.

76. Fornage BD, Schernberg FL: Sonographic diagnosis of foreign bodies of the distal extremities. *AJR* 147:567–569, 1986.

77. Crawford R, Matheson AB: Clinical value of ultrasonography in the detection and removal of radiolucent foreign bodies. *Injury* 20:341–343, 1989.

78. Bray PW, Mahoney JL, Campbell JP, et al.: Sensitivity and specificity of ultrasound in the diagnosis of foreign bodies in the hand. *J Hand Surg* 20:661–666, 1995.

79. Bonatz E, Robbin ML, Weingold MA: Ultrasound for the diagnosis of retained splinters in the soft tissue of the hand. *Am J Orthopedics* 27:445–459, 1998.

80. Banerjee B, Das RK: Sonographic detection of foreign bodies of the extremities. *Br J Radiol* 64:107–112, 1991.

81. Crystal CS, Masneri DA, Hellums JS, et al.: Bedside ultrasound for the detection of soft tissue foreign bodies: A cadaveric study. *J Emerg Med* 36(4):377–80, 2009.

82. Lyon M, Brannam L, Johnson D, et al.: Detection of soft tissue foreign bodies in the presence of soft tissue gas. *J Ultrasound Med* 23(5):677–681, 2004

83. Friedman DI, Forti RJ, Wall SP, et al.: The utility of bedside ultrasound and patient perception in detecting soft tissue foreign bodies in children. *Pediatr Emerg Care.* 21(8):487–492, 2005.

84. Dean AJ, Gronczewski CA, Costantino TG: Technique for emergency medicine bedside ultrasound identification of a radiolucent foreign body. *J Emerg Med* 24(3):303–308, 2003.

85. Leech SJ, Gukhool J, Blaivas M: ED ultrasound evaluation of the Index Flexor Tendon: A comparison of Water-bath Evaluation Technique (WET) versus direct contact ultrasound. *Acad Emerg Med* 10(5):573, 2003.

86. Leech SJ, Blaivas M, Gukhool J: Water-bath vs direct contact ultrasound: A randomized, controlled, blinded image review. *Acad Emerg Med* 10(5):573–574, 2003.

87. Blaivas M, Lyon M, Brannam L, et al.: Water bath evaluation technique for emergency ultra-sound of painful superficial structures. *Am J Emerg Med.* 22(7):589–593, 2004.

88. Halaas GW. Management of foreign bodies in the skin. *Am Fam Physician* 76(5);683–688, 2007.

89. Callegari L, Leonardi A, Bini A, et al.: Ultrasound-guided removal of foreign bodies: Personal experience. *Eur Radiol* 19(5):1273–1279, 2009.

90. Grassi W, Filippucci E, Busilacchi P: Musculoskeletal ultrasound. *Best Pract Res Clin Rheumatol* 18:813–826, 2004.

91. Filippucci E, Unlu Z, Farina A, et al.: Sonographic training in rheumatology: A self teaching approach. *Ann Rheum Dis* 62:565–567, 2003.

92. Finnoff JT, Smith J, Nutz DJ, et al.: A musculoskeletal ultrasound course for physical medicine and rehabilitation residents. *Am J Phys Med Rehabil* 89(1):56–69, 2010.

93. Hoglund M, Tordai P, Engkvist O: Ultrasonography for the diagnosis of soft tissue conditions in the hand. *Scand J Plast Reconstr Hand Surg* 25:225–231, 1991.

94. Cheng JW, Tank SF, Yu TY, et al.: Sonographic features of soft tissue tumors in the hand and forearm. *Chang Gung Med J* 30(6):547–554, 2007.

95. Taboury J: Etude echographique des tendons des muscles rotateurs de l'epaule. *Annales de Radiologie* 38:275–279, 1995.

96. Vick CW, Bell SA: Rotator cuff tears. Diagnosis with sonography. *AJR* 154:121–123, 1990.

97. Farin P, Jaroma H: Sonographic detection of tears of the anterior portion of the rotator cuff (subscapularis tendon tears). *J Ultrasound Med* 16:221–225, 1996.

98. Fornage BD: Musculoskeletal evaluation. In: Mittelstaedt CA, ed. *General Ultrasound*. New York, NY: Churchill Livingstone, 1992:157.

99. Robinson P: Sonography of common tendon injuries. *AJR Am J Roentgenol* 193(3);607–618, 2009.

100. McNally EG, Shetty S: Plantar fascia: Imaging diagnosis and guided treatment. *Semin Musculoskelet Radiol* 14(3):334–343, 2010.

101. Adler R, Sofka C: Percutaneous ultrasound-guided injections in the musculoskeletal system. *Ultrasound Q* 19:3–12, 2003.

102. Chen M, Lew H, Hsu T, et al.: Ultrasound-guided shoulder injections in the treatment of subacromial bursitis. *Am J Phys Med Rehabil* 85:31–35, 2006.

103. Ekeberg OM, Bautz-Holter E, Tveita EK, et al.: Subacromial ultrasound guided or systemic steroid injection for rotator cuff disease: Randomized double blind study. *BMJ* 338:a3112, 2009.

104. Gruber H, Peer S. Loizides A: The "dark tendon sign" (DTS): A sonographic indicator for idiopathic trigger finger. *Ultrasound Med Biol* 37(5):688–692, 2011.

105. Guerini H, Pessis E, Theumann N, et al.: Sonographic appearance of trigger fingers. *J Ultrasound Med* 27(10):1407–1413, 2008.

106. Bodor M, Flossman T: Ultrasound-guided first annular pulley injection for trigger finger. *J Ultrasound Med* 28(6):737–743, 2009.

107. Muir JJ, Curtiss HM, Hollman J, et al.: The accuracy of ultrasound-guided and palpation-guided peroneal tendon sheath injections. *Am J Phys Med Rehabil* 90(7):564–571, 2011.

108. Jeyapalan K, Choudhary S: Ultrasound-guided injection of triamcinolone and bupivacaine in the management of De Quervain's disease. *Skeletal Radiol* 38(11):1099–1103, 2009.

109. Bianchi S, Martinoli C, Abdelwahab I: Ultrasound of tendon tears. Part 1: General considerations and upper extremity. *Skeletal Radiol* 34:500–512, 2005.

110. Kalebo P, Sward L, Karlsson J, et al.: Ultrasonography in the detection of partial patellar ligament ruptures (jumper's knee). *Skeletal Radiol* 20:285–289, 1991.

111. Hyman GS: Jumper's knee in volleyball athletes: Advancements in diagnosis and treatment. *Curr Sports Med Rep* 7(5):296–302, 2008.

112. Mahlfeld K, Kayser R, Mahlfeld A, et al.: Wert der Sonographie in der Diagnostik von Bursopathien im Bereich der Achillessehne. *Ultraschall Med* 22:87–90, 2001.

113. Hashimoto BE, Kramer DJ, Wiitala L: Applications of musculoskeletal sonography. *J Clin Ultrasound* 27:293–318, 1999.

114. Martinoli C, Bianchi S, Zamorani M, et al.: Ultrasound of the elbow. *Eur J Ultrasound* 14:21–27, 2001.

115. Finlay K, Ferri M, Friedman L: Ultrasound of the elbow. *Skeletal Radiol* 33:63–79, 2004.

116. Howlett D: High resolution ultrasound assessment of the parotid gland. *Br J Radiol* 76:271–277, 2003.

117. Dudea SM: Ultrasonography of the salivary glands: What's new? *Med Ultrason* 12(3):173–174, 2010.

118. Katz P, Hartl DM, Guerre A: Clinical ultrasound of the salivary glands. *Otolaryngol Clin North Am* 42(6):973–1000, 2009.

119. Alyas F, Lewis K, Williams M, et al.: Diseased of the submandibular gland as demonstrated using high resolution ultrasound. *Br J Radiol* 78:362–369, 2005.

120. Lamont J, McCarty T, Fisher T, et al.: Prospective evaluation of office-based parotid ultrasound. *Ann Surg Oncol* 8:720–722, 2001.

121. Zhang L, Zhang ZY: Evaluation of the ultrasonographic features of salivary gland tumors. *Chin J Dent Res* 13(2):133–137, 2010.

122. Bialek EJ, Jakubowski W, Zajkowski P, et al.: US of the major salivary glands: Anatomy and spatial relationships, pathologic conditions, and pitfalls. *Radiographics* 26(3):745–763, 2006.

123. McCaig LF, Hughes JM: Trends in antimicrobial drug prescribing among office-based physicians in the United States. *JAMA* 273(3):214–219, 1995.

124. Piccirillo JF, Mager DE, Frisse ME, et al.: Impact of first-line vs. second-line antibiotics for the treatment of acute uncomplicated sinusitis. *JAMA* 286(15):1849–1856, 2001.

125. Hickner JM, Bartlett JG, Besser RE, et al.: Principles of appropriate antibiotic use for acute rhinosinusitis in adults: Background. *Ann Emerg Med* 37(6):703–710, 2001.

126. Geiss HK: Nosocomial sinusitis. *Intens Care Med* 25(10):1037–1039, 1999.

127. Engels EA, Terrin N, Barza M, et al.: Meta-analysis of diagnostic tests for acute sinusitis. *J Clin Epidemiol* 53(8):852–862, 2000.

128. Varonen H, Makela M, Savolainen S, et al.: Comparison of ultrasound, radiography, and clinical examination in the diagnosis of acute maxillary sinusitis: A systematic review. *J Clin Epidemiol* 53(9):940–948, 2000.

129. Puhakka T, Heikkinen T, Makela MJ, et al.: Validity of ultrasonography in diagnosis of acute maxillary sinusitis. *Arch Otolaryngol Head Neck Surg* 126(12):1482–1486, 2000.

130. Varonen H, Savolainen S, Kunnamo I, et al.: Acute rhinosinusitis in primary care: A comparison of symptoms, signs, ultrasound, and radiography. *Rhinology* 41(1):37–43, 2003.

131. Price D, Park R, Frazee B, et al.: Emergency department ultrasound for the diagnosis of maxillary sinus fluid. *Acad Emerg Med* 13(3):363–b–364, 2006.

132. Fufezan O, Asavoaie C, Chereches Panta P, et al.: The role of ultrasonography in the evaluation of maxillary sinusitis in pediatrics. *Med Ultrason* 12(1):4–11, 2010.

133. Hilbert G, Vargas F, Valentino R, et al.: Comparison of B-mode ultrasound and computed tomography in the diagnosis of maxillary sinusitis in mechanically ventilated patients. *Crit Care Med* 29(7):1337–1342, 2001.

134. Kaups KL, Cohn SM, Nageris B, et al.: Maxillary sinusitis in the surgical intensive care unit: A study using bedside sinus ultrasound. *Am J Otolaryngol* 16(1):24–28, 1995.

135. Lichtenstein D, Biderman P, Meziere G, et al.: The "sinusogram," a real-time ultrasound sign of maxillary sinusitis. *Intensive Care Med* 24(10):1057–1061, 1998.

136. Vargas F, Bui HN, Boyer A, et al.: Transnasal puncture based on echographic sinusitis evidence in mechanically ventilated patients with suspicion of nosocomial maxillary sinusitis. *Intens Care Med* 32(6):858–866, 2006.

137. Vargas F, Boyer A, Bui HN, et al.: A postural change test improves the prediction of a radiological maxillary sinusitis by ultrasonography in mechanically ventilated patients. *Intensive Care Med* 33(8):1474–1478, 2007.

138. Boet S, Guene B, Jusserand D, et al.: A-mode ultrasound in the diagnosis of maxillary sinusitis in ventilated patients. *B-ENT* 6(3):177–182, 2010.

139. Sahlstrand-Johnson P, Jannert M, Strömbeck A, et al.: Computed tomography measurements of different dimensions of maxillary and frontal sinuses. *BMC Med Imaging* 11:8, 2011.

140. Gwaltney JM, Jr, Phillips CD, Miller RD, et al.: Computed tomographic study of the common cold. *N Engl J Med* 330(1):25–30, 1994.

141. Yiengpruksawan A, Ganepola GA, Freeman HP: Acute soft tissue infection in intravenous drug abusers: Its differential diagnosis by ultrasonography. *J Natl Med Assoc* 78(12):1193–1196, 1986.

142. Yeh HC, Rabinowitz JG: Ultrasonography of the extremities and pelvic girdle and correlation with computed tomography. *Radiology* 143(2):519–525, 1982.

143. vanSonnenberg E, Wittich GR, Casola G, et al.: Sonography of thigh abscess: Detection, diagnosis, and drainage. *AJR Am J Roentgenol* 149(4):769–772, 1987.

144. Sandler MA, Alpern MB, Madrazo BL, et al.: Inflammatory lesions of the groin: Ultrasonic evaluation. *Radiology* 151(3):747–750, 1984.

145. Gitschlag KF, Sandler MA, Madrazo BL, et al.: Disease in the femoral triangle: Sonographic appearance. *AJR Am J Roentgenol* 139(3):515–519, 1982.

146. Peleg M, Heyman Z, Ardekian L, Taicher S: The use of ultrasonography as a diagnostic tool for superficial fascial space infections. *J Oral Maxillofac Surg* 56(10):1129–1131, 1998; discussion 1132.

147. Srinivas K, Sumanth KN, Chopra SS. Ultrasonographic evaluation of inflammatory swellings of the buccal space. *Indian J Dent Res* 20(4):458–462, 2009.

148. Tayal VS, Hasan N, Norton HJ, et al.: The effect of soft-tissue ultrasound on the management of cellulitis in the emergency department. *Acad Emerg Med* 13(4):384–388, 2006.

149. Squire BT, Fox JC, Anderson C: Abscess: Applied bedside sonography for convenient evaluation of superficial soft tissue infections. *Acad Emerg Med* 12(7):601–606, 2005.

150. Page-Wills C, Simon B, Christy D: Utility of ultrasound on emergency department management of suspected cutaneous abscess. *Acad Emerg Med* 7:493, 2000.

151. Sivitz AB, Lam SH, Ramirez-Schrempp D, et al.: Effect of bedside ultrasound on management of pediatric soft tissue infection. *J Emerg Med* 39(5):637–643, 2010.

152. Gaspari RJ, Resop D, Mendoza M, et al.: A randomized controlled trial of incision and drainage versus ultrasonographically guided needle aspiration for skin abscesses and the effect of methicillin-resistant Staphylococcus aureus. *Ann Emerg Med* 57(5):483–491, 2011.

153. Maze MJ, Pithie A, Dawes T, et al.: An audit of venous duplex ultrasonography with lower limb cellulitis. *N Z Med J* 124(1329):53–56, 2011.

154. Huang MH, Chang YC, Wu CH, et al.: The prognostic values of soft tissue sonography for adult cellulitis without pus or abscess formation. *Intern Med J* 39(12):841–844, 2009.

155. Adhikari S, Blaivas M: Utility of bedside sonography to distinguish soft tissue abnormalities from joint effusions in the emergency department. *J Ultrasound Med* 29(4):519–526, 2010.

156. Gaspari RJ: Bedside ultrasound of the soft tissue of the face: A case of early Ludwig's angina. *J Emerg Med* 31(3):287–291, 2006.

157. Schechter E, Lazar J, Nix ME, et al.: Identification of subcutaneous myiasis using bedside emergency physician performed ultrasound. *J Emerg Med* 40(1):e1–3, 2011.

158. Sharma P, Neupane S, Shrestha M, et al.: An ultrasonographic evaluation of solitary muscular and soft tissue cysticercosis. *Kathmandu Univ Med J* 8(30):257–260, 2010.

159. Frazee BW, Fahimi J, Lambert L, et al.: Emergency department sonographic probe contamination and experimental model of probe disinfection. *Ann Emerg Med* 58(1):56–63, 2011.

160. Marin JR, Alpern ER, Panebianco NL, et al.: Assessment of a training curriculum for emergency ultrasound for pediatric soft tissue infections. *Acad Emerg Med* 18(2):174–182, 2011.

161. Heiner JD: A new simulation model for skin abscess identification and management. *Simul Heathc* 5(4):238–241, 2010.

162. Loyer EM, DuBrow RA, David CL, et al.: Imaging of superficial soft-tissue infections: Sonographic findings in cases of cellulitis and abscess. *AJR Am J Roentgenol* 166(1):149–152, 1996.

163. Craig JG: Infection: Ultrasound-guided procedures. *Radiol Clin North Am* 37(4):669–678, 1999.

164. Bureau NJ, Chhem RK, Cardinal E: Musculoskeletal infections: US manifestations. *Radiographics* 19(6):1585–1592, 1999.

165. Loyer EM, Kaur H, David CL, et al.: Importance of dynamic assessment of the soft tissues in the sonographic diagnosis of echogenic superficial abscesses. *J Ultrasound Med* 14(9):669–671, 1995.

166. Lille ST, Sato TT, Engrav LH, et al.: Necrotizing soft tissue infections: Obstacles in diagnosis. *J Am Coll Surg* 182(1):7–11, 1996.

167. Yen ZS, Wang HP, Ma HM, et al.: Ultrasonographic screening of clinically-suspected necrotizing fasciitis. *Acad Emerg Med* 9(12):1448–1451, 2002.

168. Chao HC, Kong MS, Lin TY: Diagnosis of necrotizing fasciitis in children. *J Ultrasound Med* 18(4):277–281, 1999.

169. Wronski M, Slodkowski M, Cebulski W, et al.: Necrotizing fasciitis: Early sonographic diagnosis. *J Clin Ultrasound* 39(4):236–239, 2011.

170. Morrison D, Blaivas M, Lyon M: Emergency diagnosis of Fournier's gangrene with bedside ultrasound. *Am J Emerg Med* 23(4):544–547, 2005.

CHAPTER 19

Ocular

Matthew Lyon and Dietrich von Kuenssberg Jehle

Ultrasound of the globe and orbit can be very helpful in evaluating ED and critical care patients with serious eye complaints or potentially elevated intracranial pressure. In many acute ocular conditions, the physical examination is difficult and may be unreliable. Specialized equipment and ophthalmologic expertise are frequently unavailable in the ED, especially on nights, evenings, weekends, and holidays. In these circumstances, ultrasound is more accurate than traditional examination techniques for assessing a wide variety of ocular and orbital diseases, including penetrating globe injuries, retinal detachment, and papilledema.[1–4]

The eye is an ideal structure for ultrasound interrogation since the anterior chamber and vitreous cavity are fluid filled. With ultrasound, the globe, orbit, and retrobulbar structures can be evaluated accurately and safely.[2] While ophthalmologists typically use highly specialized ultrasound transducers, ocular ultrasound is performed using transducers readily available to emergency providers.[5–8] This technology can accurately differentiate between pathology requiring immediate ophthalmologic consultation and that which can be followed up on an outpatient basis.

► CLINICAL CONSIDERATIONS

Physical examination incorporating ophthalmoscopic and slit lamp examination is the primary diagnostic approach to most ocular complaints. There are many situations in which the physical examination may be limited and imaging is required. Ultrasound examination of the eye is potentially useful in many situations encountered in emergency and acute care settings. Since physical examination requires a clear visual axis to examine the structures of the eye, any obstruction, such as blood in the anterior chamber or vitreous, obscures visualization and limits physical examination. Ultrasound allows imaging beyond the obstruction. There is little attenuation of the ultrasound signal. Detailed, high-resolution images of posterior structures can be obtained even when direct visualization is difficult or impossible.

Situations in which direct visualization of intraocular structures may be difficult or impossible include lid abnormalities due to facial trauma, severe edema, subcutaneous air, or previous surgeries. In cases of facial trauma and swelling, it may be difficult to assess the eye without significant manipulation, which may be painful and even harmful if there is globe perforation. Visual axis obstruction can also occur in the presence of corneal scars, cataracts, hyphema, or hypopyon, or with vitreous hemorrhage. Furthermore, normal conditions such as miosis make visualization of the retina difficult without pharmacologic agents.

Ultrasound may also be helpful in situations where physical examination alone is inadequate. An example is peripheral retinal detachment. Patients presenting with a history consistent with retinal detachment may have an unremarkable ophthalmologic examination, and performing an examination with a dilated pupil is not always feasible. Ultrasound allows for visualization of the entire retina without dilation of the pupil.

CT is frequently employed to evaluate the globe after trauma. CT is highly sensitive for orbital fractures, foreign bodies, and retrobulbar hematomas. Fine-cut CT scans with 2-mm sections are able to localize foreign bodies as small as 0.7 mm.[9] In contrast, ultrasound has been demonstrated to have a slightly lower sensitivity but a comparable positive predictive value for detecting similar size metal foreign bodies in a porcine model.[10] Patients with a potential foreign body and a negative ultrasound examination will require an orbital CT scan.

► CLINICAL INDICATIONS

The clinical indications for ocular ultrasound are as follows:

- Eye trauma
- Acute change in vision
- Headache, head trauma, or altered mental status (potentially elevated intracranial pressure)

EYE TRAUMA

Trauma is one of the leading causes of unilateral loss of vision in the United States and accounts for an estimated cost of $200 million per year.[11] Vision-threatening injuries include retrobulbar hematoma, retinal detachment, lens dislocation, traumatic optic neuropathy, and globe injuries.[12] The most common presentation for a vision-threatening injury is blindness after the injury. However, vision loss may occur gradually because of unrecognized trauma or the patient may not be able to report vision loss due to lid swelling or alteration in mental status. As a consequence, ocular injuries are often missed in these patients. A retrospective review of trauma patients with potential ocular injury demonstrated that nonophthalmologists frequently missed or underestimated potential eye trauma, diagnosing only 72% of eye injuries and referring only 27% for ophthalmologic evaluation.[13]

Significant swelling of the periorbital tissues can be encountered with midface or craniofacial fractures, injuries that increase the risk of concomitant ocular injury. One study found that of 283 patients presenting with facial fractures, 71 had an ocular injury, with 32 (12%) suffering a serious ocular injury.[14] While it is ideal for all facial trauma patients with suspected eye injury to have an examination performed immediately by an ophthalmologist, this is commonly not feasible. There are often more serious and life-threatening injuries that require emergent evaluation and treatment.

Ocular ultrasound can be performed at the bedside. It is noninvasive, so there is little risk for exacerbating an injury when it is performed correctly. Ocular ultrasound is useful even when medication, drugs, or hypoxia alter pupillary function. This is important in the initial clinical assessment of the eye, where pupil size, reaction to light, and the presence or absence of a relative afferent papillary defect are assessed.[12]

Retrobulbar hemorrhage can be diagnosed clinically when a significant hematoma is present.[15] However, this vision-threatening emergency often goes unrecognized, especially in trauma victims with a decreased level of consciousness, and delayed diagnosis may result in irreversible damage to the optic nerve. CT typically reveals stretching of the optic nerve and a tented posterior sclera. Retrobulbar hematoma may cause damage to the optic nerve either through direct compression leading to ischemia or through traction by propelling the globe forward and stretching the nerve. The hematoma occurs as a result of bleeding within or around the cone formed by the extraocular muscles. This cone of muscles combined with the bony orbit forms a compartment in which ongoing hemorrhage leads to elevated intraorbital pressure. As the pressure rises, compression of the ophthalmic and retinal vessels can occur, resulting in ischemia and ultimately blindness.[12] Any potential injury must be treated rapidly because irreversible damage may occur after only 60 minutes of ischemia.[16]

An open globe injury is defined as a full thickness wound involving the corneoscleral wall of the eye. This type of injury is typically caused either by blunt force, particularly to the anterolateral part of the orbit, or due to laceration by a foreign body.[12,17] While some open globe injuries are obvious with vitreous extrusion, a significant proportion are not readily apparent. Clues to an open globe injury include bloodstained tears, lid lacerations, presence of a significant subconjunctival hemorrhage, or hyphema. However, none of these are pathognomonic for globe rupture. Furthermore, in cases involving small high-velocity projectiles, there may be no external signs of perforation.[12] Standard CT evaluation for open globe injury has been shown to have a sensitivity and specificity of 75% and 93%, respectively.[18] Ultrasound sensitivity is similar to a standard CT scan. The best test for identifying globe injury is thin slice CT (2-mm) with reconstructions, which can identify subtle findings such as scleral discontinuity.

Thin slice CT is also the test of choice for intraocular foreign body localization.[9] Ultrasound has limitations when used for the detection of intraocular foreign bodies. In animal models, the sensitivity and specificity were 87.5% and 95.8%, respectively.[10] One study compared CT with ultrasound in a prospective study of patients with opaque intraocular foreign bodies. Ultrasound had complete concurrence with surgical or clinical follow-up in 90% of 61 cases. The study concluded that ultrasound was useful, even though CT was more accurate in detecting the intraocular foreign bodies, because ultrasound was superior to CT in demonstrating intraocular damage associated with the foreign bodies.

ACUTE CHANGE IN VISION

Acute change in vision is a fairly common complaint in emergency and acute care settings. Symptoms may include floaters, flashing lights, double vision, and even complete blindness. Although these symptoms may be indicative of nonocular problems, they require rapid attention to exclude such processes as lens dislocation, vitreous hemorrhage, retinal detachment, and vitreous detachment.

Lens dislocation is a condition frequently caused by blunt trauma. In a series of 71 consecutive patients presenting with ocular trauma, 12 were noted to have a lens dislocation.[19] Lens dislocation can also occur without trauma and be idiopathic or hereditary (Marfan's syndrome). Ultrasound easily identifies the lens due to its anterior location. Using ultrasound, the clinician is able to evaluate the lens-supporting structures to determine whether the lens is subluxed or completely dislocated. Subtle lens subluxation can be a difficult diagnosis, even for experienced clinicians.

The incidence of spontaneous vitreous hemorrhage is about 7 cases per 100,000 people.[20] Proliferative diabetic retinopathy, posterior vitreous detachment with or without a retinal tear, and retinal detachment are the most common causes. Symptoms of a spontaneous vitreous hemorrhage typically include floaters or clouded vision. Other symptoms such as flashes of light may be present, but these symptoms are usually due to the underlying cause of the hemorrhage, such as retinal detachment. As a vitreous hemorrhage ages, a membrane may form with attachments to the retina. When this membrane contracts, a retinal detachment may occur, usually weeks after the initial hemorrhage. Ultrasound allows for visualization of the hemorrhage as well as the potential cause. In fact, there is no other imaging modality that can reliably ascertain the anatomic position of the retina.[20]

Retinal detachments and retinal tears (Figure 19-1), which may be a precursor to detachment, are common causes of vitreous hemorrhage. Both represent a separation between the retinal sensory and the pigment layers. There are three types of retinal detachment: rhegmatogenous, tractional, and exudative. Most cases of rhegmatogenous retinal detachment are associated with a posterior vitreous separation; the detachment is caused by fluid seeping into a break in the sensory layer of the retina. Tractional retinal detachments occur when fibrous membranes in the vitreous pull the retina from the underlying retinal pigment epithelium, and they are typically seen with proliferative diabetic retinopathy or

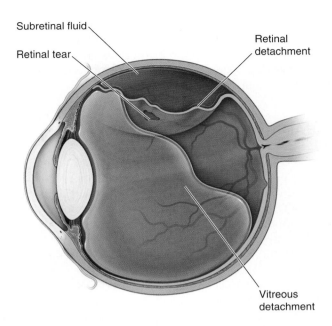

Figure 19-1. Eye with retinal and posterior vitreous detachment.

as a common sequela of aging. However, this condition is also associated with retinopathy of prematurity, sickle cell retinopathy, and prior vitreous hemorrhage. Exudative retinal detachment occurs with inflammatory, infectious, or neoplastic conditions that disturb the blood–retina barrier. This allows fluid to collect underneath the layers of the retina causing a separation. In most cases of retinal detachment, patients will complain of flashing lights, floaters, or a curtain-like vision loss.[21] As the retinal tear progresses, retinal vessels may tear, producing a vitreous hemorrhage. This is a common association and is why patients with retinal detachments typically complain of floaters prior to the onset of peripheral or total vision loss.

Posterior vitreous detachment is a separation of the vitreous humor from the retina (Figure 19-1). The separation is painless and usually abrupt; patients complain of new floaters in conjunction with the onset of flashing lights. The clinical history can be similar to retinal detachment as patients with both problems complain of flashing lights at onset. This entity is a common presentation for acute visual change in the urgent care and emergency settings as it is a normal consequence of aging. The condition occurs often in older adults and over 75% of those greater than age 65 develop it.[22] Vitreous detachment often has a benign clinical course that does not significantly threaten visual acuity; however, in approximately 15–30% of cases of vitreous detachment, a retinal hole is created that may lead to retinal detachment. Posterior vitreous detachment can also be associated with vitreous hemorrhage.[23] Ultrasound is the modality of choice for evaluating the retina and vitreous. Ultrasound may be the only method for detecting posterior vitreous detachment and is also more accurate for identifying potential associated complications (retinal detachment or hemorrhage).

HEADACHE, HEAD TRAUMA, OR ALTERED MENTAL STATUS

Headache, head injury, and altered mental status are common presentations in the ED. These complaints may be associated with elevated intracranial pressure. While many modalities are available to evaluate potential elevated intracranial pressure, each has significant limitations. In the acute trauma patient, evaluating the presence of papilledema with an ophthalmoscope is difficult. Furthermore, papilledema can take hours to develop. CT is the most common initial diagnostic modality, but it may be unavailable or obtained early in the patients course before elevated intracranial pressure develops. When unstable patients are taken directly to the operating room for abdominal injuries, there may not be time for a head CT. In these patients, ocular ultrasound can provide a method for grossly assessing the intracranial pressure. In addition, multiple examinations can be readily performed on the same patient with an evolving clinical picture.

A direct communication between the subarachnoid space of the ventricles and the optic nerve sheath has been described in cadavers and an animal model. In an experimental model using rhesus monkeys, change in the optic nerve sheath diameter in response to changing intracranial pressure was demonstrated by varying the pressure in balloons placed in the subarachnoid space.[24] Multiple clinical studies have demonstrated this effect in actual patients. One study comparing CT to ultrasound measurement of the optic nerve sheath diameter in patients with suspected intracranial hemorrhage showed a sensitivity and specificity of 100% and 95%, respectively.[25] This procedure has also been described in pediatric patients.[26]

▶ ANATOMICAL CONSIDERATIONS

The globe is an oblong structure with a mean vertical diameter of 23.5 mm and mean anteroposterior diameter of 24 mm. The eye is embedded in the orbit and covered by the eyelids. On ultrasound evaluation, the surrounding facial bones appear as bright reflectors with deep posterior shadowing. The lid is echogenic and divided by the hypoechoic tarsal plate.

The eye is divided into anterior and posterior segments. The anterior segment consists of the cornea, anterior chamber, iris, posterior chamber and lens. The

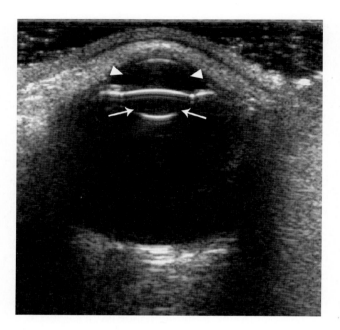

Figure 19-2. Normal ultrasound of the eye. The anterior chamber (arrow heads) and the lens (arrows) are clearly seen. The vitreous appears black.

posterior segment consists of the structures posterior to the lens; the vitreous chamber, retina, choroid, and optic nerve. The cornea appears as a thin, hyperechoic structure attached to the sclera at the periphery. The sclera is a dense membrane to which the extraocular muscles attach, but is indistinguishable from the lateral structures of the eye by ultrasound. Anechoic aqueous humor fills the anterior chamber, and echoes in the anterior chamber are seen only in pathologic states. The iris and pupil can often be visualized between the anterior chamber and the lens. The lens appears as a hyperechoic reflector, which is concave, and may show reverberation artifact at the anterior surface (Figure 19-2).

The posterior segment comprises the majority of the globe, about 80%. It contains the vitreous body, which consists of a colorless, structureless transparent gel, approximately 99% of which is water. The normal vitreous body is echolucent (dark on ultrasound); however, ultrasound artifacts may occasionally be seen.

The posterior layers of the eye consist of the retina and choroid, which are bounded by the sclera. The retina is the neural, sensory stratum of the globe. It is very thin, varying from 0.56 mm near the optic disk to 0.1 mm anteriorly. Its anterior surface is in contact with the vitreous body and the posterior surface is strongly adherent to the choroid. Near the center of the posterior aspect of the retina is the oval macula, where visual resolution is the greatest. At the macula, the retina is only a few cell layers thick. The choroid is a thin, highly vascular membrane lining the posterior globe. It is firmly

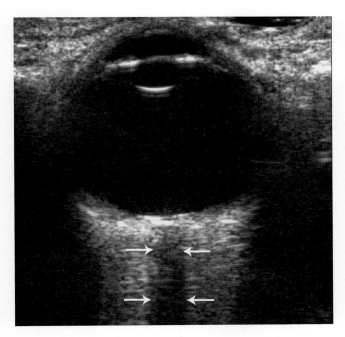

Figure 19-3. The optic nerve is seen posterior to the globe and is hypoechoic (arrows). Minimizing the gain is advisable to decrease echoes that can result in difficulty defining borders of the optic nerve sheath.

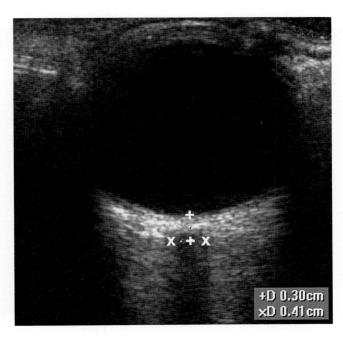

+D 0.30cm
xD 0.41cm

Figure 19-4. Normal measurement of the optic nerve sheath is shown. The measurement should take place 3 mm behind the globe.

adherent to the sclera and is thicker posteriorly where it is penetrated by the optic nerve. Its internal surface is firmly attached to the pigmented layer of the retina. On ultrasound interrogation of the normal eye, the three posterior layers (retina, choroid, and sclera) blend into one homogeneous structure. If separation occurs as with retinal detachment, the layers may be distinguished from one another.

The optic nerve and sheath may be seen posterior to the globe, traveling toward the optic chiasm. The nerve appears homogeneous on ultrasound, with low internal reflectivity (Figure 19-3). This is in contrast to the more reflective sheath.[27] Measurement of the sheath is made 3 mm posterior to the globe (Figure 19-4). Normal measurements vary by age from 5 mm and less in adults, 4.5 mm in children (1–15 years), and 4 mm or less in children less than 1 year of age.[25–27] Since the optic nerve sheath is connected to the subarachnoid space and is easily distensible, conditions that elevate the intracranial pressure lead to dilation of the optic nerve sheath.

Arterial and venous structures of the eye can be identified using color Doppler. The largest artery in the orbit is the ophthalmic artery, which runs parallel to the optic nerve.[28] The central retinal artery is located in the anterior part of the optic nerve shadow. The central retinal vein is found near the central retinal artery and is distinguishable from the central retinal artery with pulsed wave Doppler (PWD) examination.[29]

▶ GETTING STARTED

Patient positioning will vary, with trauma patients typically supine while other patients may be partially reclined or upright. Patients with a potential penetrating injury may be reclined at 45°. Make the patient comfortable with oral or parenteral medications. When a ruptured globe is suspected, consider administering antiemetics to prevent retching and a resultant rise in intraocular pressure. Topical anesthetic and cycloplegic medications are not necessary for sonographic examination of the globe.

Set the ultrasound machine with the ocular presets, which will help limit the amount of energy exposure to the ocular tissue. Always practice the ALARA (as low as reasonably achievable) principle to ensure that the total ultrasound energy is maintained below a level at which bioeffects are generated while diagnostic information is preserved. Use a linear array transducer in the 7.5–15 MHz frequency range (the same transducer utilized for line placement, soft tissue examinations, and musculoskeletal studies). Higher transducer frequencies may produce better images, but decreased penetration may limit visualization of retro-orbital structures. Use an endocavity transducer if a linear transducer is not available[1]; however, manipulating an endocavity transducer over the eye can be awkward and imaging is somewhat limited. Color and spectral Doppler capabilities allow for the evaluation of orbital vasculature and may be helpful in specific cases. An ocular or small parts setting is available on most machines. Other presets such as thyroid, musculoskeletal, and superficial settings may also be used. Sterile gel is typically not required but can be utilized.

The amount of ultrasound gel needed for ocular ultrasound depends on the possible pathology. If globe rupture or pathology in the very near field is suspected, then use a larger amount of gel to fill the preorbital space. With the eyelid closed during the examination (Figure 19-5), allow the transducer to "float" on the ultrasound gel while not touching the eyelid. If the lid is not touched and no pressure is transmitted to the globe, the possibility of vitreous extrusion from a perforated globe is minimal. The space between the transducer and the eyelid can be clearly visualized during the ultrasound examination as an echo-free space between the top of the screen and the lid, and confirms that no pressure was applied to the globe during the examination (Figure 19-6A). If globe rupture is suspected, it is advisable to have the patient keep both eyes closed so they are less likely to inadvertently open the eye being examined. If a ruptured globe is not suspected, then very light contact with the eyelid is permitted, but will still require a moderate amount of gel. The gel is nontoxic to ocular structures; however, removal of gel from the preorbital space may be difficult in a patient with a painful eye condition. Further, some patients complain

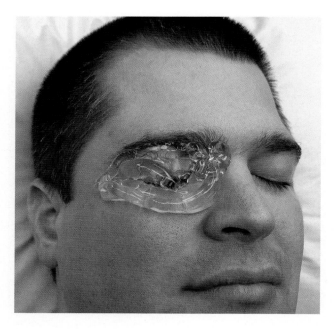

Figure 19-5. Place a generous amount of gel on top of the closed lid in the patient with suspected globe rupture. This much gel allows the clinician to make no direct contact between the transducer and the eyelid itself.

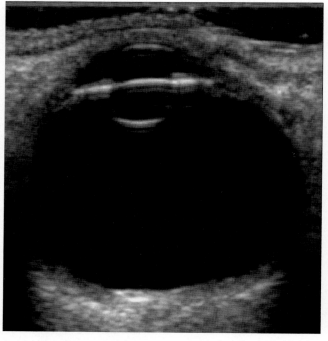

A

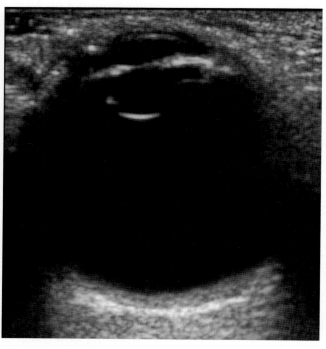

B

Figure 19-6. Image (A) shows better detail of the near-field structures because the transducer is "floated" in the ultrasound gel and does not touch the eyelid. Image (B) shows less near-field resolution of the superficial structures of the eye because the transducer is in direct contact with the eyelid.

of a burning sensation if the gel comes in contact with the cornea. When the transducer touches the eyelid, near-field structures are too close to the transducer and are not well visualized, which is in contrast to when the transducer is "floated" within the ultrasound gel (Figure 19-6B).

TECHNIQUE AND NORMAL ULTRASOUND FINDINGS

Gently place the transducer onto the closed eyelid using normal ultrasound conventions for transducer orientation (transducer indicator points to the top of the head for longitudinal views or to the patient's right for transverse views). After placing the transducer into the gel, pay particular attention to the ultrasound image, leaving a stripe of echolucent gel anterior to the eyelid. This gel separation must be maintained if there is a possibility of globe rupture. Simply suspending the transducer over the patient's eye will inevitably lead to a shaky image and compression of the globe as the clinician's arm grows tired. By resting a portion of the hand holding the transducer on a bony structure such as the ridge of the nose or the patient's eyebrow, the clinician can stabilize the transducer and avoid resting the transducer directly on the eyelid. It is common to use pressure to improve ultrasound imaging when performing abdominal ultrasound; however, with ocular ultrasound, pressure on the globe must be avoided (Video 19-1: Ocular Normal).

Adjust the gain on the ultrasound machine several times throughout the examination. If the gain is too high initially, artifacts will be created, making the examination difficult (Figure 19-7). Setting the gain too low will cause a small vitreous hemorrhage or subtle detachment to be missed. Thus, if the examination is started with normal gain settings, at some point the gain should be turned up to evaluate for subtle pathology (Figure 19-8). As the gain is increased, however, artifacts will be visualized that may mimic a vitreous hemorrhage. Comparison with the nonsymptomatic eye can help differentiate true vitreous hemorrhage from artifact associated with high gain. Adjust the focal position to the area of interest. This will change throughout the examination as the clinician examines the structures in the near field and far field.

Ultrasound imaging almost always involves visualizing structures in two orthogonal planes. Since each plane creates only a two-dimensional (2D) image, a three-dimensional (3D) mental image is created by scanning in both planes and sweeping from side to side and top to bottom. Both transverse and longitudinal imaging is necessary for an adequate examination (Figure 19-9). Sweep the transducer from side to side in both planes to demonstrate the full extent of the ocular structures, especially when the retinal periphery is being examined. If the patient is cooperative, instruct the patient to

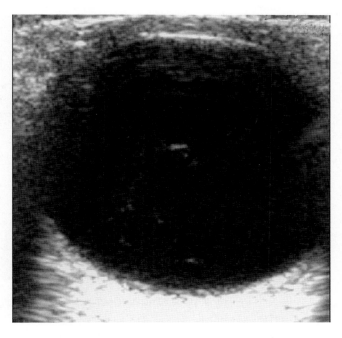

Figure 19-7. Artifacts are created by overgaining this image, and are seen in the near field as well as the periphery.

move their eye in all four quadrants to avoid missing any pathology. This allows the entire retina to be examined with less transducer movement. Also, movement of the eye is useful in classifying the type of detachment present. Movement of the detachment in response

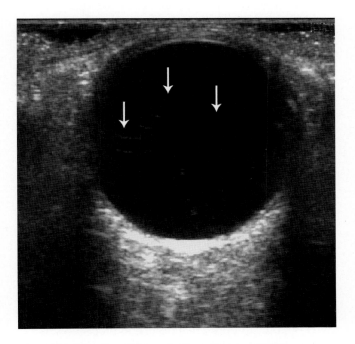

Figure 19-8. A subtle web-like abnormality is seen within the eye when the overall gain is increased (arrows).

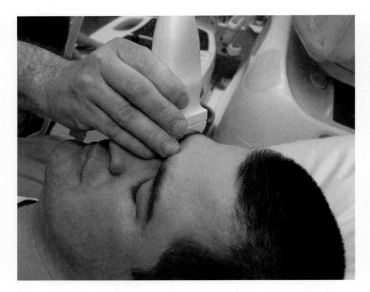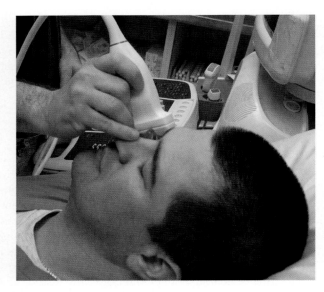

Figure 19-9. Transducer positions for longitudinal and transverse views are shown.

to rapid eye movements is referred to as "after movements." Vitreous detachments are very mobile and are often referred to as being "jiggly" in the ophthalmology literature. Retinal detachments move with eye motion, but to a lesser extent than vitreous detachments. Choroidal detachments do not demonstrate any movement with rapid eye movements.[17]

The optic nerve is seen traveling away from the globe posteriorly. The nerve itself is not seen with any great detail. Use minor changes in transducer angle to visualize the optic nerve sheath as clearly as possible. Measurement of the optic nerve sheath diameter is typically made 3 mm posterior to the optic disc. A measurement greater than 5 mm in adults is considered abnormal. Occasionally, the optic nerve sheath may appear dilated despite normal intracranial pressure. When measurements are in doubt, the 30° test can be used. Measurement of the optic nerve sheath is made in primary gaze and then after the patient shifts gaze 30° from primary. In cases of elevated intracranial pressure, the nerve and sheath are stretched with this maneuver and the fluid is distributed in the extended nerve sheath resulting in a smaller diameter than in primary gaze. If nerve sheath enlargement is secondary to parenchymal infiltration or thickening of the optic nerve, there will be no change in the nerve sheath measurement with a shift in gaze.

Color and spectral Doppler measurements are helpful in the diagnosis of several conditions. Blood flow in the retina and the region just posterior to the eye is readily identified with color or power Doppler. With PWD, graphical representation of the blood flow is depicted. When blood flow is evaluated the optic nerve is first located, then the vessels are identified using color Doppler followed by individual assessment with PWD,

as each vessel will have a typical waveform.[28] When interrogated with PWD, the ophthalmic artery tracing has a similar pattern to that of the internal carotid artery, containing a dicrotic notch. The central retinal artery waveform is more rounded and flat compared with that of the ophthalmic artery. Since Doppler ultrasound is a higher energy mode, it is recommended that these exams be as brief as possible, although no adverse effects have been reported.

► COMMON AND EMERGENT ABNORMALITIES

IRIS AND ANTERIOR CHAMBER EVALUATION

In some patients with facial trauma, assessing ocular and pupillary movements is difficult because of facial swelling. Using ultrasound, the iris is easily evaluated if the patient is able to cooperate with the examination. Ask the patient to look superiorly and place the transducer on the inferior portion of the globe in a transverse position. By sweeping the imaging sector cephalad, a frontal plane of the iris and pupil can be acquired. Measure the pupillary size and assess the function of the iris by shining a light in the uninjured eye (Video 19-2: Ocular Abnormal).

With a high-frequency transducer and the appropriate noncontact technique (see above), anterior chamber pathology can be visualized. A hyphema or hypopyon may display an echogenic area within the aqueous (Figure 19-10). Slit lamp examination is the preferred method for diagnosis, but ultrasound may have a role in patients with severe blepharospasm or swelling.

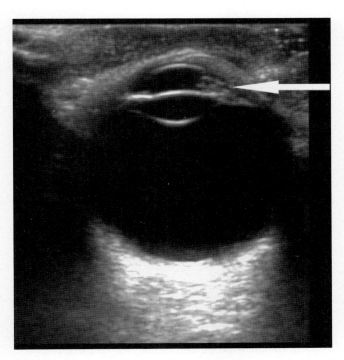

Figure 19-10. Hyphema. Longitudinal view of the eye shows an echogenic area (arrow) of settled blood within the inferior aqueous (dependent area in a sitting patient). Note: Scan carefully in the patient with a known hyphema as minimal pressure from exam or removing gel could potentially increase intraocular pressure and worsen bleeding. On the other hand, ultrasound may provide the only way to evaluate the posterior elements of the eye in the patient with a significant hyphema as these structures may not be visualized with the ophthalmoscope in this setting. (Courtesy of Charlotte Derr, MD)

EXTRAOCULAR MOVEMENTS

By visualizing eye movement in the orbit, extraocular muscle function can be assessed. If a muscle is entrapped by a fracture, movement will be limited.

VITREOUS HEMORRHAGE

Vitreous hemorrhage frequently accompanies major trauma to the face but can also be idiopathic or associated with retinal detachment, coagulopathy, diabetes mellitus, or central vein occlusion. The ultrasound appearance of vitreous hemorrhage depends on the age and severity of the hemorrhage. In fresh mild hemorrhages, small areas of mildly echogenic mobile vitreous opacities are seen (Figure 19-11). As the hemorrhage ages, particularly with severe hemorrhages, the blood first organizes (Figure 19-12) and then may form membranes. Sonographically, this appears as a vitreous filled with multiple large echogenic opacities. These opacities

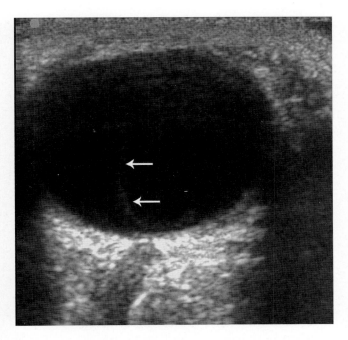

Figure 19-11. This vitreous hemorrhage could not be seen at normal gain settings. Turning the gain up significantly helped identify this strand of hemorrhage (arrows), which moved to and fro with eye movements.

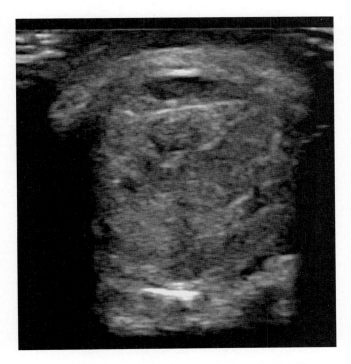

Figure 19-12. Severe intraocular hemorrhage. The posterior chamber contains a large organized hematoma. The anterior chamber also shows a hyphema. (Courtesy of Robert Reardon, MD)

may layer due to gravity. Occasionally, with a penetrating foreign body, a membrane will form over the tract. This tract may assist in localizing the foreign body.

GLOBE PERFORATION

Globe perforation is typically associated with some type of trauma. Sonographically, the globe may be decreased in size, indicating loss of pressure or vitreous. Buckling of the sclera may be seen posteriorly and vitreous hemorrhage is frequently present (Figure 19-13). Subtle perforations may be missed if little vitreous has been lost. A careful look at the anterior chamber is warranted as it may be collapsed from a small perforation.

FOREIGN BODIES

Ocular foreign bodies are easily identified with ultrasound in most cases. Even if previously detected with another imaging modality, foreign bodies can be more precisely localized with ultrasound.[30] Intraocular foreign bodies typically appear as highly reflective objects that may be located in the vitreous (accompanied by a vitreous hemorrhage), in the retina, or in the posterior orbital fat (Figure 19-14A). If embedded in the posterior orbital fat, the foreign body may be missed because of other highly echogenic structures in that region.[17] A strongly

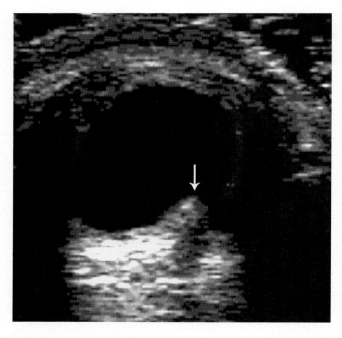

Figure 19-13. A collapsed globe from a penetrating injury showing a posterior fold (arrow).

reflective foreign body may produce a "twinkling" artifact with color Doppler (Figure 19-14B), which appears as a rapidly changing mixture of red and blue.[31] Twinkling occurs with any strong reflector including calcifications.

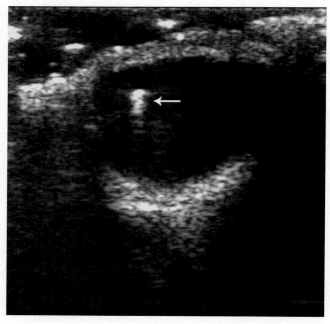

A

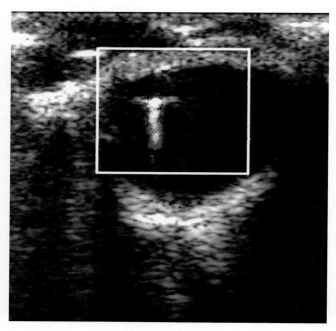

B

Figure 19-14. (A) A metallic foreign body (arrow) is seen in an eye that is starting to lose some of its shape due to vitreous extrusion. (B) The same foreign body is outlined with color Doppler, making detection much easier due to the comet-tail artifact.

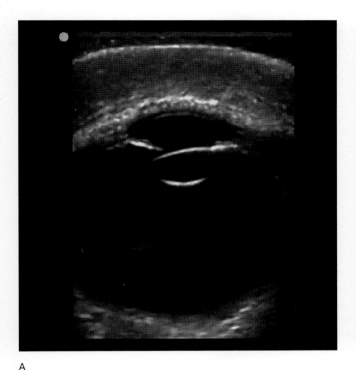

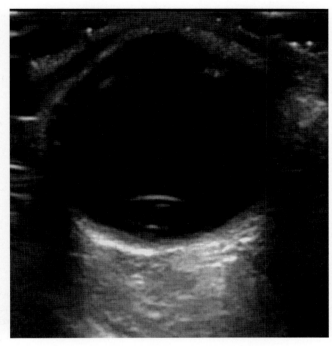

A   B

Figure 19-15. Lens dislocation. (A) Partial: An obvious subluxation of the lens is noted. A subtle finding may be enhanced by eye movements or consensual pupillary constriction. (B) Complete: The lens is located in the posterior vitreous. (Courtesy of Robert Reardon, MD)

DISLOCATION OF THE LENS

Dislocation of the lens is easily visualized when it is significant. Dislocations may be partial (subluxation) or complete (Figure 19-15). With a subluxation, the lens may initially appear to be normal. However, with eye movement, the lens appears to move independently of the surrounding structures. A complete dislocation is more obvious as the lens will be out of its usual position.

VITREOUS DETACHMENT

Vitreous detachment occurs most commonly as a normal consequence of aging, but may also occur from trauma or after intraocular surgery. A vitreous detachment often has a C-shaped, concave upward appearance sonographically. The vitreous membrane appears "jiggly" with eye movements, is thinner than a retinal detachment (may be a subtle difference), and is not attached to the margins of the optic disc. This latter point helps to differentiate this condition from posterior retinal detachment (Figure 19-16). If associated with a retinal detachment or tear, these can also occasionally result in a posterior hemorrhage.[17] A fibrinous vitreous membrane is sometimes seen when a vitreous hemorrhage leads to a retinal detachment.[17]

RETINAL DETACHMENT

Retinal detachments are important to recognize early as they may progress to full detachments and loss of vision if untreated. Retinal tears, the precursor to detachments, are difficult to see unless they are substantial. When visualized, retinal tears appear to be short, reflective, linear structures protruding into the vitreous.[17] Another clue to a retinal tear is the identification of subretinal fluid. Retinal detachments appear as a highly reflective membrane, which seems to "float" in the vitreous (Figure 19-17, Figure 19-18). In contrast to choroidal detachments, where the membrane does not change with eye movements, fresh or recent retinal detachments are mobile with eye movements.[17] As the retinal detachment ages, this flexibility is lost and the membrane becomes stiff and slightly thickened (Figure 19-19) When a retinal detachment becomes complete, a connection to the ora serrata is maintained anteriorly as well as posteriorly to the optic disc, and the membrane will have a V or funnel shape within the vitreous cavity. An incomplete retinal detachment that spans the posterior globe will

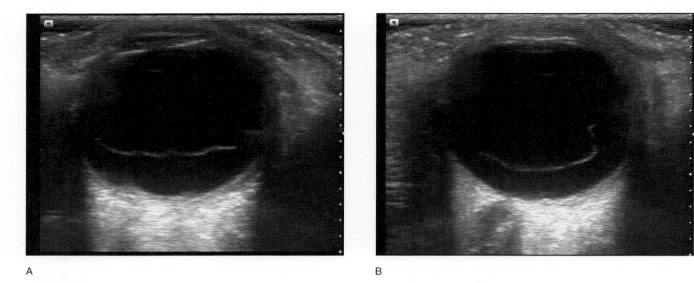

A   B

Figure 19-16. Posterior vitreous detachment. (A) A fine, lacy membrane stretches across the posterior globe. This structure was noted to float to and fro with eye movements. (B) Same patient after eye movement. The optic nerve is seen exiting the posterior globe. The vitreous membrane is *not* tethered to the margins of the optic disc. (Courtesy of James Mateer, MD)

also demonstrate tethering to the margins of the optic disc. This finding helps differentiate a retinal detachment from a vitreous detachment (Figures 19-1 and 19-16).

CHOROIDAL DETACHMENT

Choroidal detachment is the separation of the choroid from the sclera due to blood accumulation from ruptured vessels. This condition is occasionally seen after trauma to the eye or face. It occurs most frequently after intraocular surgery. Choroidal detachment appears as a smooth, dome-shaped, thick structure (or structures, if multiple hemorrhages occur simultaneously) separated from the posterior aspect of the eye (Figure 19-20). If these domes become large enough to touch in the vitreous, this is referred to a "kiss." Although the choroid itself does not display motion (after movement) with eye movement, echogenic blood inside the choroidal detachment may move with eye movements.

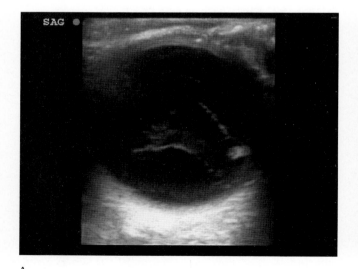 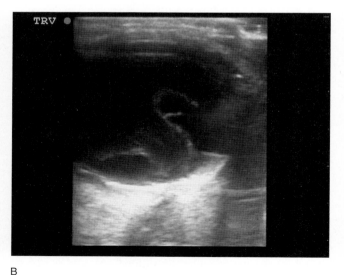

A   B

Figure 19-17. Retinal detachment, acute. (A) Funnel-shaped retinal detachment is noted with associated vitreous hemorrhage. The detached retina floats to different positions with eye movements. (B) In a different plane, optic nerve is now visible and the tethering point to the optic disc is visible. (Courtesy of Charlotte Derr, MD)

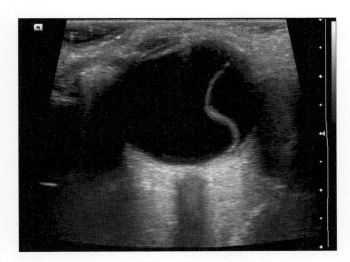

Figure 19-18. Retinal detachment, acute. The floating membrane is notably thicker than a typical posterior vitreous detachment and also does not include the area anterior to the optic disc. (Courtesy of Mark Schultz, DO)

RETROBULBAR HEMATOMA/HEMORRHAGE

A retrobulbar hematoma is seen as an echolucency just posterior to the globe. Since the orbit is a closed space, pressure may be exerted on the posterior globe by the hematoma. This pressure can be seen sonographically

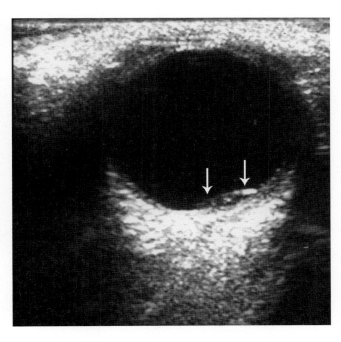

Figure 19-20. A small choroid detachment is seen posteriorly in the eye (arrows).

as a distortion in the posterior aspect of the eye (Figure 19-21). As the blood accumulates, retinal vasculature may become compressed and changes in the spectral Doppler pattern of the retinal vessels may also be seen. While ultrasound imaging can be very useful in

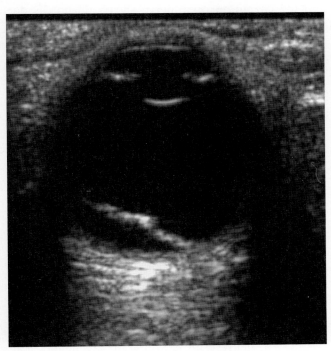

Figure 19-19. Retinal detachment, chronic. An incomplete retinal detachment is seen across the posterolateral globe. The optic nerve is not visible in this view. (Courtesy of Charlotte Derr, MD)

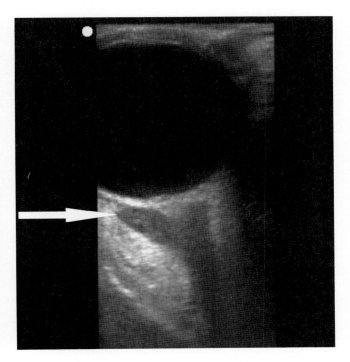

Figure 19-21. Retrobulbar hematoma. An ovoid hematoma (arrow) is located adjacent to the distal optic nerve sheath. (Courtesy of Robert Reardon, MD)

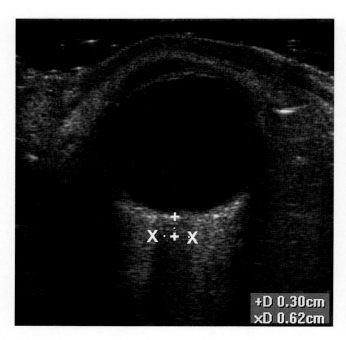

Figure 19-22. A wide optic nerve sheath is measured posterior to the globe (0.62 cm).

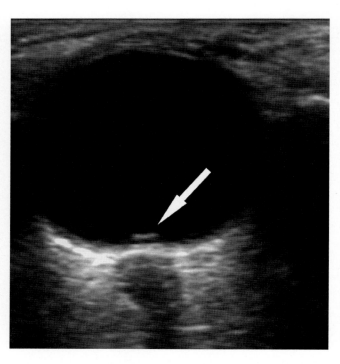

Figure 19-23. The "crescent sign" is the sonographic equivalent of papilledema.

suspected cases of retrobulbar hematoma, hemorrhage may be difficult or impossible to visualize because the blood may be isoechoic to the other posterior structures. There is a paucity of research concerning the sensitivity and accuracy of ultrasound for determining the presence of a retrobulbar hematoma in the emergency setting.

OPTIC NERVE

The optic nerve and its surrounding sheath are located posterior to the globe (Figure 19-3). When assessing for possible elevated intracranial pressure, optic nerve sheath diameter measurements are taken 3 mm posterior to the optic disc (Figure 19-4). Maximum measurements vary with age. As mentioned previously, the upper limit in adults is 5 mm, children is 4.5 mm, and infants is 4 mm.[2,27] Increasing optic nerve sheath diameter correlates well with increasing intracranial pressure (Figure 19-22). Measurements typically plateau at approximately 7.5 mm even with extremely high intracranial pressure. In cases where the intracranial pressure has been elevated for some time, one can see an echolucent circle within the optic nerve sheath separating the sheath from the optic nerve. This is referred to as the "crescent sign" (Figure 19-23) and is a corollary to funduscopic papilledema. Cadaveric-based research has shown that dilation of the optic nerve sheath occurs simultaneously with elevation of the intracranial pressure. However, the amount of dilation of the optic nerve sheath is not initially proportional to the change in intracra-

nial pressure.[32] It is assumed that variation in the rate of change between the intracranial pressure elevation and the change in optic nerve sheath dilation is due to a redistribution of the cerebrospinal fluid. Furthermore, the development of the crescent sign does not occur immediately with elevated intracranial pressure. The amount of time required to develop the crescent sign is not known. However, this sign is often seen in conditions with chronically elevated intracranial pressure such as pseudotumor cerebri.

▶ COMMON VARIANTS AND SELECTED ABNORMALITIES

MASSES

During the emergency ocular ultrasound examination, other nonemergent abnormalities may be encountered. One example is the incidental discovery of a mass. Symptoms of primary ocular cancer or metastatic disease involving the eye include blurry vision, distorted vision, blind spots, white pupils, red eye, eye pain, and vision loss. Many of these symptoms are neither specific nor sensitive for cancer. Furthermore, many ocular tumors produce no symptoms at all. The review and description of ocular tumors are beyond the scope of this chapter. The detection of a potential mass requires ophthalmologic follow-up.

RETINOSCHISIS

Retinoschisis is a separation in the layers of the retina and may occasionally be encountered in the emergency setting. Differentiating retinoschisis from a retinal detachment is difficult. By ultrasound, retinoschisis is more focal, smooth, and dome-shaped than a retinal detachment. In the emergency setting, differentiation between the two processes is not as critical as identifying the abnormality on ultrasound and obtaining ophthalmologic consultation.

CENTRAL RETINAL ARTERY AND VEIN

Central retinal vein or artery occlusion may present as painless visual loss that may or may not be complete. Utilizing color and PWD just behind the globe will allow an evaluation of the blood supply to the eye (Figure 19-24). Color Doppler typically shows two directions of blood flow (usually red toward and blue away from the transducer). Placing a PWD gate over each flow direction will allow observation of venous and arterial flow patterns (Figure 19-25A,B). The absence of either arterial or venous flow on the PWD strongly suggests a vascular cause in the patient with sudden and painless loss of vision. The use of Doppler ultrasound to evaluate these conditions generally requires significant experience, however, since abnormalities are usually unilateral, comparison of flow in the affected and unaffected eyes may allow relatively inexperienced providers to obtain valuable information.[28]

AGE-RELATED VITREOUS CHANGES

With age, syneresis (shrinkage of the vitreous humour) often leads to posterior vitreous detachment, which is benign unless hemorrhage or a retinal tear occurs. As

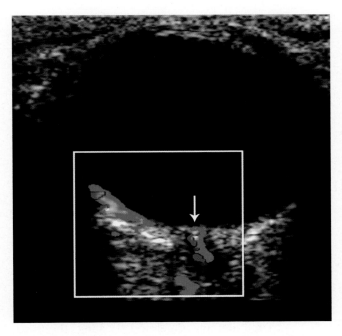

Figure 19-24. Normal arterial and venous flow is detected posterior to the globe (arrow).

a result of syneresis, or contraction and degeneration of the vitreous gel, a posterior vitreous separation may occur. Another benign condition occasionally detected by ultrasound is asteroid hyalosis. This appears as multiple pinpoint and highly reflective vitreous opacities due to reflective calcium salts that are accumulated in the vitreous.

INTRAOCULAR PRESSURE ELEVATION

Elevated intraocular pressure may be noted with PWD. As the intraocular pressure rises, the central retinal artery

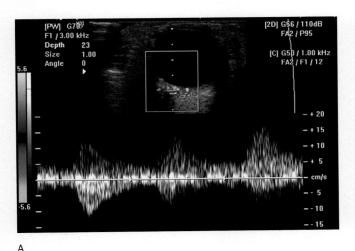

A

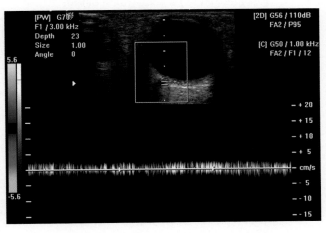

B

Figure 19-25. Pulsed wave Doppler is utilized to confirm normal arterial (A) and (B) venous flow posterior to the globe.

is compressed. With progressive compression, the peak systolic velocity (PSV) and the end-diastolic velocity (EDV) of the central retinal artery decrease. In addition, the resistive index (RI) of the central retinal artery increases. The RI is the ratio of the difference in the PSV and the EDV divided by the PSV $\{RI = (PSV - EDV)/PSV\}$.[29] One study that evaluated a healthy eye model showed that these measured differences in flow could accurately predict the presence of elevated intraocular pressure.[33]

▶ PITFALLS

1. **Safety issues.** From the standpoint of worsening an underlying injury, an ultrasound examination of the eye is safe if the techniques described in this chapter are followed. In patients with a potential globe perforation, ocular ultrasound may be safely performed by using a large amount of gel and "floating" the transducer on the gel, so that the transducer does not make contact with the eyelid or create any pressure on the globe. This can be verified and documented during the examination by visualizing an anechoic gap on the ultrasound image between the transducer surface and the skin surface of the eyelid. Like any ultrasound examination, the amount of energy exposure of any tissue should be limited to what is necessary for the examination. This is especially true when using Doppler ultrasound. PWD in particular is of higher intensity than normal B-mode ultrasound. Modern diagnostic ultrasound machines are manufactured with a maximum output power that is very unlikely to produce heating or damage to the tissues; however, there are no long-term data available with regard to the absolute safety of ocular ultrasound.

2. **Inadequate amount of gel.** Ultrasound gel is essential for an adequate examination and should be used liberally. The gel acts as a medium to couple the transducer to the skin surface, decreasing the impedance between these two interfaces. When an inadequate amount of gel is used, artifacts are more frequent and image quality deteriorates. Furthermore, the clinician may be tempted to push harder on the globe to increase contact. With a perforated globe, this can exacerbate the injury.

3. **Confusing pathology.** In clinical practice, there can be overlap in sonographic findings among various retinal abnormalities. A retinal detachment can be confused on ultrasound with a posterior vitreous detachment. Both have similar initial presentations. However, posterior vitreous detachments are often a benign process, whereas a retinal detachment can be an ophthalmologic emergency. The development of a fixed visual field deficit suggests retinal detachment. The presence (retinal detachment) or absence (posterior vitreous detachment) of tethering of the membrane to the margins of the optic disc can also be very helpful for differentiating these two entities.

4. **Retinal tears.** Ocular ultrasound is more sensitive than direct visualization for the detection of retinal detachments. This is also true for the detection of vitreous hemorrhage. However, retinal tears can be quite small and difficult to locate. Therefore, when the history is indicative of a retinal tear or detachment, but none is visualized using ultrasound, the emergency physician should consider ophthalmologic consultation or urgent referral.

▶ CASE STUDIES

CASE 1

Patient Presentation

A 32-year-old woman presented to the ED from the scene of a motor vehicle crash. She was intoxicated and was the unrestrained driver of a car that collided head on with another car. The patient was unconscious and hypotensive on arrival despite 3 L of IV crystalloid en route. Shortly after the primary survey, a trauma ultrasound examination was performed and showed a large amount of free intraperitoneal fluid. Obvious facial trauma and a midface fracture were noted just prior to endotracheal intubation. The pupils were 6 mm and sluggishly reactive bilaterally. There was concern about the possibility of severe head injury, but the trauma surgeon wanted to take the patient to the operating room immediately.

Management Course

An ocular ultrasound examination was performed and revealed normal ocular structures. The optic nerve sheaths measured 6.4 mm on the right and 6.3 mm on the left. Given this information, the trauma surgeon elected to obtain a head CT while the patient received a rapid blood and plasma infusion. Head CT showed a large epidural hematoma and the neurosurgeon joined the operating team. The patient was found to have a large splenic laceration and her spleen was removed. The epidural hematoma was evacuated. Despite repeated setbacks and two more trips to the operating room, the patient recovered, left the hospital 5 weeks later, and was able to care for herself and resume her office job.

Commentary

Case 1 illustrates a very high-risk and unstable patient. Risking a trip to the radiology suite for CT could have been disastrous if the patient had uncontrolled intraperitoneal hemorrhage. However, an expanding epidural hematoma would also have rapidly led to the patient's demise if not treated expeditiously. A rapid and noninvasive evaluation of intracranial pressure through optic nerve sheath measurement allowed the treating physicians to suspect a space-occupying lesion that required immediate attention.

CASE 2

Patient Presentation

A 35-year-old man presented to the ED with complaints of left visual difficulties. He stated that for the last 12 hours his vision in the left eye had been considerably worse than before. He was not specific about any deficits. He denied trauma or prior visual problems. He did not wear glasses and denied any other medical problems.

Management Course

Visual acuity testing revealed 20/200 vision in the left eye and 20/20 in the right eye. Ophthalmoscopic examination showed a normal-appearing fundus and generally normal-appearing retina. No detachment was noted. A point-of-care ultrasound examination was performed on the affected eye. The anterior chamber and lens appeared to be normal. The retina was obviously detached on the nasal side of the eye with the central portion extending toward but preserving the macula. An ophthalmologist was contacted. The ophthalmologist examined the patient in the ED, reviewed the ultrasound images, and agreed with the diagnosis. The patient was taken to the ophthalmology suite for urgent repair of the retinal detachment.

Commentary

Case 2 demonstrates how ocular ultrasound can significantly add vital information in the ED. The globe is an ideal organ to scan, and ophthalmologists rely heavily on ocular ultrasound in many cases. A rapid and reliable diagnosis can be made.

CASE 3

Patient Presentation

A 59-year-old diabetic woman presented to the ED complaining of waxing and waning vision in her right eye. It started approximately 12 hours before the presentation. The patient denied any similar symptoms in the past. She had not had any facial or head trauma. The patient did not wear corrective lenses and normally had good vision. Physical examination revealed 20/20 vision in the left eye with normal fields. With the right eye the patient was only able to see light and some general shapes, but could not read the Snellen chart. There was no tenderness on palpation of the globe, corneal staining did not reveal any abnormalities, and intraocular pressures were normal.

Management Course

An ocular ultrasound examination was performed and showed no structural abnormality in the right eye. The lens was in good position and there was no retinal or vitreous detachment. Color Doppler interrogation posterior to the globe revealed blood flow in the area of the central retinal vein and artery. However, only one color (blue) was noted and denoted flow away from the globe (Figure 19-26). PWD was added and showed an obvious venous tracing but no arterial flow could be located. The ophthalmologist was consulted and agreed with the diagnosis of central retinal artery occlusion. The patient was treated urgently by the ophthalmologist and regained partial vision.

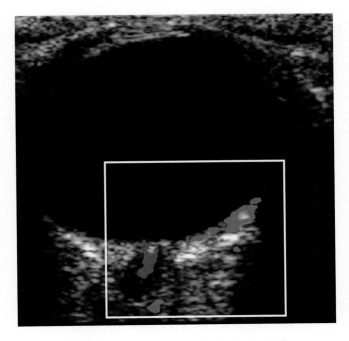

Figure 19-26. This patient had only venous flow visualized on color Doppler (blue, or leading away from the transducer). Pulsed wave Doppler interrogation confirmed absence of arterial waveforms.

Commentary

Case 3 demonstrates the expanded diagnostic capability of the ocular ultrasound. Structures posterior to the globe lend themselves readily to color and power Doppler interrogation as well as evaluation with pulsed Doppler, allowing for confirmation of appropriate blood flow to and from the eye.

► ACKNOWLEDGMENT

The authors thank Dr. Michael Blaivas for his contribution on the previous edition of this chapter.

REFERENCES

1. Blaivas M: Bedside emergency department ultrasonography in the evaluation of ocular pathology. *Acad Emerg Med* 7:947–950, 2000.
2. Blaivas M, Theodoro D, Sierzenski P: A study of bedside ocular ultrasonography in the emergency department. *Acad Emerg Med* 9:791–799, 2002.
3. Orawiec B, Gralek M, Stefanczyk L, et al.: Applicability of ultrasound in ocular tumors in children and adolescents. *Klin Oczna* 107:437–441, 2005.
4. Jehle D (Senior Editor), Bouvet S, Braden B, et al.: *Emergency Ultrasound of the Eye and Orbit.* Buffalo, NY: Grover Cleveland Press, 2011.
5. Costantino TG, Parikh AK, Satz WA, et al.: Ultrasonography-guided peripheral intravenous access versus traditional approaches in patients with difficult intravenous access. *Ann Emerg Med* 46:456–461, 2005.
6. Brannam L, Blaivas M, Lyon M, et al.: Emergency nurses' utilization of ultrasound guidance for placement of peripheral intravenous lines in difficult-access patients. *Acad Emerg Med* 11:1361–1363, 2004.
7. Theodoro D, Blaivas M, Duggal S, et al.: Real-time B-mode ultrasound in the ED saves time in the diagnosis of deep vein thrombosis (DVT). *Am J Emerg Med* 22:197–200, 2004.
8. Lizzy F, Coleman D: History of opthalmic ultrasound. *J Ultrasound Med* 23:1255–1266, 2004.
9. Papadopoulos A, Fotinos A, Maniatis V, et al.: Assessment of intraocular foreign bodies by helical-CT multiplanar imaging. *Eur Radiol* 11:1502–1505, 2001.
10. Shiver SA, Lyon M, Blaivas M: Detection of metallic ocular foreign bodies with handheld sonography in a porcine model. *J Ultrasound Med* 24:1341–1346, 2005.
11. Larian B, Wong B, Crumley RL, et al.: Facial trauma and ocular/orbital injury. *J Cranio-Maxillofacial Trauma* 5:15–24, 1999.
12. Perry M, Dancey A, Mireskandari K, et al.: Emergency care in facial trauma—A maxillofacial and ophthalmic perspective. *Injury, Int J Care Injured* 36:875–896, 2005.
13. Pelletier CR, Jordan DR, Braga R, et al.: Assessment of ocular trauma associated with head and neck injuries. *J Trauma* 44:350–354, 1998.
14. Grossman MD, Roberts DM, Carr CC: Ophthalmologic aspects of orbital injury. *Clin Plast Surg* 19:71–85, 1992.
15. Rosdeutsher JD, Stadelmann WK: Diagnosis and treatment of retrobulbar hematoma resulting from blunt periorbital trauma. *Ann Plastic Surg* 41:618–622, 1998.
16. Bailey WK, Kuo PC, Evans LS: Diagnosis and treatment of retrobulbar haemorrhage. *J Oral Maxillofac Surg* 51:780–782, 1993.
17. Fielding J: Ultrasound imaging of the eye through the closed lid using a non-dedicated scanner. *Clin Radiol* 38:131–135, 1987.
18. Joseph DP, Pieramici DJ, Beauchamp NJ: Computed tomography in the diagnosis and prognosis of open-globe injuries. *Ophthalmology* 107:1899–1906, 2000.
19. Kwong JS, Munk PL, Lin DTC, et al.: Real-time sonography in ocular trauma. *Am J Roentgenol* 158:179–182, 1992.
20. Rabinowitz R, Yagev R, Shoham A, et al.: Comparison between clinical and ultrasound findings in patients with vitreous hemorrhage. 18:253–256, 2004.
21. Gariano R, Kim C: Evaluation and management of suspected retinal detachment. *Am Fam Physician* 69:1691–1698, 2004.
22. Yonemoto J, Noda Y, Masuhara N, et al.: Age of onset of posterior vitreous detachment. *Curr Opin Ophthalmol* 7(3):73–76, 1996.
23. Brod RD, Lightman DA, Packer AJ, et al.: Correlation between vitreous pigment granules and retinal breaks in eyes with acute posterior vitreous detachment. *Ophthalmology* 98:1366–1369, 1991.
24. Hayreh S: The sheath of the optic nerve. *Ophthalmologica* 189:54–63, 1984.
25. Blaivas M, Theodoro D, Sierzenski P: Elevated intracranial pressure detected by bedside emergency ultrasonography of the optic nerve sheath. *Acad Emerg Med* 10:376–381, 2003.
26. Tsung J, Blaivas M, Cooper A, et al.: A rapid noninvasive method of detecting elevated intracranial pressure using bedside ocular ultrasound: Application to 3 cases of head trauma in the pediatric emergency department. *Pediatr Emerg Care* 21:94–98, 2005.
27. Newman W, Holliman A, Dutton G, et al.: Measurement of optic nerve sheath diameter by ultrasound: A means of detecting acute raised intracranial pressure in hydrocephalus. *Br J Ophthalmol* 86:1009–1113, 2002.
28. Williamson T, Harris A: Color Doppler ultrasound imaging of the eye and orbit. 40:255–267, 1996.
29. Martini E, Guiducci M, Campi L, et al.: Ocular blood flow evaluation in injured and healthy fellow eyes. *Eur J Ophthalmol* 15:48–55, 2005.
30. McNicholas MM, Brophy DP, Power WJ, et al.: Ocular trauma: Evaluation with US. *Radiology* 423–427, 1995.
31. Ustymowicz A, Krejza J, Mariak Z: Twinkling artifact in color Doppler imaging of the orbit. *J Ultrasound Med* 21:559–563, 2002.
32. Lyon M, Ganapathy P, Burbacher T, et al.: Time correlation of optic nerve sheath diameter to increasing intracranial pressure in a cadaveric model. *Annals of Emergency Medicine* 58(4):S273, 2011.
33. Chung H, Harris A, Evans D, et al.: Vascular aspects in the pathophysiology of glaucomatous optic neuropathy. *Survey Ophthalmol* 43:s43–s50, 1999.

CHAPTER 20

Pediatric Applications

Jason W. Fischer, Adam B. Sivitz, and Alyssa M. Abo

The role of point-of-care ultrasound in the emergent care of ill and injured pediatric patients continues to evolve and mature. Ultrasound technology is ideally suited for infants and children as it allows real-time visualization of anatomic structures without causing pain, requiring sedation, or exposing developing tissues to ionizing radiation.

There are numerous indications for emergency ultrasound common to both adult and pediatric emergency care. This has led to a greater understanding of the differences that exist when the same applications are used for both pediatric and adult patients. In addition, the functionality of emergency ultrasound has been further expanded by recent innovation and the development of several pediatric-specific applications.

▶ TRAUMA

Trauma remains one of the leading causes of morbidity and mortality in children. In the United States, traumatic injuries result in hospital admission for approximately 600,000 children each year.[1] In the pediatric age group, blunt trauma is more prevalent than penetrating trauma, and 20–30% of pediatric trauma cases involve the abdomen.[2]

The history and physical examination form the foundation of the patient evaluation; however, they may be difficult to obtain in children who have altered mental status, CNS trauma, or distracting injuries. In one study of children with blunt abdominal trauma, an initial physical examination was considered reliable in only 41% of cases.[3] Furthermore, the exam may be misleading in up to 45% of injured children.[4,5]

The use of ultrasound in pediatric trauma with the focused assessment with sonography for trauma (FAST) examination has increased over the past decade, but it has not been as well accepted or widely used as it has for adult trauma care. In a survey of general emergency physicians, pediatric emergency physicians, and trauma surgeons, 91% of the respondents considered abdominal ultrasound to be "somewhat to extremely useful."[6] However, with regard to pediatric trauma patients, 73% of all respondents considered abdominal ultrasound to be useful, while only 57% of pediatric emergency physicians considered it so. Furthermore, only 14% of pediatric emergency physicians routinely use abdominal ultrasound for evaluation of their trauma patients.[6]

Numerous advantages exist for using ultrasound in pediatric trauma, mirroring its benefits in adult trauma (see Chapter 5, "Trauma"). In pediatrics, limiting the exposure of ionizing radiation is especially appealing.[7] The results of a large prospective multicenter trial were recently reported, and showed that pediatric trauma patients with a low-to-moderate clinical suspicion for intra-abdominal injury were significantly less likely to undergo abdominal CT scanning if they underwent a FAST exam.[8]

CLINICAL CONSIDERATIONS

The 1980s saw a transition away from diagnostic peritoneal lavage toward the use of abdominal CT. CT is still the most commonly used modality in evaluating pediatric abdominal injuries.[9–18] The primary advantage of CT is that it accurately and reliably identifies and characterizes most intraperitoneal and retroperitoneal

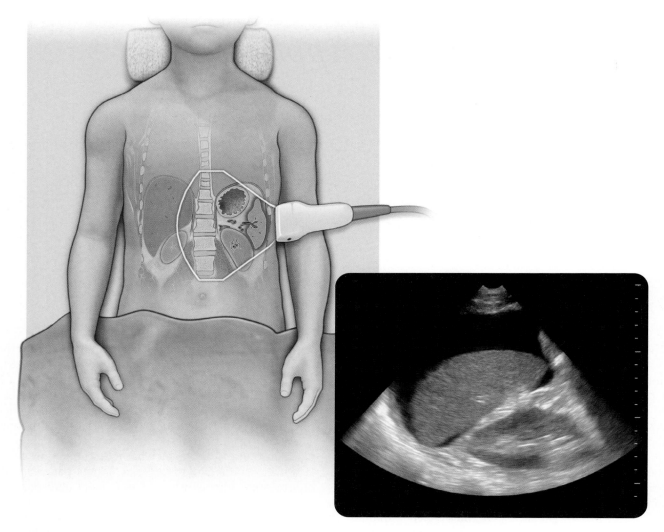

Figure 20-1. Hemoperitoneum. Ultrasound techniques and findings are outlined in the corresponding sections of this chapter.

injuries. A major disadvantage of CT is that it exposes patients to significant doses of ionizing radiation. Children are 10 times more sensitive to the induction of cancer than adults, and one study estimates that a single abdominal CT in a young girl results in a risk of fatal cancer later in life of approximately 1 in 1,000.[19] Some physicians have questioned the widespread use of CT and advocate the use of ultrasound for screening pediatric blunt trauma patients.[20–22]

The FAST examination is a noninvasive diagnostic tool for detecting hemoperitoneum, hemopericardium, and hemothorax (Figure 20-1).[6] A systematic review assessed 25 studies consisting of 3838 children undergoing abdominal ultrasound after sustaining trauma. All studies were observational and the methodology, ultrasound protocols, and outcome definitions were all highly variable. The meta-analysis showed that the FAST exam had a sensitivity of 80% for identifying hemoperitoneum.[23]

The sensitivity fell to 66% when patients with intra-abdominal injuries, but without hemoperitoneum, were included.[23] Over one-third of pediatric solid organ injuries are not associated with free intraperitoneal fluid,[26,27] and failure to identify patients with intra-abdominal injury without hemoperitoneum is a known limitation of the abdominal ultrasound examination and is not considered a reasonable outcome measure for FAST by most providers.[26,28]

A prospective observational study evaluated the test characteristics of the FAST examination to detect any amount of fluid as well as clinically significant fluid in pediatric patients who suffered blunt abdominal trauma.[24] Test characteristics for detection of *significant* intra-abdominal fluid show a sensitivity of 52% and a specificity of 96%. Clinically significant fluid was defined as moderate free fluid on abdominal CT scans or if patients went directly to the operating room for intra-abdominal injury. When evaluating the test characteristics of the FAST for detection of any intraperitoneal fluid the sensitivity dropped to 20%, while the specificity remained high at 98%. These data suggest that the FAST exam is useful when positive; however, when it is negative, it does not exclude the presence of intra-abdominal injury.

The clinical utility of the FAST exam as a screening tool that can potentially decrease the use of CT is not addressed in the pediatric trauma literature. But as in adults, the FAST exam is very sensitive for hemoperitoneum in pediatric patients who are hypotensive as the result of intraperitoneal blood loss.[25]

The E-FAST or "extended" FAST examination includes evaluation of the lungs for pneumothorax. Use of the E-FAST examination has been well established in adults (see Chapter 5, "Trauma"). Ultrasound evaluation for pneumothorax has been shown to be more sensitive (98%) than a supine chest radiograph (76%) in adult trauma patients, when compared to CT as the gold standard.[29] A case report from a neonatal special care nursery had a similar finding.[30] The E-FAST examination can be performed at the bedside in 3 minutes or less[31,32] and is easily repeatable.

CLINICAL INDICATIONS

An extended point-of-care ultrasound examination is indicated in children with:

- Significant abdominal or thoracic trauma
- Patients with unexplained hypotension
- Patients with altered mental status

Significant Abdominal or Thoracic Trauma

A complete E-FAST exam should be performed on all pediatric patients with significant blunt or penetrating thoracoabdominal trauma as part of the secondary survey. In hemodynamically unstable pediatric trauma patients, the E-FAST examination may rapidly identify an abdominal or thoracic source of hypotension and assist with decision making regarding timing of diagnostic testing versus operative intervention. The abdominal portion of the E-FAST exam has the best test performance in children who are hemodynamically unstable with significant hemoperitoneum.[25] If free intraperitoneal fluid is identified, and the patient remains hypotensive after a bolus of IV fluid, the decision to perform exploratory laparotomy should be considered. If the patient stabilizes with a fluid bolus, abdominal CT scanning may be considered to guide selective laparotomy.

The E-FAST examination may also allow for prioritization of imaging studies in hemodynamically stable patients after initial evaluation and resuscitation. Patients with positive E-FAST examinations are typically triaged to abdominal CT with greater expediency than those patients with normal E-FAST examinations. E-FAST may also be useful in evaluating alert, hemodynamically stable pediatric trauma patients without abdominal tenderness, who would otherwise not routinely undergo abdominal CT, and who may occasionally have intra-abdominal injuries.

In hemodynamically stable patients, the information provided by a negative E-FAST examination may be sufficient for the clinician to decide against abdominal CT.[8,23] It may be prudent to admit such patients for observation and serial ultrasound and physical exams. Patients who are hemodynamically stable and have a negative E-FAST examination should undergo abdominal CT scanning if they demonstrate peritoneal signs, abdominal distention, seat belt abrasion, hematuria, or persistent tachycardia.

The E-FAST examination is also indicated in pediatric patients with penetrating trauma. The main benefit of using the E-FAST exam in penetrating thoracoabdominal trauma is not necessarily to rule out injury and avoid CT scanning, but to quickly identify which body cavity is injured to guide the sequence of surgical exploration or management.

ANATOMICAL CONSIDERATIONS

The FAST examination was designed to assess the three primary dependent areas of the peritoneal cavity (right upper quadrant, left upper quadrant, and pelvis) along with the thoracic cavity. The location of the fluid depends primarily on the source of the bleeding, but may be affected by the position of the patient. For the purpose of understanding the anatomy as it relates to the FAST examination, the abdomen is divided into quadrants by the mesentery of the transverse colon horizontally and by the spine vertically (see Figure 5-6A). Relevant anatomy needs to be identified in order to evaluate for surrounding intra-abdominal, thoracic, or pericardial fluid. There are some pediatric considerations, which are discussed below.

In the right upper quadrant, Morison's pouch is the potential space between the liver and the right kidney and represents the most dependent supramesocolic area. Blood from a liver laceration will accumulate in this area; blood from a splenic injury may also spill over the lumbar spine into Morison's pouch. Blood from an inframesocolic injury can spread over the sacral promontory into Morison's pouch as well via the right paracolic gutter. Since most major blunt abdominal injuries involve the liver and spleen, the view of Morison's pouch is regarded as the most important of the four views in the FAST examination in adults.[33] Alone, it has been found to be 51–82% sensitive in detecting free fluid.[34–36] In pediatric patients, however, free fluid tends to accumulate in the pelvis.[37]

Blood from a splenic injury will accumulate first in the left subphrenic space. There is no equivalent of Morison's pouch as the splenorenal ligament attaches the spleen and kidney. Therefore, intraperitoneal fluid accumulates circumferentially around the spleen: commonly below the diaphragm, at the inferior pole of the spleen, and less so in the splenorenal fossa. Blood from this area can flow into Morison's pouch, and will preferentially reach the pelvis by spilling down the right paracolic gutter because the left upper quadrant is separated from the left paracolic gutter by the phrenicocolic ligament.[38]

Blood from inframesocolic injuries will accumulate first in the rectovesicular pouch in boys and the retrouterine pouch of Douglas in girls. These areas are the most dependent portions of the peritoneal cavity.[38] One study found an isolated pelvic view to be 68% sensitive in detecting free intraperitoneal fluid.[34] In children, the pelvis view is the region most likely to be positive if a patient has intra-abdominal free fluid due to an isolated liver or spleen laceration.[37]

Ultrasound examination of pneumothorax is based on observation of sliding of the visceral pleura of the lung on the parietal pleura of the chest wall. In a supine trauma patient, thoracic air tends to accumulate between the anterior chest wall and the lung, separating the parietal and visceral pleurae.

The classic FAST view of the heart is the subxiphoid view. In children, this view may be limited due to air in the stomach, from crying, or from bag mask ventilation. If the subxiphoid view is insufficient, consider the parasternal long-axis view of the heart. This view will visualize the right and left ventricles, left atrium, aortic and mitral valves, the pericardium, and the descending aorta. The descending aorta is the landmark used to differentiate pericardial from pleural effusions posterior to the heart.

TECHNIQUE AND NORMAL ULTRASOUND FINDINGS

The FAST examination of pediatric patients consists of subxiphoid, right and left upper quadrant, and suprapubic views, which are identical to those in adults (Figure 20-2; Video 20-1: Pediatric Considerations). The E-FAST examination adds bilateral lung views to assess for pneumothorax. Views of the hemidiaphragms and caudal thorax, to assess for hemothorax, should be obtained with the right and left upper quadrant views. Use a low-frequency transducer between 2 and 6 MHz (includes the phased-array transducer and curvilinear or convex transducers) in children. Phased-array transduc-

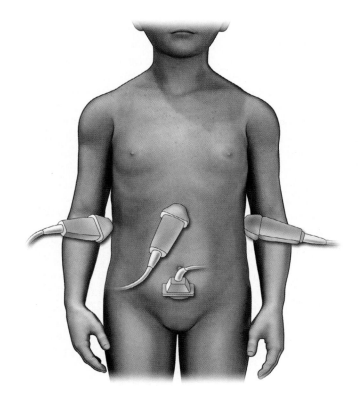

Figure 20-2. FAST examination transducer placement.

ers are preferred for younger children as the flat, small footprint allows for better imaging between the ribs. Some authors recommend using a 5.0 MHz (or even 7.5–10 MHz) transducer for finer resolution.[21,39] The E-FAST examination should be performed with the patient supine, which is how the patient is transported on a backboard after blunt trauma. By convention, the index marker on the transducer should be directed cephalad or to the patient's right. Move the transducer up or down one or more rib spaces to optimize the view.

Splenic or hepatic injuries account for 74% of cases of hemoperitoneum in pediatric blunt trauma.[40] With the index marker cephalad, place the transducer in a coronal plane in the mid to anterior axillary line at the 10th intercostal space or below (Figure 20-3). The kidney lies retroperitoneal, so direct the transducer dorsally to maximize the view of the liver–kidney interface. Rotate the transducer counterclockwise and align it with the intercostal space to minimize shadowing. Sliding or tilting the transducer cephalad brings the lower thorax into view, displaying the mirror image artifact of the liver above the diaphragm (Figure 20-4).

Visualize the diaphragm superiorly and the tip of the liver inferiorly. Scan the inferior pole of the kidney to

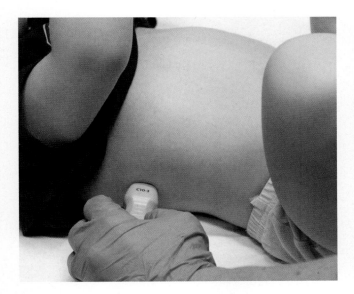

Figure 20-3. FAST examination transducer placement for RUQ.

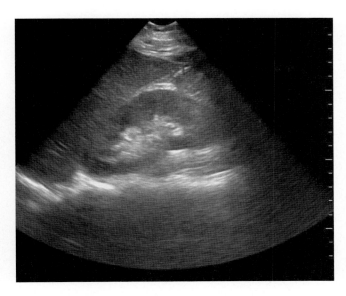

Figure 20-5. Ultrasound: Normal RUQ view, including inferior pole of the liver.

assess for free intraperitoneal fluid in the right paracolic gutter. Visualization of the inferior pole of the liver is necessary since free fluid may accumulate there before progressing to Morison's pouch (Figure 20-5).

The goal of the left upper quadrant view is to examine the potential space around the spleen, between the spleen and the diaphragm, and around the inferior pole of the spleen. With the index marker cephalad, place the transducer in the posterior axillary line in the coronal plane at the 9th intercostal space or below

(Figure 20-6). Rotate the transducer clockwise and align it with the intercostal space to minimize rib shadows. Inspect the lower left thorax for intrathoracic blood, as described above. Visualize the diaphragm superiorly and the lower pole of the spleen inferiorly (Figure 20-7). Scan the inferior pole of the left kidney to evaluate for intraperitoneal fluid in the paracolic gutter.

Scan the pelvis for free intraperitoneal fluid with both transverse and sagittal views. The bladder is used as a landmark to evaluate for hemoperitoneum.

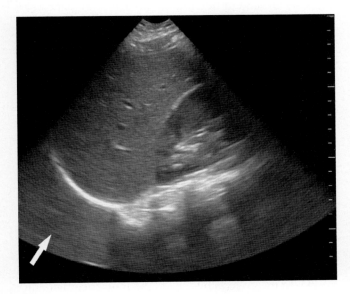

Figure 20-4. Ultrasound: Normal RUQ view with mirror image artifact (arrow).

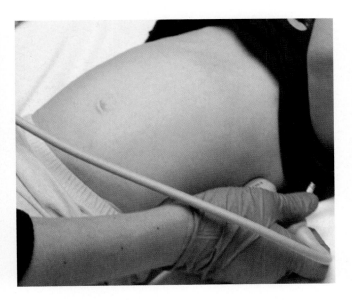

Figure 20-6. FAST examination transducer placement for LUQ.

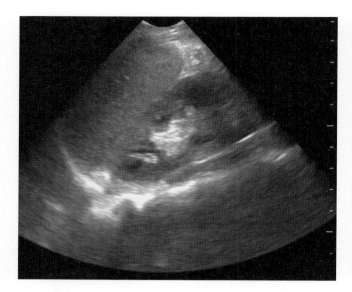

Figure 20-7. Ultrasound: Normal LUQ view.

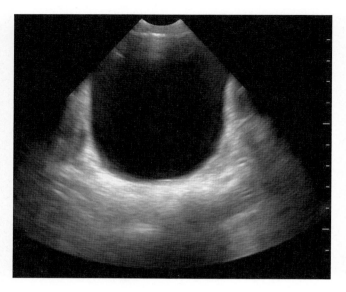

Figure 20-9. Ultrasound: Normal pelvic transverse view.

Intraperitoneal fluid accumulates cephalad and posterior to the bladder. Ideally, scan the suprapubic view prior to insertion of a Foley catheter. Urine in the bladder provides an important acoustic window. Place the transducer just cephalad to the symphysis pubis in the midline sagittal plane with the index marker cephalad and in the transverse plane with the index marker to the patient's right (Figure 20-8). Urine appears hypoechoic or anechoic and is well circumscribed by the bladder wall (Figure 20-9). The uterus in girls and prostate in boys can be seen posterior to the bladder. The transition in tissue densities between urine in the bladder and

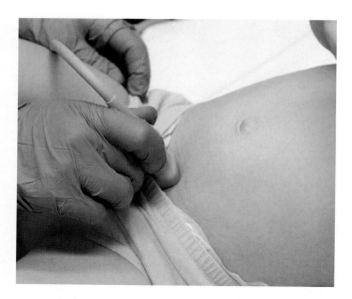

Figure 20-8. FAST examination transducer placement for the pelvis.

the surrounding soft tissue can produce bright echoes, so reducing the far gain will enhance subtle soft tissue details and help avoid missing free fluid in this area.

Obtain a midline sagittal view first to get an overview of the pelvic anatomy. In the midline sagittal view, the posterior angle of the bladder divides the intraperitoneal space containing the bowel (and the uterus in girls) from the pelvic structures (prostate and seminal vesicles in boys, vagina in girls) (Figure 20-10). Free intraperitoneal fluid only accumulates cephalad (to the left) to the posterior angle of the bladder, so it is an important anatomic landmark to recognize.

The amount of free intraperitoneal fluid that can be reliably detected in children has not been studied. In adults, 400 mL is a reasonable estimate.[41,42] One study suggests that placing the patient in Trendelenburg or decubitus positions allows for the detection of intraperitoneal fluid with only two-thirds of the amount of fluid required in the supine position.[43] The reverse Trendelenburg position may help with identification of pleural or pelvic free fluid.

Always begin the FAST examination with the subxiphoid view of the heart for penetrating trauma patients in whom cardiac injury is suspected. Place the transducer in the subxiphoid region in the coronal plane with the index marker to the patient's right. Direct it toward the left shoulder at a steep angle (relative to the abdominal skin) using the liver as an acoustic window (Figure 20-2). This provides a four-chamber view of the heart surrounded by a hyperechoic pericardium (Figure 20-11). In the crying child, slide the transducer laterally, slightly to the right of the midline, to avoid the air in the stomach by using the liver as an acoustic window.

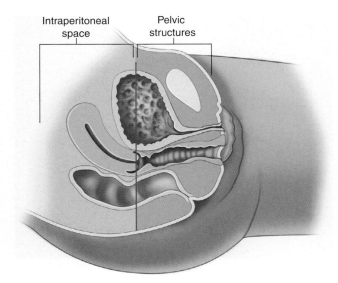

Figure 20-10. Midline sagittal view of the pelvis. This drawing demonstrates a simple technique for understanding where free intraperitoneal fluid may be seen in the pelvic views. An imaginary line (in red) drawn from the posterior angle of the bladder separates the intraperitoneal space (pink shading) from the pelvic structures (gray shading). In girls, the uterus projects into the peritoneal space (to the left) and may be surrounded by free fluid in trauma patients. In boys, free fluid will be adjacent to the bladder. Structures posterior and caudad to the bladder (to the right) include the vaginal stripe in girls, and prostate and seminal vesicles in boys, and free intraperitoneal fluid will not be seen in this region.

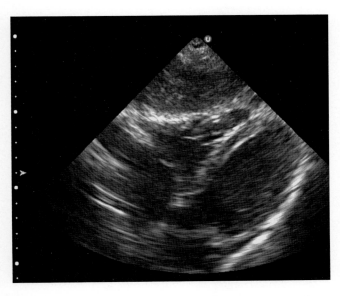

Figure 20-11. Normal subxiphoid four-chamber view of the heart using a phased-array transducer.

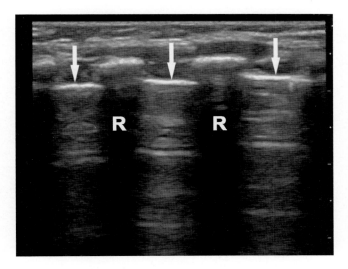

Figure 20-12. Ultrasound: Normal lung with rib shadowing (R), and location of the pleural line indicated (arrows).

If this view is insufficient, consider the parasternal long-axis view. Place the transducer along the axis of the heart from the right shoulder to the left hip. This approach will visualize the right and left ventricles, left atrium, aortic and mitral valves, as well as the pericardium surrounding the heart and the descending aorta. The descending aorta is the landmark used to differentiate pericardial from pleural effusions.

Perform the lung ultrasound examination with a linear transducer or any transducer with a higher frequency selected. Place the transducer in a longitudinal orientation with the hyperechoic ribs as landmarks on either side of the image. Decrease the depth to optimize the view of the pleural interface. Rapidly assess both sides of the chest for the presence or absence of lung sliding by scanning in the midclavicular line in the second or third intercostal space bilaterally. The interface of the visceral and parietal pleura is a thin line just deep to the ribs and appears bright and echogenic (Figure 20-12). Pleural sliding is seen in real time as scintillating, to-and-fro movement at the level of the pleural line. If pleural sliding is not obvious, observe the pleural line for at least three respiratory cycles and examine other sites on the chest wall. M-mode or color Doppler is commonly used to help assess and document pleural movement (Figure 20-13, and also see Chapter 5, "Trauma"). When evaluating the lungs in infants and toddlers, the pleura may be visible through the ribs (as a continuous hyperechoic line) because the ribs are primarily cartilage (Figure 20-14). In younger children, the ribs produce anechoic shadows but they are not as strong as the rib shadowing in adolescents and adults because the ribs are not yet completely ossified (Figure 20-15).

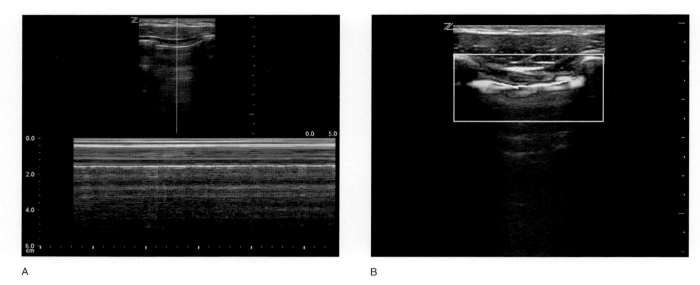

A   B

Figure 20-13. Ultrasound: Lung. M-mode (A) and color Doppler (B) used as adjuncts. M-mode displays the "seashore sign."

COMMON AND EMERGENT ABNORMALITIES

Hemoperitoneum

A small amount of intraperitoneal fluid may be visible just at the inferior portion of the liver, whereas a large amount of fluid will separate the liver from the kidney and produce a thick anechoic stripe in Morison's pouch (Figure 20-16,B). Blood most often accumulates circumferentially around the spleen and below the left

diaphragm because the splenorenal ligament maintains the integrity between the spleen and the kidney (Figure 20-17). Nonclotted blood in the pelvic region appears as anechoic free fluid posterior and cephalad to the bladder in boys (Figure 20-18A) and both anterior and posterior to the uterus in girls (Figures 20-18B).

Hemopericardium

Unclotted blood in the pericardial space will appear as an anechoic stripe lying between the two brightly,

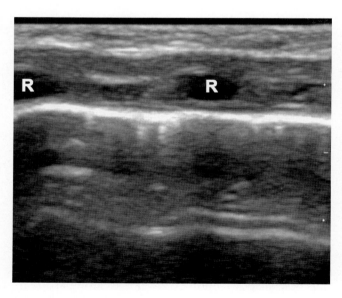

Figure 20-14. Ultrasound: Normal lung of a neonate. The ribs (R) are hypoechoic and have minimal shadowing artifacts.

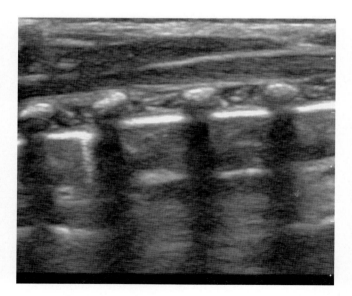

Figure 20-15. Ultrasound: Normal lung of a young child. Ribs and associated shadows are more easily identified.

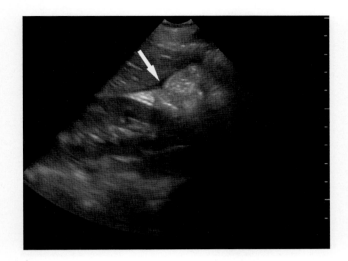

A

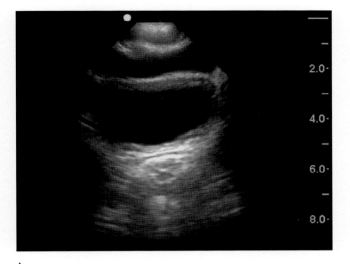

A

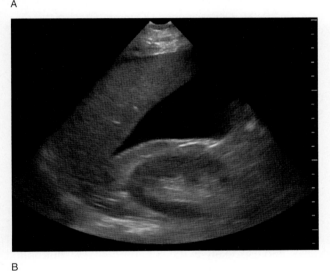

B

Figure 20-16. Ultrasound: RUQ. Hemoperitoneum including example of small (A) fluid collection (arrow), and large hemoperitoneum (B).

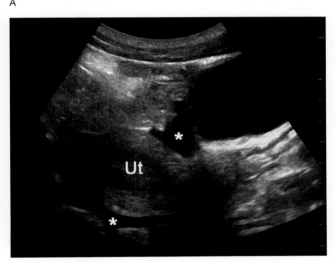

B

Figure 20-18. Ultrasound: Pelvis hemoperitoneum. Transverse view (A) shows fluid anterior to the bladder. Longitudinal view (B) reveals fluid (∗) in both the anterior and posterior cul-de-sac areas. Ut = uterus.

echogenic layers of the pericardium (Figure 20-19). Clotted blood is more complex and echogenic. Small pericardial effusions may be visible anteriorly, posteriorly, or at the apex so it is important to scan through all of these areas, especially in patients who may have a penetrating cardiac injury (Figure 20-20).

Hemothorax

Blood in the chest appears as an anechoic area cephalad to the hemidiaphragm (Figure 20-21), and eliminates the mirror artifact. A large left sided hemothorax can sometimes be seen behind the heart on cardiac views (Figure 20-20).

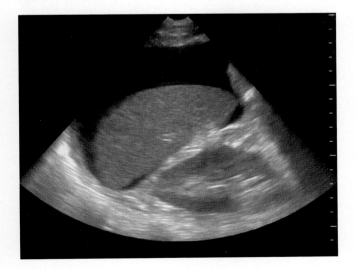

Figure 20-17. Ultrasound: LUQ hemoperitoneum.

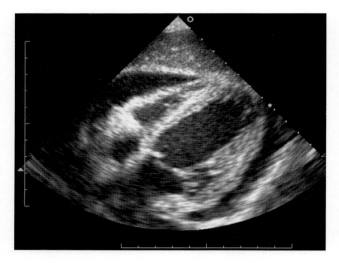

Figure 20-19. Ultrasound: Subxiphoid four-chamber view. Hemopericardium.

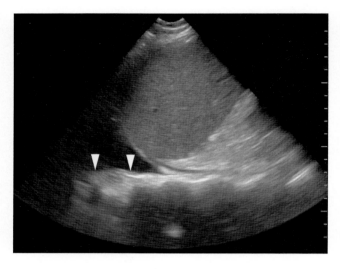

Figure 20-21. Ultrasound: LUQ view. Fluid in the chest allows visualization of the posterior chest wall (arrowheads) or spine above the level of the diaphragm.

Pneumothorax

Absence of lung sliding, visualization of a lung point, and the "stratosphere" sign with M-mode may be seen when a pneumothorax is present (Figure 20-22). The lung point is the transition point between the pneumothorax and the normal lung and is highly specific for a pneumothorax. Absence of color Doppler scanning and linear, laminar lines deep to the pleura in M-mode resembling those of the overlying stationary anterior chest wall supports the diagnosis of pneumothorax (see Chapter 5, "Trauma," for additional examples).

COMMON VARIANTS AND SELCTED ABNORMALITIES

Certain aspects of normal anatomy can be easily mistaken for positive findings. In the upper quadrant views, dark rib shadows must not be interpreted as anechoic blood. Since all fluid appears black (anechoic) on ultrasound, bile in the gallbladder and blood in the inferior vena cava (IVC) or aorta can be erroneously interpreted as free intraperitoneal fluid. In each of the abdominal views, and especially in the suprapubic view, fluid-filled loops of bowel can be mistaken for free intraperitoneal

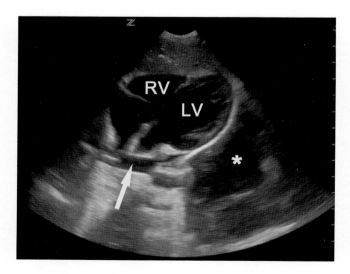

Figure 20-20. Thoracic fluid. Subcostal four-chamber view demonstrates a small pericardial effusion at the base of the heart (arrow). Pt also has a larger hemothorax (∗) adjacent to the left ventricle. LV = left ventricle, RV = right ventricle.

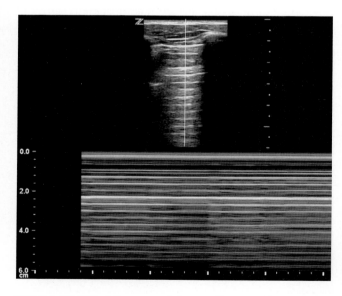

Figure 20-22. Ultrasound: Lung. Pneumothorax on M-mode, "stratosphere sign."

fluid.[28] Holding the transducer still and observing for peristaltic movements often help differentiate free fluid from intraluminal fluid.

Perinephric adipose tissue, which may be present in pediatric patients of all ages, may be hypoechoic relative to surrounding structures and can be mistaken for free fluid or clotted blood. Comparison with the area around the other kidney may help distinguish this normal variant; additionally, perinephric fat does not move separately from the kidney with respirations and is more homogenous than clotted blood.

A subcapsular hematoma may be visible between the bright reflection of the splenic capsule and the homogenous parenchyma, which may be disrupted by injury. Blood is often clotted, appearing more echogenic, but may be distinguished from the splenic parenchyma. Intraparenchymal blood is often isoechoic with the splenic parenchyma on initial evaluation.[44] Over time, a hematoma will become primarily hypoechoic.

Ascites is rarely an issue in children, and free fluid identified in the chest or abdomen in an injured child is regarded as blood until proven otherwise.

PITFALLS

1. There is no contraindication to performing an E-FAST exam unless it interferes with more important diagnostic tests or urgent patient management. Subcutaneous emphysema, gas-filled bowel, or morbid obesity may render the examination indeterminate.

2. The E-FAST examination is one data point in a continuum of clinical decision making. Repeat exams are often very helpful.

3. The E-FAST examination may not detect all intraperitoneal bleeding or significant injury. CT is generally used to characterize significant abdominal injuries, but most injuries will be managed nonoperatively in children.

4. Air scatters sound waves and makes images difficult to interpret. The inability to obtain standard views should raise the suspicion for free air or subcutaneous air.

5. Subtle free fluid may be missed if care is not taken to identify all the potential spaces. The view of Morison's pouch is generally the easiest to identify and interpret. In children, however, this view is often more caudad than in an adult. In the left upper quadrant view, clinicians often fail to place the transducer far enough posteriorly. The perisplenic region is also more cephalad than Morison's pouch. Missed subcapsular hematomas and blood between the spleen and the diaphragm are often the causes of false-negative scans; so it is recommended that at

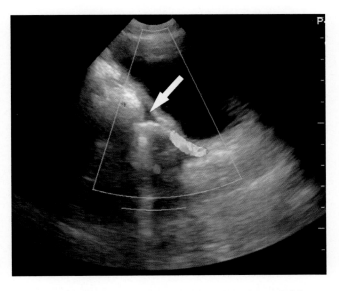

Figure 20-23. Ultrasound: Pelvic view. Free fluid (arrow) is distinguished from vessels by using color Doppler.

least 50% of the left hemidiaphragm be visualized to avoid missing blood in this area.

6. The pelvic views yield the most errors.[28,45,46] A bladder containing little urine provides a poor acoustic window. The introduction of normal saline, in quantities appropriate for the patient's age, into the bladder through a Foley catheter may be necessary to obtain good pelvic images. Also, care should be taken not to confuse free fluid with iliac vessels or other anechoic structures in the pelvis (Figure 20-23).

7. Adequate visualization of the heart in the subxiphoid view can be challenging, especially when the child is obese, crying, tachypneic, or has abdomen tenderness. Flattening the angle of the transducer and having the patient inspire may bring the heart into view. Another option is to move the transducer laterally toward the liver using the liver as an acoustic window. If adequate visualization is still not possible, a parasternal long- or short-axis view of the heart is recommended.

CASE STUDY

Patient Presentation

A 3-year-old healthy girl was transported to the ED by EMS after collapsing in her home. Her mother stated the girl came inside from playing in the yard and said, "Ow. Mommy, help," and then fell to the ground. Her mother called 911 immediately. Per EMS the girl had altered mental status on scene and a serum glucose of

200 mg/dL. She was noted to be tachycardic and hypotensive.

Upon arrival, she had a blood pressure of 70/40 mm Hg, heart rate 150 beats per minute, respiratory rate 40 per minutes, and an oxygen saturation of 98% on room air. Her mental status waxed and waned, but she opened her eyes to painful stimuli. She had an unremarkable physical exam with no signs of trauma. Her abdomen was soft but moderately tender to palpation. Her repeat blood glucose was 500 mg/dL.

Management Course

Access was established with intraosseous needles in both tibias and the team prepared to intubate the patient due to worsening vital signs and deteriorating mental status. An E-FAST exam was performed and revealed a small amount of free fluid at the inferior portion of the liver and a large amount of fluid in the pelvis (Figure 20-24). The remainder of the E-FAST exam revealed normal lung sliding (no pneumothorax) and mirror artifact above the diaphragm (no hemothorax) bilaterally. The cardiac exam revealed a hyperdynamic heart and no pericardial effusion. Surgery was immediately consulted. A repeat E-FAST 5 minutes later revealed free fluid accumulating in Morison's pouch as well as the pelvis (Figure 20-25). The patient was taken to the operating room, where the surgical team found a liver laceration and controlled the bleeding.

Commentary

This case demonstrates the utility of the E-FAST exam in young children with altered mental status, abnormal vitals signs, and no history or evidence of trauma. This patient could have been mismanaged as a patient

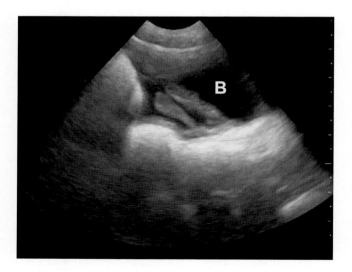

Figure 20-24. Case study-Trauma. Ultrasound: Pelvis longitudinal view. Free fluid visible superior to the bladder (B).

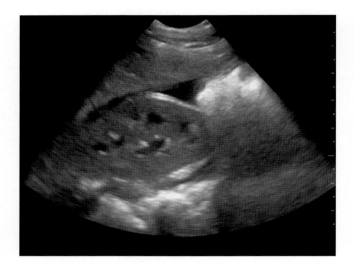

Figure 20-25. Case study—Trauma. Ultrasound: RUQ. Repeat examination showed increased free fluid compared with the initial RUQ view.

with presumed diabetic ketoacidosis had it not been for the identification of hemoperitoneum. Emergency ultrasound rapidly revealed the cause of her hypotension and directed her care appropriately to surgical intervention. Given that she was too unstable for a CT scan, emergency ultrasound was the only appropriate imaging modality.

▶ SKULL FRACTURE

The role of neuroimaging for pediatric patients presenting to the ED after a closed head injury continues to evolve. Ultrasound has become an attractive alternative to skull radiographs and CT for imaging the skull, as it is rapid, reliable, inexpensive, and without ionizing radiation.

CLINICAL CONSIDERATIONS

The identification of an intracranial injury is critical to minimize morbidity and potential mortality. Pediatric patients, especially younger children, with intracranial injury may be asymptomatic on clinical exam.[47] However, the presence of a scalp hematoma in asymptomatic infants with a head injury is predictive of skull fractures, which are in turn predictive of intracranial injury.[48]

Ultrasound has been shown to be an effective modality to identify skull fractures in a porcine model, with an accuracy of 97%.[49] A recent case series highlighted the clinical value of this same technique in pediatric patients.[50] The authors suggested three potential roles for emergency ultrasound: replacement of skull radiographs, rapid identification of a skull fracture prompting expedited management, and ruling out a skull fracture, hence potentially eliminating the need for CT. Further study is needed to fully assess the characteristics of this application and its integration with validated age-specific prediction rules.

CLINICAL INDICATIONS

An emergency ultrasound is indicated in stable pediatric patients with a scalp hematoma in whom the identification of a skull fracture will prompt further imaging or change clinical management.

ANATOMICAL CONSIDERATIONS

The cortex of the skull appears as a hyperechoic curvilinear line under the normal scalp soft tissue appearance (Figure 20-26). When overlying soft tissue edema is present, it will have a heterogeneous sonographic appearance that disrupts the normal fascial architecture.

GETTING STARTED

The presence of a skull fracture can be accurately identified with the patient in any position. For this reason, place the patient in a position of comfort, such as a caregiver's lap, in order to decrease anxiety and facilitate image acquisition. Rarely the head may need to be gently restrained. Use copious amounts of gel to minimize painful contact with the hematoma and to maximize image quality. Warm gel may also be beneficial in keeping the patient comfortable and calm throughout the exam.

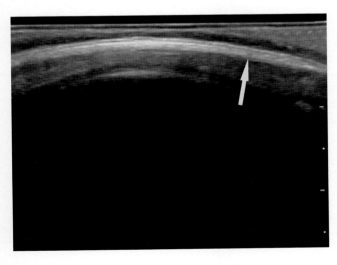

Figure 20-26. The cortex of the skull appears as a hyperechoic curvilinear line (arrow).

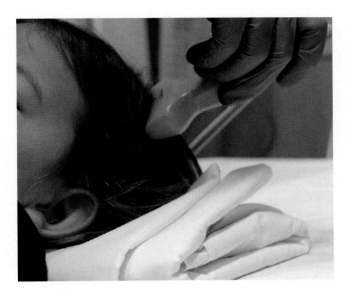

Figure 20-27. The patient is placed in a position of comfort while the transducer is placed over the area of swelling and scanned in two orthogonal planes. A large amount of gel (not shown) may be needed to overcome air artifact associated with thick hair.

TECHNIQUE AND NORMAL ULTRASOUND FINDINGS

The ideal transducer for this application is a high-frequency linear array transducer. The transducer is placed over the area of swelling and scanned in two orthogonal planes (Figure 20-27). The cortex should appear continuous with the exception of the cranial sutures and fontanelles.

COMMON ABNORMALITIES

A scalp hematoma will be identified as a distinct, homogenous hypoechoic area adjacent to the cortex (Figure 20-28). A skull fracture appears as a hypoechoic break in the contour of the hyperechoic skull (Figure 20-29). The fractured bone may appear inline or depressed depending on the character of the fracture. Comparison with the opposite side of the skull can help to distinguish cranial sutures from linear fractures.

PITFALLS

1. The sensitivity and specificity of ultrasound to detect skull fractures are currently unknown. Although this application has been demonstrated to be effective in case series, its limitations have yet to be fully documented. Care should be taken when using this application for clinical decision making.

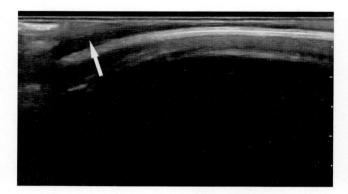

Figure 20-28. Overlying soft tissue may be edematous or demonstrate distinct hematoma formation (arrow) adjacent to the cortex.

2. Cranial sutures may be misidentified as fracture. Understanding the position and normal appearance of the cranial sutures is needed to correctly distinguish pathology. Normal cranial sutures may have an end-to-end, beveled, or overlapping appearance.[51] (Figure 20-30, Figure 20-31) A fracture or injury along a suture line must also be considered with a hematoma overlying a cranial suture and interpreted within the context of the clinical scenario.

CASE STUDY

Patient Presentation

An 8-month-old baby boy presented to the ED after a fall from his highchair onto hardwood floor 1 hour prior to admission. The mother saw the boy fall and strike

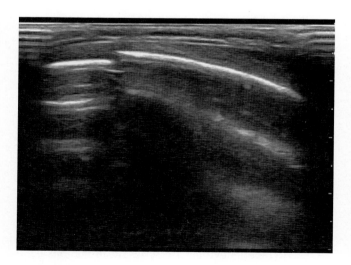

Figure 20-29. A skull fracture appears as a hypoechoic break in the contour of the hyperechoic skull.

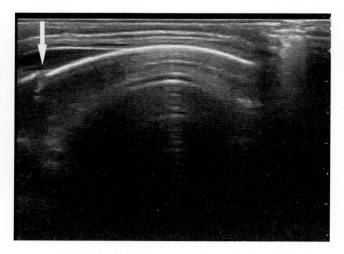

Figure 20-30. Normal cranial sutures may have a beveled appearance (arrow).

the right side of his head on impact. She denied loss of consciousness, vomiting, or abnormal behavior since the fall. His blood pressure was 90/60 mm Hg, heart rate 90 beats per minute, respiratory rate 26 per minute, and an oxygen saturation of 100% on room air. The patient was alert and appropriate, with normal tympanic membranes and no Battle's sign. He had a hematoma in the right temporoparietal area measuring 3 × 3 cm. Palpation of the underlying skull was limited due to pain and significant swelling at the site. The exam was otherwise normal.

Management Course

An emergency ultrasound confirmed the absence of a skull fracture under the area of swelling. The patient was appropriately observed in the ED and then discharged home with return precautions.

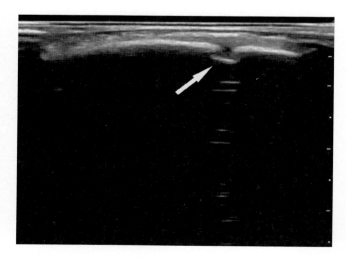

Figure 20-31. Normal cranial sutures may have an end-to-end appearance (arrow).

Commentary

This case demonstrates the advantage of using emergency ultrasound to assess for skull fracture in closed head trauma. Unnecessary imaging and radiation exposure can be avoided.

▶ INTRAOSSEOUS NEEDLE CONFIRMATION

Intraosseous access is widely used in the emergent resuscitation of pediatric patients. This life-saving technique allows for rapid fluid resuscitation and the administration of medications when peripheral IV access cannot be achieved.[52] The traditional role of the intraosseous needle (ION) has been further expanded by automated technologies that facilitate its insertion. In addition, the ION is increasingly used in the prehospital setting[53] as well as in the resuscitation of neonates.[54]

CLINICAL CONSIDERATIONS

A misplaced ION can create confusion and delay the delivery of essential fluids and medications during resuscitation. Although serious complications are rare,[55], they include extravasation of fluid, compartment syndrome, and muscle necrosis.[56] Conventional methods used to confirm needle position may be unreliable. These methods include observing a bone marrow aspirate, the presence of blood on the tip of the needle stylet, the ION standing firmly upright, and the ability to infuse fluid easily without visible extravasation or swelling. Based on current experience, ION confirmation by ultrasound is feasible and can be rapidly performed during resuscitation.[57] Ultrasound confirmation of ION placement ensures reliable delivery of the therapeutic agents while minimizing the risk of complications from a misplaced needle.

CLINICAL INDICATIONS

All patients with an ION placed in the ED or in the prehospital setting should undergo ultrasound confirmation to ensure correct needle position. Patients transferring from one ED to another are at risk of having an ION dislodged during transport. They should have needle position determined on arrival and while en route if possible. Patients with ongoing resuscitative efforts, which rely on an appropriately positioned ION, should have needle position confirmed on a serial basis to ensure continued efficacy.

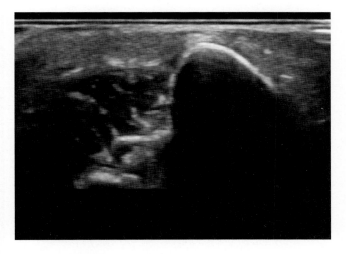

Figure 20-32. Transverse view of the infant long bone. The cortex of the target long bone in an infant should appear as a hyperechoic linear structure present below the heterogeneous soft tissue.

ANATOMICAL CONSIDERATIONS

The cortex of the target long bone should appear as a hyperechoic linear structure present below the heterogeneous soft tissue (Figure 20-32). The hyperechoic character of the cortex increases as the bone matures. For this reason, an older patient's cortex appears more distinct than a younger patient's cortex (Figure 20-33).

GETTING STARTED

The majority of ION confirmation occurs during resuscitation. Therefore, preparation is key as it minimizes

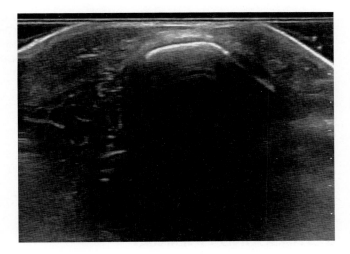

Figure 20-33. Transverse view of adolescent long bone. The hyperechoic character of the cortex increases as the bone matures as demonstrated in this adolescent.

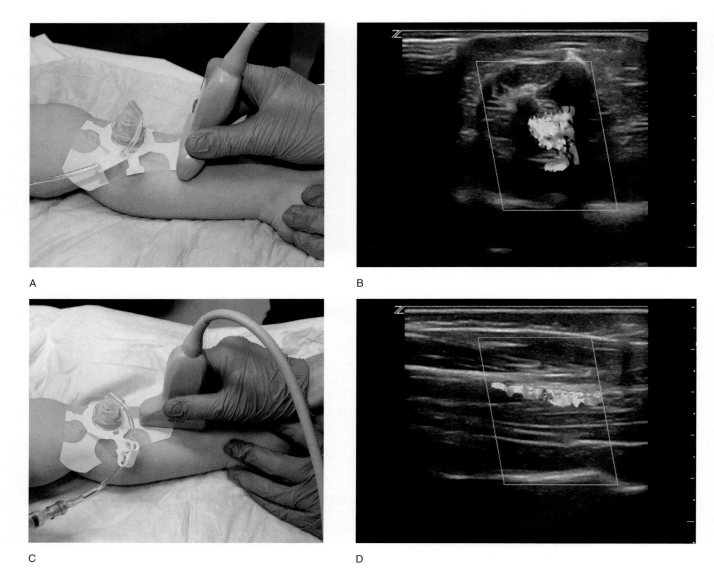

A

B

C

D

Figure 20-34. ION confirmation. (A) The transducer is placed proximal or distal to the ION in the transverse plane for visualization in a short-axis view. (B) Marrow flow is demonstrated in the transverse plane. (C) The transducer is placed in a sagittal or longitudinal plane for visualization in the long-axis view. (D) Marrow flow is demonstrated in the longitudinal plane. ION = intraosseous needle.

disrupting the tasks of other team members. The ultrasound system should have preestablished settings, gel on the transducer, and a location at the bedside that is predetermined. A system preset for ION confirmation further improves efficiency by limiting the time needed to acquire adequate images.

TECHNIQUE AND NORMAL ULTRASOUND FINDINGS

The ideal transducer for this application is a high-frequency linear array transducer, although needle confirmation may be determined with a variety of transducer types and frequencies. The transducer is placed proximal or distal to the ION in the transverse plane and the accessed long bone is then visualized in a short-axis view (Figure 20-34,C).[58] The transducer may also be positioned in a sagittal or longitudinal plane, which enables visualization in the long-axis.

Color or power Doppler may be used to identify flow below the cortex of the target site and within the bone marrow (Figure 20-34B,D). An initial 5–10 mL flush given following ION insertion can be recognized using color Doppler. Serial examinations to monitor ongoing fluid or medication infusions may require the low flow velocity sensitivity of power Doppler.

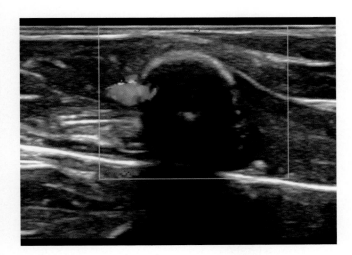

Figure 20-35. Extraosseous flow is demonstrated in the transverse plane.

COMMON ABNORMALITIES

The identification of flow in the soft tissue and not in the marrow suggests a misplaced ION. Extraosseous flow in the soft tissue may appear between the cortex and the transducer or outside the lateral margins of the target long bone (Figure 20-35, Figure 20-36).

COMMON VARIANTS AND OTHER ABNORMALITIES

There is a theoretical risk of bony fracture or a partially placed ION. Although not reported in the literature, it is possible that flow could be present both within the marrow and in the soft tissue in both these scenarios. If recognized, an alternative site of access would

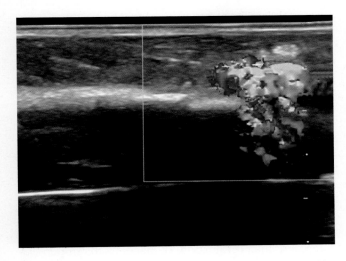

Figure 20-36. Extraosseous flow is demonstrated in the longitudinal plane.

be preferred to ensure proper fluid and medication delivery.

PITFALLS

1. Care should be taken while scanning the ION to reduce the risk of dislodging the needle during the ultrasound scan. The ION should be appropriately secured and efforts made not to bump the transducer against the needle.
2. A higher probability of error may exist when scanning with the transducer in sagittal or longitudinal view. Long-axis visualization of the cortex can lead to erroneous interpretation of flow due to inadvertent visualization off axis or visualization of the fibula.[57]
3. Low velocity flow should be considered if color Doppler fails to identify any flow during the initial manual push or subsequent infusion. A color Doppler scale adjustment or the use of power Doppler may be necessary to correctly assess needle position in this setting.[59]
4. A single determination of needle placement during resuscitation may not be adequate to ensure ongoing efficacy of the ION. The potential for needle dislodgement as a result of inadvertent movement may occur at anytime during the resuscitation. Serial examinations may be required.

CASE STUDY

Patient Presentation

A 6-month-old female child with a history of developmental delay, seizure disorder, and a gastric tube presented to the ED with 48 hours of severe vomiting and diarrhea. She had no urine output for 6 hours and had become increasingly lethargic despite ongoing hydration through the gastric tube.

Her initial blood pressure was 68/40 mm Hg, heart rate 200 beats per minute, respiratory rate 60 per minute, temperature 37.0 C, and an oxygen saturation of 96% on room air. The patient was minimally responsive to voice, mucous membranes were dry, and her eyes were sunken. Capillary refill was 3 seconds. There was severe diaper dermatitis on the buttocks. Large volume diarrhea was ongoing during the examination without blood or mucous.

Management Course

Two attempts to place peripheral IV access failed and an ION was immediately placed in the right tibia. No marrow or blood was aspirated following insertion. The ION was upright and appeared to be infusing without visible soft tissue swelling. The ION was secured and emergency ultrasound immediately confirmed correct needle placement by identifying flow within the marrow using color Doppler. Aggressive IV rehydration was immediately started and vital signs normalized.

Commentary

This case demonstrates the importance of fast and accurate ION placement in resuscitation. Emergency ultrasound confirms needle placement while conventional methods of confirmation prove unreliable. Hypovolemic shock can then be treated aggressively.

▶ APPENDICITIS

Acute appendicitis is the most common surgical emergency in children. The diagnosis is made in 60,000–80,000 children each year in the United States and accounts for 0.6% of pediatric ED visits.[60–64] While the appendix has appeared in anatomic texts for hundreds of years, the linkage with an acute inflammatory process was first noted in 1711 by Heister, followed by the intervention of an appendectomy by Melier in 1827.[65] The incidence of appendicitis is highest in the adolescent years, which correlates closely with the peak amount of lymphoid tissue present within the GI tract.[66] Appendicitis is thought to result from luminal obstruction by lymphoid hyperplasia, fecal impaction, or appendiceal calculi. The lumen subsequently distends, leading to venous congestion, wall ischemia, and bacterial translocation. Uncorrected this may lead to perforation, abscess formation, or peritonitis in 36–48 hours[67]; however, there are reports of spontaneously resolving appendicitis.[68–70]

Delays in diagnosis have been associated with higher rates of perforation and an increase in the rate of overall morbidity from 6% to 36%.[71] Studies of preschool-aged children report a perforation rate of 30–60% at laparotomy,[72–74] with 100% perforated when aged 3 and under.[75] If the diagnosis is delayed, the perforation rate increases to 65% or higher, and mortality increases as well.[76] Failure to diagnose appendicitis is one of the most frequent malpractice claims against emergency physicians.[77–79] In pediatric patients, the diagnosis is often elusive for even the most astute clinician, with misdiagnosis rates up to 100% in infants, 57% for toddlers, 28% for school aged children, and 15% for adolescents.[80]

CLINICAL CONSIDERATIONS

Acute appendicitis should be considered in any patient with right lower quadrant abdominal pain, nau-

sea, vomiting, anorexia, and fever. Together, these signs and symptoms have been found to be highly sensitive for appendicitis.[81] However, children are often unable to adequately express themselves and the physical examination may be nondiagnostic. Children with equivocal findings represent 25–30% of all cases of acute appendicitis.[82,83] Although frequently ordered, the WBC count[84] and plain abdominal radiograph[85,86] are neither sensitive nor specific for appendicitis and have a low positive likelihood ratio.[87] Because of these limitations, negative laparotomy rates as high as 20% have been reported, with rates of 10–15% accepted historically.[88–90] Negative laparotomies come at significant costs, both financially and in terms of morbidity. Morbidity includes adhesions, prolonged or return hospitalization, and time away from school.

Clinical scoring models have been proposed to identify patients who may appropriately receive surgical intervention without diagnostic imaging. Two studies proposed scoring models based on common clinical and laboratory features, with respective sensitivities of 75% and 100% and specificities of 84% and 92%.[91,92] However, attempts to validate these models in other settings have been unsuccessful.[93–97] A low-risk clinical screening model showed that patients with a low absolute neutrophil count, no nausea, and no right lower quadrant tenderness have a very low risk of appendicitis, but this model does not apply to most patients.[98] As would be expected, patients who score at the extremes of these models pose little diagnostic dilemma. These studies, however, highlight that there are many patients with equivocal signs and symptoms who need diagnostic imaging.

Currently, ultrasound and CT are commonly used to help diagnose acute appendicitis in patients with equivocal presentations. The first demonstration of an inflamed appendix by ultrasound was reported in 1981.[99] Development of the graded compression examination in 1986 established a technique and criteria for the diagnosis of appendicitis.[89]

The right lower quadrant examination of appendicitis is one of the more technically difficult ultrasound examinations. Studies of ultrasound use in children for detecting appendicitis have sensitivities ranging from 44% to 98% and specificities from 88% to 100%.[62,89,100–110,238] The wide range of sensitivity reflects the operator-dependent nature of ultrasound, particularly for this examination. This is again demonstrated by the wide range of normal appendix visualization rates, from 2% to 99%.[62,125]

Nonradiologists have also looked at employing right lower quadrant sonography in their evaluation of acute appendicitis. Emergency physicians in Taiwan compared their evaluation of patients for appendicitis using ultrasound to the surgeons' clinical impressions without sonographic examinations and found sensitivities of 94.6% and 86.2%, respectively, for the diagnosis of appendicitis.[111] Another study found a sensitivity of 65% and specificity of 90% utilizing primarily emergency medicine residents in the evaluation of appendicitis.[112] Swiss surgeons achieved a sensitivity of 91% with ultrasound for detecting appendicitis.[113] An investigation used "specially trained pediatricians" in addition to a pediatric radiologist and achieved 90% sensitivity.[101]

Studies of the use of helical CT for the diagnosis of appendicitis in children have produced sensitivities of 84–97% and specificities of 89–98%.[62, 102, 109, 110, 240] Although these ranges of sensitivity and specificity overlap with those of ultrasonography, the reliability of sonography is less consistent. When CT and ultrasonography are compared directly, CT has been superior in each study,[62, 83, 102, 109, 110, 240] except for one study in which patients undergoing noncontrast CT were compared to a historic cohort who underwent graded compression sonography.[110] In a meta-analysis comparing ultrasound to CT in children, there was no statistically significant difference found in the specificity, but with a significant difference in sensitivity of 6% in favor of CT.[114]

While CT has overall greater accuracy than ultrasound, there has been growing concern over the increased use of diagnostic imaging tests with ionizing radiation exposure.[115–119] This is particularly troubling for pediatric patients, given the greater risks of children exposed to ionizing radiation.[7, 120–123] While rates of CT use have dramatically increased, the reduction in negative appendectomies or missed appendicitis remains unclear.[115–118, 124–126] To address this concern, several authors have analyzed maximizing the specificity of the ultrasound examination in proposing a staged algorithm for diagnostic imaging for acute appendicitis. One protocol utilizing ultrasound prior to CT reduced negative appendectomies from 14% to 4% and had an accuracy of 94%.[62, 127] Another study found that the implementation of a staged protocol reduced CT usage by 50% without an increase in morbidity.[128] It is because of this safety and accuracy that the American College of Radiology has reaffirmed that the initial imaging modality for the evaluation of acute appendicitis in patients under 14 years remain graded compression ultrasonography, with CT reserved for equivocal or negative studies.[129]

MRI has also been utilized in selected patient populations, such as pregnancy, and found to be a potentially useful adjunct.[130, 131] When used in a general population sensitivities and specificities have been reported as high as 95–100%.[132, 133] The limitations of utilizing MRI in children would include cost, equipment, technician availability, and patient cooperation. Modern MRI protocols utilizing ultrafast spin echo sequences require 20 seconds of breath holding by the patient to minimize motion artifact.[132] MRI could eventually replace CT for patients with equivocal or negative ultrasound studies,

but further research is needed, since trials to date have been small.[134, 135]

CLINICAL INDICATIONS

An ultrasound examination is indicated when there is clinical suspicion for appendicitis. It should be considered in a child with all or part of a constellation of symptoms that includes migratory right lower quadrant pain, vomiting, nausea, anorexia, pain with cough or hop, rebound tenderness, abdominal distention, or peritoneal signs.

ANATOMICAL CONSIDERATIONS

The vermiform appendix is a hollow lymphoid organ whose function is not well understood. The blind-ended appendix typically arises from the cecum, 1–2 cm distal to the ileum in the right lower quadrant (Figure 20-37). It is rarely congenitally absent.[136] The classic teaching is that the maximum pain from an inflamed appendix localizes to McBurney's point, at the midpoint of an imaginary line between the umbilicus, and the anterior–superior iliac crest. However, a 1933 study reported that the classic pelvic orientation of the appendix occurred in only 31% of 10,000 autopsies and retrocecal in 65%.[137] Also, in a retrospective review on appendiceal positioning using ultrasound visualization, only 39% of patients with appendicitis had the appendix found in the classic mid-pelvic region, with 26% retrocecal.[238]

The appendix averages 6–9 cm in length, but it may be much longer. The normal diameter is <6 mm.[67]

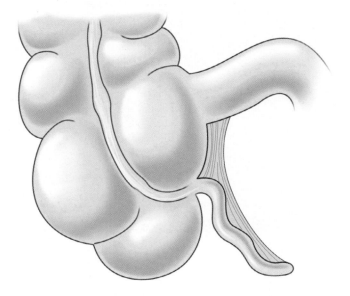

Figure 20-37. Line drawing: Normal appendix.

From outer to inner, the appendiceal wall is composed of the serosa, muscularis propria, submucosa including the muscularis mucosa, and luminal mucosa. These layers are typical of the intestinal wall except that in the appendix the submucosa is heavily infiltrated with lymphoid tissue. The appendix is partially covered by a peritoneal fold known as the mesoappendix, which contains the appendicular artery, a branch of the ileocolic artery. The fold is often short, so the appendix may be folded or kinked.[136]

TECHNIQUE AND NORMAL ULTRASOUND FINDINGS

Visualization of the normal appendix can be difficult and varies greatly with the patient and experience of the examiner (see discussion under Pitfalls, below).

A high-frequency linear array transducer is ideal for this application in children, while lower-frequency curved array transducers should be reserved for larger patients. Point the index marker cephalad or to the patient's right by convention. The graded compression technique is now the standard technique for the evaluation of appendicitis.[89] Gradual, gentle compression with the transducer displaces gas and compresses bowel loops, improving visualization by eliminating artifacts caused by the bowel (Figure 20-38A,B). Adequate compression has been achieved when the landmark iliac vessels and/or psoas muscle are visualized.[67] Since the appendix may lie in a variety of positions within the abdominal pelvic cavity, there is no single transducer position that provides consistent visualization.

There are two approaches for finding the appendix with ultrasound. First, in a patient with well-localized pain, the examiner may start in that patient-identified location.[67] Alternatively, the examiner may scan the right lower quadrant in an organized fashion with the ultimate goal of distinguishing cecum from small bowel, and then to identify the appendix as it arises off the cecum. With the transducer in transverse plane along the lateral abdomen, the examiner should note the aperistaltic loops of ascending colon and progress caudad through the cecal fossa. Moving medially from the proximal cecum should bring the actively peristalsing loops of small bowel into view, as well as the psoas muscle and iliac vessels. Moving further medially across the psoas and iliac vessels brings the pelvic contents into view. Here, there is no structure to compress loops of bowel, so a filled bladder may also be used as a window into the pelvis. From the pelvis, move cephalad again along the medial psoas up toward the level of the umbilicus. Further evaluation of the cecal fossa with the transducer in the sagittal plane starting laterally and moving medial through the fossa over the psoas may help to identify and visualize the cecum and the appendix. Considering the frequency of retrocecal position of the appendix, use alternate coronal views (as needed) between the mid and anterior axillary line with the transducer sliding along the top of the iliac crest. The patient may need to be rolled into the left lateral decubitus position to optimize retrocecal imaging. These views may avoid gas shadowing from the air-filled cecum.

A normal appendix appears ovoid and may exhibit compressibility.[138] Once the appendix is identified, measure the diameter from outer wall to outer wall

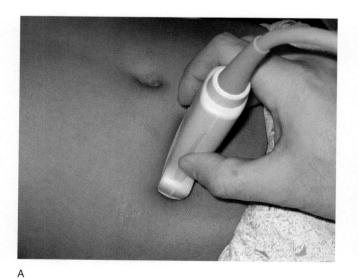

A

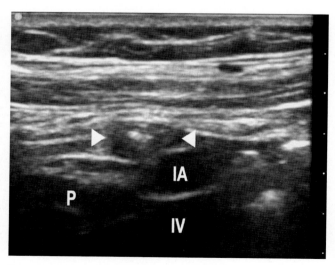

B

Figure 20-38. Transducer positioning in transverse view (A). Ultrasound RLQ: Short-axis view with compression shows a normal appendix with targetoid appearance (B). P = psoas muscle, IA = iliac artery, IV = iliac vein, arrowheads = appendix.

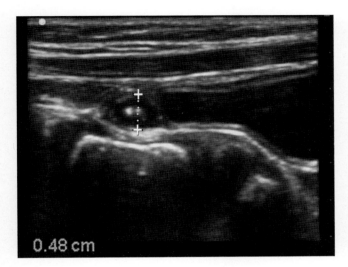

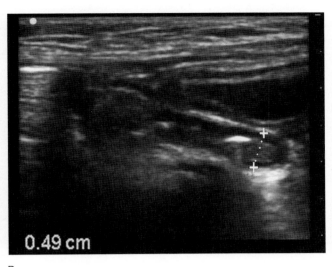

0.48 cm

A

0.49 cm

B

Figure 20-39. Normal appendix (calipers) in short (A) and long (B) axis views. A partially compressed fluid-filled viscus is adjacent to this normal appendix.

in an anterior–posterior alignment perpendicular to the long axis. If the appendix appears ovoid in transverse view, measure at the narrowest segment.[138] Trace the appendix from the origin off the cecum and document a blind-ending loop to ensure that the structure is not small bowel (Figure 20-39).

A noncompressible, nonperistalsing, tubular structure measuring ≥6 mm in anterior–posterior diameter is the most specific sign for acute appendicitis. While a normal appendix may measure >6 mm (Figure 20-40), one can exclude appendicitis with a smaller diameter. Note these findings on both the transverse and long-axis views. The transverse view gives a characteristic target-shaped appearance that may change with advancing disease. Luminal contents are variable and may appear collapsed, containing mucus, air, or some combination of both.

COMMON AND EMERGENT ABNORMALITIES

Appendicitis is diagnosed when the following findings are present (Figure 20-41):

- Target shape: Inflammation gives the appendix a classic targetoid or "bull's eye" appearance when

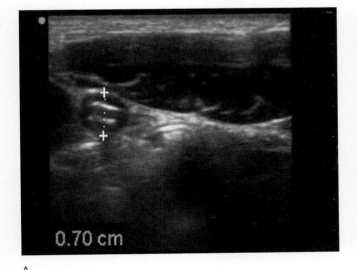

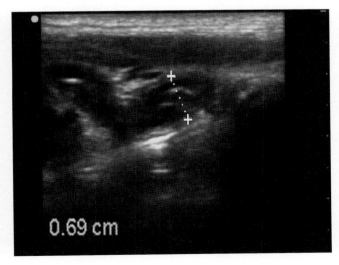

0.70 cm

A

0.69 cm

B

Figure 20-40. (A) Short-axis view of a normal appendix (calipers) with a 7 mm diameter and no signs of periappendiceal inflammation. (B) Long-axis view at tip (calipers).

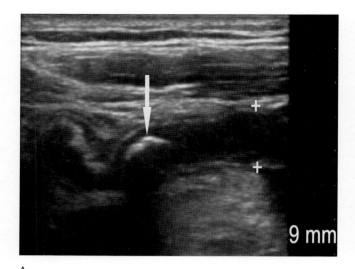

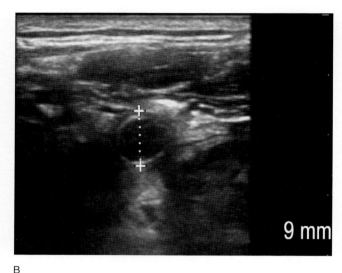

A

B

Figure 20-41. Long (A) and transverse (B) views of acute appendicitis (9 mm) with appendicolith (arrow) and periappendiceal inflammation.

viewed transversely. This results from anechoic fluid in the lumen, surrounded by an echogenic rings of mucosa, submucosa, and serosa separated by hypoechoic muscularis layers.[139]

- Diameter >6 mm: The diameter from outer wall to outer wall will be >6 mm due to inflammation.
- Noncompressible: Inflammation and appendicoliths prevent the appendix from compressing into an oval shape.
- No peristaltic activity: The appendix does not have peristalsis, as opposed to sometimes similarly appearing thickened small bowel.
- Periappendiceal inflammation: Acute appendicitis implies an active inflammatory process. This can be visualized on ultrasound as the increased echogenicity in the periappendiceal fat around an inflamed appendix, correlating with fat-stranding noted on CT. This is very similar to the sonographic changes noted in the soft tissue with cutaneous abscesses.

COMMON VARIANTS AND SELECTED ABNORMALITIES

An appendicolith, when seen with an enlarged inflamed appendix, helps make the diagnosis of appendicitis. Like renal calculi or gallstones, an appendicoltith appears as a brightly echogenic structure producing dense, anechoic shadowing. Differentiate this echogenicity from air within the lumen, which may produce a "dirty" shadowing artifact of mixed echogenicity (Figure 20-42). The finding of an appendicolith on CT has been shown to have a sensitivity of 65% and specificity of 86% for the diagnosis of appendicitis.[140] However, patients with just an isolated finding of an appendicolith without an en-

larged appendix or periappendiceal inflammation are at low risk of developing appendicitis.[141]

A ruptured appendix may be difficult to identify by ultrasound.[142,143] It may be surrounded by anechoic fluid or a developing abscess, which may be the only abnormal findings. A pericecal abscess usually demonstrates anechoic fluid with bright, hyperechoic debris (Figure 20-43). The appearance often varies, and the abscess may be loculated and more complex.

PITFALLS

1. Normal appendix. The most important variant is that the diameter of a normal appendix may

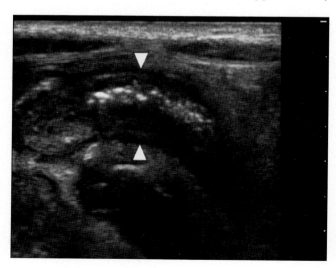

Figure 20-42. Gangrenous appendix (arrowheads) with poor differentiation between wall layers. Bright echoes within the lumen are consistent with small collections of gas.

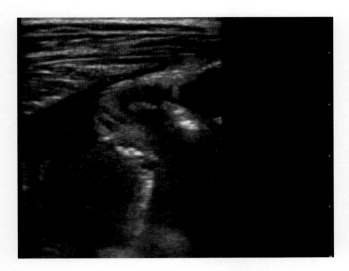

Figure 20-43. Abscess. Ill-defined fluid collection. Unable to appreciate typical anatomic landmarks.

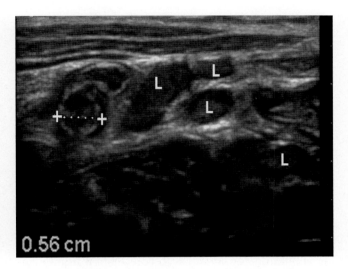

0.56 cm

Figure 20-44. Lymph nodes and bowel. Proximal appendix (calipers) with adjacent mesenteric lymph nodes.

overlap with what is considered abnormal, so that an appendiceal diameter <6 mm is better at ruling out appendicitis.[144] It has been suggested that increasing the normal measurements to 7 mm, or including an outer wall thickness measurement >1.7 mm would increase ultrasound's diagnostic accuracy by decreasing false-positive studies based on size alone.[145]

2. Visualization of the appendix is heavily dependent on the examiner, and visualization rates are variable. In his original research, Puylaert never identified a normal appendix.[89] One study reported that only 2% of normal appendices were seen on ultrasound,[62] while another was able to identify a normal appendix in 67% of healthy controls.[108] A study looking at healthy controls found a visualization rate of 82%,[146] and a study using experienced GI radiologists and advanced techniques reported a visualization rate of 99% in a group of 675 patients.

3. Visualization of proximal portions of the appendix without evaluation to the tip may miss cases with isolated distal inflammation. Furthermore, visualization in a single plane may mistake regional lymph nodes or compressed small bowel for an appendix (Figure 20-44).

4. Sonography has a much lower sensitivity for recognizing appendicitis once perforation has occurred.[142,147,148] Peritonitis associated with perforation may inhibit adequate compression, and necrosis of the appendix may render it difficult to visualize.[142]

5. Air and adipose tissue scatter sound waves and make the ultrasound image difficult or impossible to interpret. In an obese child, a 5.0 MHz transducer may be required to improve tissue penetration. An ultrasound examination may be complicated by an overlying gas-filled bowel or a location that is difficult to visualize, such as the retrocecal region. Positioning the transducer along the flank or even posteriorly may improve visualization of the retrocecal appendix, as does using a free hand positioned behind the patient lifting upward while the anteriorly placed transducer compresses downward.[149,238]

CASE STUDIES

CASE 1

Patient Presentation

A 5-year-old boy presented with a 2-day history of vomiting and diarrhea. The pediatrician told the family over the phone the day prior to start Pedialyte and come to the ED if he did not tolerate oral fluids. On presentation, he appeared uncomfortable and had abdominal distention on examination. There was no identifiable point of maximal tenderness, but he was visibly uncomfortable during the entire exam. He vomited during attempts at oral hydration.

Management Course

IV fluids were started and laboratory tests were drawn. After morphine sulfate was given for pain control, a focused emergency ultrasound exam of the right lower quadrant was performed. Free fluid and diffusely dilated bowel loops were noted on graded compression examination, but the appendix could not be visualized. The psoas muscle and iliac vessels were also difficult to visualize. The radiology department repeated the ultrasound exam. This exam noted the free fluid and measured the appendix at 6 mm, but the tip was not definitively identified and acute appendicitis could not be ruled out. At the request of the surgical consultant, a CT with oral and IV contrast was performed. The CT revealed a ruptured appendix and the patient was transported to the operating room.

Commentary

This case demonstrates both the difficulty of definitive visualization of the appendix by ultrasound and the high frequency of perforation in young children with acute appendicitis. Complete visualization necessitates localizing the blind end of the appendix, which may be the only site of inflammation. If clinical suspicion remains high after an equivocal sonographic exam, further imaging should be considered with consultation from a surgeon. Nonvisualization of the appendix on ultrasound should only be considered a negative study when done by an experienced clinician in a patient with a low probability of disease. In these select cases, the patient may be admitted for observation or discharged with instructions to return for a repeat imaging test if clinical conditions worsen.

CASE 2

Patient Presentation

A 12-year-old girl presented to the ED with abdominal pain that localized to the right lower quadrant. The pain began on the previous day as a constant vague pain around the umbilicus. She was unable to eat and had vomited twice prior to arrival. She started menstruating 2 years ago and her last menstrual period was 3 weeks ago. She was found to be afebrile and examination revealed a soft abdomen with tenderness in the right lower quadrant and pain on passive extension of the right leg.

Management Course

An IV line was established with fluids and morphine sulfate administered. Blood was drawn and sent to the laboratory for analysis. Surgery was consulted. A focused examination of the right lower quadrant revealed a tubular, blind-ended, noncompressible structure in the right lower quadrant, arising from the cecum. Midway along its course a brightly echogenic structure with dense shadowing was noted, distal to this the appendix dilated to an outer wall to outer wall diameter of 9 mm. Free fluid and an echogenic inflammatory reaction were noted around the appendix (Figure 20-42). The WBC count was 10,000 cell/μL; however, the surgeon agreed with the diagnosis of acute appendicitis based on the physical examination and ultrasound findings. A nonperforated appendix was removed laparoscopically.

Intraoperative and pathology findings confirmed the diagnosis of acute appendicitis.

Commentary

Abdominal pain in the adolescent female may be difficult to diagnose. Ovarian torsion, ectopic pregnancy, pelvic inflammatory disease, and tubo-ovarian abscess are potential diagnoses. In this case, a focused ultrasound examination showed definitive findings of appendicitis, which expedited appropriate surgical management. Overreliance on the WBC count can cause diagnostic errors.

► HYPERTROPHIC PYLORIC STENOSIS

Hypertrophic pyloric stenosis (HPS) is the most common cause of intestinal obstruction and the most common surgical cause of vomiting in infants. Overgrowth of the muscle around the pyloric channel causes a progressive gastric outlet obstruction. It is seen in 3:1000 live births, and males, (particularly first born males), are affected 5 times more often than females.[150]

HPS is a pathologic hypertrophy of the gastric pylorus muscle that occurs for unknown reasons. The disorder has been associated with elevated gastrin levels as well as dysfunction of the pyloric ganglion cells.[151,173] Exposure to erythromycin has been associated with the development of HPS.[152] It does not appear to be a congenital disease.[153] The hypertrophied muscle obstructs outflow from the stomach, leading to persistent projectile vomiting. While the typical age range of presentation is between 3 and 6 weeks, HPS has been reported as early as 10 days of age and as late as 20 weeks of age.

In 1912, Ramstedt performed the first successful pyloromyotomy, which, a century later, continues as the standard surgical treatment. Pyloromyotomy is curative and long-term sequelae are rare.[154,155] Atropine has been successfully used in Japan to reverse pyloric stenosis nonoperatively, but this treatment requires a prolonged hospital stay and a course of oral medication as an outpatient and is not standard of care in the United States.[156,157] Left untreated, HPS is typically fatal, as infants continue to vomit and become severely dehydrated with a hypochloremic, hypokalemic metabolic alkalosis.[158,173]

CLINICAL CONSIDERATIONS

Classically, the diagnosis of HPS was made in the appropriate age group by palpation of an olive-sized mass in the right upper quadrant in combination with the history of vomiting and metabolic derangement.[154,159,160] The number of patients presenting with these classic findings has declined over the last few decades, although it is unclear whether easier and earlier ultrasound access or increased physician awareness is the cause.[161–163]

Ultrasound has become the standard for diagnosing HPS. It remains an operator dependent examination, but one with an accuracy near 100%.[164,165] In cases where the ultrasound examination is nondiagnostic or negative but the patient's signs and symptoms persist, it may be appropriate for the ultrasound to be followed by an upper GI series. Sensitivity by this approach is 100%.[159] Another approach is to repeat the ultrasound if the initial study is nondiagnostic or symptoms persist. This approach has a sensitivity of 97%.[166]

Despite the potential benefits of an upper GI series as the initial diagnostic study, ultrasound predominates as the study of choice for suspected HPS.[167,168] Ultrasound is a rapid and noninvasive means of assessing for a hypertrophic pyloric segment using measurements of the pyloric width and length. Unlike an upper GI series, which only implies a hypertrophied muscle by visualization of a thinned channel of barium through the pylorus, the ultrasound examination visualizes the hypertrophied muscle itself. Infants are excellent candidates for ultrasound imaging because of their small size and limited body fat, which allows for the use of a high-frequency transducer producing high-resolution images. Pyloric sonography has been shown to be accurate by both pediatric surgery residents and emergency medicine physicians in several small studies and case series.[169–172]

CLINICAL INDICATIONS

An ultrasound examination of HPS is indicated in any patient aged 10 days to 20 weeks who presents with nonbilious projectile vomiting. Patients may have a palpable olive-sized mass in the right upper quadrant or visible peristaltic stomach waves. The hypertrophic pylorus may be found during palpation by locating the inferior border of the liver in the right upper quadrant, following it to the mid-epigastrium, then moving the hand caudally while pressing against the vertebral column. The olive-sized mass should roll under the finger tips.[173] However, most patients in this era present without long-standing symptoms, and have a normal physical examination.

ANATOMICAL CONSIDERATIONS

The pylorus is contiguous with the stomach and usually lies just to the right of the midline and just caudal to the gallbladder. In cases when the stomach is distended with fluid, the pylorus may become displaced posteri-

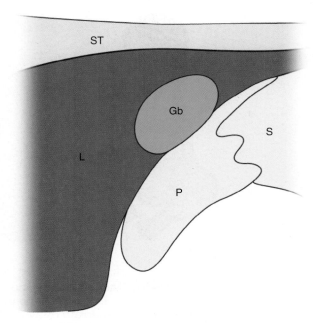

Figure 20-45. Line drawing of pylorus in abdomen. ST = soft tissue, L = liver, Gb = gallbladder, P = pylorus, S = stomach.

orly, sometimes appearing to curve beneath the stomach and toward the left (Figure 20-45).

GETTING STARTED

The examination is well tolerated and can be done at the bedside with the parent holding the infant, if necessary. Using warm gel and allowing the child to use a pacifier dipped in glucose–water solution may decrease the infant's fussiness during exam. Attempts at breast, formula, or rehydration solution feeding may be deferred until determining if fluid distention is already present in the stomach.

TECHNIQUE AND NORMAL ULTRASOUND FINDINGS

The ultrasound examination of HPS consists of identifying the pyloric wall and measuring the muscle wall thickness (MWT) as well as observing the dynamic function of the pylorus over 5–10 minutes.[151] The normal pylorus is a ring of muscle separating the pyloric antrum from the duodenum, with a MWT of <3 mm and a length <14 mm.[174] As the pyloric muscle pathologically hypertrophies, it both lengthens and thickens.

Perform the examination with a high-frequency linear array transducer in a transverse plane from an anterior approach on the supine patient (Figure 20-46). Using the liver as an acoustic window, begin in a subxiphoid position and trace the anterior gastric wall

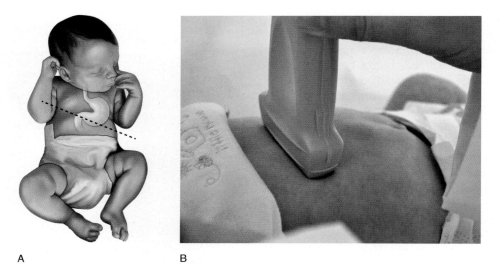

A B

Figure 20-46. Transducer position for the pylorus. (A) Orientation line for pylorus. The plane for imaging the pylorus along its length (represented by dotted line) is intermediate between the transverse and sagittal planes. (B) Initial probe position. A high-frequency linear array probe is started in the transverse body plane, and aligned with the long-axis view of the pylorus.

laterally. Identify the beginning of the pyloric antrum by the incisura angularis, which appears as a notch in the gastric wall. The pyloric muscle, viewed in long axis, will have a slightly thickened appearance, even in the normal patient. The end of the pyloric channel where it meets the first portion of the duodenum is identified by the sudden change in the thickness of the muscle wall, or curved appearance of the pyloric ring (Figure 20-47). The shape and length of the chan-

nel changes with peristalsis and may appear differently during different times of the examination. Gastric contents may be seen passing through a dilated channel or air may be present, obscuring views of the posterior pyloric wall. In cases of pylorospasm, the pyloric channel appears collapsed, but should distend again within 5–10 minutes.

Only measure the hypoechoic muscle layer and not the more echogenic mucosa. Measure only on a

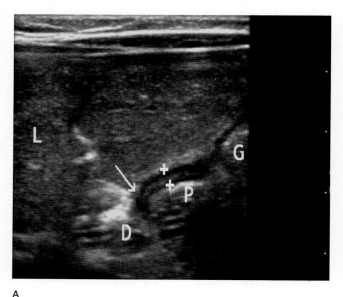

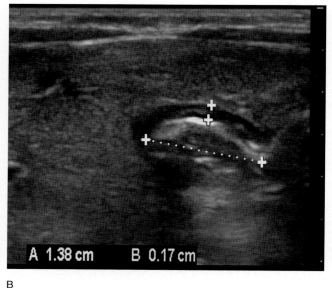

A B

Figure 20-47. Normal pylorus. (A) The pylorus (P) and pyloric sphincter (arrow) visualized using the liver (L) as an acoustic window. (B) Pyloric channel length (calipers A), MWT (calipers B). The posterior pyloric wall is obstructed by gas within the canal. MWT=muscle wall thickness (calipers), G = gastrum, D = duodenum. Arrow points to the pyloric sphincter.

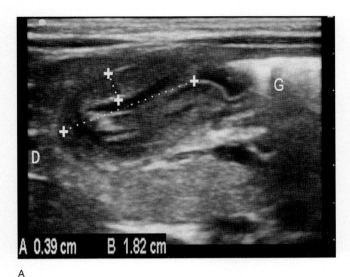

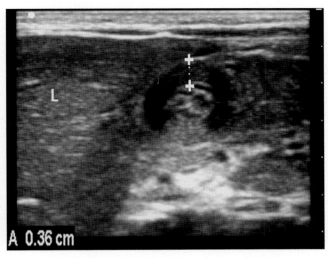

A B

Figure 20-48. HPS. (A) Long-axis view of thickened pyloric muscle wall (caliper A) and elongated channel (caliper B) situated between gastrum (G) and duodenum. (B) Short axis view. L = liver, D= duodenum.

perpendicular cross section of the pylorus in the midline on a longitudinal section. A changing MWT between 2 and 3 mm with obvious passage of gastric contents into the duodenum indicates a normal pylorus in pylorospasm and not HPS.

COMMON AND EMERGENT ABNORMALITIES

The pyloric MWT remains the most widely accepted diagnostic standard with high accuracy.[168,175] A pyloric MWT >3 mm that does not vary over time is considered diagnostic for HPS (Figure 20-48). In addition, a func-

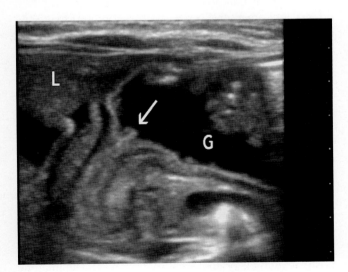

Figure 20-49. Antral nipple sign. The nipple-shaped mass (arrow) is protruding into the fluid-filled gastric antrum (G). L = liver.

tional assessment may support or refute the diagnosis of HPS.[158,176] In HPS, gastric contents will not be visualized moving through a distensible pylorus. Another finding with HPS includes the "antral nipple sign," noted when opposed gastric mucosa within the thickened pyloric cylinder project back into the fluid-filled antrum (Figure 20-49).

COMMON VARIANTS AND OTHER ABNORMALITIES

The most important normal variant to exclude is pylorospasm. The MWT in pylorospasm may exceed 3 mm transiently, but observed over time the muscle wall relaxes and allows passage of gastric contents. Fluid in the colon or small bowel may appear to represent the stomach, leading to the presumption that a portion of the bowel is the pylorus.

Gastric air may obscure visualization of the pylorus. Positioning an infant in a right lateral decubitus position allows gastric fluid to preferentially fill the pyloric antrum creating a better window, while gastric air moves away toward the fundus. In the child with gastric fluid overdistention and a posteriorly positioned pylorus, placing the infant in a left posterior oblique position may elevate the pylorus into a more anterior position closer to the transducer.

PITFALLS

1. The difference between normal and abnormal may be 1 mm or less, so accurate measurement is key. In one study, seven of eight

false-negative examinations were due to inaccurate measurements from poor technique.[166] Measure only the hypoechoic muscle layer, not the hyperechoic mucosa. Measure only on a perpendicular cross section of the pylorus or in the midline on a longitudinal section.

2. Bilious vomiting suggests obstruction more distally than the pylorus. Consider malrotation with volvulus in such cases.

3. Observe a pylorus with a borderline increased MWT for 5–10 minutes to ensure that the MWT does not vary into the normal range, indicating pylorospasm and not HPS.

4. The esophagus, duodenum, or gastric walls may be mistaken for the pylorus if they are thickened or inflamed. The esophagus may be mistaken for the pylorus, but can be correctly identified by its deep position near the aorta.

CASE STUDY

Patient Presentation

A 20-day-old female infant presented to the ED with 7 days of intermittent vomiting, described as projectile by her mother. Her mother was concerned that she was not producing enough breast milk, so she was supplementing breast-feeding with bottle feeds. The child was vomiting with the bottle feeds and appeared constantly hungry.

On physical examination, the child's vital signs included a blood pressure of 75/50 mm Hg, heart rate 160 beats per minute, respiratory rate 36 per minute, and temperature 37.0°C rectally. The infant was alert and active with a normal physical examination.

Management Course

An emergency ultrasound examination revealed a thickened, elongated pylorus, with gastric peristalsis noted, but no fluid was observed passing through the channel. Surgery was consulted and a confirmatory ultrasound by radiology revealed a thickened elongated pylorus. IV fluids were started. The patient underwent surgical correction the following morning with an uneventful course.

Commentary

This case demonstrates the often-confusing history of vomiting offered by a caregiver. It is estimated that up to 75% of ultrasound examinations for HPS will be negative, which highlights the low accuracy of clinical suspicion for this disease.[177]

▶ INTUSSUSCEPTION

Intussusception is the most common cause of intestinal obstruction in children between 3 months and 6 years of age, with a peak incidence at 10–14 months and 65% of patients presenting under 1 year of age.[178] It occurs in about 50 per 100,000 children per year and is more common in the Caucasian population.[179,180]

The etiology in most cases of intussusception is unknown. It occurs when one piece of bowel invaginates and telescopes into a more distal segment, causing intermittent pain whenever the bowel peristalses on itself. The inciting event is sometimes an anatomical mass or "lead point," such as a Meckel's diverticulum or a lymphoma that is pushed into the distal segment of bowel by peristalsis. A lead point can be identified in only about 20% of cases of intussusception in children. It is hypothesized that because a common site of intussusception in children is the ileocecal junction, where lymphoid hyperplasia in Peyer's patches may serve as a lead point.[181]

Patients classically present with a history of severe, intermittent, abdominal pain and intervening periods of lethargy. Although up to 75% of patients have some blood in the stool, the classic triad of intermittent abdominal pain, vomiting, and "currant jelly" stools occurs in <20% of cases.[178,182,183] Also, only about half of pediatric patients with intussusception have a palpable abdominal mass, usually in the right upper quadrant. A large prospective study showed that patients have a very low risk of intussusception if they are younger than 5 months of age and have a negative abdominal radiograph, or if they are older than 5 months of age and have a negative radiograph, no bilious vomiting, and the presence of diarrhea.[184]

Delays in diagnosis lead to increasing bowel wall edema, ischemia, and bowel perforation, and make the need for surgical intervention more likely.[185] During the 19th century, intussusception was usually a fatal disorder, but with current diagnostic and treatment tools mortality has been reduced to <1%. If diagnosed early, intussusception can be easily treated with hydrostatic or pneumatic enema reduction under fluoroscopic or ultrasound guidance.[186] Short-term recurrence rates of intussusception are between 5% and 10%. Surgical intervention is indicated in cases of suspected bowel ischemia, perforation, or clinical instability.[187]

CLINICAL CONSIDERATIONS

The clinical examination has poor specificity, and diagnostic imaging is often necessary.[184,188–191] The imaging modalities commonly used in the evaluation of intussusception include plain abdominal radiographs, contrast enemas, and ultrasound.

Typical plain radiograph findings include a "target" or "crescent" shaped soft tissue mass in the right side of the abdomen, lack of cecal gas, or a small bowel obstructive pattern.[183,192,193] Plain radiograph specificity is poor, with one study only having 3% of images read as positive as opposed to probable or negative.[184] While normal radiographs in combination with low risk history and exam findings may be reassuring, a normal radiograph may miss intussusception in up to 45% of patients.[194,195] Obtaining three radiographic views may significantly increase the sensitivity of plain radiographs.[188] Plain films are especially helpful if free air is detected since liquid contrast studies are contraindicated in the case of bowel perforation and surgical exploration is mandatory. Unfortunately, free air is not usually seen on plain radiographs of children with intussusception and proven perforation.[181]

The gold standard for the diagnosis of intussusception has been a contrast enema using barium or air. A contrast enema is both diagnostic and therapeutic. Reduction in the intussusception involves infusing fluid or air rectally, under fluoroscopic or ultrasound guidance, and pushing the telescoped segment out of the bowel into which it is invaginated. Despite being mildly invasive, enema studies are relatively safe, with minimal radiation exposure and a risk of perforation <1%.[182]

The use of air enemas is currently favored over barium or other liquid enemas due to the increased reported success rates; however, its use is institution dependent.[187,196] Air enemas are less messy and require less radiation. They have a slightly higher perforation rate than barium enemas (1.4% vs. 0.2%), but the perforations associated with air enemas are smaller. Leakage of air into the peritoneal space also causes fewer problems than barium leakage.[192] When enemas are not initially successful, they may be repeated up to 3 times in selected cases.[197–199]

Ultrasound has recently gained favor over enema studies as the initial diagnostic study for suspected intussusception. It has the distinct advantage of being entirely noninvasive, requiring no radiation exposure, and can be performed at the bedside if needed.

Multiple studies have demonstrated ultrasound to be 100% accurate in the diagnosis of intussusception (Pracros 1987).[154,182,183,192,200,246] Despite the operator variability with ultrasound, one study showed equal accuracy of the sonographic examination between staff radiologists and junior radiology residents.[201] In addition, an ultrasound examination can locate pathologic lead points responsible for the intussusception, whereas contrast enemas usually cannot. Ultrasound can also identify signs that may predict failure in enema reduction, such as trapped free fluid,[202,203] intramural air,[204] or absence of blood flow on Doppler imaging.[205–207] None of these findings are contraindications to attempting an enema reduction in a stable patient.

The major disadvantage of ultrasound is that if intussusception is diagnosed, the patient still requires a contrast enema for reduction. Ultrasound guidance has been used with enema reduction with success rates comparable to fluoroscopy.[186,208,243]

Some controversy remains as to whether an ultrasound examination or a contrast enema study should be the initial imaging modality for intussusception.[209]

CLINICAL INDICATIONS

An ultrasound examination is indicated in any patient suspected of having intussusception. These patients usually present with severe, intermittent abdominal pain, often associated with vomiting, a right upper quadrant mass, or guaiac-positive stool.

ANATOMICAL CONSIDERATIONS

The most common type of intussusception in the typical age range (6 months to 2 years) is an ileocolic intussusception. The cecum is located in the right lower quadrant and is the gas-filled structure sandwiched between the anterior abdominal musculature and the large posterior psoas muscle. Telescoping of terminal ileum into the cecum gives rise to the classically described mass. In 45% of cases of intussusception in children age 5 years or younger, the sigmoid colon loops into the right lower quadrant, and should not be confused with the cecum.[181]

TECHNIQUE AND NORMAL ULTRASOUND FINDINGS

Use a high-frequency linear array transducer to assess for intussusception. Scan the child in the supine position. Use warmed conducting gel if available.

Begin the examination in the transverse plane at the hepatic flexure, identifying the transverse and ascending colon. From there, the ascending colon can be traced down the lateral abdomen toward the cecum in the right lower quadrant. Identifying the actively peristalsing terminal ileum transitioning into a normal cecum rules out an ileocolic intussusception.

The normal colon is differentiated from small bowel by its larger size and aperistalsis. Large bowel will also have regular haustral markings, best seen on the ascending colon in sagittal view in the right abdomen (Figure 20-50). Normal bowel may contain air (bright echoes with shadowing artifact just under the anterior wall or mixed with fecal matter), fluid (anchoic), or stool (mixed or speckled echogenicity).

If an abdominal mass can be palpated by physical exam, this area should be imaged in multiple planes.

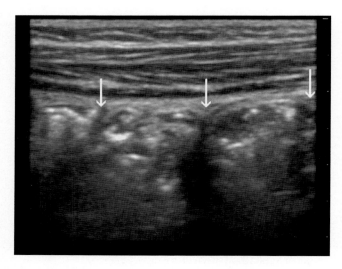

Figure 20-50. Normal ascending colon in sagittal view with regular haustral markings (arrows).

If no mass is palpated and a normal ileocecal junction is not appreciated in the right lower quadrant (added), then the path of colon should be followed from the cecum and terminal ileum to as far distally as possible, looking for a mass just deep to the abdominal wall.

COMMON AND EMERGENT ABNORMALITIES

An ileocolic intussusception is most commonly found in the right upper quadrant.[243] When imaged along its longitudinal plane, the segment of intussuscepted bowel may appear to have multiple thick hypoechoic layers that are distinctly different from normal proximal and distal bowel, or may have the general appearance of a kidney ("pseudokidney sign") (Figure 20-51A).

Another well-described finding is of a sonodense center (bowel contents) surrounded by a sonolucent ring (bowel wall), which is known as the "target sign." This is seen on transverse views of the bowel (Figure 20-51B). The typical intussusception is 3–5 cm in diameter, which will nearly fill the image on the ultrasound display making it relatively easy to identify.[181]

COMMON VARIANTS AND OTHER ABNORMALITIES

Another diagnosis is made in up to 20% of cases of suspected intussusception. In a quarter of these cases, the ultrasound examination will find alternate abnormalities, including nonspecific bowel wall thickening (Crohn's disease, Henoch–Schönlein purpura, or enterocolitis), dilated loops of bowel filled with fluid, free intra-abdominal fluid, enlarged mesenteric lymph nodes, ovarian cysts, or volvulus. Free intraperitoneal fluid does not necessarily imply perforation and may be seen in up to 50% of patients with intussusception.[210,211]

In 5% of pediatric intussusception cases, a lead point exists and may be seen on an ultrasound examination.[212] Meckel's diverticula, duplication cysts, polyps, or lymphoma may serve as lead points. An ultrasound examination may identify other masses, such

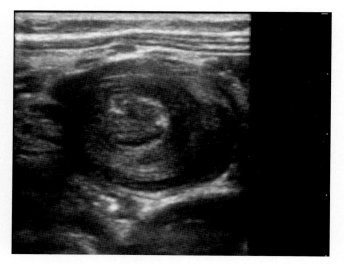

A
B

Figure 20-51. Intussusception. (A) Longitudinal image of intussusception demonstrating the "pseudokidney sign." Hypodense areas of intussusception are edematous bowel wall. Hyperechoic central area is caused by bowel contents (and possibly intussuscepted mesenteric fat). (B) Transverse scan through ascending colon demonstrates the "donut" appearance of intussusception. The outer ring is the intussuscipiens, while the central echoes are the intussusceptum.

as a polycystic kidney or Wilm's tumor, or identify complications such as pneumoperitoneum.

PITFALLS

False-positive ultrasound examinations are usually due to clinician inexperience. In one study, the most common imitator of intussusception was fecal matter in the colon.[200] Other reported false-positive findings include hematoma of the bowel wall associated with Henoch–Schönlein purpura and nonspecific bowel wall edema or inflammation.[200]

CASE STUDY

Patient Presentation

A healthy 2-year-old boy was brought to the ED by his parents after experiencing 24 hours of severe intermittent abdominal pain. The parents reported that the episodes lasted for a few minutes and then subsided. He had vomited twice. On physical examination, his vital signs were normal. He appeared tired, but in no distress. The patient's abdomen was soft and nontender on examination. Rectal examination revealed guaiac-positive stool.

Management Course

An initial plain radiograph showed a nonobstructive bowel gas pattern, but with no bowel gas noted in the right lower quadrant. An emergency ultrasound examination demonstrated a mass in the RUQ with typical multilayered hypoechoic rings consistent with intussusception (Figure 20-52). Reduction by air enema was successful.

Commentary

This case demonstrates the appropriate use of emergency ultrasound in suspected intussusception. The patient was stable with a normal physical exam. A plain radiograph was nondiagnostic. Normal single view radiographs should be interpreted with caution in a patient with suspected intussusception. The choice to proceed to emergency ultrasound versus contrast enema depends on the level of suspicion. In patients with a classic history of colicky pain, vomiting and bloody stool, with a mass palpated in the right abdomen on exam providers may decide to start with a contrast enema. In patients with equivocal findings, it may be best to limit radiation exposure, avoid discomfort, and save time by starting with an ultrasound examination.

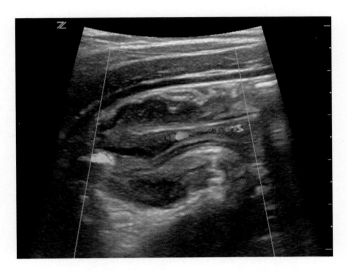

Figure 20-52. Case: Abdominal mass consistent with intussusception.

▶ HYDRATION STATUS

An accurate clinical determination of hydration status has historically been difficult to obtain in pediatric patients presenting to the ED with suspected dehydration. The gold standard measure of dehydration is change in body weight over the course of illness, which is often not available in the acute setting. Historical information such as oral intake and stool and urine output is often imprecise. Alternative methods of assessment, which rely on a constellation of signs, symptoms, and laboratory values, often prove subjective and inaccurate as well.[213,214]

CLINICAL CONSIDERATIONS

Significant dehydration, which is defined as a deficit of 5% or more of body weight, can be identified objectively by comparing the maximum diameter of the IVC to the aorta. This rapid and noninvasive method has been found to be relatively accurate.[215] A comparison of IVC/aorta ratio to the World Health Organization dehydration scale and to IVC inspiratory collapse showed that IVC/aorta ratio performed better in correctly determining severe dehydration in children.[216] In addition, this simple application allows physicians with varying levels of ultrasound training to reliably obtain comparable measurements of hydration status.[216]

Determining the IVC/aorta ratio can help clinicians identify patients with significant dehydration who may otherwise go unrecognized. This application may also reduce unnecessary interventions and the use of medical resources by identifying patients who can be safely treated with oral rehydration therapy alone. This is especially important in resource-limited settings.[216]

CLINICAL INDICATIONS

Ultrasound determination of hydration status is indicated in pediatric patients who may have significant dehydration. A similar technique may also be used to determine hypovolemic shock in pediatric patients.

ANATOMICAL CONSIDERATIONS

The IVC and aorta are both visible in the transverse plane just anterior to the vertebral bodies in the upper abdomen. The IVC appears as a nonpulsatile structure posterior to the liver, located to the right of the pulsatile aorta. The shape of the IVC ranges from circular to oval to flat depending on the patient's hydration status. The IVC normally collapses with inspiration.

GETTING STARTED

The IVC/aorta ratio can be accurately measured with the patient in the supine position, either on the bed or on the caregiver's lap, which may decrease anxiety and facilitate image acquisition. Warmed gel may also be beneficial in keeping patients comfortable and calm throughout the examination.

TECHNIQUE AND NORMAL ULTRASOUND FINDINGS

A high-frequency linear array or microconvex transducer is best for neonates and infants, and a phased-array transducer is best for larger children and adolescents. Adjustments to depth, frequency, and gain may further improve image quality and the accuracy of the measurements.

To acquire a transverse image of the IVC and aorta, place the transducer in the subxiphoid region in the midline. Obtain measurements of the anterior–posterior diameter of both vessels by freezing the image and scrolling back through the cine loop to apply the calipers (Figure 20-53). Measure the maximal width of the IVC (in the expiratory phase of the respiratory cycle) and the maximal width of the aorta (in systole).[217]

Alternatively, scan the vessels in the longitudinal plane. Identifying the IVC in the longitudinal plane may be more challenging in dehydrated patients, but it allows the operator to visualize the specific location of the

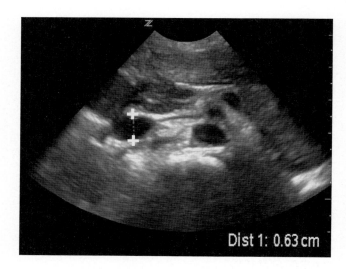

Figure 20-53. Transverse view IVC and aorta. Caliper measurements of the anterior–posterior diameter of the IVC.

IVC measurement. The IVC is most commonly measured about 2–3 cm caudal to the hepatic vein inlet (Figure 20-54), and it should not be measured at the junction of the right atrium.[218]

COMMON ABNORMALITIES

An IVC/aorta ratio of ≤ 0.8 suggests significant dehydration. This cutoff yields a sensitivity of 86–93% and a specificity of 56–59%.[215,216]

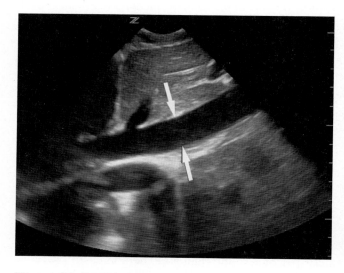

Figure 20-54. The IVC should be measured in the parallel section that is generally located 2–3 cm distal to the hepatic vein inlet (arrows).

COMMON VARIANTS AND OTHER ABNORMALITIES

An IVC/aorta ratio of 1.2 or greater, and no collapse of the IVC with inspiration or sniffing, suggests fluid overload (also see Chapter 6, "Cardiac").[219]

PITFALLS

1. Ultrasound evaluation of hydration status using the IVC/aorta ratio can only determine the current hydration status of the patient. The prognostic value of this measurement and its role in guiding rehydration therapy are unknown.

2. Care must be taken when measuring the anterior–posterior diameter of both the IVC and aorta in the longitudinal view. The transducer must be parallel and centered above the vessel to assure that the true diameter is measured. For this reason, measurements in the transverse plane may be more accurate.

3. Measure the IVC caudal to the hepatic vein inlet and cephalad to the renal vein. Measurements at the junction of the right atrium and IVC may be erroneous due to the attachment of the muscular diaphragm, which decreases vessel compliance.[218] Transitioning from a longitudinal view, in which the hepatic vein is well visualized, to a transverse view for measurement may be the best approach.

4. The accuracy of the IVC/aorta ratio is dependent on normal cardiac function and normal pulmonary pressures. Decreased cardiac function or increased pulmonary pressures can alter the caliber of the IVC and cause an overestimation of hydration status.

5. A reversal of IVC respiratory changes occur in mechanically ventilated patients and the IVC distends during insufflation. Significant distention during insufflation (>18%) is a predictor of fluid responsiveness (see Chapter 8, "Critical Care," and Chapter 6, "Cardiac").

CASE STUDY

Patient Presentation

A 2-year-old male child presented with a 5-day history of severe diarrhea. The stool was nonbloody and watery, and required a diaper change every 30 minutes. He was tolerating minimal fluids by mouth and did not produce urine for 8 hours. He was afebrile. His blood pressure was 90/60 mm Hg, heart rate 118 beats per minute, respiratory rate 28 per minute, and oxygen saturation 98% on room air. On physical exam, the patient had low-energy, mucous membranes were dry, and his eyes appeared sunken. Capillary refill was 3 seconds. There was diaper dermatitis on his buttocks. The diaper was clean and dry.

Management Course

Oral rehydration therapy was initiated at triage and well tolerated. Emergency ultrasound showed an IVC/aorta ratio of 1.0. The patient was discharged on oral therapy and made a full recovery without further medical intervention.

Commentary

This case demonstrates the benefits of using emergency ultrasound as a diagnostic tool in determining hydration status in patients at risk of significant dehydration. An accurate noninvasive measure can be achieved rapidly.

▶ URINE COLLECTION

CLINICAL CONSIDERATIONS

Urine collection for the purpose of urinalysis and culture is a common procedure in pediatric patients who are unable to voluntarily provide a urine sample. The current preferred method for collecting urine is urethral catheterization due to its minimally invasive nature. Nursing staff typically performs this safe, accurate, and rapid procedure at the bedside.[220]

An equally effective alternative to urine catheterization is bladder aspiration. This technique is typically reserved for patients in whom a urethral catheterization cannot be performed due to an anatomical barrier or is contraindicated due to urethral pathology. Suprapubic aspiration may also be necessary for bladder drainage in the setting of traumatic urethral injury or urinary retention.

Complication rates with either procedure are reported at the very low rate of 0.2%.[221] The most common complication of urethral catheterization is microhematuria, which resolves spontaneously. Other complications such as cystitis are rare. The most common complication of suprapubic aspiration is also microhematuria, which occurs in up to 4% of cases and typically resolves within 24 hours.[222] Other complications such as bowel perforation and gross hematuria seldom occur and often resolve without further sequelae.[223,224]

The use of ultrasound improves the success rates of both techniques.[59] Urethral catheterization success rises from 70% to 95% with the addition of ultrasound [225,226]. Ultrasound also increases suprapubic aspiration success rates from about 60% to as high as 96%.[222,226,227]

CLINICAL INDICATIONS

An ultrasound-assisted urethral catheterization or ultrasound-guided suprapubic aspiration is indicated for pediatric patients who are unable to voluntarily void and need an uncontaminated urine specimen and for patients who have urinary retention or obstruction. The clinical scenario will dictate which procedure is appropriate.

ANATOMICAL CONSIDERATIONS

The bladder is located in the midline of the lower abdomen and is posterior to the symphysis pubis when empty. It expands spherically above the symphysis pubis when filled with urine. In younger infants the bladder enlarges posteriorly as it fills (as opposed to cephalad), which may make suprapubic aspiration more challenging. The bladder is anterior to the peritoneal space and, when full or partially full, is the first abdominal structure encountered when passing from anterior to posterior at a level just above the symphysis pubis. This relationship makes it possible to insert a needle into the bladder from the anterior abdomen without placing any of the other abdominal organs at risk of puncture.

GETTING STARTED

Identification of the bladder and assessment of bladder volume can be achieved with the patient in nearly any position. Perform ultrasound-guided bladder aspiration with the patient in the supine position. Patients undergoing aspiration may benefit from age-appropriate restraints and the use of noninvasive anxiolytic adjuncts or medications.

TECHNIQUE AND NORMAL ULTRASOUND FINDINGS

Use a linear array, microconvex, or phased-array transducer to scan the bladder depending on the size of the patient. Place the transducer in a sagittal orientation just above the symphysis pubis in the midline of the lower abdomen (Figure 20-55). The transducer is correctly placed if caudal movement of the transducer causes the symphysis pubis to shadow most of the screen. Identify the bladder in the midline as a triangular-shaped cystic structure. The corners appear more rounded when the bladder is full.

Urethral Catheterization

Use ultrasound to assist with urethral catheterization by viewing the bladder just prior to the procedure. This ensures that there is sufficient urine in the bladder so that an unsuccessful ("dry") catheterization can be avoided.

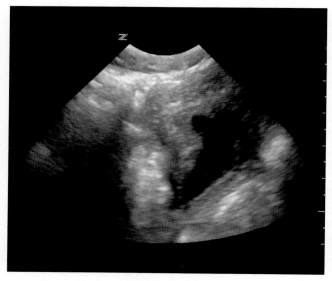

A B

Figure 20-55. Urinary bladder. (A) The transducer should be placed in a sagittal orientation, just above the symphysis pubis in the midline of the lower abdomen. (B) Corresponding longitudinal ultrasound image of a partially filled bladder.

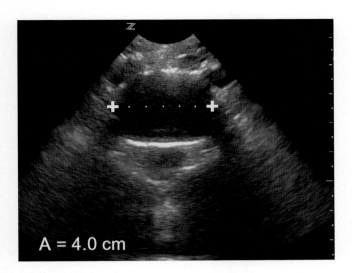

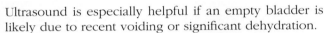

A = 4.0 cm

Figure 20-56. Volume estimation for urine collection. Transverse view of the bladder measures 4.0 cm. Urine volume is generally adequate for collection when transverse diameter is >2 cm.

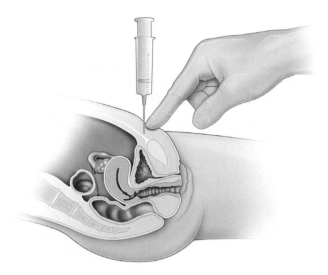

Figure 20-57. Suprapubic aspiration. The needle is generally inserted directly over the bladder and perpendicular to the skin, one fingerbreadth above the symphysis pubis. Ultrasound guidance (indirect or direct) provides a more accurate location for puncture.

Ultrasound is especially helpful if an empty bladder is likely due to recent voiding or significant dehydration.

Several methods have been described for estimating adequacy of bladder volume for urine collection, which is defined as a minimum 2.5 mL of urine. One-dimensional, two-dimensional, and three-dimensional measurement techniques result in approximately the same success rates, ranging from 94% to 100%.[225,228,229] Sample sizes in these studies are too low to show any real differences between techniques. The simplest technique is to measure the transverse bladder diameter and postpone catheterization until the diameter is ≥2 cm (Figure 20-56).[228] Rehydration therapy for 30 minutes is usually sufficient to adequately fill the bladder.

Suprapubic Aspiration

Ultrasound can be used in two distinct fashions when performing a suprapubic aspiration. *Ultrasound-assisted* means that ultrasound is used primarily to determine whether sufficient urine exists in the bladder to perform a successful suprapubic aspiration, and secondarily to confirm the best location to insert the needle; however, ultrasound is not used during the needle insertion. *Ultrasound-guided* implies continuous real-time visualization of the needle during placement. For the initial attempt at the procedure, there appears to be no significant advantage of choosing ultrasound-guided over an ultrasound-assisted suprapubic aspiration in terms of success rate.[226]

Sufficient volume must be present prior to an attempt at needle aspiration. Successful urine collection

is expected if the transverse diameter measurement exceeds 3.5 cm, while failure is likely if the measurement is <3.0 cm.[230] If the bladder diameter is inadequate, it can be rechecked in about 30 minutes.

Prior to needle insertion, scan the bladder in the transverse plane to confirm midline position. After using sterile precautions, insert a 22- or 23-gauge needle of adequate length directly over the bladder and perpendicularly to the skin, one fingerbreadth above the symphysis pubis (Figure 20-57). Maintain constant negative pressure on the syringe while the needle is advanced toward the bladder. Advance the needle until it enters the bladder and urine fills the syringe. Determine the maximal depth of needle placement by the depth markers on the ultrasound image. If no urine is returned after a single ultrasound-assisted attempt, then use real-time ultrasound-guidance for the second attempt.

PITFALLS

1. Infants may spontaneously void if startled by cold ultrasound gel or pressure on their bladder. For this reason, warmed gel and minimal transducer pressure are preferred.[220]

2. Suprapubic aspiration has the potential for serious iatrogenic injury, although complications are exceedingly rare.

3. Other fluid-filled structures may be misidentified as the bladder. Thorough visualization of

the bladder and surrounding anatomy will decrease this risk. The characteristic walls of the bladder help differentiate it from free intra-abdominal fluid that tracks around adjacent structures. Fluid-filled bowel will have intermittent peristalsis and heterogenous content.

CASE STUDY

Patient Presentation

A 14-month-old baby girl presented with 5 days of fever. She had been vomiting and unable to tolerate fluids for the past 2 days. She had no urine output for 6 hours prior to arrival. On physical examination, her initial blood pressure was 70/40 mm Hg, heart rate 160 beats per minute, respiratory rate 50 per minute, rectal temperature 38.6°C, and an oxygen saturation of 100% on room air. The patient was tender to palpation in the suprapubic region of the abdomen. She was alert, mucous membranes were dry, and her eyes were sunken. Capillary refill was 2 seconds.

Management Course

IV access was established and IV fluids were started. Point-of-care ultrasound revealed an empty bladder. A repeat ultrasound exam after 30 minutes of IV rehydration showed a partially filled bladder with a transverse diameter measurement of 3.8 cm. A successful urethral catheterization was then performed. Urinalysis confirmed a urinary tract infection and antibiotic therapy was initiated.

Commentary

This case demonstrates the advantage of ultrasound assistance in performing a successful urethral catheterization. An unsuccessful ("dry") urethral catheterization was avoided.

► ACKNOWLEDGMENTS

The authors acknowledge the contributions of Daniel Price and Michael Peterson, who authored this chapter in the second edition.

REFERENCES

1. Centers for Disease Control and Prevention. Ten leading causes of death and injury. Available at http://www.cdc.gov/injury/wisqars/LeadingCauses.html. Accessed February 21, 2012.

2. Childhood injuries in the United States. Division of injury control, center for environmental health and injury control, centers for disease control. *Am J Dis Child* 144(6):627–646, 1990.

3. Patel JC, Tepas JJ, III: The efficacy of focused abdominal sonography for trauma (FAST) as a screening tool in the assessment of injured children. *J Pediatr Surg* 34(1):44–47; discussion 52–44, 1999.

4. Jaffe D, Wesson D: Emergency management of blunt trauma in children. *N Engl J Med* 324(21):1477–1482, 1991.

5. Rodriguez A, DuPriest RW, Jr Shatney CH: Recognition of intra-abdominal injury in blunt trauma victims. A prospective study comparing physical examination with peritoneal lavage. *Am Surg* 48(9):457–459, 1982.

6. Baka AG, Delgado CA, Simon HK: Current use and perceived utility of ultrasound for evaluation of pediatric compared with adult trauma patients. *Pediatr Emerg Care* 18(3):163–167, 2002.

7. Brenner D, Elliston C, Hall E, et al.: Estimated risks of radiation-induced fatal cancer from pediatric CT. *AJR Am J Roentgenol* 176(2):289–296, 2001.

8. Menaker J, Blumberg S, Wisner D, et al.: Use and Impact of the FAST Exam in Children with Blunt Abdominal Trauma. Abstract - Pediatric Academic Societies Annual Meeting, Boston, MA, April 29, 2012.

9. Taylor GA, Fallat ME, Potter BM, et al.: The role of computed tomography in blunt abdominal trauma in children. *J Trauma* 28(12):1660–1664, 1988.

10. Taylor GA, Kaufman RA: Commentary: Emergency department sonography in the initial evaluation of blunt abdominal injury in children. *Pediatr Radiol* 23(3):161–163, 1993.

11. Meyer DM, Thal ER, Coln D, et al.: Computed tomography in the evaluation of children with blunt abdominal trauma. *Ann Surg* 217(3):272–276, 1993.

12. Turnock RR, Sprigg A, Lloyd DA: Computed tomography in the management of blunt abdominal trauma in children. *Br J Surg* 80(8):982–984, 1993.

13. Feliciano DV: Diagnostic modalities in abdominal trauma. Peritoneal lavage, ultrasonography, computed tomography scanning, and arteriography. *Surg Clin North Am* 71(2):241–256, 1991.

14. Goldstein AS, Sclafani SJ, Kupferstein NH, et al.: The diagnostic superiority of computerized tomography. *J Trauma* 25(10):938–946, 1985.

15. Mohamed G, Reyes HM, Fantus R, et al.: Computed tomography in the assessment of pediatric abdominal trauma. *Arch Surg* 121(6):703–707, 1986.

16. Richardson MC, Hollman AS, Davis CF: Comparison of computed tomography and ultrasonographic imaging in the assessment of blunt abdominal trauma in children. *Br J Surg* 84(8):1144–1146, 1997.

17. Sivit CJ, Kaufman RA: Commentary: Sonography in the evaluation of children following blunt trauma: Is it to be or not to be? *Pediatr Radiol* 25(5):326–328, 1995.

18. Stylianos S: Commentary: The role of sonography in the initial evaluation of children after blunt abdominal trauma. *Pediatr Radiol* 23(3):164, 1993.

19. Hall EJ: Lessons we have learned from our children: Cancer risks from diagnostic radiology. *Pediatr Radiol* 32(10):700–706, 2002.

20. Taylor GA, Eich MR: Abdominal CT in children with neurologic impairment following blunt trauma. Abdominal CT in comatose children. *Ann Surg* 210(2):229–233, 1989.

21. Akgur FM, Aktug T, Olguner M, et al.: Prospective study investigating routine usage of ultrasonography as the initial diagnostic modality for the evaluation of children sustaining blunt abdominal trauma. *J Trauma* 42(4):626–628, 1997.

22. Akgur FM, Tanyel FC, Akhan O, et al.: The place of ultrasonographic examination in the initial evaluation of children sustaining blunt abdominal trauma. *J Pediatr Surg* 28(1):78–81, 1993.

23. Holmes JF, Gladman A, Chang CH: Performance of abdominal ultrasonography in pediatric blunt trauma patients: A meta-analysis. *J Pediatr Surg* 42(9):1588–1594, 2007.

24. Fox JC, Boysen M, Gharahbaghian L, et al.: Test characteristics of focused assessment of sonography for trauma for clinically significant abdominal free fluid in pediatric blunt abdominal trauma. *Acad Emerg Med* 18(5):477–482, 2011.

25. Holmes JF, Brant WE, Bond WF, et al.: Emergency department ultrasonography in the evaluation of hypotensive and normotensive children with blunt abdominal trauma. *J Pediatr Surg* 36(7):968–973, 2001.

26. Taylor GA, Sivit CJ: Posttraumatic peritoneal fluid: Is it a reliable indicator of intraabdominal injury in children? *J Pediatr Surg* 30(12):1644–1648, 1995.

27. Partrick DA, Bensard DD, Moore EE, et al.: Ultrasound is an effective triage tool to evaluate blunt abdominal trauma in the pediatric population. *J Trauma* 45(1):57–63, 1998.

28. Coley BD, Mutabagani KH, Martin LC, et al. Focused abdominal sonography for trauma (FAST) in children with blunt abdominal trauma. *J Trauma* 48(5):902–906, 2000.

29. Blaivas M, Lyon M, Duggal S: A prospective comparison of supine chest radiography and bedside ultrasound for the diagnosis of traumatic pneumothorax. *Acad Emerg Med* 12(9):844–849, 2005.

30. Liu DM, Forkheim K, Rowan K, et al.: Utilization of ultrasound for the detection of pneumothorax in the neonatal special-care nursery. *Pediatr Radiol* 33(12):880–883, 2003.

31. Price DD, Wilson SR, Murphy TG: Trauma ultrasound feasibility during helicopter transport. *Air Med J* 19(4):144–146, 2000.

32. Soundappan SV, Holland AJ, Cass DT, et al.: Diagnostic accuracy of surgeon-performed focused abdominal sonography (FAST) in blunt paediatric trauma. *Injury* 36(8):970–975, 2005.

33. Hilty W, Snoey ER: Trauma ultrasonography. In: Simon BC, Snoey ER, eds. *Ultrasound in Emergency and Ambulatory Medicine*. St Louis, MO: Mosby, 1997:151–189.

34. Ma OJ, Kefer MP, Mateer JR, et al.: Evaluation of hemoperitoneum using a single- vs multiple-view ultrasonographic examination. *Acad Emerg Med* 2(7):581–586, 1995.

35. Jehle D, Guarino J, Karamanoukian H: Emergency department ultrasound in the evaluation of blunt abdominal trauma. *Am J Emerg Med* 11(4):342–346, 1993.

36. Hilty W, Wolfe RE, Moore EE, et al.: Sensitivity and specificity of ultrasound in the detection of intraperitoneal fluid (abstract). *Ann Emerg Med* 22(5):921, 1993.

37. Nance ML, Mahboubi S, Wickstrom M, et al.: Pattern of abdominal free fluid following isolated blunt spleen or liver injury in the pediatric patient. *J Trauma* 52(1):85–87, 2002.

38. Meyers MA: The spread and localization of acute intraperitoneal effusions. *Radiology* 95(3):547–554, 1970.

39. Krupnick AS, Teitelbaum DH, Geiger JD, et al.: Use of abdominal ultrasonography to assess pediatric splenic trauma. Potential pitfalls in the diagnosis. *Ann Surg* 225(4):408–414, 1997.

40. Taylor GA, Sivit CJ: Computed tomography imaging of abdominal trauma in children. *Semin Pediatr Surg* 1(4):253–259, 1992.

41. Branney SW, Wolfe RE, Moore EE, et al.: Quantitative sensitivity of ultrasound in detecting free intraperitoneal fluid. *J Trauma* 39(2):375–380, 1995.

42. Frezza EE, Solis RL, Silich RJ, et al.: Competency-based instruction to improve the surgical resident technique and accuracy of the trauma ultrasound. *Am Surg* 65(9):884–888, 1999.

43. Abrams BJ, Sukumvanich P, Seibel R, et al.: Ultrasound for the detection of intraperitoneal fluid: the role of Trendelenburg positioning. *Am J Emerg Med* 17(2):117–120, 1999.

44. Lupien C, Sauerbrei EE: Healing in the traumatized spleen: Sonographic investigation. *Radiology* 151(1):181–185, 1984.

45. Corbett SW, Andrews HG, Baker EM, et al.: ED evaluation of the pediatric trauma patient by ultrasonography. *Am J Emerg Med* 18(3):244–249, 2000.

46. Ingeman JE, Plewa MC, Okasinski RE, et al.: Emergency physician use of ultrasonography in blunt abdominal trauma. *Acad Emerg Med* 3(10):931–937, 1996.

47. Gruskin KD, Schutzman SA: Head trauma in children younger than 2 years: Are there predictors for complications? *Arch Pediatr Adolesc Med.* 153:15–20, 1999.

48. Greenes DS, Schutzman SA: Clinical indicators of intracranial injury in head-injured infants. *Pediatrics.* 104:861–867, 1999.

49. Heendeniya K, William C, Chana S: Rapid bedside ultrasonic evaluation of depressed skull fractures. *Academic Emergency Medicine: Official journal of the Society for Academic Emergency Medicine* 10:476 [abst], 2003.

50. Ramirez-Schrempp D, Vinci RJ, Liteplo AS: Bedside ultrasound in the diagnosis of skull fractures in the pediatric emergency department. *Pediatr Emerg Care.* 27(4):312–314, 2011.

51. Sobeski D, McCloskey D, Mussari B, et al.: Sonography of normal cranial sutures. *AJR Am J Roentgenol* 168(3):819–821. 1997.

52. Hafeez, W, Ronca, L, Maldonado T: Pediatric advanced life support update for the emergency physician: Review of 2010 guideline changes. *Clin Pediatr Emerg Med* 12(4):255–265, 2011.

53. Reades R, Studnek JR, Vandeventer S, et al.: Intraosseous versus intravenous vascular access during out-of-hospital cardiac arrest: A randomized controlled trial. *Ann Emerg Med* 58(6):509–516, 2011.

54. Rajani AK, Chitkara R, Oehlert J, et al.: Comparison of umbilical venous and intraosseous access during simulated neonatal resuscitation. *Pediatrics* 128(4):e954–8, 2011.

55. Hansen M, Meckler G, Spiro D, et al.: Intraosseous line use, complications, and outcomes among a population-based cohort of children presenting to California hospitals. *Pediatr Emerg Care* 27(10):928–932, 2011.

56. Moscati R, Moore GP: Compartment syndrome with resultant amputation following intraosseous infusion. *Am J Emerg Med* 8(5):470–471, 1990.

57. Tsung JW, Blaivas M, Stone MB: Feasibility of point-of-care colour Doppler ultrasound confirmation of intraosseous needle placement during resuscitation. *Resuscitation* 80(6):665–668, 2009.

58. Stone MB, Teismann NA, Wang R: Ultrasonographic confirmation of intraosseous needle placement in an adult unembalmed cadaver model. *Ann Emerg Med* 49(4):515–519, 2007.

59. Werner H, Levy J: Procedural applications of bedside emergency ultrasound. *Clin Pediatr Emerg Med* 12(1):43–52, 2011.

60. Lund DP, Folkman J: Appendicitis. In: Walker WA, Durie PR, Hamilton JR, et al., eds. *Pediatric Gastrointestinal Disease: Pathophysiology, Diagnosis and Management.* 2nd ed. St Louis: Mosby, 1996:907–915.

61. Lund DP, Murphy EU: Management of perforated appendicitis in children: A decade of aggressive treatment. *J Pediatr Surg* 29(8):1130–1133; discussion 1133–1134, 1994.

62. Garcia Pena BM, Mandl KD, Kraus SJ, et al.: Ultrasonography and limited computed tomography in the diagnosis and management of appendicitis in children. *JAMA* 282(11):1041–1046, 1999.

63. Guthery SL, Hutchings C, Dean JM, et al.: National estimates of hospital utilization by children with gastrointestinal disorders: Analysis of the 1997 kids' inpatient database. *J Pediatr* 144(5):589–594, 2004.

64. Bachur RG, Hennelly K, Callahan MJ, et al.: Advanced radiologic imaging for pediatric appendicitis, 2005-2009: Trends and outcomes. *J Pediatrics* 160:1034–1038, 2012.

65. Williams GR: Presidential address: A history of appendicitis. With anecdotes illustrating its importance. *Ann Surg* 197(5):495–506, 1983.

66. Burkitt DP: The aetiology of appendicitis. *Br J Surg* 58(9):695–699, 1971.

67. Sivit CJ: Acute appendicitis. In: Cohen HL, Sivit CJ, eds. *Fetal and Pediatric Ultrasound: A Casebook Approach.* New York, NY: McGraw-Hill, 2001:444–449.

68. Migraine S, Atri M, Bret PM, et al.: Spontaneously resolving acute appendicitis: Clinical and sonographic documentation. *Radiology* 205(1):55–58, 1997.

69. Cobben LP, de Van Otterloo AM, Puylaert JB. Spontaneously resolving appendicitis: Frequency and natural history in 60 patients. *Radiology* 215(2):349–352, 2000.

70. Abes M, Petik B, Kazil S: Nonoperative treatment of acute appendicitis in children. *J Pediatr Surg* 42(8):1439–1442, 2007.

71. Savrin RA, Clatworthy HW, Jr: Appendiceal rupture: A continuing diagnostic problem. *Pediatrics* 63(1):36–43, 1979.

72. Graham JM, Pokorny WJ, Harberg FJ: Acute appendicitis in preschool age children. *Am J Surg* 139(2):247–250, 1980.

73. Jess P, Bjerregaard B, Brynitz S, et al.: Acute appendicitis. Prospective trial concerning diagnostic accuracy and complications. *Am J Surg* 141(2):232–234, 1981.

74. Nance ML, Adamson WT, Hedrick HL: Appendicitis in the young child: A continuing diagnostic challenge. *Pediatr Emerg Care* 16(3):160–162, 2000.

75. Alloo J, Gerstle T, Shilyansky J, et al.: Appendicitis in children less than 3 years of age: A 28-year review. *Pediatr Surg Int* 19(12):777–779, 2004.

76. Hartman GE: Acute appendicitis. In: Behrman RE, Kliegman RM, Alvin AM, eds. *Nelson Textbook of Pediatrics.* 16th ed. Philadelphia, PA: WB Saunders, 1996:1109–1111.

77. Rusnak RA, Borer JM, Fastow JS: Misdiagnosis of acute appendicitis: Common features discovered in cases after litigation. *Am J Emerg Med* 12(4):397–402, 1994.

78. Brown TW, McCarthy ML, Kelen GD, et al.: An epidemiologic study of closed emergency department malpractice claims in a national database of physician malpractice insurers. *Acad Emerg Med* 17(5):553–560, 2010.

79. Trautlein JJ, Lambert RL, Miller J: Malpractice in the emergency department—Review of 200 cases. *Ann Emerg Med* 13(9, Pt 1):709–711, 1984.

80. Rothrock SG, Pagane J: Acute appendicitis in children: Emergency department diagnosis and management. *Ann Emerg Med* 36(1):39–51, 2000.

81. Reynolds SL, Jaffe DM: Diagnosing abdominal pain in a pediatric emergency department. *Pediatr Emerg Care* 8(3):126–128, 1992.

82. Rothrock SG, Skeoch G, Rush JJ, et al.: Clinical features of misdiagnosed appendicitis in children. *Ann Emerg Med* 20(1):45–50, 1991.

83. Horton MD, Counter SF, Florence MG, et al.: A prospective trial of computed tomography and ultrasonography for diagnosing appendicitis in the atypical patient. *Am J Surg* 179(5):379–381, 2000.

84. Bolton JP, Craven ER, Croft RJ, et al.: An assessment of the value of the white cell count in the management of suspected acute appendicitis. *Br J Surg* 62(11):906–908, 1975.

85. Fee HJ, Jr, Jones PC, Kadell B, et al.: Radiologic diagnosis of appendicitis. *Arch Surg* 112(6):742–744, 1977.

86. Lewis FR, Holcroft JW, Boey J, et al.: Appendicitis. A critical review of diagnosis and treatment in 1,000 cases. *Arch Surg* 110(5):677–684, 1975.

87. Bundy DG, Byerley JS, Liles EA, et al.: Does this child have appendicitis? *JAMA* 298(4):438–451, 2007.

88. White JJ, Santillana M, Haller JA, Jr: Intensive in-hospital observation: A safe way to decrease unnecessary appendectomy. *Am Surg* 41(12):793–798, 1975.

89. Puylaert JB: Acute appendicitis: US evaluation using graded compression. *Radiology* 158(2):355–360, 1986.

90. Bell MJ, Bower RJ, Ternberg JL: Appendectomy in childhood. Analysis of 105 negative explorations. *Am J Surg* 144(3):335–337, 1982.

91. Alvarado A: A practical score for the early diagnosis of acute appendicitis. *Ann Emerg Med* 15(5):557–564, 1986.

92. Samuel M: Pediatric appendicitis score. *J Pediatr Surg* 37(6):877–881, 2002.

93. Bond GR, Tully SB, Chan LS, et al.: Use of the MANTRELS score in childhood appendicitis: A prospective study of 187 children with abdominal pain. *Ann Emerg Med* 19(9):1014–1018, 1990.

94. Macklin CP, Radcliffe GS, Merei JM, et al.: A prospective evaluation of the modified Alvarado score for acute appendicitis in children. *Ann R Coll Surg Engl* 79(3):203–205, 1997.

95. Schneider C, Kharbanda A, Bachur R: Evaluating appendicitis scoring systems using a prospective pediatric cohort. *Ann Emerg Med* 49(6):778–784, 784 e771, 2007.

96. Bhatt M, Joseph L, Ducharme FM, et al.: Prospective validation of the pediatric appendicitis score in a Canadian pediatric emergency department. *Acad Emerg Med* 16(7):591–596, 2009.

97. Escriba A, Gamell AM, Fernandez Y, et al.: Prospective validation of two systems of classification for the diagnosis of acute appendicitis. *Pediatr Emerg Care* 27(3):165–169, 2011.

98. Kharbanda AB, Taylor GA, Fishman SJ, et al.: A clinical decision rule to identify children at low risk for appendicitis. *Pediatrics* 116(3):709–716, 2005.

99. Deutsch A, Leopold GR: Ultrasonic demonstration of the inflamed appendix: Case report. *Radiology* 140(1):163–164, 1981.

100. Crady SK, Jones JS, Wyn T, et al.: Clinical validity of ultrasound in children with suspected appendicitis. *Ann Emerg Med* 22(7):1125–1129, 1993.

101. Hahn HB, Hoepner FU, Kalle T, et al.: Sonography of acute appendicitis in children: 7 years experience. *Pediatr Radiol* 28(3):147–151, 1998.

102. Karakas SP, Guelfguat M, Leonidas JC, et al.: Acute appendicitis in children: Comparison of clinical diagnosis with ultrasound and CT imaging. *Pediatr Radiol* 30(2):94–98, 2000.

103. Lessin MS, Chan M, Catallozzi M, et al.: Selective use of ultrasonography for acute appendicitis in children. *Am J Surg* 177(3):193–196, 1999.

104. Rice HE, Arbesman M, Martin DJ, et al.: Does early ultrasonography affect management of pediatric appendicitis? A prospective analysis. *J Pediatr Surg* 34(5):754–758; discussion 758–759, 1999.

105. Roosevelt GE, Reynolds SL: Does the use of ultrasonography improve the outcome of children with appendicitis? *Acad Emerg Med* 5(11):1071–1075, 1998.

106. Siegel MJ, Carel C, Surratt S: Ultrasonography of acute abdominal pain in children. *JAMA* 266(14):1987–1989, 1991.

107. Sivit CJ, Applegate KE, Stallion A, et al.: Imaging evaluation of suspected appendicitis in a pediatric population: Effectiveness of sonography versus CT. *AJR Am J Roentgenol* 175(4):977–980, 2000.

108. Zaki AM, MacMahon RA, Gray AR: Acute appendicitis in children: When does ultrasound help? *Aust N Z J Surg* 64(10):695–698, 1994.

109. Kaiser S, Frenckner B, Jorulf HK: Suspected appendicitis in children: US and CT—A prospective randomized study. *Radiology* 223(3):633–638, 2002.

110. Lowe LH, Penney MW, Stein SM, et al.: Unenhanced limited CT of the abdomen in the diagnosis of appendicitis in children: comparison with sonography. *AJR Am J Roentgenol* 176(1):31–35, 2001.

111. Chen SC, Wang HP, Hsu HY, et al.: Accuracy of ED sonography in the diagnosis of acute appendicitis. *Am J Emerg Med* 18(4):449–452, 2000.

112. Fox JC, Solley M, Anderson CL, et al.: Prospective evaluation of emergency physician performed bedside ultrasound to detect acute appendicitis. *Eur J Emerg Med* 15(2):80–85, 2008.

113. Allemann F, Cassina P, Rothlin M, et al.: Ultrasound scans done by surgeons for patients with acute abdominal pain: a prospective study. *Eur J Surg* 165(10):966–970, 1999.

114. Doria AS, Moineddin R, Kellenberger CJ, et al.: US or CT for diagnosis of appendicitis in children and adults? A meta-analysis. *Radiology* 241(1):83–94, 2006.

115. Partrick DA, Janik JE, Janik JS, et al.: Increased CT scan utilization does not improve the diagnostic accuracy of appendicitis in children. *J Pediatr Surg* 38(5):659–662, 2003.

116. Frei SP, Bond WF, Bazuro RK, et al.: Appendicitis outcomes with increasing computed tomographic scanning. *Am J Emerg Med* 26(1):39–44, 2008.

117. Coursey CA, Nelson RC, Patel MB, et al.: Making the diagnosis of acute appendicitis: Do more preoperative CT scans mean fewer negative appendectomies? A 10-year study. *Radiology* 254(2):460–468, 2010.

118. Raja AS, Wright C, Sodickson AD, et al.: Negative appendectomy rate in the era of CT: An 18-year perspective. *Radiology* 256(2):460–465, 2010.

119. Kocher KE, Meurer WJ, Fazel R, et al.: National trends in use of computed tomography in the emergency department. *Ann Emerg Med* 58(5):452–462 e453, 2011.

120. Brenner DJ, Hall EJ: Computed tomography—An increasing source of radiation exposure. *N Engl J Med* 357(22):2277–2284, 2007.

121. Brenner DJ, Hricak H: Radiation exposure from medical imaging: Time to regulate? *JAMA* 304(2):208–209, 2010.

122. Brody AS, Frush DP, Huda W, et al.: Radiation risk to children from computed tomography. *Pediatrics* 120(3):677–682, 2007.

123. Shah NB, Platt SL: ALARA: Is there a cause for alarm? Reducing radiation risks from computed tomography scanning in children. *Curr Opin Pediatr* 20(3):243–247, 2008.

124. Applegate KE, Sivit CJ, Salvator AE, et al.: Effect of cross-sectional imaging on negative appendectomy and perforation rates in children. *Radiology* 220(1):103–107, 2001.

125. Lee CC, Golub R, Singer AJ, et al.: Routine versus selective abdominal computed tomography scan in the evaluation of right lower quadrant pain: A randomized controlled trial. *Acad Emerg Med: Official Journal of the Society for Academic Emergency Medicine* 14(2):117–122, 2007.

126. Flum DR, McClure TD, Morris A: Misdiagnosis of appendicitis and the use of diagnostic imaging. *J Am Coll Surg* 201(6):933–939, 2005.

127. Pena BM, Taylor GA, Fishman SJ, et al.: Effect of an imaging protocol on clinical outcomes among pediatric patients with appendicitis. *Pediatrics* 110(6):1088–1093, 2002.

128. Krishnamoorthi R, Ramarajan N, Wang NE, et al.: Effectiveness of a staged US and CT protocol for the diagnosis of pediatric appendicitis: Reducing radiation exposure in the age of ALARA. *Radiology* 259(1):231–239, 2011.

129. Rosen MP, Ding A, Blake MA, et al.: ACR Appropriateness Criteria(R) right lower quadrant pain—Suspected appendicitis. *J Am Coll Radiol* 8(11):749–755, 2011.

130. Cobben LP, Groot I, Haans L, et al.: MRI for clinically suspected appendicitis during pregnancy. *AJR American Journal of Roentgenology* 183(3):671–675, 2004.

131. Israel GM, Malguria N, McCarthy S: MRI vs. ultrasound for suspected appendicitis during pregnancy. *J Magn Reson Imaging* 28(2):428–433, 2008.

132. Cobben L, Groot I, Kingma L, et al.: A simple MRI protocol in patients with clinically suspected appendicitis: Results in 138 patients and effect on outcome of appendectomy. *Eur Radiol* 19(5):1175–1183, 2009.

133. Inci E, Hocaoglu E, Aydin S, et al.: Efficiency of unenhanced MRI in the diagnosis of acute appendicitis: Comparison with Alvarado scoring system and histopathological results. *Eur J Radiol* 80(2):253–258, 2011.

134. Hormann M, Paya K, Eibenberger K, et al.: MR imaging in children with nonperforated acute appendicitis: Value of unenhanced MR imaging in sonographically selected cases. *AJR American Journal of Roentgenology* 171(2):467–470, 1998.

135. Incesu L, Coskun A, Selcuk MB, et al.: Acute appendicitis: MR imaging and sonographic correlation. *AJR American Journal of Roentgenology* 168(3):669–674, 1997.

136. O'Rahilly R, Muller F: *Anatomy: A Regional Study of Human Structure.* 5th ed. Philadelphia, PA: WB Saunders, 1986.

137. Wakely CPG: The position of the vermiform appendix as ascertained by an analysis of 10,000 cases. *J Anat* 67:277, 1933.

138. Rettenbacher T, Hollerweger A, Macheiner P, et al.: Ovoid shape of the vermiform appendix: A criterion to exclude acute appendicitis—Evaluation with US. *Radiology* 226(1):95–100, 2003.

139. Abu-Yousef MM, Bleicher JJ, Maher JW, et al.: High-resolution sonography of acute appendicitis. *AJR American Journal of Roentgenol* 149(1):53–58, 1987.

140. Lowe LH, Penney MW, Scheker LE, et al.: Appendicolith revealed on CT in children with suspected appendicitis: How specific is it in the diagnosis of appendicitis? *AJR American Journal of Roentgenology* 175(4):981–984, 2000.

141. Rollins MD, Andolsek W, Scaife ER, et al.: Prophylactic appendectomy: Unnecessary in children with incidental appendicoliths detected by computed tomographic scan. *J Pediatr Surg* 45(12):2377–2380, 2010.

142. Borushok KF, Jeffrey RB, Jr, Laing FC, et al.: Sonographic diagnosis of perforation in patients with acute appendicitis. *AJR Am J Roentgenol* 154(2):275–278, 1990.

143. Ang A, Chong NK, Daneman A: Pediatric appendicitis in "real-time": The value of sonography in diagnosis and treatment. *Pediatr Emerg Care* 17(5):334–340, 2001.

144. Rettenbacher T, Hollerweger A, Macheiner P, et al.: Outer diameter of the vermiform appendix as a sign of acute appendicitis: Evaluation at US. *Radiology* 218(3):757–762, 2001.

145. Goldin AB, Khanna P, Thapa M, et al.: Revised ultrasound criteria for appendicitis in children improve diagnostic accuracy. *Pediatr Radiol* 41(8):993–999, 2011.

146. Wiersma F, Sramek A, Holscher HC: US features of the normal appendix and surrounding area in children. *Radiology* 235(3):1018–1022, 2005.

147. Puylaert JB, Rutgers PH, Lalisang RI, et al.: A prospective study of ultrasonography in the diagnosis of appendicitis. *N Engl J Med* 317(11):666–669, 1987.

148. Fa EM, Cronan JJ: Compression ultrasonography as an aid in the differential diagnosis of appendicitis. *Surg Gynecol Obstet* 169(4):290–298, 1989.

149. Lee JH, Jeong YK, Hwang JC, et al.: Graded compression sonography with adjuvant use of a posterior manual compression technique in the sonographic diagnosis of acute appendicitis. *AJR Am J Roentgenol* 178(4):863–868, 2002.

150. Hunter AK, Liascouras CA: Hypertrophic pyloric stenosis. In: Kliegman R, Nelson WE, eds. *Nelson Textbook of Pediatrics.* 19th ed. Philadelphia, PA: Elsevier/Saunders, 2011:1274.

151. Blumer SL, Zucconi WB, Cohen HL, et al.: The vomiting neonate: A review of the ACR appropriateness criteria and ultrasound's role in the workup of such patients. *Ultrasound Q* 20(3):79–89, 2004.

152. Cooper WO, Griffin MR, Arbogast P, et al.: Very early exposure to erythromycin and infantile hypertrophic pyloric stenosis. *Arch Pediatr Adolesc Med* 156(7):647–650, 2002.

153. Rollins MD, Shields MD, Quinn RJ, et al.: Pyloric stenosis: Congenital or acquired? *Arch Dis Child* 64(1):138–139, 1989.

154. Morrison SC: Controversies in abdominal imaging. *Pediatr Clin North Am* 44(3):555–574, 1997.

155. Sola JE, Neville HL: Laparoscopic vs open pyloromyotomy: A systematic review and meta-analysis. *J Pediatr Surg* 44(8):1631–1637, 2009.

156. Corner B: Intravenous atropine treatment in infantile hypertrophic pyloric stenosis. *Arch Dis Child* 88(1):87; author reply 87, 2003.

157. Nagita A, Yamaguchi J, Amemoto K, et al.: Management and ultrasonographic appearance of infantile hypertrophic pyloric stenosis with intravenous atropine sulfate. *J Pediatr Gastroenterol Nutr* 23(2):172–177, 1996.

158. Hernanz-Schulman M: Infantile hypertrophic pyloric stenosis. *Radiology* 227(2):319–331, 2003.

159. Hulka F, Campbell JR, Harrison MW, et al.: Cost-effectiveness in diagnosing infantile hypertrophic pyloric stenosis. *J Pediatr Surg* 32(11):1604–1608, 1997.

160. Olson AD, Hernandez R, Hirschl RB: The role of ultrasonography in the diagnosis of pyloric stenosis: A decision analysis. *J Pediatr Surg* 33(5):676–681, 1998.

161. Macdessi J, Oates RK. Clinical diagnosis of pyloric stenosis: A declining art. *BMJ* 306(6877):553–555, 1993.

162. Glatstein M, Carbell G, Boddu SK, et al.: The changing clinical presentation of hypertrophic pyloric stenosis: The experience of a large, tertiary care pediatric hospital. *Clin Pediatr (Phila)* 50(3):192–195, 2011.

163. Chen EA, Luks FI, Gilchrist BF, et al.: Pyloric stenosis in the age of ultrasonography: fading skills, better patients? *J Pediatr Surg* 31(6):829–830, 1996.

164. Hernanz-Schulman M. Imaging of neonatal gastrointestinal obstruction. *Radiol Clin North Am* 37(6):1163–1186, vi-vii, 1999.

165. Neilson D, Hollman AS. The ultrasonic diagnosis of infantile hypertrophic pyloric stenosis: Technique and accuracy. *Clin Radiol* 49(4):246–247, 1994.

166. Godbole P, Sprigg A, Dickson JA, et al.: Ultrasound compared with clinical examination in infantile hyper-trophic pyloric stenosis. *Arch Dis Child* 75(4):335–337, 1996.

167. Mendelson KL: Emergency abdominal ultrasound in children: Current concepts. *Med Health R I* 82(6):198–201, 1999.

168. Rohrschneider WK, Mittnacht H, Darge K, et al.: Pyloric muscle in asymptomatic infants: Sonographic evaluation and discrimination from idiopathic hypertrophic pyloric stenosis. *Pediatr Radiol* 28(6):429–434, 1998.

169. Malcom GE, 3rd, Raio CC, Del Rios M, et al.: Feasibility of emergency physician diagnosis of hypertrophic pyloric stenosis using point-of-care ultrasound: A multi-center case series. *J Emerg Med* 37(3):283–286, 2009.

170. McVay MR, Copeland DR, McMahon LE, et al.: Surgeon-performed ultrasound for diagnosis of pyloric stenosis is accurate, reproducible, and clinically valuable. *J Pediatr Surg* 44(1):169–171; discussion 171–162, 2009.

171. Copeland DR, Cosper GH, McMahon LE, et al.: Return of the surgeon in the diagnosis of pyloric stenosis. *J Pediatr Surg* 44(6):1189–1192; discussion 1192, 2009.

172. Boneti C, McVay MR, Kokoska ER, et al.: Ultrasound as a diagnostic tool used by surgeons in pyloric stenosis. *J Pediatr Surg* 43(1):87–91; discussion 91, 2008.

173. Letton RW, Jr: Pyloric stenosis. *Pediatr Ann.* 30(12):745–750, 2001.

174. John SD, Swischuk LE: Pediatric abdomen and pelvis. In: Brant WE, Helms CA, eds. *Fundamentals of Diagnostic Radiology.* 3rd ed. Philadelphia, PA: Lippincott, Williams & Wilkins, 2007:1282.

175. Lowe LH, Banks WJ, Shyr Y: Pyloric ratio: Efficacy in the diagnosis of hypertrophic pyloric stenosis. *J Ultrasound Med* 18(11):773–777, 1999.

176. Blumhagen JD: The role of ultrasonography in the evaluation of vomiting in infants. *Pediatr Radiol* 16(4):267–270, 1986.

177. Alvarez SM, Poelstra BA, Burd RS. Evaluation of a Bayesian decision network for diagnosing pyloric stenosis. *J Pediatr Surg* 41(1):155–161; discussion 155–161, 2006.

178. Brown L, Jones J: Acute abdominal pain in children: "Classic" presentations vs. reality. *Emerg Med Pract* 2(12):1–24, 2000.

179. Applegate KE: Clinically suspected intussusception in children: Evidence-based review and self-assessment module. *AJR Am J Roentgenol* 185(3 suppl):S175–S183, 2005.

180. Wyllie R: Ileus, adhesions, intussusception, and closed-loop obstructions. In: Kliegman R, Nelson WE, eds. *Nelson Textbook of Pediatrics.* 18th ed. Philadelphia, PA: Saunders, 2007: p. 3147.

181. Daneman A, Navarro O: Intussusception. Part 1: A review of diagnostic approaches. *Pediatr Radiol* 33(2):79–85, 2003.

182. Harrington L, Connolly B, Hu X, et al.: Ultrasonographic and clinical predictors of intussusception. *J Pediatr* 132(5):836–839, 1998.

183. Shanbhogue RL, Hussain SM, Meradji M, et al.: Ultrasonography is accurate enough for the diagnosis of intussusception. *J Pediatr Surg* 29(2):324–327; discussion 327–328, 1994.

184. Weihmiller SN, Buonomo C, Bachur R: Risk stratification of children being evaluated for intussusception. *Pediatrics* 127(2):e296–e303, 2011.

185. Meier DE, Coln CD, Rescorla FJ, et al.: Intussusception in children: International perspective. *World J Surg* 20(8):1035–1039; discussion 1040, 1996.

186. Gu L, Zhu H, Wang S, et al.: Sonographic guidance of air enema for intussusception reduction in children. *Pediatr Radiol* 30(5):339–342, 2000.

187. Daneman A, Navarro O: Intussusception. Part 2: An update on the evolution of management. *Pediatr Radiol* 34(2):97–108; quiz 187, 2004.

188. Roskind CG, Ruzal-Shapiro CB, Dowd EK, et al.: Test characteristics of the 3-view abdominal radiograph series in the diagnosis of intussusception. *Pediatr Emerg Care* 23(11):785–789, 2007.

189. Kuppermann N, O'Dea T, Pinckney L, et al.: Predictors of intussusception in young children. *Arch Pediatr Adolesc Med* 154(3):250–255, 2000.

190. Hooker RL, Hernanz-Schulman M, Yu C, et al.: Radiographic evaluation of intussusception: Utility of left-side-down decubitus view. *Radiology* 248(3):987–994, 2008.

191. Hryhorczuk AL, Strouse PJ. Validation of US as a first-line diagnostic test for assessment of pediatric ileocolic intussusception. *Pediatr Radiol* 39(10):1075–1079, 2009.

192. Littlewood Teele R, Vogel SA: Intussusception: The paediatric radiologist's perspective. *Pediatr Surg Int* 14(3):158–162, 1998.

193. Stanley A, Logan H, Bate TW, et al.: Ultrasound in the diagnosis and exclusion of intussusception. *Ir Med J* 90(2):64–65, 1997.

194. Sargent MA, Babyn P, Alton DJ: Plain abdominal radiography in suspected intussusception: A reassessment. *Pediatr Radiol* 24(1):17–20, 1994.

195. Hernandez JA, Swischuk LE, Angel CA: Validity of plain films in intussusception. *Emerg Radiol* 10(6):323–326, 2004.

196. Applegate KE: Intussusception in children: Evidence-based diagnosis and treatment. *Pediatr Radiol* 39(suppl 2)S140–143, 2009.

197. Saxton V, Katz M, Phelan E, et al.: Intussusception: A repeat delayed gas enema increases the nonoperative reduction rate. *J Pediatr Surg* 29(5):588–589, 1994.

198. Gorenstein A, Raucher A, Serour F, et al.: Intussusception in children: Reduction with repeated, delayed air enema. *Radiology* 206(3):721–724, 1998.

199. Navarro OM, Daneman A, Chae A: Intussusception: The use of delayed, repeated reduction attempts and the management of intussusceptions due to pathologic lead points in pediatric patients. *AJR American journal of roentgenology* 182(5):1169–1176, 2004.

200. Verschelden P, Filiatrault D, Garel L, et al.: Intussusception in children: Reliability of US in diagnosis—A prospective study. *Radiology* 184(3):741–744, 1992.

201. Eshed I, Gorenstein A, Serour F, et al.: Intussusception in children: Can we rely on screening sonography performed by junior residents? *Pediatr Radiol* 34(2):134–137, 2004.

202. Gartner RD, Levin TL, Borenstein SH, et al.: Interloop fluid in intussusception: What is its significance? *Pediatr Radiol* 41(6):727–731, 2011.

203. del-Pozo G, Gonzalez-Spinola J, Gomez-Anson B, et al.: Intussusception: Trapped peritoneal fluid detected with US—Relationship to reducibility and ischemia. *Radiology* 201(2):379–383, 1996.

204. Stranzinger E, Dipietro MA, Yarram S, et al.: Intramural and subserosal echogenic foci on US in large-bowel intussusceptions: Prognostic indicator for reducibility? *Pediatr Radiol* 39(1):42–46, 2009.

205. Kong MS, Wong HF, Lin SL, et al.: Factors related to detection of blood flow by color Doppler ultrasonography in intussusception. *J Ultrasound Med* 16(2):141–144, 1997.

206. Lam AH, Firman K: Value of sonography including color Doppler in the diagnosis and management of long standing intussusception. *Pediatr Radiol* 22(2):112–114, 1992.

207. Lim HK, Bae SH, Lee KH, et al.: Assessment of reducibility of ileocolic intussusception in children: Usefulness of color Doppler sonography. *Radiology* 191(3):781–785, 1994.

208. Yoon CH, Kim HJ, Goo HW: Intussusception in children: US-guided pneumatic reduction—Initial experience. *Radiology* 218(1):85–88, 2001.

209. Cohen M: Why US should not be performed for the diagnosis of intussusception. *Pediatr Radiol* 40(5):787–788; author reply 789–790, 2010.

210. Swischuk LE, Stansberry SD: Ultrasonographic detection of free peritoneal fluid in uncomplicated intussusception. *Pediatr Radiol* 21(5):350–351, 1991.

211. Feinstein KA, Myers M, Fernbach SK, et al.: Peritoneal fluid in children with intussusception: Its sonographic detection and relationship to successful reduction. *Abdom Imaging* 18(3):277–279, 1993.

212. Navarro O, Daneman A: Intussusception. Part 3: Diagnosis and management of those with an identifiable or predisposing cause and those that reduce spontaneously. *Pediatr Radiol* 34(4):305–312, 2004.

213. Gorelick MH, Shaw KN, Murphy KO: Validity and reliability of clinical signs in the diagnosis of dehydration in children. *Pediatrics* 99:e6, 1997.

214. Steiner MJ, DeWalt DA, Byerley JS: Is this child dehydrated? *JAMA* 291:2746–2754, 2004.

215. Chen L, Hsiao A, Langhan M, et al.: Use of bedside ultrasound to assess degree of dehydration in children with gastroenteritis. *Acad Emerg Med* 17(10):1042–1047, 2010.

216. Levine AC, Shaw S, Umulisa I, et al.: Ultrasound assessment of severe dehydration in children with diarrhea and vomiting. *Acad Emerg Med* 17(10):1035–1041, 2010.

217. Chen L, Kim Y, Santucci KA: Use of ultrasound measurement of the inferior vena cava diameter as an objective tool in the assessment of children with clinical dehydration. *Acad Emerg Med* 14(10):841–845, 2007.

218. Wallace DJ, Allison M, Stone MB: Inferior vena cava percentage collapse during respiration is affected by the sampling location: An ultrasound study in healthy volunteers. *Acad Emerg Med* 17(1):96–99, 2010.

219. Kosiak W, Swieton D, Piskunowicz M: Sonographic inferior vena cava/aorta diameter index, a new approach to the body fluid status assessment in children and young adults in emergency ultrasound—Preliminary study. *Am J Emerg Med* 26(3):320–325, 2008.

220. Baumann BM, Welsh BE, Rogers CJ, et al.: Nurses using volumetric bladder ultrasound in the pediatric ED. *Am J Nurs* 108(4):73–76, 2008.

221. Kimmelstiel FM, Holgersen LO, Dudell GG: Massive hemoperitoneum following suprapubic bladder aspiration. *J Pediatr Surg* 21(10):911–912, 1986.

222. Ozkan B, Kaya O, Akdag R, et al.: Suprapubic bladder aspiration with or without ultrasound guidance. *Clin Pediatr (Phila)* 39(10):625–626, 2000.

223. Saccharow L, Pryles CV: Further experience with the use of percutaneous suprapubic aspiration of the urinary bladder. Bacteriologic studies in 654 infants and children. *Pediatrics* 43(6):1018–1024, 1969.

224. Simon G: Suprapubic bladder puncture in a private pediatric practice. *Postgrad Med* 72(1):63–64, 66, 1982.

225. Chen L, Hsiao AL, Moore CL, et al.: Utility of bedside bladder ultrasound before urethral catheterization in young children. *Pediatrics* 115(1):108–111, 2005.

226. Kiernan SC, Pinckert TL, Keszler M: Ultrasound guidance of suprapubic bladder aspiration in neonates. *J Pediatr* 123(5):789–791, 1993.

227. Gochman RF, Karasic RB, Heller MB: Use of portable ultrasound to assist urine collection by suprapubic aspiration. *Ann Emerg Med* 20(6):631–635, 1991.

228. Witt M, Baumann BM, McCans K: Bladder ultrasound increases catheterization success in pediatric patients. *Acad Emerg Med* 12(4):371–374, 2005.

229. Milling TJ, Jr, Van Amerongen R, Melville L, et al.: Use of ultrasonography to identify infants for whom urinary catheterization will be unsuccessful because of insufficient urine volume: Validation of the urinary bladder index. *Ann Emerg Med* 45(5):510–513, 2005.

230. Garcia-Nieto V, Navarro JF, Sanchez-Almeida E, et al.: Standards for ultrasound guidance of suprapubic bladder aspiration. *Pediatr Nephrol* 11(5):607–609, 1997.

231. Karam O, Sanchez O, Chardot C, et al.: Blunt abdominal trauma in children: A score to predict the absence of organ injury. *J Pediatr* 154(6):912–917, 2009.

232. Poletti PA, Mirvis SE, Shanmuganathan K, et al.: Blunt abdominal trauma patients: Can organ injury be excluded without performing computed tomography? *J Trauma* 57(5):1072–1081, 2004.

233. Liu M, Lee CH, P'Eng FK: Prospective comparison of diagnostic peritoneal lavage, computed tomographic scanning, and ultrasonography for the diagnosis of blunt abdominal trauma. *J Trauma* 35(2):267–270, 1993.

234. Tso P, Rodriguez A, Cooper C, et al.: Sonography in blunt abdominal trauma: A preliminary progress report. *J Trauma* 33(1):39–43; discussion 43–34, 1992.

235. Rozycki GS, Ochsner MG, Jaffin JH, et al.: Prospective evaluation of surgeons' use of ultrasound in the evaluation of trauma patients. *J Trauma* 34(4):516–526; discussion 526–517, 1993.

236. Boulanger BR, McLellan BA, Brenneman FD, et al.: Emergent abdominal sonography as a screening test in a new diagnostic algorithm for blunt trauma. *J Trauma* 40(6):867–874, 1996.

237. Kirkpatrick AW, Sirois M, Laupland KB, et al.: Hand-held thoracic sonography for detecting post-traumatic pneumothoraces: The extended focused assessment with sonography for trauma (EFAST). *J Trauma* 57(2):288–295, 2004.

238. Baldisserotto M, Marchiori E. Accuracy of noncompressive sonography of children with appendicitis according to the potential positions of the appendix. *AJR American Journal of Roentgenology* 175(5):1387–1392, 2000.

239. Zielke A, Hasse C, Sitter H, et al.: "Surgical" ultrasound in suspected acute appendicitis. *Surg Endosc* 11(4):362–365, 1997.

240. Sivit CJ, Applegate KE, Berlin SC, et al.: Evaluation of suspected appendicitis in children and young adults: Helical CT. *Radiology* 216(2):430–433, 2000.

241. Pena BM, Taylor GA: Radiologists' confidence in interpretation of sonography and CT in suspected pediatric appendicitis. *AJR Am J Roentgenol* 175(1):71–74, 2000.

242. Hernanz-Schulman M: Infantile hypertrophic pyloric stenosis. *Radiology* 227(2):319–331, 2003.

243. Wang GD, Liu SJ: Enema reduction of intussusception by hydrostatic pressure under ultrasound guidance: A report of 377 cases. *J Pediatr Surg* 23(9):814–818, 1998.

244. Schmit P, Rohrschneider WK, Christmann D: Intestinal intussusception survey about diagnostic and nonsurgical therapeutic procedures. *Pediatric Radiol* 29(10):752–761, 1999.

245. Ein SH, Stephens CA: Intussusception: 354 cases in 10 years. *J Pediatr Surg* 6(1):16–27, 1971.

246. Pracros JP, Tran-Minh VA, Morin de Finfe CH, et al.: Acute intestinal intussusception in children. Contribution of ultrasonography (145 cases). *Ann Radiol* 30:525–530, 1987.

CHAPTER 21

Vascular Access

John S. Rose, Aaron E. Bair, and Aman K. Parikh

Establishing reliable vascular access in an emergency situation is of critical importance. Many factors, including body habitus, volume depletion, shock, history of injection drug use, congenital deformity, and cardiac arrest, can make obtaining vascular access in the critically ill or injured patient extremely difficult. The introduction of point-of-care ultrasound into emergency and acute care settings has been an important advance for facilitating rapid and successful vascular access.

► CLINICAL CONSIDERATIONS

For central access, the use of an anatomic landmark-guided approach has been the traditional practice. Internal jugular vein location traditionally relies on the sternocleidomastoid muscle and clavicular landmarks; the femoral vein relies on the inguinal ligament and femoral artery pulsation landmarks; and the subclavian vein relies on clavicular landmarks. In many patients, however, these landmarks may be distorted, obscured, or nonexistent. In addition, normal variations in the anatomic relationship of the internal jugular vein may make cannulation difficult.[1] In the emergent situation, attempting central vascular access with poor external landmarks is frequently approached using a "best guess" estimate of the vessel location. This may lead to multiple needle passes to locate the vessel. Excessive bleeding, inadvertent arterial puncture, vessel laceration, pneumothorax, and hemothorax are some of the potential complications of central vascular access. The incidence of complications increases when multiple attempts are required for cannulation.[2–5] In patients with an underlying coagu-

lopathy (pathologic or therapeutic), multiple attempts can carry significant morbidity due to hemorrhage.[6,7]

The introduction of point-of-care ultrasound has been very effective in assisting with the placement of central venous access catheters. For internal jugular vein cannulation, ultrasound use has been described by numerous disciplines, including emergency medicine, critical care medicine, anesthesiology, obstetrics/gynecology, nephrology, surgery, and radiology.[2,3,8–10] When compared to the external landmark approach, ultrasound-guided internal jugular vein cannulation results in fewer complications and is more effective in time-to-cannulation and first-attempt success.[2,6,11–15] For femoral vein cannulation, the ultrasound-guided approach was found to be more successful than the landmark approach in patients presenting in cardiac arrest.[16]

Peripheral venous access is less invasive and is used more commonly in the emergency and acute care settings than central access. The inability to find an adequate peripheral vein generally requires that the clinician consider central venous access. Traditionally, successful peripheral venous cannulation requires that a vein first be visualized or palpated. Some peripheral veins that are not readily apparent on the skin surface can be clearly visualized with the use of ultrasound, which may obviate the need for central access.[16,17] The basilic and cephalic veins of the arm are superficial veins that are not generally visible but are readily cannulated using ultrasound guidance. Basilic vein cannulation has been shown to be very successful in the ED setting in patients in whom it was difficult to obtain other peripheral vascular access.[18] Basilic vein cannulation is readily learned by novice users.[19] In addition, basilic veins have been cannulated using ultrasound in patients requiring prolonged outpatient IV access.[20]

Evidence supporting the use of ultrasound for vascular access has become overwhelming. In 2001, a report published by the Agency for Healthcare Research and Quality (AHRQ) on patient safety in health care included a chapter strongly advocating the use of ultrasound in central venous catheterization.[21] The resulting scientific and policy positions favor the use of ultrasound for central venous access stronger than any other point-of-care ultrasound application. The National Institute for Clinical Excellence (NICE) has also recommended that central venous catheters be inserted under ultrasound guidance.[22]

▶ CLINICAL INDICATIONS

Indications for ultrasound guidance for vascular access are as follows:

- **To confirm vessel location prior to landmark-based approach.** This is termed as the *static* approach with ultrasound for IV access. The patient is positioned and the ultrasound transducer is placed on the patient to confirm the predicted landmark-based anatomy. The transducer is then removed, and the patient is prepped for vascular access via the standard landmark-based technique. This can be performed by a single operator and does not require additional adjunctive equipment such as a sterile transducer sleeve. This approach is particularly useful when the patient is unable to assume the standard position for cannulation, when time is of the essence, or when the target vessel is discovered to be large and superficial during the pre-scan phase. One randomized trial demonstrated that the static technique is superior to the traditional landmark technique for central venous cannulation.[14]
- **To assist in real-time cannulation under direct ultrasound visualization.** This is termed as the *dynamic* approach. The ultrasound transducer is inserted into a sterile sleeve and placed on the patient after the sterile prep. The operator can then watch the needle entering the vessel under real-time ultrasound guidance. This technique can involve one or two operators.[23] With two operators, real-time vessel visualization can be maintained throughout the entire procedure. With a single operator, ultrasound guidance stops prior to guidewire insertion in order to free up the nondominant hand. The dynamic technique

takes full advantage of the benefits of ultrasound-assisted vascular access, and is the approach advocated in the AHRQ report. It should be emphasized that the fine motor skills required for this procedure are not automatic. Practice on models and/or phantoms is recommended in order to achieve steady control of the transducer (with the nondominant hand) while aligning the needle and target within the narrow imaging sector of the probe. Although this method may require more training and patient preparation time, it can save precious minutes when routine landmarks are not evident in the critically ill or injured patient.

- **To minimize the number of vascular access attempts.** In certain clinical situations, definitive access is needed in patients at risk for significant complications from multiple vascular attempts. Patients with therapeutic anticoagulation, disseminated intravascular coagulation, thrombocytopenia, hemophilia, or any condition that adds significant risk to vascular access attempts can benefit from the higher first-attempt success rate afforded by ultrasound.
- **To assist in alternative peripheral access.** Alternative peripheral vascular access is important in many patients. Either static or dynamic ultrasound techniques can be used to locate and facilitate cannulation of peripheral vessels. Saphenous, basilic, and cephalic veins are all easily located with ultrasound but difficult to locate with surface visualization. External jugular veins may also be located with ultrasound when anatomic limitations make surface visualization difficult. Some clinical situations require vascular access but choosing a central approach may add unwarranted risk. Ultrasound-guided approach to peripheral veins allows for reliable access without the need for central venous access. This has been shown to be helpful in both adults and children.[16,24]
- **To facilitate arterial puncture or cannulation.** Ultrasound can be used to locate arteries for puncture or cannulation. Radial, brachial, and femoral arteries are easily located with ultrasound. Both dynamic and static techniques can be used to facilitate arterial puncture.

▶ ANATOMICAL CONSIDERATIONS

At times it may not be easy to distinguish veins from arteries with B-mode ultrasound. Recognition of key sonographic characteristics can help distinguish veins from arteries. In comparison to arteries, veins have several distinct sonographic features: (1) they are more easily compressed, (2) have thinner walls, and (3) have no arterial pulsation. In addition, central veins possess characteristic triphasic venous pulsations that can be distinguished from arteries. The addition of color flow is a useful adjunct on ultrasound units used for vascular access.

CANNULATION OF THE INTERNAL JUGULAR VEIN

Ultrasound allows for easy localization of the internal jugular vein (Videos 21-1: Central Vascular Access Tips and 21-2: Central Vascular Access Examples). In addition, the carotid artery can be distinguished from the adjacent internal jugular vein. The internal jugular vein lies deep to the sternocleidomastoid muscle and is lateral and superficial to the carotid artery. Using the sternocleidomastoid muscle as the external landmark, the internal jugular vein sits below the bifurcation of the sternal and clavicular heads of the muscle (Figures 21-1 and 21-2). It is important to note that the relative relationship of the carotid artery with the internal jugular vein may change with head position. Specific technical details of internal jugular vein cannulation are provided below.

CANNULATION OF THE SUBCLAVIAN VEIN USING A SUPRACLAVICULAR APPROACH

Placement of a central venous catheter into the subclavian vein at the junction with the internal jugular vein is possible using ultrasound guidance (Figure 21-3A,B).

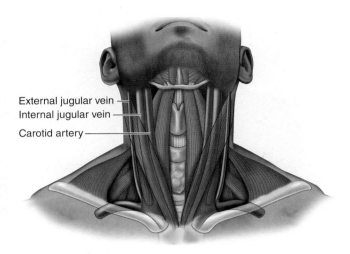

External jugular vein
Internal jugular vein
Carotid artery

Figure 21-1. The anterior superficial structures of the neck.

The use of ultrasound for the traditional infraclavicular approach to subclavian vein catheter placement is limited by the large acoustic shadow created by the clavicle in some patients. In contrast, the supraclavicular approach allows for adequate sonographic visualization of the proximal subclavian vein anatomy, and the internal jugular/innominate vein confluence.

CANNULATION OF THE SUBCLAVIAN/ AXILLARY VEIN USING AN INFRACLAVICULAR APPROACH

For this approach, place the ultrasound transducer initially just below and in contact with the clavicle. Orient

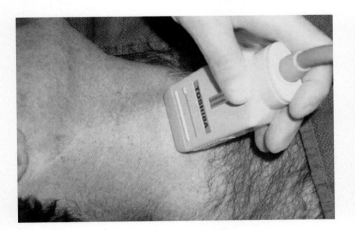

A

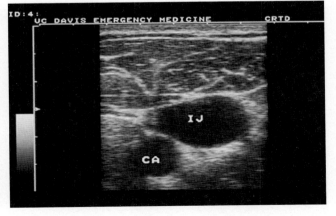

ID:4: UC DAVIS EMERGENCY MEDICINE CRTD

IJ

CA

B

Figure 21-2. Ultrasound image of the large internal jugular vein and deeper carotid artery. Transducer position (A) and corresponding ultrasound image (B). CA = Carotid artery, IJ = Internal jugular vein.

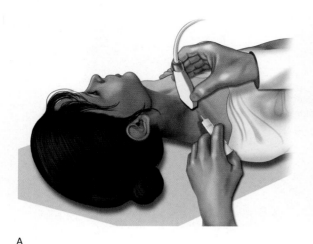

A

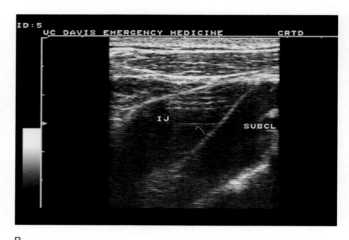

B

Figure 21-3. Placement of the transducer to facilitate visualization of the internal jugular/subclavian vein junction using a supraclavicular approach (A). The transducer should be angled to sweep the view into the upper thorax below the clavicle. Transverse view of the "venous lake" created by the combined subclavian vein and internal jugular vein (B).

the transducer in long axis over the proximal axillary vein, which travels parallel to the deltopectoral groove. Approach the axillary vein from a more peripheral location near the anterior axillary line if the vein is prominent. Alternately, a more central approach (at the midclavicular line area) will allow the needle/catheter to enter the vein just before it courses below the clavicle to become the subclavian vein. The later approach often requires that the transducer be placed partially over the clavicle so that needle entry for longitudinal (in-plane) visualization is closer to the clavicle (Figure 21-4).

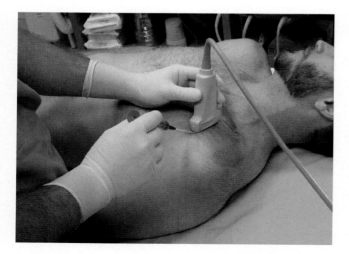

Figure 21-4. Transducer placement for cannulation of the subclavian/axillary vein using the infraclavicular approach. (Courtesy of Michael Blaivas, MD)

CANNULATION OF THE FEMORAL VEIN

Place the transducer in a transverse position just below the mid-portion of the inguinal ligament. Identification of the key vascular structures begins just below the inguinal ligament and medial to the femoral arterial pulsation. Use the compression technique to distinguish the readily compressible vein from the less compressible artery (Figure 21-5). In addition, appreciating the variable relationships of the vascular structures with respect to limb position is important. Utilize either the static or dynamic technique for femoral vein cannulation. Limit the use of the femoral vein for central venous access in adults to emergency situations because of higher complication rates.[21]

PERIPHERAL VENOUS CANNULATION

Ultrasound will permit localization of veins that often do not have consistent anatomic relationships or are too deep to be readily palpable (Video 21-3: Peripheral Vascular Access). Of note, the superficial venous structures are easily collapsed with even slight pressure of the transducer on the skin. This feature of collapsibility is useful for distinguishing between veins and arteries. Superficial veins may not be identified, however, if they are collapsed by inadvertent excessive pressure on the transducer. Placing a tourniquet on the extremity to maximize vein dilation is also advisable. Once a suitable vein is identified, the process of IV catheter placement is largely unchanged from standard practice using routinely available venous catheters. With respect to

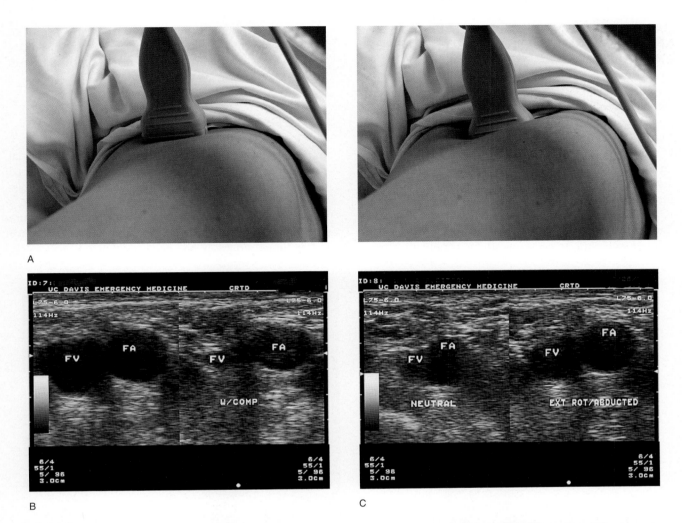

Figure 21-5. Femoral vein (FV): Gentle pressure is applied to the transducer to identify venous structures by their easy compressibility. (A) FV collapses with compression, and the femoral artery (FA) retains its shape even with compression. (B) FV position is seen to vary with hip abduction and external rotation. (C) In neutral position (left frame), the vein is closely opposed to the FA; however, when the hip is abducted and rotated, the vein is displaced from the artery (right frame). (A, Courtesy of Michael Blaivas, MD)

ultrasound guidance in peripheral venous access, either the static or dynamic technique may be successfully utilized. Ultrasound use for peripheral IV access has been shown to decrease the number of needle sticks and time to successful cannulation, and can be readily employed by novice users.[16,17]

CANNULATION OF THE EXTERNAL JUGULAR VEIN

Since the external jugular vein is superficial, it is often readily identified by visualization and palpation without ultrasound assistance (Figure 21-6). However, limited range of motion (i.e., cervical spine precautions) or adiposity may make this vessel difficult to cannulate without ultrasound guidance.

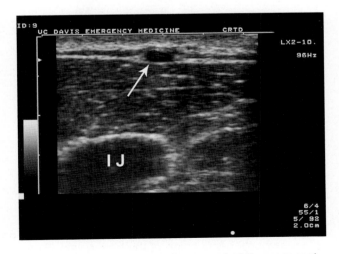

Figure 21-6. Transverse ultrasound of the external jugular vein (arrow) and internal jugular vein (IJ).

CANNULATION OF THE BRACHIAL AND CEPHALIC VEINS OF THE UPPER EXTREMITY

The antecubital veins of the arms are commonly used for venous access in the emergency setting, as are the more proximal cephalic and brachial veins (Figure 21-7A). The cephalic and brachial veins lie deeper in the structures of the upper arm and are not readily palpable; consequently, these veins are not generally used for IV catheter placement in the absence of ultrasound guidance. Be cautious with the more proximal brachial vein since it lies immediately adjacent to the ulnar and median nerves. In most patients, the depth of these vessels and angle required for cannulation man-

dates that a longer catheter (2.5 inches) be used. An example of transducer placement and vessel visualization for proximal vein cannulation is demonstrated in Figure 21-7.

ARTERIAL CANNULATION

In the absence of color flow Doppler, real-time arterial pulsation, thickness of arterial wall, and lack of arterial compressibility are all sonographic features that help distinguish arterial from venous anatomy. The mechanics of placing an arterial catheter or simple arterial puncture can proceed along traditional technical guidelines once the pertinent anatomy has been recognized.

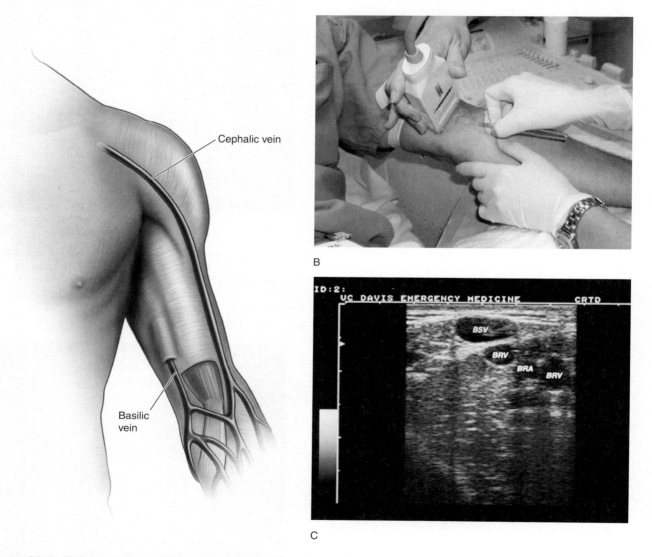

A

B

C

Figure 21-7. The superficial veins of the proximal upper extremity (A) Demonstration of transducer placement for cannulation of the basilic vein (B) An image demonstrating transverse ultrasound orientation (C) of the relatively superficial basilic vein (BSV) with deeper lying brachial artery and veins (BRV, BRA). Note the proximity of the brachial artery to its venous counterpart makes inadvertent arterial puncture a possibility.

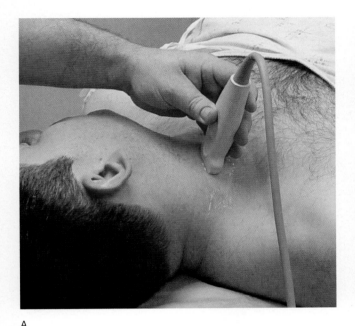

A

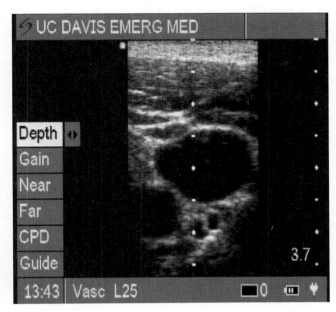

B

Figure 21-8. First P-Prescan of internal jugular vein (A) Transverse orientation of right internal jugular vein and right carotid artery (B) Note needle guide present.

▶ TECHNIQUE AND NORMAL ULTRASOUND FINDINGS

The dynamic technique can be summarized by the Four Ps: Pre-scan, Preparation, Poke, and Path. Use a 7.5 or 10 MHz linear array transducer.

The purpose of the **pre-scan** is to survey the underlying vessels, confirm the target vessel appropriately, and optimize patient and machine positions and settings in advance of the actual procedure (Figure 21-8). For internal jugular vein cannulation, observe for three structures during the pre-scan: thyroid gland, internal jugular vein, and carotid artery. Visualize all three structures before proceeding. The internal jugular vein can be easily compressed, especially in volume-depleted patients; confirming its presence in relationship to the other structures will ensure verification of the proper target vessel. When standing at the head of the bed, point the transducer position marker toward the patient's left side and the monitor located at the patient's hip and facing you. This will ensure the proper relationship of the underlying anatomy with the ultrasound image anatomy. For example, when cannulating the patient's right internal jugular vein, the thyroid, carotid artery, and internal jugular vein will be from left to right anatomically as well as on the ultrasound monitor. Thus, when moving the needle more medially, or to the left, it will move left on the monitor. When moving the needle more lateral, or to the right, it will move to the right on the monitor.

If possible, elevate the exam table to a comfortable height and tilt to allow venous distention. Lower the room lights and adjust the monitor gain (brightness) and image depth before any sterile preparation is begun.

The second P stands for **preparation** (Figure 21-9). Prepare the patient's skin for a sterile procedure in the standard fashion. For dynamic cannulation, prepare the transducer with a sterile sleeve and gel. Several types of sleeves are available for ultrasound transducers. Sleeves

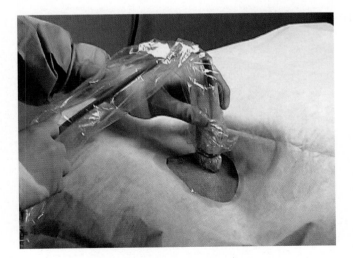

Figure 21-9. Second P-Preparation. Note the transducer with long sterile sleeve allowing easy use in a sterile field.

that cover the transducer and cable are preferred since they can be placed on the sterile field and easily located for single operator use. Careful application of coupling gel to the transducer prior to placement in a sterile sleeve is necessary to avoid entrapment of air bubbles. Secure the sterile sleeve with elastic bands and apply sterile coupling gel to the outside of the transducer sleeve prior to further imaging. With the sterile barrier in place, the transducer is ready for use.

The **poke** refers to the initial skin puncture (prior to actual venipuncture), which places the needle in the SC tissues where it is identified before further advancement. The initial insertion of the needle and its subsequent localization is an important step. Advancing the needle prior to localization can result in a misdirected path. Figure 21-10 demonstrates proper needle position for the initial insertion. Note how close the needle is to the transducer. Use a thick pool of sterile gel to prevent interference from air as the skin is pushed downward.

Following the **path** of the needle and adjusting the course are keys to successful placement. Tissue motion during initial real-time imaging of the procedure can help localize the area of the needle prior to visualization of the needle itself. The needle will be detected as a bright spot echo and ring-down artifact (short axis) or a reflection from the shaft and shadowing or reverberation artifact (long axis) (Figure 21-11A,B). Direct the needle toward the vessel while using the monitor display to locate the needle tip. Ensure that the needle *tip* has been located prior to each advancement of the needle. A common error involves mistaking the needle shaft for the needle tip and thereby misjudging the

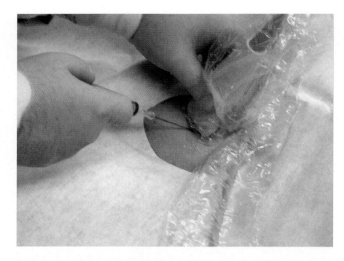

Figure 21-10. Third P-Poke. Note how close the needle is to the transducer in order to locate the needle tip immediately after the puncture.

actual tip location. Figure 21-12 illustrates scanning with different needle vectors and imaging planes. Note the convergence of the shafts of all three needle paths in the transverse plane. However, each needle tip is in a different location in relation to the vessel. Accurate needle guidance in the transverse plane requires a sweeping motion of the scan plane to localize the needle tip as it is advanced. The long-axis view of the needle has the potential advantage of visualization of the entire shaft of the needle from skin to vein; however, if the transducer is angled slightly during the procedure, the clinician risks

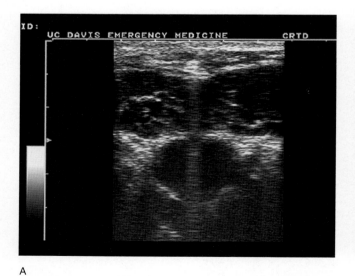

A

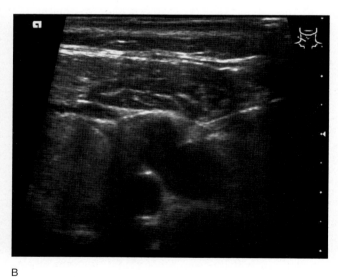

B

Figure 21-11. Transverse view of the vein and needle. (A) Ring-down artifact of needle after the initial puncture. This is used to localize the needle prior to advancing. (B) Transverse view of the vessels, with longitudinal (in-plane) view of the needle. The needle is seen approaching from the right side and the tip is just entering the vein. (B, Courtesy of James Mateer, MD)

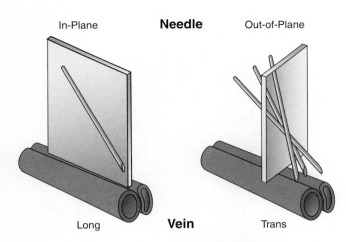

Figure 21-12. Diagram illustrating pitfall during the fourth P-Path. Note how in the transverse plane (B) all the three needles converge in one point, although their vectors are different. The needle approaches are outside the plane of the transverse image and will only produce a spot echo where they cross. In the longitudinal plane (A), the entire shaft and tip of the needle can be seen within the scanning plane, but keeping the image sector centered can be challenging. This illustrates why accurate needle visualization from skin to target is important.

guiding the needle to an adjacent incorrect target (such as the carotid artery).

Prior to successful cannulation, the vein will be seen to deform with the pressure of the advancing needle (Figure 21-13). Confirmation of successful venipuncture proceeds as usual with a flash of venous blood

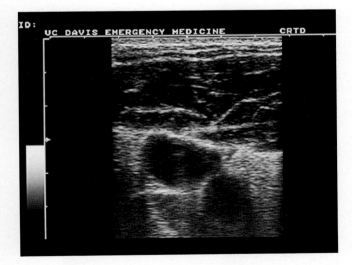

Figure 21-13. Tenting or deformity of the vessel will occur prior to needle penetration. In this example, the vessel is slightly collapsed. In real time, the vessel wall may briefly indent, then quickly rebound as the needle enters.

into the syringe. With either static or dynamic technique, the mechanics of catheter placement (i.e., using the Seldinger technique) proceeds unchanged from standard technique.

TRANSDUCER AND NEEDLE ORIENTATION: LONGITUDINAL VERSUS TRANSVERSE VERSUS OBLIQUE

Figure 21-12 illustrates the most common approaches to needle guidance where the scan plan is longitudinal or transverse to both the structure of interest and to the shaft of the needle. Certain approaches, however, require a combination of views. For example, the imaging plane for the vessel could be primarily transverse, while the needle shaft is directed within the longitudinal axis of the imaging plane (or vice versa). As this terminology can be confusing, some have begun to describe a long-axis needle approach as an "In-Plane" view, while a short-axis needle view is considered an "Out-of-Plane" view. Variations in transducer positioning will yield different information relative to vessel and needle placement. Transverse transducer positioning gives information related to lateral orientation. The longitudinal transducer position gives depth and slope information (Figure 21-14). The authors generally rely primarily on transverse short-axis imaging to assist with venous cannulation. The transverse short-axis orientation is most helpful in demonstrating relationships with other adjacent anatomy (Figure 21-8). Novice operators should use the transverse short-axis approach since time for vascular access is shorter when compared to the longitudinal axis approach.[25] The longitudinal orientation will help with needle orientation in the long axis of the vessel of interest (Figure 21-15). A potential danger with the short-axis approach is unseen penetration of the deep wall of the vein and any structure that lies deep to it. There is preliminary evidence that long access may be effective in decreasing vessel penetration through the deep wall in novice users[26] Long-axis orientation can be helpful when difficulty is encountered with the guidewire. The long-axis view may demonstrate the location of resistance and allow for subtle readjustments.

The oblique view is an alternative approach that has been developed to capitalize on the advantages of both the short- and long-axis techniques[27] This view allows better visualization of the needle shaft and tip but also offers the safety of being able to visualize all relevant anatomically significant structures at the same time and in the same plane (Figure 21-16). The transducer orientation is halfway between the short and the long axis of the vessel, and the transducer is placed over the portion of the vessel that is most superficial and/or accessible.

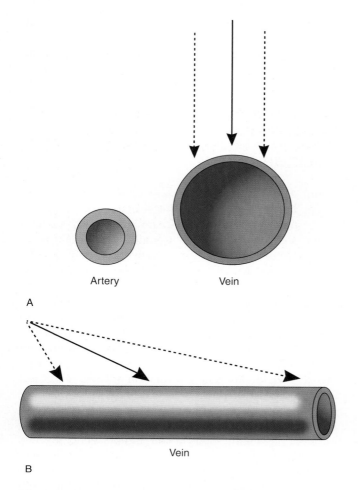

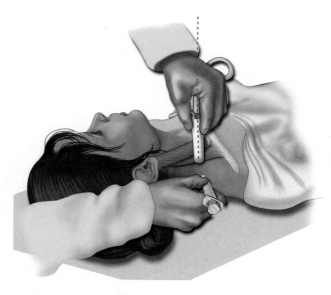

Figure 21-16. Diagram illustrating orientation and approach for the oblique view of the internal jugular vein. The ultrasound probe indicator is pointed toward the patient's left.

Figure 21-14. Diagram illustrating transverse and longitudinal orientation. Transverse gives better lateral/medial positioning (A). Longitudinal gives better slope and depth positioning (B).

This often requires a slightly more coronal position of the transducer (side of the neck). By aligning the edge of the transducer close to the posterior border of the sternocleidomastoid, the needle can enter and track just below the muscle. Avoiding muscle puncture is advantageous for patient comfort, and it avoids bleeding complications. An in-plane approach for the needle is used to direct the tip into the oval shaped internal jugular vein,

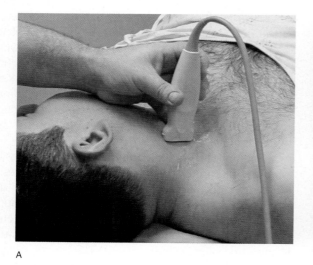

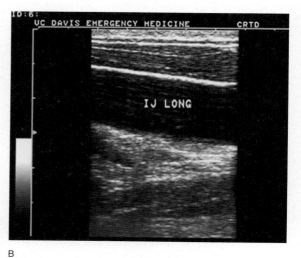

Figure 21-15. Transducer placement (A) and ultrasound image (B) of the longitudinal or long-axis plane of the internal jugular vein.

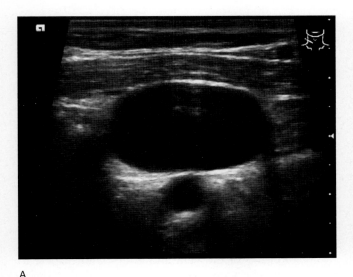
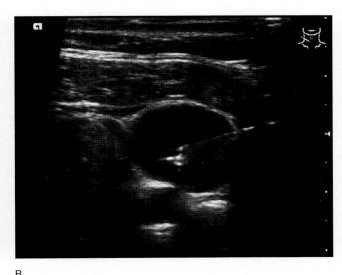

A   B

Figure 21-17. Oblique approach to the internal jugular vein. When the transducer is rotated approximately 45° to the internal jugular vein, the vessel appears larger and oval shaped (A). The carotid artery is noted directly posterior to the internal jugular vein in this case, so an anterior tranverse approach may not be optimal. The needle approach is in-plane (B), is tracking just below the SCM muscle, and is directed above the carotid artery. (Courtesy of James Mateer, MD)

while keeping the carotid artery in view (Figure 21-17). The oblique approach has great potential for infants or other patients where neck access is limited and where increased distance from the lung pleura is needed for safety (COPD patients).

STATIC VERSUS DYNAMIC PLACEMENT TECHNIQUE

Techniques utilizing ultrasound-assisted venous cannulation may vary depending on the clinical scenario and the availability of assistance as well as the necessity for strict sterile technique. The advantage of the dynamic technique is that it allows for real-time observation of the needle position and target vascular structures. The logistical simplicity of the static technique may be advantageous in the case where the landmark-based anatomy is straightforward. The static technique allows a brief inspection and confirmation of the vessel location without the reliance on a second operator. Both static and dynamic approaches have been found to be superior to the traditional landmark-based approach.[14]

NEEDLE VISUALIZATION

As clinicians gain experience with ultrasound needle guidance, it becomes more evident that accuracy for these techniques requires that the position of the needle

tip is clearly visible on the monitor during the entire procedure. There are specific adjustments in the image that can improve needle visualization. Adjust the ultrasound frequency, focus, and gain to optimize resolution in the near field. If possible, tilt the transducer to align the beam more perpendicular to the needle, which results in a stronger echo (brighter needle tip or shaft). Manufacturers have recognized this need with echo-enhanced needles. Although one study did not find improved efficiency with echo-enhanced needles for novice users, [28] anecdotal information from experienced users suggests these may be helpful. Newer machines are adding enhanced needle visualization options and some transducers are designed for use with needle guides that ensure the needle is steady and will advance only within the plane of the image.

Whatever method is used, the importance of accurately visualizing the needle from skin to target vessel cannot be stressed enough.

STERILE TECHNIQUE

There are several different options for maintaining sterile technique. The best option is to use prepackaged sterile transducer sleeves that are manufactured solely for the purpose of handling the transducer and transducer cord in a sterile fashion (Figure 21-18). Alternatively, the use of a large sterile glove, positioning the transducer and adequate amounts of conductive gel into the thumb of the glove, can also be effective (Figure 21-19). If using

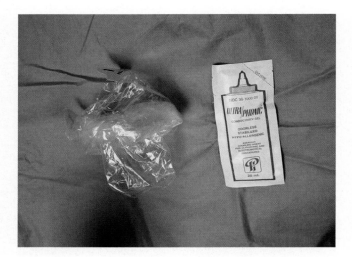

Figure 21-18. Sterile transducer cover and sterile coupling gel in prepack setup.

the glove option, care must be taken to avoid compromising sterility by puncturing one of the "extra" fingers of the glove during the process of venipuncture. Sterile lubricant is sufficient as a conductive medium between the sleeve and the skin.

► COMMON VARIANTS AND OTHER ABNORMALITIES

VARIABILITY OF NORMAL VENOUS ANATOMY

The large central venous structures of the body have fairly constant anatomy, whereas the peripheral veins are extremely variable in their position. It is helpful,

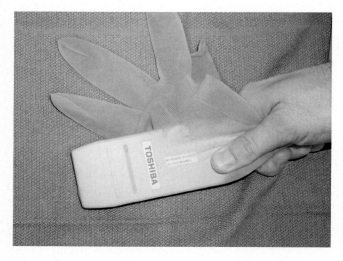

Figure 21-19. Using a sterile glove as an improvised transducer cover.

however, to keep in mind the typical course of the veins and the important adjacent structures while using ultrasound to assist in vessel identification and cannulation.

EFFECT OF PATIENT POSITIONING

The usual considerations apply for patient preparation for central or peripheral venous cannulation. The Trendelenburg position is useful to provide slight venous distention in the veins of the head and neck. Furthermore, the use of ultrasound may help determine optimal patient position with respect to surrounding arterial anatomy.[29] It is apparent in individual patients that rotation or abduction of a limb will significantly alter the relationship of the vein and artery with respect to the skin. It merits emphasizing that in certain individuals leg position alone can cause the femoral artery to directly overlie the femoral vein. Hence, the use of a standard (nonultrasound-assisted) technique, given certain patient positioning, may result in arterial injury or failed venous cannulation (Figure 21-5C).

► PITFALLS

There are no absolute contraindications to the use of ultrasound for vascular access; however, there are a few common pitfalls.

1. **Failure to identify the needle in tissue.** When using ultrasound for dynamic venous access, it is important to accurately view the needle ring-down artifact or venous tenting to confirm position. Whether using the transverse or longitudinal approach, it is important to identify the needle with ultrasound visualization before advancing into deeper structures. This is important to ensure successful cannulation while minimizing complications. Transverse orientation allows for better lateral positioning of the needle, while longitudinal orientation provides better depth and needle slope positioning.

2. **Failure to distinguish between vein and artery through compression testing or color flow Doppler.** Since arterial pulsations at times may be subtle, veins and arteries may initially appear very similar (especially in the hypotensive patient). In the absence of color flow Doppler capability, confirm that the vessel is a vein by using compression maneuvers. A vein will easily collapse with gentle external pressure. While color or power Doppler may be of some use, pulse wave Doppler will enable the clinician to actually interrogate the vessel of

choice and determine if venous or arterial flow is present.

3. **Locating the vessel with the static approach prior to the patient being in proper position.** Locate the vessel *after* the clinician has the patient properly positioned for the cannulation attempt. As emphasized earlier, many vessels will move slightly and change relationship depending on the patient's position.

4. **Failure to angle the transducer beam into the needle puncture area.** Since ultrasound provides a two-dimensional image, angle the beam toward the needle tip as the needle is advanced. Figure 21-12 demonstrates how in the short axis the needle can appear over the vessel while the tip is not within the vessel. Note how three different needle vectors intersect over the vessel although the ultimate needle tip may be in a very different location.

▶ CASE STUDIES

CASE 1

Patient Presentation

A 50-year-old man who was morbidly obese presented complaining of chest pain. On examination, he was hypotensive and diaphoretic. A 12-lead EKG revealed him to be in complete heart block. Multiple attempts at peripheral access failed. The transcutaneous pacemaker was intermittently capturing but had little effect on the patient's hemodynamic status. There were no good external anatomic landmarks due to his adiposity.

Management Course

The patient's right internal jugular vein was easily visualized under ultrasound guidance using a 7.5 MHz linear transducer. A dynamic real-time ultrasound-guided cannulation of the right internal jugular vein was successful on the first attempt. An IV pacemaker wire was then successfully placed (also under ultrasound visualization). Upon improved ventricular capture, the patient's blood pressure normalized.

CASE 2

Patient Presentation

An 18-year-old woman who was severely scarred and contractured from old burns to the neck, chest, arms, and legs, presented after ingesting a lethal quantity of a tricyclic antidepressant in a suicide attempt. On examination, the patient was hypotensive and lethargic. Nu-

merous attempts at peripheral access failed. There were no appreciable anatomic landmarks for central access due to her old scars.

Management Course

Although a femoral arterial pulsation was difficult to palpate for the landmark-based approach, the femoral vein was easily visualized under ultrasound guidance. An ultrasound-guided femoral vein catheter was inserted on the first attempt. The patient was then administered induction agents for orotracheal intubation and successfully resuscitated.

CASE 3

Patient Presentation

A 40-year-old man with a long history of injection drug use presented for drainage of a deltoid abscess. It was determined that the abscess could be drained as an outpatient with the use of systemic sedation and analgesia. Numerous attempts at routine peripheral venous access failed. The patient was refusing a central venous line.

Management Course

The patient had a large right basilic vein easily visualized with ultrasound. A 2-inch 18-gauge catheter was inserted without difficulty. The patient's abscess was successfully drained after receiving adequate IV sedation and analgesia.

Commentary

Anatomic landmarks in patients may be distorted, obscured, or nonexistent. In the three cases, each patient presented with anatomic variations that made it difficult to obtain rapid peripheral venous access or landmark-based central venous access. Venous access was facilitated by the use of ultrasound in each case, thereby expediting patient resuscitation and care. Ultrasound use allowed the clinicians to obtain venous access on the first attempt and helped prevent complications associated with delays in obtaining venous access or multiple attempts to obtain central venous access.

REFERENCES

1. Denys BG, Uretsky BF: Anatomical variations of internal jugular vein location: Impact on central venous access. *Crit Care Med* 19:1516–1519, 1991.
2. Bagwell CE, Salzberg AM, Sonnino RE: Potentially lethal complications of central venous catheter placement. *J Pediatr Surg* 35:709–713, 2000.

3. Conz PA, Dissegna D, Rodighiero MP: Cannulation of the internal jugular vein: Comparison of the classic Seldinger technique and an ultrasound guided method. *J Nephrol* 10:311–313, 1997.

4. Lee W, Leduc L, Cotton DB: Ultrasonographic guidance for central venous access during pregnancy. *Am J Obstet Gynecol* 161:1012–1013, 1989.

5. Trottier SJ, Veremakis C, O'Brien J: Femoral deep vein thrombosis associated with central venous catheterization: Results from a prospective, randomized trial. *Crit Care Med* 23:52–59, 1995.

6. Farrell J, Gellens M: Ultrasound-guided cannulation versus the landmark-guided technique for acute haemodialysis access. *Nephrol Dial Transplant* 12:1234–1237, 1997.

7. Gallieni M, Cozzolino M: Uncomplicated central vein catheterization of high risk patients with real time ultrasound guidance. *Int J Artif Organs* 18:117–121, 1995.

8. Hudson PA, Rose JS: Real-time ultrasound guided internal jugular vein catheterization in the emergency department. *Am J Emerg Med* 15:79–82, 1997.

9. Meredith JW, Young JS, O'Neil EA: Femoral catheters and deep venous thrombosis: A prospective evaluation with venous duplex sonography. *J Trauma* 35:187–190, 1993.

10. Vucevic M, Tehan B, Gamlin F: The SMART needle. A new Doppler ultrasound-guided vascular access needle. *Anaesthesia* 49:889–891, 1994.

11. Karakitsos D, Labropoulos N, De Groot E, et al.: Real-time ultrasound-guided catheterization of the internal jugular vein: A prospective comparison with the landmark technique in critical care patients *Critical Care* 10(6):R162, 2006.

12. Caridi JG, Hawkins IF, Wiechmann BN: Sonographic guidance when using the right internal jugular vein for central vein access. *AJR Am J Roentgenol* 171:1259–1263, 1998.

13. Slama M, Novara A, Safavian A: Improvement of internal jugular vein cannulation using an ultrasound-guided technique. *Intensive Care Med* 23:916–919, 1997.

14. Milling TJ, Rose JS, Briggs WM, et al.: Randomized, controlled clinical trial of point-of-care limited ultrasonography assistance of central venous cannulation: The Third Sonography Outcomes Assessment Program (SOAP-3) Trial. *Crit Care Med* 33:1764–1769, 2005.

15. Hilty WM, Hudson PA, Levitt MA: Real-time ultrasound-guided femoral vein catheterization during cardiopulmonary resuscitation. *Ann Emerg Med* 29:331–336, 1997.

16. Costantino TP, Parikh A: Ultrasonography-guided peripheral intravenous access versus traditional approaches in patients with difficult intravenous access. *Ann Emerg Med* 46:456–661, 2005.

17. Brannam L: Emergency nurses' utilization of ultrasound guidance for placement of peripheral intravenous lines in difficult-access patients. *Acad Emerg Med* 11:1361–1363, 2004.

18. Keyes LE, Frazee BW, Snoey ER: Ultrasound-guided brachial and basilic vein cannulation in emergency department patients with difficult intravenous access. *Ann Emerg Med* 34:711–714, 1999.

19. Rose JS, Norbutas CM: A randomized controlled trial comparing one-operator versus two-operator technique in ultrasound-guided basilic vein cannulation. *J Emerg Med* 35:431–435, 2008.

20. Parkinson R, Gandhi M, Harper J: Establishing an ultrasound guided peripherally inserted central catheter (PICC) insertion service. *Clin Radiol* 53:33–36, 1998.

21. Rothschild JM: Ultrasound guidance of central vein catheterization: Making healthcare safer: A critical analysis of patient safety practices. Available at http://www.ahrq.gov/clinic/ptsafety/chap21.htm.

22. National Institute for Clinical Excellence: Guidance on the use of ultrasound locating devices for placing central venous catheters. *NHS* 49:1–24, 2002.

23. Milling TJ: Randomized controlled trial of single-operator vs. two-operator ultrasound guidance for internal jugular central venous cannulation. *Acad Emerg Med* 13:245–247, 2006.

24. Bair AE, Rose JS, Vance C, et al.: Ultrasound assisted peripheral intravenous access in pediatric emergency department patients: A randomized clinical trial. *Acad Emerg Med* 12:325–328, 2005.

25. Blaivas M: Short-axis versus long-axis approaches for teaching ultrasound-guided vascular access on a new inanimate model. *Acad Emerg Med* 10:1307–1311, 2003.

26. Blaivas M: Video analysis of accidental arterial cannulation with dynamic ultrasound guidance for central venous access. *J Ultrasound Med* 28:1239–1244, 2009.

27. Phelan M, Hagerty D: The oblique view: An alternative approach for ultrasound-guided central line placement. *J Emerg Med* 37(4):403–408, 2009.

28. Phelan, MP: Do echo-enhanced needles improve time to cannulate in a model of short-axis ultrasound-guided vascular access for a group of mostly inexperienced ultrasound users? *Int J Emerg Med* 2(3):167–170, 2009.

29. Armstrong PJ, Sutherland R, Scott DH: The effect of position and different maneuvers on internal jugular vein diameter size. *Acta Anaesthesiol Scand* 38:229–231, 1994.

CHAPTER 22

Additional Ultrasound-Guided Procedures

Andreas Dewitz, Robert A. Jones, Jessica G. Resnick, and Michael B. Stone

Invasive procedures are frequently performed in the ED. Traditionally, these procedures have been performed by emergency physicians who relied on physical assessment for making the correct diagnosis and surface landmarks for determining the correct approach. In recent years, the use of point-of-care ultrasound has been incorporated into the practice of many emergency physicians to guide or assist in the performance of a variety of invasive procedures.

The use of ultrasound guidance (dynamic guidance) or ultrasound assistance (static guidance) to perform certain procedures can decrease complications when utilized correctly. Before performing any procedure under ultrasound guidance, it is imperative that clinicians have a thorough understanding of sonographic anatomy, know the basic principles of ultrasound, and have practical training with phantoms or models to develop the hand–eye coordination required. Lack of familiarity with ultrasound and the orientation of the image on the screen can lead to complications even in the hands of a physician skilled at performing the procedure in a "blind" fashion.

► PHYSICIAN TRAINING

Ultrasound is a highly operator-dependent technology and the success of an ultrasound-guided or -assisted procedure will depend on the skill of the physician performing the procedure. The amount of training required to successfully perform these procedures has not been well defined in the literature. In the 2008 American College of Emergency Physicians (ACEP) Emergency Ultrasound Guidelines, performance of a minimum of ten ultrasound-guided procedures or completion of a module on ultrasound-guided procedures with simulation on a high-quality ultrasound phantom is recommended for hospital privileging.[1] However, it is acknowledged that the training process for emergency ultrasound should move beyond strict numbers and should include experiential and competency components.

► GENERAL PRINCIPLES

DYNAMIC GUIDANCE AND STATIC GUIDANCE

Procedures can be performed using either ultrasound guidance (dynamic) or ultrasound assistance (static). Ultrasound guidance entails performing the procedure while imaging the target and needle in real-time during the procedure. Ultrasound assistance entails performing the procedure in the traditional fashion after the anatomy and any pathology has been mapped by ultrasound and the entry point marked.

The decision to perform a procedure under ultrasound guidance or ultrasound assistance is based on the procedure itself. Procedures involving small target structures or procedures requiring precise placement of the needle are best performed under ultrasound guidance. Procedures such as paracentesis, thoracentesis, and abscess drainage are frequently performed using ultrasound assistance since the fluid collections tend to be larger, and once anatomy and pathology are marked out, it is typically safe to proceed blindly.

NUMBER OF OPERATORS

Ultrasound-guided procedures can be performed using either a one-operator or two-operator technique. In a one-operator technique, the operator controls the transducer while simultaneously performing the procedure. In a two-operator technique, a second operator (assistant) controls the transducer while the first operator simultaneously performs the procedure. For those just learning to perform ultrasound-guided procedures, it is recommended that the one-operator technique be emphasized. In a study involving ultrasound guidance for internal jugular central venous cannulation, the one-operator technique appeared to be equivalent to the two-operator technique for successful ultrasound-guided internal jugular central venous catheterization with respect to overall success.[2] The hand–eye coordination and neural feedback obtained by the single operator is much more accurate than the verbal communication that occurs between two operators. Changes in transducer placement or orientation by an assistant may go unnoticed by the operator performing the procedure until it is too late. This mishap may result in the need for another attempt or more significantly may result in the inadvertent puncture of an adjacent structure.

TRANSDUCER SELECTION

Transducer selection is based on the size of the scanning area and the depth of the target structure. The depth of the target structure determines the frequency selection. Superficial target structures are best imaged using high-frequency transducers, while deeper structures are best imaged using low-frequency transducers. Array transducer choice is based on the size of the surface scanning area. Easy to access superficial structures are best imaged using a high-frequency linear transducer, while difficult to access superficial structures are best imaged using a high-frequency, small footprint curvilinear transducer. Peritonsillar abscesses are best imaged using a high-frequency endocavitary transducer. Easy to access deeper structures are best imaged using a low-frequency curvilinear transducer.

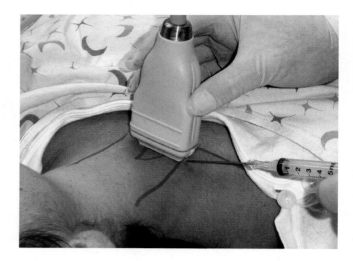

Figure 22-1. Long-axis approach. Note that the needle is in line with the transducer beam.

SPATIAL ORIENTATION

Ultrasound-guided procedures can be performed using an infinite combination of imaging and needle axis planes. When describing the approach, it is most accurate to define both the imaging plane (long, short or oblique axis to the target structure) and also define the plane of the needle path. With respect to the transducer, the needle can travel parallel to the image slice or perpendicular to the image slice. Clinicians commonly refer to these needle paths as either an "in-plane" (long-axis) or "out-of-plane" (short-axis) approach. When the imaging plane is not defined, a "long-axis approach" indicates that the transducer is in plane with the needle (Figure 22-1). A "short-axis approach" indicates that the transducer is 90° to the long axis of the needle (Figure 22-2).

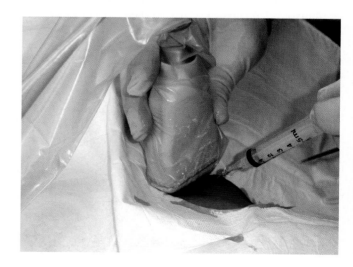

Figure 22-2. Short-axis approach. Note that the needle is perpendicular to the transducer beam.

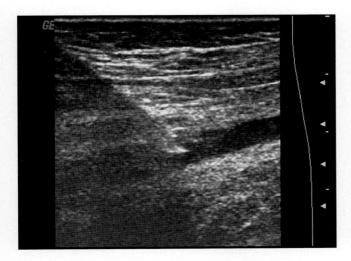

Figure 22-3. Long-axis approach with the needle tip visualized within the vessel lumen.

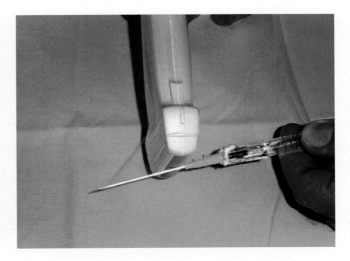

Figure 22-5. Short-axis approach. Note that the needle is perpendicular to the axis of the transducer beam.

The long-axis approach provides the advantage of allowing the needle to be visualized in its long axis, so the location of the needle tip in relationship to the target structure can be identified with certainty throughout the entire path taken by the needle (Figure 22-3). The main disadvantage of this approach is that the needle must be kept in line with the ultrasound beam and this requires reasonable hand–eye coordination, a steady hand, and significant practice. Failure to keep the beam in line with the needle can result in complete loss of visualization of the needle (Figure 22-4A,B).

The short-axis approach relies on the centering of the vessel or target structure on the screen and using the center of the long face of the transducer as the entry point (Figure 22-5). The transducer indicator is always directed to the operator's left so that transducer adjustments correlate with the direction of movement visualized on the screen. Using this approach, the shaft of the needle will be seen only in its short axis (Figure 22-6). The main disadvantage of this approach is that the tip of the needle may be hard to localize. When using this technique to perform ultrasound-guided vascular access, it is not uncommon to penetrate the anterior and posterior wall of the vessels and occasionally unintended structures posterior to the target vessel (Figure 22-7).[3,4] Therefore, the presence of key structures, such as adjacent arteries or nerves, posterior to the target structure should be noted when performing a short-axis approach in order to minimize the risk of inadvertent puncture.

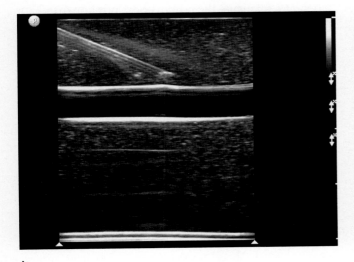

A

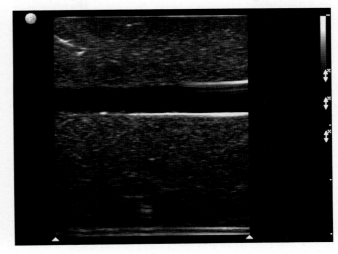

B

Figure 22-4. (A) Long-axis approach with the needle visualized. (B) Long-axis approach with complete loss of visualization of the needle due to slight movement of the transducer.

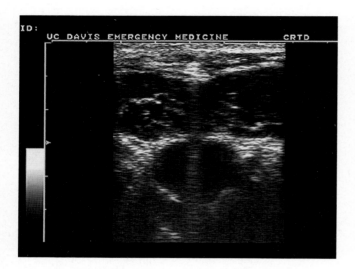

Figure 22-6. Image obtained using short-axis approach. Note needle artifact centered above vein. (Courtesy of John S. Rose, MD)

Regardless of the approach taken and the instrument used, the operator should always know where on the ultrasound screen the instrument should appear once under the skin. In the case of a long-axis approach, it is prudent to decide whether the needle will appear from the right or left side of the screen. This can be accomplished by setting the transducer in the desired orientation on whatever body surface the procedure will take place. Using a finger, disturb the skin on the side of the transducer from which the instrument will penetrate the skin. The resulting disturbance on the ultrasound screen will indicate where on the screen the instrument will appear under the skin as long as the

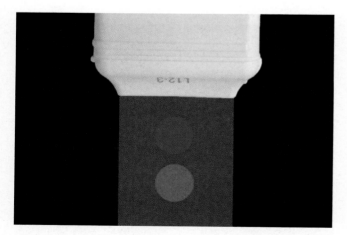

Figure 22-7. Target structure (blue circle) placed under the center of the long face of the linear transducer. Note the presence of structure (red circle) directly posterior to the target structure. Avoid approaches in which a key structure is present posterior to the target structure.

same orientation is maintained. For short-axis approach, the structure of interest should be aligned under the center of the transducer and the needle puncture done under the center of the transducer face with the transducer indicator always to the operator's left side. Some find it useful to place a permanent mark on the center of the linear array transducer to mark this location. Others use a technique of placing the needle flat between the transducer face and the skin to align the needle artifact with the intended structure before tilting the needle up to the intended puncture angle.

TECHNICAL ASPECTS

For ultrasound guidance or assistance to be successful, the desired structure must be easily and clearly visible with ultrasound. Difficulty in visualizing a structure that is normally readily imaged with ultrasound can be due to numerous technical factors such as difficult scanning plane, body habitus, inadequate gel use, and interference from adjacent structures. In these difficult patients, developing an alternative plan may be the best option if the target structure cannot be imaged despite addressing the pitfalls just listed. Trying to target a structure that cannot be clearly visualized decreases the success rate and increases the complication rate of the procedure.

Once an initial scouting ultrasound examination confirms that the target is accessible, the next step involves procedure preparation and setup. These are essential aspects of an invasive procedure. The patient should be optimally positioned prior to beginning the procedure. Experiment with different patient positions prior to beginning in order to see which position will improve the chance of success. If ultrasound assistance is used to mark a location, it will be important for the patient to maintain the same body position used for marking the skin and needle entry. An obvious example of this is fluid marking for paracentesis. If the patient moves, fluid may shift away from the path of the needle and bowel penetration may occur. A more subtle example is the slight but important realignment of vascular structures that may occur with movement (Figure 22-8).

The location of the ultrasound machine in relationship to the operator and the patient must be carefully considered. Place the machine in a location where the operator can easily visualize the screen, ideally without turning his or her head and simply by glancing up or slightly to the side (Figure 22-9). Placing the machine in a location where the operator is forced to turn around or be in an awkward position will make the process less comfortable and increase the likelihood of failure (Figure 22-10). Make correct ultrasound image adjustments before the final preparations for the procedure so that both hands are free and can remain gloved and sterile.

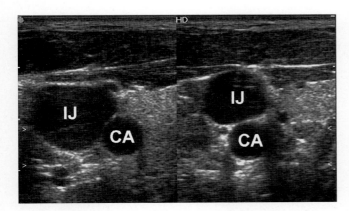

Figure 22-8. Split-screen image demonstrating the effect of head turning on the relationship of the internal jugular vein and the carotid artery. This emphasizes the importance of performing the procedure in the same position that the scan was performed. IJ = internal jugular vein, CA = carotid artery.

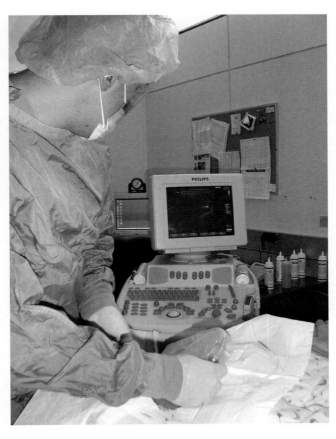

Figure 22-10. Inappropriately positioned equipment. Note that the operator has to turn his head to see the screen.

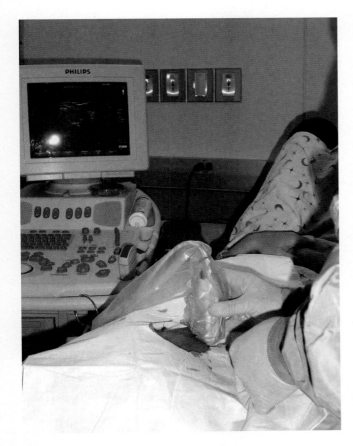

Figure 22-9. Appropriately positioned equipment. Note that the screen is in direct line with the operator's vision.

▶ GETTING STARTED IN PROCEDURAL GUIDANCE

HOLDING THE TRANSDUCER

The development of good hand–eye coordination and control of the transducer are essential for success. Poor technique may not lead to failure in straightforward cases such as an abdomen filled with 10 L of ascites. However, in the case of a small peritonsillar abscess, poor technique will lead to failure and possibly iatrogenic injury.

When scanning a patient, always have a comfortable grasp of the transducer and maintain light hand contact with the patient. Holding the transducer too close to the cable will limit fine motor control and make it difficult to keep the transducer in one position on the patient's skin. This loss of fine motor control will cause the operator to apply more pressure on the skin with the transducer and may compress or distort the target structure (Figure 22-11). The ability to maintain alignment of the ultrasound beam and instrument requires that the transducer be held steadily, which is

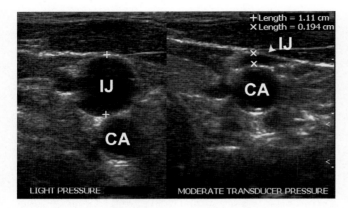

Figure 22-11. Split-screen image demonstrating the effect of compression of the internal jugular vein (arrowhead) by heavy transducer pressure. IJ = internal jugular vein, CA = carotid artery.

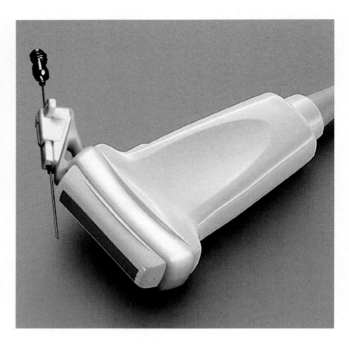

Figure 22-12. Mechanical needle guide (in plane).

made possible by keeping a finger or edge of the hand in contact with the patient's skin.

CONTROLLING THE INSTRUMENT

Move the needle, hemostat, or other instrument in a slow, controlled fashion during an ultrasound-guided procedure. Fast movements may result in loss of instrument visualization or result in operator confusion. Using short, controlled movements is usually the best way to advance the instrument through the soft tissue. Occasionally, a short jab may be called for to move the instrument through soft tissue. However, this must be performed with control to avoid over penetration and damage of vital tissues. One example is in the case of an interscalene nerve block where a noncutting spinal needle is used to avoid cutting nerve tissue and must be gently thrust to penetrate the sheath surrounding the brachial plexus. Without sheath penetration, delivery of anesthetic will be compromised. At the same time uncontrolled jabbing with the needle may result in nerve injury, even with a noncutting needle.

PROCEDURE GUIDES

Mechanical guides are commercially available to assist in ultrasound-guided procedures and can be used for both out-of-plane (short axis) and in-plane (long axis) approaches (Figure 22-12). The utility of mechanical guides in ultrasound-guided procedures is controversial.[5,6] Mechanical guides can minimize challenges associated with needle-beam alignment and may be helpful for the less experienced operator, but they also restrict needle redirection. These guides are useful for keeping the needle

in a predictable path so that intersection of the needle and ultrasound beam occurs at a known depth in case of a short-axis needle guide. Studies looking at the use of mechanical guides (out-of-plane approach) in ultrasound-guided needle biopsies found that procedure time was significantly reduced with the use of mechanical guides, especially for less experienced operators.[7] However, for biopsies of smaller targets <3 cm in diameter, the freehand technique fared better than a short-axis needle guide suggesting that the precision of needle tip placement with these guides may be inadequate.[8] For guides that place the needle in an in-plane orientation to the transducer, a needle will travel directly under the ultrasound beam for its full length, eliminating the requirement for some hand–eye coordination and adjustments. The main disadvantage of using mechanical guides is that the angle of entry is fixed on some guides (Figure 22-13). Furthermore, in the case of deep structures, the needle guide itself typically uses up a considerable length of the common needle, thus making it difficult to reach areas over 2–4 cm deep.

FACTORS AFFECTING INSTRUMENT VISUALIZATION

Instrument visualization is critical in ultrasound-guided procedures, regardless of whether the instrument is a needle, hemostat, trocar, or some kind of transducer. Despite what appears to be good alignment of the

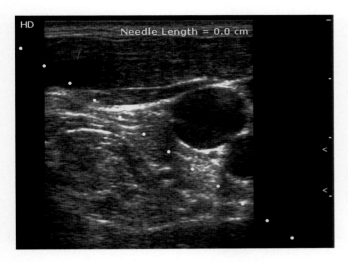

Figure 22-13. Note the fixed trajectory for needle entry when using a mechanical needle guide. The path of the needle is indicated by the dotted line. If the internal jugular vein was the desired target, then the transducer would need to be repositioned since the internal jugular vein is not currently in the path of the needle.

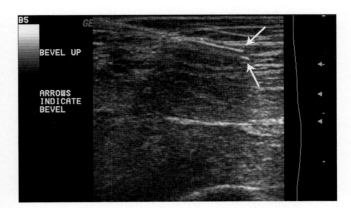

Figure 22-14. Good visualization of the needle tip (arrows) is noted with the needle bevel directed toward the transducer.

instrument and the ultrasound beam, visualization can occasionally be surprisingly difficult. Composition of the soft tissue, instrument type, needle gauge, bevel position, instrument movement, and the ultrasound beam angle all affect visualization.[9,10–13]

Needle visualization will be improved by using a larger diameter needle and by keeping the needle as close to perpendicular to the axis of the ultrasound beam as possible.[11–13] Unfortunately, an operator may not always be in a position to place the needle or other instrument perpendicular to the ultrasound beam in all situations. In these cases, keeping the ultrasound beam to instrument angle close to 60° will improve visualization (see Figure 22-13).[11] Echogenic needles are commercially available and are engineered to increase the reflection of the ultrasound waves back toward the transducer. These devices can be used to aid in needle visualization when traditional needles provide poor visualization.[10]

A needle tip will be better visualized if the bevel of the needle faces either toward or away from the sound beam (Figure 22-14).[10] When the bevel of the needle is rotated 90° in either direction, the needle tip will not be clearly visualized. It has been suggested that scattering of the beam away from the transducer when the bevel is in the 90° position from the ultrasound beam results in the return of fewer echoes to the transducer. In difficult patients or in cases where the needle angle is suboptimal, the use of an echogenic needle may be beneficial (Figure 22-15). Traditional needles with a smooth surface will demonstrate significantly fewer returning echoes (and poor needle visualization), espe-

cially when the needle angle is not perpendicular to the ultrasound beam.

LOCATING THE INSTRUMENT UNDER THE SKIN

When the instrument is difficult to visualize or cannot be visualized, first reassess the relationship of the instrument to the ultrasound beam. In long-axis procedures, the most common reason for not visualizing a needle is lack of alignment of the needle and ultrasound beam. Continued advancement of the needle is inadvisable since needle advancement will not improve needle visualization if the needle and ultrasound beam are not aligned. Gently reposition the transducer, either panning or rocking from side to side, until the instrument is visualized. If the instrument cannot be clearly visualized at this point, gently wiggle the instrument to see if this improves visualization. Avoid large motions since this

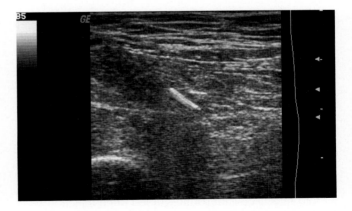

Figure 22-15. Echogenic needle with a roughened surface at the tip. Note the improved echogenicity at the tip.

may allow a sharp instrument to lacerate deep structures. In cases where the needle tip cannot be clearly identified, inject a small amount of sterile saline rapidly into the soft tissue so a small anechoic collection of fluid develops. Once the instrument is visualized, move the transducer in the same plane toward the target. Redirect the instrument toward the target while keeping in mind which direction the transducer was moved. Attempting the procedure from another entry location, changing the instrument angle after withdrawing it, or the use of a more echogenic instrument may be considered at this time if the instrument is still not visualized.

► ARTHROCENTESIS

CLINICAL CONSIDERATIONS

Emergency and acute care physicians are commonly called upon to evaluate patients with a painful or swollen joint where definitive diagnosis and treatment will depend on joint fluid being obtained for analysis. Some patients will benefit from simply having their effusion drained for therapeutic reasons, and many patients will be appropriate candidates for intra-articular steroid injections. While many acute care physicians feel comfortable tapping a knee effusion using standard clinical-examination based techniques, the comfort level for performing arthrocentesis in other joints is often much lower. The provider's discomfort with the procedure may be due to any one of a number of factors, including lack of experience with joint aspiration at a given location, lack of familiarity with the regional anatomy around a given joint or with techniques traditionally relied on for the procedure, or absence of recognizable landmarks secondary to patient obesity. Arthrocentesis of less commonly tapped joints such as the elbow, ankle, shoulder, hip, acromioclavicular, or metatarsophalangeal joints have traditionally been referred to rheumatologists, interventional radiologists, or orthopedists for further care. The use of point-of-care ultrasound for procedural applications is changing this historical pattern. Arthrocentesis of any of these joints can be added to the armamentarium of procedures performed by emergency and acute care providers who understand basic procedural principles and ultrasound anatomy. Point-of-care ultrasound is becoming more common in the field of rheumatology.

Numerous studies have documented improved performance characteristics and outcomes when ultrasound is used for arthrocentesis and/or intra-articular steroid injection. Ultrasound-guided knee injection with hyaluronic acid in patients with osteoarthritis had a significantly greater accuracy rate than blind injection (95.6% vs. 77.3%, $p = 0.01$) in a series of 89 patients.[14] In a study comparing ultrasound-guidance with palpation-guided knee arthrocentesis and steroid injection, ultrasound use was associated with 183% greater aspirated fluid volume, 48% less procedural pain, and improved clinical outcome at 2 weeks, in a series of 64 patients.[15] A study on the management of knee effusions noted less pain, a shorter procedure time, more fluid removed, and greater provider comfort when ultrasound guidance was used for the procedure.[16] A study evaluating the cost-effectiveness of ultrasound guidance for intra-articular injection of the osteoarthritic knee reported a 13% reduction in cost per patient per year when ultrasound was used for the procedure.[17] Studies on other joints reported similar improved performance characteristics when ultrasound guidance was used for the procedure. Patients injected with steroids for shoulder pain were noted in one review to have significant improvement in pain and function at 6 weeks when ultrasound-guidance was used compared with landmark-guided injection.[18] In a related report, ultrasound-guided injections for subacromial bursitis resulted in significant improvement in shoulder range of motion when compared with a blind injection technique.[19] In a study of steroid injection of many different joints, ultrasound-guided injection by rheumatology residents was found to be more accurate than clinical examination-guided injections performed by more experienced rheumatologists (83% vs. 66%, $p = 0.010$). More accurate injections were also noted to lead to greater improvement in joint function at 6 weeks.[20] In a series of 148 painful joints randomized to steroid injection by palpation versus an ultrasound-guided technique, sonographic guidance was noted to result in a 43% reduction in procedural pain, a 58.5% reduction in absolute pain scores at 2 weeks, and a 25.6% increase in the responder rate. Sonography also increased detection of effusion by 200% and volume of aspirated fluid by 337%.[21] Increased procedural success has also been noted when ultrasound guidance was utilized for aspiration of PIP and MCP joints. Intra-articular needle placement was noted in 96% of ultrasound-guided injections as opposed to 59% with a palpation-guided technique.[22]

In summary, most performance characteristics for arthrocentesis are improved when ultrasound is used for the procedure (better effusion detection, more accurate diagnosis, decreased procedural pain, more fluid removed). Additionally, ultrasound-guided intra-articular steroid injections are associated with significantly improved pain and range of motion outcomes compared with palpation-guided techniques.

CLINICAL INDICATIONS

- Diagnostic fluid sampling from a joint for laboratory testing
- Therapeutic fluid drainage from a joint
- Intra-articular steroid injection

ANATOMICAL CONSIDERATIONS

Joints in the human body, while built on similar principles, vary in their individual design and size. Sampling fluid from each requires knowledge of the particular anatomy of the specific joint. The following section contains a brief discussion of the sonographic anatomy of joints that are commonly aspirated or injected.

TECHNIQUE AND ULTRASOUND FINDINGS

Most ultrasound machines in point-of-care settings are outfitted with a linear array transducer suitable for performing arthrocentesis. Use a 5–12 MHz linear array transducer for most joints except the hip, where a curvilinear 5 MHz or lower frequency transducer may be utilized. Adjust image depth appropriately for the joint in question (the 80/20 rule applies: 80% of the image should focus on the anatomic area of interest, with 20% left over in the far field so as to see adjacent anatomy) and optimize image focus for the joint in question. Perform Doppler evaluation to identify any vascular structures surrounding the effusion or along the planned aspiration approach in order to avoid inadvertent vascular puncture.

For precise localization, map the joint fluid collection in two orthogonal planes and mark the skin with an indelible skin marker on either side of the middle of the transducer. A squeezable gentian violet skin marker that expresses the marking ink even when in contact with ultrasound gel is preferable; other markers will frequently cease to function once the coupling gel contacts the marker tip. Connecting the lines will create a target with the aspiration site in the center of the " + ". In addition, determine the optimal aspiration angle. Appreciate the depth from the skin surface to the deepest portion of the effusion so that an appropriate length needle can be chosen for the procedure. Most effusions will be mapped and marked, and subsequently aspirated using a freehand technique. If real-time guidance is used, skin marking will not be required. Prepare the site in a sterile manner, as with all procedures, and cover the ultrasound transducer with a sterile adhesive dressing or a sterile transducer cover. Guiding the needle to a joint effusion in real-time is similar to ultrasound-guided vascular access or abscess drainage techniques.

Graded compression and power Doppler can help distinguish complex synovial fluid or clot from synovial proliferation. A color flow signal may be noted at the border between synovium and where joint fluid is moving due to compression caused by the transducer. Freely mobile loose bodies will occasionally be seen within a joint effusion and will typically reveal themselves by

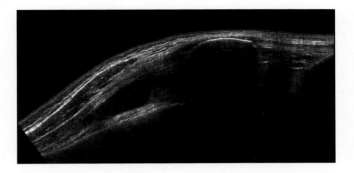

Figure 22-16. Midline longitudinal panorama image of a patient with a large knee effusion. This large volume hypoechoic collection high above the knee joint represents the distended suprapatellar bursa. The hyperechoic surface of the patella, patellar ligament, and the proximal tibia are seen in the near field on the right half of the sonogram. A dense posterior acoustic shadow is noted beneath the patella.

virtue of their hyperechoic acoustic profile and accompanying posterior acoustic shadowing. They are typically found in the suprapatellar bursa of the knee or in the elbow joint and they can be seen to move with either gentle palpation of the effusion or pressure on the transducer.

Knee

The suprapatellar bursa is a large synovium-lined pouch that is really an extension of the joint space of the knee. It is located at the anterior distal femur extending about a hand breadth above the adult knee joint, bounded superiorly by skin, subcutaneous tissue, and quadriceps tendon and inferiorly by prefemoral fat and the femur. When the knee joint is distended with fluid, the deepest collections will be found in the suprapatellar bursa (Figure 22-16) or where the suprapatellar bursa bulges out on either side of the quadriceps tendon particularly at the lateral suprapatellar recess (Figure 22-17). The suprapatellar bursa is the largest bursa in the body and can distend to accommodate a large volume of fluid. Numerous other bursae also surround the knee joint. Two that are of clinical relevance are the gastocnemius-semimembranosus bursa (found in the medial popliteal fossa) and the subcutaneous prepatellar bursa. The former often communicates with the knee joint, when distended can cause pain and swelling in the popliteal fossa, and is commonly known as a Baker's cyst. The subcutaneous prepatellar bursa lies immediately below the skin over the lower patella and proximal patellar ligament, does not communicate with the knee joint, and may become swollen and infected due to local trauma.

The normal knee joint will have little or no fluid visible within the joint space (Figure 22-18). The highest

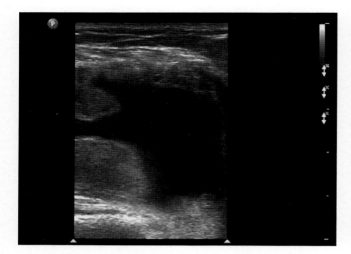

Figure 22-17. Transverse sonogram of a knee effusion at the lateral suprapatellar recess. The anechoic suprapatellar bursa is surrounded by a very thickened synovial lining, consistent with a chronic arthritic process.

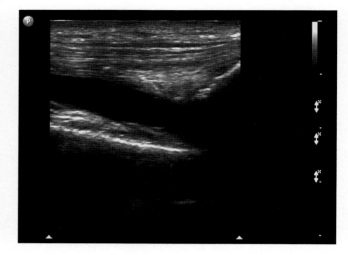

Figure 22-19. Midline longitudinal sonogram of a simple knee effusion. The image is centered over the suprapatellar bursa; echogenic femur and prefemoral fat are noted in the far field; a portion of the superior patella is seen on the right side.

yield sites for detection of an effusion will be in the lateral and medial recesses of the suprapatellar bursa, and compression on the contralateral recess will help increase fluid detection if the effusion is small. A simple effusion appears as a hypoechoic fluid collection separated from the brightly echogenic femoral cortex

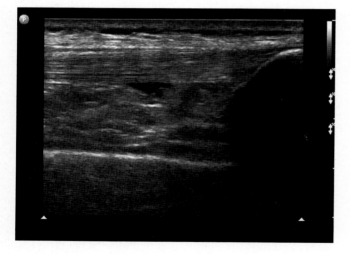

Figure 22-18. Midline longitudinal sonogram of a normal knee. Beneath skin and scant subcutaneous tissue, the striated appearing quadriceps tendon is seen to insert on the superior patella. A scant amount of physiologic joint fluid is noted; the anterior suprapatellar fat pad can be seen on the immediate right of the fluid collection. The echogenic anterior surface of the femur is noted below; a layer of prefemoral fat will always be seen just anterior to the femur on this view.

by a thin layer of hyperechoic prefemoral fat (Figure 22-19). With a more chronic process, inflammatory synovial changes (pannus) may be appreciated and will appear as a thickening of the synovium or hyperechoic lobulations within the joint space (Figure 22-20A–C). An effusion due to intra-articular hemorrhage may initially appear echo-free but later exhibit a homogenous midlevel gray echotexture consistent with clotted or partially clotted blood (Figure 22-21). A knee joint effusion should not be confused with other fluid collections that can be found around this joint. A prepatellar bursitis appears as a hypoechoic fluid collection that is seen in the subcutaneous tissue just anterior to the inferior patella and proximal patellar ligament and will typically be surrounded by hyperechoic edematous soft tissue typical of cellulitis (Figure 22-22). A Baker's cyst communicates with the knee joint and classically appears as a hypoechoic stomach-shaped fluid collection in the medial posterior fossa of the knee. On occasion this bursa may exhibit complex echogenicity due to synovial thickening and appear more like a complex cyst (Figures 22-23 and 22-24).

Scan the knee with the patient supine and with the slightly flexed knee supported from behind with a sheet or towel for patient comfort. Scanning is most easily performed in a paramedian longitudinal plane just above the patella. Small volumes of fluid will first be seen in the lateral or medial recesses of the suprapatellar bursa. Detection and aspiration of smaller effusions will be enhanced by placing pressure on the contralateral side of the knee so as to maximally distend the suprapatellar bursal recess at the chosen scanning/aspiration site. Longitudinal and transverse scanning of the fluid

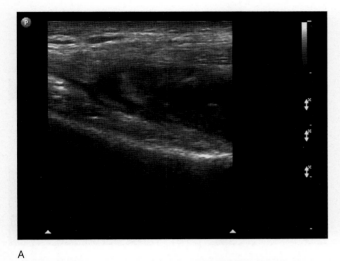

A

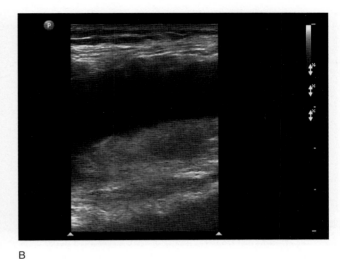

B

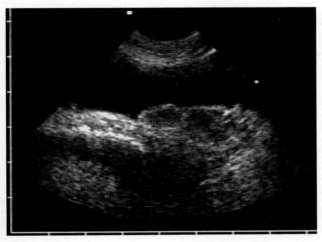

C

Figure 22-20. (A,B,C) Evidence of chronic inflammation is apparent in all these knee effusions; synovial hypertrophy may appear layered, smooth and thickened, or lobulated depending on the chronicity of the process.

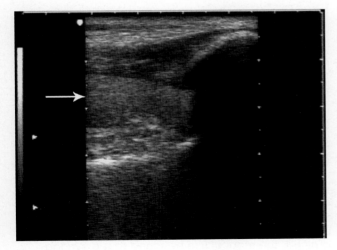

Figure 22-21. Midline sagittal sonogram of a knee hemarthrosis. The curved shadow of the patella is seen on the right side of the image and the bright echo of the anterior femoral cortex below. Just above the prefemoral fat there is a homogenous mid-gray echotexture layer (arrow) consistent with hematoma.

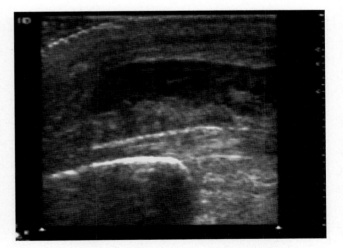

Figure 22-22. Sagittal midline sonogram of a prepatellar bursitis. Note the thickened hyperechoic skin, some debris within the fluid-filled prepatellar bursa, the shadow from the echogenic patella on the left inferior border of the image, and a portion of the fibrillar proximal patellar ligament.

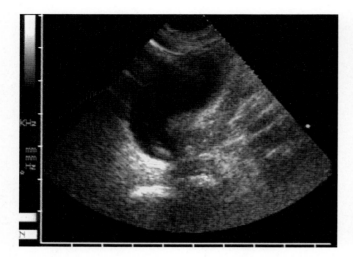

Figure 22-23. Transverse sonogram at the medial popliteal fossa demonstrating the characteristic stomach-shaped fluid collection of a Baker's cyst.

collection is followed by marking of the skin with indelible ink to form a "+" designating the optimal site for aspiration (Figure 22-25). Note the depth from the skin surface to the effusion and the optimal aspiration angle. Perform the aspiration freehand; from this point, the procedure does not differ from a blind aspiration technique. If real-time guidance is preferred, dress the transducer in a sterile sheath and use sterile coupling gel. An in-plane approach allowing for long-axis visualization of the aspirating needle is best and is identical to other needle guidance techniques. Since many patients with large knee effusions have chronic arthritic conditions, the joint aspiration may frequently be coupled with an

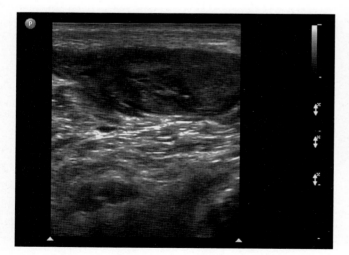

Figure 22-24. Synovial hypertrophy and chronic inflammation make this Baker's cyst appear sonographically similar to a soft tissue abscess. Several popliteal vessels are noted in cross section in the left far field of the sonogram.

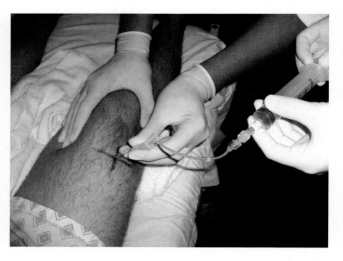

Figure 22-25. Knee aspiration technique at the lateral suprapatellar recess: two-person technique where pressure is applied to the contralateral recess for maximal joint cavity distension and maximal fluid removal. Sterile drape omitted for purposes of illustration.

intra-articular steroid injection. If a steroid injection is being simultaneously performed, a double syringe and needle setup with 80 mg of methylprednisolone acetate suspension and a local anesthetic agent can facilitate the aspiration and injection process (Figure 22-26).

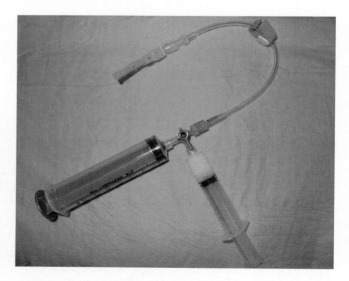

Figure 22-26. Equipment setup for combined knee effusion aspiration and intra-articular steroid injection. Several large volume syringes may be filled in the case of large effusions. When the fluid is maximally drained, the stopcock is switched to the syringe containing the steroid and local anesthetic and the medication is then instilled into the joint. A two-person technique is optimal so that the needle remains in the correct location. Knee range of motion after the injection helps distribute the medication throughout the joint.

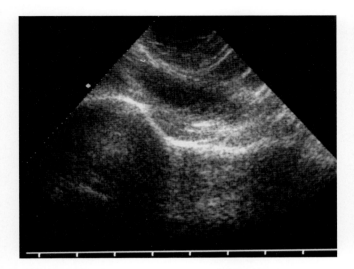

Figure 22-27. Ventral oblique sonogram of the normal hip. The prominent curve of the femoral head is seen on the left side of the image and leads to a concave region along the femoral neck where an effusion will preferentially collect.

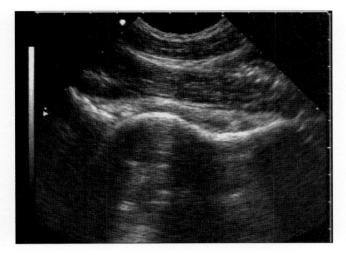

Figure 22-28. Ventral oblique sonogram of the hip. The joint capsule is seen as a hyperechoic, horizontally oriented layer extending from the acetabular labrum to the femoral neck. A small amount of joint fluid is noted below the joint capsule.

Hip

Sonographic evaluation of the hip joint can be successfully accomplished with a variety of transducers, ranging from a 3–5 MHz curved array or sector transducer to a 7.5–10.0 MHz linear array transducer. With the transducer aligned along the long axis of the femoral neck (orientation marker pointing toward the umbilicus), the normal hip will appear as a brightly curved line about 3–6 cm below the skin surface, convex along the surface of the femoral head on the left side of the image, and then gently concave along the femoral neck to the right. The area just anterior to the femoral neck is termed the anterior synovial recess and represents the potential space between the femoral neck and the joint capsule where a hip effusion will preferentially collect (Figure 22-27). A thin line of hypoechogenicity may be noted adjacent to the cortex of the femoral head; this line corresponds to the articular hyaline cartilage. The acetabular labrum will often be seen as an echogenic area to the immediate left of and slightly superior to the femoral head. The joint capsule is of variable echogenicity, sometimes difficult to identify, other times clearly visible as an echogenic layer 3–8 mm in thickness extending from the acetabular labrum to the base of the femoral neck (Figure 22-28). The joint capsule is usually readily identified when an effusion is present. The commonly accepted sonographic criteria for defining a hip effusion in a native hip include[14] a convex bulging joint capsule with a fluid stripe >5–6 mm, or[15] when compared with the asymptomatic joint, a >2 mm increase in the distance from the cortical echo to the joint capsule. A perpendicular measurement of the effusion is taken at its widest anteroposterior di-

mension between the surface of the femoral neck and the inner surface of the joint capsule. Comparison with the contralateral hip should be routine (Figure 22-29).

In the prosthetic hip, the sonographic landmarks will obviously be different. Transducer alignment should still be along the long axis of the prosthetic femoral neck aiming toward the umbilicus. A series of four horizontally oriented hyperechoic lines will be noted. First, a short segment to the left of the image may be seen that corresponds to the acetabular component of the prosthesis. Adjacent to this line is a somewhat wider,

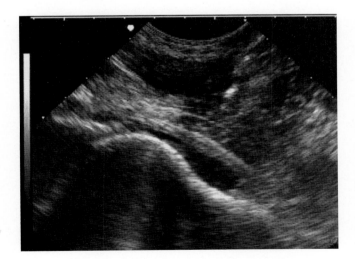

Figure 22-29. Ventral oblique sonogram of a hip effusion in a patient with reactive arthritis. The anterior synovial recess is distended with fluid and the capsule is seen to bulge anteriorly. The hyperechoic echo from the approaching aspirating needle is seen in the upper right of the image.

more superficially located horizontal line that represents the head of the prosthesis. A prominent metallic reverberation or ring-down artifact will be seen behind the prosthesis during real-time scanning. To the immediate right, a longer and somewhat deeper echogenic horizontal line will be seen, corresponding to the neck of the hip prosthesis, and a metallic ring-down artifact will be noted here as well. Finally, a bright and somewhat thicker echo will be noted to the far right of the image. This echogenic line is located a few millimeters superficial to the echo from the prosthetic femoral neck and represents the anterior surface of the most proximal portion of the remaining native femur into which the prosthesis has been inserted. It is typical to see a small amount of hypoechoic fluid surrounding the neck of the prosthesis. Of note, the native joint capsule will no longer be present since it will have been removed during hip replacement surgery (Figure 22-30). A perpendicular measurement is taken of the width of the fluid collection located between the superior surface of the most proximal edge of the remaining native femoral cortex and the edge of the pseudocapsule above. A fluid collection with a width of >3.2 mm at this location is considered to be abnormal (Figure 22-31).[23]

In children, the sonogram of the hip appears somewhat different from that of the adult. The growth plate of

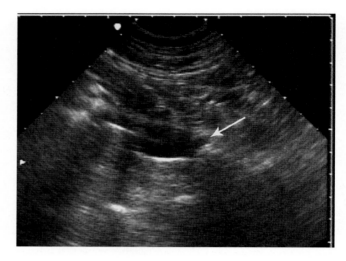

Figure 22-31. Ventral oblique sonogram of a septic prosthetic hip. A reverberation artifact is seen emanating from the prosthetic femoral head. A large fluid collection is seen anterior to the prosthetic femoral neck. A 5-mm fluid collection was measured between the most proximal native femur and the pseudocapsule above (arrow) (>3.2 mm is considered abnormal).

the femoral capital epiphysis produces a curved notch in the convexity of the femoral head and, depending on the degree of ossification, a linear lucency in the anterior head of the femur. The hypoechoic region anterior to the notch represents the cartilaginous acetabulum and should not be mistaken for an effusion (Figure 22-32).

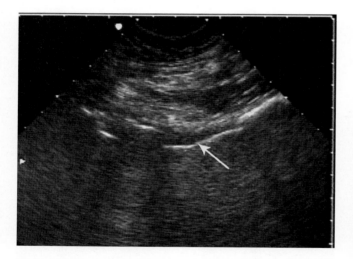

Figure 22-30. Ventral oblique sonogram of a normal prosthetic hip. Four echogenic lines are noted. From left to right: a short segment that corresponds to the acetabular component of the prosthesis; next, a wider more superficially located line that corresponds to the femoral head (a prominent metallic reverberation is noted below it); next, the long prosthetic femoral neck; and finally, a somewhat more anterior and more echogenic line that corresponds to the most proximal portion of the remaining native femur. A small amount of fluid is normally seen anterior to the prosthetic femoral neck (arrow).

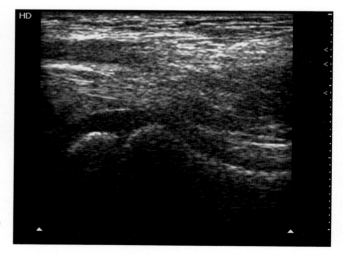

Figure 22-32. Ventral oblique sonogram of a pediatric hip. A notch is seen in the femoral head that corresponds to the growth plate of the femoral capital epiphysis. The hypoechoic area adjacent to this notch corresponds with the still cartilaginous acetabulum and should not be mistaken for an effusion.

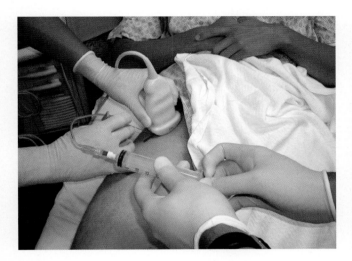

Figure 22-33. Ultrasound-guided hip aspiration technique. The needle is advanced in line within the long-axis scan plane of the transducer and its characteristic reverberation artifact is used to guide the needle tip into the effusion. For purposes of illustration, the sterile drape and transducer cover are not shown.

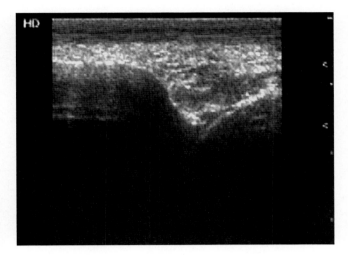

Figure 22-34. Sagittal midline sonogram of a normal ankle joint. The V-shaped recess is formed by the distal tibia on left and the talar dome on the right, and is filled by the anterior intracapsular fat pad. No fluid is seen in this example.

To aspirate a hip effusion, one can either employ a "map and mark" technique with a subsequent free-hand aspiration or perform the aspiration under real-time guidance. With the "map and mark" approach the widest portion of the effusion is mapped, marked with indelible ink, prepped, anesthetized, and then aspirated. If a real-time aspiration technique is employed, a sterile sheath is placed over the transducer and sterile gel utilized. Align the transducer along the long axis of the femoral neck as described previously and note the location of the femoral vessels in order that they may be avoided. Once the effusion is identified, center its most bulging portion on the monitor. Using sterile technique, insert the aspirating needle at inferior edge of the transducer and visualize it "in-plane" as it is advanced toward and into the effusion (Figure 22-33).

Ankle

Scan the ankle with a 5–10 MHz linear array transducer. In a sagittal scan plane over the distal tibia, a brightly echogenic horizontal line that corresponds to the anterior tibial cortex will be noted about 1 cm below the skin surface. As the transducer is moved further distally, a V-shaped recess will appear on the right side of the image, formed by the distal tibia on the left and the dome of the talus on the right. This location is the region where the anterior synovial recess of the ankle joint is found and is normally filled by an anterior intracapsular fat pad (Figure 22-34). A small amount of echo-free fluid may be seen at the base of this recess, and a collection of

<3 mm in anteroposterior height is considered normal. In sagittal midline orientation, an ankle effusion will appear as a prominent triangular area of sonolucency that fills this V-shaped recess. The joint capsule will be seen as a distinct echogenic structure lying horizontally just anterior to the upper border of the effusion (Figure 22-35). More medially, the effusion will often take on a rectangular configuration (Figure 22-36). On occasion, there may be associated soft tissue swelling of the overlying

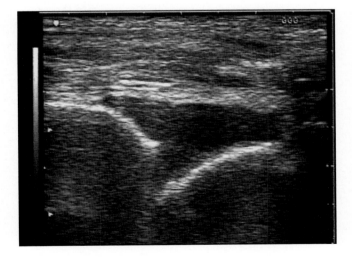

Figure 22-35. Sagittal midline sonogram of an ankle effusion. The joint capsule is seen as somewhat echogenic structure just above the hypoechoic effusion. The cortical echoes from the distal tibia and talar dome outline the posterior surface of the triangular effusion.

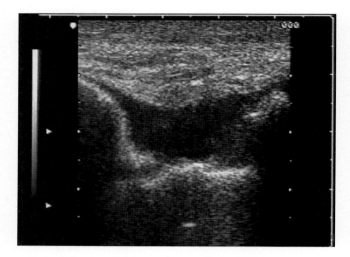

Figure 22-36. Sagittal medial paramedian sonogram of an ankle effusion. The ankle effusion in this location appears more rectangular in configuration.

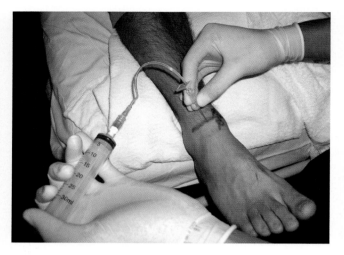

Figure 22-38. Freehand ankle aspiration technique. The location of both the deepest portion of the anterior recess and the anterior tibial/dorsalis pedis artery junction has been marked on the skin. Needle entry is lateral to the artery. When fluid is obtained, the needle can be held fixed in place with one hand while the syringe aspirates the effusion with the other. Sterile drape omitted for purposes of illustration.

skin accompanying the inflammatory process within the joint. On a transverse image through the joint line, the anterior tibial/dorsalis pedis artery junction will be located somewhat medial to the midline and appear as a hypoechoic circle just above the hypoechoic effusion (Figure 22-37).

Once a fluid collection has been identified in long-axis orientation, position the transducer so that the deepest portion of this V-shaped recess is located in the exact center of the image. A horizontal line drawn on the skin with an indelible marker on either side of the trans-

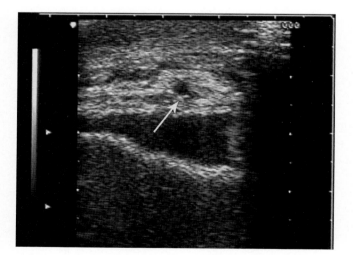

Figure 22-37. Transverse sonogram of an ankle effusion. The location of the hypoechoic anterior tibial/dorsalis pedis artery junction (arrow) should be marked on skin with a "ø" so that it may by avoided during the aspiration. The deep peroneal nerve is located just medial to the artery.

ducer's midline will then correspond to the deepest portion of the effusion. Next, obtain a transverse view and mark the location of the anterior tibial/dorsalis pedis artery junction on the skin with a "ø" so that it may be avoided during the aspiration. Note the angulation of the transducer, if any, as well as the degree of ankle plantar flexion. This information will be useful for aiming the needle in the appropriate direction during the aspiration. After sterile preparation of the patient, perform the aspiration using a freehand technique (Figure 22-38). If a real-time technique is desired, obtain the largest subjective image of the effusion in a transverse orientation with simultaneous visualization of the artery. Insert the needle under direct visualization lateral to the artery using a superior or inferior approach. This technique requires additional preparation and a sterile transducer cover, and is less commonly employed.

Elbow

Ideally, position the patient on a stretcher with the elbow held in 90° of flexion and the forearm resting in neutral position on a folded towel on the patient's lap. Scan the posterior lower arm in a transverse plane from behind the patient with the orientation marker facing left. The curved echogenic posterior surface of the humerus flattens at the level of the medial and lateral epicondyles (Figure 22-39) and then, somewhat more distally, forms a centrally located echogenic "U"-shaped depression that corresponds to the olecranon fossa (Figure 22-40). This space is normally filled with a fat pad

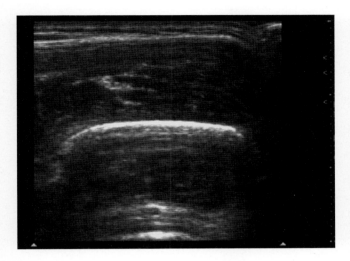

Figure 22-39. Transverse sonogram of posterior humerus just above medial and lateral epicondyles. Skin and hypoechoic triceps muscle are seen in the near field. The brightly echogenic posterior humerus transitions from its rounded profile above to the flat profile as seen here. As the transducer is moved a bit further distally, a U-shaped depression will appear in the humeral cortex, corresponding with the olecranon fossa.

that exhibits a mid-level gray echotexture with some regions of increased internal echogenicity. In a longitudinal midline orientation over the distal elbow (orientation marker now cephalad), the echogenic posterior surface of the humerus will be seen on the left side of the image,

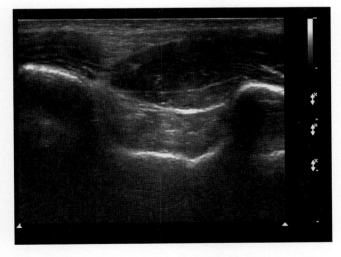

Figure 22-40. Transverse sonogram of the normal posterior elbow at the level of the olecranon fossa (also known as the posterior recess). The hyperechoic posterior surfaces of the medial and lateral epicondyles are seen on each side of the image; the U-shaped depression in the center of the humerus corresponds with the olecranon fossa and is filled by the posterior fat pad. Hypoechoic triceps muscle is seen in short axis above the fossa.

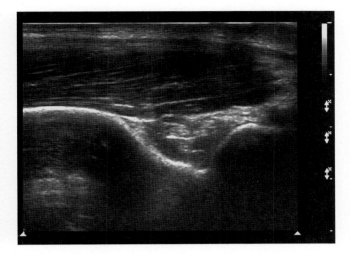

Figure 22-41. Sagittal sonogram of the normal posterior elbow. The posterior surface of the midline humerus is seen as a horizontal line in the left midfield, before it descends to the olecranon fossa on the right. The fossa is V-shaped in this orientation and the somewhat echogenic posterior fat pad is seen filling the recess. Triceps muscle is noted in long axis in the near field. The olecranon process is not seen in this image.

the olecranon fossa and the posterior fat pad will appear in a "V"-shaped recess in the center, and the echogenic posterior surface of the olecranon may be noted more superficially on the right side of the image. The triceps muscle will be apparent as a hypoechoic striated layer whose thickness depends on patient fitness and habitus. The triceps tendon will be seen just below the skin as a horizontal, somewhat hyperechoic structure with a fibrillar echotexture, but only if the transducer is in a true midline location. The distal portion of the triceps muscle appears at that location as a hypoechoic structure just beneath the tendon, superficial to the posterior fat pad (Figure 22-41).

In a transverse scan plane, an elbow effusion will be visualized as a predominantly hypoechoic collection filling the olecranon fossa and at times spreading over the posterior surfaces of the medial and lateral epicondyles (Figure 22-42). In a longitudinal posterior midline orientation, the elbow effusion will appear as an anechoic fluid collection that pushes the posterior fat pad superiorly (to the left of the image) and distends the joint capsule posteriorly (Figure 22-43). When this fat pad is pushed superiorly by an effusion, it becomes apparent on a lateral elbow radiograph creating the posterior fat pad sign. Loose bodies and synovial thickening may occasionally be seen in a swollen elbow joint (Figure 22-44). An effusion may appear hypoechoic or exhibit complex echogenicity depending on its etiology (Figure 22-45).

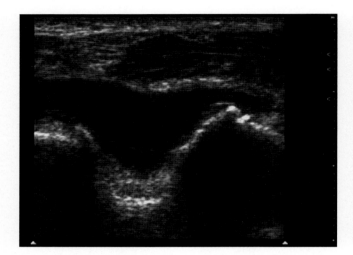

Figure 22-42. Transverse sonogram of a large elbow effusion filling the olecranon fossa and extending over the posterior epicondyles. The contour of the epicondyles is irregular.

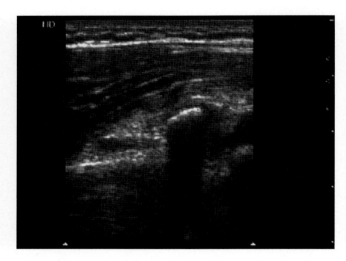

Figure 22-44. Same patient as in Figure 22-42; paramedian long-axis posterior elbow sonogram demonstrating a hyperechoic loose body with dense posterior acoustic shadowing. The joint capsule at that location is filled with inflamed echogenic synovium and almost no effusion is noted.

Screening for an elbow effusion is best accomplished in a transverse scan plane. If a fluid collection is noted, position the horizontally aligned transducer so that the largest subjective image of the fluid collection in the olecranon fossa is centered on the monitor. Mark the skin with indelible ink at both ends of the transducer and connect the ends with a horizontal line. Alternatively, the line may be constructed by scanning in a midline sagittal position (orientation marker facing up) and marking the deepest portion of the recess on either side of the center of the transducer. These mapped

lines will determine the optimum vertical location for the aspiration. The needle insertion site should always be 1–2 cm lateral to the midline, thereby remaining remote from the medially located ulnar nerve and avoiding the centrally located triceps tendon. Aim the aspirating needle toward the midline, however, in order to access the deepest portion of the centrally located olecranon fossa. After prepping the skin, perform the aspiration

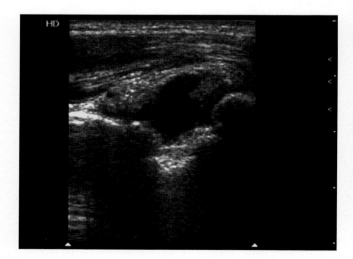

Figure 22-43. Long-axis sonogram of the same patient in Figure 22-42. The effusion has pushed the posterior fat pad superiorly. The posterior joint capsule is noted to be lined by thickened synovium.

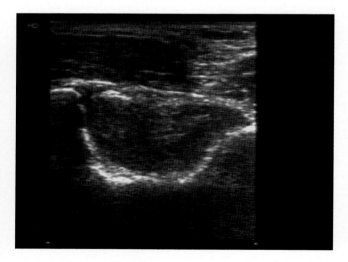

Figure 22-45. Transverse sonogram of the posterior elbow of a patient on warfarin with atraumatic elbow pain and an elevated INR. The olecranon fossa is filled with clotted blood. The bony outline of the fossa is brighter than usual because of posterior acoustic enhancement.

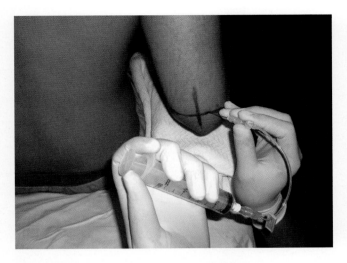

Figure 22-46. Elbow arthrocentesis technique—Posterior approach. The effusion has been mapped and marked. Needle insertion is *lateral* to the midline to avoid the triceps tendon and to stay well remote from the ulnar nerve ("Medial is madness!"). The needle should be medially angulated, however, so that it will reach the deepest portion of the centrally located olecranon recess.

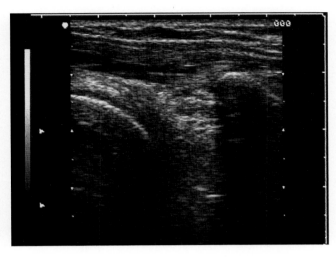

Figure 22-47. Transverse sonogram of the right anterior shoulder. The deltoid muscle is seen as a thin hypoechoic layer just below the skin. The curved medial humeral head appears on the left, and the coracoid process with its pronounced posterior acoustic shadow is seen on the right.

freehand (Figure 22-46). If a real-time technique is preferred, orient the transducer in a transverse scan plane with the needle tip inserted from the lateral aspect of the elbow using an in-plane approach.

Shoulder

On the transverse sonogram of the anterior shoulder at the level of the coracoid process, an echogenic layer of skin and subcutaneous tissue will be seen overlying a thicker, hypoechoic, and horizontally striated layer that corresponds to the anterior portion of the deltoid muscle. Deep to the deltoid muscle lie two distinct, brightly echogenic lines that represent the medial humeral head (seen as a large, smoothly curved echo in the lateral portion of the image) and the anterior surface of the coracoid process (seen as a somewhat flatter, anterior echo in the medial portion of the image). The thin hypoechoic rim surrounding the humeral head represents hyaline cartilage and should not be mistaken for a layer of fluid. The coracoid process is distinctive by virtue of the dense posterior acoustic shadow that it casts (Figure 22-47). If the profile of the medial humerus appears flattened (Figure 22-48), slightly externally rotate the arm to obtain the more desirable rounded profile of the humeral head. The middle of the space between these two bony echoes will identify the vertical line along which an intra-articular shoulder effusion can be aspirated, usually several centimeters inferior to the level of the coracoid. A shoulder joint effusion will appear as a

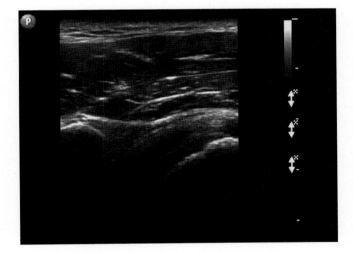

Figure 22-48. Transverse sonogram of the left anterior shoulder. The hypoechoic deltoid muscle in the near field appears much thicker in this muscular individual. The echogenic coracoid process is seen on the left side of the image and the humeral head to the right. The profile of the medial humerus appears somewhat flat because the arm is too internally rotated. With slight external rotation, a more desirable curved profile of the humeral head can be obtained. The midline space between these two structures represents the sagittal plane where the aspiration should occur. The actual aspiration site should be several centimeters below the level of the coracoid process, however, at the level of the axillary recess.

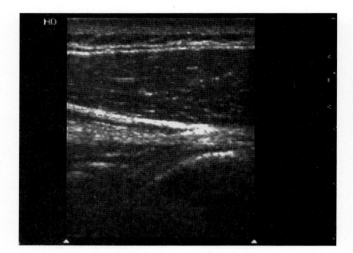

Figure 22-49. Transverse sonogram of the right posterior shoulder. The deltoid muscle is seen below the skin in the near field as a thick hypoechoic layer. The triangular or beak-shaped infraspinatus muscle (hypoechoic) and tendon (hyperechoic) are seen pointing to the right over the curved echogenic humeral head. The glenoid rim is seen as an indistinct echogenic line medial to the humeral head.

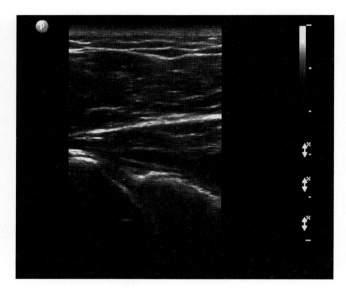

Figure 22-50. Transverse sonogram of a left posterior shoulder just below the acromion process. A thick layer of hypoechoic deltoid muscle is seen just beneath skin and subcutaneous tissue. A triangular layer of infraspinatus muscle points laterally. The curved posterior humeral head is seen in the left far field. The echogenic surface of the glenoid labrum is noted in the right far field. Intra-articular fluid, if present, will be seen in the space between the glenoid labrum and the humeral head.

hypoechoic collection that extends past the midline into the axillary recess of the joint capsule.

On the transverse sonogram of the *posterior* shoulder just below the posterior angle of the acromion, the echogenic layer of skin and hypoechoic subcutaneous tissue will be seen overlying a substantially thicker hypoechoic layer that represents the posterior portion of the deltoid muscle. Deep to the deltoid, the triangular or beak-shaped infraspinatus muscle (hypoechoic) and tendon (hyper or hypoechoic, depending on the angle of insonation) will be seen pointing laterally over the curved echogenic line that corresponds to the humeral head (Figure 22-49). A thin rim of hypoechoic hyaline cartilage may be noted lining the head of the humerus. Medial to the humeral head, two additional lines may be noted: a slightly more superficial echogenic line corresponding to the dorsal glenoid labrum and a somewhat deeper horizontal echogenic line corresponding to the posterior surface of the scapula. If a narrow aperture transducer is used, only the humeral head and glenoid labrum may be seen (Figure 22-50). An intra-articular effusion will appear as an anechoic region in the groove between the humeral head and the dorsal glenoid labrum (Figure 22-51). External rotation of the arm will enhance visualization of a small intra-articular fluid collection. Finally, a subacromial/subdeltoid bursal effusion that frequently occurs in patients with chronic shoulder bursitis appears as a hypoechoic or slightly complex fluid collection immediately beneath the deltoid muscle but superficial to the supraspinatus tendon

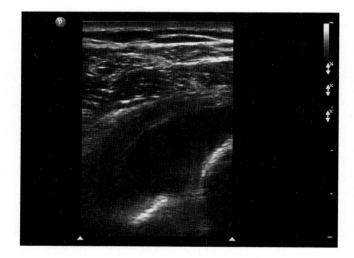

Figure 22-51. Transverse sonogram of a right posterior shoulder. A large hypoechoic effusion is seen centered in the area between the humeral head and the glenoid labrum. The joint capsule is seen as a thickened layer just above the effusion. Arthrocentesis can be best accomplished with ultrasound guidance in this case; the needle would be seen coming in from the right and should be targeted in the space between the glenoid labrum and humeral head.

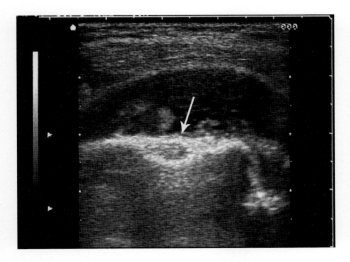

Figure 22-52. Transverse sonogram of a right anterior shoulder in a patient with a chronic subacromial (subdeltoid) bursitis. A large, complex hypoechoic collection is seen immediately beneath the deltoid muscle. The bursal fluid contains some echogenic debris and the synovium appears thickened and lobulated below. The echogenic anterior surface of the proximal humerus is seen beneath the effusion with the hypoechoic rounded biceps tendon resting within the bicipital groove (arrow). The bursal sac is seen to extend somewhat medial to the proximal humerus on the right side of the image.

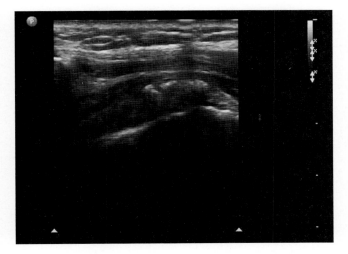

Figure 22-53. Anterior sonogram of a shoulder with calcific tendonitis. Skin, subcutaneous tissue, and a thin layer of deltoid muscle are seen in the near field. A thin layer of fluid is noted in the subacromial bursa between the deltoid muscle and the supraspinatus tendon below. Echogenic calcifications are seen within the substance of the supraspinatus tendon. The echogenic and irregularly contoured humeral head is seen beneath the tendon.

(Figure 22-52). The effusion will best be seen from an anterior transverse approach at the level of the coracoid process (similar to the scan technique employed when assessing the biceps tendon for peritendinous fluid). Calcific tendonitis and a small bursal fluid collection may also be noted at this site (Figure 22-53). The fluid collection seen with a subacromial/subdeltoid bursitis will not extend significantly inferior to the coracoid process; this characteristic can help distinguish it from an intra-articular effusion on an anterior view of the shoulder.

Shoulder arthrocentesis is typically performed from either an anterior or a posterior approach and can be ultrasound-assisted or ultrasound-guided. For the seated or supine patient, an anterior approach may be used (Figure 22-54). Extend the arm in slight abduction with the palm facing up. Place a 7.5–12 MHz linear array transducer in transverse orientation at the level of the coracoid process. Align the "V"-shaped recess seen between the medially located coracoid process and the laterally located medial head of the humerus in the center of the image. Mark the skin on both sides of the middle of the transducer with an indelible skin marker at the precise location of the base of this recess and draw a vertical line along this axis. The optimal site for aspiration will be on this line, but several centimeters inferior

to the level of the coracoid process where the axillary recess will be found. If performed blindly, advance the needle perpendicular to the skin surface.

For the posterior approach, place the patient in a sitting position with the elbow flexed and with the

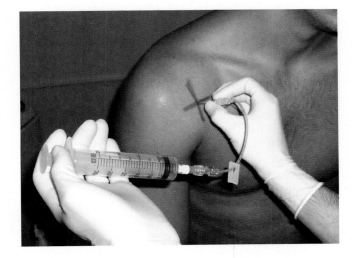

Figure 22-54. Shoulder arthrocentesis technique—Anterior approach. The space midway between coracoid process and the medial humeral head has been mapped and marked with a vertical line. The aspiration should occur perpendicular to the skin several centimeters below the level of the coracoid (at the horizontal line) and the needle should always remain lateral to the coracoid process.

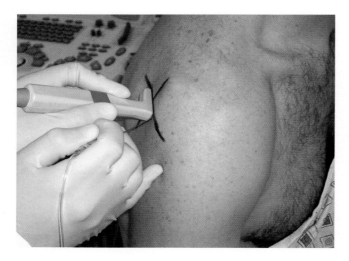

Figure 22-55. Shoulder arthrocentesis technique—Ultrasound-guided posterior approach. The effusion is mapped and marked several centimeters inferior and medial to the bulge of the posterior angle of the acromion. The aspiration needle is guided to the space between the glenoid rim and the medial humeral head under ultrasound guidance. Sterile drape and probe cover are omitted for purposes of illustration. Flipping the hockey stick transducer's orientation marker would have allowed the probe to be held with the tip pointing to the right. This would have moved the probe handle out of the way of the hand with the advancing centesis needle.

forearm resting at the side in neutral position (Figure 22-55). Place the transducer in transverse orientation approximately 2–3 cm inferior and 1–2 cm medial to the bulge of the posterior acromion. Obtain the optimal image of the joint space by tilting the lateral edge of the transducer slightly inferiorly from the horizontal plane. The triangular or beak-shaped infraspinatus muscle and tendon will be seen overlying the echogenic curve of the medial humeral head. Slightly deeper and just medial to the humerus will be a less distinct echo that corresponds to the dorsal glenoid labrum. An effusion will appear as an anechoic or hypoechoic collection adjacent to the curved head of the humerus, filling the groove between it and the medially located glenoid labrum.

The needle entry site should be from the lateral edge of the transducer in the plane of the ultrasound beam. Cover the transducer with a sterile sheath, and after a sterile prep, aim the needle toward the fluid collection in the groove between the medial humeral head and the glenoid rim. The aspiration path is fairly horizontal; this will enhance visualization of the needle and help guide precise placement of the needle tip. Puncture the joint capsule along the medial border of the humeral head, slightly lateral to the glenohumeral joint so as to avoid contact with the circumflex scapular vessels and

the suprascapular nerve that are located medial to the glenoid rim.

Other Joints and Bursae

Patients will occasionally present with joint pain that is due to a pathologic process affecting the acromioclavicular, sternoclavicular, or the metacarpophalangeal or metatarsophalangeal joints. Ultrasound allows for a quick determination of the presence of an effusion and precise mapping of these superficially located joints. The acromioclavicular and sternoclavicular joints are located on the lateral and medial end of the clavicle, respectively, and contain an articular disc that separates and cushions the clavicle from the abutting acromion or sternal articular surfaces. The fibrous capsule of the joint is inserted on the bone immediately adjacent to the articular surfaces. The capsule of the first metatarsophalangeal joint surrounds the joint, extending from the nonarticular bony surfaces of the distal metatarsal bone to the proximal portion of the proximal phalanx.

The acromioclavicular and sternoclavicular joints are most easily scanned by first placing the transducer sagittally over the upper chest in order to identify the bright superficial echo from the clavicle. Slide the transducer either medially or laterally, and once at the AC joint, rotate along the long axis of the clavicle spanning the joint space. Mark the hypoechoic "V"-shaped recess that corresponds to the joint space on either side of the transducer, and then mark again with the transducer turned orthogonally. Connect the two lines and mark the center of the " + " as the location for the aspiration. A gouty AC joint is shown in Figure 22-56. Scan

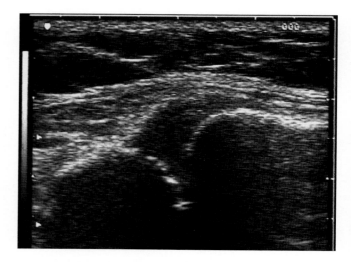

Figure 22-56. Longitudinal sonogram across the right acromioclavicular joint in a patient with gout. The hypoechoic V-shaped recess between the acromion on the left and the clavicle on the right represents the site where an aspiration or steroid injection would be directed.

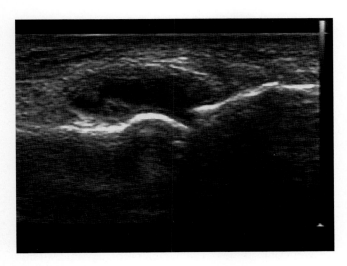

Figure 22-57. Longitudinal sonogram of a gouty first MTP joint. The dorsal surface of the metatarsal head is seen in the center of the sonogram and the dorsal proximal phalanx to the right. The synovial cavity of the MTP joint is normally very flattened and barely visible; here it is very distended and fluid-filled, with a thickened and irregular synovial lining. The collection was mapped and marked, easily tapped from a paramedian location, and gout crystals were identified on fluid analysis.

the first metatarsophalangeal joint axially over the dorsal joint space and utilize a similar mapping technique. Alternatively, use the acoustic shadow of a paper clip here to map the desired puncture site. After the usual sterile prep, vertically puncture and aspirate at the mapped sites. Perform the aspiration slightly off midline to avoid puncturing the extensor tendon. A distended gouty 1st MTP joint is shown in Figure 22-57.

PITFALLS

1. **Inadvertent puncture of an adjacent vessel or nerve.** This can be avoided with basic knowledge of the regional anatomy and an understanding of which structures are to be avoided at each arthrocentesis site.
2. **Failure to aspirate fluid after mapping and marking an effusion may occasionally occur.** Reevaluation with Doppler imaging may help clarify if the apparent fluid collection actually represents synovial hypertrophy. In other cases, procedural success may require real-time needle guidance.
3. **Vasovagal reactions may on occasion occur with needle penetration.**
4. **Iatrogenic joint infection is extremely rare, but a possibility.**

► LUMBAR PUNCTURE

CLINICAL CONSIDERATIONS

Lumbar puncture (LP) is a commonly performed procedure in any ED or intensive care unit. In skilled hands, it is usually successfully performed without the need for imaging assistance. There remains, however, a challenging subset of patients in which even a skilled practitioner will be unable to successfully perform an LP. Procedural failure in these patients often occurs because of the inability to identify bony landmarks or because of degenerative changes in the interspinous structures. Ultrasound imaging can be used to assist with landmark localization, potentially obviating the need for fluoroscopic guidance, and thereby facilitating successful performance of the procedure at the bedside.

The traditional landmark technique for performance of an LP relies on the identification of midline lumbar spinous processes and the intercristal or Tuffier's line, an imaginary line drawn on the back between the highest points of the two iliac crests. The intersection of these two lines is purported to represent the location of the L4 spinous process or the L4/L5 interspace. An LP needle inserted at the intersection of Tuffier's line and the closest midline interspace is thought to be sufficiently remote from the conus medullaris (typically found at T12/L1, but on occasion as high as T12 and as low as the L3/L4 disc).[24] The accuracy of the landmark technique has been questioned by many investigators, most recently in a series of 114 adult subjects where a curved array ultrasound transducer was placed in a paramedian location and the interspaces identified sonographically. The intercristal line was noted to be at the L3/L4 interspace in 75%, at the L4/L5 interspace in 14%, and at the L2/L3 interspace in 13% of the subjects.[25] In another report that calls landmark localization techniques into question, a comparison of the physical exam versus ultrasound localization of the intervertebral level was undertaken in a series of 50 patients undergoing radiographs of the lumbar spine, with the lumbosacral spine radiograph as the gold standard. Palpation was successful in identifying the correct interspace in only 30% of cases, whereas ultrasound correctly identified the location of the interspace in 71% of cases. Distant outliers (defined as two spaces too high or too low) were seen only in the palpation group.[26]

For well over a decade, ultrasound has been used by anesthesiologists for localizing landmarks of the lumbar spine prior to epidural anesthesia. In one report on a series of 300 parturients receiving epidural anesthesia, prepuncture ultrasound of the lumbar spine created conditions that allowed for a more focused "puncture process" and for a significant reduction in the number of puncture attempts. Determination of an optimal skin puncture site, the ideal direction of needle advancement, and most importantly, knowledge of the depth from skin to the epidural space were the factors that were felt to have contributed to improved procedural success.[27] In another report on 120 orthopedic patients with either morbid obesity or difficult spinal landmarks, ultrasound imaging was compared with a traditional landmark localization technique for performing spinal anesthesia. In the ultrasound group, first attempt spinal anesthesia success was noted to be more than double that obtained in the landmark group (65% vs. 32%, p <0.001).[28]

Ultrasound has also been found to be useful in the assessment of failed neonatal LPs. Because the relevant anatomic structures are more superficial and the posterior elements of the spine poorly ossified in this group of patients, high-resolution images of both intra- and extraspinal anatomy can frequently be obtained.[29] In a series of 32 patients age 3–86 days referred for fluoroscopy after failed blind LP attempts, the authors emphasized the value of ultrasound for assessing the thecal sac for a possible epidural or intrathecal hematoma. Because success rates in obtaining spinal fluid are low in patients with no definable cerebrospinal fluid (CSF) space, a fluoroscopic attempt would therefore be avoided or delayed.[30]

The use of ED ultrasound for spinal landmark localization prior to an LP was first described in 2005.[31] In one report, the utility of ultrasound for identifying pertinent landmarks for LP was found to be inversely related to body mass index (BMI). Notwithstanding, in patients with difficult to palpate landmarks ultrasound allowed for identification of pertinent landmarks for LP in 76% of the subjects.[32] In another study, the ability of emergency physicians to identify relevant spinal anatomy using ultrasound was investigated in 76 subjects with a mean BMI of 31.4. High-quality scans were obtained in <1 minute in 88% of the subjects and in 100% of subjects within 5 minutes.[33] One study found the use of ultrasound for LP significantly reduced the number of failures in all patients and improved the ease of the procedure in obese patients.[34] In a case report, an ultrasound-assisted LP was performed in a patient with a BMI of 34 where surface landmarks were difficult to palpate. Using a curved array transducer in a midline longitudinal position, the relevant spinal anatomy (spinous processes and ligamentum flavum) was identified and marked, after which an uneventful LP was performed.[35] Finally, ultrasound was used as the primary means of determining the site of skin puncture, angle of needle advancement, and depth needed to access the subarachnoid space in a series of 39 patients undergoing diagnostic LP in the ED. CSF was obtained in 92% of the subjects in the first interspinous space attempted. Sonographically measured depth of the dura mater was found to correlate strongly with the final needle depth.[36]

ANATOMICAL CONSIDERATIONS

When approaching the dural space through the midline, the sequence of anatomic layers traversed by the LP needle are as follows: skin, subcutaneous fat (the thickness of which will obviously vary with the habitus of the patient), the supraspinous ligament (connects the posterior tips of the spinous processes together), the interspinous ligament (a thin flat band of ligament running between the spinous processes), and the ligamentum flavum or "yellow ligament," a band of predominantly elastic tissue, up to 10 mm in thickness in the midline and 5 mm laterally, that runs vertically from lamina to lamina, allowing for separation of the lamina during flexion of the spine and serving to close in the spaces between the vertebral arches. The ligamentum flavum extends from the anterior–inferior surface of the lamina above to the posterior–superior surface of the lamina below. The most posterior midline bony structure encountered in the lumbar spine will be the curved spinous processes of the lumbar vertebrae. They are located at varying depths below the skin surface depending on body habitus, are 3–8 mm in width with a triangular configuration in coronal section (widest portion caudal), 15–20 mm in height, have a quadrilateral shape (midline sagittal orientation) with a caudally slanting tilt of the superior and inferior borders, and are 3–4 cm in length. Of note, the fifth lumbar vertebra has a smaller spinous process than the other lumbar vertebrae (helpful for establishing a precise level for needle entry). In a patient with a normal BMI, the lumbar spinous processes normally lie only 3–5 mm below the skin surface. They become difficult to detect by palpation when they are more than about 15 mm from the skin surface. With increasing BMI they are found at progressively greater depth and can be difficult to detect with ultrasound as well. The depth of this sonographic landmark varies linearly with BMI. One report noted that the spinous process was found on a midline sonogram at a depth of 6 cm from the skin surface in a patient with a BMI of 34. The skin to ligamentum flavum distance in this same patient was 10.5 cm [35]

In a cross-sectional view of the lumbar spine from behind, the spinous process is represented as the long handle of a "Y" that then flares out into the two broad laminal plates. The laminae form the bony posterior roof of the spinal canal, splay out 30–45° laterally to each side of the spinous process on cross section, and have an anteroposterior tilt in vertical profile like shingles on a roof. The laminae are contiguous with the superior and inferior articular processes whose facets articulate with the articular processes of adjacent lumbar vertebrae. The two transverse processes are long and slender, project horizontally and slightly posteriorly to each side, and arise from the junctions of the laminae and the pedicles in the upper lumbar vertebrae, and from the pedicles and vertebral body in the lower lumbar vertebrae. The two pedicles connect all the posterior elements of the lumbar vertebra to the body of the vertebra.

The posterior epidural space is typically 5–6 mm in thickness in the lumbar region, contains the fat and blood vessels that surround the thecal sac, and is also triangle-shaped with its apex located in the dorsal midline. These epidural blood vessels are often the source of a "traumatic tap." The range of distances from the skin surface to the epidural space in a series of 72 parturients was found to be quite broad, ranging from 20 to 90 mm, with an average distance from skin to ligamentum flavum of 51 mm.[37] With caudal progression, the distance from skin to the epidural space was noted to increase.[38]

The spinal canal itself is relatively small; early studies with A-mode ultrasound and a paramedian imaging window noted an average oblique sagittal diameter of the normal lumbar spinal canal of 1.7 cm.[39] Assuming an average ligamentum flavum thickness of 5 mm and an average posterior epidural space thickness of 5 mm, the dural sac should therefore usually be found about 1 cm deep to the echo obtained from the dorsal surface of the ligamentum flavum. In a study investigating the use of ultrasound to identify pertinent landmarks for LP, 62 patients were scanned and stratified by BMI. The distance from skin to ligamentum flavum was found to directly relate to BMI, with an average of 44 mm in the normal BMI cohort, 51 mm in the overweight cohort, and 64 mm in the obese group.[33]

CLINICAL INDICATIONS

- LP in a patient with ambiguous or absent anatomic landmarks on physical examination

TECHNIQUE AND ULTRASOUND FINDINGS

A wide range of ultrasound transducers can be used for ultrasound-assisted LP. A hockey stick transducer is commonly used in neonates where the small skin contact footprint is advantageous. A linear array transducer can be used in larger children and adults, and a curved array transducer is often the only option for landmark visualization in the obese patient. Short- and long-axis midline views, as well as left and right long-axis paramedian views, can be employed depending on body habitus. The short-axis view is best used to quickly find the spinal midline. The midline long-axis view is used to identify the lumbar spinous processes; when centered directly over the spinous processes, the skin at the superior and

inferior border of the transducer can be marked to denote the spinal midline. Identify the lumbar interlaminar space on the long-axis view as the space between adjacent spinous processes. Center the transducer over this region and then rotate 90°. Mark the skin at either edge of the now horizontally oriented transducer to denote the vertical location of the interspace being mapped. The long-axis paramedian oblique view allows for best overall imaging of the lamina, ligamentum flavum, dura mater, and epidural space.[33] Count interspaces by starting with a midline view over the sacrum, then moving the transducer superiorly to identify individual lumbar spinous processes.

Proper patient positioning is important and can help increase the width of the interspinal space. Addition of a foot support for a seated patient is said to widen lumbar interspinous space distance by as much as 21%.[40] In a series of 28 children with a median age of 5 years, the interspinous space of the lumbar spine was observed to be maximally increased when in a sitting position with flexed hips. Hip flexion in a lateral recumbent position also increased the width of the interspinous space, although less so. Neck flexion, however, did not increase the width of the interspinous space.[41]

The anatomic relationship of the spinous processes, laminae, ligamentum flavum, and dura, and the recommended transducer positions for obtaining midline and paramedian oblique longitudinal images of the lumbar spine are illustrated in Figure 22-58. Midline sagittal scans of the lumbar spine with a linear array transducer set at a depth of 4–5 cm will demonstrate the hyperechoic convex posterior surfaces of the lumbar spinous processes (Figure 22-59). The skin appears somewhat hyperechoic, the subcutaneous tissue hypoechoic and of variable thickness depending on body habitus (Figure 22-60), and the horizontally oriented thoracolumbar fascia and supraspinal ligament are seen as a hyperechoic layer that follows the course of the spinous processes. If the transducer is placed in a paramedian long-axis orientation, the longitudinally oriented hypoechoic paraspinal muscle fibers will be seen just below the echogenic layer of thoracolumbar fascia (Figure 22-61). If the transducer is placed in a similar orientation but closer to the midline, the echogenic transverse process may be noted in the far field and should not be mistaken for a spinous process (Figure 22-62).

When centered over the longitudinal midline, the transducer may be moved superiorly and inferiorly to precisely locate the interspace between adjacent spinous processes. If the aperture length of the linear array transducer is sufficiently large (50 mm), then both lumbar spinous processes can be seen at the same time and the interspace clearly identified between them (Figure 22-63A). This image is sometimes called the "batwing" sign. With a smaller aperture linear array transducer (35 mm),

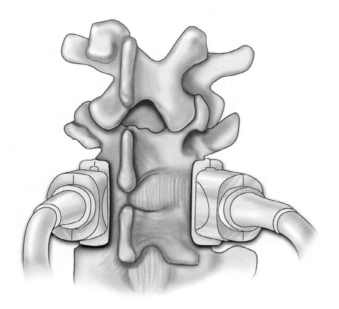

A

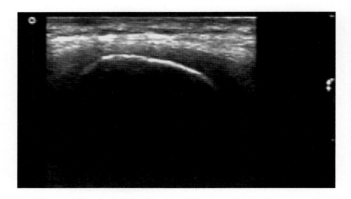

Figure 22-59. Midline sagittal linear array image of a lumbar spinous process in a patient with a normal habitus. The hyperechoic convex posterior surface of a lumbar spinous process is seen in the near field of the image, about 5 mm below the skin surface. With this small aperture transducer (35 mm), only one spinous process can be seen in the image.

the lateral portions of adjacent spinous processes will be apparent on the sonogram (Figure 22-63B).

In order to visualize the ligamentum flavum and dura, a deeper field depth will be required. The narrow acoustic window afforded by a midline imaging location and the depth of the structures can make these images somewhat difficult to obtain with a linear array transducer. In the normal BMI patient, the ligamentum flavum may be seen as a 3–4 mm wide structure with a

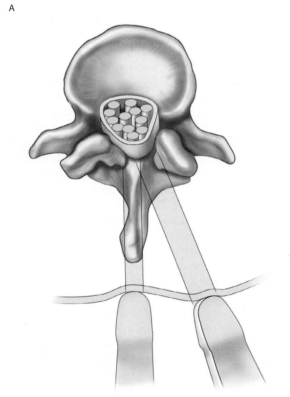

B

Figure 22-58. Sagittal (A) and transverse (B) drawings of the lumbar spine demonstrating the relationship of the spinous processes, laminae, ligamentum flavum, and dura mater as well as the recommended transducer positions for imaging the lumbar spine from both midline and paramedian locations.

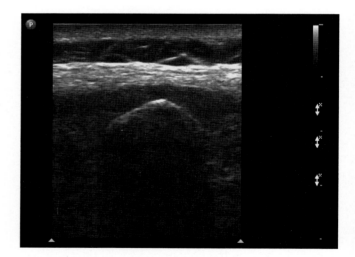

Figure 22-60. Midline sagittal linear array image of a lumbar spinous process from a patient where the spinous processes were not palpable. The skin appears slightly hyperechoic, the subcutaneous tissue hypoechoic, and the thoracolumbar fascia and supraspinal ligament appear as a very hyperechoic layer just above the echogenic contour of a lumbar spinous process located about 1.5 cm below the skin surface.

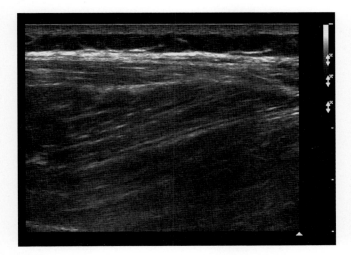

Figure 22-61. Longitudinally oriented paraspinal muscle fibers are seen just below skin, hypoechoic subcutaneous tissue, and hyperechoic thoracolumbar fascia on this sagittal sonogram that is no longer centered on the lumbar midline.

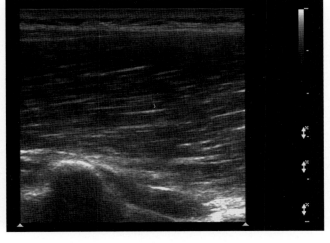

Figure 22-62. Sagittal lumbar sonogram, slightly off midline position. A portion of a transverse process is seen in cross section deep to the paraspinal muscles in the far field of the image. This structure should *not* be mistaken for a spinous process.

double wall echo, located in the well between adjacent interspaces (Figure 22-64). In a high BMI patient, a linear array transducer will be inadequate for imaging at such a field depth, and a curved array transducer using either a midline or paramedian oblique approach will need to be employed. With the better penetration and wider field of view afforded by the curved array transducer, a succession of horizontal lines may be noted

representing first the ligamentum flavum, then the posterior and anterior walls of the dural sac. Occasionally, an additional horizontal line will be noted from the posterior surface of the vertebral body (anterior wall of the spinal canal).

Paramedian oblique longitudinal imaging provides a more favorable acoustic window for visualizing the ligamentum flavum, epidural space, and the dural sac and

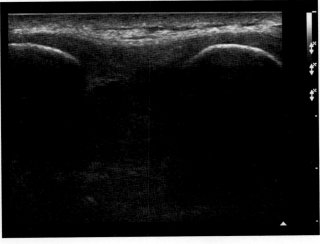

A

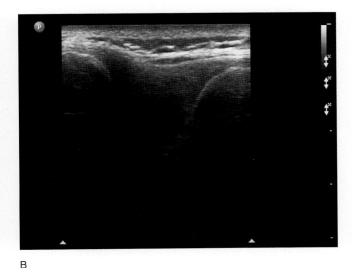

B

Figure 22-63. Midline sagittal linear array images of two adjacent spinous processes using (A) large aperture (50 mm) and (B) small aperture (35 mm) transducers. The thin echogenic supraspinal ligament is seen in the near field just beneath the skin and scant subcutaneous tissue in both images. The curved dorsal surfaces of the spinous processes are aligned on either side of the image, and the interspace is centered in the midline of the sonogram. Only a small portion of each spinous process can be seen with the smaller aperture transducer. This image is sometimes called the "batwing" sign.

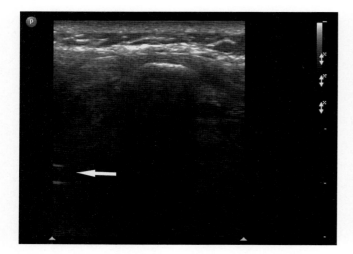

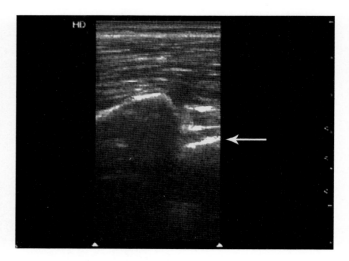

Figure 22-64. Midline sagittal linear array image of a spinous process and a portion of the ligamentum flavum. In the left far field of the image, a double wall echo is seen (arrow) from a portion of the dorsal and ventral surfaces of the ligamentum flavum.

Figure 22-65. Paramedian oblique sagittal linear array sonogram using a small aperture transducer (35 mm). The echogenic dorsal surface of a hemilamina is seen on the left side of the image, and a prominent posterior acoustic shadow is noted. The first two horizontal lines to the right of the lamina represent the dorsal and ventral surfaces of the ligamentum flavum. Immediately below lies the epidural space, followed by another echogenic horizontal line that represents the posterior wall of the dural sac (arrow). The distance from the dorsal surface of the ligamentum flavum to the posterior facing wall of the dural sac is usually about 8–10 mm.

is felt by many to be the best location for viewing spinal anatomy. Image depth can be quite variable (6–14 cm) depending on body habitus. The transducer marker is oriented cephalad as with midline imaging. The linear or curved array transducer is placed in a slightly paramedian location several centimeters off the midline and then angled in a slightly midline direction from a true sagittal imaging plane. When using a small aperture linear array transducer, only one hemilamina may be visualized. On the left side of the linear array image (Figure 22-65), a hyperechoic line is seen with distinct posterior acoustic shadowing. This echogenic line angulated downward and to the left represents the dorsal cortical surface of a hemilamina that has been scanned in a sagittal plane. Just to the right of and several millimeters deep to the posteroinferior surface of the lamina two echogenic horizontal lines are noted, representing the dorsal and ventral surfaces of the ligamentum flavum, respectively. The epidural space lies immediately below the ligamentum flavum (typically about 6–8 mm in width in the posterior midline, less so laterally) followed by another echogenic horizontal line that represents the posterior wall of the dural sac. The echo emanating from the posterior dural sac can usually be found about 8–10 mm deep to the dorsal surface of the ligamentum flavum. A depth measurement taken from the skin surface to this posterior dural sac echo will correlate highly with the depth needed to obtain CSF. If a larger aperture linear array transducer is available, two adjacent hemilamina and the ligamentum flavum, epidural space and posterior dural sac may be visualized simultaneously (Figure 22-66). With the broader field-of-view and the better penetration afforded by a curved array

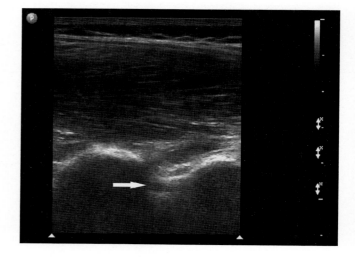

Figure 22-66. Paramedian oblique sagittal linear array sonogram using a larger aperture transducer (50 mm). Two adjacent hemilaminae, the dorsal and ventral surfaces of the ligamentum flavum, the epidural space (arrow), and the posterior dural sac are all seen on this larger field-of-view image.

transducer, several hemilamina will be seen in cross section, occasionally the ligamentum flavum, one or both walls of the dural sac, and occasionally the posterior surface of the bony spinal canal as well (Figure 22-67).

At the level of the intergluteal fold, the midline sacrum will be seen as an echogenic linear structure, 3–5 cm below the skin surface, usually tilting down toward the left portion of the image (Figure 22-68A). The small curved ridges of the three median sacral crests may be noted if one is over the exact midline. As one moves the transducer superiorly, the interspaces and spinous processes of the lower lumbar spine will come into view. Counting of the spinal interspaces can proceed using the sonographic image of the sacrum as a reference point (Figure 22-68B).

A transverse image of the lumbar spine can be used to quickly locate the midline in a patient with poorly identifiable landmarks. The hypoechoic and speckled appearing paraspinal muscles will be seen as two circular bundles on either side of the midline. As the horizontally oriented transducer is moved either superiorly or inferiorly, the spinous process will intermittently appear on the image represented as a hypoechoic inverted "V." The most dorsal bony tip of the spinous process being imaged will be seen in the midline as a 3–4 mm region of curved hyperechogenicity. The spinal lamina appears as a brightly hyperechoic region immediately beneath the paraspinal muscles. In the near field, the hyperechoic thoracolumbar fascia is seen to curve slightly downward at the midline. When centered over a spinous process, the image often has a butterfly-like appearance when a linear array transducer is used (Figure 22-69).

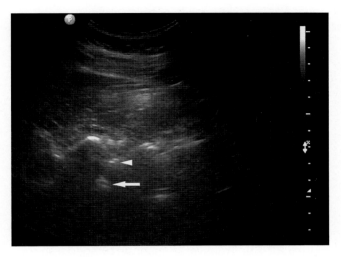

Figure 22-67. Paramedian oblique longitudinal sonogram of the lower lumbar spine. The dorsal hemilaminae of L4 and L5 are seen as echogenic angulated lines with prominent posterior acoustic shadowing. The ligamentum flavum no longer appears as a distinct structure. The posterior and anterior epidural space and both posterior (arrowhead) and anterior (arrow) walls of the dural sac are apparent in the L4/L5 window and appear as closely paired horizontal echogenic lines. The anterior dural sac, epidural space, and the anterior spinal canal are all apparent in the L5/S1 window.

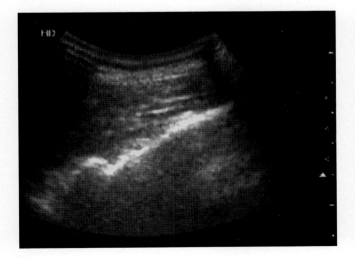

A

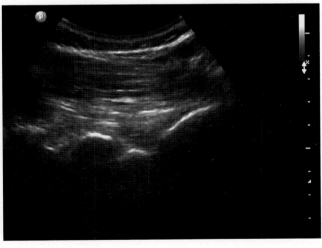

B

Figure 22-68. (A) A midline sagittal curved array image at the level of the intergluteal fold will reveal the posterior surface of the sacrum as a hyperechoic line, downsloping to the left. (B) Curved array transducer image at the lumbosacral junction. The longer curved echogenic line to the right of the mid screen corresponds to the uppermost portion of the sacrum. Immediately above lies the L5/S1 interspace, then the L5 spinous process; above that the L4/L5 interspace, then the L4 spinous process.

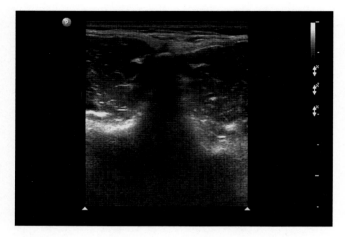

Figure 22-69. Transverse linear array sonogram of the lumbar midline centered over a spinous process. Thoracolumbar fascia is seen to curve downward at the midline. The hypoechoic speckled paraspinal muscles are seen on each side of the image. A small curved hyperechoic region in the near field corresponds to the portion of the spinous process being imaged. An inverted "V"-shaped posterior acoustic shadow follows the contour of the lamina. When centered over the spinous process, the image typically takes on the appearance of a butterfly.

A curved array transducer may be required for mapping out deeper spinal anatomy in a high BMI patient. Using a transverse scan plane, the hypoechoic circular paraspinal muscle bundles will be seen in the near field beneath skin and subcutaneous tissue. The hyperechoic but very narrow spinous process is often hard to visualize but its location can be inferred by following the inverted "V" of the acoustic shadow cast by the spinous process and laminae superiorly. When the transducer is centered below the level of the ligamentum flavum, the laminae will appear as an echogenic cape-like structure beneath the paraspinal muscles, casting a dense posterior acoustic shadow below (Figure 22-70A). When the transducer is then angled somewhat cephalad through the region of the ligamentum flavum, a series of echogenic lines will be noted that correspond to the articular and transverse processes and the posterior facing surface of the vertebral body. The spinal canal will appear as a hypoechoic circle just anterior to this vertebral body echo (Figure 22-70B).

Depending on the patient's degree of illness and ability to cooperate, and the preference of the physician performing the procedure, the patient may be placed in either a seated position leaning forward with hips flexed and feet supported, or in a lateral decubitus position with hips and back flexed. In patients where the spinous process is not readily palpable but less than about 3 cm from the skin surface, identify the spinous

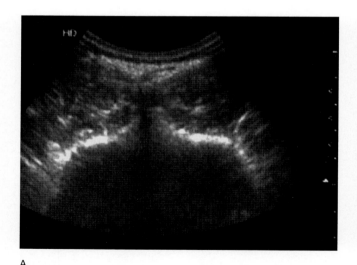

A

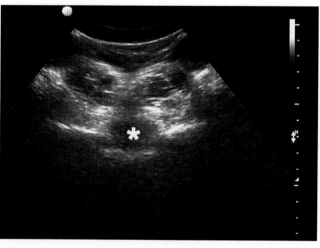

B

Figure 22-70. In this transverse curved array image (A), the lumbar spinous process is best found by following its midline posterior acoustic shadow up to the near field of the image. The paraspinal muscles appear as symmetric circular bundles on either side of the spinous process. The echogenic dorsal surfaces of the laminae appear as a cape-like structure with dense posterior acoustic shadowing below. In this somewhat more cephalad transverse curved array image (B), the hypoechoic circular paraspinal muscle bundles are seen in the near field several centimeters below the skin surface. The short paired echogenic lines immediately beneath the paraspinal muscles correspond to the articular processes, and the somewhat deeper, longer, and dorsally tilted paired echogenic lines represent the transverse processes. The slightly deeper and less echogenic line in the midline represents the posterior facing surface of the vertebral body (anterior wall of the spinal canal). The spinal canal (asterisk) appears as a circular hypoechoic region immediately above this line.

processes with the linear array transducer held in a midline sagittal orientation. When directly over the spinous process, mark the skin above and below the transducer with a skin marker to denote the midline of the spine. If a small aperture linear array transducer is used, mark the superior and inferior extent of the curve of the spinous process with a corresponding curve just lateral to the transducer. Perform this same process with the three lowest lumbar spinous processes. If a larger aperture transducer is used, then two adjacent spinous processes may be positioned to the left and right side of the sonogram, with the image now centered over the interspace. Mark the interspace with a skin marker on either side of the transducer's midline to delineate the mid-interspace location. Repeat this process for several adjacent interspaces. To determine the vertical level of each interspace, place the transducer on the midline sacrum at the level of the intergluteal fold. Note the bright echo from the surface of the sacrum and the small ridge of the superior median sacral crest. As the transducer is moved cephalad, the spinous process of L5 will be encountered, more superficially located than the superior median sacral crest below, but typically slightly smaller and deeper than the L4 spinous process above. Counting of the spinous processes can proceed accordingly from this reference point and then be correlated with the mapped interspaces. Place a horizontal line at the level of the mid-L3–L4 interspace to mark the optimal skin entry site for the LP (Figure 22-71).

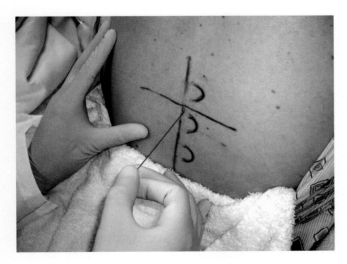

Figure 22-71. The precise location of the lumbar midline and the relative location of the curved spinous processes (and/or interspaces) can be mapped and marked with a skin marker. A horizontal line is used to indicate the location of the L3–L4 interspace. Needle entry begins in the lower half of the interspace and the needle is angled cephalad both to avoid the spinous process above and to follow the cranial slanting path to the ligamentum flavum and dural sac. For purposes of illustration, the sterile drape is not shown.

In the high BMI patient, the linear array transducer is likely to be inadequate for localizing the spinous processes and interspaces. In such cases, a curved array transducer in either a central or paramedian oblique longitudinal location can be used to map and count the interspaces. The paramedian location is likely to be the more suitable location for mapping the interspaces in such patients and will provide better visualization of the posterior dura. By starting in a paramedian oblique location near the intergluteal fold, the precise interspace location can be determined, and the depth to the dural sac measured so that an appropriate needle length can be chosen for the procedure. Perform the procedure using a "map and mark" technique from either a midline or paramedian location. Alternatively, cover the transducer with a sterile transducer cover and advance the needle to the dura at the appropriate interspace using real-time ultrasound guidance.

PITFALLS

1. **In some morbidly obese patients, the combination of excessive soft tissue and poor image quality may make detection of sonographic landmarks for LP mapping impossible.** In such cases, fluoroscopic guidance will usually be required for successful LP.

▶ NERVE BLOCKS

CLINICAL CONSIDERATIONS

Regional nerve and plexus blocks have been integral to the practice of anesthesiology for over 60 years and are commonly used for hand, arm, hip, knee, and foot surgery. Initially, training in regional anesthesia relied on identification of anatomic landmarks and the perception of various clicks and pops as fascial planes were traversed by a blunt-tipped needle. Several decades later, nerve stimulators were incorporated into the block procedure to assist with more precise placement of the anesthetic delivery needle as close to the target nerve or nerve plexus as possible. The success of these regional anesthetic blocks was highly operator dependent, however, and even with the use of a nerve stimulator in skilled hands, block failure rates of 10–30% were not uncommon, depending on the site of the block.[42,43]

Over the past 15–20 years, an emerging body of anesthesiology and emergency medicine literature has demonstrated the important role ultrasound can play in enhancing the performance characteristics and success rates of various regional blocks.[42–52] The development of more portable ultrasound equipment, higher resolution and smaller footprint transducers, and improved picture-processing technology, such as compound imaging and enhanced needle recognition software, have all helped accelerate this process. Not surprisingly, the utilization of ultrasound for performance of regional anesthetic blocks is gradually becoming the new standard of care. For the commonly performed nerve blocks, ultrasound imaging allows for real-time visualization of the target nerve(s) in most patients. With sonographic guidance, the operator can guide the anesthetic delivery needle under direct visualization and deposit the local anesthetic agent in a very precise fashion, with a lower dosing volume. This enhances all of the desirable operating characteristics of the procedure and minimizes complications.

In a series of 40 patients undergoing forearm or hand surgery, one study reported an ultrasound-guided brachial plexus block success rate of 95% at both the supraclavicular and axillary sites with no reported complications; this compares with an historical 70–80% success rate at these sites using a nerve stimulator. More importantly, the ultrasound-guided supraclavicular brachial plexus block provided the additional advantage of reliable anesthesia of the musculocutaneous nerve with a minimal risk of associated complications such as pneumothorax.[49]

In a series of 40 patients with hip fractures receiving a femoral nerve block for analgesia prior to surgery, the onset of femoral nerve sensory blockade was noted to be significantly faster in the ultrasound group (16 minutes) compared with the nerve stimulator group (27 minutes), and overall block success improved from 85% in the nerve stimulator group to 95% with ultrasound guidance.[50] In a subsequent study, 60 patients with hip fractures were randomized to receive a femoral nerve block guided by either ultrasound or nerve stimulator. The ultrasound group had a higher procedural success rate (95% with ultrasound compared with 80% with the nerve stimulator technique), an improved onset time (of sensory loss), and a smaller overall volume of anesthetic required for the block (20 mL 0.5% bupivacaine in the ultrasound-guided group compared with 30 mL 0.5% bupivacaine in the nerve stimulator group).[51]

Ultrasound guidance for regional anesthesia has been demonstrated by many investigators to result in improved nerve block success rates, more rapid onset of complete analgesia, a decreased volume of anesthetic agent required for block performance, and fewer procedural complications. A 2005 review of ultrasound utilization in the practice of regional anesthesia among 387 anesthesiology departments in Germany, Austria, and Switzerland noted that regional block success rates have increased to nearly 100%, up from a baseline of 70–80%. The authors concluded that "puncture processing" is easier and more effective when performed with ultrasound guidance in large part because it facilitates precise de-

position of the local anesthetic agent at the site of the target nerve.[52]

Complications from regional nerve and plexus blocks vary with the site being punctured and include (1) pain from needle insertion and direct nerve irritation, (2) prolonged procedure times if localization is difficult or if block onset is delayed, (3) block failure, (4) spinal cord injury with the interscalene block, (5) phrenic or recurrent laryngeal nerve paralysis, (6) inadvertent lung puncture and pneumothorax with the interscalene and supraclavicular brachial plexus blocks, (7) inadvertent vascular puncture and bleeding, (8) systemic reactions to local anesthetics, (9) infection, and (10) vasovagal reactions.

Peripheral nerve injury (PNI) occurs in 0.0003–0.0005% of blocks and was historically attributed to intraneural injection. However, studies have demonstrated that intraneural injection itself does not correlate with PNI, and have thus called into question the mechanism by which iatrogenic nerve damage occurs.[53,54] The precise mechanism remains unclear, but factors such as high injection pressures, paresthesias during the procedure, immunologic or neurohormonal effects of local anesthetic agents, and compressive nerve damage due to poor positioning of anesthetic limbs are all potential contributing factors. At this time, most authors suggest avoiding intentional intraneural injection, halting the injection and repositioning the needle tip if high injection pressures or paresthesias occur during the block, and paying careful attention to protect against compressive damage to an anesthetized limb.

ANATOMICAL CONSIDERATIONS

Physicians performing these blocks should familiarize themselves with the detailed regional anatomy of the area being punctured. The successive anatomic layers encountered in the supraclavicular region are as follows: skin, platysma muscle fibers coursing inferolaterally from the chin to the clavicle, sternocleidomastoid muscle forming the medial border, clavicle forming the anterior border, and the trapezius muscle forming the posterior border of this triangular-shaped region. The C5–T1 nerve roots that make up the brachial plexus exit from their respective vertebral foramina between the anterior and middle scalene muscles and course inferolaterally where they coalesce into the upper, middle, and lower trunks of the brachial plexus in the supraclavicular region. The trunks subsequently divide into anterior and posterior divisions, and then into the medial, lateral, and posterior cords before ending as the terminal branches of the brachial plexus (the radial, median, and ulnar nerves) in the upper axillary region. The three scalene muscles (anterior, middle, and posterior) arise from the transverse processes of the cervical spine and insert on the superior surface of the first rib. At the anterior border of the supraclavicular fossa and immediately posterior to the clavicle, the superficially located brachial plexus trunks and divisions are clustered in a fascial plane that lies immediately lateral to the subclavian artery. The anterior scalene muscle—inserting on the medial aspect of the first rib—lies just medial to the subclavian artery; the first rib lies below or in close proximity to the combined artery and plexus cluster, and the middle scalene muscle lies just lateral to the plexus. The subclavian vein courses over the flattened surface of the first rib just *medial* to the anterior scalene muscle insertion. Lung tissue lies just below the rib with the cupula of the lung rising above the level of the first rib more medially and posteriorly. The phrenic nerve runs longitudinally along the anteromedial surface of the anterior scalene muscle.

At the level of the axillary crease in the uppermost anterior axilla, the axillary artery, veins, and the branches of the brachial plexus course just below the skin surface within a neurovascular fascial sheath, resting on a fascial plane known as the medial brachial intermuscular septum. This fascial plane separates the arm flexors (biceps and coracobrachialis muscles) from the arm extensors (triceps muscle). The terminal branches of the brachial plexus (median, ulnar, and radial nerves) are found within this neurovascular fascial sheath in close proximity to the axillary vessels, typically surrounding the axillary artery. The musculocutaneous nerve will typically be located superolateral to the axillary artery, often found in the fascial plane between the coracobrachialis and biceps muscles.

At the level of the mid-wrist, the median nerve will be found immediately below the skin surface at the level of the volar proximal wrist crease superficial to the flexor tendons. The optimal site for blocking the median nerve is located 5–10 cm proximally, where the median nerve will be found lying just anterior to the fascia separating the superficial and deep flexor muscles. The ulnar nerve can be found by locating the hypoechoic ulnar artery just below the echogenic flexor carpi ulnaris tendon at the proximal volar wrist crease, then following the artery approximately three quarters the length up the forearm until the hypoechoic artery and adjacent hyperechoic ulnar nerve (located *ulnar* to the ulnar artery) separate from one another. The radial nerve is often most easily visualized at the lateral distal humeral area, about 5 cm above the elbow, anterior to the lateral epicondyle. The nerve bundle can be followed inferiorly, where it splits into superficial and deep branches at the antecubital crease. The superficial branch of the radial nerve (located *radial* to the radial artery) continues distally along the volar radial aspect of the upper forearm, beneath the brachioradialis muscle, at first somewhat separated, then in close proximity to the radial artery. About 7 cm above the wrist, the superficial branch of the radial nerve passes beneath the brachioradialis tendon.

The distribution of anesthesia provided by these nerve blocks is typically as follows. An axillary brachial plexus block will provide complete anesthesia of the elbow, forearm, and hand provided that the musculocutaneous nerve is successfully blocked at the axillary level. If the musculocutaneous nerve is not blocked, no anesthetic effect will be achieved in the region innervated by the lateral cutaneous nerve of the forearm (specifically, the radial half of the dorsal and volar forearm, from elbow to wrist). The more proximal supraclavicular brachial plexus block provides anesthesia from the upper humerus to the hand and has been called by some "the spinal of the arm" due to the dense anesthesia often obtained through the use of this technique. It is of particular value when complete anesthesia of the entire forearm or antecubital fossa is desired. This block can be employed when this larger field of anesthesia is desired as might be the case in a patient with multiple self-inflicted forearm lacerations or a large antecubital abscess. Note that neither of these two blocks provide adequate anesthesia for procedures of the shoulder; in situations where shoulder anesthesia is desired, an interscalene block would be employed. In the hand, the median nerve supplies sensation to most of the palmar surface of the hand up to the mid-ring finger, the palmar and dorsal branches of the ulnar nerve supply the little finger and the ulnar side of the ring finger, and the superficial radial nerve supplies sensation to the dorsal radial hand.

In the femoral region at the level of the inguinal crease (just inferior to the inguinal ligament), the anatomic layers of relevance for the femoral nerve block are as follows: skin, subcutaneous tissue, fascia lata (dense connective tissue that covers the muscles of the hip and thigh), and from medial to lateral, the femoral vein, artery, and nerve. The femoral artery and vein are encased in a thick connective tissue sheath. The femoral nerve is found immediately lateral and somewhat deep to the femoral artery. Proximal to the inguinal ligament, the femoral nerve lies deep to and then somewhat lateral to the psoas major muscle. As the femoral nerve comes from behind the psoas muscle and approaches the inguinal region, it then runs deep to the iliopectineal arch. Despite its immediate proximity to the femoral artery, the femoral nerve is located in a separate fascial plane, physically separated from the vessels in the femoral sheath by the iliopectineal fascia (fascia iliaca). The latter is a thick connective tissue fascial layer that arises from the psoas minor tendon, covers the medial distal portion of the iliacus muscle and the femoral nerve, and then extends medially under the adjacent femoral artery and vein to the anterior surface of the pectineus muscle found inferior and medial to the femoral vein. The pubic bone and the iliopubic eminence of the acetabulum lie just deep to the femoral vessels and nerve.

Peripheral nerves are not rigidly fixed and they may exhibit some degree of mobility within the anesthetic solution that is injected around them. The shape of a given nerve or nerve plexus in short-axis orientation may vary from round, flattened, triangular, or oval depending on its relationship to underlying bony structures or fascial planes and where in its long-axis location it is scanned. Some of the commonly blocked nerves will be found to be located at a very shallow depth below the skin surface. In a study of 15 volunteers, the mean skin-to-nerve distance of the most superficial portion of the brachial plexus in the supraclavicular area was noted to be 0.9 ± 0.3 cm. Similar results have been reported in the axillary region.

CLINICAL INDICATIONS

• Regional nerve blockade in any location

Contraindications to Nerve Block

• Altered level of consciousness (patients must be able to communicate paresthesias during the procedure and cooperate with pre- and post-block neurologic assessments).
• Infection of the overlying skin.
• Patients at significant risk of compartment syndrome should only receive blocks in consultation with physicians who will be providing ongoing inpatient care in order to assure appropriate monitoring and prompt diagnosis of compartment syndrome should it develop.
• Relative contraindications include anticoagulation and preexisting neuropathy.

TECHNIQUE AND ULTRASOUND FINDINGS

Nerve tissue may appear hypoechoic or hyperechoic relative to surrounding subcutaneous tissue and nerves as small as 2 mm in diameter (such as the digital nerves at the proximal digital crease) may be visualized with a high-frequency linear array transducer. From anatomic correlation studies, it is reported that a 15 MHz transducer will reveal approximately one-third of the fascicles that are seen on microscopy. Cervical roots exhibit a sonographic pattern that is hypoechoic; they are described as being monofascicular and in short axis appear as rounded hypoechoic structures surrounded by brightly echogenic fascial tissue. Nerves are nearly always more echoic than blood vessels and, unlike blood vessels, are not compressible. This feature, along with color or power Doppler interrogation, can help distinguish a nerve from an adjacent vessel.

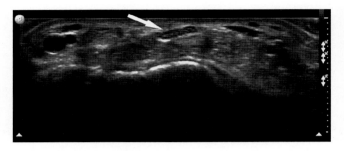

Figure 22-72. Right median nerve in cross section at the level of the volar proximal wrist crease. The nerve appears as a very superficially located hypoechoic rectangular structure in the center of the image, lying just above the more fibrillar appearing flexor tendons in the carpal tunnel. The radial artery and paired radial veins are seen on the left side of the image; the ulnar artery and paired ulnar veins are somewhat less clearly seen on the right side of the image. The echogenic volar surface of the distal radius is noted in the far field on the left half of the image.

As nerve bundles become larger or more distal, they will typically exhibit greater internal echogenicity. A more prominent internal fascicular pattern may be noted, due to the greater amount of echogenic connective tissue (epineurium and perineurium) holding the nerve bundles together. Depending on the size of the nerve being imaged and the resolution of the transducer being employed, nerve bundles will also exhibit some degree of anisotropy, although less so than tendons.

The median nerve is an excellent target nerve to image for improving one's skills at nerve recognition by ultrasound. It is readily visualized in cross section at the midline proximal volar wrist crease with a 10 MHz or higher frequency transducer. In short axis, it appears as a superficial hypoechoic flattened oval structure with an echogenic rim. Its echotexture is described as being fascicular, and is differentiated from the typically more echogenic fibrillar echotexture of the adjacent flexor tendons beneath the nerve (Figure 22-72). As one moves proximally on the arm, the median nerve assumes a more rounded or triangular shape, and can be found in the mid-wrist in the fascia separating the superficial and deep flexor muscles of the hand (Figure 22-73).

The ulnar nerve is found by locating the ulnar artery at the volar proximal wrist crease. The hypoechoic ulnar artery and the smaller paired ulnar veins will be found just beneath and radial to the flexor carpi ulnaris tendon; the ulnar nerve is located just ulnar to the artery and is often difficult to discern at this location (Figure 22-74). Following the ulnar artery proximally, the nerve can be clearly visualized adjacent to the artery in the mid-forearm, and then separating from the artery in the upper forearm (Figure 22-75).

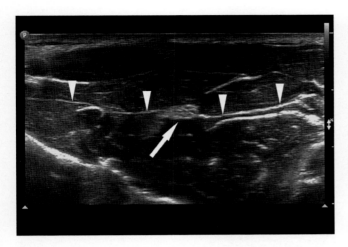

Figure 22-73. Median nerve in cross section about 5 cm above the volar wrist crease. The median nerve at the level of the mid-forearm appears as a hyperechoic oval structure (arrow). The fascial plane (arrowheads) separating the superficial and deep flexors of the forearm serves as a reliable landmark for identifying the nerve at this location.

The radial nerve can be found at the lateral epicondyle about 5 cm above the elbow. The lateral epicondyle appears as an echogenic peaked structure and the radial nerve will be seen as a rounded or flattened fascicular bundle anterior to the lateral epicondyle (Figure 22-76A). The nerve can be followed inferiorly into the upper forearm. Here the superficial radial nerve will be seen just below the brachioradialis muscle, and radial from the nearby hypoechoic radial artery (Figure 22-76B). As the artery and nerve track distally, they are located next to one another (Figure 22-76C) until the level of the distal brachioradialis muscle, at which point the nerve moves dorsally and is no longer seen next to the radial artery.

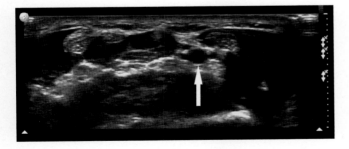

Figure 22-74. Right ulnar nerve in cross section at the volar wrist crease. The hypoechoic ulnar artery (arrow) and small paired ulnar veins are seen in the right near field just inferior and radial to the flexor carpi ulnaris tendon. The ulnar nerve lies just medial (ulnar) to the ulnar artery and is often difficult to clearly visualize at this location

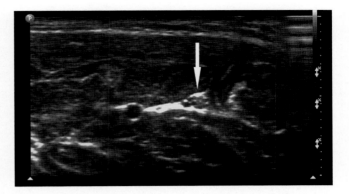

Figure 22-75. Right ulnar nerve in cross section about three quarters the way up the volar forearm. The hyperechoic ulnar nerve and hypoechoic ulnar artery are now physically separated from one another. The ulnar nerve (arrow) can be safely approached with the block needle at this location using either an in-plane or out-of-plane technique.

In the mid-supraclavicular region, the rounded anechoic subclavian artery will be seen either just above or adjacent to the echogenic superior margin of the first rib. A dense posterior acoustic shadow beneath the rib helps confirm its identification. A slightly deeper echogenic line representing the pleural surface of the cupola of the lung will also be noted; lung sliding and comet tail artifacts will commonly be seen at this interface in real time. The cluster of nerves that make up the brachial plexus at this level will always be found immediately lateral and often somewhat superior to the level of the subclavian artery. The visualized trunks and divisions of the brachial plexus appear as a cluster of many oval or rounded hypoechoic nodules (sometimes referred to as a "cluster of grapes") set off by the more hyperechoic fascial tissue that surrounds them. The fascial sheath containing the brachial plexus is situated between two hypoechoic muscle bundles: the medially located anterior scalene muscle and the laterally located middle scalene muscle (Figure 22-77). Color Doppler imaging of the supraclavicular and interscalene brachial plexus allows identification of the transverse cervical artery, which is critical for avoiding unintentional intravascular injection.

In a short-axis view of the arm at the level of anterior axillary crease, the pulsatile axillary artery will appear as an anechoic circle in the near field, located about 1–1.5 cm below the skin surface. Since the axillary vessels are quite superficial at this level, even light transducer pressure may collapse the axillary vein (or veins) and make it (or them) invisible. The axillary vein(s) may therefore only become apparent if the patient performs a Valsalva maneuver. The axillary vessels and branches of the brachial plexus rest on an echogenic fascial plane known as the medial brachial intermuscular septum; this septum separates the arm flexors above (biceps and

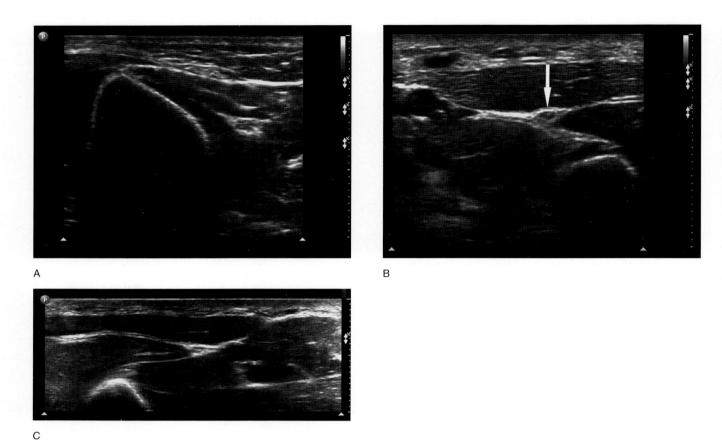

A

B

C

Figure 22-76. (A) Radial nerve above the elbow: the right radial nerve is seen in cross section as an echogenic circular structure just anterior to the hyperechoic outline of the lateral epicondyle. (B) Left radial nerve in cross section in the *upper forearm*. The hypoechoic brachioradialis muscle is seen in the near field. The radial artery and the paired radial veins are noted in the left near field and the hyperechoic superficial radial nerve (arrow) is seen as a triangular echogenic structure lying on the echogenic fascia just beneath the brachioradialis muscle. The curved volar surface of the upper shaft of the radius is seen in the right far field of the image. (C) Right radial nerve in cross section, *mid-forearm*. The curved echogenic surface of the shaft of the radius is seen in the left far field; the superficial radial nerve appears as a triangular echogenic structure immediately adjacent to the radial artery in the fascial plane separating the hypoechoic distal brachioradialis muscle above from the flexor carpi radialis muscle below.

coracobrachialis) from the extensors below (triceps muscle). In short-axis orientation at the level of the axilla, the three terminal nerve branches of the brachial plexus (the median, ulnar, and radial nerves) will typically be seen as hypoechoic circles circumferentially surrounding the axillary artery; occasionally only two nerves will be noted. The musculocutaneous nerve will typically be found more laterally, most often in the fascial plane separating the biceps and coracobrachialis muscles. It appears flattened to triangular in shape depending on where it is imaged (Figure 22-78).

In the femoral region, the femoral nerve may have a rounded, oval, or triangular shape in short-axis orientation and may exhibit somewhat greater echogenicity than the nerves seen in the brachial plexus. The femoral nerve can be found immediately lateral and somewhat deep to the anechoic common femoral artery, and is situated medial to the iliacus muscle (Figure 22-79).

High-frequency linear array transducers in the 7.5–15 MHz range are recommended for supraclavicular and axillary brachial plexus blocks, and 5–10 MHz linear array transducers have been used successfully for femoral nerve blocks. Hockey stick transducers with their combination of high frequency and small skin contact footprint are ideal for blocking smaller peripheral nerves. The usual sterile prep, drape, and transducer preparation are assumed for the performance of all nerve blocks as well as use of appropriate anesthetic agents and needles.

For single-shot injections (not involving placement of a perineural catheter), transducer preparation can be accomplished using a sterile adhesive dressing or a

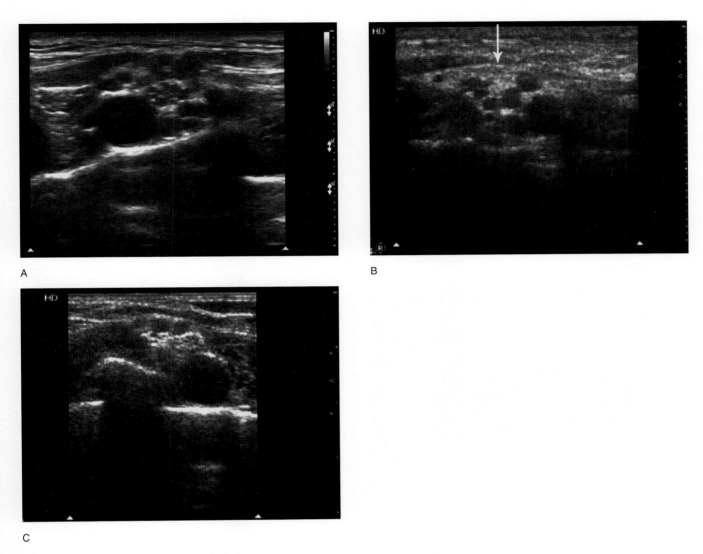

Figure 22-77. Supraclavicular brachial plexus. (A) *Left* supraclavicular brachial plexus. The hypoechoic nerve trunks and divisions are seen clustered immediately lateral and superior to the anechoic subclavian artery. The artery rests on the echogenic surface of the first rib and the pleural line is seen as an echogenic line in the right far field of the image. Lung sliding and comet tail artifacts were apparent at this location on real-time scanning. **(B)** *Right* supraclavicular brachial plexus with the nerve trunks and divisions appearing as a cluster of superficial hypoechoic circles within a more hyperechoic fascial sheath (arrow). The middle scalene muscle appears as a hypoechoic structure just lateral to the plexus (to the left on this image), the subclavian artery is seen as the largest and most hypoechoic circle near the center of the image, and the anterior scalene muscle appears as a somewhat indistinct hypoechoic structure just medial to the subclavian artery (to the right on this image). **(C)** *Right* supraclavicular brachial plexus. The first rib casts a prominent posterior acoustic shadow and the brightly echogenic pleural line is noted immediately below the anechoic subclavian artery. The brachial plexus is somewhat less distinct in this patient, and appears superolateral to the subclavian artery.

sterile transducer sheath. If a catheter is being placed, a full sterile transducer sheath is mandatory. Most anesthesiologists prefer using block needles not commonly available in EDs. While traditional cutting needles found in most EDs may be more likely to penetrate a peripheral nerve, they are also easier to position accurately,

associated with less pain and, in animal studies, have not been associated with an increased incidence of significant nerve injury. It is our practice to use standard cutting needles or Quincke-tipped spinal needles for the vast majority of blocks in our ED. We feel that needle tip placement (at a safe distance from the target nerve

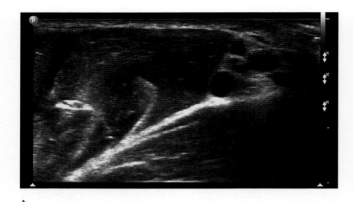

A

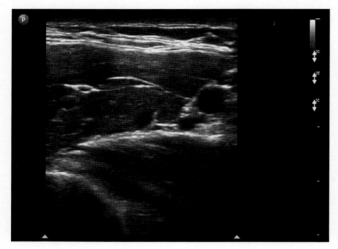

B

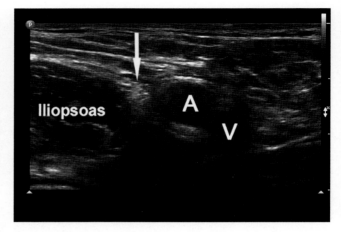

A

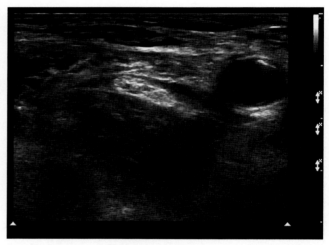

B

Figure 22-78. (A) Right axillary brachial plexus. The axillary artery, veins, and hypoechoic nerve branches (median, ulnar, and radial) are seen in the right far field of the image. Graded compression can be helpful to distinguish artery from veins and hypoechoic nerves. The echogenic fascial plane on which the vessels and plexus rest is known as the medial brachial intermuscular septum. It separates the arm extensors (biceps and coracobrachialis) above from the flexors (triceps) below. This septum may be obliquely or horizontally situated in the image depending on how the transducer is held. The musculocutaneous nerve can be seen as an echogenic oval structure in the left midfield. (B) Right axillary brachial plexus. The curved echogenic surface of the proximal humerus is seen in the left far field, and the echogenic medial brachial intermuscular septum has a more horizontal appearance in this image. The anechoic axillary artery and a portion of the plexus are seen in the right near field. The musculocutaneous nerve is seen as an ovoid structure with a hyperechoic rim in the fascial plane separating the biceps from the coracobrachialis muscle.

Figure 22-79. (A) Right femoral nerve in cross section. The femoral nerve (arrow) at the level of the inguinal crease appears as a superficially located hyperechoic oval structure lateral to the femoral artery and vein. The iliopsoas muscle is lateral and deep to the nerve, and the fascia iliaca covers the muscle and nerve superficially, then passes beneath the femoral artery. Injection of anesthetic must be deep to the fascia iliaca to ensure a successful block. (B) Close-up of the right femoral nerve in cross section. The fascia lata is seen as an echogenic horizontal band in the central near field in line with the upper border of the anechoic femoral artery. The femoral nerve appears as a flattened hyperechoic structure lateral and somewhat inferior to the artery in the center of the sonogram. The fascia iliaca (iliopectineal fascia) can be seen as a thin echogenic line located just above the femoral nerve, then continuing medially *beneath* the femoral artery. A = femoral artery, V = femoral vein.

within the appropriate fascial plane) is far more important than needle choice in avoiding iatrogenic nerve injury.

Needles may be directed using a "hand-on-needle" technique, where the needle is attached via sterile extension tubing to a syringe containing anesthetic solution. The operator holds the ultrasound transducer in the nondominant hand and the hub of the needle in the dominant hand. An assistant holds the syringe and aspirates and injects as directed by the operator. Alternatively, the needle may be connected to a syringe directly in a "hand-on-syringe" technique more familiar to most emergency physicians. The provider holds the ultrasound transducer in the nondominant hand, the syringe in the dominant hand, and aspirates and injects without the help of an assistant.

Anesthetic solutions typically used in the ED include lidocaine, bupivacaine and, more rarely, ropivacaine and mepivacaine. A detailed discussion of these agents can be found in any standard emergency medicine textbook and will not be covered in this chapter. However, it is important to realize that inadvertent intravascular injection of bupivacaine is highly cardiotoxic and may result in CV collapse. We recommend the use of lidocaine or newer amide anesthetics until significant familiarity and skill with ultrasound nerve blocks has been achieved. In addition, providers should be familiar with the management of local anesthetic systemic toxicity and the use of intravascular lipid emulsions.[55]

For providers without considerable experience with these techniques, we advise that the needle used for anesthetic deposition be advanced "in-plane" to the ultrasound beam so that precise real-time needle tip localization can be performed. This is best accomplished with needle insertion on one end of the transducer with the nerve bundle(s) visualized in short axis and the needle visualized in long axis. The tip of the advancing block needle can then be visualized throughout its course and precise delivery of anesthetic can be assured. Providers should take advantage of the fascial planes that typically surround peripheral nerves. Placement of the needle tip within the proper fascial plane will facilitate spread of anesthetic solution around the nerve without requiring placement of the needle tip in close proximity to the nerve itself. If paresthesias are elicited, high injection pressures are encountered, or local anesthetic is not visualized on the ultrasound screen during the injection, the needle should be moved slightly so that an intraneural or intravascular injection is avoided. Needle tip visualization can be further enhanced if the needle bevel is directed face up. As providers gain experience, they may find that many blocks are more easily performed out-of-plane, with the needle inserted in the middle of the transducer, crossing under the plane of the transducer perpendicular to the long axis of the transducer. This technique allows for shorter skin-to-target distances, but needle tip visualization is often more difficult than with the in-plane technique.

Special Considerations for Supraclavicular and Interscalene Blocks

Both the interscalene and supraclavicular brachial plexus blocks are associated with temporary paralysis of the phrenic nerve, causing ipsilateral hemidiaphragmatic paralysis. This occurs near-universally with the interscalene approach, and in >50% of cases with the supraclavicular approach. In healthy subjects, this phenomenon has no clinical effect on respiratory status, but these blocks must be avoided in patients with preexisting respiratory compromise. In addition, due to the expected phrenic nerve paralysis, bilateral blocks should never be performed.

Supraclavicular Brachial Plexus Block

Position the patient either supine or sitting up at about 30°, with arms at the side in neutral position and the head turned 45° away from the side of the block. Sterilize and drape the skin in the supraclavicular fossa. Cover the transducer with a sterile adhesive dressing or a sterile transducer cover, and apply a sterile conductive medium to the skin. Place the transducer just posterior to the clavicle and lateral to the sternocleidomastoid in an oblique coronal plane with the transducer orientation marker facing the provider's left. Angle the medial portion of the transducer more anteriorly than coronally, paralleling the course of the clavicle (Figure 22-80). Anesthetize the skin entry site with lidocaine under direct ultrasound visualization. Introduce the needle from the posterolateral edge of the transducer and move the needle in-plane anteromedially toward the brachial plexus nerve cluster under real-time guidance. When the needle tip is in close contact to the cluster, advance it through the fascial sheath surrounding the plexus with a well-controlled short quick jab. Hold the needle fixed in place while the provider (or an assistant if using a hand-on-needle technique) delivers a test dose of 1–2 mL of anesthetic agent after first aspirating to ensure that no intravascular injection will occur. If the agent spreads around the target nerves, continue to slowly deliver the rest of the anesthetic agent; if not, reposition the needle, deliver another test dose, and proceed accordingly. Several repositionings of the block needle under ultrasound guidance are advised to ensure even distribution of the anesthetic agent throughout the entire cross-sectional area of the plexus. Pay particular attention that the anesthetic agent reaches the inferior portion of the brachial plexus adjacent to the first rib to ensure that a successful block will occur. We recommend administering 3–5 mL aliquots every 30–60 seconds with

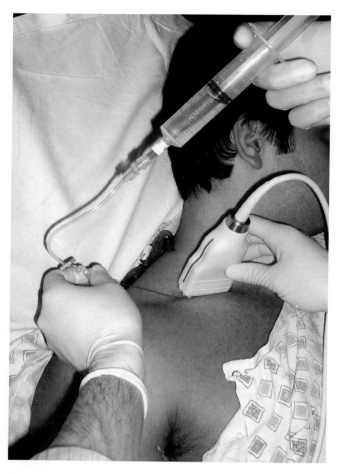

Figure 22-80. Supraclavicular brachial plexus block. "hand-on-needle" technique. The patient's head is turned to the opposite side, and the transducer is held in an oblique coronal plane just behind the clavicle. The anesthetic delivery needle is inserted on the lateral aspect of the transducer and positioned under direct ultrasound guidance. When the needle tip reaches the desired location, the operator can hold it in fixed position while an assistant delivers a test dose (1–2 cc) of the anesthetic solution to confirm adequate needle tip placement. For purposes of illustration, the sterile drape and transducer cover are not shown.

aspiration of the syringe between injections for a total of 10–15 mL of the desired anesthetic agent.

Interscalene Brachial Plexus Block

Position the patient either supine or sitting up at about 30°, turned slightly away from the side of the block (a towel roll can be used to assist with this positioning). Place the patient's arms at their side in a neutral position and turn the head 45° away from the side of the block. Sterilize and drape the skin of the lateral neck. Cover

the transducer with a sterile adhesive dressing or a sterile transducer cover, and apply a sterile conductive medium to the skin. There are two common techniques used to localize the interscalene brachial plexus. One approach involves placing the transducer over the anterior neck at the level of the cricoid cartilage and locating the carotid artery and internal jugular vein. Move the transducer posterolaterally and identify the posterior edge of the sternocleidomastoid. Just deep to the posterior edge of the sternocleidomastoid is the interscalene groove, between the anterior and middle scalene muscles. The roots of the brachial plexus appear as three anechoic circular structures arranged in a vertical pattern that has been termed "the traffic light sign." (Figure 22-81) An alternative approach involves identifying the interscalene brachial plexus by locating the supraclavicular brachial plexus as described previously, and then moving the transducer cephalad, tracing the brachial plexus proximally into the interscalene groove. Anesthetize the skin entry site with lidocaine and introduce the needle from the posterolateral edge of the transducer. Move the needle in-plane anteromedially through the middle scalene muscle toward the interscalene groove under real-time guidance. The needle can be held fixed in place while the provider (or an assistant if using a hand-on-needle technique) delivers a test dose of 1–2 mL of anesthetic agent after first aspirating to ensure that no intravascular injection will occur. If the agent spreads around the target nerves, continue to slowly deliver the rest of the anesthetic agent; if not, reposition the needle, deliver another test dose, and proceed accordingly. It is usually not necessary to reposition the needle as distribution of the anesthetic agent typically occurs with proper needle placement in the interscalene groove. We recommend administering 3–5 mL aliquots every 30–60 seconds with aspiration of the syringe between injections for a total of 10–15 mL of the desired anesthetic agent.

Axillary Perivascular Brachial Plexus Block

Position the patient either supine or sitting up at 30° with the head midline, arm abducted to 90°, and the elbow either flexed at 90–100° with the back of the hand resting on the bed facing upward ("high-5" position), or fully extended and resting on a table. Sterilize and drape the skin at the level of the anterior axillary crease. Cover the transducer with a sterile adhesive dressing or a sterile transducer cover, and apply a sterile conductive medium to the skin. Place the transducer high in the anterior axilla at the level of the anterior axillary crease (at the border between the deltoid and the biceps muscle). Place the transducer perpendicular to the long axis of the humerus with the orientation marker facing cephalad so that a short-axis view of the axillary vessels and

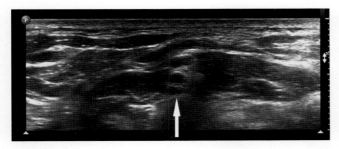

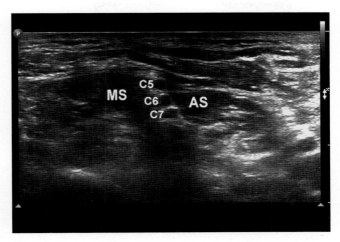

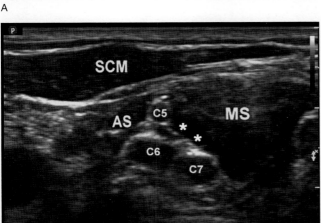

Figure 22-81. (A) *Left* interscalene brachial plexus. A portion of the flattened hypoechoic sternocleidomastoid (SCM) muscle is seen in the left near field. The three vertically oriented hypoechoic circles in the center of the sonogram represent the C5, C6, and C7 nerve roots (above arrow). They are typically arranged in a vertical pattern known as the "traffic light sign," are surrounded by a rim of hyperechoic fascia, and are located in the interscalene groove located between the anterior and middle scalene muscles. (B) *Right* interscalene brachial plexus. A portion of the hypoechoic SCM muscle is now seen in the right near field. The plexus (C5, C6, C7) is seen in the interscalene groove, surrounded by echogenic fascia, located between the anterior scalene (AS) and middle scalene (MS) muscles. (C) Left interscalene brachial plexus block. Anechoic local anesthetic solution (asterisks) is visualized in the interscalene groove adjacent to the C5, C6, and C7 nerve roots. The SCM muscle lies superficially, and the AS and middle scalene (MS) muscles define the medial and lateral borders, respectively, of the interscalene groove.

nerves will be obtained (Figure 22-82). Anesthetize the skin entry site with lidocaine under direct ultrasound visualization. Introduce the needle from the superior edge of the sagittally oriented transducer and move the needle toward the axillary artery with real-time guidance, similar to the long-axis approach for vascular access. The needle tip will typically be directed just above the axillary artery and the sheath entered close to where the median nerve typically resides. The needle can then be held fixed in place while the provider (or an assistant if using a hand-on-needle technique) delivers a test dose of 1–2 mL of anesthetic agent after first aspirating to ensure that no intravascular injection will occur. If the agent is seen to spread around the target nerves, continue to slowly deliver the anesthetic agent; if not, reposition the

needle, deliver another test dose, and proceed accordingly by administering 3–5 mL aliquots every 30–60 seconds with aspiration of the syringe between injections for a total of 10–15 mL of the desired anesthetic agent. As with the supraclavicular brachial plexus block several repositionings of the block needle with ultrasound guidance are advised to ensure an even distribution of the anesthetic agent within the entire plexus.

Femoral Nerve Block

Position the patient supine with both legs extended; the side on which the block is to be performed may be slightly externally rotated. Sterilize and drape the skin at the area of the femoral crease and femoral vessels,

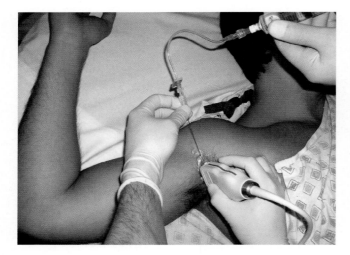

Figure 22-82. Axillary brachial plexus "hand-on-needle" technique. The patient is in a "high-5" position with transducer placed high in the anterior axilla at the level of the anterior axillary crease (at the border between the biceps and the deltoid muscle). The transducer is oriented vertically, perpendicular to the long axis of the humerus. The anesthetic delivery needle is inserted from the superior aspect of the transducer and positioned under direct ultrasound guidance. When the needle tip reaches the desired location, the operator can hold it in a fixed position while an assistant delivers a test dose (1–2 cc) of the anesthetic solution to confirm adequate needle tip placement. For purposes of illustration, the sterile drape and transducer cover are not shown.

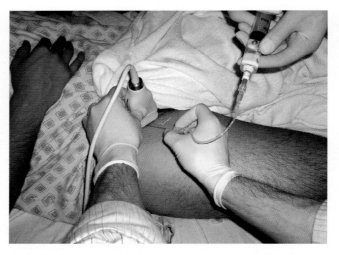

Figure 22-83. Femoral nerve block "hand-on-needle" out-of-plane technique. The transducer is placed in an oblique transverse orientation at the level of and in line with the inguinal crease, orientation marker facing left. The femoral nerve is positioned in the center of the image and the anesthetic delivery needle is inserted below the center of the transducer in an out-of-plane approach. Under ultrasound guidance, the needle tip is positioned below the iliopectineal fascia as close to the femoral nerve as possible. When the needle tip reaches the desired location, the operator can hold it in a fixed position while an assistant delivers a test dose (1–2 cc) of the anesthetic solution to confirm adequate needle tip placement. For purposes of illustration, the sterile drape and transducer cover are not shown.

and cover the transducer with a sterile transducer cover. Apply sterile conductive medium to skin. Place the transducer in an oblique transverse orientation at the level of, and in line with, the inguinal crease. The femoral nerve will be seen immediately lateral to and somewhat deep to the common femoral artery; position the nerve in the center of the image. Anesthetize the skin entry site with lidocaine under direct visualization. Insert the needle using either an in-plane or out-of-plane technique. Introduce the needle at the lateral edge of the transducer (long-axis or in-plane approach) and advance the needle under real-time guidance. The needle will need to pass through two fascial layers: the more superficially located fascia lata and the somewhat deeper fascia iliaca (iliopectineal fascia). When the needle tip has punctured the iliopectineal fascia and is in close proximity to the femoral nerve, hold the needle fixed in place while the provider (or an assistant if using a hand-on-needle technique) delivers a test dose of 1–2 mL of anesthetic agent after first aspirating to ensure that no intravascular injection will occur. If the anesthetic agent is seen to spread around the femoral nerve, continue to slowly

deliver the rest of the anesthetic agent; if not, reposition the needle, deliver another test dose, and proceed accordingly by administering 3–5 mL aliquots every 30–60 seconds with aspiration of the syringe between injections for a total of 15–20 mL of the desired anesthetic agent. Once again, needle repositioning is advised to ensure spread of the anesthetic agent around the nerve. Note that an inguinal paravascular injection technique will often fail to block the femoral nerve both because the femoral sheath impedes the lateral spread of anesthetic agent and because the femoral nerve is physically separated from this sheath by the iliopectineal fascia. Figure 22-83 illustrates the out-of-plane femoral nerve block technique.

Forearm Ultrasound Nerve Blocks (FUN Blocks)

Median, Ulnar, and Radial Nerves

Extend the forearm on a tray table and scan in short axis at the level of the proximal wrist crease. Locate the median nerve in the mid-wrist and follow it about

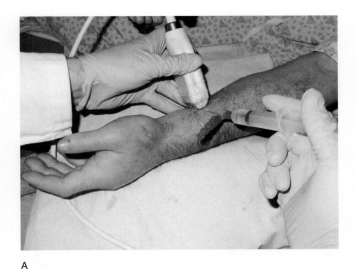
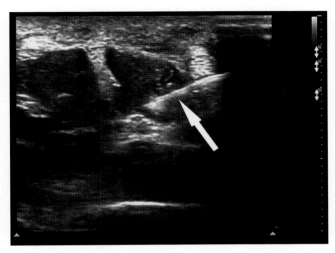

A   B

Figure 22-84. (A) Forearm median nerve block "hand-on-syringe" in-plane technique. The arm rests on a tray table, the transducer is covered with a sterile adhesive dressing, the skin has been prepped, and a sterile lubricant has been applied. The needle is advanced in plane. (B) Transverse sonogram of the same patient: the hyperechoic block needle (arrow) is seen immediately above the centrally located median nerve.

5–10 cm proximally where it assumes a more triangular configuration surrounded by the superficial and deep flexor muscles of the wrist and hand. Use a sterile skin prep, sterile conductive gel, and a sterile adhesive dressing for all the FUN blocks. Perform needle insertion either in-plane or out-of-plane with the needle tip directed to the fascial plane separating the flexor digitorum profundus and superficialis muscles, in proximity to the nerve. Deposit 3–7 mL of the desired anesthetic agent with needle redirection as needed to assure adequate circumferential spread (Figure 22-84 and Figure 22-85).

Using similar positioning and preparation as noted above, locate the ulnar nerve at the proximal wrist crease on the volar ulnar aspect of the wrist. Using a short-axis technique, the hypoechoic ulnar artery will appear as a small circular structure in the near field, immediately below the flexor carpi ulnaris tendon. The course of the artery should be followed about three quarters the way up the forearm where the ulnar nerve and artery will be seen to physically separate from one another. At this location, employ either an in-plane or out-of-plane injection technique to surround the nerve with the anesthetic agent. Ulnar nerve blockade at this proximal location will anesthetize both the dorsal and palmar branches of the nerve with a single injection (Figure 22-86).

Consider the radial nerve block in the upper forearm as a mirror image of the ulnar nerve block. Using similar equipment preparation and patient positioning as above, scan the upper radial volar forearm and identify the brachioradialis muscle, radial artery, superficial

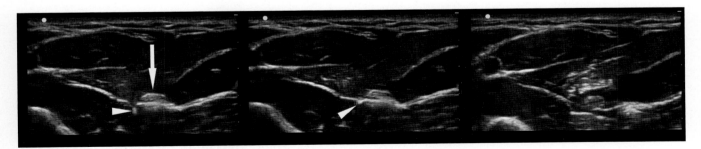

Figure 22-85. Transverse sonogram sequence for an out-of-plane median nerve block. (A) The needle tip (arrowhead) is positioned adjacent to the median nerve (arrow), slightly deep to the fascia separating the deep and superficial flexors of the forearm. (B) The needle is withdrawn slightly until the tip is located within the fascial plane. (C) After injection, anechoic local anesthetic solution is visualized surrounding the median nerve.

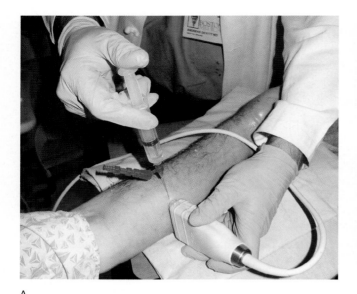

A

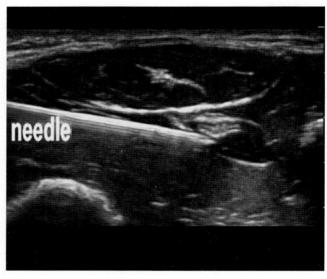

B

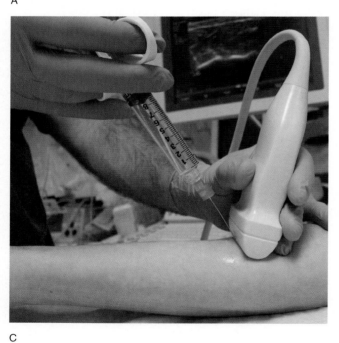

C

Figure 22-86. (A) In-plane forearm ulnar nerve block technique. The transducer is placed transversely on the ulnar aspect of the volar mid to upper forearm. Under ultrasound guidance, the needle is inserted below the lateral aspect of the transducer in an in-plane approach. (B) Transverse sonogram of an in-plane ulnar nerve block, right arm, needle entering from a lateral approach. After positioning the needle tip adjacent to the nerve, spread of local anesthetic is visualized surrounding the nerve during injection. (C) Out-of-plane ulnar nerve block technique.

radial nerve, and the proximal shaft of the radius. Either an in-plane or out-of-plane technique can be employed for this block (Figure 22-87 and Figure 22-88). If the block is performed more proximally at the level of the lateral epicondyle of the humerus, the distal sensory branches as well as the wrist extensors will be blocked.

PITFALLS

1. **Misidentification of vascular structures for nerves may lead to potential intravascular injection of a large amount of anesthetic solution, as well as a failed block.** Survey the area carefully prior to the block with a graded compression technique or Doppler interrogation to identify, and therefore avoid, all vascular structures.

2. **High injection pressures, paresthesias, and/or failure to visualize anesthetic spread during injection may indicate inadvertent intraneural or intravascular injection.** If these occur, halt the injection and reposition the needle tip before resuming the block.

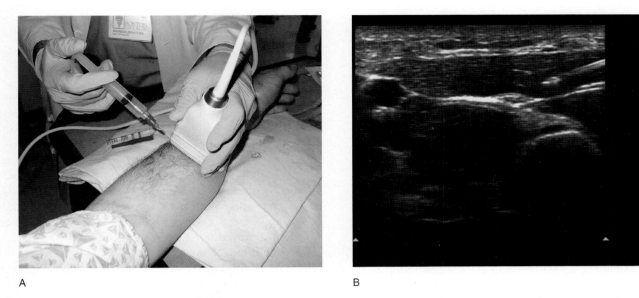

A   B

Figure 22-87. (A) In-plane superficial radial nerve block technique. The transducer is placed transversely on the radial aspect of the mid to upper forearm, and the block needle is advanced below the lateral aspect of the transducer in an in-plane approach. (B) Same patient. Transverse sonogram of a left arm superficial radial nerve block. The echogenic block needle is seen approaching the superficial radial nerve from a lateral (radial) approach. The hypoechoic radial artery is seen medially, the upper radial shaft below.

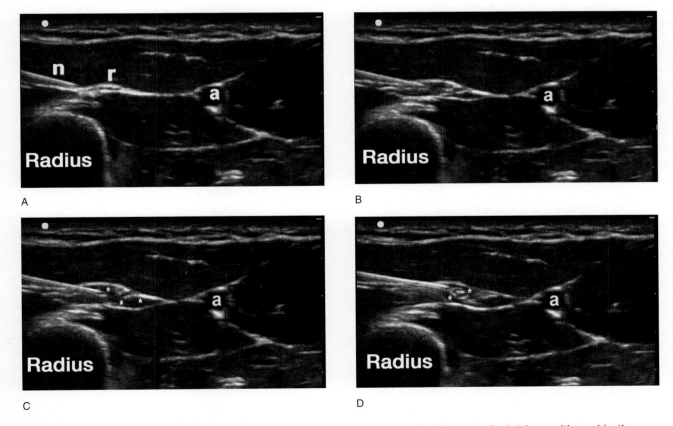

A   B

C   D

Figure 22-88. Superficial radial nerve block sequence, right arm. (A) The needle (n) is positioned in the fascial plane radial to the radial nerve (r). The radial artery (a) is located medially, and the radius is located deep to the nerve. (B) Local anesthetic is injected and begins to distend the fascial plane surrounding the nerve. (C) and (D) Anechoic local anesthetic solution (asterisks) is visualized surrounding the nerve.

▶ PARACENTESIS

CLINICAL CONSIDERATIONS

Confirming the presence and location of peritoneal fluid prior to paracentesis is simply an extension of the Focused Assessment with Sonography for Trauma (FAST) examination. Indications for performing abdominal paracentesis in the ED or acute care setting include the evaluation of the patient with new onset ascites, obtaining fluid for diagnostic purposes in the patient with suspected spontaneous bacterial peritonitis, and as a therapeutic intervention to relieve discomfort or respiratory embarrassment in symptomatic patients with massive ascites. Portable point-of-care ultrasound is also being used in the home hospice setting to diagnose and guide palliative paracentesis in patients suffering from tense malignant ascites.[56] Paracentesis may additionally play a role in clarifying the nature of intra-abdominal fluid detected in patients with a positive FAST examination but no clear history of trauma.

Ultrasound is considered the gold standard test for detecting ascites, reliably identifying as little as 100 mL of free fluid and occasionally able to detect volumes in the range of 5–10 mL around the bladder. Larger volumes are required for successful paracentesis, however, with reported success rates of only 44% when the volume of ascites is 300 mL, increasing to 78% with 500 mL.[57] While the left lower quadrant has long been considered a standard location for blind paracentesis, patients with smaller volumes of ascites may have no sonographically demonstrable fluid present in this area. Routine point-of-care ultrasonography prior to every paracentesis procedure is highly recommended. In one series of 100 ED patients undergoing abdominal paracentesis, there was a significantly higher procedural success rate for ultrasound-assisted paracentesis compared with the traditional "blind" technique (95% vs. 65%).[58]

Diagnostic paracentesis involves the collection of small volumes of fluid for laboratory analysis (often <60 mL). Small volume therapeutic paracentesis is defined as removal of <2 L of ascitic fluid. Large volume therapeutic paracentesis is commonly defined as >4 L removed. In a report on 29 patients with large volume ascites, measurement of the fluid depth measured at the paracentesis site was shown to correlate with the drained fluid volume; for every 1 cm increase in the smallest fluid depth, there was an average 1 L increase in the drained fluid volume.[59]

Complications of paracentesis are infrequent but can include abdominal wall hematoma, inferior epigastric artery pseudoaneurysm, mesenteric hematoma, intraperitoneal hemorrhage, bladder and bowel perforation, abdominal wall abscess, persistent ascitic fluid leak, and peritonitis.

ANATOMICAL CONSIDERATIONS

Although visualization of an accessible fluid pocket is paramount, guidelines for paracentesis also include a number of common-sense caveats. Avoid the upper quadrants (hepatosplenomegaly), avoid surgical scars (possible adhesions and adherent bowel loops), stay remote and lateral to the rectus muscles (the superior and inferior epigastric vessels may inadvertently be punctured), avoid large collateral venous channels visible on the abdominal wall, and use a relatively small-gauge needle. A fluid collection of at least 3 cm in depth is considered adequate for the procedure. With the goal of finding a location for paracentesis that would simultaneously offer both the deepest pocket of fluid and the thinnest portion of the abdominal wall, one study obtained ultrasound images on 62 cirrhotic patients at two standard locations: the left lower quadrant (defined as 2 finger breadths medial and 2 finger breadths cephalad to the left anterior superior iliac spine) and the midline infraumbilical area (defined as 2 finger breadths inferior to the umbilicus). The abdominal wall exhibited a wide range of thickness in both locations (0.6–9.1 cm in the left lower quadrant and 0.9–9.5 cm in the infraumbilical midline), but was noted to be consistently thinner in the left lower quadrant (a mean of 1.8 cm compared with 2.4 cm in the midline). When the patient was positioned in the left lateral oblique position, the pool of ascites was noted to increase from an average of 2.8 to 4.6 cm.[60]

CLINICAL INDICATIONS

- Diagnostic sampling of intraperitoneal fluid
- Therapeutic drainage of intraperitoneal fluid

TECHNIQUE AND ULTRASOUND FINDINGS

Simple transudative ascites will appear as an anechoic extraluminal fluid collection within the peritoneal cavity. In a midline longitudinal orientation in the lower abdomen, the echogenic bladder dome will be seen on the right of the image with anechoic fluid and bowel loops noted adjacent to the bladder (Figure 22-89). Echogenic fibrinous strands may occasionally be noted within the fluid. Loops of peristaltic small bowel will usually be seen floating within the ascitic fluid and varying degrees of "dirty" shadowing may be present depending on the amount of intraluminal bowel gas present (Figure 22-90). A mesenteric stalk attached to the bowel loops may also be noted. The presence of intraperitoneal fluid on

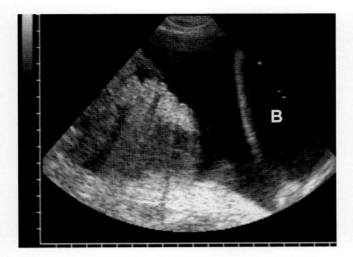

Figure 22-89. Midline sagittal view of a patient with a large amount of simple ascites. The echogenic bladder dome appears to the right of the image. Both urine and simple ascites appear similarly hypoechoic. Echogenic loops of bowel with "dirty" shadowing from intraluminal bowel gas are seen on the left side of the image. B = bladder.

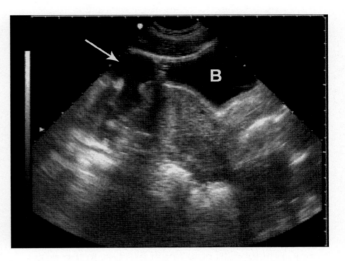

Figure 22-91. Midline sagittal view of a female with hemoperitoneum. The bladder and uterus are noted to the right of the image; the hypoechoic pocket of fluid (arrow) above the bladder dome represents unclotted blood and is sonographically indistinguishable from ascites. B = bladder.

ultrasound examination does not always signify ascites. Acute hemoperitoneum (Figure 22-91) or malignant ascites may also appear on ultrasound as an echo-free fluid collection. If any doubt exists as to the fluid identity, a diagnostic paracentesis or further imaging may be performed. The presence of a nodular, shrunken, and hyperechoic liver on the sonogram suggests a cirrhotic etiology and can be helpful in cases when the patient history is unobtainable or the diagnosis is unknown (Figure 22-92). A thickened hyperechoic omentum ("omental caking") may be the first sonographic clue to a new diagnosis of malignant ascites (Figure 22-93).

Ascitic fluid may occasionally appear particulate, exhibiting complex fluid characteristics with varying degrees of internal echogenicity that reflect the presence of either leukocytes, erythrocytes, protein particles, or fibrin within the fluid (Figure 22-94).

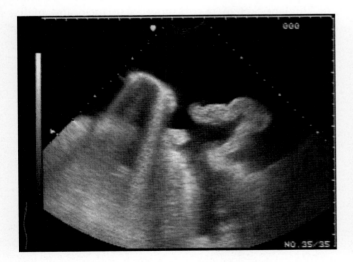

Figure 22-90. Large-volume simple ascites with hyperechoic loops of small bowel. Some "dirty" shadowing and hyperechoic reverberation artifacts from intraluminal bowel gas are noted. Gain settings have been adjusted to make the simple fluid appear uniformly black.

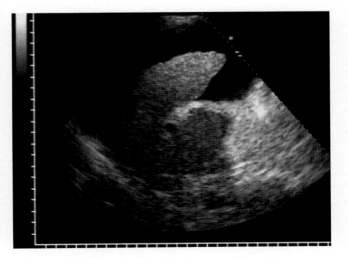

Figure 22-92. FAST orientation in the right upper quadrant. A large volume of anechoic intraperitoneal fluid is noted; given the hyperechoic, shrunken, and nodular appearance of the liver, one can reasonably assume that this fluid is ascites.

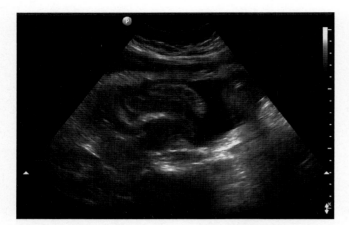

Figure 22-93. Sonogram of the upper abdomen in a female patient with new onset ascites. In the near field, a long segment of very thickened and hyperechoic omentum is seen immediately above several loops of small bowel. This "omental caking" is most typically found in abdominal or pelvic malignancies. Tuberculous peritonitis may also give rise to this sonographic finding.

Perform the ultrasound examination for ascites with a 3.5–5 MHz curved array abdominal transducer. Adjust gain settings to make the fluid appear black (assuming that the patient has simple ascites). If possible, raise the head of the bed and, if needed, turn the patient slightly to the left lateral oblique position to maximize the depth of the fluid collection in the left lower quadrant. Optimally, perform the sonogram just prior to the procedure

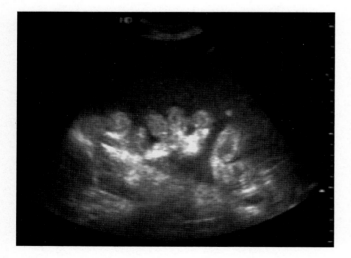

Figure 22-94. Hemorrhagic ascites; the ascitic fluid in this patient with known cirrhosis and ascites exhibits a complex pattern with increased echogenicity throughout. The patient presented with a 10-point drop in HCT from a recent prior visit; the search for a bleeding hepatoma proved positive.

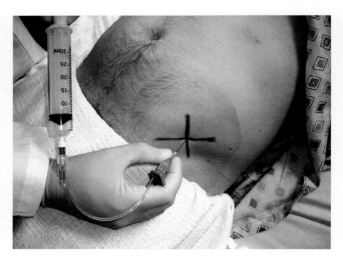

Figure 22-95. Paracentesis: Small-volume aspiration technique. The fluid pocket has been mapped and marked in two orthogonal planes, and the skin has been prepped and anesthetized down to the peritoneum. The patient remains in the exact same position for the aspiration as when mapped and is asked to protrude the abdomen during the procedure to facilitate needle insertion and prevent inadvertent puncture of deeper structures. The extension tubing allows for manipulation of the syringe, while the needle is held fixed in place. For purposes of illustration, the sterile drape is not shown.

with the patient remaining in the exact same position during the paracentesis. Note the location of the bladder dome so that it may be avoided if the planned site of paracentesis is in the midline infraumbilical region. Map the fluid pocket in two orthogonal planes, and mark the skin entry site with an indelible ink skin marker. Note the thickness of the abdominal wall, the depth of the fluid pocket until bowel or bladder is encountered, and the anticipated puncture angle. The volume of ascitic fluid being removed will dictate the type of equipment needed for the aspiration. For a diagnostic small volume aspiration, only an 18–20-gauge needle, a short piece of extension tubing, and a 60-mL syringe are needed (Figure 22-95). For a therapeutic paracentesis, use commercially available paracentesis kits with an 8 French catheter with multiple side holes and a gravity feed collection bag (or vacuum bottles) for the fluid collection (Figure 22-96). In the vast majority of paracenteses, the procedure can be successfully performed with prepuncture mapping only. Real-time guidance may be useful in patients where only a small volume of ascites has been found; in such cases, a sterile adhesive dressing over the transducer and sterile conductive medium will be needed. Finally, asking the patient to cough or protrude the abdomen during the needle insertion can facilitate the puncture process and minimize the chance of inadvertent puncture of deeper structures.

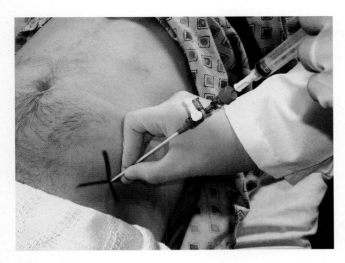

Figure 22-96. Paracentesis: Large-volume aspiration technique. Procedural details are similar to the small volume aspiration technique but with several additions. A skin stab wound is made to the beveled edge of the scalpel blade included in the centesis kit; this will facilitate passage of 8 French catheters. Once ascitic fluid is aspirated, the catheter needle is held fixed while the catheter is advanced several centimeters. The large-gauge needle is then withdrawn from the catheter assembly, and connector tubing may then be attached to the side port of the stopcock. Drainage may be passive, into a collection bag included in the kit, or vacuum assisted into evacuated glass containers. For purposes of illustration, the sterile drape is not shown.

PITFALLS

1. Allowing the patient to move after fluid mapping may lead to a shift in the location of the fluid pocket and result in a dry tap or bowel penetration.
2. Fluid-filled structures such as a large bladder, a large ovarian cyst, or a dilated fluid-filled loop of bowel could be mistaken for an intraperitoneal fluid collection. It is important to verify the nature of all fluid collections noted by performing a brief sonographic survey of the entire abdomen prior to paracentesis.

▶ THORACENTESIS

CLINICAL CONSIDERATIONS

Point-of-care chest ultrasound allows for rapid identification, characterization, and precise localization of pleural effusions. Preprocedure ultrasound assessment and marking of relevant landmarks and the location of the fluid pocket prior to thoracentesis improve the performance characteristics of a procedure that can be asso-

ciated with a complication rate as high as 20–50%.[61] Chest ultrasound has long been demonstrated to be superior to chest radiography for detecting pleural fluid and assisting in collection of an adequate fluid sample for analysis.[62] Ultrasound guidance for thoracentesis has become the standard of care and has been shown to reduce overall hospital costs and complications associated with thoracentesis.[63] In a meta-analysis of 6605 thoracenteses, the overall pneumothorax rate was noted to be 6%, and 34 % of this latter group ultimately required chest tube insertion. Ultrasound guidance was associated with a significantly lower risk of pneumothorax (odds ratio 0.3). Variables known to be associated with thoracentesis-related pneumothorax include inexperienced operators, lack of ultrasound use, and removal of large volumes of pleural fluid.[64] A steep increase in the risk of pneumothorax occurs when large volumes of pleural fluid are removed. In a series of 735 thoracenteses performed in a Swedish hospital, the pneumothorax rate was noted to 3.8 times greater if 1.8–2.2 L were removed when compared with patients in whom only 0.8–1.2 L was drained. In patients who had >2.3 L drained, the pneumothorax rate was noted to be 5.7 times higher.[65] In a review of 52 patients undergoing thoracentesis of large free-flowing pleural effusions, ultrasound guidance was associated with significantly fewer overall complications. While the pneumothorax rate was 19% overall, *none* occurred in the ultrasound-guided group.[66] In a report on 26 patients where attempts at blind thoracentesis had failed, subsequent ultrasound-guided aspiration was successful in 88% of the cases. Of note, the initial (failed) puncture site was noted to be directly over the liver, spleen, or kidney in 15 cases, underscoring the danger of relying on traditional physical diagnosis skills for preprocedure effusion "mapping."[67]

Patients who are mechanically ventilated may present a significant challenge as the inflation and deflation of the lung and their typically supine position make blind thoracentesis more hazardous. Ultrasound guidance may be especially helpful in such patients. In a report on ultrasound-guided thoracentesis in 40 mechanically ventilated patients, the procedure was safely and rapidly performed, with a success rate of 97% for obtaining >5 mL of fluid. No pneumothorax or hemoptysis was observed in this series. The authors recommended that the following guidelines be followed: the width of the fluid collection (as measured by the parietal to visceral interpleural distance) should be at least 15 mm and the fluid should be visible over at least 3 intercostal spaces. Of incidental note, pleural fluid was considered to be "absent" on the chest radiograph in 17 of 40 patients in whom fluid was subsequently identified and obtained with ultrasound.[68]

Finally, pleural fluid volume can be estimated in mechanically ventilated patients using a simplified formula as follows: the patient's trunk is elevated to 15° and the relevant hemithorax is scanned at the posterior axillary line in a transverse scan plane. The maximal separation between parietal and visceral pleura at the lung base is measured in end-expiration. The amount of pleural fluid can be measured as follows: volume (mL) = 20 × pleural separation (mm).[69]

ANATOMICAL CONSIDERATIONS

When performing thoracentesis, the anatomic area of interest will typically be located in the mid to lateral back below the level of the scapulae, or on occasion, the lateral chest wall in the mid-axillary region. The broad latissimus dorsi muscles cover most of the posterior and lateral chest wall deep to the skin and subcutaneous tissue of the back below the scapulae. Deep to this muscular layer lie the lower ribs, curving inferolaterally, with the intercostal muscles spanning adjacent ribs. Coursing along the inner surface of each intercostal space just below the parietal pleura that lines the chest cavity are the intercostal vein (closest to the inferior edge of the rib above), the intercostal artery, and the intercostal nerve. This neurovascular bundle follows the curve of the interspace and can be avoided by the aspirating needle only by paying meticulous attention while performing the thoracentesis *immediately* above the superior edge of the marked rib. From a lateral approach, the chest wall layers of the lower mid-axillary region consist of skin and subcutaneous tissue, external oblique muscle, ribs, intercostal muscles, the neurovascular bundle as noted above, and finally, the parietal pleura. Higher in the lateral mid-axillary region, the muscular layer is made up of the slips of the serratus anterior muscle instead of the external oblique. The top of the diaphragm normally rests at the level of the 10th thoracic vertebra.

Pleural fluid will initially collect along the most dependent surfaces between the inferior surface of the lower lobes and the diaphragm in a potential space called the costodiaphragmatic recess. The recess can track as low at the 12th rib posteriorly and to the level of the 8th rib laterally. The exact location of the lung will depend on the size of the pleural effusion, the degree of atelectasis, and the timing of the respiratory cycle. Even though the liver, spleen, and kidneys lie inferior to the diaphragm, inadvertent puncture of these organs can occur when a blind thoracentesis technique is employed.

CLINICAL INDICATIONS

- Obtaining pleural fluid for diagnostic purposes
- Therapeutic drainage of a pleural effusion to improve oxygenation and/or patient comfort

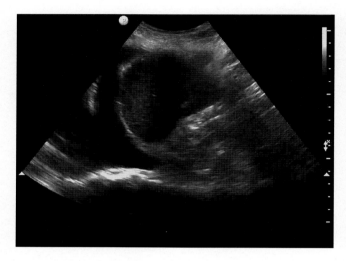

Figure 22-97. Oblique coronal view of the right upper quadrant centered over the liver. A large anechoic pleural effusion is apparent on the left side of the image. A portion of the inferior lung is seen as a curved echogenic structure at the far left side of the image. A curved echogenic vertebral body is seen in the far field just beneath the effusion.

TECHNIQUE AND ULTRASOUND FINDINGS

A pleural effusion is often first detected during the FAST exam or when performing abdominal scanning. On the oblique coronal view of the upper quadrants, a simple pleural effusion will appear as an anechoic collection superior to the liver or spleen with the echogenic diaphragm separating the fluid from the solid organs below. The echogenic inferior border of the lung may be seen within the effusion, located somewhat above the diaphragm in a location that will vary depending on the respiratory cycle and the depth of the effusion (Figure 22-97). On a transverse view of the abdomen, a simple pleural effusion will appear as an echo-free collection in the most dependent portion of the image, the costodiaphragmatic recess (Figure 22-98). The fluid collections are typically asymmetric in location and will be located on a somewhat lower scan plane on the left, and a somewhat higher one on the right. When scanning the patient in long-axis orientation from the back (with the patient sitting upright), a simple pleural effusion will appear as an echo-free collection closest to the transducer just deep to the chest wall. In the left hemithorax, the heart will be seen in short-axis orientation in the far field of the image, the lower border of the lung to the left, and the diaphragm and spleen to the right (Figure 22-99). If the transducer is moved medially, the tubular appearance of the descending aorta will be noted in the far field of the image with the inferior lung border to the left of the image and the effusion immediately below (Figure 22-100). In short-axis orientation from the back,

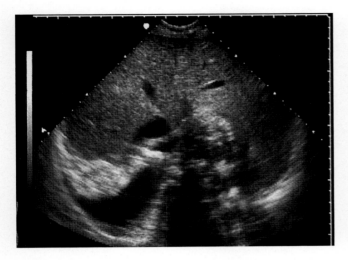

Figure 22-98. Right-sided pleural effusion seen in the costodiaphragmatic recess on transverse sonogram in this patient with hepatosplenomegaly.

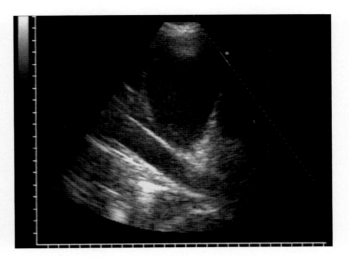

Figure 22-100. A more medially oriented longitudinal view of a left pleural effusion from the posterior chest; the tubular descending aorta is seen in the far field and the inferior lung border on the left.

the outline of the hemithorax will be apparent and lung will appear as a mid-gray region of echogenicity with a hyperechoic visceral pleura outline (Figure 22-101).

If the sonogram should reveal that a loculated pleural effusion is present, further imaging and appropriate specialist consultation is warranted. In such cases more aggressive management with either surgery or radiologically guided thoracostomy tube placement is often undertaken (Figure 22-102).

When marking the location for the thoracentesis from behind, the echogenic surface of the rib and its dense posterior acoustic shadow will be noted just deep to the subcutaneous tissue and the latissimus dorsi

muscle. Deep to the rib, the brightly echogenic pleural line will be visually apparent and its depth within the image will precisely represent the amount of chest wall that must be traversed to enter the pleural cavity (Figure 22-103).

Curved array, linear array, and phased array transducers may all be used for mapping a pleural effusion. A pleural effusion will most commonly be mapped with a curved or phased array transducer in the 2.5–5.0 MHz range. A tightly curved array transducer, if available, is optimal because the small skin contact footprint facilitates imaging through the narrow rib interspaces.

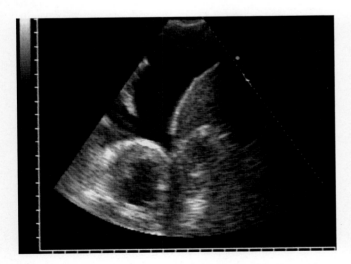

Figure 22-99. A longitudinal view of a left pleural effusion from the posterior chest. The heart is seen in short axis in the far field, the spleen to the right, the inferior lung border to the left, with the posterior chest wall closest to the transducer

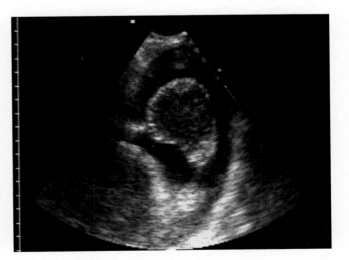

Figure 22-101. Transverse sonogram of the posterior left hemithorax. The cross-sectional outline of the entire hemithorax is clearly visible. Lung tissue is seen fully surrounded by the effusion in the center of the image.

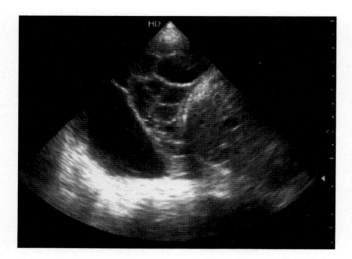

Figure 22-102. Right upper quadrant sonogram of a patient with a loculated pleural effusion. Further imaging with CT and specialist consultation is usually warranted in such cases.

Most patients requiring thoracentesis will have large effusions, are likely to be aspirated for both diagnostic *and* therapeutic purposes, and will have their aspiration performed from a dorsal approach (Figure 22-104). Position mobile and cooperative patients on the edge of a bed, sitting as vertically as possible with their arms folded and their head resting on pillows that have been placed on a tray table. Scan the relevant hemithorax from the upper lumbar region to the inferior border of

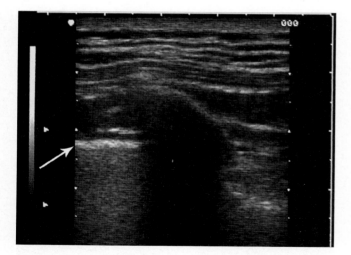

Figure 22-103. A linear array image of posterior chest wall showing skin, subcutaneous tissue, the thin muscular layer of the latissimus dorsi muscle, a rib with a prominent posterior acoustic shadow, and the brightly echogenic pleural line (arrow). Depth to the pleural line should routinely be noted when a thoracentesis is performed. No pleural effusion is seen in this image.

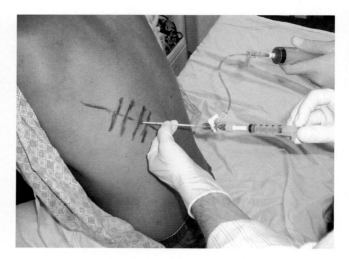

Figure 22-104. Thoracentesis procedural technique—Dorsal approach. The rib interspace for the aspiration has been marked and mapped. Needle insertion is over the center of the rib; the aspirating needle is then moved to a point immediately above the superior border of the rib into the interspace. A commercially available self-sealing thoracentesis needle is employed, and an assistant is available to aspirate the pleural fluid sample or connect the side port to a drainage bag.

the scapula and from the paravertebral region to the posterior axillary line. When an adequate fluid collection is sonographically visualized, map its location and size to determine an optimal site for aspiration. Assess the effusion in two orthogonal planes and note the superior and inferior borders of the fluid. Since transverse scanning will be performed along the rib interspaces, the ultrasound beam will be positioned somewhat obliquely to a true transverse scan plane. Note the location of the diaphragm, underlying liver or spleen, and any interposed lung. Pay particular attention to any changes in the position of the lung that occur with respiration. In order to ensure that an adequate fluid depth is maintained throughout the respiratory cycle, consider scanning the region using a combined B- and M-mode technique. Record the excursion of any lung parenchyma that may move in and out of the intended field with respiration and make measurements of the fluid pocket depth (Figure 22-105).

Mark the ribs surrounding the chosen interspace with indelible ink. The optimum depth for needle or catheter insertion can be predetermined by directly measuring the distance from the skin surface to the fluid collection or by estimation using the depth scale markers located on the ultrasound screen. In the debilitated or intubated patient, thoracentesis is commonly performed from a lateral approach with the puncture site in the lateral chest in the mid-axillary line. Less frequently, a dorsal approach can be utilized with the patient in a lateral

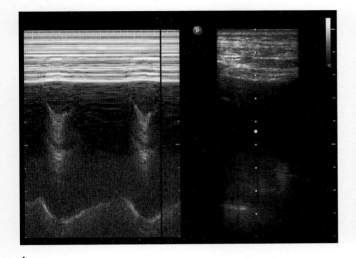

A

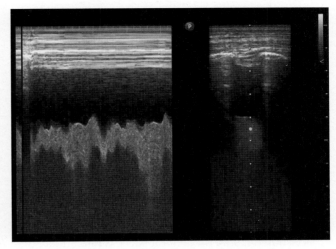

B

Figure 22-105. Combined B- and M-mode linear array sonograms of a pleural effusion at intended aspiration sites. (A) On the first image, the M-mode tracing shows that a portion of lung is moving in and out of the field during respiration leaving only about 1 cm of clearance between pleura and lung tissue. (B) On the second sonogram, the B-mode image shows two ribs and the pleural effusion through the interspace. No interposed lung tissue is seen on the M-mode tracing throughout the respiratory cycle, and the pleural effusion can be safely tapped at this location as long as the aspirating needle is not advanced more than about 3.5 cm.

decubitus position. For the lateral approach, position the patient supine with the head of the bed elevated at about 45° and the ipsilateral arm positioned as one would for a chest tube (arm abducted, elbow flexed with the hand behind the head). For the dorsal approach, place the patient in lateral decubitus position lying on the side of the effusion with the back next to the edge of the bed. Needle insertion for this position is just above the rib at the posterior axillary line. With both of these positions, it is advantageous to have intubated patients deeply sedated during the procedure. Angle the transducer in all four directions from the anticipated puncture site checking specifically for the absence of interposed lung, heart, liver, or spleen during the respiratory cycle. Again, note the distance from skin to parietal pleura, the movement of lung parenchyma in and out of the field during the respiratory cycle, and the depth of the fluid collection itself, and adjust the needle depth and approach angle accordingly.

Perform the thoracentesis immediately after the effusion is mapped with the patient remaining in the exact same position as when scanned. From this point, the procedural technique is the same as for blind aspiration. Use adequate local anesthesia at the skin, rib, and pleura to ensure patient comfort during the procedure. Alternatively, utilize real-time ultrasound guidance to actually guide the needle to the fluid collection after entering the skin. This is not typically necessary with moderate-to-large fluid collections. If real-time guidance is used, insert the needle to one side of the phased array transducer, which should be covered with a sterile sheath

during the procedure. The needle is best visualized in its long axis and the same basic principles are applied that are utilized for the in-plane approach to vascular access or nerve blocks.

PITFALLS

1. **Cellulitis involving site of desired needle entry may lead to infection of an otherwise sterile pleural effusion.** Needle puncture should not be undertaken through a site of a skin infection.
2. **Penetrating too deeply into the chest cavity with the aspirating needle can lead to lung or great vessel injury.** Make note of the thickness of the chest wall and the depth of the lung-free fluid collection at the aspiration site and do not penetrate deeper than this depth.
3. **Clear visualization of an effusion may be difficult in morbidly obese patients, thereby precluding safe performance of a thoracentesis.**

▶ PERICARDIOCENTESIS

CLINICAL CONSIDERATIONS

Cardiac tamponade is a life-threatening condition caused by the accumulation of fluid in the pericardial space, resulting in reduced ventricular filling and subsequent hemodynamic compromise. Beck's classic triad of physical findings for diagnosing cardiac tamponade (hypotension, jugular venous distention, and muffled heart sounds) applies only to patients in whom the increase in intrapericardial pressure is rapid.[70] Even in this acute population, Beck's triad appears in only 35% of patients, typically just before cardiac arrest.[71] When a pericardial effusion is suspected, ultrasound is the test of choice for making the diagnosis and the standard tool used to guide pericardiocentesis.[72–75] Blind pericardiocentesis has an estimated complication rate of 15%.[76] Echocardiography is preferentially used to guide needle placement into the pericardial space. A study examining 1127 consecutive ultrasound-guided pericardiocenteses demonstrated a 97% procedural success rate and a complication rate of only 4.7%.[77] With increased availability of ultrasound in the ED, echo-guided pericardiocentesis should replace the blind approach even for patients who are in extremis.

CLINICAL INDICATIONS

The clinical indication for pericardiocentesis is drainage of an ultrasound-diagnosed pericardial effusion in cases of:

- Cardiac arrest with pericardial effusion
- Hypotension in the setting of a moderate or large pericardial effusion

Contraindications:

- When the procedure would delay necessary thoracotomy or pericardiotomy[78,79]

ANATOMICAL CONSIDERATIONS

The two most common entry locations for pericardiocentesis are the subxiphoid and parasternal/apical approaches. The subxiphoid approach is most often used for pericardiocentesis that is performed without imaging ("blind"), while the parasternal/apical approach is a good choice for ultrasound-guided pericardiocentesis. In the parasternal/apical approach, visualization of the fluid ensures that the aerated lung and other vital organs are not in the pathway of the needle. Aerated lung tissue produces high acoustic impedance and does not permit visualization of fluid posterior to the lung. Superficial vascular structures to be avoided include internal mammary artery (3–5 cm lateral to parasternal border) and intercostal arteries (located along the inferior margin of the ribs).

TECHNIQUE AND ULTRASOUND FINDINGS

The sonographic findings of cardiac tamponade are the direct result of the progressive limitation of ventricular diastolic filling, and the reduction in stroke volume and cardiac output that occurs because of the increased intrapericardial pressure. Right ventricular diastolic collapse (Figure 22-106), right atrial collapse during systole (Figure 22-107), and dilated inferior vena cava with lack of inspiratory collapse (Figure 22-108) are seen with cardiac tamponade. The presence of isolated left atrial systolic collapse or left ventricular diastolic collapse may occur with localized left-sided compression or in patients with severe pulmonary hypertension.

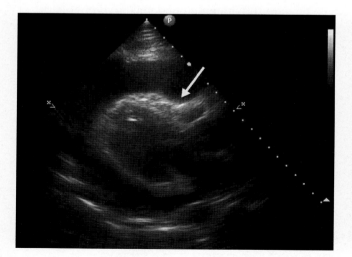

A

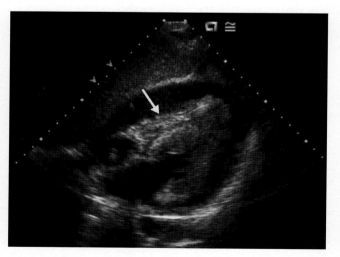

B

Figure 22-106. Cardiac tamponade. Parasternal long axis (A) and subcostal view (B) of a patient with moderate/large pericardial effusion and right ventricular diastolic collapse (arrows).

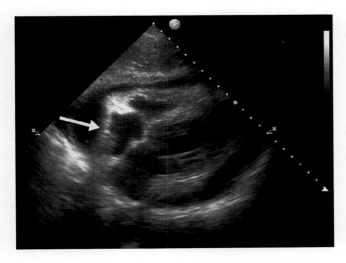

Figure 22-107. Pericardial effusion and right atrial collapse (arrow) during ventricular systole—subcostal window.

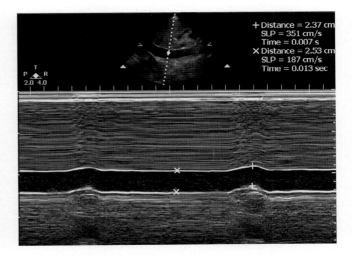

Figure 22-108. Subcostal, sagittal window with dilated inferior vena cava and M-mode showing lack of respiratory variation.

Scan the patient using the standard cardiac windows with a phased array or microconvex transducer of appropriate frequency. Choose a needle entry site that allows for the shortest path between the skin and the largest collection of fluid. One study found that the anterior thoracic approach was selected in 79% of cases and was preferred over the subxiphoid approach because of its close proximity to the largest part of the effusion and the lack of key structures within the path of the needle.[77] Once an entry site is selected, prep the skin with an antiseptic solution and place an appropriate sterile cover on the transducer.

For the parasternal/apical approach, position the patient in the left lateral decubitus position if possible. The largest pocket of fluid will often be located somewhere between the traditional transducer positions used for the standard parasternal and apical views (Figure 22-109). Long-axis views of the heart as well as longitudinal needle guidance are generally recommended for ultrasound-guided pericardiocentesis. Avoid vascular structures (described above). Infiltrate with local

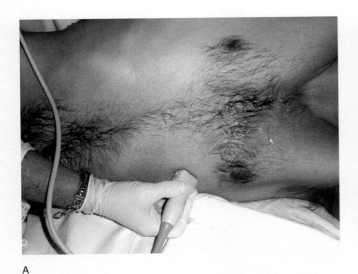

A

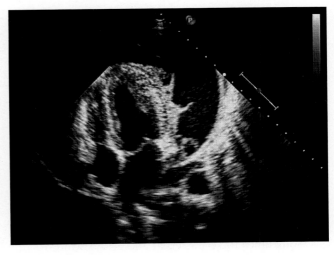

B

Figure 22-109. Transducer placement for the apical four-chamber view (A). For direct needle guidance, the transducer should be rotated 90° counterclockwise to the apical long-axis view. (B) Apical window with large echogenic pericardial effusion. The transducer is centered over the left anterior apex (and rotated for the four-chamber view in this example). The maximum fluid pocket will often be located in this area for patients who are in a left lateral decubitus position. Note the absence of lung artifact at intended area of puncture.

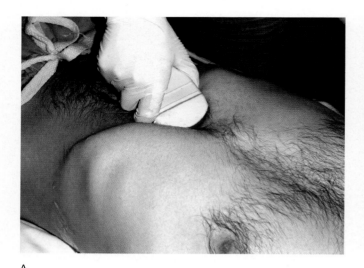

A

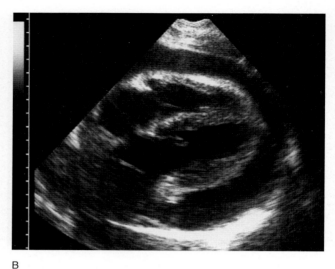

B

Figure 22-110. (A) Transducer placement for the subcostal window. (B) Four-chamber subcostal window. A moderate pericardial effusion is present. (Image B, Courtesy of James Mateer, MD)

anesthesia at the entry site and deeper along the predetermined trajectory if clinical circumstances allow. Introduce the needle adjacent to the transducer in the long-axis plane and opposite the transducer orientation indicator. Use an 18-gauge needle (larger if the patient is in extremis or cardiac arrest) with an over-the-needle Teflon-sheathed angiocatheter, or have a pigtail drain ready for placement via the Seldinger technique. Introduce the needle using an in-plane approach so that the needle will be visualized in its entirety. An 18-gauge needle is usually adequate, but a larger needle and catheter will allow for easier fluid removal if the fluid is viscous. Also, a larger needle will be visualized more easily during real-time guidance. Once the needle is visualized after initial penetration through the skin, the same guidance principles apply as for needle placement in vascular access and abscess drainage applications. Track the needle in long axis along its entire path and visualize it entering the pericardial effusion. When fluid is obtained, place the Seldinger guidewire and then the pigtail catheter, or advance the Teflon sheath, while removing the needle.

As an alternative, the transducer position, angle, and fluid depth can be noted and the procedure completed without direct needle guidance (static method). Be careful to avoid patient movement between sonographic mapping and needle insertion.

Sometimes the parasternal and apical windows are not ideal, and the best needle path is from the subcostal window. This view is obtained by placing the transducer in the subcostal space with the ultrasound beam directed into the patient's left chest and the transducer indicator directed to the patient's right, assuming an abdominal orientation preset is used (Figure 22-110A). This window

will provide a four-chamber view of the heart (Figure 22-110B). Because the liver may be prominent in the near field while the heart is located in the far field, the needle may have to traverse other structures prior to reaching the effusion when the subcostal approach is used.

If bloody fluid is obtained, a bubble test may be performed to assure that the tip of the needle is in the pericardial space. To perform a bubble test, rapidly reinject 3–5 mL of the aspirated fluid. Note that agitated saline is not needed to perform a bubble test. If echogenic contrast is visible within the effusion, the needle tip is in the pericardial space (Figure 22-111). A pigtail catheter or other type of drain may then be placed safely. If

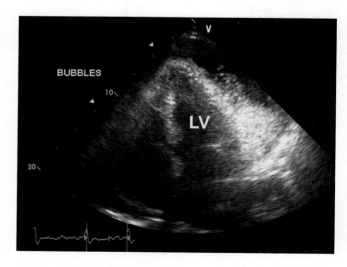

Figure 22-111. Apical four-chamber view with bubbles from agitated saline injection into the pericardial fluid. LV = left ventricle.

echogenic contrast is visualized within the cardiac chambers, or not visualized at all, withdraw the needle and start the procedure over. A single needle puncture of the myocardium is not necessarily a serious complication, and is best treated by proper placement of a pericardial drain.[77]

PITFALLS

1. Failure to consider the location of the internal mammary artery and the neurovascular bundles located on the underside of the ribs when choosing an entry point.
2. Failure to confirm location of the needle when bloody fluid is obtained if the needle tip is not adequately visualized on ultrasound.
3. Failure to consider alternative approaches if there is significant obstruction from lung tissue in the parasternal approach.

▶ TRANSVENOUS PACEMAKER PLACEMENT

CLINICAL CONSIDERATIONS

Transvenous pacing is indicated in the ED for prolonged pacing or when transcutaneous pacing is ineffective or not tolerated by the awake patient. Traditional guidance of the transvenous pacing catheter follows electrocardiographic monitoring of the pacer wire attached to one of the cardiac monitor leads. This may be too time consuming and inaccurate in an emergent situation. In hypotensive patients, a low-flow state may make it more difficult for the pacing catheter to naturally flow into the right ventricle. Ultrasound is ideal for visualizing catheter advancement into the right atrium and right ventricle.[80,81] It can also aid in confirming mechanical capture in both transcutaneous and transvenous pacing.[82,83]

CLINICAL INDICATIONS

- To assist in correct placement of transvenous pacing catheter
- To confirm pacemaker wire location in a transvenous pacemaker that is no longer capturing
- To confirm myocardial contraction from pacemaker firing

ANATOMICAL CONSIDERATIONS

The subxiphoid, parasternal, or apical windows can all be used to evaluate myocardial contraction in response to pacing. For pacemaker placement, the subxiphoid and four-chamber apical windows are most useful for adequate visualization of pacing catheter entry into the right atrium with progression into the right ventricle. A good four-chamber apical view is optimal for detecting and directing catheter placement. The clinician should be familiar with more than one approach to ensure adequate visualization.

TECHNIQUE AND ULTRASOUND FINDINGS

The transvenous pacing catheter can be seen in both the subxiphoid four-chamber and apical four-chamber views as it enters the right atrium. The catheter may appear out of plane initially, and some sonographic fanning through the atrium may be required to visualize the catheter. In the subxiphoid view, the right ventricle is at the top left of the screen (Figure 22-112). In the apical four-chamber view, the wire will appear in the bottom left as it enters the right atrium. A phased array cardiac transducer is ideal for this application, although a low-frequency convex transducer can also be used. If the pacing catheter is not visualized after an appropriate length of the pacemaker has been inserted, checking the inferior vena cava may reveal the catheter to be below the diaphragm.

When the pacing catheter first appears in the right atrium, ultrasound guidance is not yet complete because catheter coiling in the right atrium is common. Slight retraction of the catheter may be required, followed by

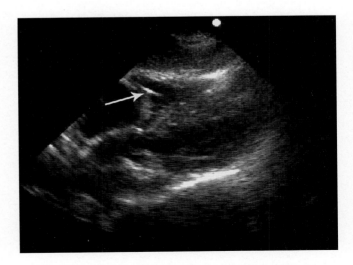

Figure 22-112. Placement of an ultrasound-guided emergency transvenous pacing catheter–subcostal 4-C view. The catheter (arrow) is visualized in real time as it passes through the tricuspid valve and into the right ventricle (Courtesy of Robert Reardon MD).

further incremental insertion. Advance the pacing catheter (with balloon up) through the tricuspid valve and into the right ventricle. Visualize the catheter as it enters the apex of the right ventricle. Mechanical capture is confirmed by directly visualizing myocardial contractions associated with pacer spikes.

PITFALLS

1. The subxiphoid window is sometimes challenging to obtain because of bowel gas or a protuberant abdomen.
2. The apical four-chamber view may be difficult in very obese patients or those with emphysema.

▶ PERITONSILLAR ABSCESS DRAINAGE

CLINICAL CONSIDERATIONS

Peritonsillar abscesses are the most common deep space infection of the head and neck. Clinical examination cannot be used to reliably distinguish between peritonsillar cellulitis and peritonsillar abscess. Diagnostic strategies include CT scan of the neck, blind needle aspiration, and, increasingly, point-of-care ultrasound. In one study comparing modalities for diagnosing peritonsillar abscess, clinical diagnosis was 78% sensitive and 50% specific, CT neck was 100% sensitive and 75% specific, and ultrasound was 89% sensitive and 100% specific.[84]

Point-of-care ultrasound for the detection of a peritonsillar abscess facilitates a rapid diagnosis while avoiding ionizing radiation and unnecessary needle aspiration. Ultrasound has emerged as an extremely valuable tool in the diagnosis and management of peritonsillar infections and is being used with increasing frequency for this application. One emergency medicine study of point-of-care ultrasound demonstrates a high positive predictive value for peritonsillar abscess: 34 out of 35 patients with a positive ultrasound exam had pus on aspiration.[85] In addition, the otolaryngology and radiology literature report low rates of false negative exams.[84,86,87]

CLINICAL INDICATIONS

The clinical indications for the use of ultrasonography in the management of peritonsillar infections include:

- Discrimination between peritonsillar cellulitis and peritonsillar abscess

- Real-time ultrasound needle guidance for peritonsillar abscess drainage

ANATOMICAL CONSIDERATIONS

The anatomy of the posterior pharynx and peritonsillar region is highly complex with numerous structures being visible on intraoral ultrasound. Structures that may be visualized by intraoral ultrasound include the palatine tonsil, the margin of the bony hard palate and styloid process of the temporal bone, the medial pterygoid muscle, various fascial planes, the internal jugular vein, and the internal carotid artery. In the sonographic evaluation of peritonsillar abscess, only the internal carotid artery and the palatine tonsil, if need be, are identified in every case. The internal carotid artery courses anterior to the internal jugular vein within the carotid sheath and is normally located posterolateral to the tonsil and within 5–25 mm of a peritonsillar abscess.

TECHNIQUE AND ULTRASOUND FINDINGS

Peritonsillar abscesses can have a variable echogenic appearance. Some will have an echogenic rim with a central area of hypoechogenicity. Depending on the composition of the purulent material, the fluid within the cavity may have an isoechoic or hyperechoic appearance (Figure 22-113). It is therefore important to recognize the relationship of the mass to the tonsil.

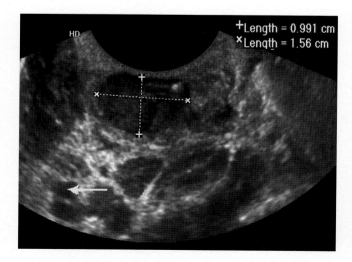

Figure 22-113. Peritonsillar abscess (right). Note the presence of the hypoechoic, purulent fluid collection within the abscess cavity (cursors) and the proximity of the carotid artery (arrow).

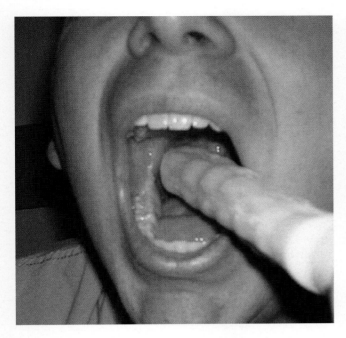

Figure 22-114. Intraoral transducer position for peritonsillar imaging.

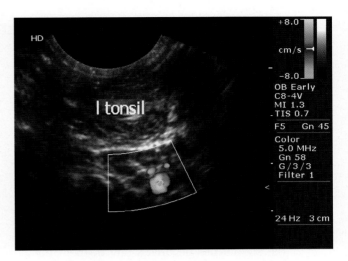

Figure 22-115. Transverse image of the posterior pharynx and left peritonsillar region with color Doppler identification of adjacent vascular structures.

Consider an echogenic mass with mass effect adjacent to the tonsil to be sonographic evidence for the presence of an abscess. Utilize gentle pressure to assess for fluid movement within the cavity, but this is not well tolerated by most patients.

Use an intracavitary transducer for this exam. Explain the procedure completely to the patient before performing it. An important aspect of intraoral ultrasound is that it requires a cooperative patient. Apply topical anesthetic spray to the back of the throat prior to the examination. Cover the transducer with a sheath and a small amount of gel, similar to an endovaginal scan. Gently insert the transducer into the mouth until it contacts the posterior pharynx (Figure 22-114). Perform the examination in a horizontal orientation, allowing visualization of much of the posterior pharynx. The relationship of the tonsil and peritonsillar abscess cavity to the internal carotid artery is best defined in the transverse plane (Figure 22-115). Scanning in a vertical orientation may be helpful in many situations to better define adjacent anatomy. In select cases, it can be helpful to scan the normal side for comparison.

When an abscess is visualized, drainage can be achieved using either ultrasound guidance, or more commonly, ultrasound assistance. Unless a biopsy guide is used on the endocavity transducer, aligning the needle with the ultrasound transducer while the transducer is in the patient's mouth can be challenging. An assistant may hold the transducer, while the operator aligns the needle just lateral to the transducer and aims to the center of the transducer tip (Figure 22-116). A safety measure sometimes practiced for novice clinicians is cutting off the tip of the needle cap to control the depth of needle penetration. With ultrasound, the precise length of needle required to enter the abscess can be determined by measuring the depth of the posterior wall of the abscess, making carotid penetration unlikely.

PITFALLS

1. **Failure to recognize an isoechoic or a hyperechoic abscess cavity.** The purulent fluid within a peritonsillar abscess cavity is typically hypoechoic in appearance. The presence of an isoechoic or a hyperechoic abscess may result in the clinician overlooking it.

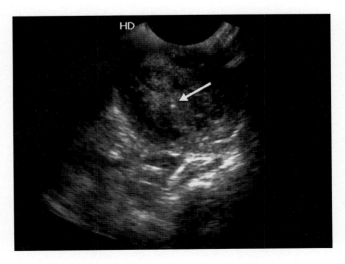

Figure 22-116. Needle (arrow) located in center of abscess with ultrasound guidance.

2. **Failure to visualize the internal carotid artery.** The relationship of the internal carotid artery to the abscess cavity must be noted before commencing with the surgical drainage. The internal carotid artery courses posterolateral to the tonsil and is typically located within 5–25 mm of the abscess cavity.

3. **An uncooperative patient.** An intraoral ultrasound examination requires that the patient be cooperative.

4. **Losing track of the needle during insertion when using ultrasound guidance.** If the needle is lost on the ultrasound screen, the clinician no longer knows where it is traveling and how deep it might be. At this point, the needle should not be driven any deeper and the ultrasound transducer should be moved up and down to locate the needle. Once it is located, the physician can then assess how far out of plane the needle is and redirect it toward the abscess.

▶ SUPRAPUBIC BLADDER ASPIRATION

CLINICAL CONSIDERATIONS

Percutaneous bladder aspiration and catheterization are emergency procedures that may be aided by ultrasound guidance. Suprapubic needle aspiration of the bladder used to be considered the gold standard method for obtaining a sterile urine culture in patients younger than 2 years of age, and may still be useful in selected rare cases. However, the American Academy of Pediatrics 2011 guidelines recommend a combination of ultrasound to verify the presence of urine followed by a urethral catheterized specimen.[88] In cases of urethral trauma or inability to pass a urethral catheter, suprapubic aspiration or catheter placement may be necessary.

CLINICAL INDICATIONS

- Urethral stricture or known false passage
- Inability to catheterize the urethra
- Suspected urethral trauma

Ultrasound can facilitate higher success rates of suprapubic aspiration by determining whether or not the bladder has sufficient urine to aspirate, guiding the needle or catheter to the greatest depth of the bladder, and identifying abnormalities or anatomic variations that may help reduce the risk of complications. Physical examination is insensitive for determining bladder fullness. Blind suprapubic aspiration has variable rates of success with esti-

mates ranging from 40% to 80%.[89–91] Complications of suprapubic aspiration or catheterization are rare but may include bowel perforation and hematuria. Ultrasound saves time, prevents multiple attempts at aspirating an empty bladder, and decreases the complication rate.

ANATOMICAL CONSIDERATIONS

The bladder is fixed inferiorly. In the neonate, the bladder is an abdominal organ and distends anteroposteriorly. As the body grows, the pelvis rises above the bladder, and in adults, the bladder is an intrapelvic organ. The bladder is a midline structure but may be shifted off the midline by pelvic or abdominal masses. Variability exists in the shape of the bladder and contributes to inaccuracy when estimating bladder volume with standard formulas. An obviously distended bladder can be easily aspirated or cannulated under direct ultrasound guidance.

TECHNIQUE AND ULTRASOUND FINDINGS

The bladder is typically a midline elliptical structure with posterior enhancement (Figure 22-117). Structures that are fluid filled but off midline may be distended loops of bowel or ovarian cysts (Figure 22-118). Limitations in bladder visualization are evident in morbidly obese patients or those with scar tissue.

Use a 2–5 MHz convex transducer for a screening ultrasound examination to confirm an adequate volume of urine (Figure 22-119). A linear transducer may be used in small children. The cutoff value for an adequate volume to attempt aspiration varies in the literature from

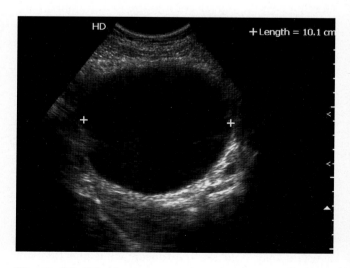

Figure 22-117. Transverse view of a full, round-shaped bladder—10 cm diameter, 9 cm height.

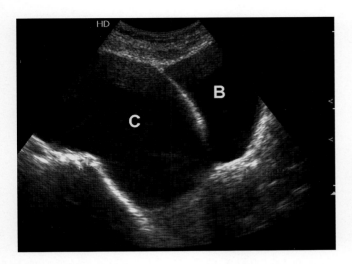

Figure 22-118. Bladder displacement due to a large ovarian cyst. B = bladder, C = cyst.

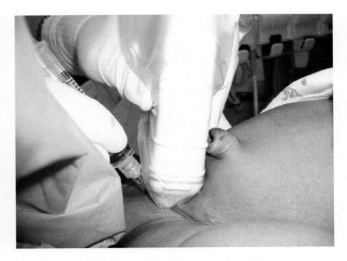

Figure 22-120. Hand and needle position for ultrasound-guided bladder aspiration (short-axis approach).

1 cm × 1 cm in the transverse plane to 3.5 cm in the transverse plane to >10 mL estimated volume when using a dedicated bladder scanner. A safe estimate is to use a minimum of 2 cm measured in at least two planes. If the bladder is empty on initial view, then repeat scanning every 15 minutes until an adequate volume of urine is identified. In neonates, apply minimal pressure to the skin to avoid irritating the bladder and having the patient urinate prior to the procedure.

Sterilize the skin and place a sterile sheath over the transducer. Much like inserting a needle into an abscess cavity, the long-axis approach to the needle, which allows visualization throughout its length, is ideal. Line up the greatest depth of the bladder with the center of the transducer in long or short axis and proceed under direct visualization. When bladder volumes are very small

(neonates), the short-axis approach may be preferred (Figure 22-120). Proper local anesthetic is required for patient comfort. Aspirating urine and visualizing the needle within the bladder should unequivocally confirm that the needle tip is within the bladder. At this point, proceed with catheterization using the Seldinger technique unless only a bladder aspiration is required.

PITFALLS

1. **Attempting to aspirate an empty bladder.** Wait for an adequately filled bladder before attempting to aspirate, especially in a neonate.
2. **Do not confuse the bladder with a distended loop of bowel or an enlarged ovarian cyst.** Examining for peristalsis and tracing the extent of all fluid-filled structures should help differentiate bowel from bladder. A large ovarian cyst that crosses midline and compresses the bladder can be quite difficult to differentiate. Noting the presence of ureteral jets should reassure the clinician. More extensive scanning may be required if the fluid-filled structure seems to extend to the adnexa.

REFERENCES

1. American College of Emergency Physicians: Emergency ultrasound guidelines—2008. *Ann Emerg Med* 53:550, 2009.
2. Milling T, Van Amerongen R, Melniker L, et al.: Randomized controlled trial of single-operator vs. two-operator ultrasound guidance for internal jugular central venous cannulation. *Acad Emerg Med* 13:245, 2006.

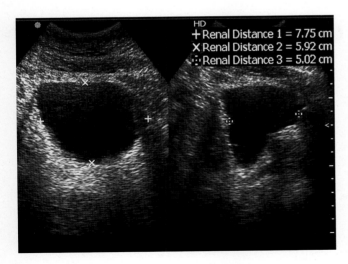

Figure 22-119. Transverse and sagittal views of bladder. The volume can be estimated using the simplified formula (length × width × height × 0.75)

3. Blaivas M, Adhikari S: An unseen danger: Frequency of posterior vessel wall penetration by needles during attempts to place internal jugular vein central catheters using ultrasound guidance. *Crit Care Med* 37:2345, 2009.

4. Stone MB, Moon C, Sutijono D, et al.: Needle tip visualization during ultrasound-guided vascular access: Short-axis vs long-axis approach. *Am J Emerg Med* 28:343, 2010.

5. Matalon TA, Silver B: US guidance of interventional procedures. *Radiology* 174:43, 1990.

6. Dodd GD, Esola CC, Memel DS, et al.: Sonography: The undiscovered jewel of interventional radiology. *Radiographics* 16:1271, 1996.

7. Phal PM, Brooks DM, Wolfe R: Sonographically guided biopsy of focal lesions: A comparison of free-hand and probe-guided techniques using a phantom. *Am J Roentgenol* 184:1652, 2005.

8. Hatada T, Ishii H, Ichii S, et al.: Ultrasound-guided fine-needle aspiration biopsy for breast tumors: Needle guide versus freehand technique. *Tumori* 85:12, 1999.

9. Culp WC, McCowan TC, Goertzen TC, et al.: Relative ultrasonographic echogenicity of standard, dimpled, and polymeric-coated needles. *J Vasc Interv Radiol* 11:351, 2000.

10. Hopkins RE, Bradley M: In-vitro visualization of biopsy needles with ultrasound: A comparative study of standard and echogenic needles using an ultrasound phantom. *Clin Radiol* 14:1553, 2003.

11. Nichols K, Wright LB, Spencer T, et al.: Changes in ultrasonographic echogenicity and visibility of needles with changes in angles of insonation. *J Vasc Interv Radiol* 14:1553, 2003.

12. Bondestam S, Kreula J: Needle tip echogenicity. A study with real time ultrasound. *Invest Radiol* 24:555, 1989.

13. Schafhalter-Zoppoth I, McCulloch CE, Gray AT: Ultrasound visibility of needles used for regional nerve block: An in vitro study. *Reg Anesth Pain Med* 29:480, 2004.

14. Im SH, Lee SC, Park YB, et al.: Feasibility of sonography for intra-articular injections in the knee through a medial patellar portal. *J Ultrasound Med* 28(11):1465–1470, 2009.

15. Sibbitt W, Kettwich L, Band P, et al.: Does ultrasound guidance improve the outcomes of arthrocentesis and corticosteroid injections of the knee? *Scand J Rheumatol* 41(1):66–72, 2012.

16. Wiler JL, Constantino TG, Filippone L, et al.: Comparison of ultrasound-guided and standard landmark techniques for knee arthrocentesis. *J Emerg Med* 39(1):76–82, 2010.

17. Sibbitt WT, Band PA, Kettwich LG, et al.: A randomized controlled trial evaluating cost-effectiveness of sonographic guidance for intra-articular injection of the osteoarthritic knee. *J Clin Rheumatol* 17(8):409–415, 2011.

18. Soh E, Li W, Ong KO, et al.: Image-guided versus blind corticosteroid injections in adults with shoulder pain: A systematic review. *BMC Musculoskelet Disord* 12:137, 2011.

19. Chen MJ, Lew HL, Hsu TC, et al.: Ultrasound-guided shoulder injections in the treatment of subacromial bursitis. *Am J Phys Med Rehabil* 85(1):31–5, 2006.

20. Cunnington J, Marshall N, Hide G, et al.: A randomized, double-blind, controlled study of ultrasound-guided corticosteroid injection into the joint of patients with inflammatory arthritis. *Arthritis Rheum* 62(7):1862–9, 2010.

21. Sibbitt WL, Peisajovich A, Michael AA, et al.: Does sono-

graphic needle guidance affect the clinical outcome of intraarticular injections. *J Rheumatol* 36(9):1892–902, 2009.

22. Raza K, Lee CY, Pilling D, et al.: Ultrasound guidance allows accurate needle placement and aspiration form small joints in patients with early inflammatory arthritis. *Rheumatology* 42(8):976–979, 2003.

23. Van Holsbeeck M, Eyler W, Sherman L, et al.: Detection of infection in loosened hip prostheses: Efficacy of sonography. *AJR* 163:381–384, 1994.

24. Hogan QH: Tuffier's line: The normal distribution of anatomic parameters (letter). *Anesth Analg* 78:194, 1994.

25. Pysyk CL, Persaud D, Bryson GL, et al.: Ultrasound assessment of the vertebral level of the palpated intercristal (Tuffier's) line. *Can J Anaesth* 57(1):46–49, 2010.

26. Furness G, Reilly M, Kuchi S: An evaluation of ultrasound imaging for identification of lumbar intervertebral level. *Anaesthesia* 57:277–280, 2002.

27. Grau T, Leipold W, Conradi R, et al.: Efficacy of ultrasound imaging in obstetric epidural anesthesia. *J Clin Anesth* 14:169–175, 2002.

28. Chin KJ, Perlas A, Chan V, et al.: Ultrasound imaging facilitates spinal anesthesia in adults with difficult surface anatomic landmarks. *Anesthesiology* 115(1):94–101, 2011.

29. Rapp H, Grau T: Ultrasound imaging in pediatric regional anesthesia (correspondence). *Can J Anesth* 51:277–278, 2004.

30. Coley BD, Shiels WE, Hogan MJ: Diagnostic and interventional ultrasonography in neonatal and infant lumbar puncture. *Pediatric Radiology* 31:399–402, 2001.

31. Peterson M, Abele J: Bedside ultrasound for difficult lumbar puncture. *J Emerg Med* 28:197–200, 2005.

32. Stiffler KA, Jwayyed S, Wilber ST, et al.: The use of ultrasound to identify pertinent landmarks for lumbar puncture. *Am J Emerg Med* 25(3):331–334, 2007.

33. Ferre RM, Sweeney TW: Emergency physicians can easily obtain ultrasound images of anatomical landmarks relevant to lumbar puncture. *Am J Emerg Med* 25(3):291–296, 2007.

34. Nomura JT, Leech SJ, Shenbagamurthi S, et al.: A randomized controlled trial of ultrasound-assisted lumbar puncture. *J Ultrasound Med* 26(10):1341, 2007.

35. Huang MY, Lin AP, Chang WH: Ultrasound-assisted localization for lumbar puncture in the ED. *Am J Emerg Med* 26(8):955–957, 2008.

36. Ferre RM, Sweeney TW, Strout TD: Ultrasound identification of landmarks preceding lumbar puncture: A pilot study. *Emerg Med J* 26(4):276–277, 2009.

37. Grau T, Leipold W, Conradi R, et al.: Ultrasound control for presumed difficult epidural puncture. *Acta Anaesthesiol Scand* 45:766–771, 2001.

38. Cork RC, Kryc JJ, Vaughan RW: Ultrasonic localization of the lumbar epidural space. *Anesthesiology* 52:513–516, 1980.

39. Porter RW, Wicks M, Ottewell D: Measurement of the spinal canal by diagnostic ultrasound. *J Bone Joint Surg Br* 1978;60:481–484.

40. Fisher A, Lupu L, Gurevitz B, et al.: Hip flexion and lumbar puncture: A radiological study. *Anesthesia* 56:262–266, 2001.

41. Abo A, Chen L, Johnston P, et al.: Positioning for lumbar puncture in children evaluated by bedside ultrasound. *Pediatrics* 125(5):e1149–e1153, 2010.

42. Grau T: Ultrasonography in the current practice of regional anesthesia. *Best Pract Res Clin Anesthesiol* 19:175–200, 2005.

43. Gray A: Ultrasound-guided regional anesthesia: Current state of the art. *Anesthesiology* 104:368–373, 2006.

44. Liebmann O, Price D, Mills C, et al.: Feasibility of forearm ultrasonography-guided nerve blocks of the radial, ulnar, and median nerves for hand procedures in the emergency department. *Ann Emerg Med* 48:558–562, 2006.

45. Stone MB, Wang R, Price DD: Ultrasound-guided supraclavicular brachial plexus nerve block vs procedural sedation for the treatment of upper extremity emergencies. *Am J Emerg Med* 26(6):706–710, 2008.

46. Blaivas M, Adhikari S, Lander L: A prospective comparison of procedural sedation and ultrasound-guided interscalene nerve block for shoulder reduction in the emergency department. *Acad Emerg Med* 18(9):922–927, 2011.

47. Beaudoin FL, Nagdev A, Merchant RC, et al.: Ultrasound-guided femoral nerve blocks in elderly patients with hip fractures. *Am J Emerg Med* 28(1):76–81, 2010.

48. Herring AA, Stone MB, Fischer J, et al.: Ultrasound-guided distal popliteal sciatic nerve block for ED anesthesia. *Am J Emerg Med* 29(6):697.e3–5, 2011.

49. Kapral S, Krafft P, Klemens E, et al.: Ultrasound-guided supraclavicular approach for regional anesthesia of the brachial plexus. *Anesth Analg* 78:507–13, 1994.

50. Marhofer PSchrogendorfer K, Koinig H, et al.: Ultrasonographic guidance improves sensory block and onset time of three-in-one blocks. *Anesth Analg* 85:854–857, 1997.

51. Marhofer PSchrogendorfer K, Wallner T, et al.: Ultrasonographic guidance reduces the amount of local anesthetic for 3-in-1 blocks. *Reg Anesth Pain Med* 23:584–588, 1998.

52. Kefalianakis F: Ultraschall zur blockade peripheren nerven. *Anesthesiol Intensivmed Notfallmed Schmerzther* 40:142–149, 2005.

53. Chan V, Brull R, McCartney C, et al.: An ultrasonographic and histological study of intraneural injection and electrical stimulation in pigs. *Anesth Analg* 104(5):1281–1284, 2007.

54. Sala Blanch X, Lopez A, Carazo J, et al.: Intraneural injection during nerve stimulator-guided sciatic nerve block at the popliteal fossa. *Br J Anesth* 102(6):855–861, 2009.

55. Neal J, Bernards C, Butterworth J, et al.: ASRA practice advisory on local anesthetic systemic toxicity. *Reg Anesth Pain Med* 35(2):152–161, 2010.

56. Mariani PJ, Setla JA: Palliative ultrasound for home care hospice patients. *Acad Emerg Med* 17(3):293–296, 2010.

57. Bard C, Lafortune M, Breton G: Ascites: Ultrasound guidance or blind paracentesis? *Can Med Assoc J* 135:209–210, 1986.

58. Nazeer SR, Dewbre H, Miller AH: Ultrasound-assisted paracentesis performed by emergency physicians vs the traditional technique: A prospective, randomized study. *Am J Emerg Med* 23:363–367, 2005.

59. Irshad A, Ackerman SJ, Anis M, et al.: Can the smallest depth of ascitic fluid on sonograms predict the amount of drainable fluid? *J Clin Ultrasound* 37(8):440–444, 2009.

60. Sakai H, Sheer TA, Mendler MH, et al.: Choosing the location for non-image guided abdominal paracentesis. *Liver Int* 25:984–986, 2005.

61. Quershi N, Momin ZA, Brandstetter RD: Thoracentesis in clinical practice. *Heart Lung* 23:376–383, 1994.

62. Kohan JM, Poe RH, Israel RH, et al.: Value of chest ultrasonography versus decubitus roentgenography for thoracentesis. *Am Rev Respir Dis* 133:1124–1136, 1986.

63. Patel PA, Ernst FR, Gunnarsson CL: Ultrasonography guidance reduces complications and costs associated with thoracentesis procedures. *J Clin Ultrasound* 40(3):135–141, 2012.

64. Gordon CE, Feller-Kopman D, Balk EM, et al.: Pneumothorax following thoracentesis: A systematic review and meta-analysis. *Arch Intern Med* 170(4):332–339, 2010.

65. Josephson T, Nordenskjold CA, Larsson J, et al.: Amount drained at ultrasound-guided thoracentesis and risk of pneumothorax. *Acta Radiol* 50(1):42–47, 2009.

66. Grogan DR, Irwin RS, Channick R, et al.: Complications associated with thoracentesis. *Arch Intern Med* 150:873–877, 1990.

67. Weingart JP, Guico RR, Nemcek AA, et al.: Ultrasound findings following failed, clinically directed thoracenteses. *J Clin Ultrasound* 22:419–426, 1994.

68. Lichtenstein D, Hulot JS, Rabiller A, et al.: Feasibility and safety of ultrasound-aided thoracentesis in mechanically ventilated patients. *Intensive Care Med* 25:955–958, 1999.

69. Balik M, Plasil P, WAldauf P, et al.: Ultrasound estimation of volume of pleural fluid in mechanically ventilated patients. *Intensive Care Med* 32(2):318–321, 2006.

70. Beck C: Two cardiac compression triads. *JAMA* 104(9):714–716, 1935.

71. Yao ST, Vanecko RM, Printen K, et al.: Penetrating wounds of the heart: a review of 80 cases. *Ann Surg* 168(1):67–78, 1968.

72. Plummer D, Brunette D, Asinger R, et al.: Emergency department echocardiography improves outcome in penetrating cardiac injury. *Ann Emerg Med* 21(6):709–712, 1992.

73. Rozycki GS, Feliciano DV, Ochsner MG et al.: The role of ultrasound in patients with possible penetrating cardiac wounds: A prospective multi-center study. *J Trauma* 46(4):543–551, 1999.

74. Rozycki GS, Ballard RB, Feliciano DV, et al.: Surgeon-performed ultrasound for the assessment of truncal injuries: Lessons learned from 1540 patients. *Ann Surg* 228(4):557–567, 1998.

75. Tsang TS, Freeman WK, Sinak LJ, et al.: Echocardiographically guided pericardiocentesis: Evolution and state-of-the-art technique. *Mayo Clin Proc* 73(7):647–652, 1998.

76. Wong B, Chang CJ, Hassenein K, et al.: The risk of pericardiocentesis. *Am J Cardiol* 44(6):1110–1114, 1979.

77. Tsang TS, Enriques-Sarano M, Freeman WK, et al.: Consecutive 1127 therapeutic echocardiographically guided pericardiocentesis: Clinical profile, practice patterns, and outcomes spanning 21 years. *Mayo Clin Proc* 77(5):429–436, 2002.

78. Isselbacher EM, Cigarroa JE, Eagle KA: Cardiac tamponade complicating proximal aortic dissection. Is pericardiocentesis harmful? *Circulation* 90(5):2375–2378, 1994.

79. Kurimoto Y, Hase M, Nara S et al.: Blind subxiphoid pericardiotomy for cardiac tamponade because of acute pericardium. *J Trauma* 61(3):582–585, 2006.

80. Macedo W Jr, Sturmann K, Kim JM, et al.: Ultrasonographic guidance of transvenous pacemaker insertion in the emergency department: a report of three cases. *J Emerg Med* 17(3):491–496, 1999.

81. Aguilera PA, Durham BA, Riley DA: Emergency transvenous cardiac pacing placement using ultrasound guidance. *Ann Emerg Med* 36(3):224–227, 2000.

82. Ettin D, Cook T: Using ultrasound to determine external pacer capture. *J Emerg Med* 17(6):1007–1009, 1999.

83. Tam MM: Ultrasound for primary confirmation of mechanical capture in emergency transcutaneous pacing. *Emerg Med (Fremantle)* 15(2):192–194, 2003.

84. Scot PM, Loftus WK, Kew J, et al.: Diagnosis of peritonsillar infections: A prospective study of ultrasound, computerized tomography, and clinical diagnosis. *J Laryngol Otol* 113(3):229–232, 1999.

85. Lyon M, Blaivas M: Intraoral ultrasound in the diagnosis and treatment of suspected peritonsillar abscess in the emergency department. *Acad Emerg Med* 12(1):85–88, 2005.

86. Araujo Filho BC, Sakae FA, Sennes L, et al.: Intraoral and transcutaneous cervical ultrasound in the differential diagnosis of peritonsillar cellulitis and abscesses. *Braz J Otorhinolaryngol* 72(3):377–381, 2006.

87. Kew J, Ahuja A, Loftus WK: Peritonsillar abscess appearance on intra-oral ultrasonography. *Clin Radiol* 53(2):143–146, 1998.

88. Subcommitte on urinary tract infection; steering committee on quality improvemetn and management. Urinary Tract Infection: Clinical Practice Guideline for the Diagnosis and Management of the Initial UTI in Febrile Infants and Children 2 to 24 Months. Pediatrics. 2011 Aug 28.

89. Munir V, Barnett P, South M: Does the use of volumetric bladder ultrasound improve the success rate of suprapubic aspiration of urine? *Pediatr Emerg Care* 18(5):346–349, 2002.

90. Chu RW, Wong YC, Luk SH, et al.: Comparing suprapubic urine aspiration under real-time ultrasound guidance with conventional blind aspiration. *Acta Paediatr* 91(5):512–516, 2002.

91. Kozer E, Rosenbloom E, Goldman D, et al.: Pain in infants who are younger than 2 months during suprapubic aspiration and transurethral bladder catheterization: A randomized, controlled study. *Pediatrics* 118(1):e51–e56, 2006.

INDEX

Note: Page number followed by f and t indicates figure and table respectively.